THE NETTER COLLECTION
of Medical Illustrations
Second Edition

Reproductive System
Endocrine System
Respiratory System
Integumentary System
Urinary System
Musculoskeletal System
Digestive System
Nervous System
Cardiovascular System

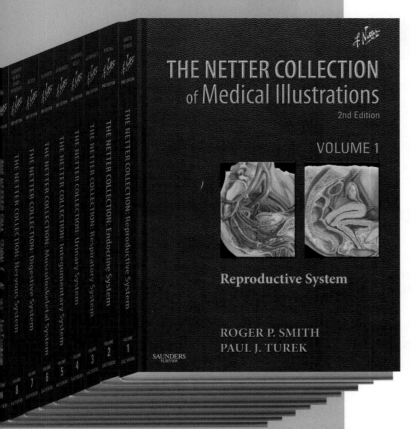

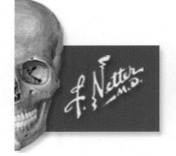
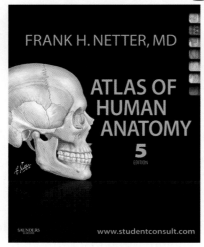
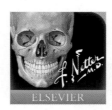
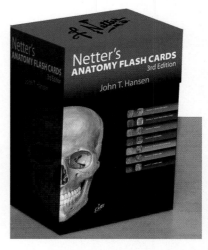

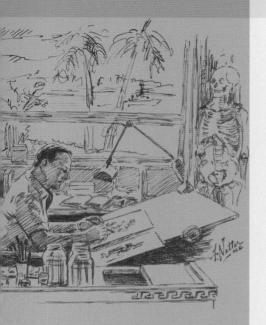

VOLUME 4

The Netter Collection
OF MEDICAL ILLUSTRATIONS
Integumentary System

2nd Edition

A compilation of paintings prepared by
FRANK H. NETTER, MD

Authored by

Bryan E. Anderson, MD

Associate Professor of Dermatology
Pennsylvania State University
College of Medicine
Hershey, Pennsylvania

Additional illustrations by Carlos A. G. Machado, MD

CONTRIBUTING ILLUSTRATORS
Tiffany S. DaVanzo, MA, CMI
John A. Craig, MD
James A. Perkins, MS, MFA
Anita Impagliazzo, MA, CMI

ELSEVIER
SAUNDERS

ELSEVIER
SAUNDERS

1600 John F. Kennedy Blvd.
Ste 1800
Philadelphia, PA 19103-2899

THE NETTER COLLECTION OF MEDICAL ILLUSTRATIONS: ISBN: 978-1-4377-5654-8
INTEGUMENTARY SYSTEM

Notices

Library of Congress Cataloging-in-Publication Data

Anderson, Bryan E.
   The Netter collection of medical illustrations : integumentary system / Bryan E. Anderson. – 2nd ed.
      p. cm.
   ISBN 978-1-4377-5654-8 (hardcover : alk. paper)
   1. Skin—Physiology—Atlases.   2. Body covering (Anatomy)—Atlases.
3. Skin—Diseases—Atlases.   I. Title.
   QP88.5.A53 2013
   612.7'90222–dc23
                                                        2011042444

Content Strategist: Elyse O'Grady
Content Development Manager: Marybeth Thiel
Publishing Services Manager: Anne Altepeter
Senior Project Manager: Doug Turner
Designer: Ellen Zanolle

Printed in China

Last digit is the print number: 9   8   7

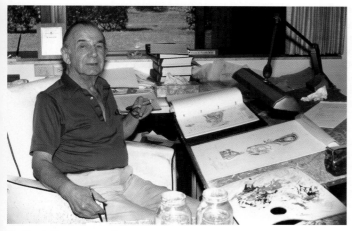

Dr. Frank Netter at work

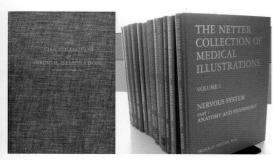

The single-volume "blue book" that paved the way for the multi-volume Netter Collection of Medical Illustrations series affectionately known as the "green books"

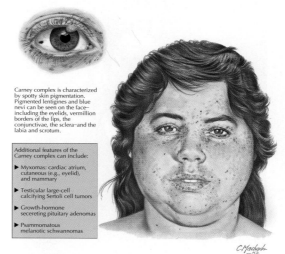

CUSHING'S SYNDROME IN A PATIENT WITH THE CARNEY COMPLEX

Carney complex is characterized by spotty skin pigmentation. Pigmented lentigines and blue nevi can be seen on the face–including the eyelids, vermillion borders of the lips, the conjunctivae, the sclera–and the labia and scrotum.

Additional features of the Carney complex can include:

▶ Myxomas: cardiac atrium, cutaneous (e.g., eyelid), and mammary

▶ Testicular large-cell calcifying Sertoli cell tumors

▶ Growth-hormone secreting pituitary adenomas

▶ Psammomatous melanotic schwannomas

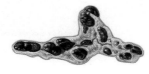

PPNAD adrenal glands are usually of normal size and most are studded with black, brown, or red nodules. Most of the pigmented nodules are less than 4 mm in diameter and interspersed in the adjacent atrophic cortex.

A brand new illustrated plate painted by Carlos Machado, MD, for *The Endocrine System*, vol. 2, 2nd ed.

Dr. Frank H. Netter exemplified the distinct vocations of doctor, artist, and teacher. Even more importantly—he unified them. Netter's illustrations always began with meticulous research into the forms of the body, a philosophy that steered his broad and deep medical understanding. He once said, "Clarification is the goal. No matter how beautifully it is painted, a medical illustration has little value if it does not make clear a medical point." His greatest challenge and greatest success was charting a middle course between artistic clarity and instructional complexity. That success is captured in this series, beginning in 1948, when the first comprehensive collection of Netter's work, a single volume, was published by CIBA Pharmaceuticals. It met with such success that over the following 40 years the collection was expanded into an eight-volume series—each devoted to a single body system.

In this second edition of the legendary series, we are delighted to offer Netter's timeless work, now arranged and informed by modern text and radiologic imaging contributed by field-leading doctors and teachers from world-renowned medical institutions, and supplemented with new illustrations created by artists working in the Netter tradition. Inside the classic green covers, students and practitioners will find hundreds of original works of art—the human body in pictures—paired with the latest in expert medical knowledge and innovation and anchored in the sublime style of Frank Netter.

Noted artist-physician, Carlos Machado, MD, the primary successor responsible for continuing the Netter tradition, has particular appreciation for the Green Book series. "*The Reproductive System* is of special significance for those who, like me, deeply admire Dr. Netter's work. In this volume, he masters the representation of textures of different surfaces, which I like to call 'the rhythm of the brush,' since it is the dimension, the direction of the strokes, and the interval separating them that create the illusion of given textures: organs have their external surfaces, the surfaces of their cavities, and texture of their parenchyma realistically represented. It set the style for the subsequent volumes of Netter's Collection—each an amazing combination of painting masterpieces and precise scientific information."

Though the science and teaching of medicine endures changes in terminology, practice, and discovery, some things remain the same. A patient is a patient. A teacher is a teacher. And the pictures of Dr. Netter—he called them pictures, never paintings—remain the same blend of beautiful and instructional resources that have guided physicians' hands and nurtured their imaginations for more than half a century.

The original series could not exist without the dedication of all those who edited, authored, or in other ways contributed, nor, of course, without the excellence of Dr. Netter. For this exciting second edition, we also owe our gratitude to the authors, editors, advisors, and artists whose relentless efforts were instrumental in adapting these timeless works into reliable references for today's clinicians in training and in practice. From all of us with the Netter Publishing Team at Elsevier, we thank you.

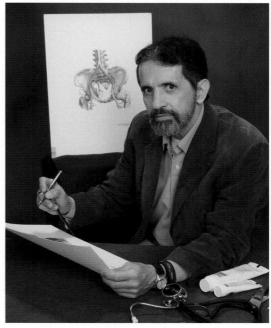

Dr. Carlos Machado at work

ABOUT THE AUTHOR

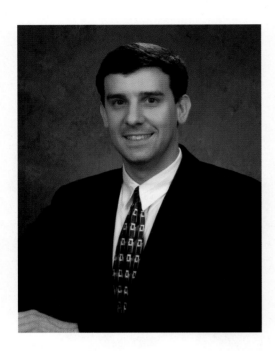

Bryan E. Anderson, MD, is Associate Professor of Dermatology at the Pennsylvania State University College of Medicine. He is proud to have received both his undergraduate and medical degrees from The Ohio State University. He completed his internship and Dermatology residency at the Pennsylvania State University College of Medicine in Hershey, Pennsylvania, where, upon completion thereof, he joined the faculty in the Department of Dermatology in 2002. There he works as a clinician, educator, and researcher. Dr. Anderson is currently the Dermatology Residency Program Director and Director of a multidisciplinary outpatient specialty clinic. He is also a part of the Hershey Medical Centers Cancer Institute's Multidisciplinary Skin Oncology Clinic. His areas of interest and research include resident education and cutaneous malignancies, with an emphasis on melanoma. He is an active member in his state medical society, the American Academy of Dermatology, and the American Contact Dermatitis Society. He has written numerous journal articles and book chapters and is coeditor of a large online dermatology resource. He currently lives in Hershey with his wife, Susan, and two daughters, Rachel and Sarah. In his leisure time he enjoys woodworking, cheering on his alma mater, and spending time with this family.

It has been both an honor and a challenge to serve as the author of *The Netter Collection: Integumentary System*. I am honored to have contributed to the legacy that The Netter Collection so deserves with its timeless quality and continued contribution to medical education. Of course, the challenge was in determining that which would and should be included in the volume, in keeping with the tradition of relevance of the series. My hope is that this volume is appreciated by those with vast experience as well as those individuals just beginning their journey of lifelong learning, which I feel so accurately describes the medical world.

My sincerest gratitude is extended to people behind the scenes at Elsevier, specifically Marybeth Thiel, as well as the artists who were able to bring the slightest nuance to life for the benefit of clinician and patient alike. Although no volume exclusively dedicated to the integumentary system existed, I attempted to incorporate as many of Frank Netter's depictions as possible. In several instances however, this simply was not possible, and I therefore had the pleasure and privilege of working with Carlos Machado, MD, and Tiffany S. DaVanzo, MA, CMI, whose talent deserves to be formally recognized. Their artwork captures the subtleties of the integumentary system. For that I am forever grateful.

I would like to thank all those who have positively influenced, taught, and mentored me, specifically, Jeffrey Miller, MD, Warren Heymann, MD, the late John Stang, MD, and James Marks, MD—your impact on my career has been immeasurable. Certainly, this list is not exhaustive. I have had the pleasure of crossing paths with so many fine people—sadly, too many to list. A special thank you goes to Ruth Howe and Cheryl Hermanson, whose help was simply incredible; I truly appreciate all you did. Additionally, I would like to thank my colleagues at the Milton S. Hershey Medical Center, whose encouragement and support have always been a part of our culture.

Finally, I would like to recognize and express appreciation for my family: my parents, sisters, Uncle Lou, and my loving Grandmother Ermandina. Your encouragement and support is the foundation from which I draw my confidence to tackle a project such as this. At the time of this writing, my wife, Susan, is in a select group of people who have read, literally, every word of text in this volume. I cannot thank Susan enough for her supportive nature, patience, and love; you are the gem of my life. Lastly, I need to acknowledge my daughters, Rachel and Sarah, of whom I am so proud. The sacrifice of your evenings for more than a year so that I could work in an environment that was productive and conducive to concentration will forever be appreciated.

Bryan E. Anderson, MD

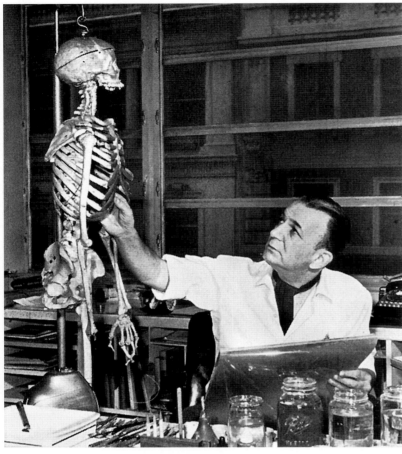

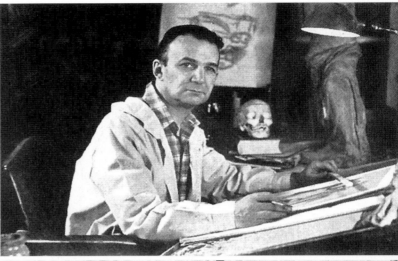

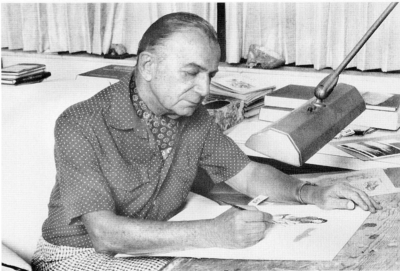

Frank H. Netter, MD
(1906-1991)
"The Medical Michelangelo"

Celebrated as the foremost medical illustrator of the human body and how it works, Dr. Frank H. Netter began his career as a medical illustrator in the 1930s when the CIBA Pharmaceutical Company commissioned him to prepare illustrations of the major organs and their pathology. Dr. Netter's incredibly detailed, lifelike renderings were so well received by the medical community that CIBA published them in a book. This first successful publication in 1948 was followed by the series of volumes that now carry the Netter name, *The Netter Collection of Medical Illustrations*. Even years after his death, Dr. Netter is still acknowledged as the foremost master of medical illustration. His anatomical drawings are the benchmark by which all other medical art is measured and judged.

"As far back as I can remember, ever since I was little tot, I studied art," said Dr. Netter during an interview in 1986. At the time he was hailed by the *New York Times* as "The Medical Michelangelo." "All I wanted to do was to make pictures," he reflected. Born in New York in 1906, Dr. Netter had already established himself as a successful commercial artist in the 1920s when, at the advice of his parents, he changed careers. "I gave up art at the urging of my family," he said. "They felt

that artists led a very dissolute life, which of course was really not true."

To find a more "dependable" career, Dr. Netter entered New York University Medical School. But even as he pursued his training as a surgeon, Dr. Netter found that it was easier for him to take notes in pictures than in words. "Mine was a graphic viewpoint. My notebooks were crammed with illustrations. It was the only way I could remember things." Soon faculty members recognized his artistic talents, and Dr. Netter began to pay for part of his medical education by illustrating lectures and textbooks.

Starting out as a young physician during the Depression, Dr. Netter found that there was more interest in his medical artwork than his surgical capabilities. "I thought I could do drawings until I had my practice on its feet," he recalled, "but the demand for my pictures grew much faster than the demand for my surgery. As a result, I gave up my practice entirely."

In 1938, Dr. Netter was hired by the CIBA Pharmaceutical Company to work on a promotional flyer for a heart medication. He designed a folder cut in the shape of and elaborately depicting a heart, which was sent to physicians. Surprisingly, many of the doctors wrote

back asking for more heart flyers—without the advertising copy. Dr. Netter went on to design similar product advertisements depicting other organs, and all were extremely well received. After that project was concluded, Dr. Netter was commissioned to prepare small folders of pathology plates that were later collected into the first *CIBA Collection of Medical Illustrations*.

Following the success of these endeavors, Dr. Netter was asked to illustrate a series of atlases that became his life's work. They are a group of volumes individually devoted to each organ system and cover human anatomy, embryology, physiology, pathology, and pertinent clinical features of the diseases arising in each system. Dr. Netter has completed volumes on the nervous system, reproductive system, lower and upper digestive tracts, liver, biliary tract and pancreas, endocrine system, kidney, ureters, urinary bladder, respiratory system, and musculoskeletal system.

Dr. Netter's beautifully rendered volumes are now to be found in every medical school library in the country, as well as in many doctors' offices around the world, and his work has helped to educate and enlighten generations of physicians. In 1988, the *New York Times* called Netter "an artist who has probably contributed more to medical education than most of the world's anatomy professors taken together."

Dr. Netter's career has spanned the most revolutionary half-century in medicine's history. He chronicled the emergence of open heart surgery, organ transplants, and joint replacements. To learn first hand about a variety of diseases and their effects on the body, Dr. Netter traveled widely. In the early 1980s, Dr. William Devries asked Netter to be present at the first artificial heart transplant, a procedure that Netter illustrated in full detail. Dr. Netter also developed a variety of unusual medical art projects, including building the 7-foot *Transparent Woman* for the San Francisco Golden Gate Exposition, which depicted the menstrual process, the development and birth of a baby, and the physical and sexual development of a woman.

When asked whether he regretted giving up his surgical practice, Dr. Netter replied that he thought of himself as a clinician with a specialty that encompasses the whole of medicine. "My field covers everything. I must be a specialist in every specialty; I must be able to talk with all physicians on their own terms. I probably do more studying than anyone else in the world," he said.

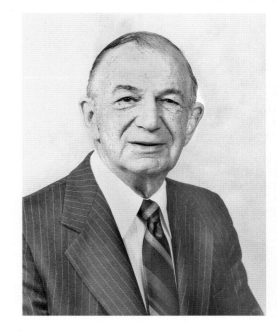

In his work, Dr. Netter made pencil sketches, which he then copied, transferred, and painted to portray gross anatomy, microscopic anatomy, radiographic images, and drawings of patients. "I try to depict living patients whenever possible," Dr. Netter said. "After all, physicians do see patients, and we must remember we are treating whole human beings."

Into his eighth decade, Dr. Netter continued to create his medical illustrations and added to the portfolio of thousands of drawings that encompass his long and illustrious career. Dr. Netter died in 1991, but his work lives on in books and electronic products that continue to educate millions of health care professionals worldwide.

ADVISORY BOARD

Walter H. C. Burgdorf, MD
Clinical Lecturer
Department of Dermatology
Ludwig Maximilian University
Munich, Germany

William D. James, MD
Paul R. Gross Professor of Dermatology
Department of Dermatology
University of Pennsylvania
Philadelphia, Pennsylvania

Dott. Bianca Maria Piraccini, MD, PhD
Professor
Department of Internal Medicine, Aging and
    Nephrological Diseases, Dermatology
University of Bologna
Bologna, Italy

Eduardo Cotecchia Ribeiro, MD, PhD
Associate Professor
Morphology and Genetic Department
Federal University of Sao Paulo—School of Medicine
São Paulo, Brazil

CONTENTS

ANATOMY, PHYSIOLOGY, AND EMBRYOLOGY

Plate 1-1   Integumentary System

EMBRYOLOGY OF THE SKIN

The human skin develops from two special embryonic tissues, the ectoderm and the mesoderm. Epidermal tissue is derived from the embryonic ectoderm. The dermis and subcutaneous tissue are derived from the embryonic mesoderm. The developmental interactions between mesoderm and ectoderm ultimately determine the nature of human skin. Interestingly, neural tissue and epidermal tissue are both derived from the ectoderm. It is believed that calcium signaling is critical in determining the fate of the ectoderm and its differentiation into either epidermis or neural tissue.

At approximately 4 weeks after conception, a single layer of ectoderm is present, surrounding a thicker layer of mesoderm. Two weeks later, this ectodermal layer has separated into two different components: an outer periderm and an inner basal layer, which is connected to the underlying mesoderm. At 8 weeks after conception, the epidermis has developed into three separate layers: the periderm, an intermediate layer, and the basal cell layer. The dermal subcutaneous tissue is now beginning to develop, and a distinct dermal subcutaneous boundary can be seen by the end of the eighth week. Between weeks 10 and 15 after conception, the beginning of the skin appendages can be seen.

The formation of hair follicles is initiated by a complex genetic mechanism that causes the dermis to direct certain basal epidermal cells to congregate and form the rudimentary hair follicle. This process occurs in a highly organized fashion beginning from the scalp and working caudally to the lower extremity. At the same time, the hair follicles are developing and the dermal papillae are beginning to form. The hair follicles continue to differentiate throughout the second trimester, and the hair of the fetus can be seen at approximately 20 weeks after conception. This first hair is known as lanugo hair and is almost always shed before delivery.

The fingernails and toenails develop from ectoderm that invaginates into the underlying mesoderm by the fourteenth week after conception. By the fifth month, the fetus has fully developed fingernails and toenails. The fingernails fully develop slightly before the toenails.

Melanocytes are specialized cells derived from neural crest tissue. These cells form along the neural tube. Melanocytes migrate in a specific pattern laterally and then outward along the trunk. Melanocytes can be seen in the epidermis by the middle of the first trimester, but they are not functional until the end of the second trimester. The density of melanocytes is highest during the fetal period and decreases thereafter until young adulthood. Melanocytes are beginning to make their first melanosomes and are capable of transferring melanin pigment to adjacent keratinocytes by approximately 5 months after conception. Melanocytes are not fully functional until birth. Langerhans cells are specialized immune surveillance cells that appear within the epidermis at approximately 40 days after conception. In contrast to melanocytes, the density of Langerhans cells increases with time.

By late in the second trimester, the periderm begins to shed. This shedding results in the vernix caseosa, a whitish, cheese-like material that covers the fetus. It is believed to have a protective function. At the beginning of the third trimester, the individual epidermal layers can be seen, including the stratum basale, stratum granulosum, stratum spinosum, and stratum corneum. Keratinization begins to occur during the

second trimester, first in the appendageal structures and then in the epidermis. The thickness of the epidermis in a newborn closely approaches that in an adult. The significant difference is that the skin barrier function in a newborn is not as fully developed as in an adult and therefore is more vulnerable to infection and external insults.

By studying the embryology of the skin, one can gain insight into the mechanisms of certain genetic

disorders. For example, one of the more studied groups of genetic diseases are the congenital blistering diseases. The various types of epidermolysis bullosa are all caused by genetic defects in proteins responsible for adhesion of keratinocytes. A firm understanding of the embryology of skin development is essential for understanding the pathogenesis of these diseases and ultimately for developing a mechanism to detect and therapeutically treat them.

Midsagittal section of folding gastrula

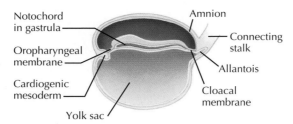

Cross section of folding gastrula

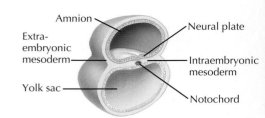

Vertebrate body plan after 4 weeks

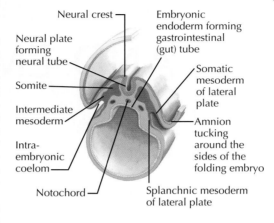

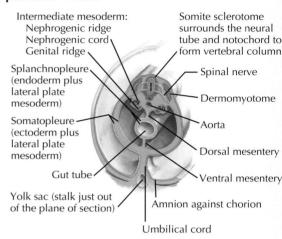

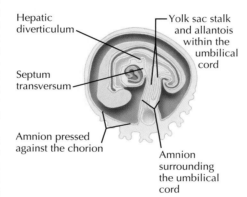

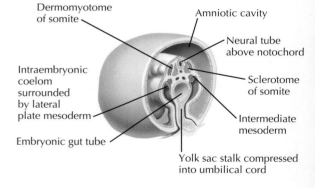

Dorsal views

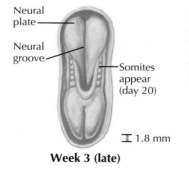

Week 3 (late)

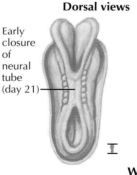

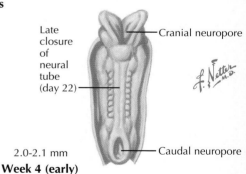

Week 4 (early)

Plate 1-2

Anatomy, Physiology, and Embryology

NORMAL SKIN ANATOMY

The human skin, taken collectively, is the largest organ in the human body. On average, it weighs between 4 and 5 kg. It is vitally important to life. The skin is made up of three distinct layers: the epidermis, the dermis, and the subcutaneous tissue; some anatomists do not include the subcutaneous tissue as part of the skin and classify it separately as the hypodermis. Each of these layers plays a pivotal role in the execution of day-to-day functions of the skin. The skin's main function is to protect the interior of the body from the exterior environment. It performs this role in many fashions: It acts as a semipermeable barrier to both hydrophilic and hydrophobic substances; it is the first line of immunological defense against invading microbes; it contains many components of the adaptive and innate immune system; and it has many physiological roles, including metabolism of vitamin D.

The majority of the epidermis is made up of keratinocytes. It also contains melanocytes, Langerhans cells, and Merkel cells. The epidermis is avascular and receives its nutrition from the superficial vascular plexus of the papillary dermis.

Melanocytes are derived from neural crest and are responsible for producing the melanin family of pigments, which are packaged in melanosomes. Melanocytes are found in equal density in all humans, but darker-skinned individuals have a higher density of melanosomes than those with lighter skin. This is the reason for color variation among humans. Eumelanin, the predominant type of melanin protein, is responsible for brown and black pigmentation. Pheomelanin is a unique variant of melanin that is found in humans with red hair.

The skin is found in continuity with the epithelial lining of the digestive tract, including the oral mucosa and the anal mucosa. Distinct transition zones are seen at these interfaces. The skin also abuts the conjunctival mucosa of the globe and the mucosa of the nasal passages. The skin and its neighboring epithelial components supply the human body with a continuous barrier to protect it from the external world.

Many appendageal structures are present throughout the skin. The major ones are the hair follicles, their associated sebaceous glands, and the eccrine glands. Most of the skin is hair bearing. Fine vellus hairs make up the preponderance of the skin's hair production. Terminal hairs are much thicker and are found on the scalp, eyebrows, and eyelashes; in the axilla and groin areas; and in the beard region in men. Glabrous skin, which is devoid of hair follicles, includes the vermilion border of the lips, the palms, the soles, the glans penis, and the labia minora.

Human skin varies in thickness. It is thickest on the back, and the thinnest areas are found on the eyelids and the scrotum. Regardless of thickness, all skin possesses the same immunological function and barrier activity.

Various appendageal structures are found in higher densities in certain regions of the skin. Sebaceous glands are located predominantly on the face, upper chest, and back. These glands play an instrumental role in the pathomechanism of acne vulgaris. Because sebaceous glands are attached to hair follicles, they are found only on hair-bearing skin. Eccrine sweat glands, on the other hand, are found ubiquitously. The highest densities of eccrine glands are on the palms and soles.

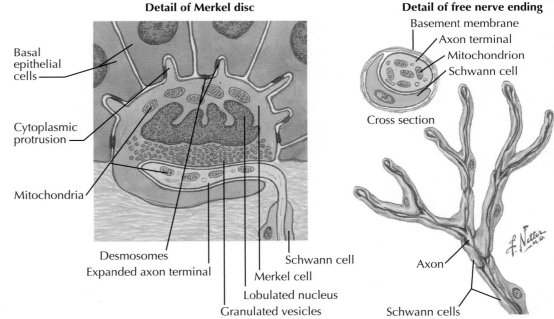

Detail of Merkel disc

Detail of free nerve ending

Cross section

The other main sweat glands of the skin, the apocrine glands, are found almost exclusively in the axillae and the groin. The apocrine glands, like sebaceous glands, are found only in conjunction with hair follicles.

Nails are composed of specialized keratin proteins. These keratins make a hard nail plate that is believed to be important for protection, grasp, and defense. Fingernails and toenails are made of the same keratin structure and in the same manner. The only difference is that the fingernails grow slightly faster than the toenails. The average thumbnail takes 6 months to replace itself, whereas the average great toenail takes 8 to 12 months.

Skin is also an important means of communication with other humans. The sense of touch is mediated through specialized receptors within the skin. One cannot underestimate the importance of this function in the formation of human relationships.

Plate 1-3

Integumentary System

NORMAL SKIN HISTOLOGY

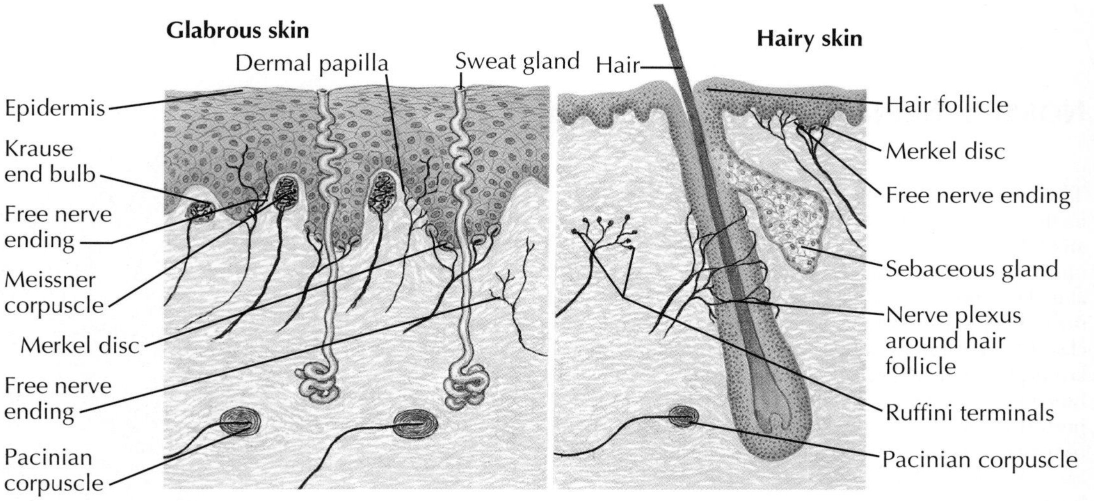

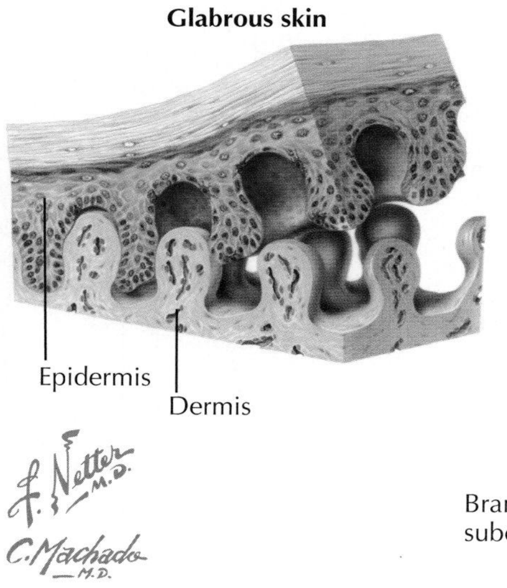

The integumentary system is composed of multiple subunits that work in unison. The skin and its appendageal structures make up the integumentary system. There are three main layers to the skin: epidermis, dermis, and subcutaneous tissue. Within the epidermis, the principal skin cell is the keratinocyte. Other cells found in the epidermis include melanocytes, Merkel cells, and Langerhans cells. The main cell type found within the dermis is the fibroblast. Fibroblasts make collagen, which forms the mechanical support for the skin. The dermis is a region of high vascularity. The subcutaneous fat tissue is found directly beneath the dermis and is composed primarily of adipocytes.

The normal human epidermis varies extensively in thickness in different regions of the body. It is thickest on the back and thinnest on the eyelids and on the scrotal skin. The epidermis can be subdivided into five components: stratum basale, stratum spinosum, stratum granulosum, stratum lucidum, and stratum corneum. The stratum lucidum is found only on the skin of the palms and soles. Each layer of the epidermis has important anatomical and physiological functions.

The stratum basale is the deepest layer. It consists of cuboidal epithelium sitting atop a basement membrane zone. The stratum basale contains the proliferating keratinocytes, which are constantly undergoing replication to replace the overlying epidermis. It takes approximately 28 days for a basal keratinocyte to progress to the outermost layer of the stratum corneum. Melanocytes and Merkel cells can also be found within the stratum basale. Melanocytes are pigment-forming cells; they transfer their pigment to neighboring keratinocytes. Merkel cells are modified nerve endings and have been found to be important as mechanoreceptors.

The stratum spinosum is many cell layers thick and is recognized by the intercellular connections among adjacent keratinocytes, which are seen on light microscopy as tiny spines. From the lower to the upper layers of the stratum spinosum, the keratinocytes progressively become flatter in appearance.

The stratum granulosum is recognized by the large number of basophilic keratohyalin granules within its keratinocytes. This stratum is typically 2 to 4 cell layers thick. The keratohyalin granules are composed primarily of the protein profilaggrin; they vary from 1 to 4 μm in diameter. Profilaggrin is the precursor to filaggrin, an essential protein that is required for the integrity of the overlying epidermis.

The stratum lucidum occurs only in the skin of the palms and soles. It is composed of a translucent eosinophilic layer. The stratum lucidum is made up of tightly packed squamous keratinocytes.

The stratum corneum, the outermost layer of skin, is made up of anucleate, cornified keratinocytes. Keratinization (cornification) is a complex process that results in the appearance of the stratum corneum. As cells progress up the stratum corneum, they are shed in the process known as desquamation.

The dermis is primarily composed of collagen, which is produced by fibroblasts. This portion of the skin contains a highly vascular network that is responsible for the nutrition of the skin and for thermoregulation. This network includes a deep dermal plexus and a superficial plexus. The superficial plexus is responsible for thermoregulation. It undergoes vasoconstriction during exposure to cold temperatures and vasodilation in times of warm temperature. The dermis can be split into two regions, called the papillary and the reticular portions. The papillary dermis is juxtaposed to the overlying epidermis and interdigitates with it. The papillary dermis and the epidermis are connected by the basement membrane zone. This zone contains many unique proteins. These proteins are the targets for the various autoantibodies that can be found in patients with autoimmune blistering diseases.

The subcutaneous tissue is composed of adipocytes. This tissue's main functions are storage of energy, insulation, and cushioning. The adipocytes are closely packed in a connective tissue septum with associated blood vessels and nerve endings.

There are many types of skin appendages, including hair follicles, sebaceous glands, eccrine glands, apocrine glands, and various nerve endings.

Glabrous skin

Epidermis
Dermal papilla
Sweat gland
Krause end bulb
Free nerve ending
Meissner corpuscle
Merkel disc
Free nerve ending
Pacinian corpuscle

Hairy skin

Hair
Hair follicle
Merkel disc
Free nerve ending
Sebaceous gland
Nerve plexus around hair follicle
Ruffini terminals
Pacinian corpuscle

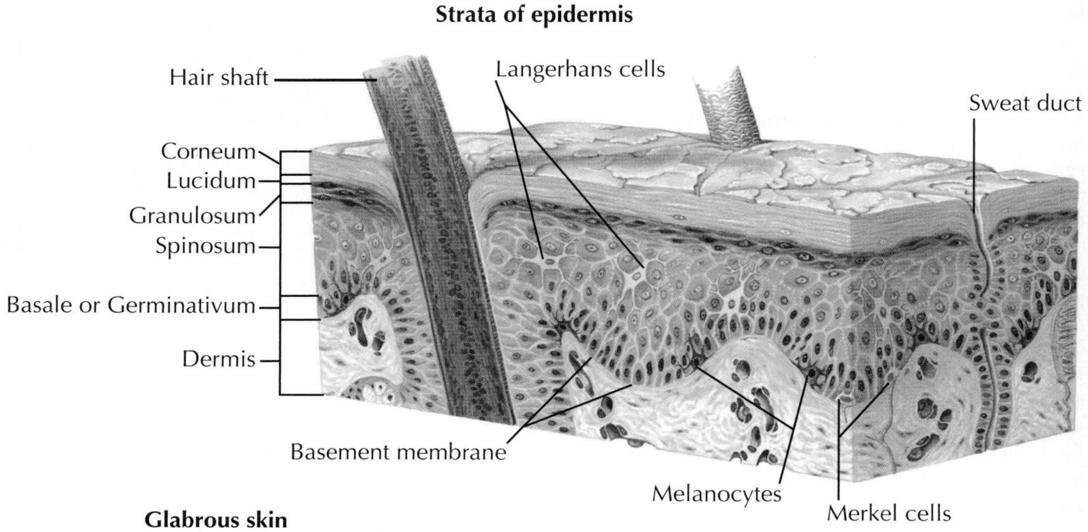

Strata of epidermis

Hair shaft
Langerhans cells
Sweat duct
Corneum
Lucidum
Granulosum
Spinosum
Basale or Germinativum
Dermis
Basement membrane
Melanocytes
Merkel cells

Glabrous skin

Epidermis
Dermis

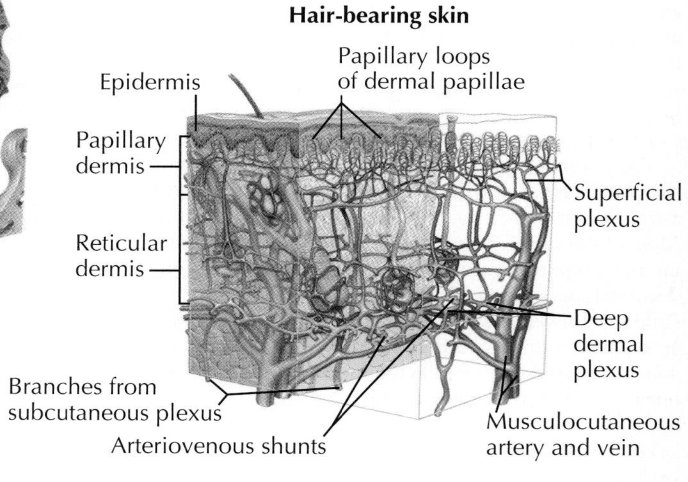

Hair-bearing skin

Epidermis
Papillary loops of dermal papillae
Papillary dermis
Superficial plexus
Reticular dermis
Deep dermal plexus
Branches from subcutaneous plexus
Arteriovenous shunts
Musculocutaneous artery and vein

Plate 1-4

Anatomy, Physiology, and Embryology

SKIN PHYSIOLOGY: THE PROCESS OF KERATINIZATION

Keratinization, also known as cornification, is unique to the epithelium of the skin. Keratinization of the human skin is of paramount importance; it allows humans to live on dry land. The process of keratinization begins in the basal layer of the epidermis and continues upward until full keratinization has occurred in the stratum corneum. The function and purpose of keratinization is to form the stratum corneum.

The stratum corneum is a highly organized layer that is relatively strong and resistant to physical and chemical insults. This layer is critically important in keeping out microorganisms; it is the first line of defense against ultraviolet radiation; and it contains many enzymes that can degrade and detoxify external chemicals. The stratum corneum is also a semipermeable structure that selectively allows different hydrophilic and lipophilic agents passage. However, the most obvious and most studied aspect of the stratum corneum is its ability to protect against excessive water and electrolyte loss. It acts as a barrier to keep chemicals out, but more importantly, it keeps water and electrolytes inside the human body. Transepidermal water loss (TEWL) increases as the stratum corneum is damaged or disrupted. The main lipids responsible for protection against water loss are the ceramides and the sphingolipids. These molecules are capable of binding many water molecules.

As keratinocytes migrate from the stratum basale and journey through the layers of the epidermis, they undergo characteristic morphological and biochemical changes. The keratinocytes flatten and become more compacted and polyhedral. The resulting corneocytes become stacked, like bricks in a wall. These corneocytes are still bonded together by desmosomes, which are now called corneodesmosomes.

The stratum granulosum gets its name from the appearance of multiple basophilic keratohyalin granules present within the keratinocytes. These granules are largely composed of the protein profilaggrin. Profilaggrin is converted into filaggrin by an intercellular endoproteinase enzyme. Filaggrin is so named because it is a filament-aggregating protein. Over time, filaggrin is broken down into natural moisturizing factor (NMF) and urocanic acid. NMF is a breakdown product of filaggrin that slows water evaporation from the corneocytes.

The intercellular space is composed of lipids and water. The lipids are derived from the release of the lamellar bodies (Odland bodies). Ceramides make up the overwhelming majority of the contents of the lamellar bodies. Other components include free fatty acids, cholesterol esters, and proteases. The lamellar bodies fuse with the cell surface and release their contents into the intercellular space. The fusion of the lamellar body with the cell surface is dependent on the enzyme transglutaminase I.

Concurrently, the cornified cell envelope (CCE) develops. The CCE proteins envoplakin, loricrin, periplakin, small proline-rich proteins, and involucrin are cross-linked in various arrangements by transglutaminase I and transglutaminase III, forming a sturdy scaffolding along the inner surface of the keratinocyte cell

Bricks (keratinocytes)

Mortar (intercellular space of the stratum corneum)

Corneodesmosomes

Cornified cell envelope cross linked with ceramides replaces plasma membrane

Corneodesmosome

Filaments of keratin

Corneocyte

Keratohyalin granules

Golgi apparatus

Lamellar bodies (LB) that are seen today as part of a branched tubular structure like the trans-Golgi network migrate to the surface of the cell of the stratum granulosum (SG) and release their content into the intercellular space (ICS). The released lipids are rearranged into lamellar membrane (LM)

The dashed lines (◄ - - ►) show the tortuous intercellular penetration pathway within the stratum corneum taken by water-soluble substances when the permeability of the skin barrier is activated

membrane. As the keratinocyte migrates upward, the cell membrane is lost, and the ceramides that are released begin cross-linking with the CCE proteins. The cells continue to move toward the surface of the skin and begin to lose their nucleus and cellular organelles. The loss of these organelles is mediated by the activation of certain proteases that can quickly degrade protein, DNA, RNA, and the nuclear membrane.

Once the cells reach the outer layers of the stratum corneum, they begin to be shed. On average, a keratinocyte spends 2 weeks in the stratum corneum before being shed from the skin surface in a process called desquamation. Shedding is achieved by the final degradation of the corneodesmosomes by proteases that destroy the desmoglein-1 protein.

Keratinization is especially important in the diseases of cornification. Many skin diseases have been found to involve defects in one or more proteins that are critical in the process of cornification. Examples are lamellar ichthyosis, which is caused by a defect in the transglutaminase I enzyme, and Vohwinkel's syndrome (keratoma hereditarium mutilans), which results from a genetic mutation in the loricrin protein and a resultant defective CCE.

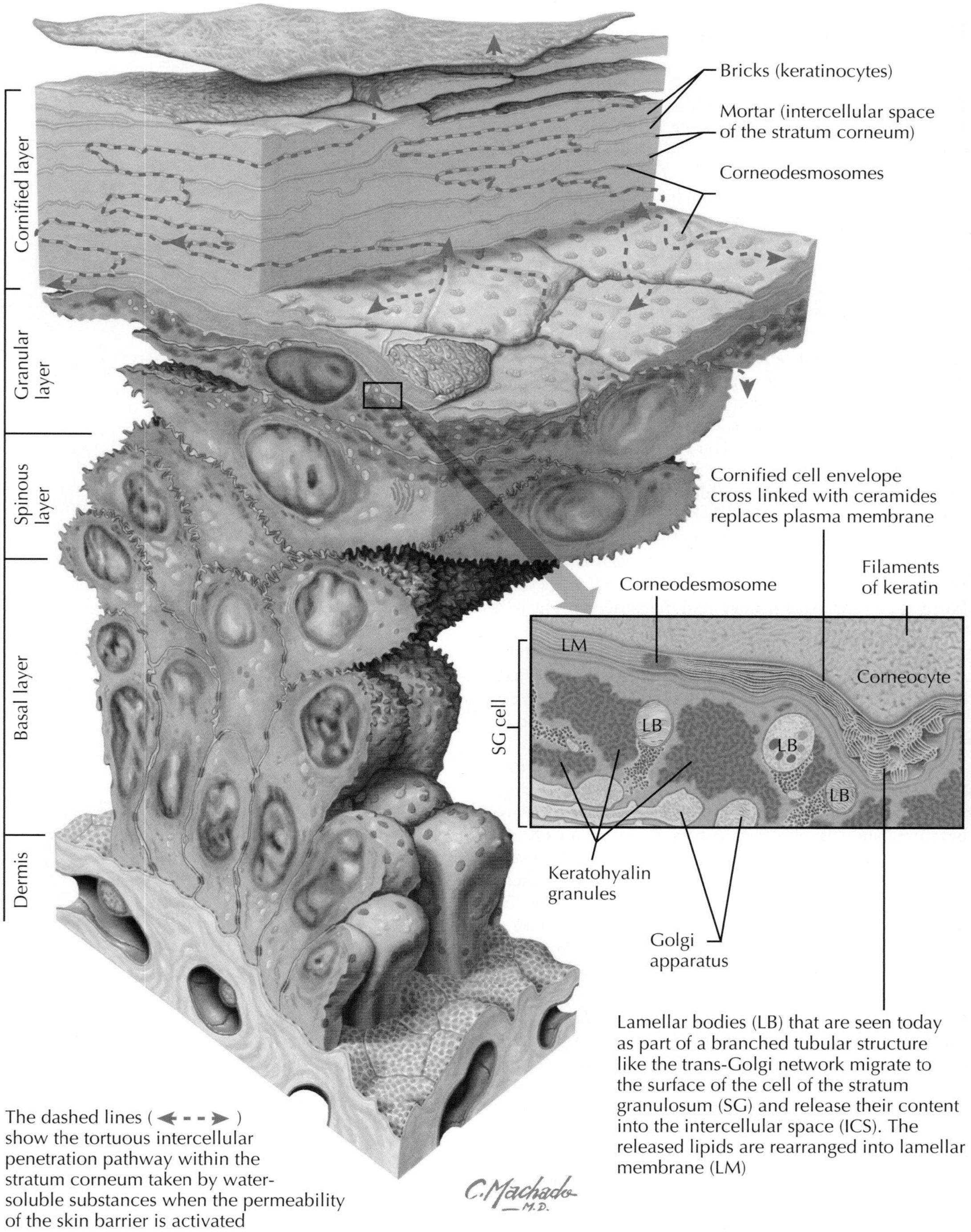

Plate 1-5   Integumentary System

NORMAL SKIN FLORA

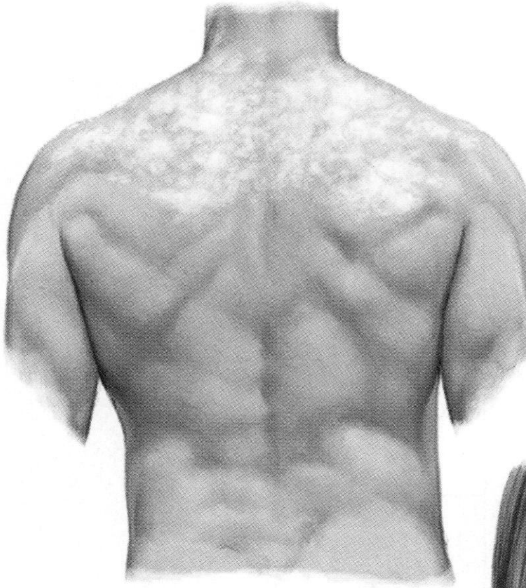

The skin contains normal microflora that are universally found on all humans. It has been estimated that the number of bacteria on the surface of the human skin is greater than the number of cells in the human body. The normal skin flora include the bacteria *Staphylococcus epidermidis*, *Corynebacterium* species, *Propionobacterium acnes*, *Micrococcus* species, and *Acetobacter* species. The demodex mites are the only parasites considered to be part of the normal flora. *Pityrosporum* species are the only fungi that are considered to be normal skin flora.

The microbes that make up the normal skin flora under most circumstances do not cause any type of disease. They are able to reproduce and maintain viable populations, living in harmony with the host. In stark contrast, transient skin flora can sustain growth only in certain skin environments. Transient microbes are not able to produce long-lasting, viable reproductive populations and therefore are unable to maintain a permanent residence. Some examples of transient skin flora are *Staphylococcus aureus*, including methicillin-resistant *S. aureus* (MRSA), *Enterobacter coli*, *Pseudomonas aeruginosa*, *Streptococcus pyogenes*, and some *Bacillus* species. Normal and transient flora can become pathogenic under the correct environmental conditions.

Normal bacterial colonization begins immediately after birth. Once newborns are exposed to the external environment, they are quickly colonized with bacteria. *S. epidermidis* is often the first colonizing species, and it is the one most commonly cultured in neonates.

The innate ability of certain bacteria to colonize the human skin is dependent on a host of contributing factors. Availability of nutrients, pH, hydration, temperature, and ultraviolet radiation exposure all play a role in allowing certain bacteria to develop a synergistic balance. The normal skin flora use these factors to their survival advantage and live in a symbiotic relationship with the human skin. These microbes have evolved a competitive advantage over the transient skin flora.

Under certain circumstances, normal skin flora can become pathogenic and cause overt skin disease. Overgrowth of *Pityrosporum ovale (Malassezia furfur)* causes tinea versicolor, an exceedingly common superficial fungal infection. Warm and humid environments are believed to be factors in the pathogenesis. Tinea versicolor manifests as fine, scaly patches with hyperpigmentation and hypopigmentation. Other *Malassezia* species have been implicated in causing neonatal cephalic pustulosis, pityrosporum folliculitis, and seborrheic dermatitis.

The common skin bacterium, *S. epidermidis*, is a gram-positive coccus that can become a pathogenic microbe under certain circumstances. Conditions that increase the chance that this bacterium will cause pathogenic skin disease include use of immunosuppressive medications, immunocompromised state (e.g., human immunodeficiency virus infection), and presence of a chronic indwelling intravenous catheter. *S. epidermidis* creates a biofilm on indwelling catheters, which can lead to transient bacteremia and sepsis in immunocompromised patients and occasionally in the immunocompetent.

P. acnes is a gram-positive organism that is found within the pilosebaceous unit. These bacteria occur in high densities in the sebum-rich regions of the face, back, and chest. It is the major species implicated in the pathogenesis of acne vulgaris. In immunocompromised individuals, it has been reported to cause abscesses.

Corynebacterium species, when in an environment of moisture and warmth, can produce an overgrowth on

The normal skin flora includes *Pityrosporum/Malassezia furfur*, which under pathologic conditions may cause tinea versicolor.

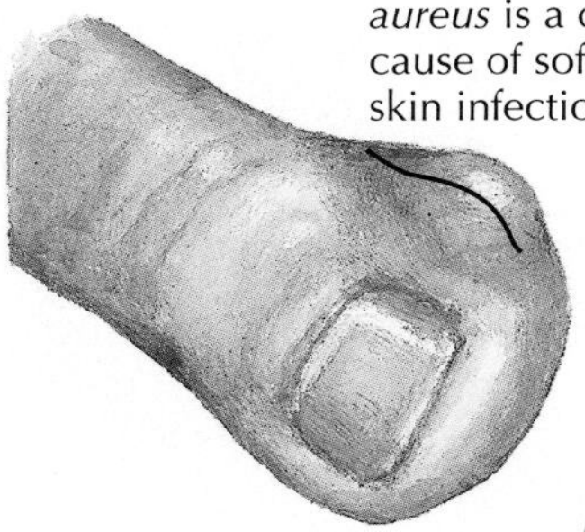

Staphylococcus aureus is a common cause of soft tissue skin infections.

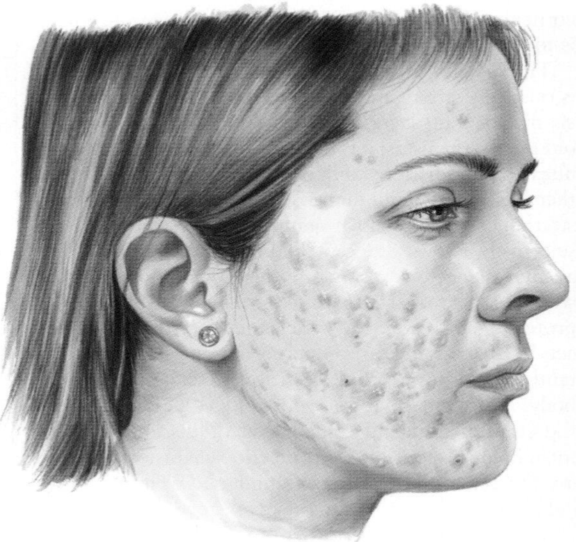

The normal skin flora *Propionibacterium acnes* is partially responsible for the pathomechanism of acne vulgaris.

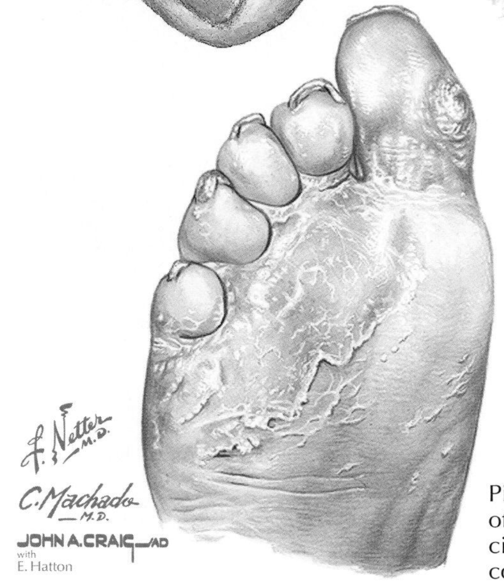

Pitted keratolysis may be caused by overgrowth of *Corynebacterium* species. Under normal circumstances, corynebacterium species are considered normal skin flora.

the terminal hairs of the axilla and groin regions, resulting in the condition known as trichomycosis axillaris. Different colonies of this bacterium can produce superficial red, yellow, or black nodules along the terminal hair shafts. Corynebacteria can also cause pitted keratolysis, a superficial infection of the outer layers of the epidermis on the soles.

The only parasites that can be found normally on human skin are the demodex mites, which live in various regions of the pilosebaceous unit. *Demodex brevis* lives within the sebaceous gland ducts, whereas *Demodex*

folliculorum lives in the hair follicle infundibulum. Demodex mites can cause demodex folliculitis. an infection of the hair follicles that manifests as superficial, follicle-based pustules.

The most important skin microbes, based on their ability to cause pathology, are the transient microbes. The best-known species is *S. aureus*. The ability of *S. aureus* to cause folliculitis, boils, abscesses, and bacterial sepsis is well documented and is a major cause of morbidity and mortality.

Plate 1-6

Anatomy, Physiology, and Embryology

VITAMIN D METABOLISM

The skin plays a critical role in the production of vitamin D and thus in calcium and phosphate hemostasis. The epidermis turns provitamin D_3 (7-dehydrocholesterol) into vitamin D_3 (cholecalciferol) through interaction with ultraviolet B (UVB) radiation. The keratinocytes within the epidermis contains enzymes that convert vitamin D_3 into 25-hydroxyvitamin D_3. The skin also can produce 1,25-dihydroxyvitamin D_3, known as calcitriol. This biologically active metabolite is critical in calcium metabolism, bone metabolism, and neuromuscular transmission and most likely is an important player in the immune system regulation of ultraviolet-induced DNA damage. Vitamin D_2 (ergocalciferol) and vitamin D_3 are both absorbed by the gastrointestinal tract; they are often collectively referred to as vitamin D.

When skin is exposed to sunlight, it immediately begins production of vitamin D_3. Ultraviolet radiation, predominantly UVB (290-320 nm), interacts with keratinocytes to convert provitamin D_3 (which is also an important precursor in the production of cholesterol) into previtamin D_3. Previtamin D_3 is further converted into vitamin D_3 via a spontaneous endothermic reaction. Vitamin D_3 produced in the skin can act locally or be absorbed into the systemic circulation and added to the concentration of vitamin D_3 absorbed by the gastrointestinal tract. An elevated level of vitamin D_3 in the general circulation causes increased absorption of calcium and phosphate through the gastrointestinal tract, increased mobilization of calcium stores from bone tissue, and increased release of parathyroid hormone (PTH), which results in a lowering of the serum phosphate concentration.

The earliest sign of vitamin D deficiency is an often subtle and transient decrease in the serum calcium level. This decrease causes the pituitary gland to secrete PTH, which acts on the kidneys to increase calcium reabsorption, decrease phosphate retention, and increase osteoclast activity. This increase in osteoclast activity also increases the serum calcium level. Vitamin D deficiency is manifested by normal serum calcium levels, increased PTH levels, and decreased phosphorous levels.

Vitamin D_3 synthesis in the skin is dependent on contact with UVB radiation. Sunscreens, clothing, and glass all block UVB radiation and diminish the local production of vitamin D_3 in the skin.

Immunologically, 1,25-vitamin D_3 has been found to regulate the maturation of dendritic cells, monocytes, and T lymphocytes. Vitamin D and its analogues are believed to inhibit tumor cell proliferation and to cause apoptosis of tumor cells. Because the vitamin D receptor (VDR) forms heterodimers with the retinoid X receptor (RXR) and other retinoid receptors, the combination of vitamin D and vitamin A analogues may ultimately be found to be responsible for the immunological effects of both of these vitamins.

Rickets is a disease of childhood that is caused by severe vitamin D deficiency. It is rarely seen in the United States in the twenty-first century, but it is not uncommon in developing countries. Vitamin D deficiency in adults more commonly manifests as osteomalacia, which occurs throughout the world. The deficiency leads to decreased bone mineralization and can cause osteopenia and osteoporosis. The normal concentration of vitamin D in serum is believed to be between 35 and 200 nmol/L.

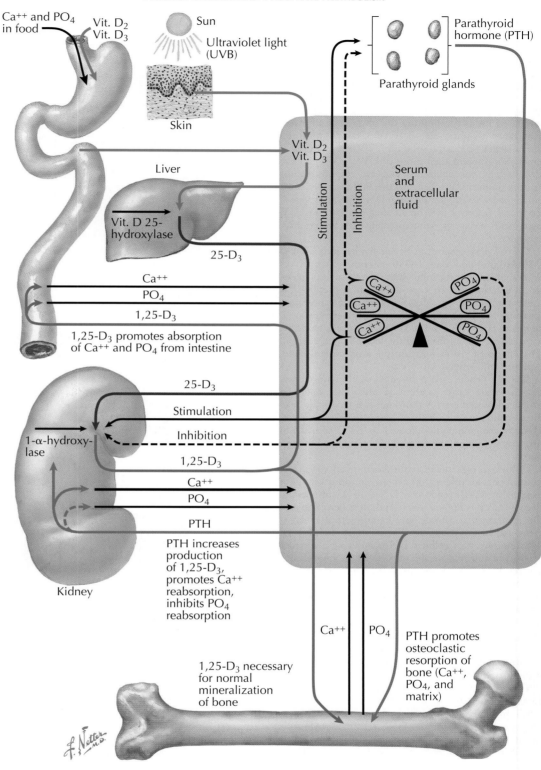

NORMAL CALCIUM AND PHOSPHATE METABOLISM

1,25-Vitamin D_3 exerts its effect by binding with the VDR and then interacting with DNA to directly modulate the transcription of specific genes. The VDR is a member of the nuclear receptor family. 1,25-Vitamin D_3 enters a cell, binds with VDR in the cytoplasm, and then enters the nucleus of the cell. There, the complex interacts with cellular DNA by binding to various regulatory sites. In this way, vitamin D_3 and the VDR are able to modulate gene transcription. The

VDR also forms heterodimers with other members of the nuclear receptor family, mainly the RXR. Most VDR signaling involves this heterodimer form.

Vitamin D is one of the fat-soluble vitamins. It is found in many foods, such as cod liver oil, many fish, egg yolks, and liver. More commonly, one encounters vitamin D as a supplement in many foods such as milk, breads, and cereals. Oral vitamin D supplements are easily obtained and well tolerated.

Plate 1-7

Integumentary System

PHOTOBIOLOGY

On a daily basis, the skin interacts with some form of light. The most abundant and physiologically relevant portion of the light spectrum is the ultraviolet range (200-400 nm). The ozone layer essentially prevents all ultraviolet C rays (200-280 nm) from reaching the surface of the earth, limiting the physiologically relevant range to ultraviolet B (UVB; 280-320 nm) and ultraviolet A (UVA; 320-400 nm). UVB rays are 1000 times more potent than those of UVA. UVB rays are absorbed by the epidermis and are responsible for causing sunburns. It is believed that 300 nm is the most potent wavelength for causing DNA photoproducts. Erythema begins 2 to 6 hours after exposure to UVB light and peaks at approximately 10 hours after exposure.

The UVA spectrum can be subdivided into UVA II (320-340 nm) and UVA I (340-400 nm). UVA II rays are responsible for the immediate but transient pigmentation that is seen after exposure to ultraviolet light. It causes melanocytes to release preformed melanosomes, resulting in a mild increase in skin pigmentation that begins to fade within a day. UVA I rays are responsible for a longer-lasting but slightly delayed pigmentation. The effects of visible light on the skin are still being explored and defined.

The sun produces vast amounts of ultraviolet light, but there are other sources of ultraviolet radiation produced by humans. A thorough history should take into account an individual's occupations and exposures. Welders are commonly exposed to UVC and, if not properly protected, can develop severe skin and corneal burns.

Ultraviolet rays interact with skin in many ways. The most important interaction is between ultraviolet light (especially UVB) and the DNA of keratinocytes. Because UVB is limited in its depth of penetration into the epidermis, it affects only keratinocytes, melanocytes, and Langerhans cells. The photons of ultraviolet light interact with cellular DNA, inducing a number of specific and nonspecific effects. These interactions can result in DNA photoproducts, which are formed between adjacent pyrimidine nucleoside bases on one strand of DNA. The most common photoproducts are cyclobutane pyrimidine dimers and the pyrimidine-pyrimidone 6,4 photoproduct. The common cyclobutane pyrimidine dimer mutation is highly specific for ultraviolet damage. These photoproducts cause a decrease in DNA replication, mutagenesis, and, ultimately, carcinogenesis.

The cell nucleus is well equipped to handle DNA damage caused by photoproducts. A series of DNA repair proteins are in constant surveillance. Once a photoproduct is found, the DNA repair mechanism is called into service. There are at least seven well-described proteins that help in recognition, removal of the damage, and repair of the DNA strand. These seven proteins were named XPA through XPG after studies of numerous patients with the photosensitivity disorder, xeroderma pigmentosum. Each is uniquely responsible for some part of the DNA repair mechanism. Defects in any of these XP proteins results in a differing phenotype of xeroderma pigmentosum. Patients with xeroderma pigmentosum are prone to develop multiple skin cancers at a young age.

Proteins within the cells are also susceptible to damage from ultraviolet light exposure. The amino acids histidine and cysteine are very susceptible to

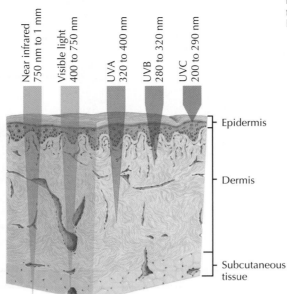

Comparison of penetration of radiation with different wavelengths into human skin

Near infrared 750 nm to 1 mm
Visible light 400 to 750 nm
UVA 320 to 400 nm
UVB 280 to 320 nm
UVC 200 to 290 nm

Epidermis

Dermis

Subcutaneous tissue

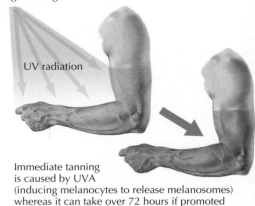

Erythema and tanning onset and duration are UV wavelength dependent. By comparison, UVA radiation induces transient erythema. The erythema from UVB takes 6–24 hours to induce and is much longer lasting.

UV radiation

Immediate tanning is caused by UVA (inducing melanocytes to release melanosomes) whereas it can take over 72 hours if promoted by UVB (increased production of melanin)

C.Machado M.D.

Nucleotide excision repair (NER) is a major DNA repair mechanism in eukaryotic cells for removing several DNA lesions caused by different agents, including UV-induced damages such as thymine-thymine dimer, the most common cyclobutane pyrimidine dimer mutation. NER comprises the following steps:

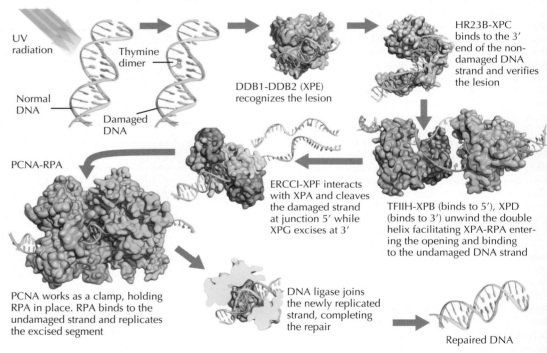

UV radiation

Thymine dimer

Normal DNA

Damaged DNA

DDB1-DDB2 (XPE) recognizes the lesion

HR23B-XPC binds to the 3' end of the non-damaged DNA strand and verifies the lesion

PCNA-RPA

ERCCI-XPF interacts with XPA and cleaves the damaged strand at junction 5' while XPG excises at 3'

TFIIH-XPB (binds to 5'), XPD (binds to 3') unwind the double helix facilitating XPA-RPA entering the opening and binding to the undamaged DNA strand

PCNA works as a clamp, holding RPA in place. RPA binds to the undamaged strand and replicates the excised segment

DNA ligase joins the newly replicated strand, completing the repair

Repaired DNA

XP (XPA XPB, XPC...) = Xeroderma pigmentosum (A, B, C...), **HR23B** or **hHRD23B** = Human Homologue of Yeast Rad23, **DDB** = Damaged DNA-binding protein TFIIH = Transcription factor iih, **PCNA** = Proliferating Cell Nuclear Antigen, **RPA** = Replication Protein A, **ERCC** = Excision repair cross-complementing

oxidation reactions after interaction with ultraviolet light. Melanin pigment also absorbs ultraviolet light, and this is one of the means by which the skin defends itself against ultraviolet assault. Absorption of ultraviolet light by cell membranes, organelles, RNA, and other components of the living cell can cause oxidative stress and cellular damage.

When exposed to ultraviolet radiation, the skin increases production of melanin, which in turn helps in photoprotection. Many organic and inorganic compounds have been used as sunscreens to help neutralize the effects of ultraviolet radiation on skin. The main protective mechanisms are absorption, reflection, and physical blockade.

Plate 1-8

Anatomy, Physiology, and Embryology

WOUND HEALING

Wound healing is a complex process that involves an orderly and sequential series of interactions among multiple cell types and tissue structures. Classically, wound healing has been divided into three phases: inflammation, new tissue formation, and matrix formation and remodeling. Each of these phases is unique, and particular cell types play key roles in the different phases.

Once a disruption of the skin barrier occurs, a cascade of inflammatory mediators are released, and wound healing begins. The disruption of dermal blood vessels allows extravasation of blood into the tissues. The ruptured vessels undergo immediate vasoconstriction. Platelets begin the process of coagulation and initiate the earliest phase of inflammation. The formation of the earliest blood clot provides the foundation for future cell migration into the wound. Many inflammatory mediators are released during this initial phase. Once initial homeostasis is achieved, the platelets discharge the contents of their alpha granules into the extravascular space. Alpha granules contain fibrinogen, fibronectin, von Willebrand's factor, factor VIII, and many other proteins. The fibrinogen is converted into fibrin, which aids in formation of the fibrin clot. Platelets also play a critical role in releasing growth factors and proteases. The best known of these is platelet-derived growth factor (PDGF), which helps mediate the formation of the initial granulation tissue.

During the late portion of the inflammatory phase, leukocytes are seen for the first time. Neutrophils make up the largest component of the initial leukocyte response. Neutrophils are drawn into the area by various cytokines and adhere to the activated vascular endothelium. They enter the extravascular space by a process of diapedesis. These early-arriving neutrophils are responsible for the recruitment of more neutrophils, and they also begin the process of killing bacteria by use of their internal myeloperoxidase system. Through the production of free radicals, neutrophils are efficient at killing large numbers of bacteria. Neutrophil activity continues for a few days, unless the wound is contaminated with bacteria. Once the neutrophil activity has cleared the wound of bacteria and other foreign particles, monocytes are recruited into the wound and activated into macrophages. Macrophages are critical in clearing the wound of neutrophils and any remaining cellular and bacterial debris. Macrophages are capable of producing nitrous oxide, which can kill bacteria and has also been shown to decrease viral replication. Macrophages also release various cytokines, including PDGF, interleukin-6, and granulocyte colony-stimulating factor (G-CSF), which in turn recruit more monocytes and fibroblasts into the wound.

At this point, new tissue formation, the proliferative phase of wound healing, has begun. This phase typically begins on the third day and ends about 14 days after the initial insult. It is marked by reepithelialization and formation of granulation tissue. Reepithelialization occurs by the movement of epithelial cells (keratinocytes) from the free edge of the wound slowly across the wound defect. The migrating cells have the distinct phenotype of basal keratinocytes. It is believed that a low calcium concentration in the wound causes the keratinocytes to take on the characteristics of basal keratinocytes. PDGF is an important stimulant for keratinocytes and is partially responsible for this migration across the wound. The migrating keratinocytes

HEALING OF INCISED, SUTURED SKIN WOUND

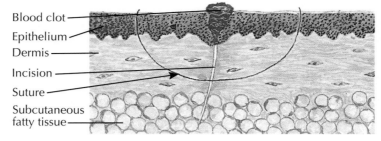

Blood clot
Epithelium
Dermis
Incision
Suture
Subcutaneous fatty tissue

Immediately after incision
Blood clot with fine fibrin network forms in wound. Epithelium thickens at wound edges.

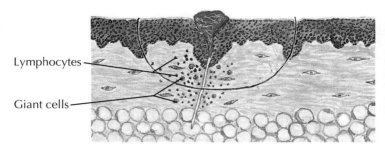

Lymphocytes
Giant cells

24-48 hours
Epithelium begins to grow down along cut edges and along suture tract. Leukocyte infiltration, chiefly round cells (lymphocytes) with few giant cells, occurs and removes bacteria and necrotic tissue.

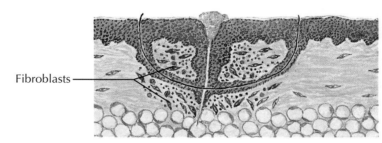

Fibroblasts

5-8 days
Epithelial downgrowth advances. Fibroblasts grow in from deeper tissues and add collagen precursors and glycoproteins to matrix. Cellular infiltration progresses.

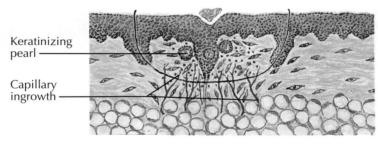

Keratinizing pearl
Capillary ingrowth

10-15 days
Capillaries grow in from subcutaneous tissue, forming granulation tissue. Epithelium bridges incision; epithelial downgrowths regress, leaving keratinizing pearls behind. Fibrosed clot (scab) is being pushed out. Collagen formation progresses and cellular infiltration abates.

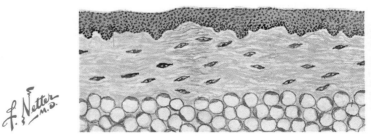

3 weeks–9 months
Epithelium is thinned to near normal. Tensile strength of tissue is increased owing to production and cross-linking of collagen fibers; elastic fibers reappear later.

contain the keratin pairs 5,14 and 6,16. They secrete vascular endothelial growth factor, which promotes the production of dermal blood vessels. At the same time the keratinocytes are migrating, the underlying fibroblasts are synthesizing a backbone matrix, made up predominantly of type III collagen and some proteoglycans. Some of the fibroblasts are converted into myofibroblasts by PDGF and tumor growth factor-β1. These myofibroblasts are important in that they cause the overlying wound to contract, decreasing its surface.

The final phase of wound healing involves scar maturation and tissue remodeling. This phase overlaps in time with the first two phases; it is said to begin with the production of the first granulation tissue. This phase extends for months and is complete when most of the collagen III and fibronectin have been replaced by mature type I collagen. In the final mature scar, the collagen fibers are oriented in large bundles running perpendicular to the basement membrane zone. The resulting scar has only 80% of the tensile strength of the uninjured skin.

Plate 1-9   Integumentary System

MORPHOLOGY: LICHENIFICATION, PLAQUES, AND FISSURES

MORPHOLOGY

The first lesson a student of dermatology must learn is how to properly describe skin diseases. Skin morphology has been well defined over the years and is the basis for all discussions about skin disorders. One must be adept at describing skin lesions before it is possible to develop a differential diagnosis. For example, once it has been determined that a rash is in the morphological category of macule, all rashes in the blistering and nodular categories can easily be excluded from the differential diagnosis. To get a firm grasp of dermatology, one must have an excellent foundation in description and morphology. The most common descriptors used in the dermatology lexicon are discussed here.

Skin lesions and rashes can be described as primary or secondary lesions. The primary category includes macules, papules, comedones, patches, plaques, nodules, tumors, hives, vesicles, bullae, and pustules. The secondary lesions are best described as scales, crusts, erosions, excoriations, ulcerations, fissures, scars, lichenification, and burrows.

Many adjectives are used in conjunction with primary and secondary descriptive terms to better characterize the lesion and to help determine a differential diagnosis and, ultimately, a diagnosis for the patient. Color is of utmost importance and is universally used in the description of skin lesions. For example, a good description of melanoma would include color, size, regularity, and the primary morphology, such as "a dark black, irregularly shaped macule with a central nodule."

Other descriptive terms often used in dermatology deal with the configuration of the lesion, such as a linear or an annular configuration. Words such as arcuate, polycyclical, nummular, and agminated are also commonly used. Some skin rashes tend to follow specific types of skin lines, most commonly Langer's lines (skin tension lines) and Blaschko's lines (embryological cleavage lines).

The distribution of skin lesions is also important, because some skin diseases have a propensity to occur in specific areas of the body. A classic example is acne, which typically affects the face, upper back, and chest. It would be inappropriate to consider acne in the differential diagnosis of a rash on the hands and feet.

Starting with the primary skin lesions, a macule is most often thought of as a well-circumscribed, flat area on the skin with a distinct color change. The macule may have an irregular or a regular border. Macules are not raised and are essentially nonpalpable. An example of a macule is vitiligo.

A papule is a well-circumscribed, small (<5 mm in diameter) elevation in the skin of variable color. A papule is solid and should not be confused with a vesicle. Papules may be described as flat-topped or umbilicated, and their consistency may be characterized as soft or firm. An example of an umbilicated papule is molluscum contagiosum.

Comedones are seen in acne and in a few less common conditions. Essentially, they come in two forms, open and closed. Open comedones are also known as blackheads. Each comedo represents a dilated follicular infundibulum with a buildup of oxidized keratin. Closed comedones are seen as tiny white papules, which are

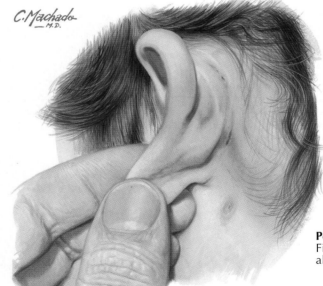

Urticaria (hives). Evanescent pink-red pruritic plaques

Lichen simplex chronicus. Lichenified excoriated plaque on the ankle, showing accentuation of the skin lines

C. Machado
M.D.

Postauricular fissures. Fissures are linear thin erosions or ulcers along skin lines.

produced when the follicular epithelium sticks together and seals the follicular orifice.

The word *patch* is sometimes used to describe a large macule. A more precise definition of a patch is an area of the skin that is not elevated but has surface change such as scale or crust. An example of a patch is tinea corporis. Depending on the source or reference review, the term *patch* can include either of these two definitions.

A plaque is a well-defined lesion that has a plateau-like elevation and is typically larger than 5 mm in diameter. The term *plaque* can also be used to describe a confluence of papules. An example of a plaque is a lesion of psoriasis.

A nodule is defined as a space-occupying lesion in the dermis or subcutaneous tissue. Its breadth is typically larger than its height. Surface changes may or may not

Plate 1-10

Anatomy, Physiology, and Embryology

MORPHOLOGY: MACULES, PATCHES, AND VESICULO-PUSTULES

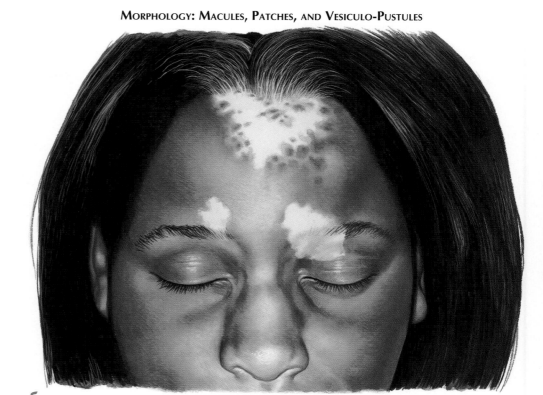

Vitiligo. Depigmented macules

MORPHOLOGY (Continued)

be present. Most authors agree that nodules are typically larger than 1 cm in diameter, and they can be much larger.

A tumor is generally considered to be larger than 2 cm in diameter, and the term should be reserved exclusively for the description of malignant neoplasms. The words *tumor* and *nodule* are sometimes used interchangeably, which has caused confusion. Tumors can be elevated from the skin and located entirely in the epidermis, or they can be space-occupying lesions in the dermis or subcutaneous tissue. Tumors often develop necrosis over time because of their neoplastic nature. A classic example of a skin tumor is a fungating tumor, as seen with mycosis fungoides.

Hives or wheals are also known as urticaria; this is a very specific term used to describe evanescent, pink-red, pruritic plaques that spontaneously develop and remit within 24 hours. They tend to be extremely pruritic. Dermatographism is commonly seen in association with hives.

Blistering disorders are common pathological conditions, and their lesions may be described as vesicles or bullae. A vesicle is defined as a fluid-filled elevation less than 1 cm in diameter. A bulla is a fluid-filled epidermal cavity larger than 1 cm in diameter. Blisters are most often filled with serous fluid, but they can be filled with a purulent exudate or a hemorrhagic infiltrate. Bullae are often described as flaccid or as firm and intact.

Pustules are small elevations in the epidermis that are filled with neutrophilic debris. The infiltrate within a pustule may be sterile or infectious in nature. An example of a sterile pustule is pustular psoriasis. An example of an infectious pustule is folliculitis.

Secondary lesions are often encountered in the dermatology clinic and are of utmost importance when describing skin lesions and rashes. The word *scale* is used to describe exfoliating keratinocytes that have typically built up in such a mass that there is obvious surface change to the skin. Normal shedding of keratinocytes occurs on a daily basis, so a small amount of scale is found on every human's skin. It is the collection in large quantities that allows one to use *scale* as a descriptive term. Scale must be differentiated from crust. Crust is produced by the drying of blood, serum, or purulent drainage. Most commonly, a crust is described as a scab.

Excoriations are secondary lesions that develop as a result of repetitive scratching. Excoriations are typically linear but can be seen in many bizarre configurations.

Erosions are seen in many skin disorders, most commonly superficial blistering diseases, in which the upper layers of the epidermis have been removed, leaving a shallow, denuded erosion. Erosions are defined as breaks in the epidermis. This is in contrast to ulceration, which is defined as a break in the skin that extends into the dermis or subcutaneous tissue or, in severe cases, muscular tissue. A fissure is often seen on the palms or soles; it is a full-thickness epidermal break that follows the skin lines. Fissures have very sharply defined borders and are typically only a few centimeters long.

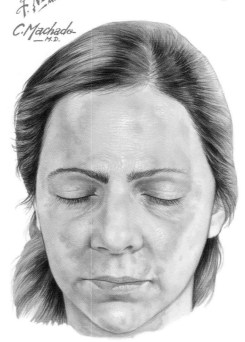

Tinea faciei. Annular scaly patches with a leading edge of scale

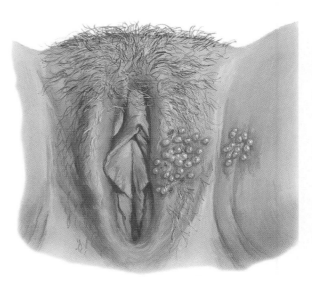

Herpes simplex virus. Tender vesiculo-pustules on a red base

Scar is another secondary descriptive term used to describe the healing of the epidermis and dermis, usually in a linear or a geographic pattern, caused by some form of trauma or end-stage inflammatory process. Fresh scars are typically pink to red; over time, they mature, becoming flattened and more pale.

Lichenification is seen as an end process in chronically rubbed skin. The skin lines become accentuated and thickened from the chronic rubbing. A classic example of lichenification is lichen simplex complex.

The last of the secondary descriptive lesions discussed here are burrows. Burrows are seen as tiny, irregularly shaped, serpiginous or linear scale, often with a tiny black dot at one end. They are pathognomonic for the diagnosis of scabies, and the tiny black dot represents the scabies mite.

BENIGN GROWTHS

Plate 2-1

Integumentary System

ACROCHORDON

Acrochordons are better known by their common name of skin tag or fibroepithelial polyp. They are found universally throughout humankind. Probably every adult has at least one skin tag located somewhere across the surface of his or her skin. Except for a few loose associations with certain syndromes, skin tags have no clinical importance and are often ignored.

Clinical Findings: Skin tags can be found throughout the adult population. They have no sex or race predilection. They are completely benign skin growths that have no malignant potential. They are most commonly located in the axillae, on the neck, in the groin area, and on the eyelids but can be found in other locations. Skin tags are almost never seen in children. The finding of a skin tag in a child should lead one to perform a biopsy to rule out a basal cell carcinoma. Basal cell carcinoma syndrome has been well documented to manifest in children, and the basal cell carcinoma has been shown in this syndrome to mimic the appearance of skin tags. If one sees a skin tag in a child, performs a skin biopsy, and discovers it is a basal cell carcinoma, the patient should immediately be evaluated for the basal cell carcinoma syndrome.

Most skin tags are minute, 1 to 5 mm in length, with a skin-colored to slightly hyperpigmented appearance. They are pedunculated papules that appear as outpouchings of the skin. They are soft and nontender. Occasionally, larger skin tags are found with a thickened or a more sessile stalk. These larger skin tags may approach 1 to 1.5 cm in length with a 5-mm base. Most individuals have more than one skin tag, and some individuals are afflicted with hundreds of them.

On occasion, a patient presents with a painful, necrotic skin tag. This is most commonly caused by trauma to the skin tag or twisting of the base that results in strangulation of the blood supply and subsequent necrosis. In these cases, removal is advised. If the appearance or clinical history is not classic, the specimen should be sent for pathological evaluation.

Many investigations have looked at the association of skin tags and underlying medical disorders with conflicting and confusing results. Patients with multiple skin tags may be at a higher risk for glucose intolerance. Some studies have even suggested that patients with multiple skin tags are at a higher risk for colonic polyps, but this is still subject to debate.

Pathogenesis: The pathogenesis of skin tags is believed to be a localized overgrowth of fibroblasts within the dermis. They may be more common during pregnancy, and they have been shown to be increased in patients with increased weight. This has led some to implicate insulin-like growth factor-1 as a possible driver of skin tag formation. The initiating factor is not completely understood.

Histology: The overlying epidermis is essentially normal. The skin tag appears as an outgrowth of the skin. The dermis appears normal, and there is a minimal inflammatory infiltrate present, if any at all. Thrombosed or strangulated skin tags show necrosis of the dermis and epidermis and thrombosis of the superficial supplying blood vessels. There is no atypia present.

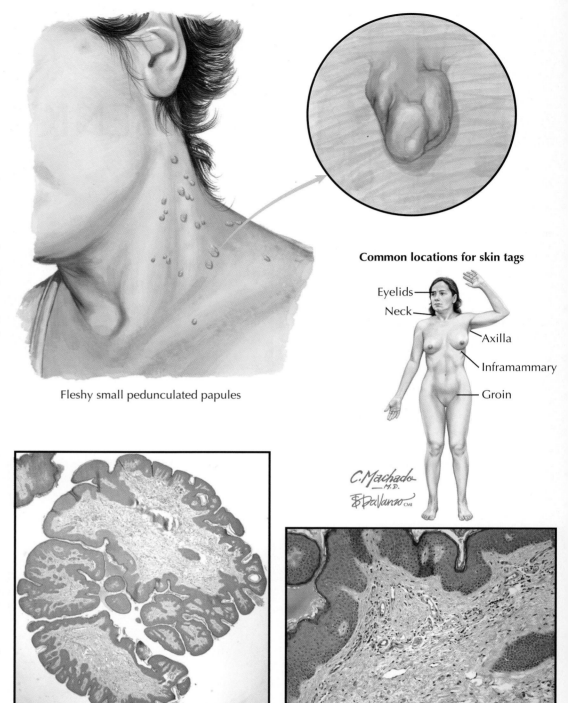

Fleshy small pedunculated papules

Common locations for skin tags

Eyelids
Neck
Axilla
Inframammary
Groin

Low power. The pedunculated skin tag is bisected horizontally. It has a symmetrical appearance with many small dermal capillaries present within a background of collagen bundles.

High power. A slightly acanthotic epidermis is seen overlying a vascular dermis with plentiful collagen.

Treatment: No therapy is necessary for these extraordinarily common skin growths. They are mostly overlooked and not even mentioned on routine skin examination. The rare strangulated or thrombosed skin tag can be removed easily with a forceps and skin tag removal scissors after injection of a local anesthetic. If cosmetic removal is desired, it can easily be done by cleaning the skin with alcohol or chlorhexidine and removing individual skin tags with a forceps and skin tag removal scissors. Application of aluminum chloride after removal causes the superficial bleeding to stop.

Screening of individuals with skin tags for errors in glucose metabolism or for colonic polyps is controversial but should be performed if other findings in the review of systems or the clinical history and physical examination suggests one of these underlying disorders.

Plate 2-2

Benign Growths

BECKER'S NEVUS (SMOOTH MUSCLE HAMARTOMA)

Becker's nevi most commonly appear on the shoulder or upper limb girdle of prepubescent boys. It is a rather common benign condition that is seen in up to 0.5% of the male population. It is less commonly seen in females. Becker's nevi are acquired nevi. Most occur before 10 years of age. Becker's nevus is classified as a smooth muscle hamartoma. It does not contain melanocytic nevus cells and is not considered to be a melanocytic nevus. It was given its name by the dermatologist Samuel Becker, who first described this condition.

Clinical Findings: Becker's nevi begin as ill-defined, slightly hyperpigmented macules on the upper limb girdle. Over time (1 year, on average), the hyperpigmented region develops hypertrichosis, resulting in its characteristic appearance. Backer's nevi may occur anywhere on the human body, but by far the most common locations are on the shoulder, upper chest, and back. The area of hypertrichosis is limited to the underlying hyperpigmented area. The clinical significance of Becker's nevi is its differentiation from large congenital nevi and café-au-lait macules. Becker's nevi confer no increased risk for development of melanoma, and they are rarely associated with any underlying abnormalities. The most common underlying abnormality is unilateral hypoplasia of the breast, which has minimal clinical significance. Rarely, a patient with a Becker's nevus has underlying hypoplasia of bone and soft tissue, the cause of which is unknown. The differential diagnosis includes a giant congenital nevus and a café-au-lait macule. These two conditions should be easily differentiated from Baker's nevus, because they both are typically apparent at birth or soon thereafter, whereas Becker's nevi are typically acquired at about the age of 10 years.

The diagnosis is typically made on clinical findings, but a skin biopsy is sometime needed to confirm the diagnosis if the nevus is in an unusual anatomical location. The punch biopsy is the best method for obtaining tissue.

Histology: The biopsy specimen shows a smooth muscle hamartoma. Multiple smooth muscle fascicles are seen within the dermis. There is an increased ratio of terminal to vellus hairs and a lack of melanocytic nevus cells. The hyperpigmentation results from increased formation of pigmentation within the melanocytes of the stratum basalis. There is no increase in the number of melanocytes. Varying amounts of acanthosis and hyperkeratosis are seen.

Pathogenesis: The pathogenesis of Becker's nevus is unclear. It is believed to be caused by the dermal presence of hamartomatous smooth muscle tissue. Research has shown that the tissue in Becker's nevi has an increased number of androgen receptors. It is thought that increased androgen levels at puberty interact with the excessive androgen receptors and cause the clinical findings.

Becker's nevus is the most common type of smooth muscle hamartoma in the skin. Smooth muscle hamartomas by themselves are rarely found within the skin.

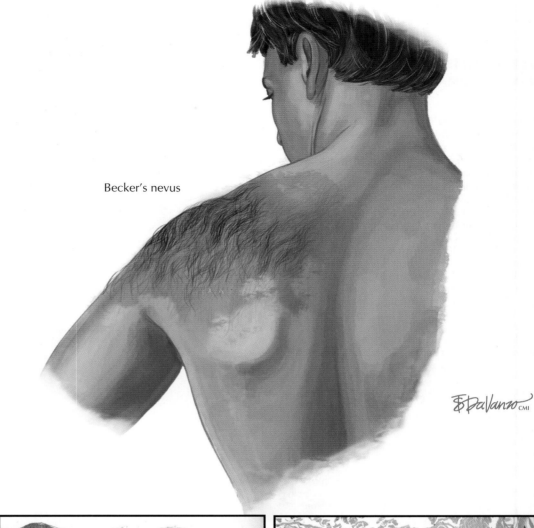

Becker's nevus

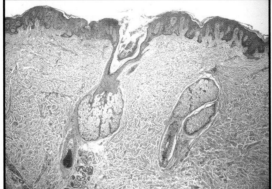

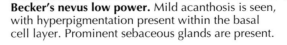

Becker's nevus low power. Mild acanthosis is seen, with hyperpigmentation present within the basal cell layer. Prominent sebaceous glands are present.

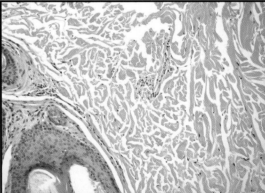

Becker's nevus high power. Collagen bundles surround the prominent adnexal structures.

Non-Becker's smooth muscle hamartomas are usually present at birth or soon thereafter and manifest as a small, flesh-colored plaque located anywhere on the body. All smooth muscle hamartomas may at some point exhibit the pseudo-Darier's sign. To clinically elicit this sign, one gently rubs the smooth muscle hamartoma; the lesion may fasciculate due to smooth muscle activity, or the region may develop an urticarial appearance. This sign has nothing to do with histamine release; rather, it is caused by a neurally mediated contraction of the underlying hamartomatous smooth muscle tissue.

Treatment: No therapy is required. Surgical excision is likely to produce a mutilating scar unless the nevus is extraordinarily small. The hypertrichosis can be treated for cosmetic purposes with any of a multitude of therapies including laser removal, shaving, and electrolysis. Most patients prefer to not treat the area.

Plate 2-3

Integumentary System

DERMATOFIBROMA (SCLEROSING HEMANGIOMA)

Dermatofibromas are among the most common types of benign skin growths. Usually, they occur on the extremities, with a predilection for the legs. There is some debate as to whether this is a true neoplasm or an inflammatory reaction.

Clinical Findings: Dermatofibromas are seen almost exclusively in adults, and females tend to be afflicted slightly more often than males. There is no race predilection. Dermatofibromas can range in diameter from 2 mm to 2 cm. They are round or oval. Most often they are solitary, but numerous dermatofibromas may be present in an individual. Dermatofibromas are usually small (4-5 mm), firm, red to slightly purple papules that dimple with lateral pressure. This "dimple sign" is often used clinically to differentiate dermatofibromas from other growths. There are many variations of dermatofibromas clinically. Elevated dome-shaped papules or plaques may be seen. The surface may or may not have a slight amount of scale, and occasionally there is an appearance of hyperpigmentation. On the lower legs of females, they are often excoriated as a result of shaving, and this is often the reason the patient presents for evaluation. Dermatofibromas are most frequently asymptomatic, but they can be slightly pruritic.

If dermatofibromas are numerous and located in many areas of the body, the clinician should consider the association with an underlying immunodeficiency state. There have been reports of multiple eruptive dermatofibromas in patients with systemic lupus erythematosus, human immunodeficiency virus infection, and other immunosuppressive states. The dermatofibromas in these patients have been shown to contain more mast cells.

The differential diagnosis of a dermatofibroma can be broad. If the dermatofibroma does not exhibit the dimple sign, the lesion is often biopsied to help differentiate it from melanocytic nevus, melanoma, basal cell carcinoma, dermatofibrosarcoma protuberans (DFSP), prurigo papules, and other epidermal and dermal tumors.

Histology: Dermatofibromas are made up of a collection of dermal spindle-shaped fibroblasts. Histiocytes and myofibroblasts are also found throughout the lesion. The synonym *sclerosing hemangioma* arises when numerous extravasated red blood cells are seen within the dermatofibroma. Characteristically, the overlying epidermis is acanthotic with broadening of the rete ridges. The rete ridges are slightly hyperpigmented, and this is sometimes referred to as "dirty feet" or "dirty fingers." This finding explains the hyperpigmentation seen clinically.

Dermatofibromas stain positively for factor XIIIa and negatively for CD34. This is the opposite of the pattern seen in DFSP. Immunohistochemical staining also provides a marker that can be used to help distinguish the benign dermatofibroma (which stains with stromelysin-3) from the malignant DFSP (which does not). In contrast to DFSP, dermatofibromas do not infiltrate the underlying adipose tissue. Dermatofibromas can push down or displace the adipose tissue, but they never truly demonstrate an infiltrative pattern as

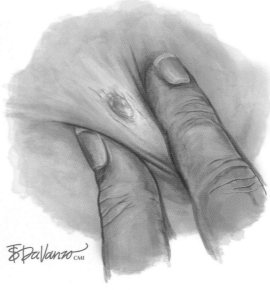

Dermatofibroma. Demonstrating the "dimple sign"

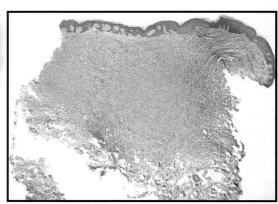

Low power. There is a dermal proliferation of spindle-shaped fibroblasts. The epidermis centrally shows acanthosis and basilar hyperpigmentation. The tumor cells do not reach to the subcutaneous tissue.

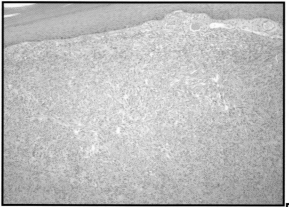

High power. Multiple spindle-shaped fibroblasts are arranged in a whorled pattern.

Dermatofibrosarcoma protuberans. The tumor is poorly circumscribed. The tumor cells are arranged in a storiform pattern. Invasion into the subcutaneous tissue is helpful in differentiating this malignant tumor from the benign dermatofibroma.

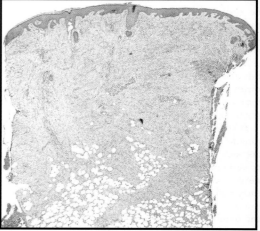

does a DFSP. There are numerous histological variants of dermatofibromas.

Pathogenesis: The precipitating factor that initiates the formation of a dermatofibroma is thought to be superficial trauma, such as from a bug bite, which causes the fibrous tissue proliferation. The exact etiology is unknown.

Treatment: Most dermatofibromas are not treated in any manner. Complete elliptical excision with a minimal 1- to 2-mm margin is curative. The resulting scar may be more noticeable than the initial dermatofibroma. There is no evidence to support the routine removal of these common tumors to prevent malignant degeneration into a DFSP.

Plate 2-4

Benign Growths

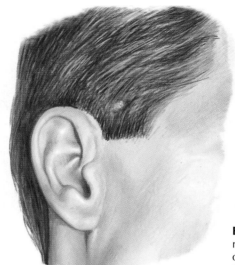

Eccrine poroma on the scalp. Glistening red papule or nodule. Can be located at any location

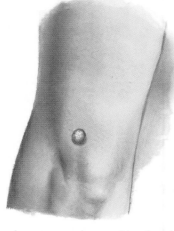

Eccrine porocarcinoma. Nondescript red papule or nodule. Ulceration may occur. A biopsy is required to diagnose this rare form of skin cancer.

ECCRINE POROMA

Eccrine poromas are the most common tumors in the poroma family of skin tumors. Other tumors in this family include the dermal ductal tumor, the poroid hidradenoma, and the hidroacanthoma. Eccrine porocarcinoma is the rare malignant counterpart to the eccrine poroma. Eccrine poromas develop from the appendageal structures of the skin. The all-encompassing term *poroma* is more accurate in that it appears that not all of these tumors are derived from eccrine structures. There is unconfirmed evidence that the cell of origin is actually apocrine. Other possibilities for the cell of origin include the sebaceous gland and the follicular epithelium.

Clinical Findings: Eccrine poromas are uncommon tumors of the skin. They occur equally in men and women and almost exclusively in the adult population. They are typically small tumors, ranging from 5 to 20 mm. They are most frequently found on the soles and palms. As many as 50% to 60% of these tumors have been found on the sole, but they have been described to occur in any skin location. Pain and bleeding are the two most common symptoms encountered. Eccrine poromas tend to have a vascular appearance and often manifest as a red or purplish papule or nodule. They are almost always solitary in nature, and they easily bleed when traumatized. On inspection, the eccrine poroma often has a slight, dell-like depression surrounding the tumor. This is more commonly seen on acral skin. This dell, when seen by the perceptive clinician, often leads to a differential diagnosis that includes an eccrine poroma. There is nothing clinically that can be used with certainty to make the diagnosis. The differential diagnosis includes vascular tumors, metastatic lesions (particularly the vascular renal cell carcinoma metastasis), pyogenic granuloma, and melanoma, because some eccrine poromas exhibit pigmentation. The diagnosis is made by histological examination after biopsy.

Histology: Eccrine poromas show varying degrees of ductal differentiation. The tumor is well circumscribed and has characteristic features. The keratinocytes have been described as cuboidal. They tend to be small and have an increased nuclear to cytoplasmic volume. Necrosis is often seen in parts of the tumor. The ductal portions of the tumor are lined by an eosinophilic layer or cuticle. The stromal portions of the tumor are rich in vascular components. This vascular element imparts the red appearance to the tumor. Eccrine poromas can be histologically classified as other members of the poroma family of tumors, based on their location in the skin. As an example, the hidroacanthoma, a member of this family, is defined as an eccrine poroma that is entirely located in the epidermis.

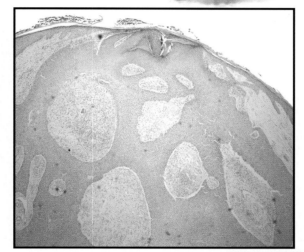

Low power. The tumor appears as an extension of the epidermis. The finger-like projections of tumor cells extend into the dermis. There is a clear difference between keratinocytes and the smaller tumor cells. Many blood vessels are present within the tumor stroma.

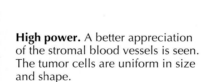

High power. A better appreciation of the stromal blood vessels is seen. The tumor cells are uniform in size and shape.

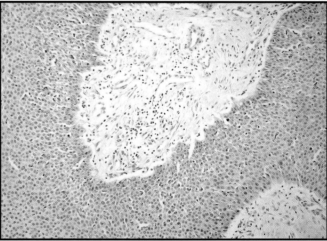

The eccrine porocarcinoma is very uncommon; histologically, it is a tumor that is poorly circumscribed and often found in conjunction with an eccrine poroma. Cells with multiple large nuclei and multiple mitoses help make the diagnosis. Eccrine porocarcinomas can mimic metastatic adenocarcinomas, and immunohistochemical staining is required to make certain of the diagnosis.

Treatment: Although they are benign tumors, eccrine poromas often are located on the sole or palm and require removal from a functional standpoint. Surgical excision with a small (1-2 mm), conservative margin is curative. The recurrence rate is very low after surgical excision. Electrodesiccation and curettage has been used successfully. Eccrine porocarcinomas require surgical excision and close clinical follow-up. Chemotherapy is reserved for cases of metastatic disease. The role of sentinel lymph node sampling in these tumors has yet to be defined.

Plate 2-5

Integumentary System

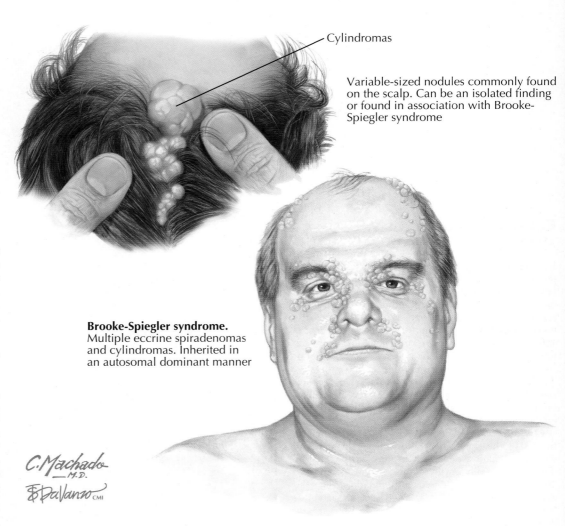

Cylindromas

Variable-sized nodules commonly found on the scalp. Can be an isolated finding or found in association with Brooke-Spiegler syndrome

Brooke-Spiegler syndrome. Multiple eccrine spiradenomas and cylindromas. Inherited in an autosomal dominant manner

ECCRINE SPIRADENOMA

Eccrine spiradenomas are uncommon benign tumors of the skin. Most often they are solitary, but they can occur in conjunction with cylindromas in the Brooke-Spiegler syndrome. They can occur in any location on the human body but are most commonly found on the head and neck. The next most common region is the ventral trunk. These tumors are uncommon on the extremities. Spiradenomas tend to appear between the ages of 15 and 40 years, although they have been reported to occur at any age. Malignant degeneration is extremely rare, but if it does occur, it is often fatal.

Clinical Findings: A spiradenoma usually manifests as a solitary dermal nodule or papule ranging from 5 to 20 mm in diameter. The average size is approximately 10 mm. They are typically seated deeply in the dermis and can be very painful to light touch. The tumors grow very slowly, and except for the pain can go unnoticed for some time. The pain tends to have a waxing and waning course, and it is more often than not the reason the patient seeks medical advice. The overlying epidermis is almost always normal. The dermal nodule sometimes takes on a purple or bluish coloration. Although they are most commonly solitary, multiple spiradenomas may be seen in association with multiple cylindromas in Brooke-Spiegler syndrome.

Brooke-Spiegler syndrome is an autosomal dominant inherited skin condition caused by a genetic defect in the *CYLD* gene. This syndrome is characterized by multiple cylindromas, spiradenomas, and trichoepitheliomas. The tumors usually begin in the third decade of life and increase in number and size throughout the patient's life. The *CYLD* gene encodes a tumor suppressor protein and is an important downregulator of the nuclear factor NF-κB pathway. The clinical phenotype varies depending on the type of mutation in this gene. Patients with familial cylindromatosis also have defects in this gene. The gene has been localized to the long arm of chromosome 16.

The eccrine spiradenoma is considered to be one of the group of unique tumors that can cause painful dermal nodules. This group also includes angiolipomas, neuromas, glomus tumors, and leiomyomas. This group of tumors makes up the differential diagnosis when evaluating these painful nodules. If the nodule is asymptomatic, lipoma and other adnexal tumors would also be considered in the differential diagnosis.

The exact cell type from which the spiradenomas are derived is still undetermined. They were originally believed to arise from eccrine tissue, but increasing evidence is pointing to a derivation from apocrine tissue.

Histology: The histological hallmark of an eccrine spiradenoma is the appearance of large nests of basophilic cells in the dermis. There are no epidermal

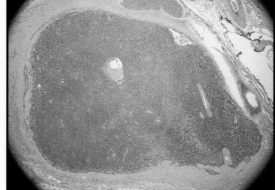
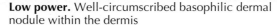

Low power. Well-circumscribed basophilic dermal nodule within the dermis

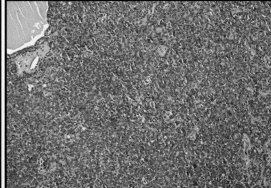

High power. Two cell populations are present, a larger pale cell type and a peripheral smaller basophilic cell type.

changes, and the multilobulated tumors do not connect with the epidermis. This gives rise to the term "blue balls in the dermis." The tumor is composed of two unique cell types. Large, pale cells predominate, with surrounding aggregates of smaller basophilic cells that contain hyperchromatic nuclei. The tumor is well circumscribed and is surrounded by a fibrous capsule.

Treatment: Surgical excision is curative. Surgical removal with carbon dioxide laser ablation has also been found to be highly successful. Because of the number and size of the tumors in patients with the Brooke-Spiegler syndrome, a multidisciplinary approach is often taken. Plastic surgeons are often the primary physicians removing these tumors.

Plate 2-6

Benign Growths

ECCRINE SYRINGOMA

Eccrine syringomas are extremely common benign skin growths. They are most often found on the lower eyelids and malar cheek regions of adults. These small tumors are of no clinical significance and are routinely ignored in clinical practice.

Clinical Findings: Eccrine syringomas are some of the most common benign skin tumors to affect human-kind. They are believed to be more common in women than in men. They typically manifest in adulthood as flesh-colored, small (2-4 mm) papules on the lower eyelids or upper cheek regions. They are usually multiple and symmetric. Some have a slight yellow or tan hue. Other areas of the body on which syringomas are seen include the upper eyelids, neck, and chest. They have been reported to occur on any region of the body.

Plaque-like syringomas have been reported to occur on the forehead, and they have the appearance of a flesh-colored to slightly yellow, broad, flat plaque with minimal to no surface change. They can be quite large, up to 4 to 5 cm in diameter. They are essentially asymptomatic, but occasionally a patient complains of slight intermittent itching or of an increase in size with strenuous physical activity. This is possibly explained by the eccrine nature of the tumors: Under conditions of activity, an increase in sweating causes the tumors to transiently appear to enlarge. There are specific variants seen in patients with diabetes mellitus and in those with Down syndrome. A form of eruptive syringoma has been described that typically afflicts the anterior trunk and the penile shaft. Linear syringomas have been reported to occur on a unilateral limb, and these have been termed *unilateral linear nevoidal syringomas.*

The clinical differential diagnosis of eccrine syringomas is relatively limited when the clinician encounters symmetric small papules on the lower eyelids. The differential diagnosis for a solitary syringoma is broad and includes other adnexal tumors as well as basal cell carcinoma. The most difficulty arises when reviewing the histological features of a syringoma that has been biopsied in a superficial manner. If the pathologist is not given a thick enough specimen, the eccrine syringoma can mimic a microcystic adnexal carcinoma. These two tumors, one benign and the other malignant, can have very similar histological features in the superficial dermis. In some cases, it is only with a full-thickness biopsy that a pathologist can confidently differentiate the two tumors.

Histology: The overlying epidermis is normal. The tumor is based within the dermis and is sharply circumscribed. The syringoma typically does not penetrate deeper than the upper third of the dermis. Clusters of cells with a pale cytoplasm are found throughout the tumor. A background of sclerotic stromal tissue is always appreciated. A characteristic finding is the "tadpole" sign. The tadpole- or comma-shaped, dilated ductal eccrine gland apparatus is pathognomonic for eccrine syringoma. Clear cell variants are associated with diabetes mellitus. A microcystic adnexal carcinoma is poorly circumscribed, is asymmetric, and infiltrates into the underlying subcutis.

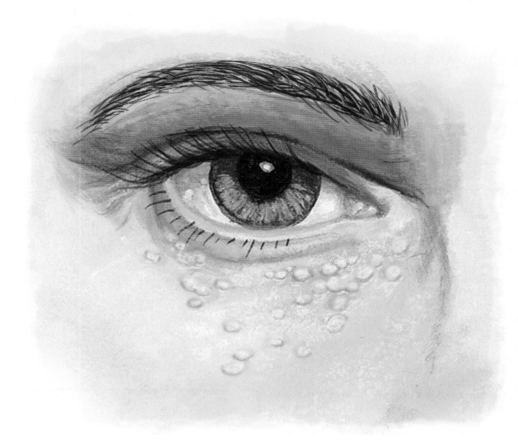

Syringoma. The most common location for syringomas is on the lower eyelid.

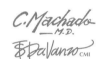

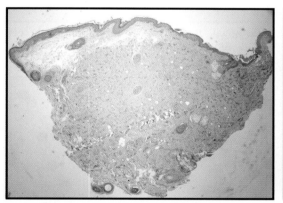

Low power. The overlying epidermis is normal. The tumor is located in the superficial dermis and is made up of comma-shaped dilated ductal eccrine glands.

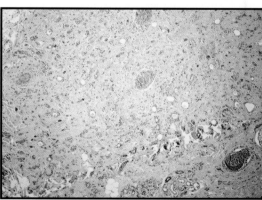

High power. Clusters of cells with a pale cytoplasm are found throughout the tumor. There is a background of sclerotic stromal tissue. The comma-shaped dilated ductal eccrine gland apparatus is apparent.

Pathogenesis: Eccrine syringomas are believed to be an overgrowth of the eccrine sweat ductal apparatus. Researchers have proposed that this proliferation is caused by an inflammatory response to an as yet undetermined antigen. The precise pathogenesis of eccrine syringomas is unclear. Familial patterns suggest a genetic predisposition, but most patients do not have a family history to support genetic transmission.

Treatment: No treatment is necessary. If one wishes to pursue therapy, it should be done with caution, because treatment experiences are anecdotal, and scarring may have a worse appearance than the syringoma itself. Electrocautery, light cryotherapy, chemical peels, laser resurfacing, dermabrasion, and excision have been reported with variable results.

Plate 2-7

Integumentary System

EPHELIDES AND LENTIGINES

Ephelides, also known as freckles, are common benign findings. They typically manifest in childhood in fair-skinned individuals, especially those with red or blonde hair color. Ephelides tend to be passed down from generation to generation in an autosomal dominant inheritance pattern.

Lentigines are sun-induced proliferations of melanocytes. They tend to occur in older people, but they may be seen in individuals at a young age after repetitive sun exposure. They can be almost impossible to differentiate from ephelides. Solar lentigines have many synonyms, including sun spots, liver spots, and lentigo senilis.

Clinical Findings: Ephelides occur at a very young age and tend to show an autosomal dominant inheritance pattern. They are accentuated in sun-exposed regions, particularly the head, neck, and forearms. Exposure to the sun or other ultraviolet source causes the ephelides to become darker and clinically more noticeable. They do not occur within the oral mucosa. They are usually uniform in coloration but can have many different sizes and shapes. Some are round or oval; others are angulated or have a bizarre shape. Their color is usually a uniform light to dark brown; they are never black. They have no malignant potential. Patients with multiple ephelides may have a higher risk for skin cancer, because their presence may be an indication of increased exposure to ultraviolet radiation. The differential diagnosis is usually very narrow and includes lentigines and common acquired nevi. The clinical location, age at onset, family history, and skin type usually make the diagnosis straightforward. The difficulty can occur when trying to differentiate a solitary lentigo from an ephelide in an adult patient.

Solar lentigines most often arise in the adult population and are distributed evenly among males and females. They can occur in anyone but are much more common in light-skinned persons. The number of lentigines typically increases with the age of the patient. Lentigines are induced by ultraviolet radiation, the most common source being chronic sun exposure. Lentigines tend to get darker with ultraviolet light exposure and lighten over time when removed from the exposure. Unlike ephelides, they never completely fade away. They are clinically highly uniform in color and size within an individual patient. They can be small (1-5 mm), but some are much larger (2-3 cm in diameter). They are most commonly located in sun-exposed areas but in some syndromes can be located anywhere on the human body, including the mucosal regions. Over time, some lentigines merge together to form rather large lentigines.

There are some important variants of lentigines. Lentigo simplex and the ink spot lentigo are two very common versions. Lentigo simplex is believed to occur at any age and to have no or minimal relationship to sun exposure. The lesions are found anywhere on the body. Ink spot lentigines are variants of lentigo simplex that are differentiated by their characteristic dark brown to almost black coloration. Under dermatoscopic evaluation, they have a characteristic uniform pigment network, with accentuation of pigment in the rete ridge regions. They are so named because they have the appearance of a tiny drop of dark ink dropped on the skin. Neither of these two forms of lentigines has malignant potential.

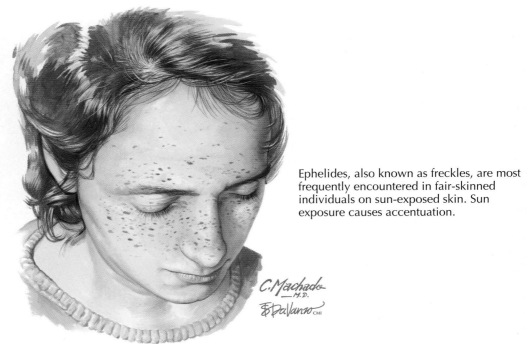

Ephelides, also known as freckles, are most frequently encountered in fair-skinned individuals on sun-exposed skin. Sun exposure causes accentuation.

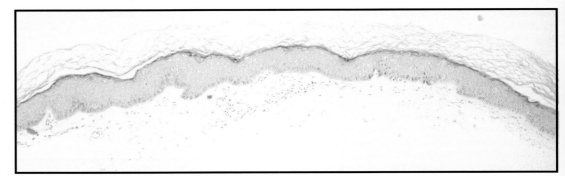

Low power. Basilar pigmentation is uniformly seen along the biopsy specimen. There is no increase in the density of melanocytes present.

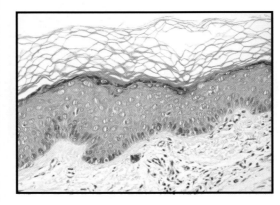

High power. Pigmentation is isolated to the basal layer. A nice basketweave stratum corneum is seen with a nicely formed granular layer.

One of the more important and unique variants of lentigines are the psoralen + ultraviolet A light (PUVA) lentigines. PUVA lentigines are iatrogenic in nature and occur after medical therapy with PUVA treatment. Patients who have undergone long-term therapy with PUVA have a high risk of developing PUVA lentigines. These lentigines are darkly pigmented macules that occur across the entire body except in the areas that were not exposed to the PUVA therapy. More than half of patients who have undergone prolonged PUVA treatment will develop PUVA lentigines. They are more common in patients with fair skin types and rarely occur in darker-skinned individuals. The lentigines induced by PUVA therapy are permanent and can have disastrous cosmetic consequences. Like all patients undergoing ultraviolet phototherapy, these patients must be routinely monitored for their entire lives, because they are at increased risk for melanoma and

Plate 2-8

Benign Growths

EPHELIDES AND LENTIGINES
(Continued)

non-melanoma skin cancer due to their chronic use of PUVA treatment.

Patients with Peutz-Jeghers syndrome have clinical findings of multiple lentigines of the oral mucosa and lips and of the hands. These patients are at increased risk for gastrointestinal carcinomas, particularly colon cancer. Peutz-Jeghers syndrome is inherited in an autosomal dominant fashion and is caused by a defect in the *STK11/LKB1* tumor suppressor gene.

LEOPARD syndrome is another of the well-described genetic syndromes associated with lentigines. This syndrome is composed of **l**entigines, **e**lectrocardiographic abnormalities, **o**cular hypertelorism, **p**ulmonary stenosis, **a**bnormal genitalia, **r**etardation of growth, and **d**eafness. It is caused by a genetic mutation in *PTPN11*, which encodes a tyrosine phosphatase protein.

Histology: Histopathological evaluation is one method to differentiate a lentigo from an ephelide. This is rarely done. The most common use of histology is to differentiate the benign lentigo from its malignant counterpart, lentigo maligna (melanoma in situ).

On histopathologic evaluation, ephelides show no change in the epidermis. There is no increase in the number of melanocytes. The only finding is an increase in the amount of melanin and an increased rate of transfer of melanosomes from melanocytes to keratinocytes.

Lentigines, on the other hand, show an increased number of melanocytes within the area of involvement. The hyperpigmentation is obvious along the club-like configuration of the rete ridges. The increase in the number of melanocytes is not associated with any nesting of those melanocytes, as is seen in melanocytic nevi. In solar lentigines, the dermis often shows signs of chronic sun damage, with a thinning of the dermis and solar elastosis. The epidermis is also thinned in some cases.

Lentigo maligna shows many more melanocytes, some large and bizarre appearing. There is pagetoid spread of the melanocytes and an asymmetry to the lesion. Lentigo simplex has also been shown to lack defects in the *BRAF* gene, in contrast to melanoma, and this may be one way to differentiate the two.

Pathogenesis: Ephelides are thought to be genetically inherited, most likely in a dominant pattern. They become more prominent with sun exposure and fade during times with less exposure to ultraviolet radiation. The increase in pigment is caused by an increase in the production of melanin and an increase in the transfer of melanosomes from melanocytes to keratinocytes. There is no increase in the number of melanocytes in ephelides. The exact reason for this has not been determined.

Lentigines are caused by an increased proliferation of melanocytes locally within the skin. The cause of this proliferation is most likely ultraviolet light in the case of solar lentigines. In the case of lentigo simplex, the cause is unknown. The increased number of melanocytes ultimately leads to an increase in the amount of melanin produced, resulting in the overlying hyperpigmentation.

The cause of lentigines in some of the genetic disorders is probably the underlying genetic defect. The exact mechanism of how the various gene defects lead

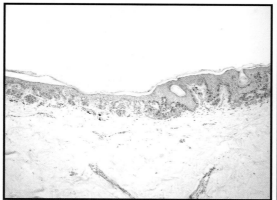

LENTIGINES

Solar lentigines

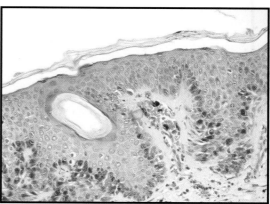

Peutz-Jeghers syndrome is well known to cause mucocutaneous lentigines.

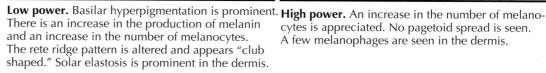

Low power. Basilar hyperpigmentation is prominent. There is an increase in the production of melanin and an increase in the number of melanocytes. The rete ridge pattern is altered and appears "club shaped." Solar elastosis is prominent in the dermis.

High power. An increase in the number of melanocytes is appreciated. No pagetoid spread is seen. A few melanophages are seen in the dermis.

to an increase in lentigines is under investigation. A better understanding of how lentigines form in certain genetic syndromes may lead to discovery of the true pathogenesis of solar lentigines and lentigo simplex.

Treatment: No therapy is needed other than to recommend sun protection, sunscreen use, and routine skin examinations in the future. For cosmetic reasons, lentigines can be removed in a myriad of ways. Light cryotherapy is effective and easy to perform. This

treatment can leave hypopigmented areas and should be used with caution in darker-skinned individuals. Many different chemical peels and dermabrasion techniques have been used to help decrease the appearance of lentigines. With the proliferation of medical laser devices in dermatology, lasers with unique wavelengths have been developed to target the melanin in lentigines. These laser devices have shown promise in lightening and removing solar lentigines.

Plate 2-9

Integumentary System

EPIDERMAL INCLUSION CYST

Epidermal inclusion cysts are the most common benign cysts derived from the skin. They are also known as epidermoid cysts or follicular infundibular cysts. The name "sebaceous cyst" has been used to describe these cysts, although this is a misnomer, because epidermal inclusion cysts are not derived from sebaceous epithelium. The cysts can occur anywhere on the body except the palms, soles, glans, and vermilion border.

Clinical Findings: Most epidermal inclusion cysts are subcutaneous nodules that vary in size from 5 mm to more than 5 cm. They have no race predilection but are seen more commonly in men than in women. Onset most commonly occurs during the third decade of life. The nodules characteristically have an overlying central punctum. From this punctum, drainage of white, cheese-like material, which represents a buildup of macerated keratin debris, can occur. Most small epidermal inclusion cysts are asymptomatic, and they rarely cause a problem.

Larger epidermal inclusion cysts can become irritated and inflamed. If the inflammation is severe enough, the cyst wall ruptures. When the cyst contents enter the dermis, the keratin sets off a massive inflammatory reaction, which manifests clinically as edema, redness, and pain. Once this has occurred, patients often seek medical advice.

The main differential diagnosis for a ruptured epidermal inclusion cyst is a boil or furuncle. Ruptured epidermal inclusion cysts are almost never infected, although infection can occur within a long-standing ruptured cyst that has not been treated. The main differential diagnosis of an unruptured, noninflamed epidermal inclusion cyst is a pilar cyst. Pilar cysts do not have an overlying central punctum, and this is the easiest means of differentiating the two cyst types. Pilar cysts are also more common on the scalp. Milia are considered to be tiny epidermal inclusion cysts.

Histology: The epidermal inclusion cyst is a true cyst with an epithelial lining of stratified squamous epithelium and an associated granular cell layer. The central cavity is filled with keratin debris. The cyst is derived from follicular epithelium.

Pathogenesis: The epidermal inclusion cyst is derived from the infundibulum of the hair follicle. Epidermal inclusion cysts occur as the result of direct implantation of epidermis into the underlying dermis; from there, the epidermal component continues to grow into the cyst lining. Many researchers have looked at the roles of ultraviolet light and human papillomavirus infection in the etiology, but no definitive conclusions on either have been drawn.

Treatment: Small cysts that are asymptomatic do not need to be treated. One should advise patients not to manipulate or squeeze the cysts. Such trauma could cause rupture of the cyst wall and set off an inflammatory reaction. Small cysts can be cured by a complete elliptical excision, making sure to remove the

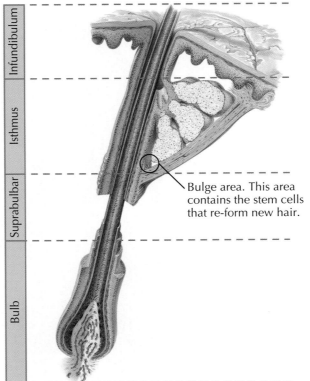

Origin of pilosebaceous unit cysts

Infundibulum

Isthmus

Suprabulbar

Bulb

Bulge area. This area contains the stem cells that re-form new hair.

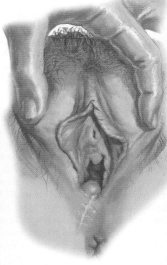

Epidermal inclusion cyst, sometimes referred to as a sebaceous cyst. The upper cyst is red and inflamed. The lower noninflamed cyst has a central punctum.

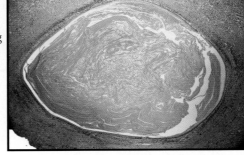

Low power. A well-circumscribed cyst is seen within the dermis. The cyst lining is formed by stratified squamous epithelium, which contains a granular cell layer. A slight amount of dermal inflammation is seen surrounding the cyst.

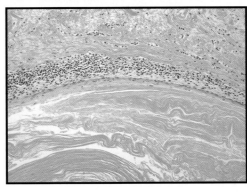

Epidermal inclusion cyst arising at the site of scar

High power. The stratified squamous lining is better appreciated in this high-power image. An intact granular layer is seen. The cyst contents appear as wavy eosinophilic material.

entire cyst wall. If a small portion of the cyst wall is left behind, the cyst is likely to recur.

Inflamed cysts should be treated initially with an incision and drainage technique. The region is anesthetized and then incised with a no. 11 blade. The resulting cheesy-white macerated keratin debris is removed with lateral pressure, and a curette is used to break apart internal loculations. The drainage material has a pungent odor. The resulting cyst cavity can be packed or left open until the patient returns in 2 to 3 weeks for definitive removal of the cyst lining by excision. Intralesional triamcinolone is very effective in decreasing the inflammation and pain in these inflamed cysts. Long-standing cysts should be cultured and the patient given the appropriate antibiotic therapy based on the culture results.

Plate 2-10

Benign Growths

EPIDERMAL NEVUS

Epidermal nevi are benign epidermal hamartomatous growths that most commonly occur as small plaques but can be widespread and can have associated systemic findings. Epidermal nevi have a tendency to follow the embryologic lines of Blaschko. The lines of Blaschko are well defined and follow a whorl-like pattern. The reason why these lesions follow Blashko's lines is not fully understood, but it is probably caused by an interruption of normal epidermal migration during embryogenesis.

Clinical Findings: The epidermal nevus typically manifests in childhood as a solitary linear plaque. Epidermal nevi do not have a race predilection, and they can be found equally in males and females. This type of nevus is not melanocytic in nature; rather, it is composed of a proliferation of keratinocytes. The nevus initially has a smooth surface and develops a mamillated or verrucal surface over time. Epidermal nevi appear to occur most commonly on the head and neck region but can occur anywhere. After puberty, the lesions do not change dramatically. Most are flesh colored to slightly hyperpigmented. If found on the scalp, an epidermal nevus can mimic a nevus sebaceus and can be associated with hair loss, but more commonly it does not cause alopecia.

The epidermal nevus is usually small and slightly linear. Some are large, encompassing the entire length of an extremity, and still others cover a large percentage of the body surface area. Rarely, there is intraoral mucosal involvement. These larger epidermal nevi are more likely to be associated with systemic findings, such as underlying bone abnormalities. The most common bony abnormality is shortening of the unilateral limb. The epidermal nevus syndrome is a rare disorder associated with a large or widespread epidermal nevus and many systemic findings.

The epidermal nevus syndrome is made up of a constellation of findings. These children often present with neurological deficits, including seizures, and developmental delay. They can have a multitude of bony abnormalities, cataracts, and glaucoma. The finding of a widespread epidermal nevus in an infant should alert the clinician to the possibility of this syndrome and the need for a multidisciplinary approach to patient care.

Pathogenesis: The epidermal nevus is a hamartomatous proliferation of the epidermal components. The exact cause is unknown. These lesions are believed to be caused by a developmental abnormality of the ectoderm. The epidermal nevus syndrome has not been shown to have any appreciable inheritance pattern and is believed to be sporadic in nature. The exact genetic defect is unknown; it is most likely a result of genetic mosaicism. The involvement of fibroblast growth factor has been studied, but no firm conclusions have been made. These lesions do not show any abnormalities of melanocytes.

Histology: The findings in this condition are all located within the epidermis. Significant acanthosis and hyperkeratosis, with papillomatosis, predominates. A variable degree of pigmentation is seen in the involved keratinocytes, but this is not a disorder of melanocytes, and the number of melanocytes is normal. The granular cell layer is expanded. Many unique histological variants of epidermal nevi have been described.

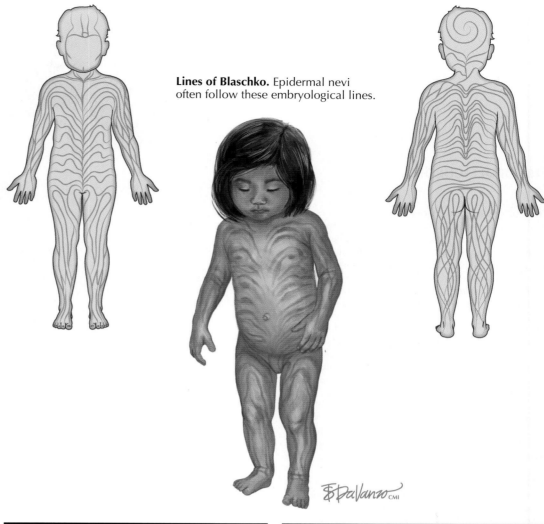

Lines of Blaschko. Epidermal nevi often follow these embryological lines.

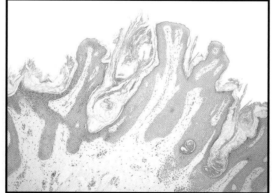

Epidermal nevus, low power. Hyperkeratosis, acanthosis, papillomatosis, and basilar hyperpigmentation are prominent.

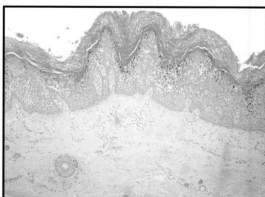

Epidermolytic hyperkeratosis, low power. The same architecture as an epidermal nevus is seen; however, prominent vacuolar changes are seen within the epidermis.

Treatment: Small, isolated epidermal nevi can be removed with shave removal technique. They have a high rate of recurrence with this technique, but recurrence may take many years. The advantages of this technique are that it is relatively easy, noninvasive, and quick, and it provides an opportunity to histopathologically evaluate the tissue for any evidence of epidermolytic hyperkeratosis. The disadvantage of shave removal is that it is appropriate only for small epidermal nevi. Cryotherapy with liquid nitrogen has been used successfully, but it may leave unsightly hypopigmentation in darker-skinned individuals and should be used with caution.

Complete surgical excision is curative for small epidermal nevi. However, it leaves a scar that may be more noticeable than the nevus was. Laser resurfacing, dermabrasion, and chemical peels have been used to help smooth out the appearance of epidermal nevi.

Plate 2-11

Integumentary System

FIBROFOLLICULOMA

Fibrofolliculomas are uncommon benign tumors of the skin. They are derived from the hair follicle epithelium and show a unique mantle differentiation. These tumors are uncommonly seen, but if they are seen in multiples, one needs to consider that they are a constellation of Birt-Hogg-Dubé syndrome.

Clinical Findings: These tumors, when seen, are often solitary skin growths on the head and neck. They are small (2-5 mm), flesh-colored to tan-yellow papules. They most commonly manifest in the third or fourth decade of life. They are asymptomatic and rarely, if ever, get inflamed or bleed spontaneously. On occasion, a small hair is seen emanating from the center of the lesion. The main differential diagnosis clinically includes compound nevus, basal cell carcinoma, fibrous papule, and other types of adnexal tumor. Definitive diagnosis is impossible without histological examination. Solitary fibrofolliculomas are usually found incidentally on routine skin examination. Some patients present with a slightly enlarging new papule, often expressing concern for or fear of skin cancer.

Multiple fibrofolliculomas are seen in association with Birt-Hogg-Dubé syndrome. This syndrome is caused by a genetic defect in the tumor suppressor gene, *folliculin (FLCN)*. This gene has been localized to the short arm of chromosome 17. Other cutaneous constellations of this autosomal dominantly inherited syndrome include trichodiscomas and skin tags. The most important aspect of diagnosing this syndrome early is to screen patients for the possibility of renal tumors, both benign and malignant. Renal oncocytomas are the most common malignant renal tumor seen in this syndrome. Another rare renal cancer, the chromophobe renal cell carcinoma, also may be seen. This very rare tumor is seen in a higher percentage of patients with Birt-Hogg-Dubé syndrome than in the general population. It has a less aggressive behavior than other forms of renal cell carcinoma. Patients with this syndrome are also at higher risk for spontaneous pneumothorax. Some believe that trichodiscomas are the same type of tumor as the fibrofolliculoma and that the difference in histological appearance is caused by sampling and processing artifact (i.e., the identical tumor processed at different tissue surface levels).

Pathogenesis: Fibrofolliculomas are believed to be derived from the upper part of the follicular epithelium. The tumors are thought to be hamartomatous processes that develop within the dermis. Mantle-like structures, as seen in sebaceous glands, are often present and may be the derivation of these tumors. Some authors even consider the manteloma (an extremely rare benign skin tumor) to be in the same spectrum of tumors as the fibrofolliculoma and the trichodiscoma.

Histology: The tumor surrounds a well-formed terminal hair shaft. The upper portion of the hair shaft is slightly dilated. Emanating from the central hair shaft

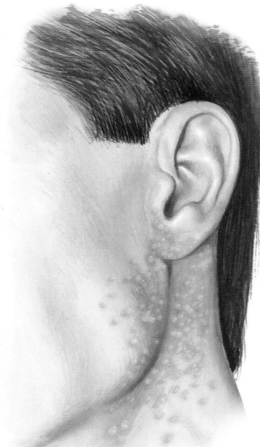

Fibrofolliculomas. Note the periauricular and retroauricular location of monomorphous papules. They are most commonly seen in association with Birt-Hogg-Dubé syndrome.

Skin Finding in Birt-Hogg-Dubé
1. Fibrofolliculomas
2. Skin tags
3. Trichodiscomas
4. Lipomas
5. Angiolipomas
6. Angiofibromas

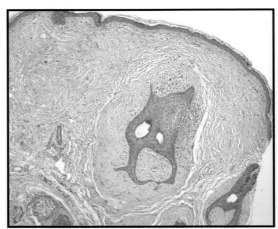

Low power. The tumor is made up of a centrally located basophilic tumor lobule with what appears to be a hair shaft forming within the lobule.

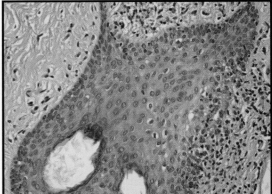

High power. Close-up view shows the basophilic tumor lobule and the fine hair shaft with keratin debris.

epithelium are cords or epithelial strands that project into the surrounding dermis. These cords interconnect at various positions and form a weave-like pattern. Trichodiscomas do not contain a hair shaft; one sees a proliferation along a hair follicle of a fibrovascular stroma akin to an angiofibroma. It is postulated that these two tumors are indeed the same but appear to be two distinct tumors due to routine processing and sampling at various tissue plane levels.

Treatment: Solitary fibrofolliculomas can be removed completely with the shave removal technique. This gives excellent cosmetic results, and the tumors are unlikely to recur. Multiple tumors are more difficult to remove; laser resurfacing, dermabrasion, and chemical peeling have all been used with varying results. The recognition of multiple fibrofolliculomas or trichodiscomas necessitates screening for Birt-Hogg-Dubé syndrome.

Plate 2-12

Benign Growths

FIBROUS PAPULE

Fibrous papules are one of the most common benign skin growths encountered. They are often overlooked or ignored during routine skin examinations. The exact incidence is unknown, but they are believed to be extraordinarily common. These skin growths are most frequently found on the nose, but they can occur anywhere, especially on the face.

Clinical Findings: Fibrous papules are typically small, 0.5 to 5 mm in diameter. They are slightly oval and dome shaped with an overlying smooth surface. Most commonly, they are flesh colored to slightly hyperpigmented. Fibrous papules can also have a hypopigmented appearance. These benign tumors are almost entirely asymptomatic. On occasion, a patient notices a slight itching sensation; less frequently, a patient may describe spontaneous bleeding or bleeding after minor trauma. These growths are most often solitary in nature, but multiple fibrous papules have been reported. Fibrous papules most commonly occur in young adults, especially in the third to fifth decades of life. The most common location is the face, with the nose and chin the two areas most commonly involved.

Fibrous papules are considered to be angiofibromas. Multiple angiofibromas can be part of a constellation known as the tuberous sclerosis syndrome. The differential diagnosis in a teenager with multiple angiofibromas should always include tuberous sclerosis. However, solitary fibrous papules are extraordinarily common and should not cause one to look for an underlying syndrome such as tuberous sclerosis. Pearly penile papules are small, dome-shaped, 1- to 2-mm papules found along the corona of the glans. These pearly penile papules are histologically indistinguishable from fibrous papules and are also considered to be angiofibromas.

The differential diagnosis of a fibrous papule can be quite broad, and a biopsy is often required to differentiate the potential mimickers. The entities most commonly included in the differential diagnosis are common acquired melanocytic nevus and basal cell carcinoma. In these cases, a shave biopsy is required to make a firm diagnosis.

Histology: A fibrous papule is considered to be an angiofibroma. There are multiple histological variants of fibrous papules. The most commonly encountered fibrous papules are typically dome shaped and small (up to 5 mm in diameter), and they show a proliferation of fibroblasts with a stroma of fibrotic collagenized material. Dilated blood vessels are often found within the papules. An inflammatory infiltrate is frequently seen, but it is typically sparse. The combination of clinical findings with the typical histopathological findings solidifies the diagnosis.

Multiple histological variants have been described, including pleomorphic, pigmented, granular cell, hypercellular, and clear cell variants. These variants are believed to be much less common than the classic type of fibrous papule. They have been described in detail and are well accepted and recognized histopathological variations.

Pathogenesis: Fibrous papules are believed to be a benign proliferation of fibroblasts and blood vessels in

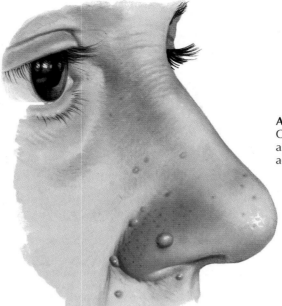

Angiofibromas. Also termed *fibrous papules.* Can be seen in isolation. Multiple angiofibromas associated with tuberous sclerosis are termed adenoma sebaceum.

Adenoma sebaceum (multiple angiofibromas) over both cheeks and nasal bridge. This is a sign of tuberous sclerosis.

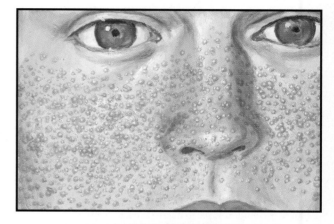

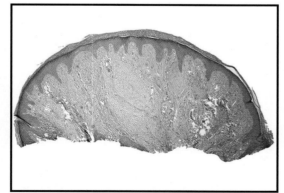

Low power. Well-circumscribed dermal tumor with multiple small blood vessels can be seen within a fibrous stroma.

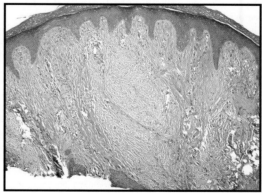

High power. Fibroblasts are the main cell type along with the blood vessels.

a collagen-filled stroma. Immunohistochemical staining has shown that the dermal dendrocyte is the most likely precursor cell to the abnormal fibroblasts seen in fibrous papules. The underlying cause has yet to be determined. The multiple angiofibromas of tuberous sclerosis are directly related to an underlying defect in the tumor suppressor gene, *tuburin (TSC2).* Patients with tuberous sclerosis also have angiofibromas in a periungual location, as well as hundreds to thousands

of angiofibromas located symmetrically on the face and nose.

Treatment: No treatment is necessary, although a small shave biopsy is often all that is required to remove the fibrous papule with an excellent cosmetic result. Most fibrous papules are removed because they are mistaken for basal cell carcinomas or for relief of some underlying irritation, such as itching or bleeding.

Plate 2-13

Integumentary System

Extensor tendon retracted

Firm, rubbery, sometimes lobulated swelling over carpus, most prominent on flexion of wrist. *Broken line* indicates line of skin incision.

Carpal ligaments and capsule

Excision of ganglion via transverse incision. Excision is one of the therapies with the lowest recurrence rate. The surgeon must expose the entire cyst and remove the entire lining to limit recurrence.

Intralesional steroid injections have been used with success.

Loss of strength can be diagnosed on physical exam. Muscle weakness may occur from pressure on an underlying nerve by the cyst.

GANGLION CYST

Ganglion cysts are commonly encountered in the general population. They are fluid-filled cavities that occur most commonly on the dorsal aspect of the hands. They are believed to be derived from the synovial lining of various tendons. They typically manifest as asymptomatic, soft, rubbery nodules below the skin.

Clinical Findings: Ganglion cysts are common benign growths that occur on the distal upper extremity in most cases; they are almost always located on the dorsal aspect of the hand or wrist. Ganglion cysts are almost always solitary, but some patients present with more than one, and occasionally the individual ganglion cysts coalesce into one large area. Most are relatively small, 1 cm in diameter, but some can get very large (2-3 cm). The overlying epidermis is normal, and the cyst is located in the subcutaneous space below the adipose tissue. They are smooth, dome-shaped, fluid-filled cysts that are slightly compressible. The cyst is a direct extension of the synovial lining of the tendon. The cysts form by various mechanisms and fill with synovial fluid. This fluid is critical in the normal lubrication of the tendon space to decrease friction and allow the tendon to easily slide back and forth within its synovial covering. These cysts can occur at any age, but they are much more common in the younger population and often manifest in the third or fourth decade of life. Women are much more likely than men to develop these cysts.

Most cysts are asymptomatic, but they can cause discomfort and pain if they become large enough to press on underlying structures. Rarely, the cyst compresses an underlying nerve, resulting in symptoms of numbness or muscle weakness. The differential diagnosis is limited, and most often the diagnosis is made clinically. Occasionally, a biopsy is required to differentiate ganglion cysts from giant cell tumors of the tendon sheath. Giant cell tumors of the tendon sheath are much more likely to be firm in nature. Ganglion cysts have no malignant degeneration potential. In difficult cases, an ultrasound examination can be performed; it is highly sensitive in detecting these fluid-filled cysts.

Pathogenesis: Ganglion cysts are believed to be caused by an outgrowth of the underlying synovial lining of the tendon sheath. Trauma is likely the leading culprit in initiating the formation of these cysts. Patients with osteoarthritis are also at increased risk for development of ganglion cysts, most likely because of the mechanical trauma that the synovial lining repetitively undergoes when it rubs against osteoarthritic bone.

Histology: Ganglion cysts are not true cysts in that they do not have a well-formed epithelial lining that surrounds the entire cystic cavity. The lining is a loose

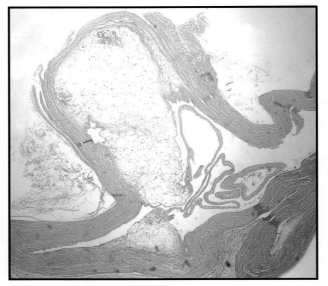

Ganglion cyst. No epidermis is appreciated. The ganglion cyst does not have a true epithelial lining; rather, it is surrounded by a loose collection of collagen and fibrous material. The cyst contains mucopolysaccharides.

collection of fibrous connective tissue composed mostly of collagen. The cyst lining is multilobulated in most cases and typically has no connection to the underlying joint capsule or tendon sheath. The contents of the cyst are made of mucopolysaccharides.

Treatment: No therapy is required for small, asymptomatic ganglion cysts. If a patient desires removal or if the cyst is causing symptoms, especially weakness and numbness, therapy is needed. Needle aspiration is often used as a first-line treatment option; a pressure bandage is applied to try to keep the cyst from reexpanding. After the aspiration, intralesional injection of triamcinolone is used to try to scar the lining of the cyst. This has shown excellent results. If aspiration and injection are not successful, surgical excision is necessary. It is important to have a hand surgeon evaluate and treat these cysts because of their proximity to multiple vital nerve and tendon structures.

Plate 2-14

Benign Growths

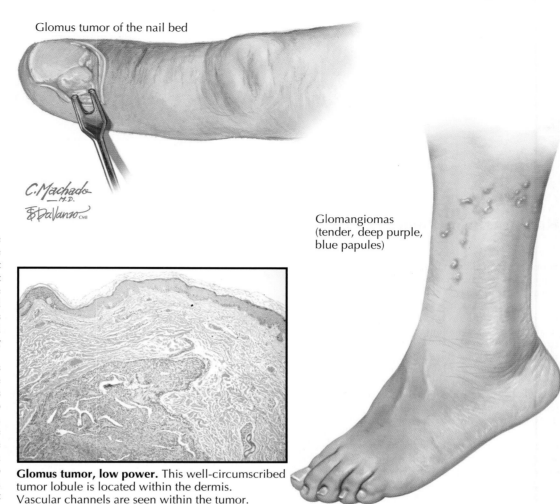

Glomus tumor of the nail bed

C. Machado
M.D.
B. DaVanzo CMI

Glomangiomas
(tender, deep purple,
blue papules)

GLOMUS TUMOR AND GLOMANGIOMA

Glomus tumors are benign tumors derived from the glomus body. The glomus body is a component of the vascular thermoregulatory unit. These tumors are most frequently encountered in early adulthood and are most commonly found on the digits. Glomus tumors are solitary in nature, and the term *glomangioma* is used when describing the glomuvenous malformation. This usually manifests as a congenital defect in infants and young children and appears to be a multifocal grouping or mass of coalescent glomus tumors.

Clinical Findings: The solitary glomus tumor is often found on the digit in a subungual location. The tumors occur equally in men and in women. Lesions have been described in all regions of the skin and also in extracutaneous locations. These tumors are small, well localized, and almost always tender or painful. The glomus tumor is in the differential diagnosis of the painful dermal nodules. On examination, one often observes a 1- to 2-cm, well-circumscribed, blue to purple dermal nodule. It is tender to palpation and can be extremely painful with changes in the ambient temperature.

Glomangiomas are frequently congenital and manifest as a multifocal cluster of coalescing, blue-purple nodules and papules. There is occasionally some surface change over the top of the tumors. The Hildreth sign is a diagnostic maneuver that can be used to help make the diagnosis. The sign is positive if the pain from the glomus tumor decreases or disappears when a blood pressure cuff is placed proximal to the tumor and inflated to a pressure greater than the patient's systolic blood pressure. Glomangiomas can be confused with hemangiomas or other vascular malformations. The differential diagnosis of a solitary glomus tumor includes angiolipoma, neuroma, eccrine spiradenoma, leiomyoma, and vascular tumors. The differential diagnosis of a glomangioma includes hemangiomas and other vascular malformations.

Histology: The tumor manifests as a well-circumscribed nodule of glomus cells surrounding a number of small capillaries. The glomus cells are distinctive and uniform. They appear round and have round nuclei. The cytoplasm is scarce and eosinophilic. The background stroma is myxoid, and there is often a fibrous capsule surrounding the entire tumor.

Pathogenesis: Glomus tumors arise from the Sucquet-Hoyer canal. This canal is an arteriovenous shunt found in the small vasculature of the skin. These canals have been found in a higher density within the blood vessels of the digits. They are responsible for thermoregulation and cause shunting of blood in response to neurological and temperature changes. The exact initiating factor is unknown. Anecdotal reports of glomus tumors occurring after trauma have led some to believe that trauma is causative. This may explain the preponderance of the

Glomus tumor, low power. This well-circumscribed tumor lobule is located within the dermis. Vascular channels are seen within the tumor.

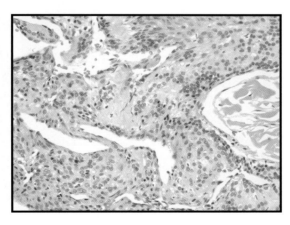

Glomus tumor, high power. The uniform-appearing glomus cells are seen surrounding the vascular structure. The glomus cells are eosinophilic in nature with uniformly basophilic nuclei.

tumors on the digits, where they are prone to trauma. Trauma is unlikely to be the true initiating factor, because these tumors are quite rare and trauma to the digits occurs frequently.

Some glomangiomas have been described to be inherited in an autosomal dominant fashion. These cases are caused by a deletion defect in the *glomulin (GLMN)* gene, which is located on the short arm of chromosome 1. The exact function of the protein encoded by this gene or how its defect causes glomangiomas is still not understood.

Treatment: Glomus tumors are successfully treated with complete surgical excision. Glomangiomas, because of their size, can be excised in a staged approach or with the help of tissue expanders. Reports of treatment with laser ablation, electrocauterization, and sclerotherapy, with some success, have been documented in the literature.

Plate 2-15

Integumentary System

HIDRADENOMA PAPILLIFERUM

Hidradenoma papilliferum is a rare benign tumor of the genital and perianal regions. It is most commonly located on the vulva, although extragenital locations have been described. It has a predilection for women in the fourth and fifth decades of life. Typically, these are small tumors a few millimeters in diameter, but some large tumors have been described. There is no connection to the overlying epidermis or mucosa.

Clinical Findings: Hidradenoma papilliferum is an extremely rare benign tumor located in the dermis. It seen almost exclusively in middle-aged women. The lesions are almost always located in the genital region. They typically manifest as asymptomatic nodules that are discovered incidentally. There are usually no overlying epidermal changes, and the tumor is well circumscribed, freely movable, and firm in consistency. They do not have a connection with the overlying epithelium. In rare instances, they can be tender or pruritic and can bleed or ulcerate. Most of these tumors are found on routine gynecological examination. The most common location is the labia majora. The differential diagnosis of a solitary, firm dermal nodule in the genital region is very broad, and a biopsy for histopathological examination is required in all cases to make the diagnosis. It is essential for dermatologists and gynecologists to be aware of this tumor and the common locations in which it is found.

Pathogenesis: Hidradenoma papilliferum is a tumor that is believed to be derived from apocrine tissue. For this reason, it is considered to be a type of apocrine adenoma. Apocrine glands are found in higher density in the anogenital region, and that may be one reason for the unequal cutaneous distribution of this tumor. The tumor is benign and is closely related to another benign adnexal tumor, the syringocystadenoma papilliferum. The latter tumor is more common on the head and neck, with a predilection for the scalp. Histologically, these two tumors are almost identical, with the major differentiating factor being that the syringocystadenoma papilliferum has a connection to the overlying epidermis. Clinically, the syringocystadenoma papilliferum usually manifest as an ulcerated papule or plaque. Both of these tumors can develop within a nevus sebaceus.

Histology: Hidradenoma papilliferum is a well-circumscribed dermal tumor. It almost never has any overlying epithelial abnormalities. The syringocystadenoma papilliferum, on other hand, has a connection with the overlying epidermis. They both commonly arise in conjunction with a nevus sebaceus. On closer inspection, the hidradenoma papilliferum is composed of vascular papillary projections into the center of the tumor lobule. These projections are lined by cells with

Hidradenoma papilliferum is most frequently located on the external genitalia of women.

Syringocystadenoma papilliferum arising within a nevus sebaceous. Transformation of a nevus sebaceous into various tumors, including syringocystadenoma papilliferum and basal cell carcinoma, occurs most frequently after puberty.

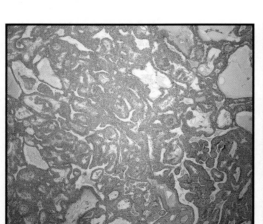

Low power. Symmetrically arranged dermal tumor, with multiple papillary projections.

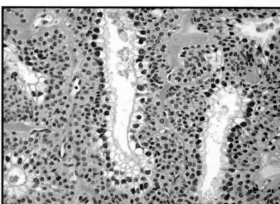

High power. Close-up of the papillary projections. The projections are lined by cells with an apocrine origin. Apocrine secretion (decapitation secretion) is often noted in various sections of the tumor.

an apocrine origin that have a columnar configuration. Apocrine secretion (decapitation secretion) is often noted in various sections of the tumor. There is also a thin layer of myoepithelial cells. Within the papillary projections is a background stroma composed of many vascular spaces and lymphocytes.

Syringocystadenoma papilliferum has almost identical central characteristics. Compared with the hidradenoma papilliferum, it has a more dense plasma cell infiltrate and has an attachment to the overlying epidermis, which usually manifests as an invagination of the epidermis into the tumor lobule.

Treatment: A complete excision is diagnostic and curative at the same time. Often, a biopsy is performed to ascertain the diagnosis, followed by the curative complete excision. These are rare and benign tumors. There have been reports of malignant degeneration, but this is exceedingly rare.

Plate 2-16

Benign Growths

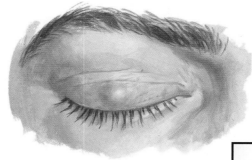

Hidrocystomas of the eyelid may appear similar to a chalazion or a basal cell carcinoma. They may appear translucent and easily rupture. They are almost always asymptomatic.

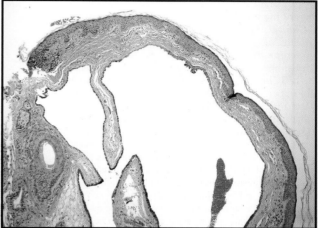

Low power. A well-circumscribed cystic lining is seen in the dermis. Minimal surrounding inflammation is present.

HIDROCYSTOMA

Hidrocystomas, also known as eccrine hidrocystomas, are common benign skin tumors that are most frequently found along the eyelid margin. These benign tumors have a typical appearance and no malignant potential. Most often, they manifest as solitary, asymptomatic papules.

Clinical Findings: Eccrine hidrocystomas manifest as solitary, translucent, pale, clear to blue or light purple papules. They have a smooth surface and a dome shape. Eccrine hidrocystomas are soft; they feel as if pressure could easily rupture their cystic wall. Puncturing of the cyst wall with a 30-gauge needle causes drainage of a thin, watery fluid. These tumors are almost always asymptomatic. They can occur at any age but are far more common after the fourth decade of life. No difference in incidence has been observed based on race or gender. Lesions are typically small, 5 mm to 1 cm in diameter, and can fluctuate in size. It is not uncommon for a patient to relate that the tumor enlarges during physical exercise, only to shrink after a few days. If ruptured, these tumors drain a thin, watery liquid, and the cystic cavity deflates. Although they are almost always solitary, there are reports of hundreds of these tumors developing in some patients. Large eccrine hidrocystomas occurring in atypical locations have also been described.

The main differential diagnosis is between eccrine hidrocystoma and basal cell carcinoma. Cystic basal cell carcinomas can have an identical appearance; however, the patient history will be quite different. Basal cell carcinomas typically enlarge over time and ulcerate, causing bleeding of the ulcerated papule. Hidrocystomas rarely, if ever, ulcerate or bleed. If left alone, they only transiently increase in size and never get much larger than 1 cm in diameter, and usually they are much smaller. A biopsy for pathological evaluation is diagnostic.

Pathogenesis: Hidrocystomas develop from the eccrine apparatus. It is believed that a portion of the eccrine duct within the dermis becomes occluded. This occlusion causes a buildup of eccrine secretions proximal to the blockage. Once enough fluid collects, a translucent papule becomes evident on the surface of the skin. No genetic abnormalities of the involved eccrine duct have been discovered, and this cystic formation is most likely caused by damage from superficial trauma to the skin and the underlying eccrine ducts. Sun damage to the eccrine ducts has been theorized to play a role, although this theory has yet to be vigorously tested.

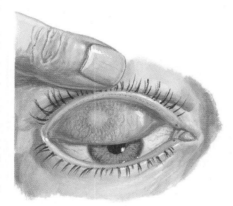

Chalazion; lid everted. Tender nodule of the eyelid.

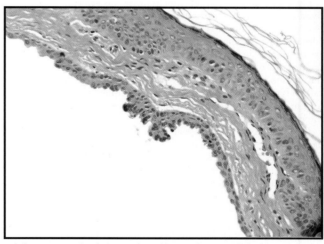

High power. The lining is made up of two cell layers of cuboidal epithelium. There is a small amount of dermis between the cyst and the overlying epidermis.

Histology: A lone cystic space is seen within the dermis. The cyst is well circumscribed, and the lining of the cyst contains two layers of cells. The cells are cuboidal and have an eosinophilic cytoplasm. The cell wall has no myoepithelial cell component. The cysts are found near eccrine gland structures. There is minimal to no inflammatory infiltrate surrounding the cyst. The central cavity of the cyst contains an small amount of lightly eosinophilic material that is consistent with eccrine gland secretions. There is no evidence for sebaceous gland or apocrine gland secretion or derivation.

Treatment: Most eccrine hidrocystomas are biopsied to make sure they are not actually basal cell carcinomas. They rarely recur after biopsy. If they do recur, no treatment is required. Surgical excision is the definitive treatment and is curative. Hidrocystomas almost never recur after excision.

Plate 2-17

Integumentary System

KELOID AND HYPERTROPHIC SCAR

Keloids are common benign skin tumors that consist of excessive scar tissue that forms after trauma or inflammatory skin conditions such as acne vulgaris. The keloid proliferates uncontrolled and expands beyond the borders of the underlying scar produced by the traumatic event. Hypertrophic scars, on the other hand, are exuberant scar formation that stays within the confines of the original scar border.

Clinical Findings: Keloids are often large overgrowths of scar tissue that expand over the original border of the underlying scar and affect previously normal-appearing skin. They may occur anywhere on the body but are more common on the earlobe, chest, and upper arms. They can affect any age group and affect males and females equally. Dark-skinned individuals have a higher incidence of keloid-type scarring. Almost all keloids manifest after a preceding traumatic event such as a cut, ear piercing, burn, or surgical excision. Many other causes have been found to initiate the formation of keloids, including acne lesions and bug bites. Keloids often start as small, red, itchy papules that quickly enlarge into plaques and nodules. They usually have a smooth surface with firm consistency. Itching is a frequent complaint and often precedes the growth stage. Keloids are diagnosed clinically in a patient with the appropriate history. The differential diagnosis of early keloids includes hypertrophic scars. Difficulty sometimes arises when a patient presents with a firm, enlarging plaque or nodule but no preceding history of trauma. In these cases, a biopsy is prudent to rule out a dermatofibrosarcoma protuberans. The histopathological findings easily differentiate the two lesions.

Hypertrophic scars occur after trauma and are confined to the area of the original trauma or scar. Hypertrophic scars, unlike keloids, do not grow into the adjacent normal skin. They can be quite large and often are pink to red in color and pruritic. Hypertrophic scars tend not to reach the size or extent of keloids, and for that reason they are a bit easier to manage therapeutically. Hypertrophic scars are diagnosed clinically in a patient with a typical history of preceding trauma and the characteristic clinical findings.

Pathogenesis: Keloids appear to be more common in dark-skinned individuals during the first 3 decades of life. Keloids may have a genetic pathogenesis that has yet to be discovered. Certain areas of the body are more prone to keloid formation, including the chest and earlobes, and there may be some local skin cytokine profile that allows for their formation. Biological studies have looked at various cytokines, and transforming growth factor-β (TGF-β) has been found in elevated levels in keloids. TGF-β causes recruitment of fibroblasts into the region and induces them to produce more collagen. Local blockade of this cytokine may be developed as a therapy in the future.

Histology: Keloids show an increase in collagen production, and the collagen is arranged in a disorganized fashion. The overlying epidermis is typically thin due to the mass effect of the keloid tumor pressing on the undersurface of the epidermis, which causes attenuation of the surface epithelium. Mucopolysaccharides are found between the collagen fibers.

Hypertrophic scars are smaller and not exophytic in nature, and the collagen bundles are arranged parallel to the epidermis. There may be an increase in mast cells in both hypertrophic scars and keloids.

Hypertrophic scars

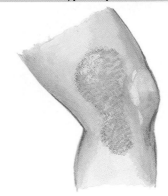

Hypertrophic scars do not extend beyond the border of the original injury.

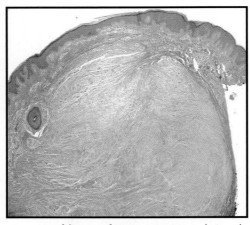

Hypertrophic scar, low power. Non-elevated scar made of numerous collagen bundles, fibroblasts, and blood vessels

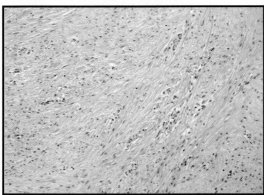

Hypertrophic scar, high power. Numerous fibroblasts with an increased number of vascular channels. The collagen bundles are arranged in the same direction.

Treatment: Hypertrophic scars do not need to be treated, because most will eventually flatten and blend with the surrounding skin. Intralesional triamcinolone may be used to help speed the process along, but care should be taken not to inject too much and thereby cause atrophy. Daily massage by the patient has also been shown to be effective in decreasing the outward appearance of the scar. The redness of both hypertrophic and keloid scars can be treated successfully with pulsed dye laser.

Keloids

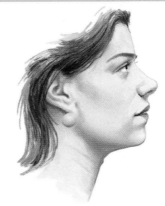

One of the most common locations for a keloid is the earlobe, and it can occur after ear piercing.

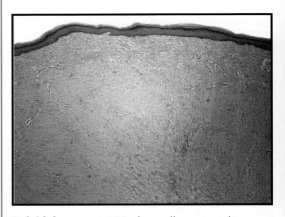

Keloid, low power. Haphazardly arranged collagen bundles. Thick eosinophilic bundles of collagen with surrounding fibroblasts

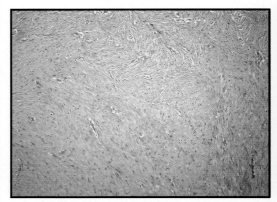

Keloid, high power. Thickened eosinophilic collagen bundles

Keloids are more challenging to treat. They have a high rate of recurrence after excisional removal, and for this reason adjunctive therapy should always be used after excision. Serial injections with intralesional triamcinolone monthly for 4 to 6 months may help avoid a recurrence after surgery. Postoperative radiation therapy has also been very successful in decreasing the recurrence rate. There are anecdotal reports of treatment with imiquimod and cryotherapy, but they are of questionable value.

Plate 2-18

Benign Growths

LEIOMYOMA

Cutaneous leiomyomas are uncommon benign tumors of the arrector pili muscle of the skin. They can occur as a solitary tumor or as multiple lesions. Both types can be associated with underlying genetic defects. This occurs more commonly in multiple cutaneous leiomyomatosis, and one needs to look for systemic findings in affected patients. Other muscle sources of cutaneous leiomyoma formation include the smooth muscle of blood vessel walls and the dartos muscle. These rare forms of cutaneous leiomyomas are named angioleiomyomas and solitary genital leiomyomas, respectively.

Clinical Findings: Leiomyomas manifest as dermal papules or nodules with a slight hyperpigmentation of the overlying epidermis. They can also have a reddish or brownish hue. The tumors are 1 to 2 cm in diameter. They occur equally in males and females and affect all races. They may occur anywhere on the skin, but the anterior chest and the genital region are two of the more common areas of involvement. They typically are tender, and they can be painful. Most leiomyomas become more painful and more sensitive over time. Cold temperatures have been shown to exacerbate the pain. The leiomyomas exhibit the pseudo-Darier's sign. This sign is elicited by rubbing the leiomyoma; on manipulation, the lesion begins to twitch or fasciculate. It does not form an urticarial plaque as would be seen with a true Darier's sign (e.g., in cutaneous mastocytosis). Malignant transformation is exceedingly rare.

Multiple cutaneous leiomyomas occur most commonly on the trunk and proximal extremities. They are the same size as their solitary counterparts, but they can become so numerous that they appear to coalesce into large plaques. In most patients, onset occurs in the third to fifth decades of life. There is a definite autosomal dominant inheritance pattern to multiple cutaneous leiomyomas. These patients have a genetic defect in the *FH* gene (also called *MCUL1*), which encodes the Krebs cycle protein fumarate hydratase. The fumarate hydratase protein has been found to have tumor suppressor functions. Many different types of mutations have been described, ranging from frameshift mutations to deletion of entire genes. This most likely explains the variety of phenotypes seen. The most concerning and lifethreatening aspect of this mutation is the possibility of developing an aggressive and deadly form of papillary renal cell carcinoma. This tumor in patients with multiple cutaneous leiomyomas tends to be highly aggressive and metastasizes early. Early screening of the patient and genetic screening of family members may help decrease the risk of metastatic renal carcinoma. Patients should be evaluated routinely for kidney disease.

The term *Reed syndrome* is used to denote women with cutaneous leiomyomas and uterine leiomyomas.

Pathogenesis: Solitary leiomyomas not associated with the fumarate hydratase protein defect are believed to be caused by an abnormal proliferation of myocytes. The cause for this proliferation is unknown. Fumarate hydratase mutations result in a lack of tumor suppressor function. The role of this tumor suppressor protein in the production of multiple leiomyomas has yet to be determined.

Histology: The tumor is located within the dermis and is composed of interconnected fascicles of spindle-shaped cells. The cells are arranged in a whorl-like pattern. The cells are uniform and bland appearing. Mitosis should be absent. The cells have been described as cigar shaped, meaning that they have a long, plump central region with blunt tip ends. The cell of origin is

the myocyte. Immunohistochemical staining can be used to help differentiate difficult tumors. Leiomyomas stain with muscle markers such as smooth muscle actin. The overlying epidermis is usually normal.

Treatment: Surgical excision of the solitary form of leiomyoma is curative. Multiple cutaneous leiomyomatosis can be treated with a number of medications to help control the discomfort and pain. Use of α_1-adrenergic receptor blockers has been reported most frequently. Doxazosin and phenoxybenzamine have both been successful. Calcium channel blockers such as nifedipine have also been successful anecdotally. Gabapentin and botulinum toxin have been reported to help. Surgical excision is warranted for any lesion that is painful and not responding to therapy. Patients with multiple cutaneous leiomyomas should be evaluated for the genetic defect in the fumarate hydratase protein and should have appropriate screening for kidney disease.

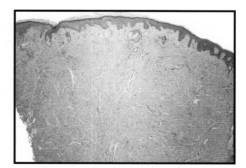

Low power. Tumor is located within the dermis and is composed of interlacing fascicles of spindle-shaped muscle cells.

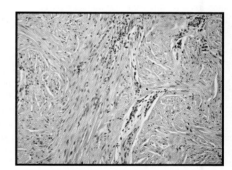

High power. Spindle cells are bland appearing with blunt-tipped ends.

Plate 2-19

Integumentary System

LICHENOID KERATOSIS

Lichenoid keratoses are common benign skin growths also known as lichen planus–like keratoses. These are most often solitary, benign skin tumors and may be found anywhere on human skin. They are more common during adulthood. The keratosis may be misdiagnosed as a non-melanoma skin cancer, most commonly a superficial basal cell carcinoma.

Clinical Findings: Lichenoid keratoses are most frequently found on the upper trunk and upper extremities. The incidence is equal in males and females, and there is no race predilection. They are rare in childhood. They typically manifest as pruritic, red to slightly purple patches and thin plaques. Occasionally, a patient notices that the area arises in a preexisting seborrheic keratosis or solar lentigo. Most lichenoid keratoses are 1 cm or smaller in their largest diameter. Most patients present to their physician with a chief complaint of tenderness, itching, or bleeding secondary to scratching or rubbing of the lesion. The lesions may have a striking resemblance to the rash of lichen planus; the differentiating factor is that a lichenoid keratosis is solitary, whereas lichen planus includes a multitude of similar skin lesions. These skin growths have no malignant potential. It can be difficult to differentiate lichenoid keratoses from inflamed seborrheic keratoses, basal cell carcinomas, actinic keratoses, or squamous cell carcinomas. Therefore, a biopsy of the lesion is prudent to discern a pathological diagnosis.

There are a few unusual clinical variants, including an atrophic form and a bullous type of lichenoid keratosis. The differential diagnosis of these two variants includes conditions such as lichen sclerosis for the former and autoimmune blistering diseases for the latter. The dermatoscope has become an indispensable tool and can be helpful in diagnosing lichenoid keratosis. Lichenoid keratoses have been shown to have a localized or diffuse granular-type pattern under dermatoscopic viewing. This finding should help differentiate these tumors from melanocytic tumors.

Histology: On histological examination, a lichenoid keratosis has a symmetric, well-circumscribed area of intense lichenoid inflammation along the basement membrane region. There is disruption of the basilar keratinocytes. This leads to the appearance of a number of necrotic keratinocytes, also called Civatte bodies. Civatte bodies are seen in almost all cases of lichenoid keratosis and also in lichen planus. There is pronounced sawtooth hypergranulosis and pronounced acanthosis. There is no atypia of the involved keratinocytes, thus ruling out an inflamed actinic keratosis. The underlying inflammatory infiltrate is made up almost entirely of lymphocytes. However, it is not uncommon to find a rare eosinophil or plasma cell anywhere throughout the infiltrate. The pathological differential diagnosis includes lichen planus. The clinical history is very important: Whereas a lichenoid keratosis is a solitary lesion, the same findings in a biopsy specimen taken from a widespread rash of purple, flat-topped papules would be more consistent with the diagnosis of lichen planus. This example illustrates the importance of including the clinical history on a pathology report.

Pathogenesis: The exact etiology of a lichenoid keratosis is unknown. It is believed to be caused by an inflammatory response to a lentigo or a thin seborrheic

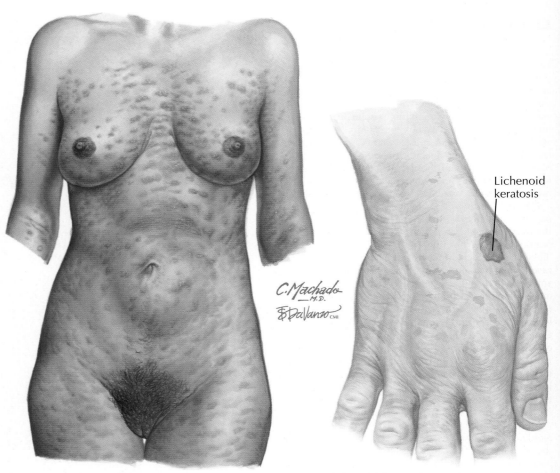

Lichen planus. Widespread pruritic purpilsh papules and plaques, some with Wickham striae.

Lichenoid keratosis

Lichenoid keratosis. A solitary growth in comparison to the widespread nature of lichen planus. Histology can be identical.

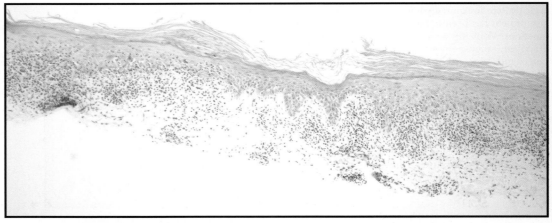

A lichenoid lymphocytic infiltrate is seen along the dermal-epidemal junction. Disruption of the dermal-epidermal junction is prominent. Necrotic keratinocytes are seen in the epidermis.

keratosis. The specific precipitating factor may be trauma. Chronic rubbing has been implicated in inducing lichenoid keratoses from lentigines. The role of human papillomavirus (HPV) in causing lichenoid keratoses has been studied, but no firm conclusions have been made.

Treatment: Most biopsies of a lichenoid keratosis result in complete resolution of the lesion. Even if the

entire lesion was not removed with the biopsy specimen, no treatment is necessary. Use of a topical corticosteroid cream or ointment twice daily for 1 to 2 weeks after healing of the biopsy site is likely to lead to complete resolution of the lichenoid keratosis. Other treatment options include light cryotherapy or a light curettage after anesthesia. Benign lichenoid keratoses rarely if ever recur.

Plate 2-20

Benign Growths

LIPOMA

Lipomas are common benign skin growths that can be seen as solitary lesions and frequently as multiple dermal nodules scattered about the skin. The lipoma is an overgrowth of the fibrofatty adipose tissue in the subcutaneous tissue plane. Patients with multiple lipomas often describe a familial inheritance pattern.

Clinical Findings: Lipomas are often small (1-2 cm), soft, subcutaneous nodules that are slow growing and freely moveable underneath the skin. Some lipomas become quite large (>5 cm in diameter), and they can be a cause for concern due to interference with movement and the possibility of malignant degeneration into a liposarcoma. There are no overlying epidermal changes, and there is no connection to the epidermis. Most often they are asymptomatic, but they can become painful if traumatized.

In stark contrast, a rare variant called the angiolipoma is almost always tender and multiple in nature. Angiolipomas contain a much higher percentage of blood vessels throughout the lobule of adipose tissue, and the diagnosis is made based on this histopathological finding. These tumors are benign and have no familial inheritance pattern.

The differential diagnosis of a lipoma is broad and can include other dermal tumors; however, the clinical examination findings are often diagnostic. Occasionally, a small lipoma can be confused with an epidermal inclusion cyst, pilar cyst, lymph node, or adnexal tumor. Large, freely movable, rubbery nodules that are slow growing are easily diagnosed clinically as lipomas.

Lipomas occur most commonly on the trunk and extremities. They most often affect women in their third through fifth decades of life but can affect people of any age and sex. There is no race predilection. They rarely affect the face, except for the subfrontalis lipoma, which occurs underneath the frontalis muscle on the forehead.

Rare syndromes of adipose tissue have been described, including benign symmetric lipomatosis, adiposis dolorosa (Dercum's disease), and familial multiple lipomatosis. The best described of these syndromes is benign symmetric lipomatosis, also known as Madelung's disease. In this condition, there is massive proliferation of adipose tissue on the neck and upper arms of men. The patients take on the appearance of a body builder.

Pathogenesis: The exact cause is unknown. Lipomas are believed to be an overgrowth of normal tissue in a normal location. The tumor lobules are indistinguishable from normal adipose tissue. A genetic pattern of inheritance has been described, but no specific gene defect has been located.

Histology: Lipomas are composed of mature adipose tissue. The lobules are separated by fibrous septa that contain the blood supply for the adipose cells. Lipomas

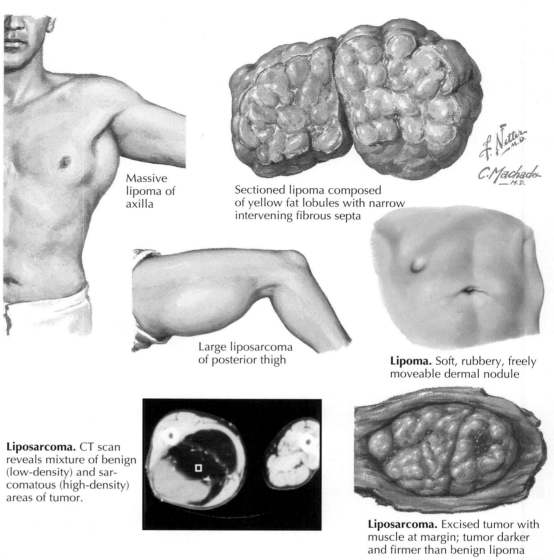

Massive lipoma of axilla

Sectioned lipoma composed of yellow fat lobules with narrow intervening fibrous septa

Large liposarcoma of posterior thigh

Lipoma. Soft, rubbery, freely moveable dermal nodule

Liposarcoma. CT scan reveals mixture of benign (low-density) and sarcomatous (high-density) areas of tumor.

Liposarcoma. Excised tumor with muscle at margin; tumor darker and firmer than benign lipoma

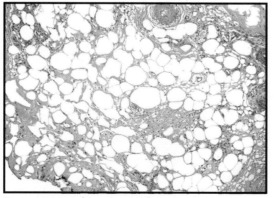

Low power. Adipocytes with varying amounts of fibrous tissue and blood vessels

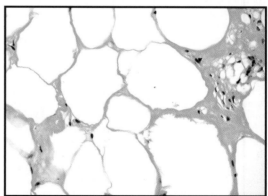

High power. Mature adipocytes are the main component of the tumor.

have a fibrous capsule enclosing the adipose lobules. Angiolipomas are described as those fatty tumors in which 10% to 50% of the mass is composed of blood vessels. The various rare lipomatosis variants are identical in appearance histologically to a common lipoma.

Treatment: No therapy is required for these benign skin tumors. Solitary lipomas can be treated with a simple excision or with liposuction. Subfrontalis lipomas are more difficult to remove, because the surgeon must dissect below the frontalis muscle to locate the lipoma. Small lipomas have been treated with intralesional steroid injection to take advantage of the steroid's atrophogenic effects. Injections with deoxycholate have also been effective. Large, fast-growing lipomas should be removed to rule out malignant transformation into a liposarcoma. Compared with lipomas, liposarcomas are typically faster growing, firmer, and tender in nature.

Plate 2-21   Integumentary System

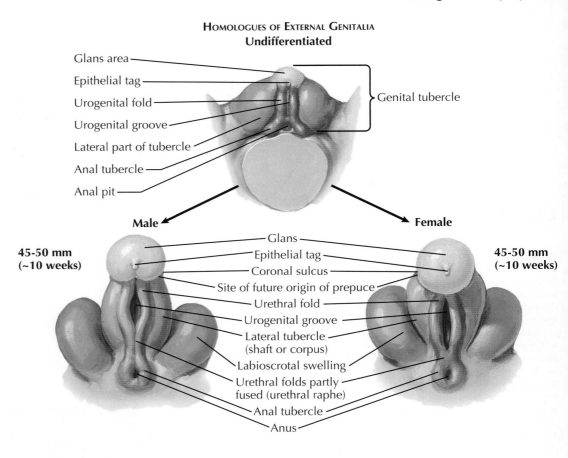

HOMOLOGUES OF EXTERNAL GENITALIA
Undifferentiated

Glans area
Epithelial tag
Urogenital fold
Urogenital groove
Lateral part of tubercle
Anal tubercle
Anal pit
Genital tubercle

Male

45-50 mm
(~10 weeks)

Female

45-50 mm
(~10 weeks)

Glans
Epithelial tag
Coronal sulcus
Site of future origin of prepuce
Urethral fold
Urogenital groove
Lateral tubercle
(shaft or corpus)
Labioscrotal swelling
Urethral folds partly
fused (urethral raphe)
Anal tubercle
Anus

MEDIAN RAPHE CYST

Median raphe cysts are uncommon benign cysts that form in the midline region of the perineum. They most commonly occur on the ventral shaft of the penis but can occur anywhere from the urethral opening along the ventral surface of the penis, in the midline across the scrotum, and to the anus. This cyst is considered to be formed from a congenital abnormality of the genitalia. An abnormal folding of the urethral folds is believed to be the cause of these developmental cysts.

Clinical Findings: Most median raphe cysts are found in young boys on the ventral surface of the penis and midline scrotum. They have no race predilection. They are present at birth but may go unnoticed for some time, even into adulthood. They appear as small (0.5-1 cm), solitary, soft, translucent cystic nodules. They are almost always asymptomatic. On occasion, they can rupture and drain serous fluid. The cyst rarely connects to the underlying urethra or other structures. The clinical differential diagnosis can be very broad, and the only way to make a definitive diagnosis is to perform a biopsy or complete excision.

Pathogenesis: These cysts are believed to be caused by an abnormal folding or fusing of the paired urogenital/urethral folds during embryological development. These folds normally combine and fuse to form the external genitalia at about the eighth to tenth weeks of gestation. In the male the folds form the shaft of the penis, and in females they form the labia minora. Hypospadias is another congenital abnormality caused by improper folding of these embryological tissues. The cause of the abnormal folding has yet to be determined.

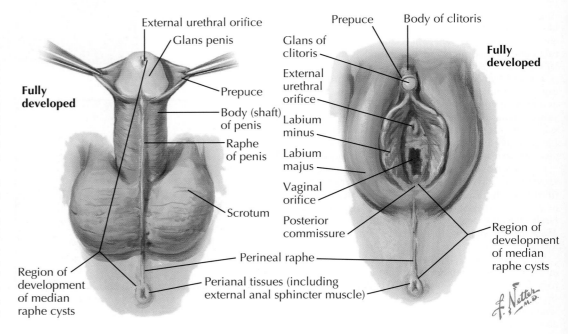

External urethral orifice
Glans penis
Fully developed
Prepuce
Body (shaft) of penis
Raphe of penis
Scrotum
Region of development of median raphe cysts

Prepuce   Body of clitoris
Glans of clitoris
Fully developed
External urethral orifice
Labium minus
Labium majus
Vaginal orifice
Posterior commissure
Region of development of median raphe cysts

Perineal raphe
Perianal tissues (including external anal sphincter muscle)

Histology: The cysts are lined with a pseudostratified or stratified columnar epithelium. The epithelium can closely approximate the appearance of transitional urethral cell epithelium. The lining surrounds a central cavity filled with serous fluid. Large mucinous cells are scattered throughout the columnar epithelium. The luminal cells have been shown to stain with cytokeratin 7, cytokeratin 13, epithelial membrane antigen (EMA), and carcinoembryonic antigen (CEA). Histologically, these cysts have a very characteristic appearance. The main pathological differential diagnosis is between the median raphe cyst and an apocrine cystadenoma. Immunohistochemical staining can be used to differentiate the two.

Treatment: Simple surgical excision is all that is required for cure. They will not recur, because they are developmental cysts. Care should be taken not to damage underlying structures, and often a urological surgeon performs the procedure.

Plate 2-22

Benign Growths

MELANOCYTIC NEVI

There are numerous types of melanocytic nevi, including the benign congenital melanocytic nevi, the blue nevi, and the common acquired melanocytic nevi. Atypical and dysplastic nevi are discussed with melanoma in the section on malignant growths. Evaluation of melanocytic nevi is one of the dermatologist's most common and important tasks. Every patient who enters a dermatologist's office should be offered the opportunity to have a full-body skin examination, specifically evaluating melanocytic nevi for any signs of malignant transformation and or de novo melanoma production. The importance of evaluating melanocytic nevi is to screen for melanoma. Melanoma is a life-threatening skin cancer that, if discovered early, can be cured. Different types of melanocytic nevi have varying rates of malignant transformation, and it is critical for the clinician to be aware of those nevi that are likely to be encountered on a daily basis.

Clinical Findings: Melanocytic nevi can be classified both clinically and histopathologically. The common acquired melanocytic nevus is a clinical diagnosis, and if the lesion is biopsied, it may show some evidence of atypia or dysplasia of melanocytes. It is for this reason that a universally accepted classification of melanocytic nevi has yet to be adopted.

Benign melanocytic nevi are extremely common. Virtually all humans have some form of these growths on their body. Common acquired melanocytic nevi are universally found and can have varying morphologies. They affect males and females equally. They are uncommon at birth but increase in number over the first 4 decades of life, after which the number typically stabilizes. As one ages, the nevi tend to slowly involute. They can be macular or papular in appearance. Most are uniform and symmetric in size and color. They can be flesh colored or slightly brown in coloration. They tend to grow proportionally as a child grows or as an adult gains weight. They also can become slightly larger and darker during pregnancy.

There is a risk for malignant degeneration into melanoma, and changes in color, size, symmetry, or border should be assessed. Nevi that become symptomatic, especially pruritic, and nevi that spontaneously bleed should be evaluated and biopsied appropriately.

Blue nevi are unique benign melanocytic tumors that have a characteristic clinical and histological pattern. These nevi tend to be small, to be located on the dorsal aspect of the hands or feet, and to have a bluish to blue-gray coloration due to their location within the dermis. The blue color is believed to result from the Tyndall effect. This is a process by which various wavelengths of light are absorbed preferentially, and the reflected light or color that is seen depends on the material and depth of the substance being illuminated. Blue nevi share similar histological characteristics with the nevus of Ota, nevus of Ito, and Mongolian spots. However, the clinical appearance is so different that these lesions are not considered in the differential diagnosis of a blue nevus.

Blue nevi can occur at any age, and they appear equally often in men and in women. They typically manifest as small (2-5 mm), oval or round macules or papules. They are well circumscribed with nice, distinct borders. They are commonly located on the dorsal aspect of the hands and feet but have been reported to

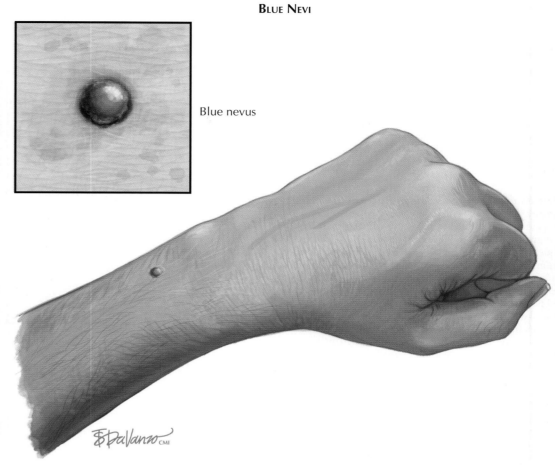

Blue nevus

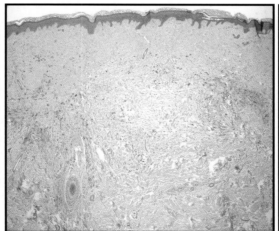

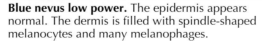

Blue nevus low power. The epidermis appears normal. The dermis is filled with spindle-shaped melanocytes and many melanophages.

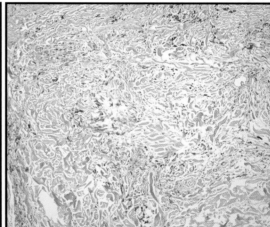

Blue nevus high power. Elongated pigmented melanocytes are appreciated with multiple dermal melanophages. The melanocytes are interspersed between the collagen bundles.

occur anywhere, including the mucous membranes. They are frequently biopsied because of their unusual coloration. They are small and usually can be removed easily with a punch biopsy that is 1 mm larger than the lesion. Patients often give a history of having been stabbed with a pencil during childhood and believe that the lesion is a graphite tattoo. This occasionally

is the case, but most of these lesions are actually blue nevi. Malignant transformation of blue nevi is extremely rare.

Multiple blue nevi can be seen in the Carney complex, also known as the NAME or LAMB syndrome. This complex of clinical findings includes multiple blue nevi, lentigines, ephelides, myxomas, atrial myxomas,

Plate 2-23   Integumentary System

COMMON ACQUIRED NEVI AND GIANT CONGENITAL MELANOCYTIC NEVI

MELANOCYTIC NEVI
(Continued)

testicular tumors, pituitary tumors, psammomatous melanotic schwannomas, and adrenal tumors. This is a rare syndrome that has been determined to be caused by a genetic defect in the gene *PRKAR1A*. This is a tumor suppressor gene that encodes a protein kinase A subunit.

Congenital melanocytic nevi can be divided clinically into distinct subtypes based on size (small, medium, and giant). Small congenital nevi are the most common type; they are defined as those nevi smaller than 2 cm in greatest diameter. These nevi occur with equal frequency in males and females and have no race predilection. Some authors estimate their prevalence at about 1% of the population. These nevi are typically described as well-defined macules, papules, or plaques. They are hyperpigmented compared with the normal surrounding skin. They are almost always uniform in color and symmetric. Over time, some 50% develop terminal hair growth within the nevi. The risk of malignant transformation in these small congenital nevi is low and approaches that of the common acquired melanocytic nevi. Melanoma can arise in these nevi at any point in the patient's life but usually after puberty.

Medium-sized congenital melanocytic nevi are defined as those that have a diameter between 2 and 20 cm. They have the same risk of malignant transformation as small congenital nevi. They occur equally in males and females and can be seen in about 1% of the population. They can occur anywhere on the body.

Giant or large congenital melanocytic nevi, also known as "bathing trunk" nevi, are important clinically in many ways. First, they have an increased risk of malignant transformation. This transformation can be difficult to discern clinically until the lesions are quite large. Most melanomas develop in a dermal or subcutaneous location, which make them difficult to assess clinically. Melanomas typically occur before puberty, and they have been reported to occur in as many as 15% of giant congenital nevi. The risk of malignant transformation is higher in axial nevi than in acral nevi. For this reason, these lesions are treated more aggressively, and patients with large congenital melanocytic nevi need lifelong, frequent routine follow-up. These nevi occur equally in men and women and in any racial group. They affect the truncal region more often than any other region of the body.

The significant finding of neurocutaneous melanosis occurs at a higher rate in patients with large congenital nevi of the trunk. These nevi almost always occur over the majority of the trunk, and they can have any number of satellite melanocytic nevi. Patients with large truncal congenital melanocytic nevi should undergo magnetic resonance imaging (MRI) of the nervous system to evaluate for neurocutaneous melanosis. Patients with neurocutaneous melanosis are at a high risk (almost 50%) for development of leptomeningeal melanoma, which is almost always fatal. A multidisciplinary approach to care for these patients is required, including the patient's pediatrician, dermatologist, neurologist, and neurosurgeon.

Histology: In common acquired melanocytic nevi, the melanocytes are arranged symmetrically in a lateral fashion. They are arranged in nests. The nested melanocytes do not have the typical dendritic appearance of

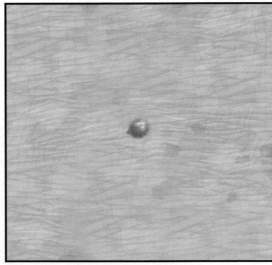

Common acquired nevus

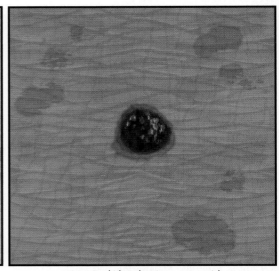

Atypical/dysplastic nevus with surrounding solar lentigines

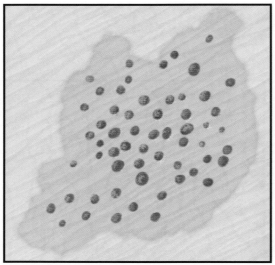

Nevus spilus

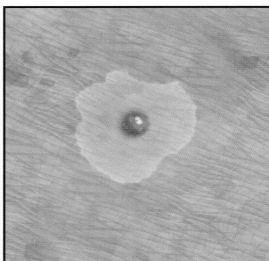

Halo nevus

normal melanocytes found within the stratum basalis. They are round and uniform in shape and show increasing maturation with depth in the dermis. Maturation of nevi cells implies a decrease in the ratio of nuclear to cytoplasmic volume and an overall decrease in the size of the melanocytes. The melanocytes are still uniform in size and shape at various depths within the dermis; they are not symmetric vertically. Many forms are seen

histologically. Based on the location of the melanocyte nests, they can be classified as junctional, intraepidermal, dermal, or compound nevi. A junctional nevus has its nests arranged along the basement membrane zone, whereas a compound nevus has epidermal and dermal nests.

Blue nevi are located entirely within the dermis. These nevi are made of melanocytes that resemble

Plate 2-24

Benign Growths

CONGENITAL NEVI

MELANOCYTIC NEVI
(Continued)

dendrites. The dendritic processes contain melanin pigment, and this pigment is responsible for the coloration of the lesion. Collagen is interwoven between the dermally located melanocytes. Melanophages are almost always seen in and around the lesion. A grenz zone is sometimes appreciated above the melanocytic lesion. Numerous histological subtypes of blue nevi have been described, including the dendritic blue nevus (common blue nevus), amelanotic blue nevus, cellular blue nevus, and epithelioid blue nevus.

Small, medium, and large congenital nevi all show the same histological characteristics, and they cannot be distinguished on pathological evaluation. The major criteria used to separate congenital nevi from other types of nevi are size and location. The nests are found deep within the dermis and can also be found within the subcutaneous tissue, fascia, and underlying muscle. Infiltration of muscle is unusual and is more likely to be seen in large congenital nevi. The nests of nevus cells accumulate around adnexal structures and are frequently seen juxtaposed to hair follicles, sebaceous glands, and eccrine glands. The melanocytes can penetrate the arrector pili muscles. The nevus cells show proper maturation and are uniform in appearance.

Pathogenesis: There are many conflicting theories as to the pathogenesis of common acquired melanocytic nevi and blue nevi. Some think that there is an abnormal migration of melanocytes embryologically, whereas others believe that stem cells are located within the dermis or epidermis and melanocytes migrate upward or downward to form the nevi. Perhaps a combination of these processes occurs, but no definitive pathogenic mechanism has been universally accepted.

Congenital melanocytic nevi are thought to be caused by an embryological malfunction of melanocyte migration. The precise mechanism that causes the disrupted or abnormal migration of melanocytes into the involved areas has not been determined. Migration in these cases is believed to be controlled by a complex but abnormal growth and regulatory signaling pathway.

Treatment: Common acquired melanocytic nevi do not need to be treated. They can be removed by various means for cosmetic purposes. Shave removal and punch biopsy removal are two highly successful techniques. Elliptical excision should be reserved for larger lesions in areas where the scar can be camouflaged. Only highly skilled physicians should consider removing pigmented lesions with laser therapy, because there is no tissue left for histological evaluation.

Blue nevi are easily removed by punch biopsy or elliptical excision. They are often removed for cosmetic reasons, and a small excision gives an excellent cosmetic result.

Removal of small and medium congenital nevi should be done with surgical excision. This removes the entire lesion and allows for pathological evaluation. Most of these small and medium congenital melanocytic nevi can be observed over time and removed if there are changes. Serial photographs are invaluable in monitoring these nevi for changes. Some of these lesions occur in cosmetically sensitive areas, such as the face, and

patients should be referred to a plastic surgeon for evaluation. The social and psychological well-being of the child can be enhanced by having a disfiguring congenital nevus removed.

Large congenital nevi present the biggest treatment difficulty because of the high rate of malignant transformation. If possible, serial excisions to remove large nevi are the best option. Tissue expanders are often used to help decrease the need for skin grafting. The

goal should be 100% removal, although in some cases this is not feasible. If the nevi cover 10% to 30% or more of body surface area, they become almost impossible to remove. In these cases, as in all the others, the importance of lifelong surveillance needs to be taught to the parents, the afflicted individuals, and the participating physicians. The goal in these cases is to biopsy and remove any changing areas of the nevi in an effort to prevent metastasis if a melanoma were to develop.

Medium congenital nevus

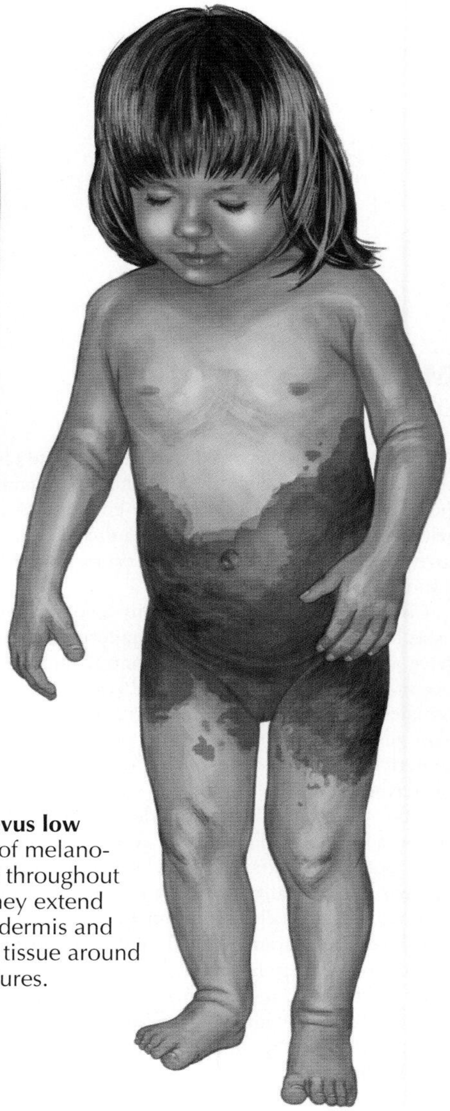

Small congenital nevus

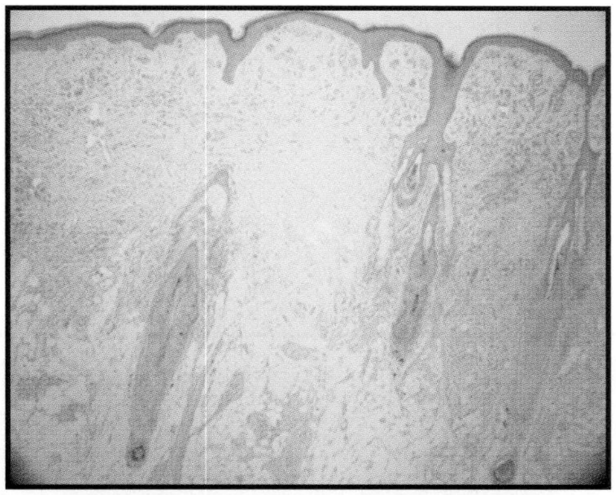

Congenital nevus low power. Nests of melanocytes are seen throughout the dermis. They extend deep into the dermis and subcutaneous tissue around adnexal structures.

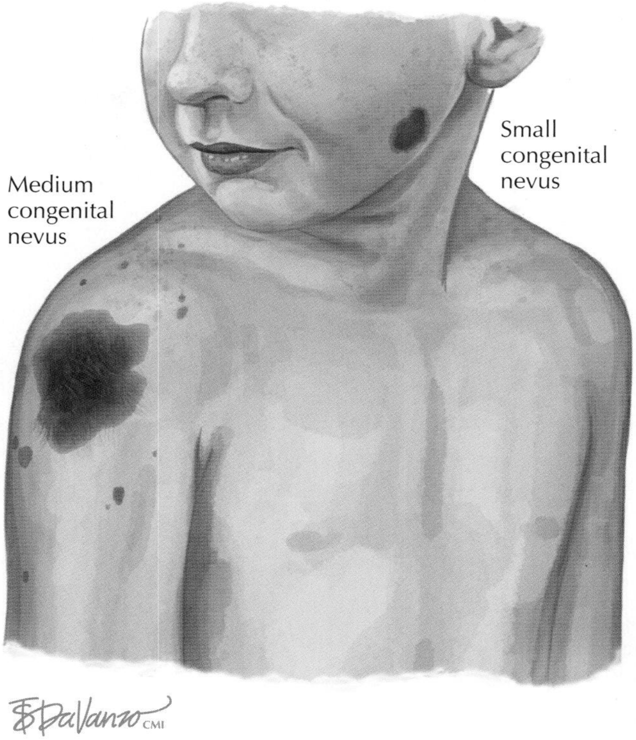

Giant congenital bathing trunk nevus

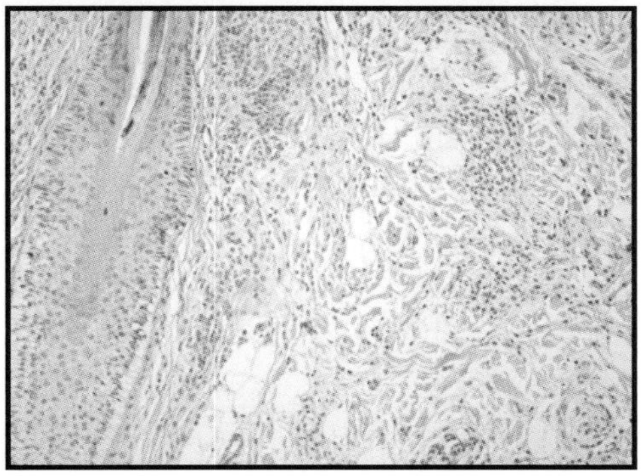

Congenital nevus high power. Melanocytes are seen adjacent to adnexal structures. This is one characteristic finding in congenital nevi.

Plate 2-25

Integumentary System

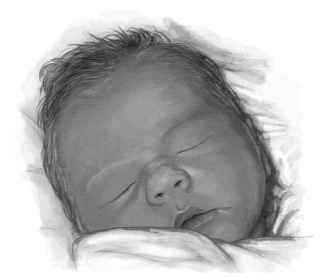

Congenital milia in a newborn. This is a common incidental finding.

MILIA

Milia are tiny (1-3 mm), superficially located epidermal inclusion cysts. They typically have a characteristic porcelain-white color. One often encounters a patient with a solitary milium or multiple milia. These tiny skin growths are entirely benign and cause no harm to the patient.

Clinical Findings: Milia are tiny epidermal inclusion cysts located superficially in the epidermis. They do not have an appreciable overlying central punctum. They occur in all races, at all ages, and equally in males and females. Primary milia occur without an underlying skin disorder. Secondary milia occur because of an underlying skin disorder, most often a subepidermal blistering condition. As the subepidermal blister heals, it is not uncommon to see the development of milia in the area of the previous blister. As an example, patients with porphyria cutanea tarda develop subepidermal blisters and typically heal with scarring and milia formation. Occasionally, a milium can have a somewhat translucent appearance and should be biopsied to rule out a basal cell carcinoma or an intradermal nevus.

In adults, milia most commonly occur on or around the eyelids. Up to half of all newborns have milia. These are typically located on the head and are termed more specifically *congenital milia*. They almost always resolve on their own without therapy, and therapy should be withheld to provide time for spontaneous resolution. Unique forms of milia eruptions have been described in the literature, including eruptive multiple milia, grouped milia, and generalized milia. Eruptive milia manifest over a period of weeks, with the appearance of 10 to 100 milia. This has been described in teenagers and adults. Grouped milia and milia en plaque are rare; these terms are used, respectively, to describe a nodular grouping and a plaque-like grouping of milia.

Certain genetic syndromes show an association with milia, the best recognized one being Bazek's syndrome. This syndrome is defined as a constellation of milia, basal cell carcinomas, hypotrichosis, and follicular atrophoderma. A few other genetic syndromes that have milia are the Rombo syndrome, familial milia syndrome, and atrichia with papular lesions. Many other syndromes with milia have been reported.

Histology: Milia are tiny cysts in the superficial epidermis. The cyst has a true lining of stratified squamous epithelium. A granular cell layer is present in the cyst wall lining. The center of the cyst is filled with a small

Milia in an adult. Small white papules just underneath the epidermis. They represent small cysts and are very commonly located on the eyelids.

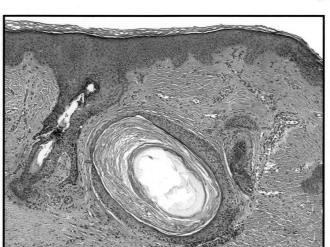

A small well-circumscribed cyst is seen within the dermis. The lining is stratified squamous epithelium with a granular cell layer.

amount of keratin debris. There is typically no surrounding inflammation in a primary milium.

Pathogenesis: The cause is unknown, but the cysts are believed to be derived from the hair follicle, sebaceous gland, or eccrine gland epithelium. Secondary milia occur after subepidermal blistering or trauma that interrupts the epidermal-dermal junction.

Treatment: No therapy is required. Most milia are found during routine skin examinations and are brought to the attention of the patient for education. Patients are often unaware of the milia. If a patient is bothered by the appearance of the cyst, extraction with a comedone extractor after creating a tiny (1-mm) incision with a no. 11 blade is all that is required for removal. Once the cyst is removed, it almost never recurs, although other milia may develop after extraction. Treatment of congenital milia in infants is not required because they almost all resolve spontaneously.

Plate 2-26

Benign Growths

NEUROFIBROMA

Neurofibromas are uncommon benign skin tumors that can be solitary but are more commonly found in multiples in patients with neurofibromatosis. Neurofibromatosis is one of the more common genodermatoses, afflicting 1 in every 3000 to 4000 individuals. It is caused by a defective tumor suppressor gene.

Clinical Findings: Neurofibromas are small (up to 1 cm on average) papules or nodules that have a soft, rubbery feel. They are flesh colored to slightly hyperpigmented. When pressed, they show a characteristic "buttonholing" phenomenon, in which the neurofibroma invaginates into the underlying dermis and subcutaneous fat. The neurofibroma returns to its natural location once it is unconfined. Most solitary neurofibromas are asymptomatic. The clinical differential diagnosis is between a neurofibroma and a common acquired melanocytic nevus (compound or intradermal nevus). When multiple neurofibromas are seen in an individual patient, the clinician should look for other signs of neurofibromatosis.

Neurofibromatosis type 1 (previously known as von Recklinghausen disease) is a common genetic systemic disease with cutaneous findings. It is inherited in an autosomal dominant pattern but can also result from a spontaneous mutation. The gene that has been implicated, known as *NF1*, is located on the long arm of chromosome 17 and encodes the tumor suppressor protein, neurofibromin. This guanosine triphosphatase (GTPase) protein is critical in the regulation of the Ras cell signaling pathway. Other forms of neurofibromatosis have been described and show variations of the clinical phenotype. Neurofibromatosis type 2 is caused by a defect in *NF2*, a gene on the long arm of chromosome 22.

Patients with neurofibromatosis type 1 begin developing neurofibromas at puberty, and the lesions increase in number dramatically over their life span. They are often larger than solitary neurofibromas and can range from a handful to thousands. The sheer number of neurofibromas can cause significant disfigurement and can affect social and psychological well-being. In this genetic disease, neurofibromas can occur not only in the skin but along any nerve in the body. Neurofibromas that occur in areas where there is minimal room for expansion (e.g., in the intervertebral foramen) can cause significant morbidity and need for surgical intervention.

Patients with neurofibromatosis type 1 have many other skin findings, including multiple café-au-lait macules, axillary freckling, and plexiform neurofibromas. Plexiform neurofibromas are a unique variant of the neurofibroma and are considered pathognomonic for this disease. They are composed of multiple individual neurofibromas grouped into a large plaque. Systemic findings seen in neurofibromatosis include optic gliomas, Lisch nodules on the iris, multiple bony findings, various impairments of the central nervous system, and a number of endocrine disorders. The varying phenotypes of this disease may result from different mutations in the involved gene. These patients are also at much higher risk for malignancy than non-afflicted controls.

Pathogenesis: Solitary neurofibromas have not been found to contain defects in the neurofibromin protein. They arise as a result of unknown factors that cause proliferation within the dermis of all the components of a nerve filament. The neurofibromas found in neurofibromatosis are believed to be caused by the genetic

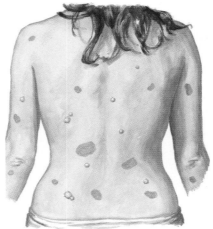

Multiple café-au-lait spots and neurofibromas are the most common manifestations of NF.

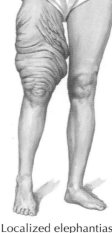

Localized elephantiasis of thigh with redundant skin folds

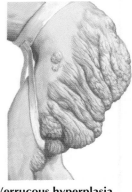

Verrucous hyperplasia. Maceration of velvety-soft skin may cause weeping and infection in crevices.

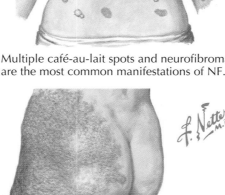

Plexiform neurofibroma. Characteristically localized to one side of trunk and thigh

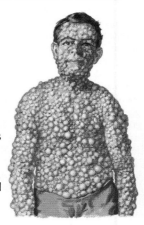

von Recklinghausen disease. One of von Recklinghausen's original patients, who had extensive neurofibromas but no neurologic symptoms. Fortunately, such widespread skin involvement is uncommon.

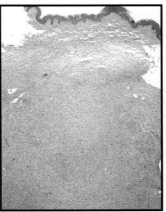

Low power. A non-encapsulated dermal tumor of cells with spindle-shaped nuclei. A small grenz zone is appreciated.

High power. Wavy-appearing nuclei seen within the center of the tumor. Mast cells are often found in the tumor.

defect in the tumor suppressor gene. How this defect ultimately regulates the formation of neurofibromas is not fully understood.

Histology: Individual neurofibromas have a well-circumscribed, spindle-shaped proliferation within the dermis. No capsule is present. Schwann cell proliferation and proliferation of the axonal components of the nerve are seen. Many mast cells are present in these tumors. The epidermis is uninvolved, and a small grenz zone is often appreciated.

Treatment: Definitive treatment of a solitary neurofibroma is complete excision. This is curative and results in a very low recurrence rate. No treatment is necessary, because the transformation into malignancy is extremely low.

Any neurofibroma that starts growing or becomes hard or tender should be removed to look for degeneration into neurofibrosarcoma.

Patients with neurofibromatosis require a multidisciplinary approach and need to see a good internist to coordinate all the potential systemic complications. The neurofibromas may be removed surgically. This approach is not ideal, because the number of lesions typically precludes removal of only the bothersome ones. Plexiform neurofibromas should be removed by a plastic surgeon, because they can have large subcutaneous extensions that are not visible clinically. There is no cure for this genetic disease; lifelong screening and follow-up are required, and the patient should be referred for genetic counseling before reaching child-bearing age.

Plate 2-27

Integumentary System

NEVUS LIPOMATOSUS SUPERFICIALIS

Nevus lipomatosus superficialis is a not-uncommon benign skin growth that is considered to be a hamartomatous proliferation of adipose tissue located in the dermis. It was originally named nevus lipomatosus cutaneous superficialis of Hoffman-Zurhelle. There are no known systemic associations with this benign skin growth, and no inheritance pattern has been described.

Clinical Findings: These nevi are most commonly found along the pelvic girdle. They have no sex or race predilection. They may occur at any age but are most common before the third decade of life. The lesions usually have a soft, bag-like appearance, often mimicking a large skin tag, and are flesh colored to yellow-tan. They are soft, nontender, easily moveable papules with a sessile base or pedunculated plaques with a thick stalk-like projection. The main differential diagnosis includes a skin tag, a compound nevus, and a connective tissue nevus. However, these lesions are much larger on average than the common skin tag.

Although the diagnosis can be considered clinically, the definitive diagnosis can be ascertained only after pathological evaluation. These lesions are often solitary, but reports of multiple lesions have been described in the literature. In the case of multiple tumors, the lesions are typically described as flesh-colored to slightly red dermal nodules that tend to coalesce into larger plaques. Some of the tumors have a cerebriform appearance to their surface. They can become very large (>10 cm in diameter) if left untreated. However, most never grow larger than 1 to 2 cm in diameter. A generalized variety of this condition has been described, but it is exceedingly uncharacteristic.

Children present after their parents notice the growth or growths, and a skin biopsy is often used to determine the diagnosis. Adults often present because of a slowly enlarging plaque that has an unsightly appearance or has become eroded or ulcerated due to trauma from the size of the lesion.

Pathogenesis: This condition is believed to be a hamartomatous process of adipose tissue located in the dermis. For some unknown reason, this normal-appearing adipose tissue proliferates within the dermis, often causing an outward herniation of the overlying epidermis, which ultimately leads to the distinctive clinical findings. The exact mechanism has not been elucidated. No genetic abnormalities of the adipose tissue have been established, and there is no known malignant potential.

Histology: Nevus lipomatosus superficialis has a characteristic pathology. It shows mature normal adipose tissue within the dermis. The one key finding is lack of connection of the abnormally located dermal adipose tissue with the normally located subcutaneous

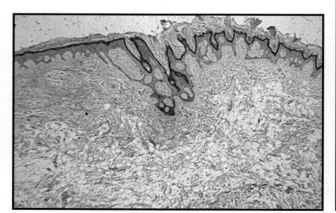

Fleshy plaquelike benign growth that is diagnosed by histopathological analysis

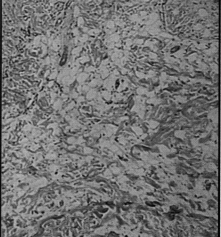

Pedunculated lesion. These tumors are soft, typically asymptomatic, and removed for cosmetic purposes or because of chronic irritation.

C. Machado
—M.D.
B.DaVanzo CMI

Low power. The dermis is almost entirely replaced with adipose tissue.

High power. The adipose tissue is normal in appearance.

adipose tissue. Variable amounts of fat tissue make up the individual lesions. No definitive percentage has been established to make the diagnosis, but as little as 10% to more than 50% of each lesion is made up of adipose tissue. The overlying epidermis can be normal or can exhibit acanthosis and papillomatosis. The more cerebriform appearing the lesion is clinically, the more likely it is that epidermal changes will be seen on pathological examination. Skin tags do not

have adipose tissue present, and this is a key discriminating factor.

Treatment: These solitary lesions are best excised surgically; this gives the best cosmetic result and the best cure rate. Multiple lesions can be left alone after a diagnosis is made. If the group of lesions is amenable to surgical excision without the potential for disfiguring scarring, or if the scarring would result in a better cosmetic outcome, surgical excision can be undertaken.

Plate 2-28

Benign Growths

NEVUS OF OTA AND NEVUS OF ITO

Both nevus of Ota (oculodermal melanocytosis, nevus fuscoceruleus ophthalmomaxillaris) and nevus of Ito (nevus fuscoceruleus acromiodeltoideus) are considered to be benign hamartomatous overgrowths of melanocytes. These two processes are located on the face and upper shoulder, respectively. They share a common pathogenesis and histology with Mongolian spots and are most likely caused by abnormal embryological migration of melanocytes.

Clinical Findings: The diagnosis of these conditions is most often made on clinical grounds, and a skin biopsy is rarely, if ever, needed to make the diagnosis. Nevus of Ota and nevus of Ito have characteristic locations, and this helps the clinician make the ultimate diagnosis. The closely related Mongolian spot is located on the lower back of infants and manifests as a deep blue, asymptomatic macule that almost always fades away slowly until it disappears completely by adulthood. It has a higher prevalence in children of Asian or Mayan Indian descent.

Nevus of Ota occurs in a periocular location and can affect the bulbar conjunctiva. It is almost always unilateral in nature. Nevus of Ota manifests as a bluish to blue-gray macule with indistinct borders that fade into the surrounding normal-colored skin. It is usually located over the distribution of the first two branches of the trigeminal nerve. If the bulbar conjunctiva is involved, the color may vary from bluish gray to dark brown. This condition occurs much more commonly in women and in patients of Asian descent. Nevus of Ota is most often seen in isolation, but on occasion it can be seen with a coexisting nevus of Ito.

Nevus of Ito has a similar clinical appearance; however, the location is on the shoulder girdle and neck. Unilateral lesions are the rule. The blue to blue-gray macules can be large and can cause the patient considerable dismay. These lesions are asymptomatic but can be a major cosmetic concern for patients and can cause considerable psychological and social difficulties.

Both nevus of Ota and nevus of Ito are more prevalent in the Asian population. Nevus of Ota appears to have a very small malignant potential. It is believed that Caucasian females with a nevus of Ota are at higher risk for transformation into malignant melanoma. Nevus of Ito does not appear to have a malignant potential.

Histology: The histological findings in nevus of Ota, nevus of Ito, and Mongolian spots are identical and resemble those of common blue nevi. Within the lesion, nodular collections of melanocytes are found in the dermis, with noticeable elongation of the melanocytes in the superficial dermis. There is surrounding fibrosis in the dermis with a number of melanophages present.

Pathogenesis: Under normal circumstances, melanocytes migrate during embryogenesis from the neural crest outward to their final locations (e.g., skin, retina). Nevus of Ota and nevus of Ito are believed to be caused by abnormal migration of these melanocytes. During their migration, some unknown signal causes the melanocytes to collect on the face or on the shoulder, respectively. There does not appear to be a genetic inheritance pattern.

Treatment: These are benign lesions that require no therapy. It is not unreasonable to monitor them clinically for the rare development of malignant transformation. Most patients present for therapy because they are bothered by the appearance of the lesions.

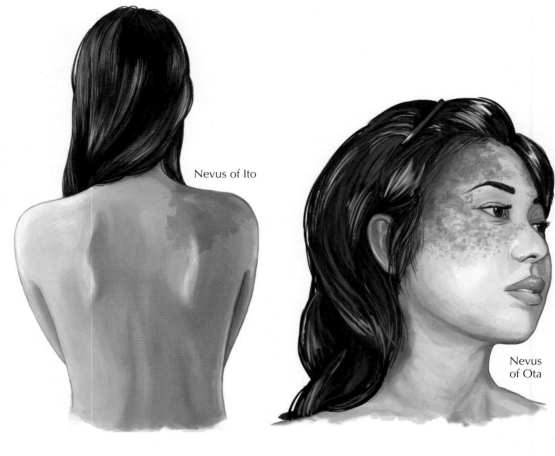

Nevus of Ito

Nevus of Ota

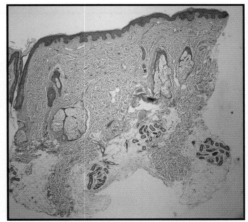

Nevus of Ota low power. Pigmented melanocytes are spread out within the dermis.

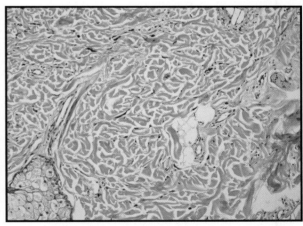

Nevus of Ota high power. Pigmented melanocytes with elongated dendritic processes are seen amongst the dermal collagen bundles.

Because of the psychological and social hardships engendered by these cosmetically disfiguring lesions, therapy is appropriate, albeit difficult. If only small areas are involved, cosmetic makeup may be used to camouflage the region. Topical therapies with hydroquinone and tretinoin have shown minimal to no effect on the pigmentation.

Use of the 1064-nm neodymium:yttrium-aluminumgarnet (Nd:YAG) laser has resulted in the most success in treating these lesions, and it can be used in patients of almost any skin type. Q-switching of the laser is a method that has been shown to increase its efficacy. Q-switched ruby, alexandrite, and 1064-nm Nd:YAG lasers have all been used successfully.

Plate 2-29   Integumentary System

Nevus Sebaceus

Nevus sebaceus, also known as organoid nevus or nevus sebaceus of Jadasshon, is a benign tumor that manifests in infancy or early childhood. This tumor has a risk of malignant transformation after puberty, and basal cell carcinoma is the malignant tumor that most frequently develops within these lesions.

Clinical Findings: Most of these growths are very small, and some escape detection for years. Others can be obvious at birth. They show a large range in dimensions. Most are solitary. The most common location in which to find a nevus sebaceus is within the scalp. Together, the scalp and face are overwhelmingly the areas of involvement, and it is rare to find a lesion any other place on the body. At or soon after birth, an area of the scalp is seen to be obviously affected. Nevus sebaceus typically start off as a thin, yellowish-brown patch or plaque. The area is almost universally devoid of terminal hair shafts. With time, the area becomes more cobblestoned in appearance. These nevi are usually asymptomatic but can be a cosmetic problem depending on their size and exact location. They occur in males and females with equal frequency. The lesions enlarge in proportion to the growing child. Before puberty, the risk of malignant transformation is very low. After puberty, approximately one third of these lesions develop a secondary growth, which usually manifests as a new nodule within the nevus sebaceus. The nodule can vary in color, but a light, translucent purple color is not infrequently seen. It is also common for a bleeding nodule or papule to develop within the underlying nevus sebaceus.

Most commonly, these growths that occur within the nevus sebaceus are benign in nature. The syringocystadenoma papilliferum is the most common benign tumor to develop within a nevus sebaceus. Because of the connection to the epidermis, these growths usually manifest as a draining or bleeding nodule that is slowly enlarging. The most common malignant growth to develop in a nevus sebaceus is a basal cell carcinoma. These usually manifest as a pearl-colored papule with a central ulceration and varying amounts of bleeding or crusting. The transformation to malignancy has been shown to increase with the age of the patient. It is estimated that about 1% of nevus sebaceus lesions will develop a malignant growth over the patient's lifetime. There have been multiple reports of various tumors arising within a nevus sebaceus, and there have also been reports of multiple tumors arising within the same nevus sebaceus.

The nevus sebaceus syndrome is a very rare finding. It is similar in nature to the epidermal nevus syndrome. This syndrome can have a varying phenotype. The neurological system, including the eye, and the musculoskeletal, cardiovascular, and genitourinary systems can all be involved to varying degrees. Patients with this syndrome usually have abnormally large areas of cutaneous involvement. The lesions can be found anywhere on the body and are often multiple.

Pathogenesis: Nevus sebaceus is considered to be a hamartomatous process of the epidermis and adnexal structures of the skin. The exact mechanism and cause have not been discovered.

Histology: The histological picture is dependent on the age of the patient. Before puberty, the findings are more subtle than after puberty. Prepubertal lesions most commonly show undeveloped adnexal structures. After puberty, the lack of terminal hair follicles is a universal finding. Fine vellus hair follicles are often

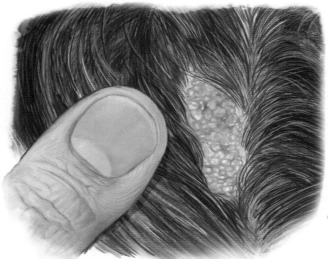

Nevus sebaceus. Flesh- to yellow-colored plaque, typically on the scalp with associated overlying alopecia

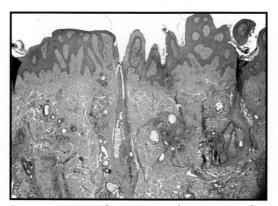

Low power. Acanthosis seen with an increased number of sebaceous glands and hair follicles

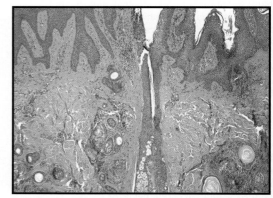

High power. Characteristic finding of the emptying of a sebaceous gland directly onto the surface of the epidermis

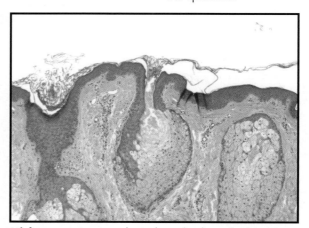

High power. Increased number of enlarged sebaceous glands, with the central sebaceous gland emptying onto the surface of the skin

present but in reduced numbers. Prominent sebaceous glands are seen. Many of the sebaceous glands empty directly onto the surface of the epidermis. The overlying epidermis shows acanthosis and papillomatosis. The presence of apocrine glands is often appreciated.

Treatment: If treatment is undertaken, complete surgical excision is the treatment of choice. This not only removes the lesion but also removes the risk of malignant potential. Another approach is to watch and wait,

with routine observation. If the nevus sebaceus develops any areas of change, a prompt biopsy is warranted. The timing of the surgical removal is controversial, and because the risk of malignancy is low, it is acceptable to wait until the patient is old enough to make the decision. The size and location of the nevus sebaceus dictates the type of surgical excision and repair required. Treatment of the rare nevus sebaceus syndrome requires a multidisciplinary team approach.

Plate 2-30

Benign Growths

OSTEOMA CUTIS

Osteoma cutis is a rare benign tumor in which bone formation occurs within the skin. There are two types of osteoma cutis, primary and secondary. Primary osteoma cutis is idiopathic in nature, whereas secondary osteoma cutis is caused by bone formation in an area of trauma or another form of cutaneous inflammation. It can also be seen secondary to abnormalities of parathyroid hormone metabolism, and this form of osteoma cutis is called metastatic ossification. Secondary osteoma cutis is much more common than the primary idiopathic form.

Clinical Findings: Primary osteoma cutis is not associated with any defined underlying disorder and can manifest as a solitary nodule, plaque, or plate-like hardening of the skin. Some are quite small, whereas others are large and cause discomfort. Males and females are equally affected, and there is no race predilection. The age at onset is variable. Plate-like or plaque-like osteoma cutis is a form of primary osteoma cutis that occurs during the first few months of life and can even be present at birth. The acral regions are most commonly affected. Over time, these osteomas tend to develop ulcerations or erosions of the overlying epidermis. With this ulceration, small parts of the osteoma are extruded from the underlying dermis and expelled from the skin. This may be the cause for presentation to the clinician. Most patients present with a thickened or hardened area of skin with no preceding trauma or inflammatory condition. There is no malignant potential.

Primary osteomas of the skin may be seen in the genetically inherited disease, Albright's hereditary osteodystrophy. This condition is characterized by a constellation of findings including short stature, osteoma cutis, mental and physical delay, and brachydactyly. Varying degrees of obesity and a round appearance to the face are also seen. This condition is caused by an underlying defect in the *GNAS* gene. This gene encodes a stimulatory G protein (G$_s$) that is responsible for cell signaling through the eventual production of cyclic adenosine monophosphate (cAMP). Albright's hereditary osteodystrophy has been reported to manifest with resistance to parathyroid hormone, but other Albright's patients have not shown this resistance. These differences are likely due to the complex inheritance pattern and whether the defective gene was inherited from the maternal or paternal side or both. Most patients have associated hypocalcemia and hyperphosphatemia.

Secondary osteoma cutis is far more common than the primary form, by a ratio of about 9:1. Bone formation may occur in any area of previous skin trauma, acne cysts, or epidermal inclusion cysts and are commonly seen in pilomatricomas. Pilomatricomas are benign tumors that most often manifest in childhood. Inflammatory conditions associated with osteoma cutis include dermatomyositis and scleroderma.

Fibrodysplasia ossificans progressiva is a rare genetic condition in which connective tissue is turned into bone after minor trauma, causing secondary osteomas. The skin can be involved, but so can the muscle and other

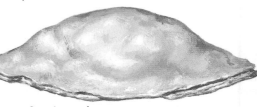

Painless bony mass protrudes from anterior aspect of tibia. Scars due to repeated skin abrasions

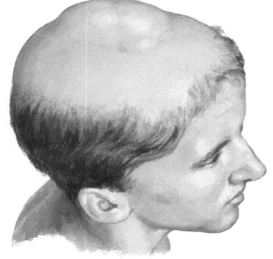

Radiograph reveals globular outgrowth on tibial cortex with sloping extensions (Codman's triangles)

Specimen demonstrates continuity of tumor with overlying periosteum.

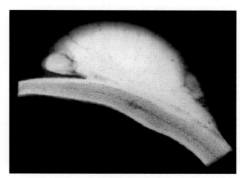

Radiograph of excised tumor reveals densely ossified cortical mass protruding from outer table of skull.

Slowly enlarging, asymptomatic bony mass on dome of head

High power. A well-circumscribed nodule of bone formation just underneath the epidermis. A few haversian canals are present.

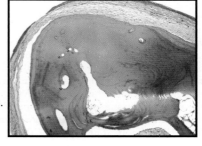

underlying tissue. This disease is progressive and can result in premature death. This condition is unique in that it is caused by endochondral bone formation.

Pathogenesis: Primary forms of osteoma cutis show intramembranous ossification that is centered within the dermis. There is no preceding cartilage formation to act as a scaffolding for the bone to form. The exact cause is unknown. The G protein that is defective in Albright's hereditary osteodystrophy has been found to be important in bone regulation. The precise reason why some areas of skin are involved while others are left intact in this genetic disease is not well understood.

Histology: Areas of bone formation are seen ectopically in the dermis or subcutaneous tissue. The bone is formed by an intramembranous mechanism without the assistance of a preceding cartilage scaffolding.

Treatment: Secondary osteoma cutis can be removed with a number of surgical techniques. Creation of a small, nick-like incision over the area of osteoma formation and removal with a small curette or laser resurfacing has produced the best results. This treatment can be very time-consuming and labor intensive in cases of multiple secondary osteoma cutis (e.g., in some cases of acne-associated osteoma cutis).

The treatment of primary plaque-like osteoma cutis is surgical removal. Albright's hereditary osteodystrophy and fibrodysplasia ossificans progressiva are rare diseases that require a multidisciplinary approach at centers with experience treating these conditions.

Plate 2-31

Integumentary System

PALISADED ENCAPSULATED NEUROMA

The palisaded encapsulated neuroma (PEN) is an uncommon benign tumor that is derived from nerve tissue. It is also known as solitary circumscribed neuroma of the skin. Most of the tumors occur on the head and neck.

Clinical Findings: The lesions of PEN most often manifest on the head and neck region of patients in the fourth and fifth decades of life. They afflict men and women equally and have no race predilection. They are firm, dome-shaped papules or dermal nodules. They are almost always solitary in nature. The overlying epidermis is unaffected and is flesh colored. These benign tumors tend to grow slowly over a period of years until they reach a size (often <1 cm in diameter) that makes them worrisome to the patient. They are commonly misdiagnosed as compound nevi or basal cell carcinomas, and it is not until they are biopsied that the true diagnosis is made. These tumors have a propensity to develop on the eyelid margin and at the interface between keratinized skin and the mucous membranes. Many are seen and removed by ophthalmologists. Most of these tumors are completely asymptomatic. On occasion, they are tender. This tumor is not associated with any underlying neural or systemic symptoms. In contrast, traumatic neuromas occur at sites of trauma, especially at amputation stump sites, and are caused by hypertrophy and proliferation of the damaged nerve ending. These tumors are solid, hard dermal nodules that cause pain on palpation.

Pathogenesis: The PEN tumor is derived from neural tissue. The Schwann cell is believed to be the cell type of origin for this growth. The proliferation of Schwann cells forms the tumor lobule. The exact mechanism or signal that causes this proliferation has not yet been discovered. Schwann cell origin is important to recognize and helps differentiate this tumor from other neurally derived tumors. The capsule is derived from perineural cells and collagen bundles. The capsule is believed to occur as a reaction to the underlying Schwann cell proliferation.

Histology: The PEN has a clear and well-demarcated capsule lining that is derived from collagen and perineural cells. The tumor is located entirely within the dermis, and the overlying epidermis is normal in appearance. There is no inflammatory infiltrate. The tumor is composed of spindle-shaped cells that form a tight, interweaving pattern. Immunohistochemical staining is often used to help differentiate these tumors form other neurally derived tumors such as schwannomas, neurofibromas, and traumatic neuromas. Neurofibromas do not have a true capsule circumventing the tumor. The capsule stains with epithelial membrane antigen (EMA). This stain helps indicate the location of the perineural capsular cell components. The tumor proper stains with S100, vimentin, and type IV

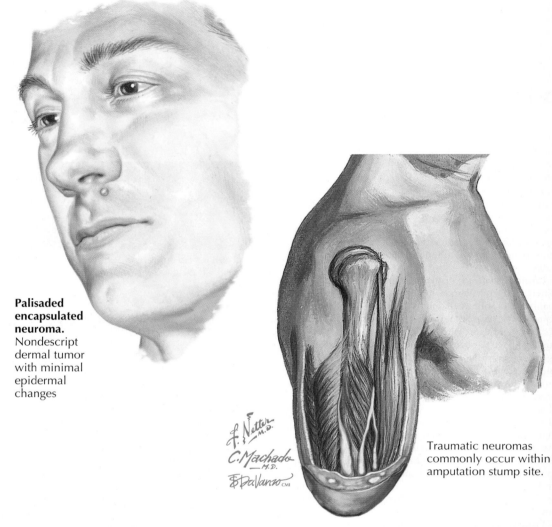

Palisaded encapsulated neuroma. Nondescript dermal tumor with minimal epidermal changes

Traumatic neuromas commonly occur within amputation stump site.

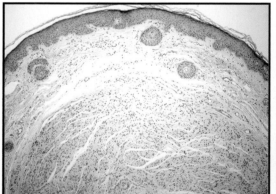

Palisaded encapsulated neuroma, low power. Well-circumscribed dermal tumor of spindle cells

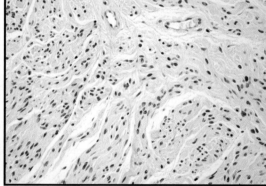

Palisaded encapsulated neuroma, high power. Close-up of the fascicles that make up the tumor

collagen. This staining pattern has been described for Schwann cells, so a positive result helps to determine the derivation of this tumor. Schwannomas are differentiated by their characteristic Antoni A and B regions and their subcutaneous location. Traumatic neuromas are not encapsulated and are composed of all the individual components that make up the previously normal traumatized nerve tissue.

Treatment: Complete excision is diagnostic and curative. The tumors rarely recur after elliptical excision. They have no malignant potential, and patients can be reassured that they do not have any possibility of an underlying neural syndrome. Traumatic neuromas can be cured by surgical removal. There is a small risk of recurrence. Pain control is also critical in the management of traumatic neuromas.

Plate 2-32

Benign Growths

PILAR CYST (TRICHILEMMAL CYST)

Pilar cysts are relatively common benign growths that occur most frequently on the scalp. They go by many names, including wen, trichilemmal cyst, and isthmus-catagen cyst. Most are solitary, but it is not uncommon to see multiple pilar cysts in a single individual. Their appearance is similar to that of epidermal inclusion cysts, but the pathogenesis is completely different. There is a malignant counterpart called a metastasizing proliferating trichilemmal cyst. The malignant transformation of a pilar cyst is exceedingly rare. Subsets of these growths are inherited.

Clinical Findings: Pilar cysts occur most frequently on the scalp. They can be mistaken for epidermal inclusion cysts. The main clinical differentiating points are that pilar cysts do not have an overlying central punctum, and they tend to be a bit firmer to touch. These cysts occur more commonly in adults, and they have a tendency to affect women more often than men. They typically manifest as slowly growing, firm dermal nodules with no overlying epidermal changes and no central punctum. These cysts do not drain, as epidermal cysts sometimes do. They also rarely get inflamed. Almost exclusively found in the scalp, they are for the most part asymptomatic. Patients present to the clinician because of an enlarging nodule. As opposed to the epidermal inclusion cyst, which essentially has no malignant potential, the pilar cyst does have a small proliferating and malignant potential. This risk is very low.

Some families show an autosomal dominant inheritance pattern. The exact gene defect has yet to be determined, but a possible gene has been mapped to chromosome 3. Most patients with the hereditary version of this condition have solitary lesions. Numerous lesions are infrequently encountered in the inherited form.

Pathogenesis: Pilar cysts are also called trichilemmal cysts, because they are derived from the outer root sheath of the hair follicle, which undergoes trichilemmal keratinization. This form of keratinization is unique in that there is no granular layer. The hereditary version of this disease was originally thought to be caused by a defect in the gene encoding β-catenin. This has been disproven, and the familial gene has been mapped to the short arm of chromosome 3, although the exact genetic defect has yet to be elucidated. These cysts are believed to be derived from the isthmus of anagen-type hairs. They are formed from deeper elements of the hair shaft apparatus than the epidermal inclusion cyst are.

Histology: Pilar cysts are composed of compact layers of stratified squamous epithelium without a granular cell layer. The cysts are found within the dermis, and

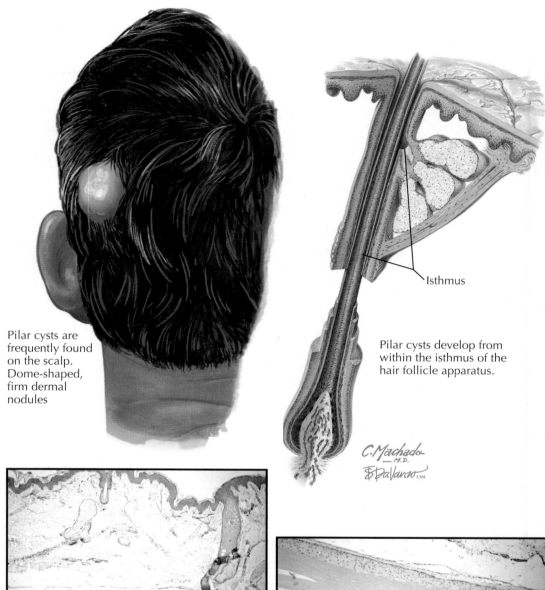

Pilar cysts are frequently found on the scalp. Dome-shaped, firm dermal nodules

Isthmus

Pilar cysts develop from within the isthmus of the hair follicle apparatus.

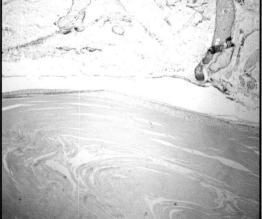

Low power. Dermal cyst with compacted central keratin. The epidermis is unaffected.

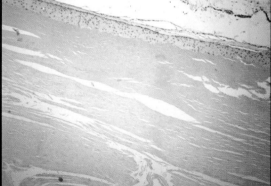

High power. The epithelial lining does not contain a granular cell layer and is composed of stratified squamous epithelium.

the overlying epidermis is unaffected. These cysts show an absence of intercellular adhesion molecules. The cysts can become calcified or ossified. The cysts have a unique peripheral rim of keratinocyte nuclei, which is very helpful in classifying them. The central aspect of the cyst contains homogenous pale, eosinophilic, compressed keratin.

Treatment: Simple surgical excision is curative. The recurrence rate is minimal. These cysts typically are removed very easily after excision through the overlying skin into the cyst wall. The cyst almost always "pops" out with slight lateral pressure, and only a small incision is needed. After removal, care needs to be taken to decrease the amount of dead space left, to avoid seroma formation. This can be prevented by removing some of the redundant overlying epidermis and suturing the deeper tissues together to close the space left by the removed cyst.

Plate 2-33

Integumentary System

POROKERATOSIS

The porokeratoses are a group of benign epidermal proliferations. The most common and best-described clinical variants include disseminated superficial actinic porokeratosis (DSAP), porokeratosis of Mibelli, porokeratosis palmaris et plantaris disseminata, and punctuate porokeratosis. The underlying disease state is the same for all variants, as are the characteristic and diagnostic histopathological findings. There are many other clinical variants that are infrequently seen.

Clinical Findings: Porokeratoses are typically inherited in an autosomal dominant fashion. They manifest beginning in the third to fourth decades of life and are more common in sun-exposed areas. The lesions can be minute to a few centimeters in diameter. They usually are 1- to 2-cm, thin, flesh-colored to slightly pink or hyperpigmented patches with a characteristic hyperkeratotic surrounding rim. This rim encompasses the entire lesion and is almost pathognomonic for porokeratosis.

The DSAP form is the most common and most easily recognized clinical variant. Patients present with a family history of similar skin growths. The lesions are almost entirely located in sun-exposed regions of the body. Patients who have had more ultraviolet light exposure over their lifetime are more likely to have multiple and more noticeable lesions. Most porokeratoses are asymptomatic, and patients typically present because of the appearance of the lesions and the fact that they continue to develop more lesions over time. Most lesions are flesh colored to slightly pink or red. Some can be frankly inflamed, with redness and crusting. Transformation into squamous cell carcinoma has been reported. and patients should be counseled to be reevaluated if they develop growths or ulcerations within the porokeratosis. The lesions of DSAP are much more likely to affect the skin on the extremities than the facial skin.

The porokeratosis of Mibelli is a solitary lesion, or a group of lesions with a linear array that have an identical morphology of a thin patch with a thin hyperkeratotic rim. They may occur anywhere on the body.

Porokeratosis palmaris et plantaris disseminata is a unique variant that affects the skin of the palms and soles initially and then can disseminate into a generalized pattern. The lesions of the palms and soles can be tender. This variant is also inherited in an autosomal dominant manner. The lesions begin on the palms and soles during the third to fourth decades of life and slowly spread to other areas of the skin in a generalized pattern.

Punctate porokeratosis of the palms and soles is a rare clinical variant that is localized to the palms and soles. The lesions tend to be 0.5 to 1 cm in diameter and have a well-defined rim of hyperkeratosis. Occasionally, they can be mistaken for plantar warts.

Pathogenesis: The pathogenesis of porokeratosis, no matter which variant, is believed to be an abnormality of keratinocyte proliferation. A clonal expansion of the abnormal keratinocytes leads to development of the expanding rim of hyperkeratotic tissue. This rim of hyperkeratosis is recognized histopathologically as the cornoid lamella. No genetic defect has been identified. Porokeratosis is more commonly found in patients taking chronic immunosuppressive medications (e.g., after solid organ transplantation) and in those infected with the human immunodeficiency virus. This is indirect evidence that chronic immunosuppression may lead to a lack of tumor surveillance and the development of porokeratosis.

Histology: On biopsy, the hallmark of porokeratosis is recognition of the cornoid lamella. The cornoid lamella is the pathological representation of the hyperkeratotic peripheral rim of tissue seen on clinical examination. The cornoid lamella is positioned at an angle away from the center of the lesion. The granular cell layer underneath the cornoid lamella is often absent or severely thinned. The appearance of the center of the lesion is dependent on the clinical variant seen. The area can be atrophic or acanthotic. It is not uncommon to see an inflammatory infiltrate underneath the lesion, composed predominantly of lymphocytes.

Treatment: Treatment is difficult and often unsuccessful for widespread areas such as those involved in DSAP. Sun protection and sunscreen use are recommended. Solitary lesions can be removed surgically. Multiple disseminated lesions can be ablated with carbon dioxide laser ablation, 5-fluorouracil, or dermabrasion. These therapies are not always effective and may be associated with scarring. It is imperative to continue to monitor these patients with routine skin examinations, because porokeratoses have a potential for malignant degeneration.

Disseminated superficial actinic porokeratosis (DSAP). Thin patches with a thin rim of epidermal hyperkeratosis on sun-exposed skin

Types of Porokeratosis
▶ Disseminated superficial actinic porokeratosis (DSAP)
▶ Porokeratosis palmaris et plantaris disseminata
▶ Linear porokeratosis
▶ Punctate porokeratosis
▶ Porokeratosis of Mibelli (solitary porokeratosis)

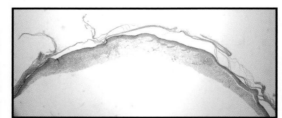

Low power. An atrophic epidermis with a scant amount of dermal inflammation is seen. A peripherally located cornoid lamella is appreciated.

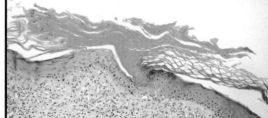

High power. The cornoid lamella is made of compacted stratum corneum. It overlies an area that has lost its granular cell layer. The cornoid lamella is oriented with its distal ends pointing inward.

Plate 2-34

Benign Growths

PYOGENIC GRANULOMA

Pyogenic granulomas are common benign skin tumors. They frequently occur after trauma and can be induced by certain classes of medications. They are also seen in increased frequency during pregnancy. Pyogenic granulomas are vascular tumors or proliferations of vascular tissue. They occur in all races, and there is no age or gender predilection, although they are more commonly seen in pregnancy.

Clinical Findings: Patients often present with a bleeding papule or nodule that is beefy red and has a collarette of scale. Pyogenic granulomas are friable and bleed easily when manipulated. There is often a preceding history of trauma. The lesions are usually small (5 mm) papules, but some have been reported to be 1 to 2 cm in diameter. These benign growths can also occur on the mucosa, and another common but unique location is in a periungual position. They can be tender and occasionally can become superinfected. A characteristic finding is the "band-aid" sign. This sign represents the surrounding skin findings of a contact dermatitis caused by the frequent use of bandages to cover the pyogenic granuloma due to its propensity to bleed, sometimes profusely. Pyogenic granulomas are more common during pregnancy and can be seen on the gingival mucosa. The most frequent oral location of involvement is the gingival mucosa. They rarely resolve spontaneously. The differential diagnosis is usually between pyogenic granuloma and other vascular-appearing tumors including metastatic carcinoma, particularly renal cell carcinoma, bacillary angiomatosis, and amelanotic melanoma. Pyogenic granulomas are almost always removed and the diagnosis is confirmed by histopathologic evaluation.

Pathogenesis: Pyogenic granulomas are thought to arise after trauma or secondary to medications and to be caused by a hyperplastic proliferation of vascular tissue. Chronic localized trauma can cause the release of vascular growth factors that may induce the proliferation. Pyogenic granulomas have not been shown to have any genetic inheritance pattern and are considered to be sporadic. The exact mechanism of formation is not well understood. The fact that they are more commonly seen in pregnancy suggests that certain hormonal regulations play a role in the formation of these tumors.

Histology: Pyogenic granulomas are also known as lobular capillary hemangiomas. This is an excellent descriptive name. The lesion is an exophytic growth that has a lobular configuration to its growth pattern. The tumor is typically well circumscribed and

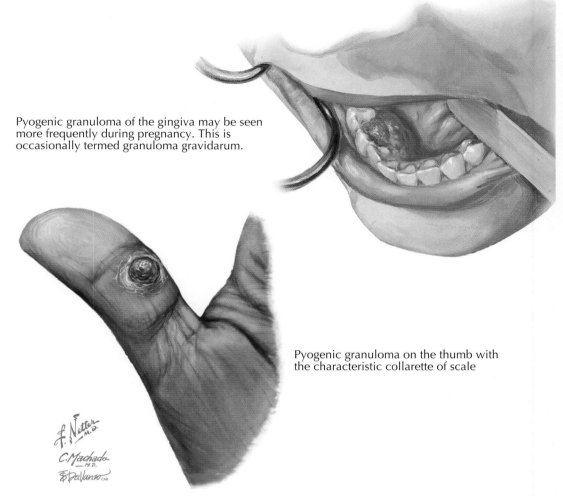

Pyogenic granuloma of the gingiva may be seen more frequently during pregnancy. This is occasionally termed granuloma gravidarum.

Pyogenic granuloma on the thumb with the characteristic collarette of scale

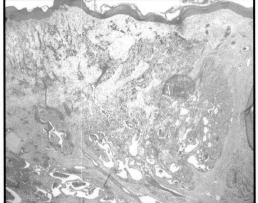

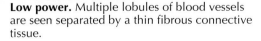

Low power. Multiple lobules of blood vessels are seen separated by a thin fibrous connective tissue.

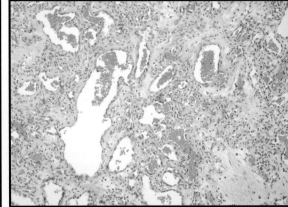

High power. Proliferation of capillary vessels is prominent in the center of the tumor lobules.

surrounded by a collarette of hyperplastic epithelium. Multiple capillary loops are found within each of the tumor lobules. Strands of fibrous tissue divide the tumor into individual lobules of varying size. Many of these lesions show evidence of surface ulceration resulting from thinning of the overlying epidermis. The cells involved are bland appearing.

Treatment: Most pyogenic granulomas resolve after shave removal and curettage with cautery of the base of the lesion. These tumors do have a propensity to recur, and occasionally an elliptical excision is required for removal. Application of silver nitrate and laser ablation with the pulsed dye laser have been used successfully. If the pyogenic granulomas are drug induced, stopping the offending medication is sometimes effective in resolving them. However, many cases of medication-induced pyogenic granulomas require some method of surgical removal.

Plate 2-35

Integumentary System

RETICULOHISTIOCYTOMA

Reticulohistiocytomas, also called solitary epithelioid histiocytomas, are conglomerations of large eosinophilic histiocytes within the dermis. The cytoplasm of these cells has been described as "glassy" in appearance. Reticulohistiocytomas are a subset of the histiocytoses group of diseases. In contrast to the other histiocytoses, patients with reticulohistiocytoma have normal lipid levels.

Reticulohistiocytomas can occur as a solitary growth or as multiple growths in a condition known as multicentric reticulohistiocytosis. The solitary variant is more often seen. On histopathological examination, the two clinical variants are identical in nature. Multicentric reticulohistiocytosis is a rare disease with systemic involvement. It can often be a marker of internal malignancy, and patients are afflicted with a severe arthritis.

Clinical Findings: Solitary lesions are typically small, firm dermal nodules ranging from 1 to 2 cm in diameter. They are usually asymptomatic. Their coloration may vary, but most often they are slightly pink to red-brown. They are found most commonly on the head and neck region of the body but have been described in all locations. They occur with similar frequency in males and females and have no age or race predilection.

Multicentric reticulohistiocytosis is unique in that it occurs in an older population, with a higher percentage of females affected. The number of lesions is in the hundreds to thousands. The multiple reticulohistiocytomas found in this condition are most often localized to the dorsal aspect of the hands and to the face. A distinctive finding is that of small papules along the lateral and proximal nail folds. This finding has been described as "coral beading," and it is highly specific for multicentric reticulohistiocytosis. These patients also have a severe arthropathy, and this diagnosis should lead one to look for an underlying malignancy. The arthropathy almost always affects the interphalangeal joints, particularly the distal interphalangeal joints. Multicentric reticulohistiocytosis is believed to be a paraneoplastic condition in up to 25% of the cases. The type of malignancy is variable, with no predominant type more prevalent than any other. For this reason, age-appropriate cancer screening is recommended. In about one third of patients with multicentric reticulohistiocytosis, the joint symptoms precede the growths; in one third, they appear at the same time; and one third of the patients develop only clinically minor or no arthropathy. This arthropathy is a severe inflammatory arthropathy that is symmetric and polyarticular. A mutilating arthritis may develop, sometimes very quickly. Early recognition and treatment has helped decrease the progression into severe mutilating arthritis. This truly is a multisystem organ disease. Many patients have cardiac involvement, and almost all organ systems have been reported to be affected, some with fatal outcomes.

Pathogenesis: Multicentric reticulohistiocytosis and solitary reticulohistiocytoma are believed to represent a rare disorder of histiocytes. The cause of the histiocytic proliferation is unknown.

Histology: The tumor shows a well-circumscribed dermal infiltrate without a capsule. The infiltrate is made up almost entirely of histiocytes with a "ground-glass"

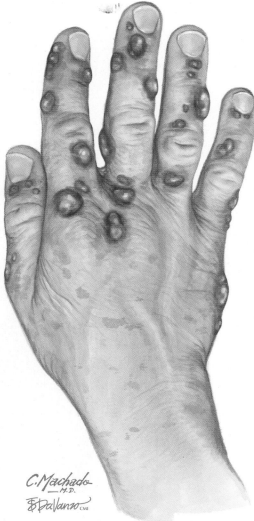

Multicentric reticulohistiocytomas. Coral red papules on the fingers. Can be associated with severe disabling arthritis.

Organs Involved in Reticulohistiocytoma
▶ Inflammatory arthritis (hands, knees, shoulders) ▶ Lungs ▶ Bone marrow ▶ Eyes ▶ Heart

Associated Autoimmune Diseases and Malignancy	
▶ Systemic lupus erythematosus	▶ Lymphoma
▶ Breast cancer	▶ Lung cancer
▶ Colon cancer	
▶ Primary biliary cirrhosis	

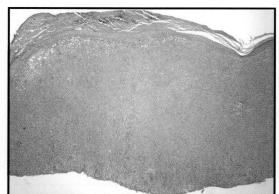

Low power. A diffuse dermal infiltrate of "ground-glass" histiocytes

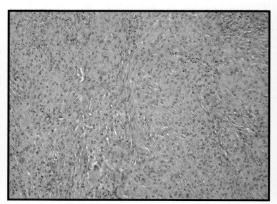

High power. A few multinucleated giant cells are seen within the tumor.

appearance of the cytoplasm. Multinucleate giant cells are always seen. They contain more than three nuclei, which can be arranged in many variations. The cells stain with the immunohistochemical stains CD45 and CD68, but do not stain with S100. On electron microscopy, no Langerhans cells are found in the infiltrate.

Treatment: Solitary reticulohistiocytomas are cured with a simple elliptical excision. They rarely recur.

Patients with multicentric reticulohistiocytosis require systemic therapy. Screening and constant vigilance for an underlying malignancy is required in all cases. Corticosteroids, methotrexate, hydroxychloroquine, and cyclophosphamide have all been used. Anti–tumor necrosis factor (anti-TNF) agents have been used. The goals are to prevent or suppress the arthropathy and to screen for malignancy.

Plate 2-36

Benign Growths

SEBORRHEIC KERATOSIS

One of the most commonly encountered of all benign skin growths is the seborrheic keratosis. These growths come in all sizes and shapes and invariably can be found on any human older than 40 years of age. They commonly begin in the fourth decade of life and tend to increase in number over one's lifetime. They have no malignant potential but are often brought to the attention of physicians because they can mimic other skin growths, most importantly malignant melanoma.

Clinical Findings: Seborrheic keratoses are found equally in males and females, and they are seen in all races. They begin to manifest in the third to fifth decade of life and continue to increase in number thereafter. They come in various sizes and shapes. Some are quite small, whereas others can be 5 to 6 cm in diameter. They occur almost exclusively in sun-exposed regions of the body. The classic description is that of a 1- to 2-cm plaque with a "stuck-on" appearance and small horn cysts. Most commonly flesh colored, they can also be tan, brown, or almost black. It is for this reason that they are occasionally mistaken for melanoma. Most individuals have a few scattered keratoses, but not infrequently a patient has thousands of these skin growths.

Many clinical variants of seborrheic keratosis can be seen. Stucco keratoses are small (1-5 mm), gray-tan papules with a stuck-on appearance or thin patches on the lower extremities. Dermatosis papulosis is a condition in which multiple seborrheic keratoses occur on the face and neck. This condition has a definite inheritance pattern.

Some seborrheic keratoses are smooth surfaced, but more commonly they have a pebbly or dry, rough surface. They have a characteristic stuck-on appearance, and in some instances they are easily removed by gently peeling from one side. These growths can easily become irritated or inflamed. The resulting pain, itching, or bleeding often brings the patient to medical treatment.

The sign of Leser-Trélat is the rapid onset of multiple seborrheic keratoses associated with an underlying internal malignancy. This sign has not been validated and is not a reliable indicator of an internal malignancy.

Histology: There is a well-circumscribed proliferation of keratinocytes. They have an exophytic growth pattern. The keratinocytes show acanthosis and hyperkeratosis. Marked papillomatosis is also commonly encountered. Two types of cysts are seen within the seborrheic keratosis. The horn cyst develops within the epidermis and is made of a keratin-filled cystic space with a surrounding granular cell layer. A pseudo-horn cyst is formed by an invagination of the stratum corneum into the underlying epidermis. Multiple histological subtypes have been described.

Pathogenesis: The formation of this benign epidermal tumor is not fully understood. It is caused by a proliferation of keratinocytes within the epidermis. The location in sun-exposed skin and the increasing number of lesions with increasing age has led some to believe that they are caused by a local suppression of the immune system that results in the epidermal proliferations. A definitive inheritance pattern has not been discovered, but these keratoses show some genetic predisposition. Chromosomal analysis of these tumors has not revealed any chromosomal defects. A link with the

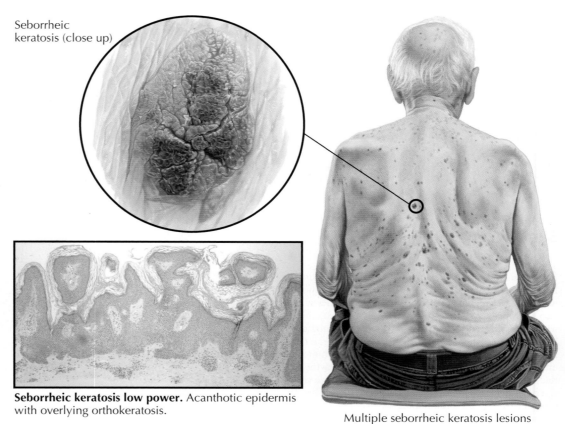

Seborrheic keratosis (close up)

Seborrheic keratosis low power. Acanthotic epidermis with overlying orthokeratosis.

Multiple seborrheic keratosis lesions

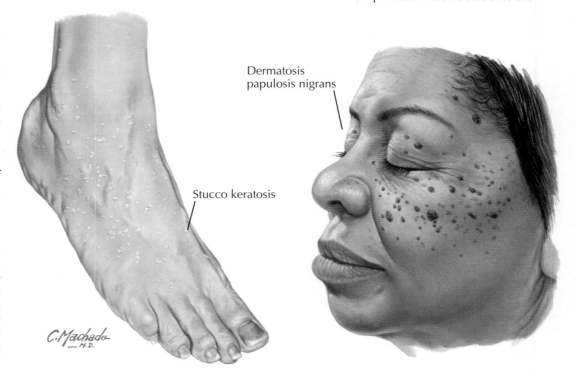

Dermatosis papulosis nigrans

Stucco keratosis

human papillomavirus has been proposed but has yet to be proven.

Treatment: These keratoses require no therapy. If they become inflamed or irritated, a simple shave biopsy removal is curative. Cryotherapy and curettage are often used to treat these benign skin growths, and both are extremely effective. After cryotherapy treatment, a blister usually forms at the base of the seborrheic keratosis, and within a day or two the keratosis falls off.

Another extremely effective method of removal that can be done in the office is cryotherapy followed by a light curettage; this also allows for histological evaluation. Occasionally, dark brown or black seborrheic keratoses can mimic melanoma, and in other cases a melanoma may arise adjacent to a seborrheic keratosis and mislead the clinician. If there is ever a doubt that the growth could be a melanoma, a biopsy is required. This allows for pathological confirmation of the diagnosis.

Plate 2-37

Integumentary System

SPITZ NEVUS

Spitz nevi are acquired nevi that occur most commonly in children. The classic Spitz nevus is a benign growth with minimal malignant potential. The Spitz nevus is also known as a spindle-cell nevus. In the past, they were also referred to as "benign juvenile melanoma," but that name should be avoided, because the term *melanoma* should be used to describe malignant tumors only. The difficulty with these melanocytic growths is that they do not always have the classic appearance and can be difficult to differentiate from melanoma. This is especially true in the adult population, where Spitz nevi are uncommon. For this reason, the terms *atypical Spitzoid melanocytic lesion, atypical Spitz nevus,* and *Spitzoid tumor of undetermined potential* have made their way into the dermatology lexicon to describe these difficult-to-classify cases.

Clinical Findings: The classic Spitz nevus occurs in childhood and has a characteristic reddish-brown color. It has even coloration and regular borders. It is typically dome shaped and smooth. It occurs equally in boys and girls and is more commonly found in the Caucasian population. The most common location has been reported to be the lower limb. The size is variable, but they are usually 5 to 10 mm in diameter. Spitz nevi are almost always solitary, but multiple Spitz nevi in an agminated pattern have been described. The clinical differential diagnosis of a Spitz nevus includes the common acquired nevus, pilomatricoma, dermatofibroma, adnexal tumors, and juvenile xanthogranuloma. Most Spitz nevi are asymptomatic and are brought to the clinician's attention as an incidental finding. Classic Spitz nevi rarely, if ever, spontaneously bleed or change in color.

Pathogenesis: The Spitz nevus is a melanocytic lesion derived from spindle-shaped or epithelioid melanocytes. The initiating factor or factors that cause this melanocytic proliferation to arise are unknown. They are unique melanocytic lesions, and their pathogenesis is likely to be entirely different from that of congenital melanocytic or common acquired melanocytic nevi.

Histology: The classic Spitz nevus is symmetrically shaped, without shouldering. It shows the proper benign maturation of melanocytes from top to bottom of the lesion. The melanocytes do not show pagetoid spread (single melanocytes) within the epidermis. Spitz nevi melanocytes in general have a spindle shape or epithelioid morphology. Another helpful finding is the presence of eosinophilic Kamino bodies. These can be either solitary or coalescing into large globules. Kamino bodies are found in juxtaposition to the basement membrane zone and are composed of elements of the basement membrane, specifically type IV collagen. There is

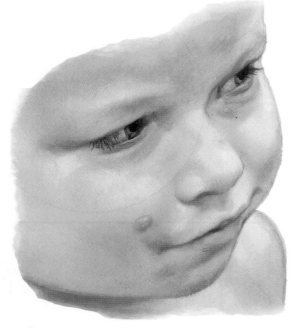

Solitary Spitz nevus. Reddish-brown dermal papule

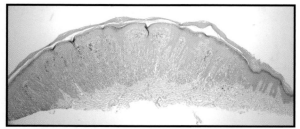

Low power. Symmetric melanocytic tumor, with maturation of the melanocytes

Agminated Spitz nevi

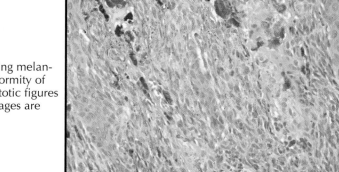

High power. Bland-appearing melanocytes predominate. A uniformity of cell size is seen, and no mitotic figures are appreciated. Melanophages are present.

no immunohistochemical stain that can definitively differentiate a Spitz nevus from melanoma. As alluded to earlier, the classic Spitz nevus is usually a straightforward diagnosis. However, many difficult-to-classify melanocytic lesions have overlapping features of Spitz nevus and melanoma and can be exceedingly challenging diagnostically.

Treatment: Complete excision for a classic Spitz nevus is curative and allows for a complete histological evaluation. Indeterminate lesions should be reexcised with conservative margins to make sure they have been completely removed. Spitz nevi in adults should all be excised to allow for complete histopathological examination. Unclassifiable or difficult to classify melanocytic tumors with features of both Spitz nevus and melanoma are best treated as if they were melanoma. The Breslow depth should be used to plan for appropriate therapy.

MALIGNANT GROWTHS

Plate 3-1

Integumentary System

ADNEXAL CARCINOMA

Adnexal carcinomas are a diverse group of malignant skin tumors that are derived from the various components of the skin appendageal structures. These tumors are extremely rare and comprise well less than 1% of all skin cancers diagnosed annually. They are difficult to diagnosis clinically because they can all mimic the more common types of skin cancer, particularly basal cell carcinoma and squamous cell carcinoma. They can be diagnosed with certainty only after histological examination. These tumors are believed to be derived from hair follicle, sebaceous gland, apocrine gland, or eccrine gland epithelium. They are thought to arise de novo and can also arise from a preexisting benign precursor. An example is an eccrine porocarcinoma developing within an eccrine poroma.

Clinical Findings: These tumors are very rare, and one is unlikely to consider them in the differential diagnosis when evaluating an individual with an undiagnosed skin growth. There are few clues to their origin, which makes diagnosis of these cancerous tumors almost impossible based on clinical findings alone. Most manifest as a solitary papule, plaque, or dermal nodule. Most are asymptomatic, but pruritus, bleeding, and pain may be present.

The diagnosis of these tumors requires tissue sampling. A punch or excisional biopsy is the best method to biopsy these lesions, because it allows the pathologist to get a large enough piece of tissue to evaluate. A punch biopsy is especially important to help differentiate microcystic adnexal carcinoma from a benign syringoma. The latter is very superficial in nature, whereas the microcystic adnexal carcinoma displays a deep infiltrative growth pattern that will not be appreciated with a superficial shave biopsy.

Pathogenesis: The pathogenesis of these tumors is poorly understood. In contrast to basal and squamous cell carcinomas, they are unlikely to be caused by ultraviolet light exposure. The rarity of the tumors makes them difficult to study. There appears to be no genetic inheritance to these malignant tumors, with the lone exception of the sebaceous carcinoma. Sebaceous carcinoma can be seen in the Muir-Torre syndrome, which is inherited in an autosomal dominant pattern.

Histology: Each tumor is unique histologically. The tumors can be subdivided according to the type of epithelium from which they are derived: sebaceous, hair follicle, eccrine, or apocrine. The pathologist is able to differentiate these tumors based on certain criteria. The tumors show varying amounts of cellular atypia and an invasive growth pattern. They are usually poorly circumscribed with varying amounts of mitotic figures, necrosis, and abnormal-appearing cells. Various gland-like structures can be seen in some tumors, which can be helpful in making the diagnosis. Often, special immunohistochemical stains are used to help differentiate the subtypes of these tumors.

Treatment: These tumors should all be surgically excised with clear surgical margins. The Mohs surgical technique has been used successfully to treat these tumors, as has a standard wide local excision. Sentinel node removal and evaluation is not routinely performed, but some clinicians advocate its use, especially

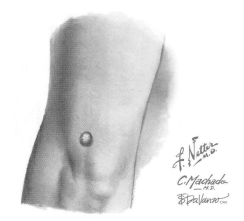

Eccrine porocarcinoma. Nondescript red papule or nodule. Ulceration may occur. A biopsy is required to diagnose this rare form of skin cancer.

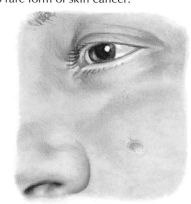

Microcystic adnexal carcinoma. Small plaque on cheek. Slow-growing tumor that can become quite large by the time of diagnosis

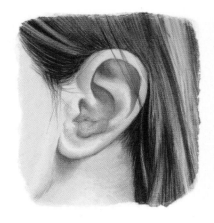

Spiradenocarcinoma, presenting as a plaque on the ear. Adnexal tumors are rare, and a biopsy for histological evaluation is required for diagnosis.

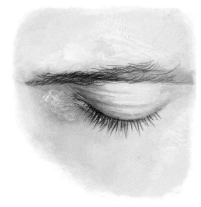

Sebaceous carcinoma. Yellowish patch often located around the eye, in this case near the medial canthus. These tumors may be seen in association with the Muir-Torre syndrome.

Cutaneous Adnexal Tumors	
Apocrine gland derived	**Eccrine gland derived**
Adenocarcinoma of Moll's glands Apocrine carcinoma Ceruminous adenocarcinoma Cribriform apocrine carcinoma Extramammary Paget's disease	Adenoid cystic carcinoma Aggressive digital papillary adenocarcinoma Clear cell eccrine carcinoma Hidradenocarcinoma Eccrine ductal adenocarcinoma Eccrine porocarcinoma Malignant chondroid syringoma Malignant cylindroma Malignant eccrine spiradenoma Microcystic adnexal carcinoma Mucinous adenocystic carcinoma Mucoepidermoid carcinoma Polymorphous sweat gland carcinoma Signet-ring cell carcinoma of the eyelid Syringoadenocarcinoma papilliferum Syringoid eccrine carcinoma
Hair follicle derived	
Malignant proliferating trichilemmal tumor Pilomatrix carcinoma Trichilemmal carcinoma Trichoblastic carcinoma	
Sebaceous gland derived	
Sebaceous carcinoma	

in some of the more aggressive subtypes such as the eccrine porocarcinoma. Sentinel node removal and evaluation has not shown any survival benefit to date. Mohs surgery may lead to a decrease in recurrence rate and is tissue sparing. Because of the rare nature of these tumors and the lack of prospective randomized studies, it is difficult to determine the best removal method. For the same reasons, the ultimate prognosis and the

recurrence rate of these tumors are unknown. After diagnosis and removal of these tumors, the patient should have long-term follow-up to evaluate for recurrence.

Adnexal tumors that have metastasized are treated with chemotherapy with or without radiotherapy. The prognosis is poor for patients who develop metastatic adnexal carcinoma.

Plate 3-2

Malignant Growths

ANGIOSARCOMA

Angiosarcoma is a rare, aggressive, malignant tumor of vascular or lymphatic vessels. These tumors can be seen as a solitary finding or secondary to long-standing lymphedema, such as after radiation therapy or an axillary or inguinal lymph node dissection. This latter form tends to occur years after the radiation or surgical procedure. Soft tissue sarcomas are very rare and make up a small percentage of all malignancies reported.

Clinical Findings: Angiosarcomas are most common in the older male population. They have no race predilection. The tumors most commonly arise in the head and neck region and can manifest in many fashions. They often appear as a red to purple plaque with ill-defined borders. They can often look like a bruise, and the diagnosis can be delayed. The tumor continues to expand, forms satellite foci of involvement, and eventually ulcerates and bleeds. For some reason, the scalp and face of older men are most commonly involved. The tumor has a propensity to involve sun-exposed areas of the face and scalp. The tumors typically show an aggressive growth pattern and have a tendency to metastasize early in the course of disease.

Angiosarcomas can also arise in regions of previous long-standing lymphedema caused by radiation exposure or surgical procedures. Any procedure that can result in abnormal lymphatic drainage can lead to chronic lymphedema. It is believed that long-standing lymphedema can result in the development of angiosarcoma. Common surgical procedures that cause chronic lymphedema are radical mastectomies and lymph node dissections of the axilla or groin after a diagnosis of lymph node involvement by breast cancer or melanoma. Angiosarcomas arising in areas of chronic lymphedema were first described by Stewart and Treves and have been given the eponym *Stewart-Treves syndrome.* This type of angiosarcoma is highly aggressive and portends a poor outcome. The Stewart-Treves type of angiosarcoma has been reported most commonly in women who have undergone radical mastectomy or lymph node dissection for treatment of breast cancer. After years of chronic lymphedema in the ipsilateral limb, the patient may develop a reddish, bruise-like area on the limb. This area slowly enlarges and develops plaque-like areas or nodules within the affected region. At this point, the diagnosis is often entertained, and the diagnosis is made with a skin biopsy. These tumors tend to be large at diagnosis, which most likely accounts for the poor prognosis.

Radiation-induced angiosarcomas may occur at the site of the radiation therapy or as a result of long-standing chronic lymphedema if the radiation therapy interrupts the lymphatic drainage. These tumors also tend to be diagnosed after they have become quite large, and this portends a poor prognosis. These tumors tend to occur 4 to 10 years after the initial radiation therapy.

Pathogenesis: Angiosarcomas are soft tissue tumors that are derived from the endothelial lining of small blood or lymphatic vessels. Some tumors are found to have elevated levels of vascular endothelial growth factor (VEGF), which is critical in the regulation of vessel growth. Other potential players in the pathogenesis of this tumor are mast cells, which cause an increase in stem cell factor; Fas and Fas ligand expression; and lack of the vascular endothelial cadherin protein. All of these factors may interact in an unknown way to induce tumorigenesis. The exact mechanism of formation of angiosarcoma is unknown. Radiation-induced angiosarcoma may result from a direct mutagenic effect of the

Stewart-Treves syndrome. Plaque on chronic edematous arm. The chronic lymphedema is secondary to prior mastectomy and axillary lymph node dissection.

Angiosarcoma arising from the scalp of a 65-year-old man. Red indurated plaque with a central crust due to underlying ulceration of the tumor. These tumors can be very aggressive.

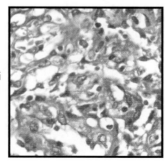

Hemangiopericytoma. Eccentric hyperchromatic nuclei of pericytic cells surrounding vascular spaces. (H&E stain)

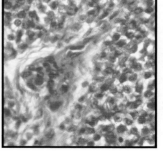

Hemangioendothelioma. Central hyperplastic capillary surrounded by malignant endothelial cells. (H&E stain)

radiation on the endothelial DNA. No relation with human herpesvirus-8 infection has been proven.

Histology: All angiosarcomas share the same pathological features. The tumor lobules are poorly circumscribed and have an infiltrative growth pattern. They contain large amounts of vascular tissue in a disorganized arrangement. The lining of the vascular spaces contains atypical-appearing endothelial cells. Mitoses are frequently encountered, as are intracytoplasmic lumina. The same tumor can contain well and poorly differentiated regions.

Treatment: The standard treatment is wide local excision with the goal of obtaining clear margins. This is usually followed by postoperative radiation therapy. The 5-year survival rate is low (15%-20%). Tumors that are metastatic or nonoperable can be treated palliatively with various chemotherapeutic regimens. The median survival time in these cases is 3 to 6 months.

Plate 3-3   Integumentary System

BASAL CELL CARCINOMA

Basal cell carcinoma (BCC) is the most common malignancy in humans. Its true incidence is unknown, but the number of BCCs diagnosed each year easily surpasses the number of all other malignancies combined. It is estimated to affect approximately 25% to 33% of the U.S. Caucasian population over their lifetimes. The yearly number of BCCs diagnosed is quickly approaching 1 million. BCC rarely metastasizes or causes mortality. The real crisis it presents is in the significant morbidity and cost to the health care system. The vast majority of these lesions are located on the head and neck region and are of considerable cosmetic concern. The major morbidity involved is the significant disfigurement that these locally invading tumors can inflict.

Clinical Findings: The prototypical BCC is described as a pearly red papule with telangiectasias that has a rolled border and a central dell or ulceration. They occur with highest frequency in sun-exposed areas of the skin. Most BCCs start as a small red macule or papule and slowly enlarge over months to years. Once this occurs, the tumor may be friable and may bleed easily with superficial trauma. The tumors most commonly range in size from 1 mm to 1 cm. However, neglected tumors can be enormous and have been reported to cover areas up to 60 cm² or more. They affect males and females with equal frequency. BCCs are more common in individuals with Fitzpatrick type I skin and decrease in frequency as one moves across the skin type spectrum. Fitzpatrick type VI skin has the lowest incidence of BCC, but these individuals still can develop these tumors. BCCs occur with an increasing frequency with age. They are uncommon in childhood, with the exception of the association of childhood BCCs with the nevoid BCC syndrome (also called basal cell nevus syndrome or Gorlin's syndrome).

The tumors are most likely to occur (>80%) on the head and neck region. The trunk is the next most common area. The vermilion border, the palms and soles, and the glans theoretically should not develop BCCs because these areas are devoid of hair; however, they can be affected by direct extension from a neighboring tumor. These tumors rarely metastasize, and those that do are most often neglected large tumors or tumors in immunosuppressed patients. BCC most commonly metastasizes to regional lymph nodes and the lung.

Many clinical variants of BCC exist, including superficial, pigmented, nodular, and sclerotic or morpheaform variants. There are many other histological variants. Clinically, a superficial BCC manifests as a very slowly enlarging, pink or red patch without elevation or ulceration. If left alone for a long enough period, it will develop areas of nodularity or ulceration. Nodular BCCs are probably the most common variant; they manifest as the classic pearly papule with telangiectasias and central ulceration. The pigmented variant can mimic melanoma and is often described as a brown or black papule or plaque with or without ulceration. Early on, these types of BCCs can appear as pearly papules or plaques with minute flecks of brown or black pigmentation. Patients with the sclerotic or morpheaform version often have larger tumors at presentation because of their slow, inconspicuous growth pattern. These slow-growing tumors are almost skin colored and have ill-defined borders. They tend not to ulcerate until they have become large, and this often delays the seeking of

medical advice. These tumors can mimic the appearance of scar tissue, which can also hinder making the diagnosis. Eventually, the tumor enlarges enough to cause ulceration or superficial erosions, and the diagnosis is made. The sclerotic BCC is often much larger than the other variant types at the time of diagnosis.

The most important genetic syndrome associated with the development of BCCs is the nevoid BCC

Basic Facial Anatomy

- Epicranial aponeurosis (galea aponeurotica)
- Frontal belly (frontalis) of epicranius muscle
- Procerus muscle
- Corrugator supercilii muscle
- Orbital part
- Palpebral part } of orbicularis oculi muscle
- Levator labii superioris muscle
- Transverse part
- Alar part } of nasalis muscle
- Levator labii superioris muscle
- Auricularis anterior muscle
- Zygomaticus minor muscle
- Zygomaticus major muscle
- Levator anguli oris muscle
- Depressor septi nasi muscle
- Buccinator muscle
- Risorius muscle
- Orbicularis oris muscle
- Depressor anguli oris muscle
- Depressor labii inferioris muscle
- Platysma muscle
- Mentalis muscle

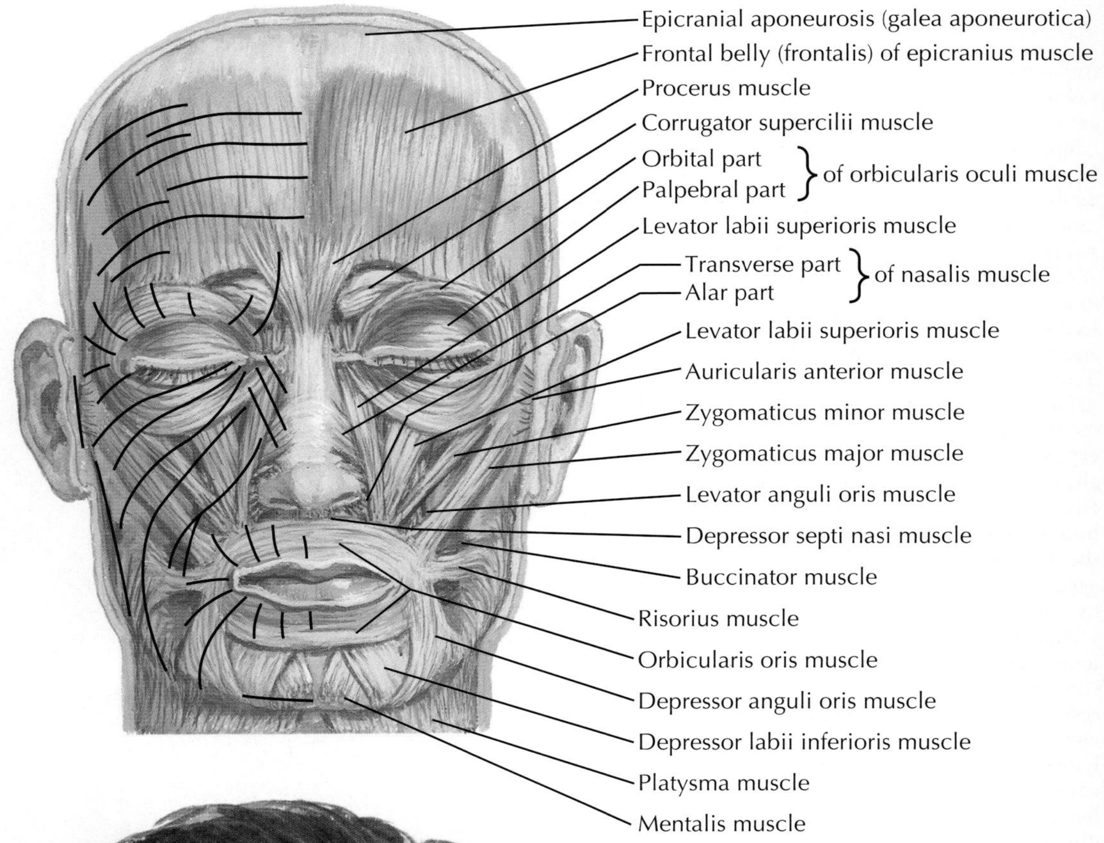

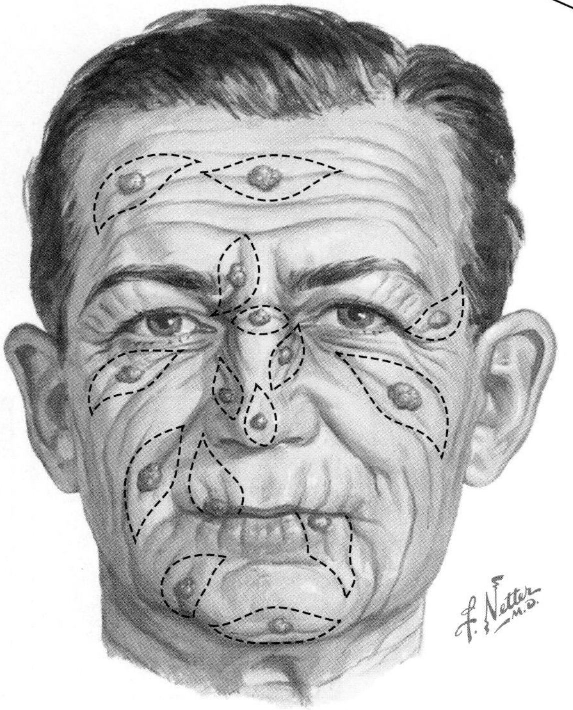

Course of wrinkle lines of skin is transverse to fiber direction of facial muscles. *Elliptical incisions* for removal of skin tumors conform to direction of wrinkle lines.

syndrome. This syndrome is inherited in an autosomal dominant fashion and is caused by a defect in the *patched 1* gene, *PTCH1*. This gene is located on chromosome 9q22. It encodes a tumor suppressor protein that plays a role in inhibition of the sonic hedgehog signaling pathway. A defect in the patched protein allows for uncontrolled signaling of the smoothened protein and an increase in various cell signaling pathways,

Plate 3-4

Malignant Growths

BASAL CELL CARCINOMA
(Continued)

ultimately culminating in the development of BCCs. Patients with nevoid BCC syndrome also may have odontogenic cysts of the jaw, palmar and plantar pitting, various bony abnormalities, and calcification of the falx cerebri. Frontal bossing, mental delay, and ovarian fibromas are only a few of the associated findings that can be seen in this syndrome.

Other rare syndromes in which BCCs can be seen include xeroderma pigmentosa, Bazek's syndrome, and Rombo syndrome.

Pathogenesis: Risk factors associated with the development of BCC include cumulative exposure to ultraviolet radiation and ionizing radiation. In the past, arsenic exposure was a well-recognized cause of BCCs, and arsenic pollution is still a concern in some areas of the world. Since the advent of organ transplantation, there has been an increase in the development of skin cancers in immunosuppressed organ recipients. The incidences of BCC, squamous cell carcinoma, and melanoma are all increased in these chronically immunosuppressed patients. Mutations of various genes have also been implicated in the pathogenesis of BCCs, including *PTCH1, p53 (TP53), sonic hedgehog (SHH), smoothened (SMO),* and the *glioma-associated oncogene homolog 1 (GLI1).* However, it is still believed that most BCCs are sporadic in nature.

The greatest amount of information is known about the pathogenesis of BCC in the nevoid BCC syndrome. The genetic defect in the *PTCH1* gene allows for uncontrolled signaling of the smoothened signaling pathway. This pathway initiates uncontrolled signaling of the *GLI1* transcription factors, which ultimately leads to uncontrolled cell proliferation.

Histology: Many histological subtypes have been described, and a tumor can show evidence of more than one subtype. The most common subtypes are the nodular and superficial types. These tumors arise from the basaloid cells of the follicular epithelium. The tumor always shows an attachment to the overlying epidermis. The tumor extends off the epidermis as tumor lobules. These lobules are basophilic in nature and show clefting between the basophilic cells and the surrounding stroma. The cells have a characteristic peripheral palisading appearance. The cells in the center of the tumor lobules are disorganized. The ratio of nuclear to cytoplasmic volume in the tumor cells is greatly increased. Mitoses are present, and larger tumors usually have some evidence of overlying epidermal ulceration. The tumor is contiguous and does not show skip areas. The nodular form of this tumor extends into the dermis to varying degrees, and its depth of penetration is dependent on the length of time it has been present.

The superficial type is also quite common. The tumor does not extend into the underlying dermis but appears to be hanging off the bottom edge of the epidermis. It has not yet penetrated the dermal-epidermal barrier. There are numerous other histological subtypes of BCC including micronodular, adenoid, cystic, pigmented, infiltrative, and sclerosing varieties.

Treatment: Various surgical and medical options are available, and the therapy should be based on the location and size of the tumor and the wishes of the patient. Tumors on the face are most often treated with Mohs micrographic surgery. This surgical technique allows

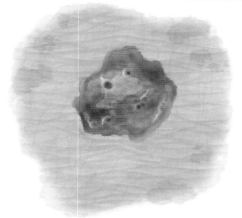

Superficial basal cell carcinoma. Slightly scaly pink to red patch. These tumors are slow growing and occur on chronically sun-exposed skin.

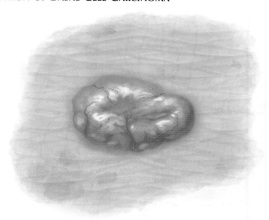

Nodular basal cell carcinoma. Pearly plaque with telangiectatic central ulceration, and rolled border

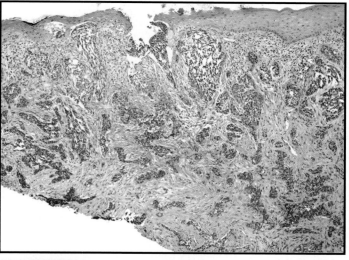

Basophilic tumor lobules and strands extending from the epidermis into the dermis

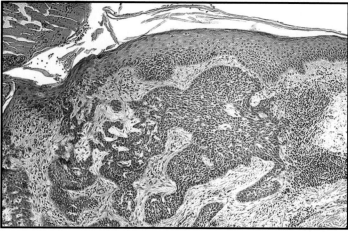

Basophilic tumor lobules within the dermis showing slight retraction artifact and peripheral palisading

for the highest cure rate and is tissue sparing, resulting in the smallest possible scar. It is more labor intensive than a routine elliptical excision. Most BCCs can be treated with an elliptical excision or electrodessication and curettage.

Medical therapy with imiquimod or 5-fluorouracil has also been shown to be useful in selected BCCs, usually the small, superficial type. One of the newest treatments is photodynamic therapy. It is performed by applying aminolevulinic acid to the skin tumor and then exposing the area to visible blue light. An oral inhibitor of the smoothened protein, called GDC-0449, has shown excellent results in patients with the nevoid BCC syndrome.

Plate 3-5

Integumentary System

BOWEN'S DISEASE

Bowen's disease is a variant of cutaneous squamous cell carcinoma (SCC) in situ that occurs on non–sun-exposed regions of the body. That strict definition is not always followed, and the term *Bowen's disease* is often used interchangeably with *squamous cell carcinoma in situ*. SCC in situ is often derived from its precursor lesion, the actinic keratosis. Actinic keratosis is differentiated from SCC in situ and Bowen's disease by its lack of full-thickness keratinocyte atypia, which is the hallmark of Bowen's disease and SCC in situ.

Clinical Findings: Bowen's disease can occur on hair-bearing and non–hair-bearing skin, and the clinical appearance in various locations can be entirely different. Bowen's disease on hair-bearing skin often starts as a pink to red, well-demarcated patch with adherent scale. Women are most commonly affected, and it occurs later in life. Multiple lesions can occur, but it is far more common to see this as a solitary finding. Erythroplasia of Queyrat is a regional variant of Bowen's disease that occurs on the glans penis. These lesions tend to be glistening red with crusting. The area is often well circumscribed. The diagnosis is often delayed because the lesion is easily confused with dermatitis, psoriasis, and cutaneous fungal infections. A biopsy should be performed on any nonhealing lesion or rash in the genital region. It has been estimated that up to 5% of untreated Bowen's disease lesions will eventually develop an invasive component.

The relationship between Bowen's disease and internal malignancy has come under scrutiny; if it exists at all, it is likely a consequence of the use of arsenic in the past. Patients with a history of arsenic ingestion are at a higher risk of developing Bowen's disease and internal malignancy. Now that arsenic exposure is limited in most developed countries, the association between Bowen's disease and internal malignancy is thought to be unlikely.

Most SCCs in situ are found on sun-exposed areas of the skin and develop directly from an adjacent actinic keratosis. Some SCCs in situ eventually develop into an invasive form of SCC. This is clinically evident by increased thickness, bleeding, and pain associated with the lesion.

Pathogenesis: Exposure to arsenic and other carcinogens has been implicated in the development of Bowen's disease. Certainly, ultraviolet radiation and other forms of radiation play a role in the its pathogenesis. Human papillomavirus (HPV) has been implicated in causing many forms of SCC. The oncogenic viral types 16, 18, 31, and 33 are notorious for causing mutagenesis and malignancy in cervical and some other genital SCCs. HPV vaccines may decrease the incidence of these tumors dramatically in the future. HPV can cause cellular transformations to occur and is directly responsible for tumorigenesis.

Histology: Bowen's disease shows full-thickness atypia of the keratinocytes within the epidermis. No dermal invasion is present. The underlying dermis may show a lymphocytic perivascular infiltrate. The atypia of the keratinocytes extends down to involve the hair

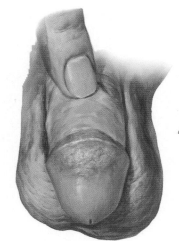

Erythroplasia of Queyrat

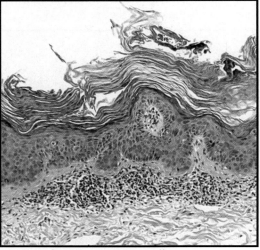

Bowen's disease (squamous cell carcinoma in situ) showing full-thickness atypia of the epidermal keratinocytes. Note that the tumor does not invade the dermis.

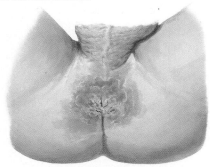

Perianal Bowen's disease can have an insidious onset and be misdiagnosed as tinea or dermatitis. Biopsy of any rash not responding to therapy should be a consideration for the treating clinician.

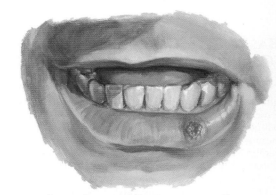

Early carcinoma of lip. Squamous cell carcinoma in situ is common on the lower lip.

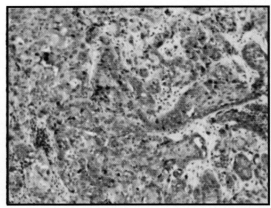

Squamous cell carcinoma. Tumor invading the dermis.

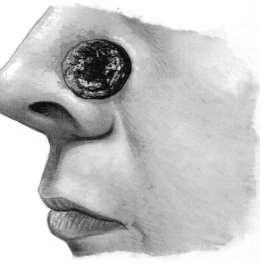

Large crateriform squamous cell carcinoma. These tumors can be locally invasive and destructive. On occasion they can also metastasize.

follicle epithelium, and care must be taken when evaluating these lesions histologically not to mistake this finding for dermal invasion. Various amounts of cellular atypia are present.

Treatment: Treatments can be divided into surgical and nonsurgical forms. The choice depends on various factors, most importantly the location and size of the lesion. Some tumors are best treated surgically, whereas others are best treated medically.

Simple excision or electrodessication and curettage are highly effective treatments. Cryotherapy is another destructive method that can be selectively used with good success. Medical therapies include the application of 5-fluorouracil, imiquimod, or 5-aminolevulinic acid followed by exposure to blue light. These all have been reported to be successful. The risk of recurrence is between 3% and 10% depending on the type of therapy used.

Plate 3-6

Malignant Growths

BOWENOID PAPULOSIS

Bowenoid papulosis is considered to be a special variant of squamous cell carcinoma (SCC) in situ that is caused by the human papillomavirus (HPV) and is located predominantly in the genital region, particularly on the penile shaft. As with other HPV-induced genital skin cancers, HPV 16, 18, 31, and 33 are the more common viral types, although many other subtypes have been found in these lesions. Bowenoid papulosis is considered by some to be a precancerous lesion with a low risk of developing invasive properties and by others as a true SCC in situ. This lesion does have a low risk of invasive transformation; if it is treated, the prognosis is excellent. It is believed that approximately 1% of all bowenoid papulosis lesions will develop into invasive SCC.

Clinical Findings: Bowenoid papulosis is most commonly found in men in the third through sixth decades of life. There is no racial preference. It is believed to be more common in patients who have had multiple sexual partners because of their increased risk for exposure to HPV. It is too soon to determine whether vaccination against HPV has resulted in any changes in the incidence of bowenoid papulosis. The lesions are most common in males on the shaft of the penis and in females on the vulva. They are typically well-circumscribed, slightly hyperpigmented macules and papules that occasionally coalesce into larger plaques. Minimal surface change is noted. They are often found in association with genital warts and can be difficult to distinguish from small genital warts. The cause of bowenoid papulosis is thought to be transformation of the keratinocyte caused by HPV, and therefore lesions of bowenoid shed HPV and are contagious.

The lesions are rarely symptomatic and are usually brought to a physician's attention because of the patient's concern for genital warts. For undefined reasons, circumcision appears to help prevent penile cancer. It has been theorized that the uncircumcised male is at higher risk for penile carcinoma because of retention of smegma and chronic maceration, which can provide a portal for HPV infection, in conjunction with chronic low-grade inflammation.

Pathogenesis: Almost all lesions of bowenoid papulosis have evidence of HPV. HPV subtype 16 is by far the most predominant HPV type found in bowenoid papulosis. Cells of the genital region that are chronically infected with HPV express various proteins that are critical in the transformation into cancer. The best-studied HPV oncoproteins, the E6 and E7 proteins, can disrupt normal cell signaling in the p16 (TP16) and retinoblastoma (RB) pathways. This disruption can lead to a loss of control of cell signaling and loss of normal apoptosis. These alterations eventually result in loss of the normal cell processes and the development of cancer.

Histology: The histology is almost the same as that of SCC in situ. There is full-thickness atypia of the epidermis with involvement of the adnexal structures and a well-intact basement membrane zone. Varying amounts of epidermal acanthosis and hyperkeratosis are seen. The cells are often enlarged and pleomorphic

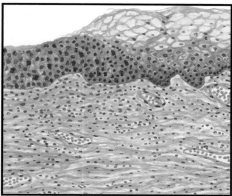

Cancer in situ showing oblique line of transition

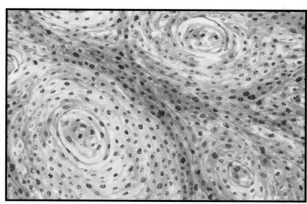

Squamous cell cancer showing pearl formation

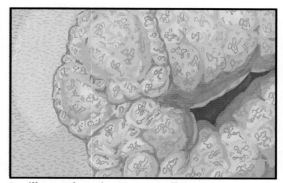

Papilloma of cervix. Some papillomas may predispose to cervical malignancy.

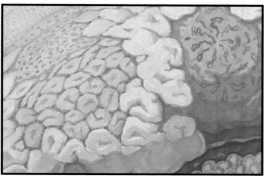

Changes suggestive of carcinoma in situ. Abnormal vasculature with leukoplakia, mosaicism, and punctation

Bowenoid papulosis. Slightly hyperpigmented papules on the shaft of the penis

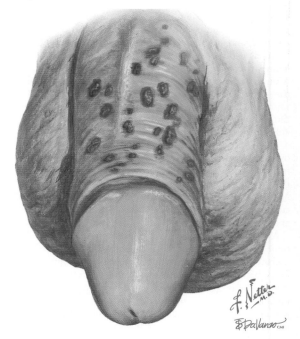

with visible mitoses. Evidence of HPV infection is almost universally seen as cells mimicking vacuolated koilocyte cells. Special techniques such as polymerase chain reaction (PCR) can be used to look for HPV subtyping.

Treatment: After biopsy has ruled out an invasive component to this tumor, the main treatment of bowenoid papulosis is to clinically remove the areas of involvement. The importance of decreasing HPV transmission to the patient's sexual partners must be addressed. Condoms should be used at all times to help decrease the risk of transmission. Topical therapy with 5-fluorouracil or imiquimod has been advocated as the first-line therapy. Surgical treatment with electrocautery, cryotherapy, or laser ablation has also been reported to be successful. Both patients and their sexual partners should be seen for routine follow-up examinations.

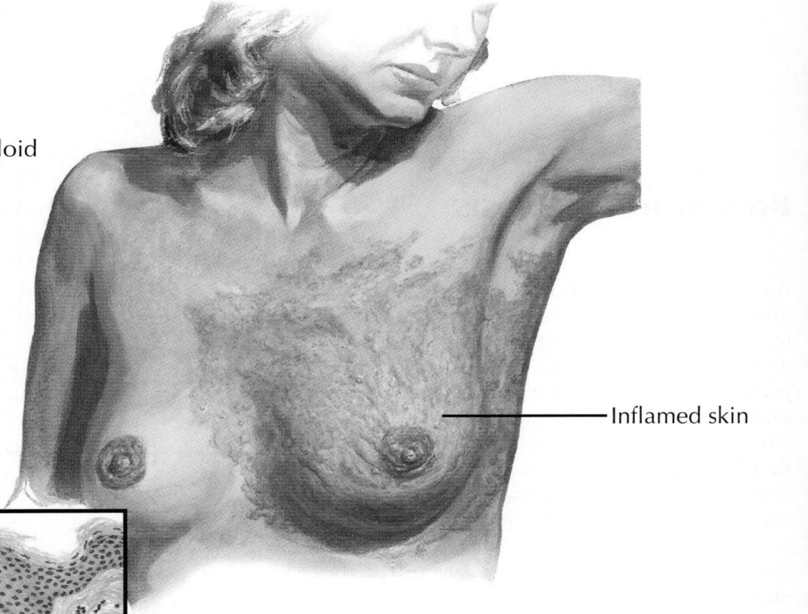

Plate 3-7

Integumentary System

CUTANEOUS METASTASES

Metastasis to the skin is an uncommon presentation of internal malignancy. Cutaneous metastases are far more likely to be seen in a patient with a diagnosis of previously metastatic disease. The frequency of cutaneous metastasis is dependent on the primary tumor. Almost all types of internal malignancy have been reported to metastasize to the skin; however, a few types of cancers account for the bulk of cutaneous metastases. The distribution of the metastases is also dependent on the original tumor. The most common form of skin metastasis is from an underlying, previously metastatic melanoma.

Clinical Findings: Most cutaneous metastases manifest as slowly enlarging, dermal nodules. They are almost always firm and have been shown to vary in coloration. Some nodules eventually develop necrosis, ulcerate, and spontaneously bleed. Skin metastasis can occur as a direct extension from an underlying malignancy or as a remote focus of tumor deposition. Although skin metastasis often arises in the vicinity of the underlying primary malignancy, the location of tumor metastases is not a reliable means of predicting the primary source. The scalp is a common site, probably because of its rich vascular flow.

Sister Mary Joseph nodule is a name given to a periumbilical skin metastasis from an underlying abdominal malignancy. This is a rare presentation that was first described by an astute nun at St. Mary's Hospital at the Mayo Clinic. This has been described to occur most commonly with ovarian carcinoma, gastric carcinoma, and colonic carcinoma.

Melanoma metastases are usually pigmented and tend to occur in groups. Cutaneous metastasis from melanoma can manifest with the rapid onset of multiple black papules and macules that continue to erupt. As the tumors progress, patients can develop a generalized melanosis. This is a universally fatal sign that occurs late in the course of disease. It is believed to be caused by the systemic production of melanin with deposition in the skin.

Breast carcinoma is another form of malignancy that frequently metastasizes to the skin. Breast carcinoma tends to affect the skin within the local region of the breast by direct extension.

Pathogenesis: The exact reason why some tumors metastasize to the skin is unknown. This is a complex biological process that is dependent on many variables. Metastases are likely to be dependent on size, ability to invade surrounding tissues (including blood and lymphatic vessels), and ability to grow at distant sites far removed from the original tumor. This is an intricate process that depends on the production of multiple growth factors and evasion of the patient's immune system.

Histology: The diagnosis of cutaneous metastasis is almost always made by the pathologist after histological review. Each tumor is unique, and the histological picture depends on the primary tumor.

Treatment: Solitary cutaneous metastases can be surgically excised. The risk of recurrence is high, and adjunctive chemotherapy and radiotherapy should be considered. Palliative surgical excision can be undertaken for any cutaneous metastases that are painful, ulcerated, or inhibiting the patient's ability to function. The prognosis for patients with cutaneous metastasis is poor. The overall survival rate for multiple cutaneous metastases has been reported to be 3 to 6 months. The length of survival is increasing now because of improved treatments.

Fulminant erysipeloid cancer from an underlying breast carcinoma

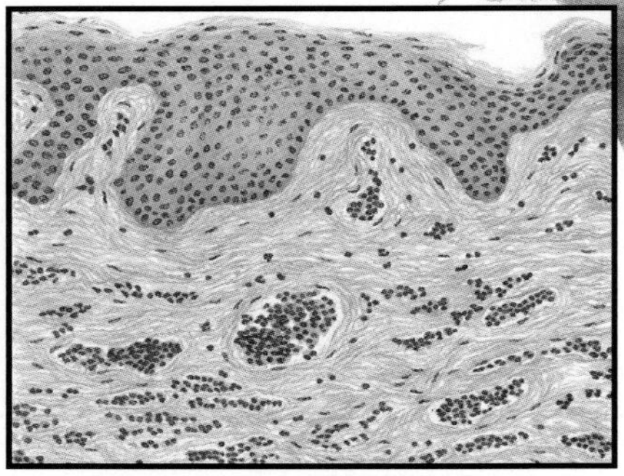

Inflamed skin

Invasion of dermal lymphatics and lining up of tumor cells between collagen bundles

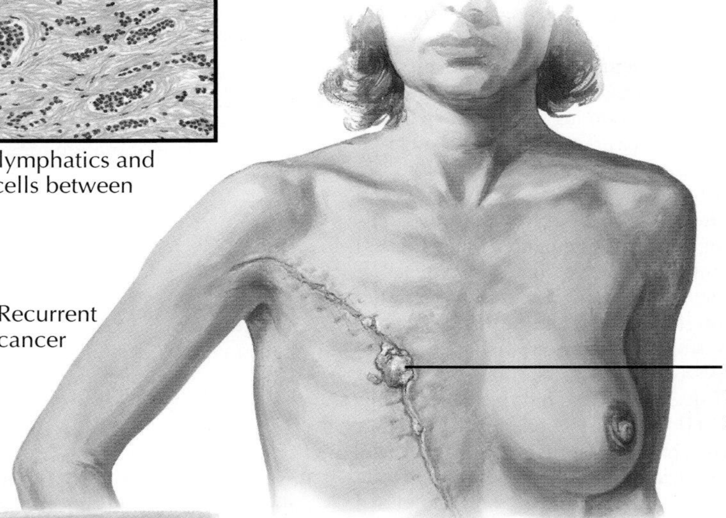

Recurrent cancer

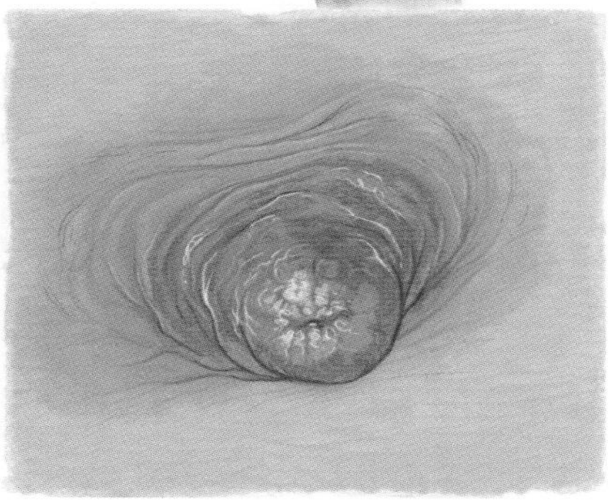

Carcinoma forming along surgical wound

Colonic adenocarcinoma metastatic to the flank

Plate 3-8

Malignant Growths

DERMATOFIBROSARCOMA PROTUBERANS

Dermatofibrosarcoma protuberans is a rare cutaneous malignancy that is locally aggressive. The tumor is derived from the dermal fibroblast, and it is not believed to arise from previously existing dermatofibromas. Dermatofibrosarcoma protuberans rarely metastasizes, but it has a distinctive tendency to recur locally.

Clinical Findings: Dermatofibrosarcoma protuberans is a slow-growing, locally aggressive malignancy of the skin. These tumors are low-grade sarcomas and make up approximately 1% of all soft tissue sarcomas. The tumor is found equally in all races and affects males slightly more often than females. Most tumors grow so slowly that the patient is not aware of their presence for many years. The tumor starts off as a slight, flesh-colored thickness to the skin. Over time, the tumor enlarges and has a pink to slightly red coloration. It slowly infiltrates the surrounding tissue, particularly the subcutaneous tissue. If the tumor is allowed to grow long enough, the malignancy will grow into the fat and then back upward in the skin to develop satellite nodules surrounding the original plaque. This is often the reason a patient seeks medical care. The tumor tends to grow slowly for years, but it can hit a phase of rapid growth. This rapid growth phase allows the tumor to grow in a vertical direction, and hence the term *protuberans* is applied. If medical care is not undertaken, the tumor will to continue to invade the deeper structures, eventually invading underlying tissue, including fascia, muscle, and bone.

Dermatofibrosarcoma protuberans is, for the most part, asymptomatic in the initial phases of the tumor. As it enlarges, the patient may notice an itching sensation or, less frequently, a burning sensation or pain. As the tumor enlarges, patients often notice tightness of the skin or a thickening sensation; however, this development is so slow that most patients ignore it for many more months or even years. The differential diagnosis is often between dermatofibrosarcoma protuberans and a keloid or hypertrophic scar. The atrophic variant can often be confused with morphea. One clue to the diagnosis of dermatofibrosarcoma is the loss of hair follicles within the tumor region. The adnexal structures are crowded out by the ever-expanding tumor. If the tumor is allowed to enlarge enough, it will begin to outgrow its blood supply, and ulceration and erosions develop thereafter. The tumors have ill-defined borders, and determining the extent of the tumor clinically can be challenging or impossible. A punch biopsy of the tumor leads to the appropriate pathological diagnosis. Metastatic disease is uncommon; however, local recurrence after surgical excision remains an issue.

Pathogenesis: The exact pathogenesis is unknown. By genetic chromosomal tissue analysis, these tumors have been found to have a reciprocal translocation, t(17;22)(q22;q13.1), which is believed to be pathogenic in causing the tumor. The exact reason for this translocation is unknown. The translocation causes fusion of

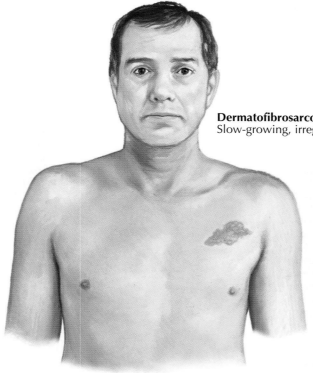

Dermatofibrosarcoma protuberans.
Slow-growing, irregularly shaped tumor

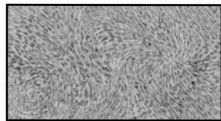

Dermatofibrosarcoma protuberans.
Ill-defined, slow-growing tumor.
Red-orange plaque with nodular and atrophic regions

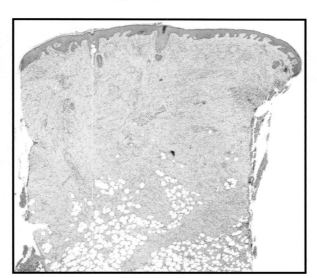

Low power. The tumor is seen invading the underlying subcutaneous tissue. The storiform pattern is seen throughout the dermal portions of the tumor.

High power. Malignant spindle cells make up the bulk of the tumor.

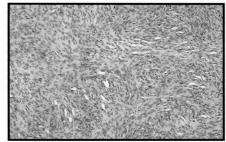

Medium power. The storiform or cartwheel-arranged cells

the *platelet-derived growth factor B-chain (PDGFB)* gene with the *collagen type I α1 (COL1A1)* gene. This translocation directly causes the *PDGFB* gene to be under control of the *COL1A1* gene. PDGFB is then overexpressed, and it drives a continuous stimulation of its tyrosine kinase receptor.

Histology: Dermatofibrosarcoma protuberans shows an infiltrative growth pattern. It invades the subcutaneous fat tissue. The tumor cells can be seen encasing adipocytes. The tumor is poorly circumscribed, and its borders can be difficult to distinguish from normal dermis. The tumor itself is made up fibroblasts arranged in a storiform pattern. These tumors stain positively with the CD34 immunohistochemical stain and are negative for factor XIII. These two stains are often used

to differentiate dermatofibrosarcoma protuberans from the benign dermatofibroma, which has the opposite staining pattern. The stromolysein-3 stain is also used to help differentiate the two tumors; it is positive in cases of dermatofibroma and negative in cases of dermatofibrosarcoma protuberans.

Treatment: Because of the ill-defined nature of the tumors and their often large size at diagnosis, wide local excision with 2- to 3-cm margins is often undertaken. Postoperative localized radiotherapy has been used to help decrease the recurrence rate. Imatinib has shown promise in dermatofibrosarcoma protuberans as a treatment before surgery to help shrink large or inoperable tumors. There has also been anecdotal success with the use of imatinib in metastatic disease.

Plate 3-9

Integumentary System

MAMMARY AND EXTRAMAMMARY PAGET'S DISEASE

Extramammary Paget's disease is a rare malignant tumor that typically occurs in areas with a high density of apocrine glands. It is most commonly an isolated finding but can also be a marker for an underlying visceral malignancy of the gastrointestinal or genitourinary tract. Paget's disease is an intraepidermal adenocarcinoma confined to the breast; it is commonly associated with an underlying breast malignancy.

Clinical Findings: Extramammary Paget's disease is most often found in the groin or axilla. These two areas have the highest density of apocrine glands. It is believed that extramammary Paget's disease has an apocrine origin. There is no race predilection. These tumors most commonly occur in the fifth to seventh decades of life. Women are more often affected than men. The diagnosis of this tumor is often delayed because of its eczematous appearance. It is often misdiagnosed as a fungal infection or a form of dermatitis. Only after the area has not responded to therapy is the diagnosis considered and confirmed by skin biopsy.

The tumor is slow growing and is typically a red-pink patch with a glistening surface. Itching is the most common complaint, but patients also complain of pain, burning, stinging, and bleeding. The area is sore to the touch, and there are areas of pinpoint bleeding with friction. The red, glistening surface often has small white patches. This has been described as the "strawberries and cream" appearance, and it is characteristic of extramammary Paget's disease. As the cancer progresses, erosions develop within the tumor, and occasionally ulcerations form. The clinical differential diagnosis is often among Paget's disease, an eczematous dermatitis, inverse psoriasis, and a dermatophyte infection. A skin biopsy is required for any rash in these regions that does not respond to therapy.

The tumor is often a solitary finding; however, it can be seen in conjunction with an underlying carcinoma, most commonly adenocarcinoma of the gastrointestinal or genitourinary tract. Rectal adenocarcinoma has been the most frequently reported underlying tumor. The percentage of these tumors that are associated with an underlying malignancy is not known but is estimated to be low. Appropriate screening tests must be performed to evaluate for these associations. Usually, the underlying tumor is diagnosed before the extramammary Paget's disease or at the same time of diagnosis.

Pathogenesis: The exact mechanism of malignant transformation is unknown. Two leading theories exist as to the origin of the tumor. The first is that the tumor represents an intraepidermal adenocarcinoma of apocrine gland origin. The second theory is that an underlying adenocarcinoma spreads to the skin and forms an epidermal component that manifests as extramammary Paget's disease. Although most believe this tumor to be of apocrine origin, controversy surrounds this theory, and the exact cell of origin is still unknown. There are no known predisposing factors.

Histology: The histology is diagnostic of the disease; however, the pathological appearance often mimics that of melanoma in situ or squamous cell carcinoma. There are a plethora of pale-staining Paget's cells scattered throughout the entire epidermis. This type of pagetoid spread of cells is often seen in melanoma. The cells can be clustered together and can have the appearance of forming glandular structures. Immunohistochemical staining is often used to differentiate melanoma and squamous cell carcinoma from extramammary Paget's

Eczematous type of Paget's disease

Ulcerating type of Paget's disease

Extramammary Paget's disease. Glistening red plaque with superficial adherent white patches

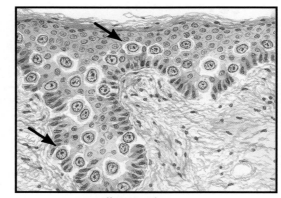

Paget cells in epidermis (*arrows*)

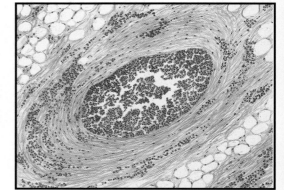

Duct invasion

disease. Extramammary Paget's disease is unique in that it stains positively with carcinoembryonic antigen (CEA) and also with some low-molecular-weight cytokeratins. It does not stain with S100, HMB-45, or melanin A. The staining pattern with cytokeratins 7 and 20 has been used with some success to predict an underlying adenocarcinoma; however, the routine use of these tests is not clinically useful at this time.

Treatment: The prognosis for extramammary Paget's disease depends on the stage of the tumor. Disease that

is localized to the skin has an excellent prognosis. The treatment of choice is wide local excision. The risk of recurrence is high, and lifelong clinical follow-up is required. The prognosis for disease associated with an underlying adenocarcinoma is dependent on the stage of the underlying tumor. Lesions associated with an underlying malignancy have a worse prognosis. Metastatic disease has a poor prognosis, and various chemotherapeutic regimens have been tried with and without radiotherapy.

Plate 3-10

Malignant Growths

KAPOSI'S SARCOMA

Kaposi's sarcoma is a rare malignancy of endothelial cells seen in unique settings. The classic variant is seen in older patients, most commonly individuals living in the region surrounding the Mediterranean Sea. Kaposi's sarcoma associated with human immunodeficiency virus (HIV) infection or with acquired immunodeficiency syndrome (AIDS) is seen predominantly in men, and the tumor is thought to be caused by human herpesvirus-8 (HHV8). There is also a variant seen in chronically immunosuppressed patients, such as those who have undergone solid organ transplantation. The African cutaneous variant of Kaposi's sarcoma is seen in younger men in their third or fourth decade of life. Kaposi's sarcoma is a locally aggressive tumor that rarely has a fatal outcome. The one exception is the very rare African lymphadenopathic form of Kaposi's sarcoma, which is distinct from the more common African cutaneous form.

Clinical Findings: The tumors are very similar in appearance across the subtypes of clinical settings. They usually appear as pink-red to purple macules, papules, plaques, or nodules. In the classic form of Kaposi's sarcoma, the tumors are most often found on the lower extremities of older men. Some tumors in this setting remain unchanged for years, and the patient often dies of other causes. Occasionally, the tumors grow and ulcerate, causing pain and bleeding. The disseminated form of classic Kaposi's sarcoma can be very aggressive, and patients require systemic chemotherapy.

AIDS-associated Kaposi's sarcoma is the most common form of the disease. It is most often seen in younger men. In comparison with the classic form, this form usually manifests as purple macules, plaques, and nodules on the head and neck, trunk, and upper extremities. This is an AIDS-defining illness. Patients with AIDS-associated Kaposi's sarcoma are at a higher risk for internal organ involvement. The small bowel has been reported to be the internal organ most commonly affected by Kaposi's sarcoma, but it can affect any organ system. Since the advent of multiple-drug therapy for HIV infection, the incidence of AIDS-associated Kaposi's sarcoma has decreased dramatically.

Tropical African cutaneous Kaposi's sarcoma is most often seen in younger men. The clinical findings are not much different from those of the classic form of Kaposi's sarcoma. These patients are much more likely to suffer from severe lower-extremity edema. The tumor also has a higher incidence of bone invasion than the other types. The main difference between the classic and the African forms of Kaposi's sarcoma is the age at onset. The aggressive form of African Kaposi's sarcoma occurs in childhood and is often fatal because of its aggressive ability to metastasize. The lymph nodes are often involved before the skin is. The reason the African forms act so differently from each other is poorly understood.

Pathogenesis: The pathogenesis of the classic and African forms of Kaposi's sarcoma is unknown. The cell of origin of this tumor is believed to be the endothelial cell. Matrix metalloproteinases 2 and 9 have been shown to increase angiogenesis and increase the tissue invasion of the affected endothelial cells. Kaposi's sarcoma associated with AIDS or other immunosuppressive states is believed to be caused by the action of HHV8 in a genetically predisposed individual. HHV8 is thought to cause dysregulation of the immune response in the afflicted endothelial cells, allowing them to proliferate uncontrolled by normal immune functions.

Histology: Biopsies of Kaposi's sarcoma show many characteristic findings. The promontory sign is often seen; it is represented by plump endothelial cells jutting into the lumen of the capillary vessel. Many slit-like spaces are also seen. These spaces represent poorly formed blood vessels, which are thin walled and easily compressed. They are filled with red blood cells. The tumor in general is very vascular, with a predominance of vascular spaces and a large amount of red blood cell extravasation into the dermis.

Treatment: For classic Kaposi's sarcoma, the mainstay of therapy has been localized radiation treatment. Many other treatments have been advocated, including topical alitretinoin, imiquimod, intralesional vincristine, and interferon. Systemic chemotherapy for disseminated and aggressive forms is indicated and is usually based on a regimen of either vinblastine, paclitaxel, bleomycin, or pegylated liposomal doxorubicin.

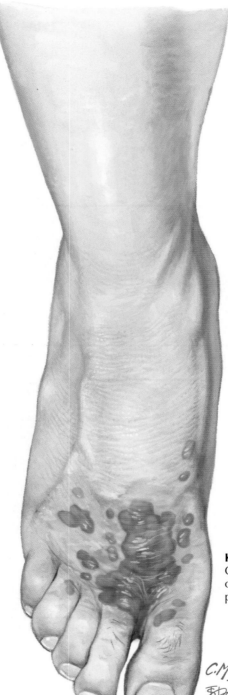

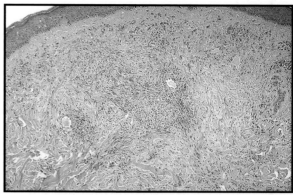

Low power. An abnormal proliferation of blood vessels with slitlike spaces and extravasation of red blood cells

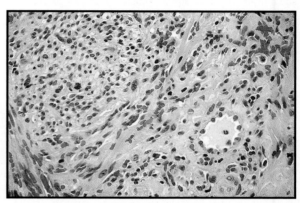

High power. Plump endothelial cells, with mutiple abnormal-appearing blood vessels in a disorganized pattern. Multiple extravasated red blood cells are appreciated.

Kaposi's sarcoma.
Classic Kaposi's sarcoma presenting on the lower extremity as purplish papules, plaques, and nodules

Plate 3-11

Integumentary System

KERATOACANTHOMA

The keratoacanthoma is a rapidly growing malignant tumor of the skin that is derived from the keratinocyte. The tumor is believed by many to be a subset of squamous cell carcinoma of the skin, but its natural history and morphology are distinct enough to merit a separate discussion. Most keratoacanthomas are solitary, but many rare variants have been well documented. These variants include the Ferguson-Smith, Witten-Zak, and Grzybowski syndromes.

Clinical Findings: The classic solitary keratoacanthoma starts as a small, flesh-colored papule that rapidly enlarges to form a crateriform nodule with a central keratin plug. The tumor is unique in that, if left alone, the keratoacanthoma will spontaneously resolve after a few weeks to months. The nonclassic form of keratoacanthoma does not spontaneously resolve, and it is inadvisable to leave these tumors alone, because a high percentage will continue to enlarge. If left alone, these tumors can behave aggressively, with local invasion as well as distant metastasis. The most common area of metastasis is the regional lymph nodes. The most common variant of keratoacanthoma is the solitary variant. This almost exclusively occurs in sun-exposed regions of the body. The peak age at onset is in the fifth to sixth decades of life. These tumors are more common in the Caucasian population, and there is slight male preponderance.

Many unique variants of keratoacanthomas exist. Keratoacanthoma centrifugum marginatum is one such variant that manifests with an ever-expanding ridge of neoplastic tissue. As the tumor enlarges, it becomes an enormous-sized plaque with a peculiar raised border. These tumors can be massive and can encompass a large portion of a limb. This subtype presents a therapeutic challenge.

Multiple keratoacanthomas occur rarely and have been divided into three distinct subtypes. The Grzybowski syndrome consists of multiple keratoacanthomas erupting in a generalized distribution, almost always in an adult. The Ferguson-Smith form consists of multiple keratoacanthomas occurring in an autosomal dominant fashion. The keratoacanthomas are uniform in appearance and also form in a generalized pattern. The onset is in childhood, and the tumors have a higher chance of spontaneously resolving. The Witten-Zak syndrome also has an autosomal dominant inheritance pattern. The tumors are more variable in size and configuration than in the Ferguson-Smith subtype. The onset of this type is also in childhood.

Pathogenesis: The exact pathogenesis is unknown; however, the tumor has a keratinocyte cell origin. There is more evidence for the keratinocytes derived from hair follicle epithelium as the primary cell responsible for the formation of this tumor. Keratoacanthomas have an increased incidence in patients with chronic ultraviolet exposure and in the chronically immunosuppressed. The classic keratoacanthoma is described as a self-resolving tumor. The reason that some of these tumors undergo autoinvolution is unknown. There is

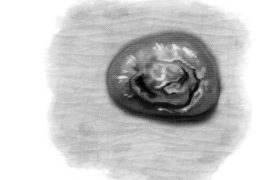

Solitary keratoacanthoma. Typical keratoacanthomas manifest as crateriform nodules with hyperkeratosis on sun-exposed skin.

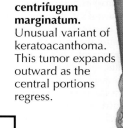

Keratoacanthoma centrifugum marginatum. Unusual variant of keratoacanthoma. This tumor expands outward as the central portions regress.

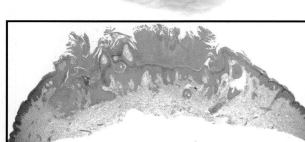

Low power. Cup-shaped invagination of the edpidermis, with a central keratin core

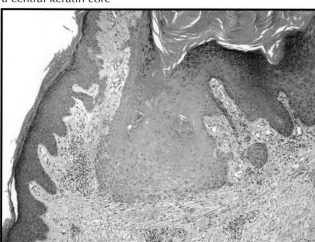

High power. Atypical keratinocytes are seen throughout the epidermis.

evidence to suggest that the tumors, like hair follicles, are under a preset growth and involution control system. The hair follicle grows to a certain point, after which a signal stops the growth of the hair, the follicle is shed, and a new hair shaft is formed. Perhaps the growth and involution of keratoacanthomas is analogous to the turnover of hair follicles. Keratoacanthomas are also seen with an increased incidence in Muir-Torre syndrome. It is possible that the genetic defect in these patients may play a role in the pathogenesis of keratoacanthomas.

Histology: The tumor is typically a cup-shaped exophytic nodule that has a prominent keratin-filled plug. The borders of the tumor are well circumscribed. The tumor is symmetric. Neutrophilic abscesses within the

outer layers of the involved epidermis are a characteristic finding in keratoacanthomas. The keratinocytes that make up the bulk of the tumor have a glassy cytoplasm with large amounts of glycogen. Other unique findings in this tumor are the presence of plasma cells and eosinophils and the elimination of elastic fibers through the overlying epidermis.

Treatment: After a keratoacanthoma has been biopsied, the treatment of choice is surgical removal. This can be done with a standard elliptical excision or with Mohs micrographic surgery. Intralesional methotrexate and oral retinoids have been used in refractory cases and in individuals who cannot tolerate surgery. The familial forms of keratoacanthoma often require long-term retinoid therapy to keep the tumors at bay.

Plate 3-12

Malignant Growths

MELANOMA

Malignant melanoma is one of the few types of cancers that has continued to increase in incidence over the past century. Currently, the incidence of melanoma in the United States is 1 in 75 Caucasians; this is projected to continue to increase over the next few decades. However, the rate of mortality from melanoma has dropped, probably as a result of early detection and surgical intervention. According to cancer registries, melanoma ranks sixth in incidence for men and seventh for women. Melanoma is the most common cancer in women aged 25 to 30 years. Approximately 700,000 cases of melanoma were diagnosed in the United States in 2009, and approximately 9000 people died from complications directly related to melanoma.

Clinical Findings: Melanoma follows a characteristic growth pattern. The tumor arises de novo from previously normal skin in approximately 60% of cases and from preexisting melanocytic nevi in the remaining 40% of cases. Melanoma is uncommon in children, the one exception being melanoma arising from giant congenital nevi. The incidence of melanoma peaks in the third decade of life and remains fairly stable over the next 5 decades. There is no gender predilection. Melanoma is more common in the Caucasian population. There are regional variances in distribution of melanoma. The back is more commonly involved in men and the posterior lower legs in women. However, melanoma has been described to occur in any area of the skin and mucous membranes. Melanoma has also been shown to develop within the retinal melanocytes, causing retinal melanoma. This rare tumor is often found incidentally on routine ophthalmological examination.

Melanoma has been described using the ABCDE mnemonic: **a**symmetric, irregular **b**order, variation in **c**olor, **d**iameter greater than 6 mm, and **e**volving or changing. These are rough guidelines and are not meant to be used to diagnose melanoma. They are intended to be used by the lay public to increase awareness and as a method to screen for melanoma. Some melanomas have all of the ABCDE characteristics, and some have only one or two of them. Some variants of melanoma do not follow the ABCDE rules at all, but these are extremely rare.

There are four main variants of melanoma. The most common one is the superficial spreading type, followed by the nodular type. Lentigo maligna melanoma and acral lentiginous melanoma make up the remaining types. Rare variants are also seen, including the amelanotic type and the nevoid type. Superficial spreading melanoma is the most common variant of melanoma seen in clinical practice. It usually manifests as a slowly enlarging, irregularly shaped macule with variegation in color. If not recognized and removed, the melanoma will continue to enlarge and will eventually develop a vertical component that clinically represents the nodular form of melanoma. Some nodular forms of melanoma can develop de novo without the preceding superficial spreading type of melanoma as a precursor lesion. Nodular lesions are often relatively large at the time of diagnosis. This type of melanoma has entered its vertical growth phase, and it is believed that at this point it has developed the ability to metastasize.

Acral lentiginous melanoma has long been thought to portend a poor prognosis. This is most likely not because of the subtype but because this type of melanoma is often diagnosed later in the course of

MUCOCUTANEOUS MALIGNANT MELANOMA

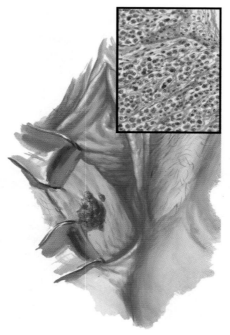

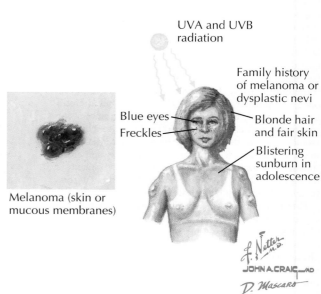

Melanoma (skin or mucous membranes)

UVA and UVB radiation

Family history of melanoma or dysplastic nevi

Blue eyes
Freckles

Blonde hair and fair skin

Blistering sunburn in adolescence

Clinical considerations

Typical clinical appearance of melanoma exhibiting features of "ABCDE" mnemonic
A) Asymmetry
B) Border irregularity
C) Color variation
D) Diameter >6 mm
E) Evolving or changing

Wide local excision of melanoma is based on the thickness of the tumor. A 1-cm border is recommended for lesions less than 2 mm thick, and a 2-cm border for lesions greater than 2 mm thick.

Excisions of lesions

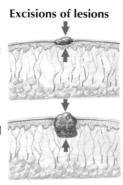

Lesions <2 mm thick

Lesions >2 mm thick

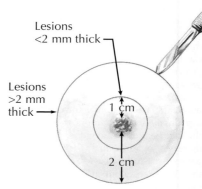

1 cm

2 cm

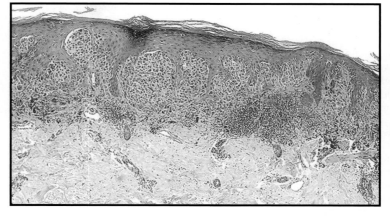

Melanoma with a Breslow depth of 0.7 mm. Dermal invasion is evident, and the tumor shows an abnormal proliferation of melanocytes within the epidermis.

its development. The lesions are often located on the soles, toes, or hands. Patients are often unaware of their presence, and they can mimic a subungual hematoma or bruise. Notably, this form of melanoma is more commonly seen in the African American population.

Lentigo maligna melanoma is most often seen on the face of patients in their fifth to seventh decades of life,

especially in those with a considerable sun exposure history. This type of melanoma can be difficult to treat and has a propensity for local recurrence. The borders of the melanoma are ill defined, and it is difficult to distinguish the background normal sun-damaged melanocytes from the tumor cells.

Amelanotic melanoma is the most difficult of all melanomas to diagnosis. These tumors often appear as

Plate 3-13   Integumentary System

MELANOMA (Continued)

slowly enlarging pink patches or plaques with no pigment. They are commonly misdiagnosed as dermatitis or tinea infections, and the diagnosis is often delayed. They can also resemble actinic keratoses. The lack of pigment takes away the clinician's most important diagnostic clue. These tumors are often biopsied because they have not gone away after being treated for something entirely different or after they have developed a papule or nodule. At that point, they are still most commonly thought to be basal cell carcinomas or squamous cell carcinomas; rarely does the clinician include amelanotic melanoma in the differential diagnosis. Patients with albinism or xeroderma pigmentosum are at a higher risk for development of amelanotic melanoma. These patients need to be screened routinely, and any suspicious lesions should be biopsied.

Pathogenesis: There is no single gene defect that can explain the development of all melanomas. The most plausible theory is that a melanocyte within the epidermis is damaged by some external event, such as chronic ultraviolet exposure, or by some internal event, such as the spontaneous mutation of a key gene in the regulation of cell proliferation or apoptosis. After this event has occurred, the abnormal melanocyte proliferates with the epidermis, starting as an in situ variant of melanoma. After time, the clonal melanoma cells begin to coalesce and form nests of melanoma cells. They then continue to proliferate and enlarge until the clinical features are evident. The tumor enters a radial growth phase at first and eventually develops a vertical growth phase with metastatic potential.

Approximately 10% of melanomas are considered to be an inherited familial form. Although no one gene explains all of these tumors, the *p16* gene *(TP16)* is likely the main susceptibility gene. This gene, when mutated, increases an individual's risk for melanoma as well as pancreatic carcinoma. *TP16* is a tumor suppressor gene that is inherited in an autosomal dominant fashion. Genetic testing for this gene is commercially available.

Histology: The diagnosis by histology of melanoma is based on multiple criteria, including symmetry, melanocyte atypia, mitosis, distribution of the melanocytes within the epidermis, lack of maturation of melanocytes as they extend deeper into the dermis, circumscription, and architectural disorder. Melanoma is believed to begin with an in situ portion, followed by an upward spread of single melanocytes within the epidermis, termed pagetoid spread. If no epidermal component of melanoma is seen, the possibility of a metastatic focus is entertained.

Treatment: When a clinician encounters a pigmented skin lesion that is believed to be a melanoma, the lesion should be biopsied promptly. The best method for biopsy of a pigmented lesion that is suspicious for melanoma is with an excisional biopsy method using a small (1-2 mm) margin of normal surrounding skin. This allows for the diagnosis and an accurate measurement of the Breslow depth. The Breslow depth is the distance from the granular cell layer to the base of the tumor. This depth is considered to be the most important prognostic indicator for melanoma.

Therapy for melanoma is based on the Breslow thickness, the presence of ulceration, and the mitotic rate of the primary tumor. The standard of care is to perform a wide local excision with varying margins of skin based on the criteria described previously. Melanoma in situ is treated surgically by wide local excision with 5-mm margins.

METASTATIC MELANOMA

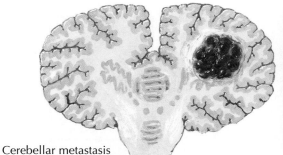

Cerebellar metastasis from cutaneous melanoma

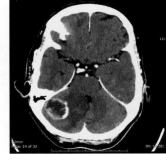

CT with contrast enhancement shows a similar large metastasis in the right cerebellum with effacement of the fourth ventricle

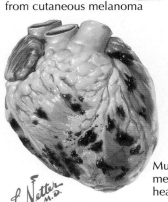
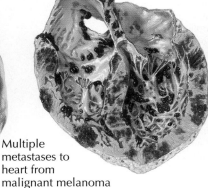

Multiple metastases to heart from malignant melanoma

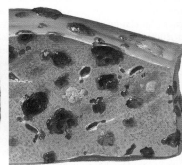

Malignant melanoma metastases to the liver

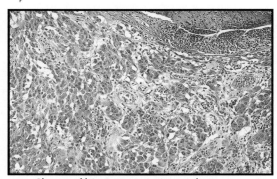

Sheets of bizarre-appearing melanocytes

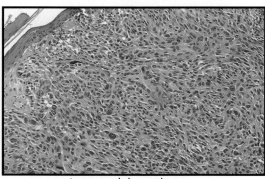

Large nodular melanoma

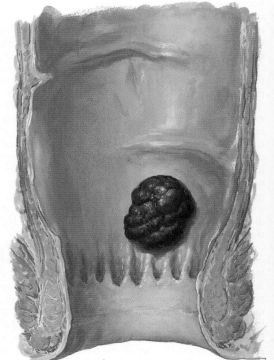

Melanoma metastasis to the large intestine

Sentinel lymph node sampling is becoming routinely performed in the care of these patients and aids in staging of the disease. If the patient has a positive sentinel lymph node biopsy for metastatic melanoma, staging is performed based on positron emission tomography/computed tomography (PET/CT) scanning and magnetic resonance imaging (MRI) of the brain. Patients with metastatic disease to local lymph nodes only are offered a localized lymph node dissection and adjunctive therapy with interferon. Those with widespread metastatic disease are given various chemotherapeutic regimens or enrolled into clinical studies. The mortality rate for stage IV melanoma is very poor. Follow-up for melanoma patients is based on the stage of disease. The National Comprehensive Cancer Network/National Cancer Institute (NCCN/NCI) has published standardized guidelines for clinicians.

Plate 3-14

Malignant Growths

MERKEL CELL CARCINOMA

Merkel cell carcinoma is an uncommonly encountered neuroendocrine malignant skin tumor that has an aggressive behavior. This tumor is derived from specialized nerve endings within the skin. The tumor promoting Merkel cell polyomavirus has been implicated in its pathogenesis. The prognosis of Merkel cell carcinoma is worse than that of melanoma. This tumor has a high rate of recurrence and often has spread to the regional lymph nodes by the time of diagnosis.

Clinical Findings: Merkel cell carcinoma is a rare cutaneous malignancy with an estimated incidence of 1 in 200,000. Merkel cell carcinoma is much more common in Caucasian individuals. The tumor has a slight male predilection. The average age at onset is in the fifth to seventh decades of life. The lesions occur most often on the head and neck. This distribution is consistent with the notion that chronic sun exposure is a predisposing factor in the development of this tumor. These tumors also occur more commonly in patients taking chronic immunosuppressive medications. The tumors often appear as red papules or plaques that quickly increase in size. They can also appear as rapidly enlarging nodules. On occasion, the tumor ulcerates. The clinical differential diagnosis is often between Merkel cell carcinoma and basal cell carcinoma, inflamed cyst, squamous cell carcinoma, or an adnexal tumor. These tumors are so rare that they are infrequently in the original differential diagnosis.

It has been estimated that up to 50% of all patients diagnosed with a Merkel cell carcinoma will develop lymph node metastasis. Other notable areas of metastasis include the skin, lungs, and liver. The staging of this tumor is based on its size (<2 cm or >2 cm), the involvement of regional lymph nodes, and the presence of metastasis. Patients with higher-stage disease have a progressively worse prognosis. Patients with metastatic disease (stage IV) have a 5-year survival rate of 0%. In contrast, the 5-year survival rate for local stage I or II disease is 65% to 75% and approximately 50% to 60% for stage III (lymph node involvement). Grouping all stages together, one third of the patients diagnosed with Merkel cell carcinoma will die from their disease.

Pathogenesis: Merkel cell carcinoma is derived from a specialized cutaneous nerve ending. The normal Merkel cells function in mechanoreception of the skin. Merkel cells, like melanocytes, are embryologically derived from the neural crest tissue. Chronic immunosuppression is believed to be one of the largest risk factors. Patients taking immunosuppressive medications after organ transplantation are at much higher risk than age-matched controls. Chronic sun exposure and its effect on downregulating local immunity in the skin have also been theorized to play an etiological role. The Merkel cell polyomavirus has been studied to assess its role in the development of Merkel cell carcinoma.

Polyomaviruses are similar in nature and structure to the better-known papillomaviruses. There are at least five polyomaviruses that cause human disease. Most of them affect patients who are chronically immunosuppressed at a higher rate than healthy matched controls. Researchers have implicated the Merkel cell polyomavirus as a potential cause of Merkel cell carcinoma. This virus has been isolated from a high percentage of Merkel cell tumors, but not from all of them. It is likely to be a player in the pathogenesis of a subset of patients with Merkel cell carcinoma, but it is unlikely to be the only explanation. The discovery of this virus may lead to therapeutic options in the future.

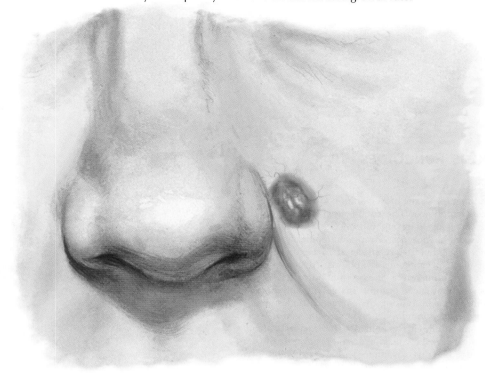

Merkel cell carcinoma. Pink-red papule on the cheek. These tumors may arise quickly and have an accelerated growth rate.

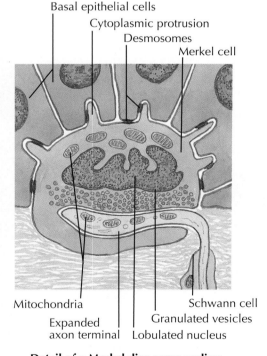

Basal epithelial cells
Cytoplasmic protrusion
Desmosomes
Merkel cell
Mitochondria
Expanded axon terminal
Schwann cell
Granulated vesicles
Lobulated nucleus

Detail of a Merkel disc nerve ending

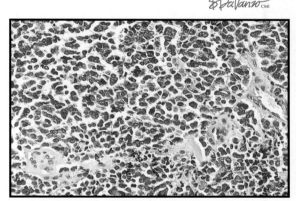

Uniform basophilic-appearing Merkel cells. Merkel cell carcinoma is classified as a small blue cell tumor. (H&E stain)

Histology: Merkel cell carcinoma is a neuroendocrine tumor. The tumor is composed of small, uniformly shaped, basophilic-staining cells. The tumor is poorly circumscribed and grows in an infiltrative pattern between dermal collagen bundles and subcutaneous fat lobules. The cells have a characteristic nuclear chromatin pattern. These tumors can be stained with various immunohistochemical stains. The most helpful one is the cytokeratin 20 stain. It has a characteristic, if not pathognomonic perinuclear dot, staining pattern.

Treatment: Surgical excision with wide (2-3 cm) margins is still the standard therapeutic treatment. Sentinel node sampling has been helpful in staging. Those patients with localized disease often undergo postoperative irradiation of the surgical removal site. Those with widespread metastatic disease are often treated with cisplatin-based chemotherapeutic regimens.

Plate 3-15

Integumentary System

CLINICAL SUBTYPES OF CUTANEOUS T-CELL LYMPHOMA

MYCOSIS FUNGOIDES

Mycosis fungoides is the most common form of cutaneous T-cell lymphoma. The cutaneous T-cell lymphomas are an assorted group of cancers with varying genotypes and phenotypes. Mycosis fungoides is a rare form of cancer, but it is considered to be the most frequent form of cutaneous lymphoma. Mycosis fungoides is predominantly a disease of abnormal CD4+ lymphocytes that have become malignant and have moved into the skin, causing the characteristic lesions. Advances with immunophenotyping and gene rearrangement studies have helped to characterize the disease and are used for diagnostic and prognostic purposes. Altogether, mycosis fungoides is a rare condition afflicting approximately 1 in 500,000 people.

Clinical Findings: Mycosis fungoides often manifests as a slowly progressing rash that occurs in double-covered areas such as the groin and breast skin. The buttocks are a very common area of involvement. There is a 2 : 1 male predominance. Mycosis fungoides is seen in all races, with a predominance in the African American population compared with the Caucasian or Asian population. It is infrequently encountered in children. Mycosis fungoides is staged based on its appearance, the body surface area (BSA) involved, and the involvement of lymph nodes, blood, and other organ systems. The most common stage of mycosis fungoides is stage IA.

Stage IA mycosis fungoides carries an excellent prognosis, with most patients leading a normal life span and dying from another cause. Stage IA disease is typically described as patches of involvement totaling less than 10% of the BSA and no lymph node involvement. The rash of stage IA disease appears as thin, atrophic patches on the buttocks, breasts, or inner thighs. There are often areas of poikiloderma (hyperpigmentation and hypopigmentation as well as telangiectasias and atrophy). The atrophy has been described as "cigarette paper" atrophy: The skin exhibits a fine crinkling similar to freshly rolled cigarette paper. The rash is often asymptomatic, but pruritus can be problematic for some. The diagnosis of mycosis fungoides is based on the clinical and pathological findings.

Patch-stage mycosis fungoides can go undiagnosed for years to decades because of its indolent nature and often bland appearance. It often appears as psoriasis, a nonspecific form of dermatitis, and initial biopsies are often nonspecific. The application of topical steroids before a skin biopsy is obtained may alter the histological picture enough to make the diagnosis of mycosis fungoides impossible. Often, serial biopsies over years are required until one shows the characteristic features of mycosis fungoides. It is best to biopsy a previously untreated area. In addition to being a very slow-developing cancer, it is possible that mycosis fungoides

may start as a form of dermatitis and over many years transform into a malignant CD4+ process.

At the other end of the spectrum is the Sézary syndrome. This is an erythrodermic variant of mycosis fungoides with peripheral blood involvement. Circulating Sézary cells are the hallmark of this syndrome. The Sézary cells are enlarged lymphocytes with cerebriform nuclei. The cerebriform nuclei can best be appreciated under electron microscopy. It is considered to be a

leukemic phase of mycosis fungoides. Sézary syndrome has a poor prognosis.

There are many varying stages of disease between these two extremes. The morphology of cutaneous lymphoma changes from patches to plaques to nodules or tumors. Varying amounts of ulceration may be present. The natural history of progression of mycosis fungoides is variable and difficult to predict clinically. The most accurate way to predict the course is based on the type of

Erythrodermic patient with erythema on greater than 90% of body surface area

Sézary cells: atypical cerebriform lymphocytes

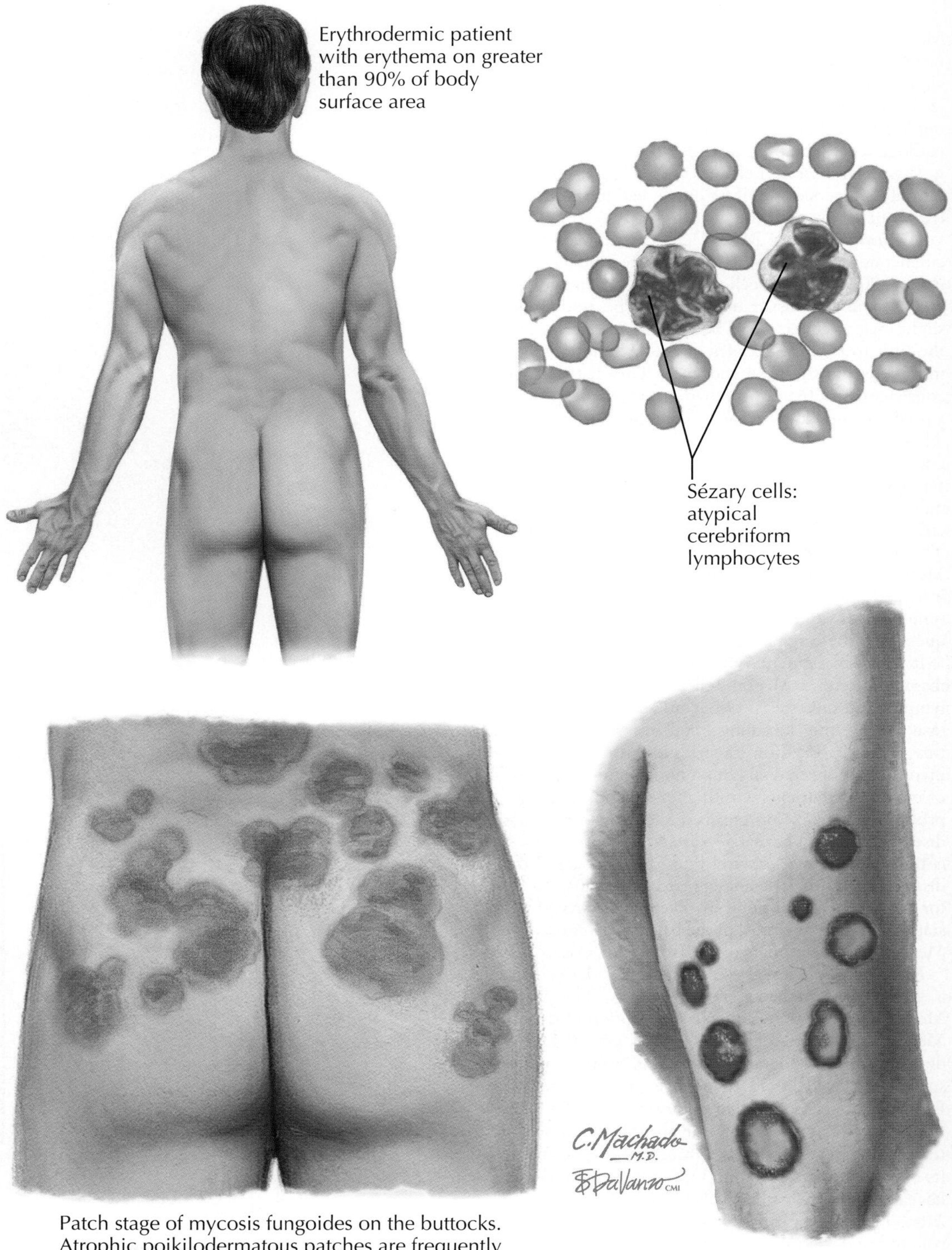

Patch stage of mycosis fungoides on the buttocks. Atrophic poikilodermatous patches are frequently encountered on the buttocks.

Annular plaques

Plate 3-16

Malignant Growths

HISTOLOGICAL ANALYSIS OF CUTANEOUS T-CELL LYMPHOMA

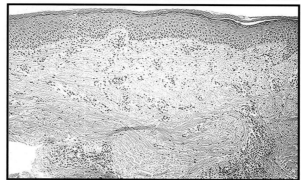

Low power. Lichenoid infiltrate of lymphocytes with epidermotropism

MYCOSIS FUNGOIDES
(Continued)

involvement and the BSA involved. The smaller the BSA of involvement, the better the prognosis. A worse prognosis is seen with the nodular form as opposed to the plaque type or the patch form of mycosis fungoides.

Pathogenesis: The etiology of mycosis fungoides is unknown. The pathomechanism that causes the responsible lymphocytes to transform into malignant cells is unknown. Significant work has looked at various causes including retroviruses, environmental insults, gene deletions, and chronic antigen stimulation. However, the exact mechanism of malignant transformation for this disease, which was originally described in 1806, remains unresolved.

Histology: Stage IA disease shows the characteristic histological findings of mycosis fungoides. There is a lichenoid infiltrate of abnormal lymphocytes with cerebriform nuclei. There are varying amounts of epidermotropism without spongiosis. The epidermotropic cells are the abnormal lymphocytes that have entered the epidermis. Occasionally, collections of the lymphocytes occur within the epidermis as small groupings called Pautrier's microabscesses. Immunophenotyping of the cells present reveals the infiltrate to be predominantly CD4+ lymphocytes with a loss of the CD7 and CD26 surface molecules. Clonality of the infiltrate can be determined by performing a Southern blot analysis. The presence or lack of clonality is not diagnostic, and this test is not routinely performed.

Peripheral blood can be analyzed by flow cytometry for the presence of circulating lymphoma cells. This is a rare finding in low-stage disease and a near-universal finding in Sézary syndrome.

Treatment: Treatment of mycosis fungoides is based on the stage of disease. Stage IA disease is often treated with a combination of topical corticosteroids, nitrogen mustard ointment, narrow-band ultraviolet B (UVB) phototherapy, or psoralen + ultraviolet A (PUVA) phototherapy. As the BSA of involvement increases, the use of creams becomes difficult. Phototherapy is often used for those with widespread patch disease.

Isolated tumors respond well to local radiotherapy. Often, systemic treatments are employed as well. These systemic agents include the retinoids (bexarotene, acitretin, and isotretinoin) and interferon, both α and γ types. Extracorporeal photopheresis has been used for all stages of mycosis fungoides, especially Sézary syndrome. The patient is given intravenous psoralen and then has peripheral blood removed and separated into its components. The white blood cells are isolated, exposed to UVA light, and then returned to the patient. The exposed leukocytes that have been damaged by the psoralen and UVA are believed to induce a vaccine-like immunological response.

Total skin electron-beam therapy can be used in special cases in institutions that have the technical

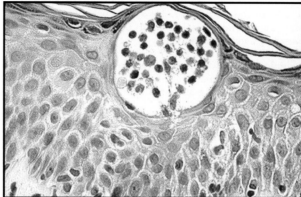

High power. Close-up of Pautrier microabscess in the epidermis

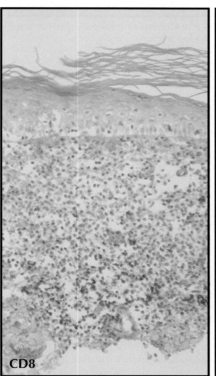

CD8

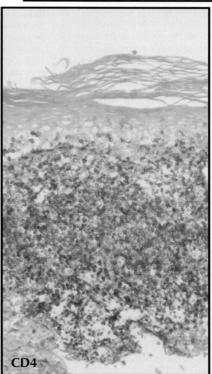

CD4

CD8 and CD4 stains showing a predominance of CD4 cells in the infiltrate

capability. Denileukin diftitox is an approved therapy for refractory disease. This drug is created by fusion of the interleukin-2 (IL-2) molecule and the diphtheria toxin. Cells that express the CD25 molecule (IL-2 receptor) are selectively killed by this medication. Denileukin diftitox can cause severe side effects and should be administered only by specialists adept at its use. Many new medications are being used with variable success in the treatment of mycosis fungoides, including

an anti-CD52 monoclonal antibody, alemtuzumab, and various investigational mediations. Bone marrow transplantation is another option for life-threatening refractory disease.

Despite the many therapies available, no treatment has been shown to increase survival in patients with mycosis fungoides. It is therefore inadvisable to treat stage IA disease with a medication that has acute, potentially life-threatening side effects.

Plate 3-17

Integumentary System

SEBACEOUS CARCINOMA

Sebaceous carcinoma is a rare malignant tumor of the sebaceous gland. These tumors are most frequently seen on the eyelids. They are most commonly found as solitary tumors but may be seen as a part of the Muir-Torre syndrome. The Muir-Torre syndrome is caused by a genetic abnormality in the tumor suppressor genes *MSH2* and *MLH1* and is associated with multiple sebaceous tumors, both benign and malignant. The syndrome is also associated with a high incidence of internal gastrointestinal and genitourinary malignancies.

Clinical Findings: These tumors are most commonly found on the eyelid skin and the eyelid margin. The reason is that the periocular skin contains many types of modified sebaceous glands, including the meibomian glands and the glands of Zeis. Many other, less common modified sebaceous glands exist, including the caruncle glands and the multiple sebaceous glands associated with the hairs of the periocular skin. It is believed that most sebaceous carcinomas arise from the meibomian glands, with the glands of Zeis the second most common site of origin. The meibomian glands are modified sebaceous glands that are located within the tarsal plate of the upper and lower eyelid.

Sebaceous carcinoma has been reported to occur in all areas of the body, but the vast majority occur on the eyelids, with the next most common area being the rest of the head and neck region, probably because the density of sebaceous glands is higher in these regions. The tumors typically start as small subcutaneous nodules or thickenings of the skin. They are initially asymptomatic and can be mistaken for a stye or chalazion. The tumor almost always has a slight yellowish coloration, which, together with the characteristic periocular location, can help with the diagnosis. The major differentiating factor is that these other two inflammatory processes are very acute in onset, are painful, and resolve within a few weeks. Sebaceous carcinoma is a slow-growing tumor that persists and continues to enlarge, eventually causing erosions and ulceration. Once this occurs, the tumor becomes painful and can easily bleed with superficial trauma. The clinical differential diagnosis is often between sebaceous carcinoma and a basal cell carcinoma or squamous cell carcinoma.

Sebaceous carcinomas occur with a higher incidence in the older female population. There is a predilection for Caucasians and for patients receiving chronic immunosuppressive therapy. Patients with the Muir-Torre syndrome are at dramatically higher risk for sebaceous carcinoma compared with age-matched controls. Previous radiation therapy for the treatment of facial or ocular tumors has also been shown to be a predisposing factor for the development of sebaceous carcinoma.

As the tumors enlarge, they exhibit an aggressive local growth pattern. They can rapidly enlarge and metastasize to regional lymph node basins.

Pathogenesis: Solitary sebaceous carcinomas arise from sebaceous glands, but the exact pathomechanism

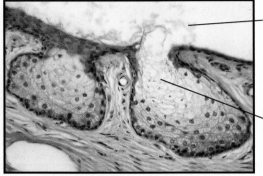

Levator palpebrae superioris muscle
Orbital septum
Superior tarsal (Müller's) muscle (smooth)
Superior conjunctival fornix
Orbicularis oculi muscle (palpebral part)
Superior tarsus
Meibomian glands of the tarsal plate
Glands of Zeis (sebaceous glands)
Eyelashes (cilia)
Openings of tarsal glands
Inferior tarsus
Orbicularis oculi muscle (palpebral part)
Inferior conjunctival fornix
Orbital septum

Sclera
Bulbar conjunctiva
Palpebral conjunctiva
Cornea
Lens
Anterior chamber
Iris
Posterior chamber

Sebaceous carcinoma most frequently arises from the meibomian glands or the glands of Zeis.

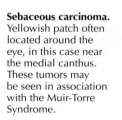

Sebaceous carcinoma. Yellowish patch often located around the eye, in this case near the medial canthus. These tumors may be seen in association with the Muir-Torre Syndrome.

Lumen of duct

Sebaceous cell

Meibomian gland

Two alveoli of a Meibomian sebaceous gland arranged in a row. The left one seems to discharge secretory product directly onto the surface into a straight opening duct. Secretory epithelial cells of the alveoli look foamy and washed out because of high lipid content.*

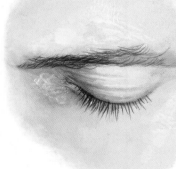

Part of a sebaceous gland. Small nucleated cells with euchromatic nuclei (*arrows*) in the periphery of the gland serve as proliferating stem cells. A thin basement membrane covers them externally. A large sebaceous cell in the center contains many prominent lipid droplets, which surround a central nucleus. The cells ultimately break down and add their contents to oily secretory product. Sebum reduces water loss from the skin surface and lubricates hair. It may also protect skin from infection with bacteria.*

Micrographs reprinted with permission from Ovalle W, Nahirney P. Netter's Essential Histology. Philadelphia: Saunders, 2008.

is not understood. Many risk factors have been determined, but how these translate into tumor development is still being studied. More is known about the sebaceous tumors associated with the Muir-Torre syndrome. This syndrome is caused by a genetic defect in the mismatch repair genes. The syndrome is inherited in an autosomal dominant fashion. The genes that are abnormal in this syndrome are responsible for microsatellite instability within the cells of the sebaceous carcinomas and may lead directly to malignant transformation of the benign sebaceous gland.

Histology: These tumors are derived from sebaceous glands and show a high degree of infiltrative growth. The tumor deeply invades the subcutaneous tissue; in the periocular area, it often invades the underlying muscle tissue. The lesions are poorly circumscribed, and mitoses are frequently seen. The tumor cells are large basaloid cells that show areas of mature sebocyte differentiation and areas that are poorly differentiated.

Treatment: The tumors are locally aggressive and have a high rate of regional lymph node metastasis. The treatment of choice is surgical removal, either with Mohs micrographic surgery or with a wide local excision, making sure to get clear tumor margins. These tumors have a high risk of recurrence, and clinical follow-up is required. The use of postoperative radiotherapy is warranted in specific cases. Patients with metastatic disease may benefit from a combination of radiotherapy and systemic chemotherapy.

Plate 3-18

Malignant Growths

SQUAMOUS CELL CARCINOMA

Squamous cell carcinoma (SCC) of the skin is the second most common skin cancer after basal cell carcinoma. Together, these two types of carcinoma are known as non-melanoma skin cancer. SCC accounts for approximately 20% of all skin cancers diagnosed in the United States. SCC can come in many variants, including in situ and invasive types. Bowen's disease, bowenoid papulosis, and erythroplasia of Queyrat are all forms of SCC in situ. A unique subtype of SCC is the keratoacanthoma. Invasive SCC is defined by invasion through the basement membrane zone into the dermis. SCC has the ability to metastasize; the most common area of metastasis is the local draining lymph nodes. Most forms of cutaneous SCC occur in chronically sun-damaged skin, and they are often preceded by the extremely common premalignant actinic keratosis.

Clinical Findings: SCC of the skin is most commonly located on the head and neck region and on the dorsal hands and forearms. These are the areas that obtain the most ultraviolet sun exposure over a lifetime. This type of skin cancer is more common in the Caucasian population and in older individuals. It is more prevalent in the fifth to eighth decades of life. The incidence of SCC increases with each decade of life. This form of non-melanoma skin cancer is definitely linked to the amount of sun exposure one has had over one's lifetime. Fair-skinned individuals are most commonly affected. There is a slight male predilection. Other risk factors include arsenic exposure, human papillomavirus (HPV) infection, psoralen + ultraviolet A light (PUVA) therapy, chronic scarring, chronic immunosuppression, and radiation exposure. Transplant recipients who are taking chronic immunosuppressive medications often develop SCCs. Their skin cancers also tend to occur on the head and on the arms, but in addition they have a higher percentage of tumors developing on the trunk and other non–sun-exposed regions.

SCCs of the skin can occur with various morphologies. They can start as thin patches or plaques. There is usually a thickened, adherent scale on the surface of the tumor. Variable amounts of ulceration are seen. As the tumors enlarge, they can take on a nodular configuration. The nodules are firm and can be deeply seated within the dermis. Most SCCs are derived from a preexisting actinic keratosis. Patients often have chronically sun-damaged skin with poikilodermatous changes and multiple lentigines and actinic keratoses. Approximately 1% of actinic keratoses per year develop into SCC.

Subungual SCC is a difficult diagnosis to make without a biopsy. It is often preceded by an HPV infection, and the area has often been treated for long periods as a wart. HPV is a predisposing factor, and with time a small percentage of these warts transform into SCC. This development is usually associated with a subtle change in morphology. There tends to be more nail destruction and a slow enlargement over time in the face of standard wart therapy. Prompt biopsy and

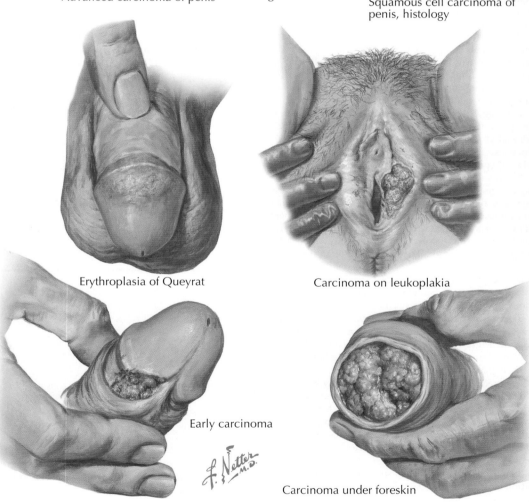

GENITAL SQUAMOUS CELL CARCINOMA

Extensive fungating carcinoma of penis

Advanced carcinoma of penis

Extensive involvement of presymphysial and inguinal nodes

Squamous cell carcinoma of penis, histology

Erythroplasia of Queyrat

Carcinoma on leukoplakia

Early carcinoma

Carcinoma under foreskin

diagnosis can be critical in sparing the patient an amputation of the affected digit.

A few chronic dermatoses can predispose to the development of SCC, including lichen sclerosis et atrophicus, disseminated and superficial actinic porokeratosis, warts, discoid lupus, long-standing ulcers, and scars. Many genetic diseases can predispose to the development of

SCC; two of the best recognized ones are epidermodysplasia verruciformis and xeroderma pigmentosum.

Pathogenesis: SCC is related to cumulative ultraviolet exposure. Ultraviolet B (UVB) light appears to be the most important action spectrum in the development of SCC. UVB is much more potent than ultraviolet A light. UVB can damage keratinocyte DNA by causing

Plate 3-19

Integumentary System

CLINICAL AND HISTOLOGICAL EVALUATION OF SUN-INDUCED SQUAMOUS CELL CARCINOMA

SQUAMOUS CELL CARCINOMA
(Continued)

pyrimidine dimers and other DNA mutations. The damaged DNA leads to errors in translation and transcription and ultimately can lead to cancer. The *p53* gene *(TP53)* is one of the most frequently mutated genes. This gene encodes a protein that is important in cell cycle arrest, which allows for DNA damage repair and apoptosis of those cells that have been damaged. If the *p53* gene is dysfunctional, this critical cell cycle arrest period is bypassed, and the cell is allowed to replicate without the normal DNA repair mechanisms acting on the damaged DNA. This ultimately leads to unregulated cell division and cancer.

Histology: Actinic keratosis shows partial-thickness atypia of the lower portions of the epidermis. The adnexal structures are spared. SCC in situ shows full-thickness atypia of the epidermis that also affects the adnexal epithelium.

SCC is derived from the keratinocytes. The pathological findings are characterized by full-thickness atypia of the epidermis and invasion of the abnormal squamous epithelium into the dermis. Variable numbers of mitoses are seen, as well as invasion into the underlying subcutaneous tissue. Horn pearls are often seen throughout the tumor. The tumors are often described as being well, moderately, or poorly differentiated. Many histological subtypes of SCC have been reported, including clear cell, spindle cell, verrucous, basosquamous, and adenosquamous cell carcinomas.

Treatment: Actinic keratoses can be treated in myriad ways. Cryotherapy with liquid nitrogen is very effective and can be used repeatedly. If this fails to clear the area, or if the actinic keratoses are numerous, medical therapy is often given with 5-fluorouracil (5-FU) or imiquimod. These creams work, respectively, by directly killing the affected cells or by causing the immune system to attack and kill the affected cells. They are both highly effective. The disadvantage is that they cause an inflammatory response that can be severe and cause erythema, crusting, and weeping during the period of application, usually 1 month or longer.

The treatment for SCC in situ is often electrodessication and curettage or simple elliptical excision. 5-FU cream is also effective but leads to a higher rate of recurrence than the traditional surgical methods. 5-FU is appropriate as a first-line agent for bowenoid papulosis. If in follow-up any residual areas are left, surgical removal is indicated. Occasionally, large areas of SCC in situ on the face are treated by the Mohs surgical technique.

Invasive SCC should be treated surgically, with Mohs surgery for lesions on the face or recurrent lesions; standard elliptical excision is adequate for most invasive SCCs. Some small, well-differentiated SCCs have been treated successfully with electrodessication and

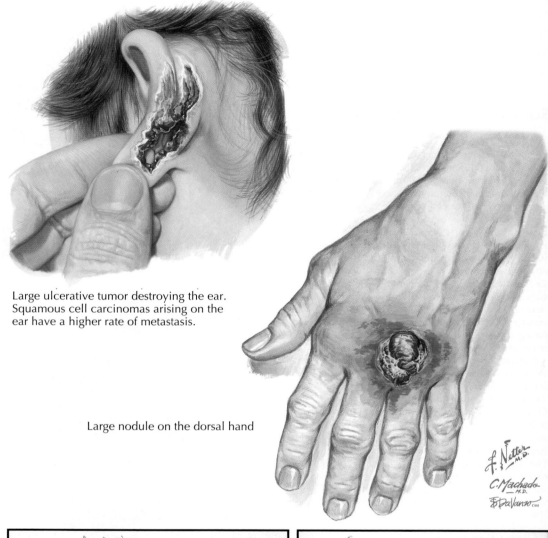

Large ulcerative tumor destroying the ear. Squamous cell carcinomas arising on the ear have a higher rate of metastasis.

Large nodule on the dorsal hand

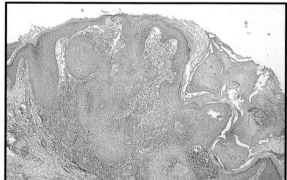

Invasive SCC, low power. Atypical squamous epithelium invading the dermis. This tumor is poorly circumscribed.

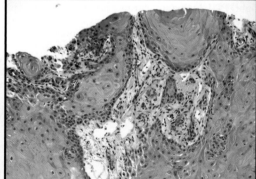

Invasive SCC, high power. Atypical keratinocytes, mitotic figures, and horn pearl formation

curettage. The metastatic rate for cutaneous SCC is low, but certain locations have a higher rate of metastasis. These areas include the lip, the ear, and areas of chronic scarring or ulceration in which the tumors develop. Recurrent SCCs, those larger than 2 cm in diameter, and those developing in patients taking chronic immunosuppressive medications pose a higher risk for the development of metastatic disease. Patients with chronic lymphocytic leukemia (CLL) are at much

higher risk for metastases; the reason is unknown but is thought to be related to the immunosuppression resulting from their CLL. The most common areas for metastasis are the local lymph nodes and lung.

Metastatic SCC of the skin should be treated with adjunctive radiotherapy and chemotherapy. However, these therapies have not shown a clear survival benefit, and the key to treatment ultimately lies in the prevention of metastasis.

RASHES

Plate 4-1

Integumentary System

ACANTHOSIS NIGRICANS

Acanthosis nigricans is a commonly encountered skin dermatosis that can be seen in various clinical scenarios. It is overwhelmingly associated with obesity but can occur secondary to medications, endocrine disorders such as the HAIR-AN syndrome (**h**yperandrogenism, **i**nsulin **r**esistance, and **a**canthosis **n**igricans), diabetes, and internal malignancies. This last type is clinically distinctive and manifests in a unique manner.

Clinical Findings: Classic cases of acanthosis nigricans affect the nape of the neck, the axillae, and the groin regions. Native Americans and African Americans are at a significantly increased risk for development of acanthosis nigricans. The slow, insidious onset of patches and plaques with a velvety, hyperpigmented, thickened, rough surface is characteristic of acanthosis nigricans. Maceration with a malodorous smell is often noted. The patients are for the most part asymptomatic, although some complain of intermittent pruritus. The clinical findings in association with obesity are enough to make the diagnosis. A thorough history should be taken to rule out a medication-induced form of acanthosis nigricans. The only routine laboratory testing performed is screening for occult diabetes. Patients with obesity are at higher risk for diabetes later in life, and lifelong follow-up and screening by their primary care physician is required.

Many medications have been shown to induce acanthosis nigricans. They include niacinamide, glucocorticoids, insulin, and some birth control pills. The medication most commonly associated with acanthosis nigricans is niacinamide. Most cases resolve or improve greatly with discontinuation of the medication. The appearance is often identical to that of classic acanthosis nigricans, but the history is suggestive, with the timing of rash onset related to the introduction of the causative medication.

Malignancy-associated acanthosis nigricans is often widespread and involves unique areas, including the mucous membranes, palms, and soles. This form has a rapid onset and affects different areas of the body than the classic form of acanthosis nigricans does. The palms and soles are often involved, and the face can be involved. Any case in which there is rapid onset of acanthosis nigricans in a widespread distribution, often in a nonobese individual, warrants proper evaluation to rule out an internal malignancy. Referral to a gastroenterologist and an internist for cancer screening is of utmost importance.

A few endocrine disorders can be associated with acanthosis nigricans, most frequently diabetes mellitus and the HAIR-AN syndrome It is associated with insulin resistance and also with hyperandrogenism.

Rare causes of acanthosis nigricans include the familial forms, which are inherited in an autosomal dominant fashion.

Pathogenesis: The skin thickening and clinical findings are possibly caused by an increase in insulin-like growth factor receptor, fibroblast growth factor receptor, and epidermal growth factor receptor and their subsequent effects on the skin. The reason it affects certain regions preferentially is unknown. Malignancy-associated acanthosis nigricans is believed to be caused by some cytokine or growth factor directly secreted by the tumor, possibly in the fibroblast growth factor receptor class of molecules. The tumor causes the clinical findings by secreting these substances. Acanthosis nigricans is believed to be a paraneoplastic process in these cases. Medication-induced acanthosis nigricans is poorly understood but is possibly related to the

Velvety hyperpigmented plaques and patches in the axilla

Acanthosis nigricans. Hyperpigmented plaques on the dorsal foot with accentuation of the skin lines

medication's local effects on the skin in genetically predisposed individuals.

Histology: Epidermal hyperplasia, acanthosis, and papillomatosis are present. There is minimal to no inflammatory infiltrate, and the dermis is essentially normal in appearance. Extensive hyperkeratosis with a mild excess of melanin production likely explains the hyperpigmentation seen in acanthosis nigricans.

Treatment: Treatment is often difficult unless the afflicted individual makes a conscious effort to get to an ideal body weight and to get his or her diabetes under excellent control. This is the only likely scenario in which the skin findings of acanthosis nigricans will resolve. Temporizing methods of therapy include the use of keratolytic agents such as lactic acid to help thin the plaques and make them less noticeable. These agents are difficult to use in the axillae because of stinging. The topical use of tretinoin cream has also been successful. Destructive laser therapies have been used with varying success.

Treatment of malignancy-associated acanthosis nigricans is directed at the underlying malignancy. Removal of the tumor may result in complete resolution of the skin disease.

Plate 4-2

Rashes

ACNE

Acne is an almost universal finding in teenagers across the globe. Acne vulgaris is the most common form of acne; it affects almost every human at some point in their lifetime. Most cases are mild and do not cause any significant disease. Most acne vulgaris is seen in the postpubertal years. Many clinical variants exist, and excellent therapeutic modalities are available to treat this skin disease.

Clinical Findings: Acne vulgaris typically begins soon after puberty. It has no racial or gender preference, although males may develop more severe cases of the disease. The first signs of acne development are the formation of microcomedones, both open and closed. Open comedones, also known as blackheads, appear as small (0.5-1 mm), dilated skin pores that are filled with a dark material, oxidized keratin. This material can be easily expressed with lateral pressure or with the help of a comedone extractor. The closed comedone, also known as a whitehead, is a small (0.5-1 mm), whitish to skin-colored papule. Comedones are believed to be the precursor lesion to the other lesions of acne. As acne progresses, inflammatory red, slightly tender papules develop, along with a variable amount of pustules. The pustules are centered on the hair follicle. More severe cases of acne, such as nodulocystic acne, show inflammatory nodule formation as well as cyst formation. These nodules and cysts can become large (2-3 cm in diameter) and can cause considerable pain. They often heal with scarring of the skin.

The face, back, upper chest, and shoulders are the predominant areas of involvement, most likely because of the higher density of sebaceous glands in these regions and the role of the sebaceous gland in the development of acne. Acne is a relentless condition: As one lesion heals, another develops simultaneously. Females often report a flare of their acne 1 week before menstruation begins, denoting hormonal influence. Acne has many clinical variants.

Adult female acne is typically seen in women between 25 and 45 years of age. They often report that they had minimal to no acne during adolescence. This form of acne is found predominantly on the cheeks, perioral region, and jaw line, and it manifests as deep-seated papules, nodules, and cysts. There is a pronounced flare around the time of menstruation.

Neonatal and infantile acne are self-limited types that are seen frequently in this population. Neonatal acne may be seen a day or two after delivery; it is caused by transplacental passage of maternal hormones. It resolves without therapy and seems to be more prevalent in male newborns. Infantile acne is seen after the first few months of life. Most cases show a few transient papules, comedones, and pustules. Most self-resolve, although a few cases last into adolescence.

Acne cosmetica and acne medicamentosa are two similar forms of acne thought to be caused by or exacerbated by the use of cosmetics and facial medications. The removal of these products usually is enough for the patient to see significant improvement. Most products implicated in this form of acne are oily in

nature; they cause follicular plugging, which allows acne production.

Acne excoriée is a form of acne that is made worse by chronic picking or manipulation of the acneiform lesions. This often leads to scarring and a worsening of the clinical appearance. It is often coexistent with an underlying anxiety disorder, obsessive compulsive disorder, or depression.

Rare forms of acne include acne fulminans, acne conglobata, and acne aestivalis. Acne fulminans is seen almost exclusively in teenage boys. It is a form of severe cystic nodular acne that heals with severe, disfiguring scarring. The cysts and nodules can easily rupture and break down, leaving multiple ulcerations. This is associated with systemic symptoms including fever,

arthralgias and arthritis, and myalgias. A peripheral leukocytosis is often seen on laboratory examination. Lytic bone lesions can be seen, with the clavicle the most commonly affected bone. This may be preceded by localized pain over the bony involvement. *Acne conglobata* is a term used to refer to severe cystic acne, which is seen mostly in young males. Patients often have multiple cysts that can be interconnected with sinus tracts. The areas involved are very painful and heal with severe scarring. This form of acne occurs in the same locations as acne vulgaris. Acne conglobata has been seen in association with hidradenitis suppurativa, and some consider these conditions to be in the same spectrum of disease processes. Acne conglobata may run a chronic course well into adulthood, with

ACNE VULGARIS

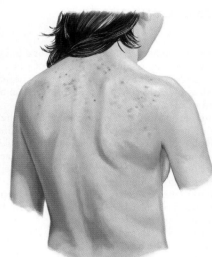

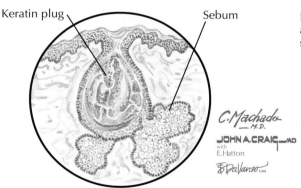

Comedones are most common lesions.

Nodular and cystic forms may result in permanent scarring.

Forehead, nose, cheeks, and chest are commonly involved in acne.

Papules, pustules, comedones, postinflammatory hyperpigmentation, and mild scarring are seen here. The upper back is commonly involved in acne.

Keratin plug

Sebum

Section of closed comedone (whitehead) showing keratin plug and accumulated sebum in sebaceous glands

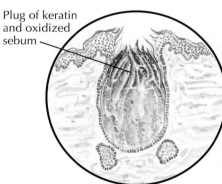

Plug of keratin and oxidized sebum

Section of open comedone (blackhead) showing plug of keratin and oxidized sebum

Plate 4-3

Integumentary System

ACNE VARIANTS

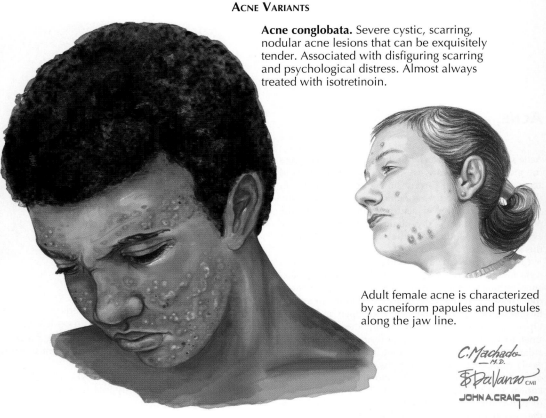

Acne conglobata. Severe cystic, scarring, nodular acne lesions that can be exquisitely tender. Associated with disfiguring scarring and psychological distress. Almost always treated with isotretinoin.

Adult female acne is characterized by acneiform papules and pustules along the jaw line.

ACNE (Continued)

persistent nodules and cysts coming and going. Acne aestivalis is one of the rarest forms of acne. It has a seasonal variation to its course. It begins in spring and resolves by early fall. It is a disease predominantly of adult women.

Steroid-induced acne occur secondary to the chronic use of oral or intravenous steroids. It manifests as a monomorphic eruption of inflammatory papules. Many other medications can be associated with acneiform eruptions, including iodides, lithium, and the epidermal growth factor inhibitors.

Pathogenesis: Acne is believed to have a multifactorial basis. Follicular keratinization appears to be faulty, and the keratinocyte adhesions do not separate as quickly as they should, leading to a follicular plug and microcomedone formation. Excessive sebaceous gland production also plays a role and is probably mediated by hormonal influences. If the sebaceous gland material is produced in an amount sufficient to cause rupture of the comedone, the contents spill into the dermis, causing an inflammatory response; clinically, this is manifested by inflammatory papules, nodules, and cysts. The third player in the pathogenesis is the gram-negative anaerobic bacteria, *Propionibacterium acnes*. This bacteria is believed to cause an activation of the immune system and results in an inflammatory infiltrate. Rare causes of acne include adrenal gland disorders that can cause virilization. These tumors are rare and often are associated with a sudden onset of acne, hirsutism, and irregular menstrual cycles. Any state of hyperandrogenism can cause acne or make preexisting acne worse. The most common cause is the polycystic ovarian syndrome in women. Less commonly, a Sertoli-Leydig cell tumor can lead to a hyperandrogenic state and resultant acne.

Histology: Biopsies of acne are not required for diagnosis. A biopsy specimen from an inflammatory acne papule shows a folliculocentric lesion with a dense inflammatory infiltrate. The follicular epithelium has signs of spongiosis. Foreign body giant cells, plasma cells, neutrophils, and lymphocytes are all seen in varying degrees. Comedones show compacted corneocytes within the sebaceous gland lumen.

Treatment: Treatment for acne vulgaris is multidimensional. One often uses a combination of a keratolytic and antibacterial agent, such as benzyl peroxide, with tretinoin (a medication that increases differentiation and maturation of keratinocytes) and an antibiotic. The antibiotics are used for their antiinflammatory and antibacterial properties. The antibiotic may be given in a topical or oral form. More severe acne, cystic acne, acne conglobata, and acne fulminans require the systemic use of isotretinoin to prevent severe scarring. Isotretinoin is given for 5 to 6 months. Significant precautions need to be taken, because this medication is a well-known teratogen. Prednisone is often advocated for these severe cases of cystic acne. It is usually used transiently, when first beginning therapy with isotretinoin, to help decrease some of the severe inflammation. It should not be used for long periods.

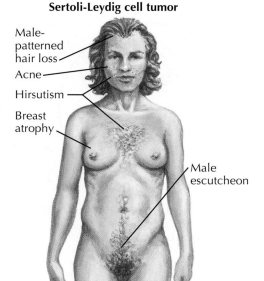

Sertoli-Leydig cell tumor

Male-patterned hair loss
Acne
Hirsutism
Breast atrophy
Male escutcheon

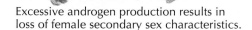

Excessive androgen production results in loss of female secondary sex characteristics.

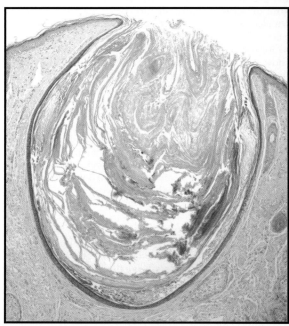

Open comedone is a common finding in acne patients. Compact keratin fills the comedone cavity.

Many other treatment options exist, including topical agents such as azelaic acid, adapalene, tazarotene, salicylic acid, and topical antibiotics. Oral medications that can be used include multiple oral antibiotics, spironolactone, and birth control pills. The latter two medications are especially helpful in the treatment of adult female acne. They work on the hormonal influence on acne and are highly successful in this type of patient.

All the medications used for acne have potential side effects, and treatment must be tailored to the individual. Comedone extraction, intralesional triamcinolone, and photodynamic therapy have shown some success in treating acne. Laser resurfacing, chemical peels, and use of artificial fillers should be reserved for the treatment of scarring after the inflammatory acne has been controlled.

Plate 4-4

Rashes

ACNE KELOIDALIS NUCHAE

Acne keloidalis nuchae is a fairly common form of inflammatory, scarring alopecia that typically occurs on the posterior occipital scalp. There is a variable spectrum of disease, ranging from very mild cases to severe scarring alopecia. The condition has psychosocial implications and is difficult to treat effectively. It is diagnosed clinically, and biopsies are rarely needed.

Clinical Findings: Acne keloidalis nuchae begins on the posterior scalp or nape of the neck as tiny, follicular, flesh-colored to red papules. The papules enlarge to form plaques, which coalesce into larger plaques. Ultimately in severe cases, the entire posterior scalp is involved. Early in the disease, no hair loss is appreciated. As the disease progresses, the hair follicles become scarred down and crowded out by the encroaching fibrosis, resulting in a variable amount of scarring alopecia.

This condition is far more common in young adult men, with a predilection for African Americans. It was originally believed to be caused by close shaving of the hair and the subsequent inflammation caused by the newly regrowing hair as it pierces the epidermis. The curly nature of the hair follicle was believed to be one of the most important factors. This theory of the pathophysiology of the disease has been questioned, and the cause of the condition is not as simple as once theorized.

The plaques, if left untreated, eventually form thickened scar tissue resembling the appearance of a keloid scar. The scarring alopecia is permanent, and the patient is left with a considerable cosmetic issue. Severe cases of this condition can cause psychological issues, as can almost any form of severe alopecia.

Pathogenesis: Originally, acne keloidalis was believed to be caused by the close haircut in African American men, which caused the hairs to penetrate the epidermis on regrowth, setting off an inflammatory reaction. It has now been determined that this is an oversimplification of the disease state. Other factors are likely to play more important roles in the pathogenesis.

Histology: Early disease often appears as a dense, mixed inflammatory infiltrate around the hair follicle and adnexal structures with plasma cells present. This appears similar to folliculitis. As the hair follicles rupture, the contents spill into the dermis and set off a dermal inflammatory reaction. There is overlying epidermal hyperplasia and acanthosis. Occasional pustule formation is seen and is composed of pools of neutrophils.

Late disease is very similar to the pathology of a keloid. There is a lack of adnexal structures and fibrosis throughout the dermis.

Treatment: Therapy for mild disease requires a multifaceted approach. If only a few papules are present with minimal hair loss, a combination of a topical and an oral antibiotic can be used for their antiinflammatory effects. The most commonly used oral antibiotics are in the tetracycline class. The topical antibiotic most often prescribed is clindamycin. Strict hair care regimens are required to help decrease the trauma to the skin. Shaving of the scalp should be avoided, and haircuts with shears should also be minimized, because the shears can cause microtrauma to the skin and potentially induce the process and scarring formation.

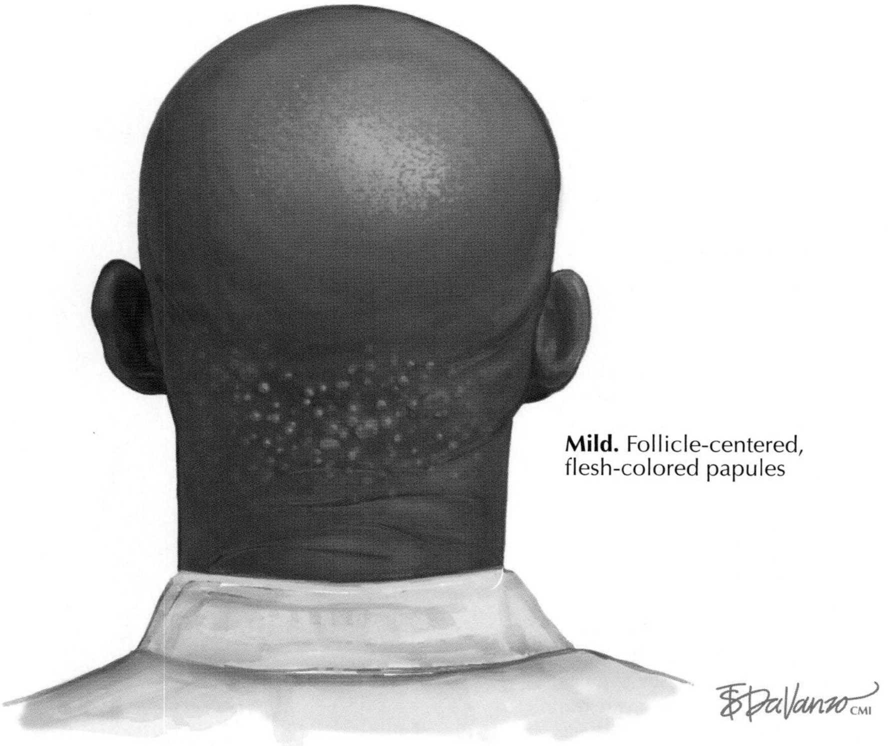

Mild. Follicle-centered, flesh-colored papules

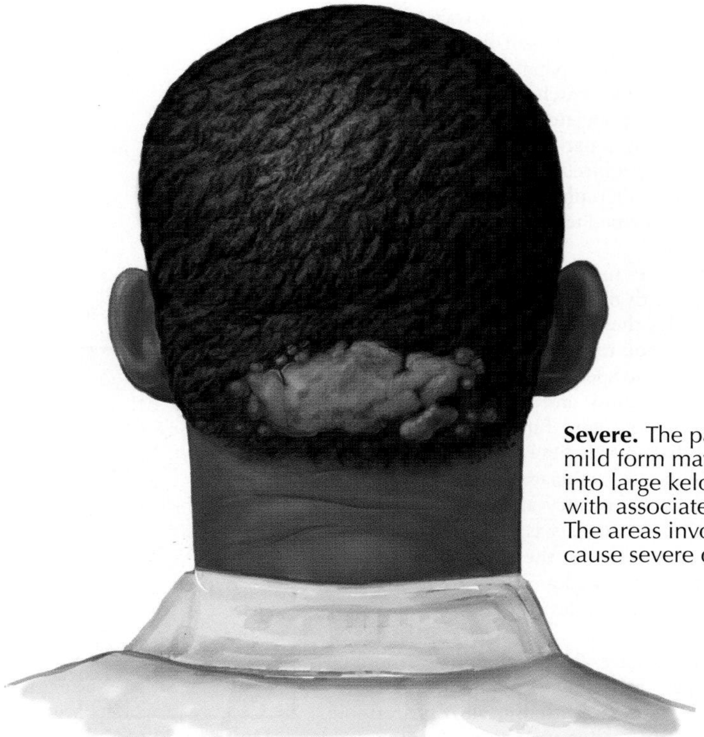

Severe. The papules of the mild form may coalesce into large keloidal plaques with associated hair loss. The areas involved can cause severe disfigurement.

Cutting the hair to a length of 3 to 5 mm is a reasonable approach that minimizes trauma to the skin. Topical retinoids such as tretinoin and tazarotene have been used with varying results. The theory is that they help the follicular epithelium mature and help correct the abnormal keratinization of the epidermis. Intralesional triamcinolone injections into the papules and plaques can also be an effective method of treating mild disease.

Severe disease is rarely responsive to medical therapy. Surgical options remain the best therapeutic choice. The goal is to remove the abnormal skin and close the wound under as little tension as possible. If the tension is too great, it is best to leave the wound open to granulate and heal by secondary intention. The scar that results is often better appearing than the thick, plaque-like scar that it is replacing.

Plate 4-5

Integumentary System

ACUTE FEBRILE NEUTROPHILIC DERMATOSIS (SWEET'S SYNDROME)

Acute febrile neutrophilic dermatosis is an uncommon rash that most often is secondary to an underlying infection or malignancy. The diagnosis is made by fulfilling a constellation of criteria. Both clinical findings and pathology results are required to make the diagnosis in a patient with a consistent history.

Clinical Findings: Acute febrile neutrophilic dermatosis is often associated with a preceding infection. The infection can be located anywhere but most commonly is in the upper respiratory system. Females appear to be more likely to be afflicted, and there is no race predilection. Patients present with fever and the rapid onset of juicy papules and plaques. Because the papules can look as if they are fluid filled, they are given the descriptive term *juicy papules.* They can occur anywhere on the body and can be mistaken for a varicella infection. Patients also have neutrophilia and possibly arthritis and arthralgias. If this condition is associated with a preceding infection, it is usually self-limited and heals without scarring, unless the papules and plaques are excoriated or ulcerated by scratching. Variable amounts of pruritus and pain are associated with this skin disease. When one is evaluating a patient with this condition, a thorough history is required. A skin biopsy must be performed. A chest radiograph, throat culture, and urinalysis should be performed to assess for the possibility of bacterial infection.

Lymphoproliferative malignancies have also been seen in association with Sweet's syndrome. The malignancy often precedes the rash, and the skin disease is believed to be a reaction to the underlying malignancy. It is important to obtain specimens from these patients for histological evaluation and culture for aerobic, anaerobic, mycobacterial, and fungal organisms. The main differential diagnosis is between an infection and Sweet's syndrome in cases associated with a malignancy. The most common malignancy associated with acute febrile neutrophilic dermatosis is acute myelogenous leukemia. The prognosis in these cases is directly related to the underlying malignancy. Often, the skin disease continues to recur unless the malignancy is put into remission.

A few medications have also been shown to induce Sweet's syndrome, including granulocyte colony-stimulating factor (G-CSF), lithium, all-*trans*-retinoic acid, minocycline, and oral contraceptives.

Pathogenesis: The pathomechanism of Sweet's syndrome is theorized to involve the secretion of a neutrophilic chemoattractant factor, which causes massive amounts of neutrophils to migrate into the skin. The exact molecule responsible for the recruitment of neutrophils into the skin is unknown. Reports of exogenous use of G-CSF have led to the theory that it is responsible for the chemoattraction of neutrophils. Other chemoattractants are possible players in the pathogenesis, including interleukin-8.

Histology: Histological examination shows massive dermal edema with a dense infiltrate composed entirely

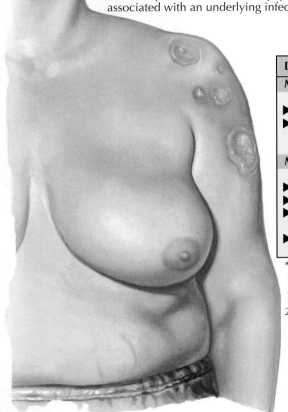

Sweet's syndrome. Edematous papules and plaques, often associated with an underlying infection or systemic illness

Diagnostic Criteria for Sweet's Syndrome*
Major criteria
▶ Abrupt onset of rash—various morphologies
▶ Histological evaluation shows diffuse neutrophilic infiltrate with papillary edema
Minor critieria
▶ Preceding infection or pregnancy or malignancy
▶ Fever >38°C
▶ Sedimentation rate >20 or elevated C-reactive protein level or leukocytosis with left shift
▶ Rapid resolution with systemic steroids

*For the diagnosis, both major criteria and one minor criterion must be present. Adapted from Odom RB, James WD, Berger T. *Andrews' Diseases of the Skin: Clinical Dermatology.* 10th ed. Philadelphia: Saunders, 2006.

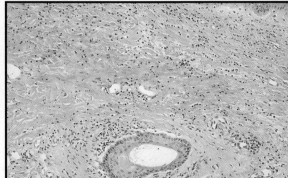

Diffuse neutrophilic infiltrate throughout the dermis

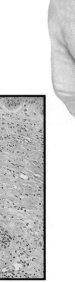

Sweet's syndrome on the dorsal hand. This can be difficult to differentiate from pyoderma gangrenosum.

of neutrophils. Varying amounts of leukocytoclasis are present. Subepidermal bulla formation is possible because of the extensive dermal edema. Special stains for microorganisms must be negative to exclude an infectious process, and these must be backed up with cultures to help disprove an infection, because the histological picture can mimic an infectious process.

Treatment: Treatment should be directed at the causative agent. Supportive care is needed for those with postinfectious Sweet's syndrome. Topical and oral steroids can dramatically shorten the course of the disease.

Sweet's syndrome that develops as a paraneoplastic process secondary to underlying leukemia should be treated with oral or intravenous steroids once an infectious process has been ruled out. This can result in a rapid response, but it is short lived once the steroids are removed. True remission occurs only if the cancer is treated and put into remission.

Plate 4-6

Rashes

MORPHOLOGY OF ALLERGIC CONTACT DERMATITIS

ALLERGIC CONTACT DERMATITIS

Allergic contact dermatitis is one of the rashes most frequently encountered in the clinician's office. It is responsible for a large proportion of occupationally induced skin disease. Urushiol from the sap of poison ivy, oak, or sumac plants is the most common cause of allergic contact dermatitis in the United States. The clinical morphology, the distribution of the rash, and results from skin patch testing are used to make the diagnosis. Patch testing is performed when the causative agent is unknown. Nickel has been the most frequent cause of positive patch testing in the world for years. Urushiol is not tested clinically, because almost 100% of the population reacts to this chemical.

Clinical Findings: Allergic contact dermatitis can manifest in a multitude of ways. The acute form may show linear streaks of juicy papules and vesicles. Variable amounts of surrounding edema can be seen. Edema is much more common in the loose skin around the eyelids and facial region. Chronic allergic dermatitis can manifest with red-pink patches and plaques with various amounts of lichenification. There are localized forms and generalized forms. One of the unique forms of allergic contact dermatitis is the scattered generalized form. Pruritus is an almost universal finding, and it can be so severe as to cause excoriations and small ulcerations.

The prototype of allergic contact dermatitis is the reaction to the poison ivy family of plants. After contact with this plant, urushiol resin is absorbed into the skin and initiates the immune system response to cause allergic contact dermatitis. The dose and the duration of contact with the allergen are important influences on the severity of the rash that develops. Between 3 and 14 days after exposure, the patient notices linear juicy papules and vesicles forming at the sites of contact. The most commonly affected areas are the extremities. Airborne contact dermatitis may be seen from burning of wood with the poison ivy vine present. These reactions are usually seen on skin that was not covered with clothing, and they can be very severe on the face and eyelids, often causing massive swelling and impeding vision.

The location of the dermatitis can be used as a clue to the diagnosis. A nurse with hand dermatitis may be allergic to a component of the gloves being worn occupationally. A young child with a lichenified rash around the umbilicus may be allergic to a metal component of a pant snap or zipper. The most common culprit in these cases is nickel. Finger dermatitis may be caused by the application of acrylic nails or nail polish. Allergic contact dermatitis can also be seen within the oral cavity, most commonly adjacent to dental amalgams or prostheses. Oral allergic contact dermatitis can mimic oral lichen planus. Lichen planus is usually widespread and affects the mucosa and gingiva both adjacent to and distant from any dental restorations.

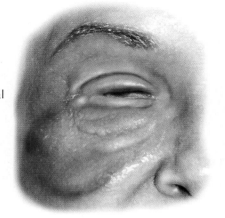

Eyelid dermatitis (red eczematous patches). Potential allergens include fragrances, thimerosal, neomycin, and various preservatives.

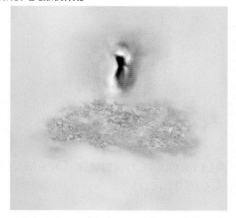

Nickel dermatitis (around the umbilicus) caused by metal snaps

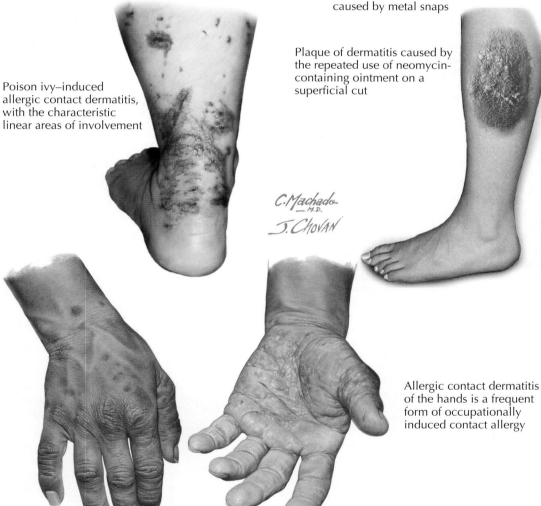

Poison ivy–induced allergic contact dermatitis, with the characteristic linear areas of involvement

Plaque of dermatitis caused by the repeated use of neomycin-containing ointment on a superficial cut

Allergic contact dermatitis of the hands is a frequent form of occupationally induced contact allergy

The diagnosis in all these cases can be made based on patch testing. Chambers loaded with specific concentrations and amounts of known allergens are applied to the back of the individual. The patches are left on for 48 hours and then removed. After an hour, the first reading is made, based on the reaction seen under the chamber. Elevation of the skin or vesiculation is considered to be a positive reaction.

The presence of only macular erythema needs to be interpreted cautiously but can be considered a positive result in certain situations. Pustular reactions are considered to be irritant reactions and not relevant. The patient must come back for a final reading 3 to 7 days after application of the patches. This is the most critical reading and gives the most valuable information.

Plate 4-7

Integumentary System

PATCH TESTING AND TYPE IV HYPERSENSITIVITY FOR ALLERGIC CONTACT DERMATITIS

Patch test

Patch test placement

Positive patch test

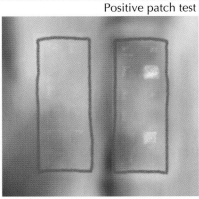

Patch testing is the best method to assess for contact allergins.

Evaluation of patch tests at 72 hours shows papular erythema.

Type IV (cell-mediated, delayed/hypersensitivity, contact dermatitis) reactions

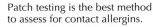

Ethylenediamine

J. Perkins
MS, MFA

Antigen-presenting cell

Edema, inflammation, fibrosis

Accumulation of lymphocytes and monocytes/macrophages

Antigen
(allergen-carrier complex)

Skin

T lymphocyte (previously sensitized to antigen)

Fibroblast

Cytokines Lymphokines

Increased vascular permeability

Expression of adhesion molecules

Blood vessel

Margination and extra-vasation of monocytes and lymphocytes

Monocyte

Lymphocyte

ALLERGIC CONTACT DERMATITIS (Continued)

Pathogenesis: Much is known about the mechanism of allergic contact dermatitis. This form of dermatitis requires a sensitization and elicitation phase for development. During the sensitization phase, the patient is exposed for the first time to the antigen. The antigen is absorbed through the skin and is phagocytosed by an antigen-presenting cell within the epidermis. The antigen-presenting cell internalizes the antigen and processes it within its lysosomal apparatus. The processed antigen is then sent to the cell surface and expressed on a human leukocyte antigen (HLA) molecule. The antigen-presenting cell migrates to the local draining lymph node and presents the antigen in association with the HLA molecule to T cells. The T cells recognize each individual antigen and proliferate locally, resulting in a clone of lymphocytes that recognize that specific antigen; these lymphocytes then remain ready for when the patient comes in contact with the same antigen in the future.

During the elicitation phase, the patient is reexposed to the antigen. The antigen-presenting cells again process the antigen and present it to the newly cloned lymphocytes, which migrate back to the skin and cause the clinical findings of edema, spongiosis, vesicles, and bullae. If the antigen is exposed in a chronic manner, the findings will be less acute in nature, and the typical findings of a chronic dermatitis are seen.

This entire process is dependent on the size and permeability of the antigen, the recognition and processing of the antigen by the antigen-presenting cell, and the complex interactions among multiple T and B cells. Antign-presenting cells and B cells are required for activation of the T cells and propagation of the allergic contact dermatitis.

Histology: The initial finding in acute allergic contact dermatitis is spongiosis of the epidermis with an associated superficial and deep lymphocytic infiltrate with scattered eosinophils. As the rash progresses, the spongiosis can worsen, and intraepidermal vesicles start to form. The vesicles may eventually coalesce into large bullae.

Chronic allergic dermatitis usually shows acanthosis with spongiosis and eosinophils within the infiltrate. A superficial and deep perivascular lymphocytic infiltrate is seen. Excoriations can also be appreciated.

Treatment: Acute localized allergic contact dermatitis can be treated with a potent topical steroid and strict avoidance of the offending agent. Oral sedating antihistamines work better for the pruritus than their nonsedating counterparts do. Soaks that help to dry the dermatitis are helpful and include aluminum acetate (Domeboro's solution). Because the most common culprit is the poison ivy plant, time should be taken to explain to the patient the appearance and nature of this plant. As a good rule of thumb, if a plant has three leaves, it could be poison ivy: "Leaves of three, let it be." Allergic contact dermatitis that is widespread or that affects the eyelids, hands, or groin region can be treated with a tapering dose of oral corticosteroid over a 2- to 3-week period. If the steroid is tapered too quickly, the patient may experience a poststeroid flare of their dermatitis, which can be resistant to further corticosteroid therapy.

Patients who do not respond to these measures should undergo patch testing to determine whether another antigen is causing or provoking the dermatitis. Without the use of patch testing, the allergen will remain unknown and the dermatitis will persist. Not infrequently, patients are found to be allergic to a fragrance or preservative that is an ingredient in one of their personal care products. Once they stop using the product, the dermatitis finally resolves.

Plate 4-8

Rashes

INFANTS AND CHILDREN WITH ATOPIC DERMATITIS

Infant with atopic dermatitis

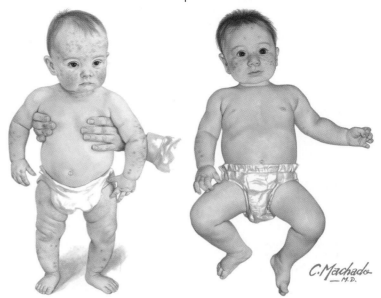

ATOPIC DERMATITIS

Atopic dermatitis is one of the most common dermatoses of childhood. It typically manifests in early life and can have varying degrees of expression. It is commonly associated with asthma and allergies. Most children eventually outgrow the condition. Atopic dermatitis has been estimated to affect up to 10% of all children and 1% of adults, and its prevalence has been steadily increasing. Patients frequently have a family history of atopic dermatitis, asthma, or skin sensitivity.

Clinical Findings: Atopic dermatitis typically begins early in life. There is no racial predilection. The clinical course is often chronic, with a waxing and waning nature. Infants a few months old may initially present with pruritic, red, eczematous patches on the cheeks and extremities as well as the trunk. The itching is typically severe and causes the child to excoriate the skin, which can lead to secondary skin infections. The skin of atopics is abnormally dry and is sensitive to heat and sweating. These children have difficulty sleeping because of the severe pruritus associated with the rash. During flares of the dermatitis, patients may develop weeping patches and plaques that are extremely pruritic and occasionally painful. With time, the patches begin to localize to flexural regions, particularly the antecubital and popliteal fossae. Severely afflicted children may have widespread disease. Patients with atopic dermatitis are more prone to react to contact and systemic allergens. Sensitivity to contact allergens is likely a consequence of the frequent use of topical medicaments and the broken skin barrier. This combination leads to increased exposure to foreign antigens that are capable of inducing allergic contact dermatitis. One should suspect a coexisting contact dermatitis if a patient who is doing well experiences a flare for no apparent reason or if a patient continues to get worse despite aggressive topical or oral therapy. Laboratory testing commonly shows an eosinophilia and an elevated immunoglobulin E (IgE) level.

Secondary infection is common in atopic dermatitis. It may manifest with the appearance of honey-colored, crusted patches in the excoriated regions, which indicates impetigo. It may also manifest as multiple follicle-based pustules, representing folliculitis, or as deep red, tender macules, indicating a deeper soft tissue infection. The rate of methicillin-resistant *Staphylococcus aureus* (MRSA) infection has increased in patients with atopic dermatitis at the same rate as in

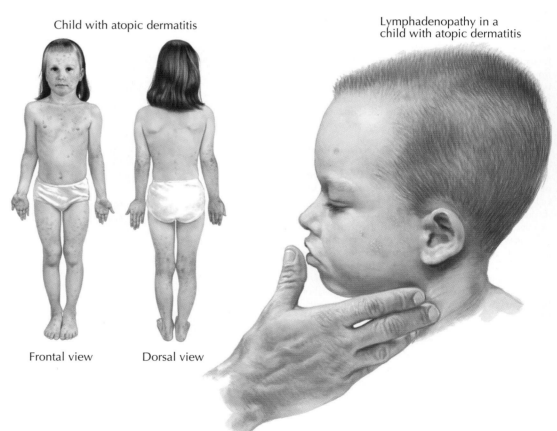

Child with atopic dermatitis

Frontal view   Dorsal view

Lymphadenopathy in a child with atopic dermatitis

the general public. The rate of colonization of atopic patients is much higher than in normal controls, most likely because of the disruption of the underlying epidermis. Colonization in certain situations may lead to infection. Acquisition of a widespread herpesvirus infection can have severe and potentially life-threatening consequences. Atopics are much more prone than others to develop eczema herpeticum. The extensive areas of abnormal, broken skin provide the

perfect environment for the development of this widespread viral infection.

Most childhood atopic dermatitis resolves spontaneously over time. It is estimated that 10% of cases will resolve by the age of 1 year, 50% by 5 years, 70% by 7 years, and so on. A small percentage of children with atopic dermatitis continue on with the rash into adulthood. These cases tend to be chronic in nature and to last for the patient's lifetime.

Plate 4-9

Integumentary System

ADOLESCENTS AND ADULTS WITH ATOPIC DERMATITIS

Scalp, facial, and truncal atopic dermatitis in a child

C. Machado
—M.D.—

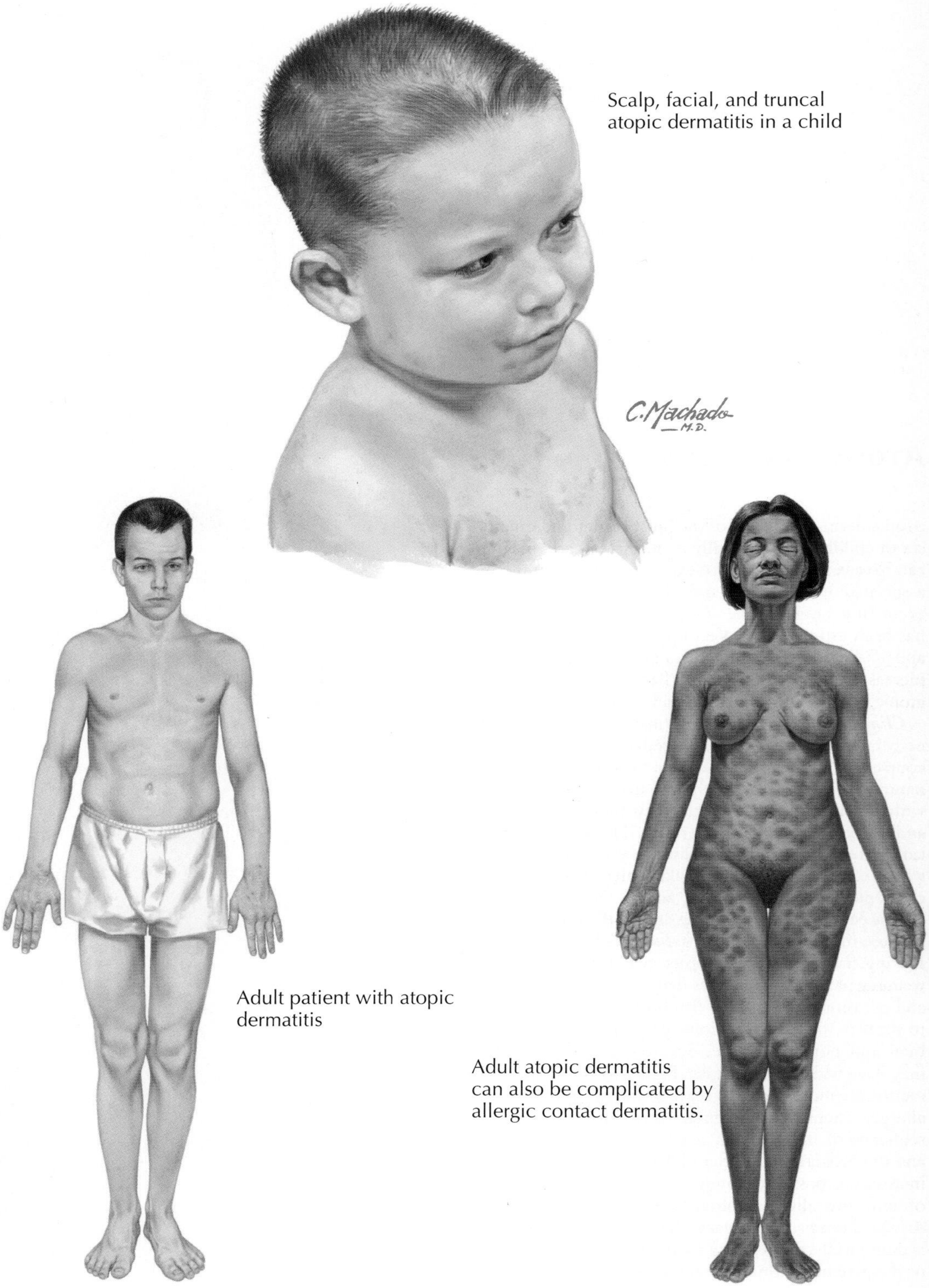

ATOPIC DERMATITIS
(Continued)

Pathogenesis: The cause of atopic dermatitis is unknown. Many exacerbating factors have been found. They include anything that irritates the skin, such as heat, sweating, stress, many chemicals, and various types of clothing. Atopic dermatitis is believed to be caused by an aberrant T-cell (Th2) response in the skin with elevated levels of Th2 cytokines. Interleukin-4 (IL-4), IL-5, and IL-13 are abnormally elevated. These cytokines are responsible for eosinophil production and recruitment and for IgE production. The concentrations of the Th1 cytokines (IL-12 and interferon-α) are below average in these patients. The reason for this response is unknown. Ultimately, the barrier of the epidermis is disrupted, and this is evident by the increase in transepidermal water loss, which can be measured.

Histology: A nonspecific lymphocytic infiltrate is seen, with associated exocytosis of lymphocytes into the epidermis with widespread spongiosis. Varying degrees of acanthosis and parakeratosis are seen. Often, bacterial elements are seen on the surface of the skin. Small intraepidermal vesicles may develop secondary to the massive spongiosis. Excoriations are frequently seen.

Treatment: Therapy consists of patient and family education about the natural history of the disease and the episodic waxing and waning. Bathing regimens must be thoroughly explained, and the use of soap should be discouraged. The patient should take shorter baths in lukewarm water, followed immediately by moisturization and application of topical steroid medications as appropriate. The intermittent use of moisturizers is also helpful. The use of topical immunomodulators, alternating with topical corticosteroids or alone, decreases the atrophogenic side effects of the topical corticosteroids. On occasion, oral steroids may be needed to calm the inflammation and give the patient some well-needed, albeit temporary, relief.

Most children do not need to avoid foods. If any question exists as to whether a food is potentially exacerbating the dermatitis, an allergist may be consulted to perform specific food allergy testing.

Prompt recognition of any bacterial or viral infection should lead to therapy that is not delayed. Impetigo, molluscum contagiosum, and eczema herpeticum are the three infections most commonly associated with atopic dermatitis. Of these, eczema herpeticum is the most important, and its recognition depends on a strong index of suspicion in any child with atopic dermatitis and new onset of a widespread, blistering rash. The differential diagnosis is varicella. A Tzanck test can help diagnosis the condition but cannot

Adult patient with atopic dermatitis

Adult atopic dermatitis can also be complicated by allergic contact dermatitis.

differentiate herpes simplex virus from varicella zoster virus. A viral culture or direct immunofluorescence antibody staining of blister fluid is required for differentiation.

Treatment is usually more successful in children than in adults. Occasionally in children and more commonly in adults, systemic therapies are used to keep the dermatitis under control. Oral antihistamines and immunosuppressive agents are not uncommonly required. A

subset of patients respond to ultraviolet phototherapy, but most are not able to tolerate the warmth and sweating that is induced by the phototherapy unit. Oral immunosuppressants are used and include cyclosporine, azathioprine, and mycophenolate mofetil. These medications have severe potential side effects and should be administered only by experienced clinicians. Routine laboratory testing is required with all of these medications.

Plate 4-10

Rashes

AUTOINFLAMMATORY SYNDROMES

The autoinflammatory syndromes are a rare group of diseases for which the specific causes have been determined. The diseases in this category include hyper-immunoglobulin D (hyper-IgD) syndrome (HIDS), the cryopyrinopathies, familial Mediterranean fever (FMF), and tumor necrosis factor (TNF) receptor–associated periodic syndrome (TRAPS). The cryopyrinopathies are a group of conditions made up of Muckle-Wells syndrome, familial cold autoinflammatory syndrome (FCAS), neonatal-onset multisystem inflammatory disease (NOMID), and chronic infantile neurological cutaneous and articular syndrome (CINCA). These groupings were first proposed in the 1990s to bring together a collection of inflammatory disorders that are distinct in nature and pathophysiology from other forms of allergic, autoimmune, and immunodeficiency syndromes. Patients with these autoinflammatory diseases lack the autoreactive immune cells (T and B cells) as well as autoantibodies. The identification of specific genes that are defective and the roles played by those genes in the development of these disorders has been critical in increasing understanding of these diverse diseases. The common link in these conditions is the fact that they all represent abnormalities of the innate immune system.

Clinical Findings: HIDS is inherited in an autosomal recessive fashion. Patients present with fever, arthralgias, abdominal pain, cervical adenopathy, and aphthous ulcers. Skin findings are consistent with a cutaneous vasculitis with palpable purpura and purpuric macules and nodules. Patients develop attacks of these symptoms with some evidence of periodicity. The attacks can last from 3 to 7 days, and typically the first attack occurs within the first year of life. As the child ages, the frequency and the severity of the attacks lessen. No reliable trigger has been found that initiates the attacks, and patients are completely normal between attack episodes.

Within the group of cryopyrinopathies, the distinctions among Muckle-Wells syndrome, FCAS, NOMID, and CINCA are not clear, and many believe that they represent a phenotypic expression spectrum of the same condition. These very rare syndromes are all inherited in an autosomal dominant fashion. Patients present with recurrent fevers, arthralgias, myalgias, and varying degrees of ophthalmic involvement with conjunctivitis and anterior uveitis. The skin findings are typically generalized and consist of red, edematous papules and plaques. The rash can appear urticarial but is less pruritic. The attack episodes almost always last less than 24 hours. The trigger for FCAS is cold exposure, but the other conditions have no known precipitating factors. Twenty-five percent of patients with Muckle-Wells syndrome develop amyloidosis later in life, which may lead to chronic renal failure. The other conditions also have been reported to lead to amyloidosis, but much less commonly than Muckle-Wells syndrome. NOMID tends to be the most severe of the cryopyrinopathies. Patients with NOMID can develop aseptic meningitis and varying degrees of mental retardation along with hepatosplenomegaly. These patients can develop a characteristic overgrowth of cartilage around the knee that is quite noticeable on physical examination.

FMF is inherited in an autosomal dominant fashion. It is the most common of all the autoinflammatory syndromes. Patients experience attacks of fever and abdominal pain along with monoarthritis. Occasionally,

PATHOPHYSIOLOGY OF AUTOINFLAMMATORY SYNDROMES

Innate immune system pathways involved in the autoinflammatory syndromes

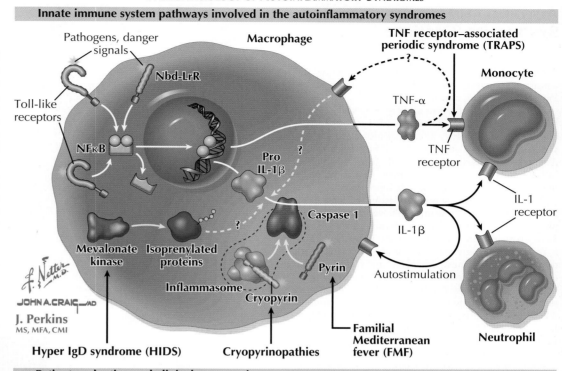

Patient evaluation and clinical presentation

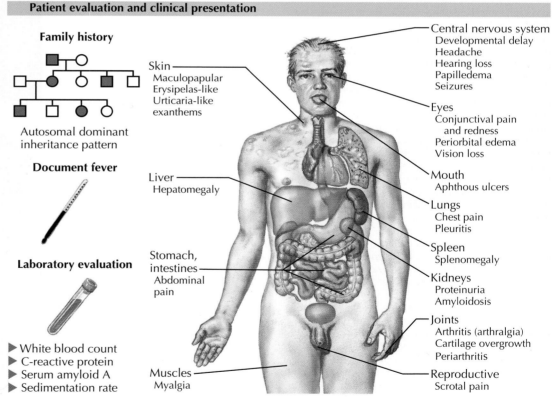

pleuritis and pericarditis are also present. The skin findings consist of an erysipelas-like rash occurring almost exclusively on the lower extremities. Lesions of palpable purpura may also be present, indicating a cutaneous vasculitis. The attacks usually last less than 3 days, with a variable length of time between attacks. Some adults develop renal dysfunction due to amyloidosis.

TRAPS is inherited in an autosomal dominant pattern and also can occur sporadically. Patients develop

attacks early in childhood, which consist of fever, abdominal pain, conjunctivitis, arthralgias, and migratory myalgias. The attacks last longer than in the other autoinflammatory syndromes. Each attack may last from days to weeks, with frequent recurrences. Attacks may be precipitated by varying amounts of stress, both physical and emotional. Again, the development of renal amyloidosis in adulthood has profound effects on the prognosis and is estimated to occur in 10% of

Plate 4-11

Integumentary System

AUTOINFLAMMATORY SYNDROMES (Continued)

TRAPS patients. Skin findings are characteristic and consist of migratory, pink to red patches and macules. Periorbital swelling may be prominent.

Histology: Each of the autoinflammatory skin lesions has a unique histology. The diagnosis cannot be made on the basis of histology alone, but histologic findings are used to rule out other conditions in the differential diagnosis and to help confirm the diagnosis of an auto-inflammatory disease. Skin biopsies should be taken during acute attacks, when a rash is present.

Cutaneous biopsy specimens from patients with HIDS typically show a neutrophilic vasculitis. Neutrophils are found throughout the dermis. A skin biopsy from a patient with one of the cyropyrinopathies shows a neutrophilic perivascular infiltrate associated with diffuse dermal edema. NOMID and CINCA also exhibit a perivascular infiltrate of lymphocytes scattered within the neutrophilic infiltrate. FMF skin biopsies show a diffuse population of dermal neutrophils. TRAPS skin biopsies are nondescript and show a bland lymphocytic infiltrate in a dermal perivascular location. Biopsy of the periorbital edema shows a perivascular lymphocytic infiltrate and dermal edema.

Pathogenesis: Remarkable success has been achieved in deciphering the pathogenesis of these disease states, which are all interconnected through the innate immune system. The defective genes and the proteins that they encode have been determined. These proteins play a critical role in regulation of the innate immune system's inflammatory response. If they are defective, they cause varying amounts of dysregulation of neutrophils and other inflammatory cells. The innate immune system is nonspecific in nature and does not rely on antibody production. Various innate pattern recognition receptors (e.g., Toll-like receptors) are able to recognize foreign molecules and directly activate the innate immune system. The normal activation of the innate immune system allows for prompt recognition of foreign elements and a proper immune reaction to those elements. The autoinflammatory conditions have been discovered to involve defects in various components of the innate immune system.

HIDS is caused by a mutation in the *MVK* gene, located on chromosome 12, which encodes the protein mevalonate kinase. This gene helps regulate cholesterol synthesis, but it is also important for production of precursors that will ultimately be isoprenylated. The lack of these isoprenylated proteins leads to dysregulation of IL-1β and ultimately to the clinical findings of HIDS. All of the cryopyrinopathies are caused by a genetic defect of the *NLRP3* gene located on chromosome 1. This gene, which is also called *CIAS1*, encodes the protein cryopyrin. The defect allows for a gain in function of the cryopyrin protein, which results in hyperactivity of the inflammasome. The inflammasome is a cytoplasmic soluble conglomeration of various proteins that is part of the innate immune system and is constantly identifying foreign material. Its stimulation ultimately increases the activity of the caspase 1 protein and the production of IL-1β. FMF has been found to be caused by a defect in the *MEFV* gene, which encodes the pyrin protein. Pyrin is also a regulator of the inflammasome, and defects in pyrin result in increased levels of IL-1β. TRAPS is caused by a defective gene on chromosome 12 named *TNFRSF1A*. This gene encodes the 55-kd TNF receptor. The defect leads to excessive

signaling due to serum TNF activation of the receptor.

Treatment: Therapy is specific to each syndrome. The molecular understanding of the pathogenesis has led to specific therapies. Because of their rarity, no randomized studies have been performed on the treatment of these conditions. HIDS has been successfully treated with nonsteroidal antiinflammatory drugs (NSAIDs), statin medications, and the interleukin

antagonist, anakinra. The cryopyrinopathies have been treated with cold avoidance in the case of FCAS, and NSAIDs, oral steroids, anakinra, and other immunosuppressants have been tried. FMF has been treated with good success with colchicine, taking advantage of its antineutrophil effect. TRAPS has been successfully treated with etanercept or anakinra. Etanercept is believed to remove the soluble TNF that is responsible for activating the mutated receptor.

CLINICAL MANIFESTATIONS OF AUTOINFLAMMATORY SYNDROMES

Cutaneous findings

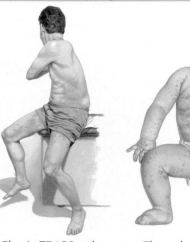

Classic TRAPS rash that migrates in a centrifugal pattern

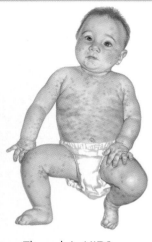

The rash in HIDS can be variable, including maculopapular and urticarial forms.

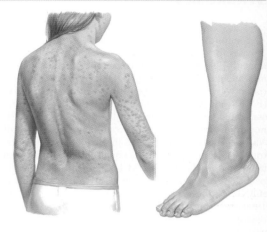

Typical appearance of urticaria-like rash of the cryopyrinopathies

Typical appearance of erysipelas-like FMF rash, often on lower extremities

Joint and central nervous system findings

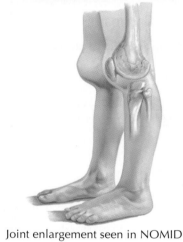

Joint enlargement seen in NOMID

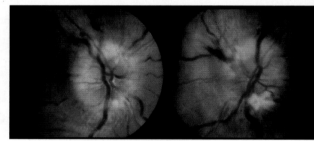

Optic fundus with papilledderma

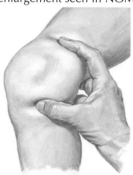

Arthritis/periarthritis

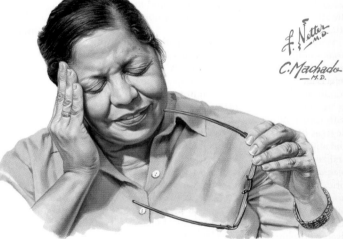

Headache

Plate 4-12

Rashes

BROWN RECLUSE SPIDERS AND SCABIES MITES

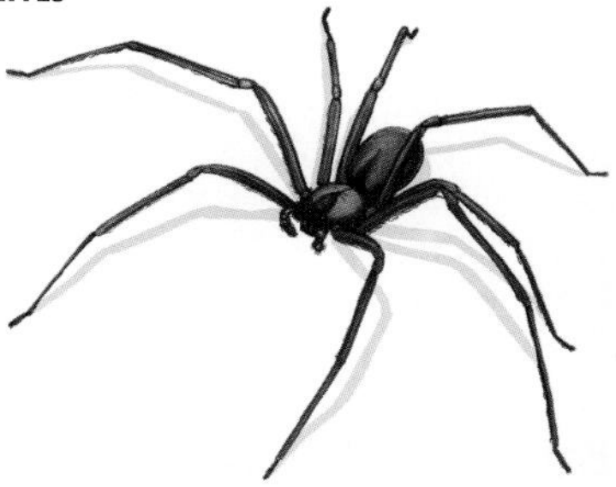

BUG BITES

Human skin is exposed to the environment on a constant basis and encounters multiple threats, including arthropods of many varieties. Each species of arthropod can inflict its own type of damage to the skin; some bites are mild and barely noticeable, and others can be life-threatening. The most common bites are those of mosquitoes, fleas, bedbugs, mites, ticks, and spiders. Not only can these bites cause direct damage to the skin, but these organisms may have the ability to transmit infectious diseases such as Lyme disease, leishmaniasis, and rickettsial diseases.

Clinical Findings: Mosquitoes are prominent insects in the spring, summer, and early fall seasons. In warmer climates, they can be seen year round. Their bite is often not noticed until after the mosquito has gone. The recently bitten person is left with a pruritic urticarial papule that typically resolves by itself within an hour or so. Some individuals are prone to severe bite reactions and develop warm, red papules and nodules that can last for a week or two and can be associated with regional lymphadenopathy. Mosquitoes are essentially a nuisance for the most part, but in some areas of the world they are the major vectors for transmission of malaria and encephalitis viruses. Sand flies are similar, but they are the major vector for leishmaniasis.

Fleas have been around since before the beginning of human civilization and were responsible in the Middle Ages for helping transmit the bubonic plague, which killed millions of people. Fleas are most commonly seen in households with pets. Individuals can be bitten after the pet transfers the fleas to bedding, carpeting, or clothing. Characteristic bites occur in groups of three, referred to as "breakfast, lunch, and dinner." Flea eggs can lay dormant for years, only to reactivate in response to movement and vibration that indicate a meal is likely to be nearby. Many flea bites occur around the ankles of adults; the fleas jump from the carpeting to the ankles, take their meal, and leave. The typical skin lesion is a small papule with a central punctum. It is self-resolving. Fleas have been known to carry organisms responsible for infectious diseases, including *Yersinia pestis* (bubonic plague) and *Rickettsia typhi* (murine typhus).

Bedbugs (*Cimex lectularius*) have made a resurgence in the United States. The are ubiquitous insects that can live in any area of the country. Households, hotels, and other sleeping quarters become infested with colonies of bedbugs. They emerge in the night, typically 1 to 2 hours before dawn, and search for a blood meal. They find their victim asleep and feed for a few minutes before retreating back to the nest. The nest is almost never in the bed; it is most likely to be located within the baseboard molding or floor boards. In the morning, the afflicted individual awakens with one to hundreds of bites. Most are small papules with a central punctum. Depending on the species of bedbug, a more inflammatory response may occur, causing vesiculation and bullae. Bedbugs have been reported to transmit hepatitis B virus.

Encounters with the large mite family of organisms are more likely to occur in the summer months in

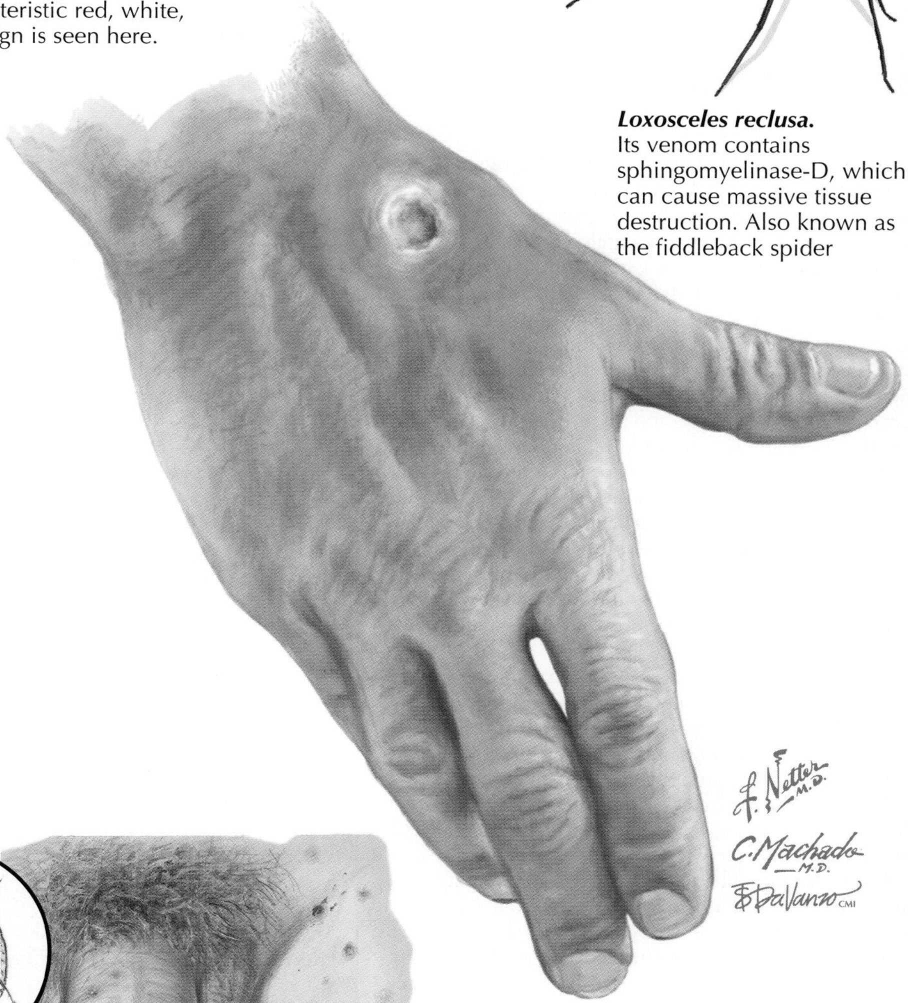

Brown recluse spider bite.
The characteristic red, white, and blue sign is seen here.

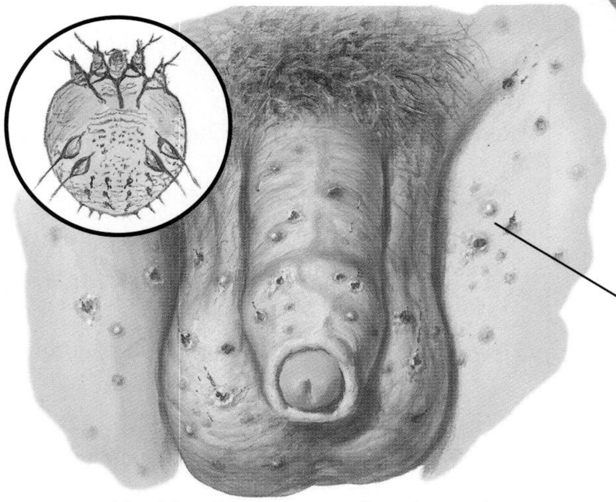

Loxosceles reclusa.
Its venom contains sphingomyelinase-D, which can cause massive tissue destruction. Also known as the fiddleback spider

Inflammatory excoriated papules (note penile involvement)

Scabies (*Sarcoptes scabiei*) in *circle*

northern latitudes but can occur at any time of the year in the southern regions. The term *chigger* refers to the larval phase of the Trombiculidae family of mites; it is one of the most common and well-recognized causes of human bites. Chiggers are small red mites, so small that they are not felt, and they bite quickly. They usually leave pinpoint red papules that can be numerous and can cause severe pruritus. Many other mites

are present in the environment and can cause similar reactions.

Most ticks bite and feed for up to 24 hours before falling off after receiving their blood meal. They can leave a tick bite granuloma, which is a small red papule with a central punctum, at the site of the bite. Many methods have been used to remove ticks; most can result in more skin damage than the actual tick bite.

Plate 4-13

Integumentary System

ARTHROPODS AND DISEASES THEY CARRY

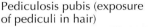

Phthirus pubis

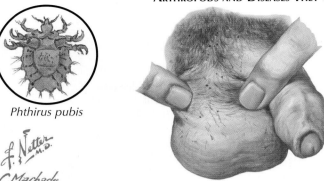

Pediculosis pubis (exposure of pediculi in hair)

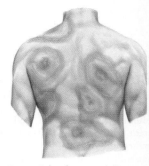

Deer ticks that carry Lyme disease can cause erythema migrans (bull's-eye rash)

BUG BITES (Continued)

These methods include burning the end of the tick with a cigarette or a match, an approach that is more likely to cause a skin burn than it is to remove the tick. The best method of removal is to grab the tick as close to the surface of the skin as possible and gently pull in a direction perpendicular to the skin. If the mouthparts are left embedded in the skin, a small punch biopsy can be performed to remove the remaining parts. Ticks are well known to transmit many infectious diseases, including Lyme disease and Rocky Mountain spotted fever.

Most spider bites are caused by jumping spiders. As with all spiders, bites frequently occurs after the spider's web or nesting location is disturbed. The bites can be painful and can leave erythema and a papule or nodular reaction. On occasion, these bites develop secondary cellulitis. Two spiders are unique in their potential to cause severe human disease: the black widow spider (*Latrodectus mactans*) and the brown recluse spider (*Loxosceles reclusa*).

The black widow spider is a web-weaving spider that paralyzes its prey with a potent neurotoxin called latrotoxin. The venom causes massive release of acetylcholine from nerve endings. In humans, this can lead to pain, fever, and symptoms of an acute abdomen.

The brown recluse spider is a solitary stalking spider that lives in dark, hidden locations. It is not aggressive and typically bites only when a human accidentally disturbs its location. The toxin released in its venom contains a mixture of sphingomyelinase-D, hyaluronidases, proteases, and esterases. Sphingomyelinase-D is the major component that is believed to be responsible for most of the tissue damage caused by the spider's bite. It can cause severe pain and aggregation of platelets and red blood cells, resulting in intravascular clotting with resultant necrosis of the skin. The characteristic pattern seen on the skin is a central bluish region with necrosis and coagulation, a surrounding vasoconstricted area that appears to be blanched white and a peripheral rim of erythema. This has been termed the "red, white, and blue" sign of a brown recluse bite. Some bites can progress rapidly and cause severe necrosis of the skin requiring surgical debridement.

Histology: Most bite reactions are not biopsied, because they are typically diagnosed clinically. The histological findings for most bug bites are very similar. There is a superficial and deep inflammatory infiltrate with many eosinophils. Superficial necrosis of the epidermis may be seen at the site of the bite. Occasionally, tick mouth parts are located in the biopsy specimen. Brown recluse spider bites show intravascular thrombosis and necrosis of the skin.

Treatment: The treatment of most bites is supportive. Pruritus can be treated with a potent topical corticosteroid and an oral antihistamine. Avoidance is the most important preventive measure. Areas of standing water provide breeding grounds for mosquitoes and should be drained routinely. Pets should be groomed

Arthropod	Disease it transmits	Appearance
Blackfly	Onchocerciasis	
Deer tick	Lyme disease, anaplasmosis, babesiosis	
Flea	Plague	
Lice	Typhus	
Lone star tick	Tularemia, anaplasmosis	
Mosquito	Malaria, yellow fever, dengue, encephalitis, West Nile virus	
Reduviid bug	Chagas disease	
Sandfly	Leishmaniasis	
Tsetse fly	African trypanosomiasis	
Wood tick	Rocky Mountain spotted fever	

and treated with preventive tick and flea medications. Flea and bedbug infestations should be treated by a professional exterminator. Proper use of bug sprays containing DEET (*N,N*-diethyl-*m*-toluamide) and staying in the center of wooded trails can help decrease one's chance of being bitten. In endemic areas, any patient with a deer tick bite that has lasted longer than 24 hours should be considered for prophylactic therapy for Lyme disease.

Narcotics (for pain control) and antivenin have been used to treat black widow spider bites and have been helpful. The antivenin is derived from horse serum, and there is a risk of an allergic reaction in susceptible patients. Brown recluse spider bites have been treated with many agents, including dapsone, to try to mitigate some of the inflammation-induced skin damage. Recognition of these spiders and avoidance is critical.

Plate 4-14

Rashes

CALCIPHYLAXIS

Calciphylaxis (calcific uremic arteriolopathy) results from deposition of calcium in the tunica media portion of the small vessel walls in association with proliferation of the intimal layer of endothelial cells. It is almost always associated with end-stage renal disease, especially in patients undergoing chronic dialysis (either peritoneal dialysis or hemodialysis). It has been reported to occur in up to 5% of patients who have been on dialysis for longer than 1 year. Calciphylaxis typically manifests as nonhealing skin ulcers located in adipose-rich areas of the trunk and thighs, but the lesions can occur anywhere. They are believed to be caused by an abnormal ratio of calcium and phosphorus, which leads to the abnormal deposition within the tunica media of small blood vessels. This eventually results in thrombosis and ulceration of the overlying skin. Calciphylaxis has a poor prognosis, and there are few well-studied therapies.

Clinical Findings: Calciphylaxis is almost exclusively seen in patients with chronic end-stage renal disease. Most patients have been on one form of dialysis for at least 1 year by the time of presentation. The initial presenting sign is that of a tender, dusky red to purple macule that quickly ulcerates. The ulcerations have a ragged border and a thick black necrotic eschar. The ulcers tend to increase in size, and new areas appear before older ulcers have any opportunity to heal. Ulcerations begin proximally and tend to follow the path of the underlying affected blood vessel. Their most prominent location is within the adipose-rich areas of the trunk and thighs, especially the abdomen and mammary regions. Patients often report that ulcerations form in areas of trauma. The main differential diagnosis is between an infectious cause and calciphylaxis. Skin biopsies and cultures can be performed to differentiate the two. Skin biopsies are diagnostic. Radiographs of the region often show calcification of the small vessels, and this can be used to support the diagnosis. Patients who develop calciphylaxis have a poor prognosis, with the mortality rate reaching 80% in some series. For some unknown reason, those with truncal disease tend to survive longer than those with distal extremity disease. Complications caused by the chronic severe ulcerations (e.g., infection, sepsis) are the main cause of mortality.

Laboratory findings often show an elevated calcium × phosphorus product. A calcium × phosphorus product greater than 70 mg^2/dL^2 appears to be an independent risk factor for development of calciphylaxis. Other risk factors are obesity, hyperparathyroidism, diabetes, and the use of warfarin. Elevated parathyroid hormone (PTH) levels are often found in association with calciphylaxis. The exact role that PTH plays is unknown, but it has been reported that parathyroidectomy, a standard treatment for calciphylaxis in the past, is not an effective means of therapy. PTH may play a role in starting the disease, but it does not appear to be necessary to exacerbate or cause continuation of calciphylaxis.

Pathogenesis: The exact mechanism of calcification of the tunica media of blood vessels in calciphylaxis is not completely understood. The fact that it is seen almost exclusively in patients undergoing chronic dialysis therapy has led to many theories on its origin. The final mechanism is a hardening of the vessel wall with calcification and intimal endothelial proliferation that leads to rapid and successive thrombosis and necrosis.

Although most commonly seen in areas of high fat content (abdomen, breast), all areas of the skin may be involved in calciphylaxis. Almost all cases are associated with underlying renal disease.

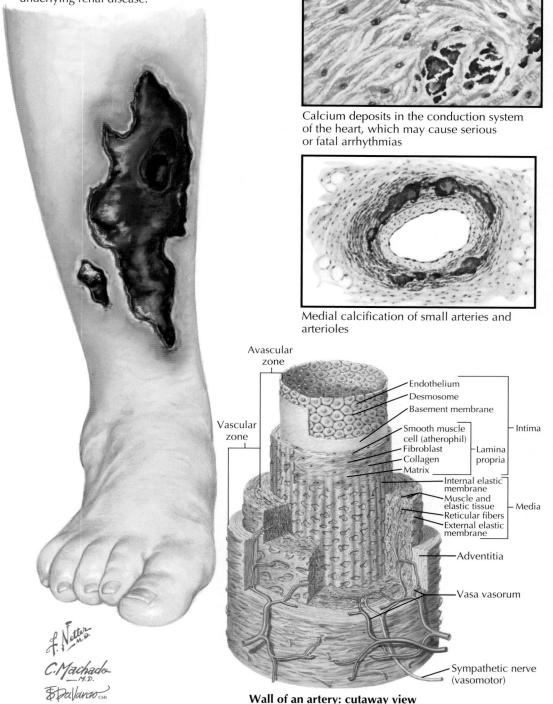

Calcium deposits in the conduction system of the heart, which may cause serious or fatal arrhythmias

Medial calcification of small arteries and arterioles

Avascular zone

Vascular zone

Endothelium
Desmosome
Basement membrane
Smooth muscle cell (atherophil)
Fibroblast
Collagen
Matrix
Intima
Lamina propria
Internal elastic membrane
Muscle and elastic tissue
Reticular fibers
External elastic membrane
Media
Adventitia
Vasa vasorum
Sympathetic nerve (vasomotor)

Wall of an artery: cutaway view

Histology: The main finding is of calcification of the medial section of the small blood vessels in and around the area of involvement. Thrombi within the vessel lumen are often observed. Intimal layer endothelial proliferation is prominent. The abnormal calcification can easily be seen on hematoxylin and eosin staining.

Treatment: No good therapy exists for calciphylaxis. Aggressive supportive care and early treatment of superinfections are critical. Surgical debridement of wounds is necessary to remove necrotic tissue that provides a portal for infection. Renal transplantation offers some hope for cure. Treatment with sodium thiosulfate has shown success in some anecdotal reports, but this is not a universal cure. The newer bisphosphonate medications have also been used with limited success. Parathyroidectomy may help initially with the ulcerations, but it does not decrease mortality.

Plate 4-15   Integumentary System

CUTANEOUS LUPUS

Lupus erythematosus is a multisystem, idiopathic connective tissue disease that can have variable and unique clinical cutaneous findings. Cutaneous lupus may be considered as a spectrum of skin disease. Many variants have been described. Discoid lupus, subacute cutaneous lupus, tumid lupus, lupus panniculitis, neonatal lupus, lupus chilblains, and systemic lupus erythematosus (SLE) all have morphologically distinctive cutaneous findings. Lupus is a heterogeneous disease with a wide continuum of clinical involvement, from purely cutaneous disease to life-threatening SLE. The cutaneous findings are often the first presenting signs, and recognition of the skin manifestations can help make the diagnosis of lupus.

SLE is the most severe form of lupus. Its clinical course and outcome vary, from mild forms to severe, life-threatening variants. In the most severe cases, the pulmonary, cardiac, neurological, and connective tissue and integumentary systems are affected. Death may occur from renal failure. Severe arthritis and skin findings are often present. SLE is diagnosed by fulfillment of criteria that have been established by the American College of Rheumatology. Variations in meeting these criteria from one patient with SLE to the next are responsible for the varying clinical spectrum of disease.

Patients with lupus can have many laboratory abnormalities. These include anemia of chronic disease and an elevated erythrocyte sedimentation rate. Antinuclear antibodies (ANA) are found in some subsets of lupus, with almost 100% of patients with the systemic form testing positive for ANA. Many other, more specific antibodies are found in patients with SLE, including anti-Smith antibodies and anti–double-stranded DNA antibodies. Patients with renal disease often have hypertension, elevated protein levels in their urine, and an elevated creatinine level.

Clinical Findings: Many variants of cutaneous lupus exist, each with its own morphological findings. Lupus is more common in women; it can be seen at any age but is most frequently observed in early adulthood. However, lupus is common enough that it is not infrequently seen in males. Neonatal lupus is a rare form that occurs in neonates born to mothers with lupus.

Discoid lupus is one of the easiest forms of cutaneous lupus to recognize. It is most commonly found on the head and neck region and has a tendency to be present within the conchal bowl of the ear. Lesions are often found in patients with SLE. Discoid lupus may occur as an entirely separate disease with no other systemic or clinical findings of lupus. Fewer than 10% of these patients eventually progress to the systemic form of lupus. Discoid lesions are exacerbated by sun exposure, more specifically by exposure to ultraviolet A (UVA) light. The lesions tend to have an annular configuration with varying amounts of scale. The lesions can produce alopecia, and there is almost always some amount of atrophy present. Follicular plugging is commonly seen in discoid lupus. It is noticed clinically as a dilation of the follicular orifices. Follicle plugs can also be seen by gently removing the scale from a discoid lesion. On close inspection of the inferior side of the scale, one will notice minute keratotic follicular plugs. This finding is specific for discoid lupus and has been termed the

"carpet tack sign," because it resembles tiny outreaching tacks. This sign can be easily missed if the scale is removed too quickly or not inspected closely enough. Discoid lesions in darker-skinned individuals may also have varying amounts of hyperpigmentation. Most patients have some erythema and hyperpigmentation. Most patients present with a few discoid lesions and are said to have localized discoid lupus. Those rare patients

with widespread disease have generalized discoid lupus. This variant is rare, and such patients are much more likely than those with localized disease to go on to fulfill the criteria for SLE at some point. The alopecia seen in discoid lupus is scarring in nature, and the hair that has been lost will not regrow even with aggressive therapy. Alopecia can be life-altering and can cause significant psychological morbidity.

CUTANEOUS LUPUS BAND TEST

A. Erythematous malar rash

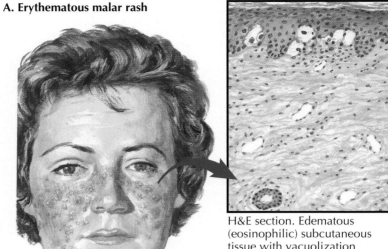

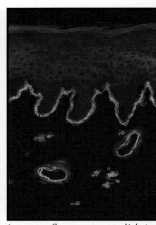

H&E section. Edematous (eosinophilic) subcutaneous tissue with vacuolization of basilar epithelium at the dermal-epidermal junction

Immunofluorescence slide*: bandlike granular deposit of gamma globulin and complement at the dermal-epidermal junction and in the walls of small dermal vessels

B. Normal-appearing (nonlesional and non–sun-exposed) skin of lupus patient

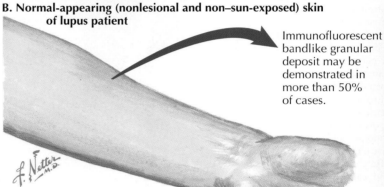

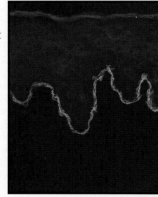

Immunofluorescent bandlike granular deposit may be demonstrated in more than 50% of cases.

C. Discoid lupus

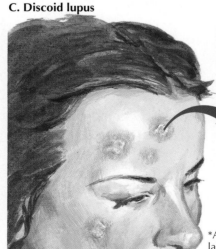

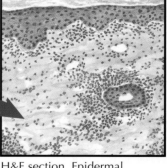

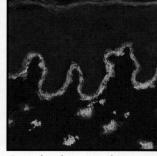

H&E section. Epidermal atrophy, hyalinization of dermis, chronic inflammation around hair follicles

Granular deposits of immune complexes at the dermal-epidermal junction and within dermis

*All fluorescence slides were stained with fluorescein-labeled rabbit antihuman gamma globulin.

Plate 4-16

Rashes

CUTANEOUS LUPUS (Continued)

Subacute cutaneous lupus erythematosus is seen in a subset of patients and has a higher incidence of developing into full-blown SLE compared with other forms of cutaneous lupus. There are variants of subacute cutaneous lupus, with the annular form and the papulosquamous form being the two most common and most important to recognize. The annular form manifests with pink to red annular patches that slowly expand and coalesce into larger, interconnected polycyclic patches. They occur most commonly on sun-exposed skin of the face and upper trunk. The papulosquamous version also manifests in sun-exposed regions. It appears as smaller, pink-red patches with overlying scale. Both forms are exacerbated by sun exposure and are pruritic. They heal with no scarring.

Neonatal lupus is an uncommon form of lupus that can manifest with or without cutaneous findings. However, cutaneous findings are the most universal clinical finding in neonatal lupus, occurring in more than 90% of those affected. The most common scenario is a child born to a mother who has not yet been diagnosed with lupus. Neonatal lupus can manifest with varying degrees of congenital heart block, and this is the most serious sequela. Some children require a pacemaker to control the arrhythmia. Thrombocytopenia is also one of the more frequent effects of neonatal lupus. Neonatal lupus is directly caused by the transplacental migration of anti-Ro (anti-SSA) antibodies and, to a lesser extent, anti-La (anti-SSB) antibodies. The antibodies are only transiently present, because the newborn does not produce any new antibodies. Therefore, neonatal lupus improves over time, and most children have no long-term difficulties. The cutaneous findings in neonatal lupus include pink to red patches or plaques, predominantly in a periorbital location. The rash resolves with time, and if any residual skin finding remains, it is that of fine telangiectases in the location of the patches and some fine atrophy. The telangiectases and atrophy tend to improve as the child enters adulthood.

Lupus panniculitis (lupus profundus) is a rare cutaneous manifestation of lupus. It manifests as a tender dermal nodule, more commonly in women. A large percentage of patients with lupus panniculitis have been reported to go on to develop SLE. The overlying skin may appear slightly erythematous to hyperpigmented, but there is no appreciable surface change. The dermal nodules tend to slowly enlarge with time. The diagnosis can be made only by biopsy, because the clinical picture is not specific. Biopsies of these dermal nodules are best performed with an excisional technique to obtain sufficient tissue for diagnosis. The inflammation is entirely confined to the subcutaneous tissue. The histological differential diagnosis of lupus panniculitis is often between lupus and cutaneous T-cell panniculitis. The diagnosis requires the use of both clinical and histological information. The histological evaluation often requires immunohistochemical staining to help differentiate the lesions from those of other mimickers. Lesions of lupus panniculitis often heal with atrophic scarring.

Tumid lupus is a rare clinical variant of cutaneous lupus that typically manifests as a red dermal plaque on a sun-exposed surface of the skin. Clinically, it can appear similar to polymorphous light eruption,

lymphoma, pseudolymphoma, or Jessner's lymphocytic infiltrate. The plaques are exacerbated by ultraviolet light exposure. They are frequently asymptomatic to slightly tender but rarely pruritic. They tend to wax and wane, with the worst outbreaks occurring in the springtime and remissions in the winter. Histologically, the infiltrate has been found to be more of a CD4+ T-cell infiltrate.

Lupus chilblains is a unique form of Raynaud's phenomenon, and it is identical in clinical presentation to pernio. It may be that this is just pernio occurring in a patient with lupus. Lupus chilblains and pernio manifest typically on the distal extremities, the toes being the most commonly affected region. The patient develops tender, cold, purplish papules and plaques. The rash is exacerbated by cold and wet environments.

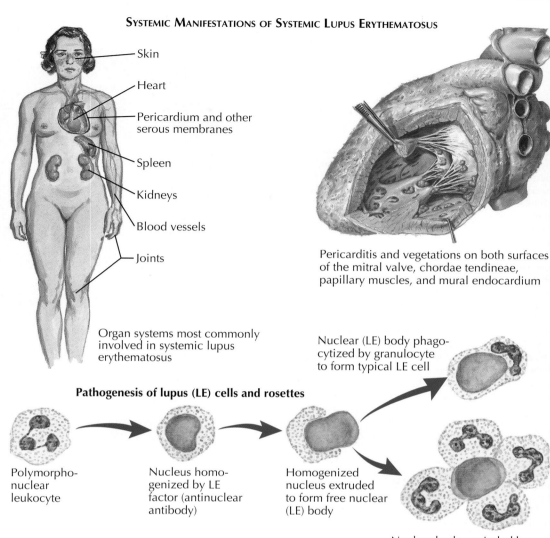

SYSTEMIC MANIFESTATIONS OF SYSTEMIC LUPUS ERYTHEMATOSUS

Skin
Heart
Pericardium and other serous membranes
Spleen
Kidneys
Blood vessels
Joints

Organ systems most commonly involved in systemic lupus erythematosus

Pericarditis and vegetations on both surfaces of the mitral valve, chordae tendineae, papillary muscles, and mural endocardium

Pathogenesis of lupus (LE) cells and rosettes

Polymorpho-nuclear leukocyte

Nucleus homogenized by LE factor (antinuclear antibody)

Homogenized nucleus extruded to form free nuclear (LE) body

Nuclear (LE) body phagocytized by granulocyte to form typical LE cell

Nuclear body encircled by granulocytes to form LE rosette

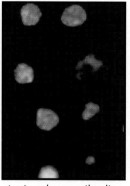

Antinuclear antibodies demonstrated by fluorescence

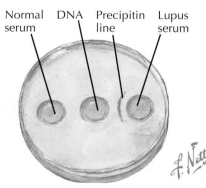

Normal serum   DNA   Precipitin line   Lupus serum

DNA antibodies demonstrated by precipitin test on agar plate

Positive   Negative

Hemagglutination of gamma globulin–coated red cells by SLE serum (tubes viewed from below). Latex agglutination test may also be done as for rheumatoid factor.

Plate 4-17

Integumentary System

CUTANEOUS MANIFESTATIONS OF LUPUS

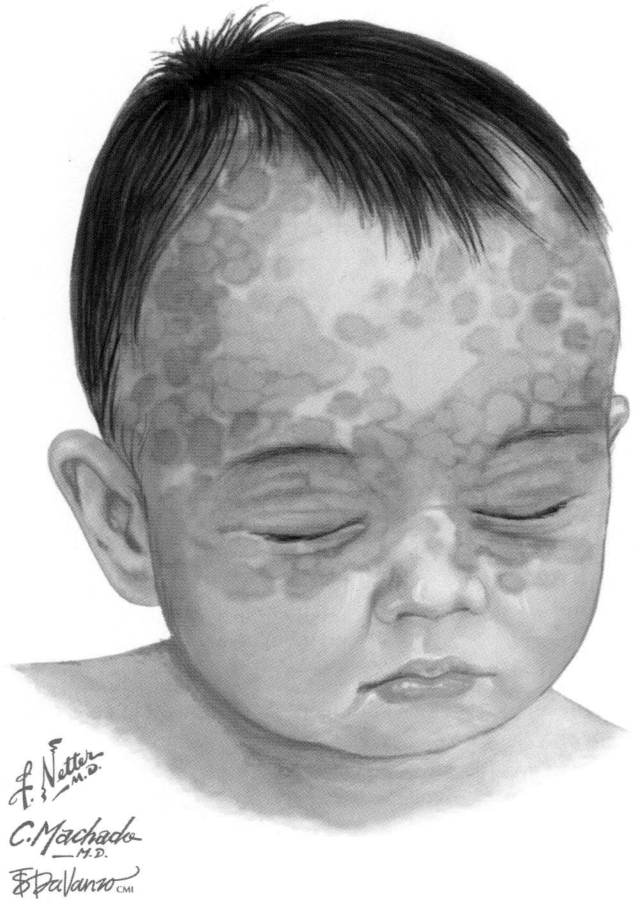

CUTANEOUS LUPUS (Continued)

Treatment includes keeping the regions dry and warm by avoiding cold exposure. Patients diagnosed with pernio probably should undergo screening for lupus, because a small percentage of them actually have lupus chilblains. Histological evaluation of lupus chilblains shows a dense lymphocytic infiltrate with some areas of thrombosis of small vessels and a lymphocytic vasculitis.

The cutaneous findings seen in SLE are vast and can overlap with other forms of cutaneous lupus. Although the systemic findings are responsible for the morbidity and mortality, the cutaneous findings are often the presenting sign, and, if the clinician is aware, they can help make the diagnosis. The most important of the cutaneous skin findings in SLE is the malar rash. This rash manifests as a tender, pink-to-red plaque or patch on the cheeks and nose, mimicking the shape of a butterfly; hence, it has been termed the "butterfly rash of lupus." It is commonly mistaken for rosacea, and vice versa. Rosacea typically affects a wider area of skin and is associated with more telangiectases and papulopustular lesions. The malar rash of lupus also spares the nasolabial fold, which is an important clinical finding and a discriminating objective discovery. It is typically more prominent during systemic flares of the underlying SLE, and patients can appear very ill. Patients are exquisitely photosensitive, and the rash is exacerbated by exposure to ultraviolet light.

Discoid lupus is also seen as a manifestation of systemic lupus, and it has the same clinical appearance as described earlier. Raynaud's phenomenon is well described, and a high percentage of patients with SLE report those symptoms. Alopecia was long used to help make the diagnosis of lupus. It is no longer part of the diagnostic criteria, but it can have significant psychological impact on the patient. Nail and capillary nail fold changes are seen if looked for. The true incidence of these findings is unknown. Nail fold telangiectases and erythema are the two most common nail findings. Nail pitting, ridging, and alterations in the color of the lunula have also been reported. Lupus patients with nail changes have been found to have a higher incidence of mucosal ulcerations, which are another of the mucocutaneous findings of SLE. Livedo reticularis is a fishnet-like pattern found typically on the lower extremities; it is a nonspecific finding but has been reported commonly in lupus. It also occurs in many other skin and systemic diseases.

Histology: The histological findings in all forms of lupus are similar, with specific forms having some unique findings. Most forms show an interface dermatitis with hydropic changes in the basilar layer of the epidermis. A superficial and deep periadnexal lymphocytic infiltrate is almost universally seen. Other connective tissue diseases (e.g., dermatomyositis) can have similar histological findings. Discoid lupus may show scarring, atrophy, and follicular plugging along with these other findings. Lupus panniculitis is unique in that the inflammation is localized to the subcutaneous tissue. The diagnosis of lupus panniculitis is difficult and requires a host of special stains and clinical pathological correlation.

Neonatal lupus. Neonatal lupus is transient in nature and is caused by maternal antibodies that cross the placenta. Newborns are at risk for developing heart block. The cutaneous findings eventually resolve spontaneously.

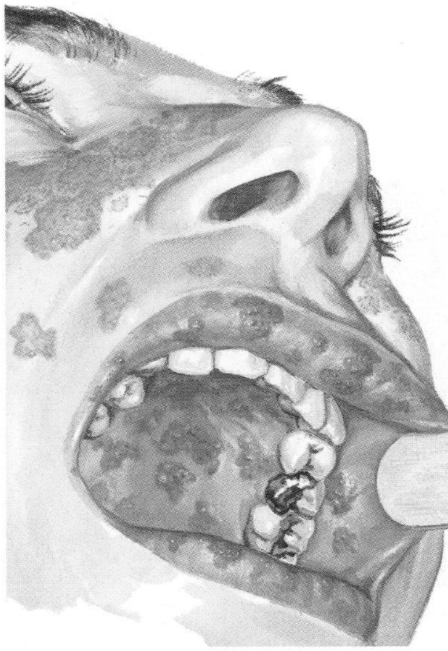

Lupus erythematosus disseminatus

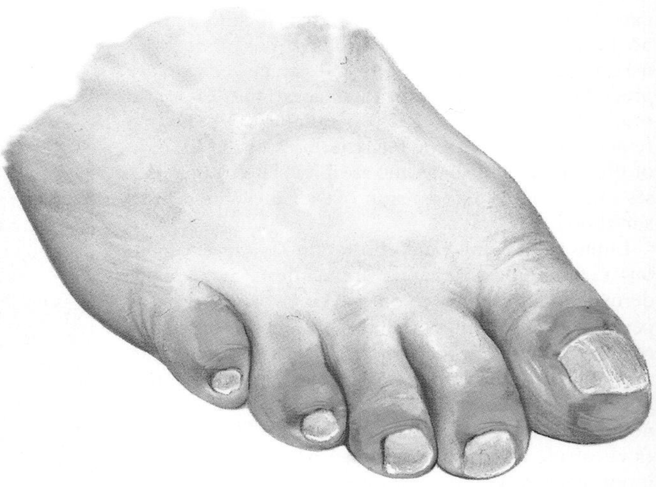

Lupus chilblains. Tender red to purple macules and papules on the feet. Exacerbated by cold and wet environments

Treatment: The treatment of cutaneous lupus is difficult and must be tailored to the patient and the specific form of lupus. Potent topical corticosteroids may work for a tiny lesion of discoid lupus, but they are not effective in lupus panniculitis. Universal treatment of cutaneous lupus requires sun protection and sunscreen use. The sunscreen used should block in the UVA range, because this is the most active form of ultraviolet light that exacerbates lupus. Smoking should be ceased immediately, and patients should be screened routinely by their family physician or rheumatologist for progression of the disease.

Specific therapies for cutaneous lupus include oral prednisone and hydroxychloroquine or chloroquine as the typical first-line agents. If these are unsuccessful, quinacrine can be added. Other agents that have been reported to be effective include dapsone, isotretinoin, and methotrexate.

Plate 4-18

Rashes

CUTIS LAXA

Cutis laxa is an unusual skin disease with multisystem complications. It has highly characteristic cutaneous findings. Laxity of the skin is the hallmark of this disease. The skin becomes easily stretched, and there is little elastic rebound. As patients age, gravity alone can make the skin droop to a disfiguring degree. Some forms of cutis laxa are incompatible with life, and those affected die in infancy. Many variants of cutis laxa have been described. With the discovery of the responsible gene defects, the phenotypes of this disease that are seen clinically have been better defined on the genetic level. Acquired variants of cutis laxa have been described.

Clinical Findings: Cutis laxa has no sexual or racial predilection. The cutaneous hallmark of the disease is loose, hanging skin with a lack of elasticity. The skin can be pulled with little resistance; the normal return of the skin to its preexisting state is delayed. The skin in the axillae and groin folds is prominently affected, as is the facial skin. The face is said to take on a "hound dog" appearance. All skin is involved to varying degrees, but the effects are most noticeable in areas of the face and in the skin folds. The overlying epidermis is completely normal, and the adnexal structures are spared.

Internal manifestations are variable and are more common with the autosomal recessive forms of the disease. The pulmonary, cardiovascular, and gastrointestinal systems can be affected by fragmentation or loss of elastic tissue, leading, respectively, to emphysema, aneurysms, and diverticula.

Those with the autosomal dominant form appear to have normal life spans, whereas those with the other variants have significantly shortened life spans secondary to severe systemic involvement.

Pathogenesis: Many modes of inheritance have been reported for cutis laxa, including autosomal recessive, autosomal dominant, and X-linked recessive forms. The X-linked form is now considered to be the same disease as Ehlers-Danlos syndrome IX. This form is caused by a defect in a copper-dependent adenosine triphosphatase (ATPase) protein found within the Golgi apparatus.

There are two autosomal recessive variants of cutis laxa. The autosomal recessive variant type I is extremely rare, and those afflicted typically die early in infancy from severe pulmonary and multisystem failure. Autosomal recessive type I cutis laxa has been found to be caused by a defect in the *fibulin-5* gene *(FBLN5)*. The product of this gene is critical in producing functional elastic fibers. Its absence is incompatible with life. Type II autosomal recessive cutis laxa is more commonly encountered than type I. The genetic defect in type II cutis laxa has yet to be defined. Patients with type II experience developmental delay and have varying amounts of joint laxity.

The most frequently seen form of cutis laxa is the autosomal dominant form, which is caused by a defect in the *elastin* gene *(ELN)*. Many different mutations in this gene have been described, and they lead to slightly different phenotypes of the disease.

All of these gene defects lead to abnormalities in the elastic fiber protein, resulting in elastolysis. Various defects lead to different irregularities in the elastic fibers, but the end result in all forms is seen clinically as cutis laxa.

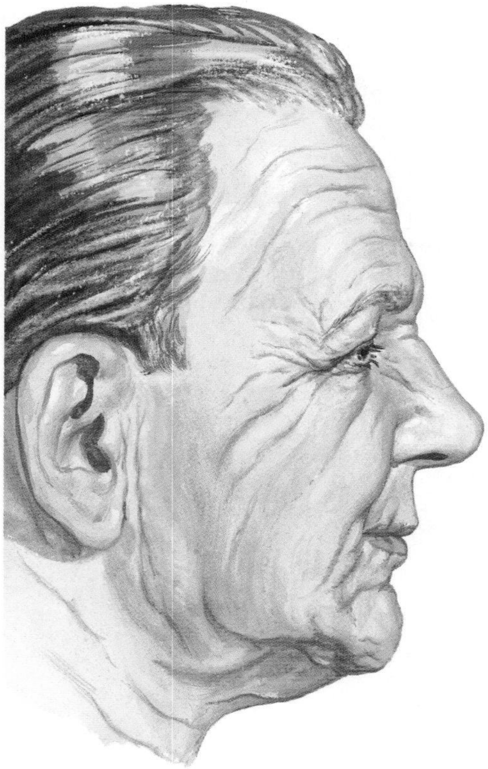

Cutis laxa. This rare disease is caused by the premature degeneration of elastic fibers. It manifests clinically with excessive sagging of the skin. The affected face may take on a "hound dog" appearance.

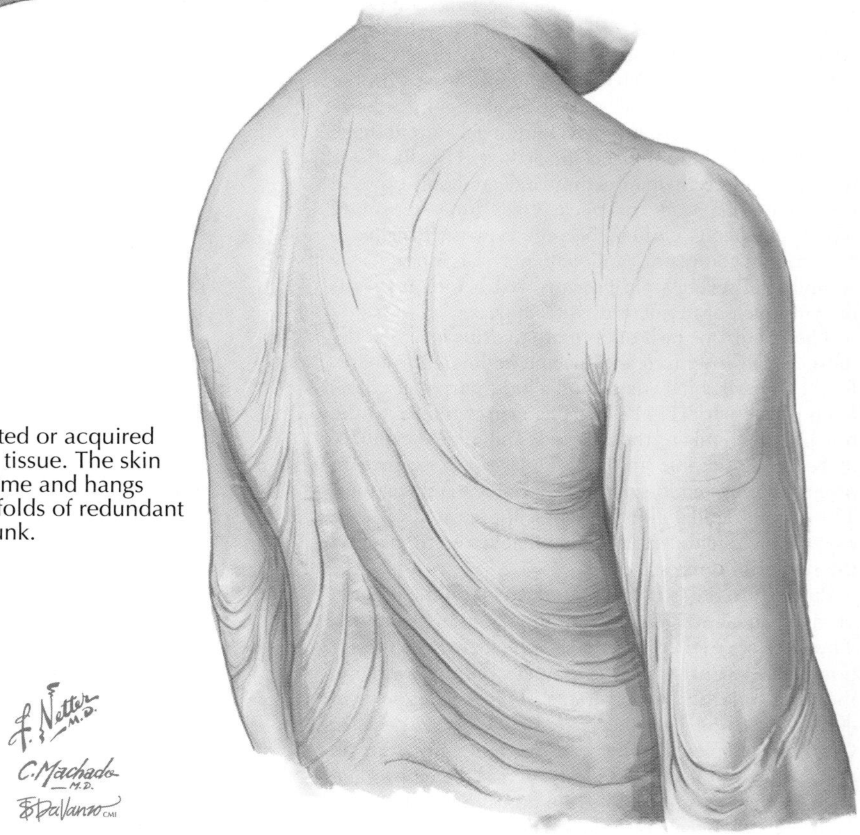

Cutis laxa is an inherited or acquired abnormality of elastic tissue. The skin becomes loose over time and hangs from the body. Large folds of redundant skin present on the trunk.

Histology: Histological examination of skin biopsies from patients with cutis laxa reveals varying degrees of elastic fiber damage and/or loss. The best way to appreciate this is with special staining to highlight elastic tissue. In some cases, there is a complete loss of elastic fibers; in others, fragmented and reduced amounts of elastic tissue are seen.

Treatment: The main goals of therapy is to screen for underlying cardiac or gastrointestinal abnormalities and for the possibility of aortic aneurysm or gastrointestinal diverticula formation. There is no medication that can reverse the genetic defect, and no gene replacement therapy is available. Excessive skin can be surgically removed to improve functionality and cosmesis.

Plate 4-19

Integumentary System

DERMATOMYOSITIS

Dermatomyositis is a chronic connective tissue disease that can be associated with an underlying internal malignancy. This connective tissue disease shares similarities with polymyositis, but the latter has no cutaneous findings. Up to one third of patients with dermatomyositis have an underlying malignancy. The myositis is often prominent and manifests as tenderness and weakness of the proximal muscle groups. The pelvic and shoulder girdle muscles are the ones most commonly affected. Dermatomyositis sine myositis is a well-recognized variant that has only the cutaneous findings; evidence of muscle involvement is absent.

Clinical Findings: Dermatomyositis has a bimodal age of onset, with the most common form occurring in the female adult population, usually between the ages of 45 and 60 years, and a smaller peak in childhood at about 10 to 15 years of age. African Americans are affected three to four times more often than Caucasians. Dermatomyositis has an insidious onset, with the development of proximal muscle weakness in association with various dermatological findings. Skin findings start slowly and are nonspecific at first. Usually, there is some mild erythema on the hands and sun-exposed regions of the head and neck. Over time, the more typical cutaneous findings become evident. Pruritus is a common complaint, and patients not infrequently complain of severe scalp pruritus well before any signs or symptoms of dermatomyositis appear.

The heliotrope rash of dermatomyositis is one of the most easily recognized and specific findings. It is manifested by periorbital edema and a light purple discoloration of the periorbital skin. The skin is tender to the touch. Hyperemia of the nail beds and dilated capillary loops are noticeable and are similar to those seen in progressive systemic sclerosis or lupus erythematous. The dilated capillary loops are best appreciated with the use of a handheld dermatoscope that serves to magnify the region of interest.

Purplish to red, scaly papules develop on the dorsum of the hands overlying the joints of the phalanges. These are not Heberden's nodes, which are a manifestation of osteoarthritis seen as dermal swellings overlying the distal interphalangeal joints. The papules seen in dermatomyositis have been termed *Gottron's papules.* Gottron's papules may be seen overlying any joint on the hands, as well as other joints such as the elbows and knees. The skin findings on the dorsal hands have led to the term "mechanic's hands." This refers to the ragged appearance of the hands in dermatomyositis; they resemble the hands of a mechanic that have suffered chronic trauma, abrasions, and erosions secondary to the occupation.

The "shawl sign" is a cutaneous finding seen on the upper back and chest. The shawl sign is so named because the location is in the same area that would be covered by a shawl garment. The skin has poikilodermatous macules and patches. There is a varying amount of skin atrophy with telangiectases, mottled hyperpigmentation and hypopigmentation, and erythema of the involved region.

MANIFESTATIONS OF DERMATOMYOSITIS

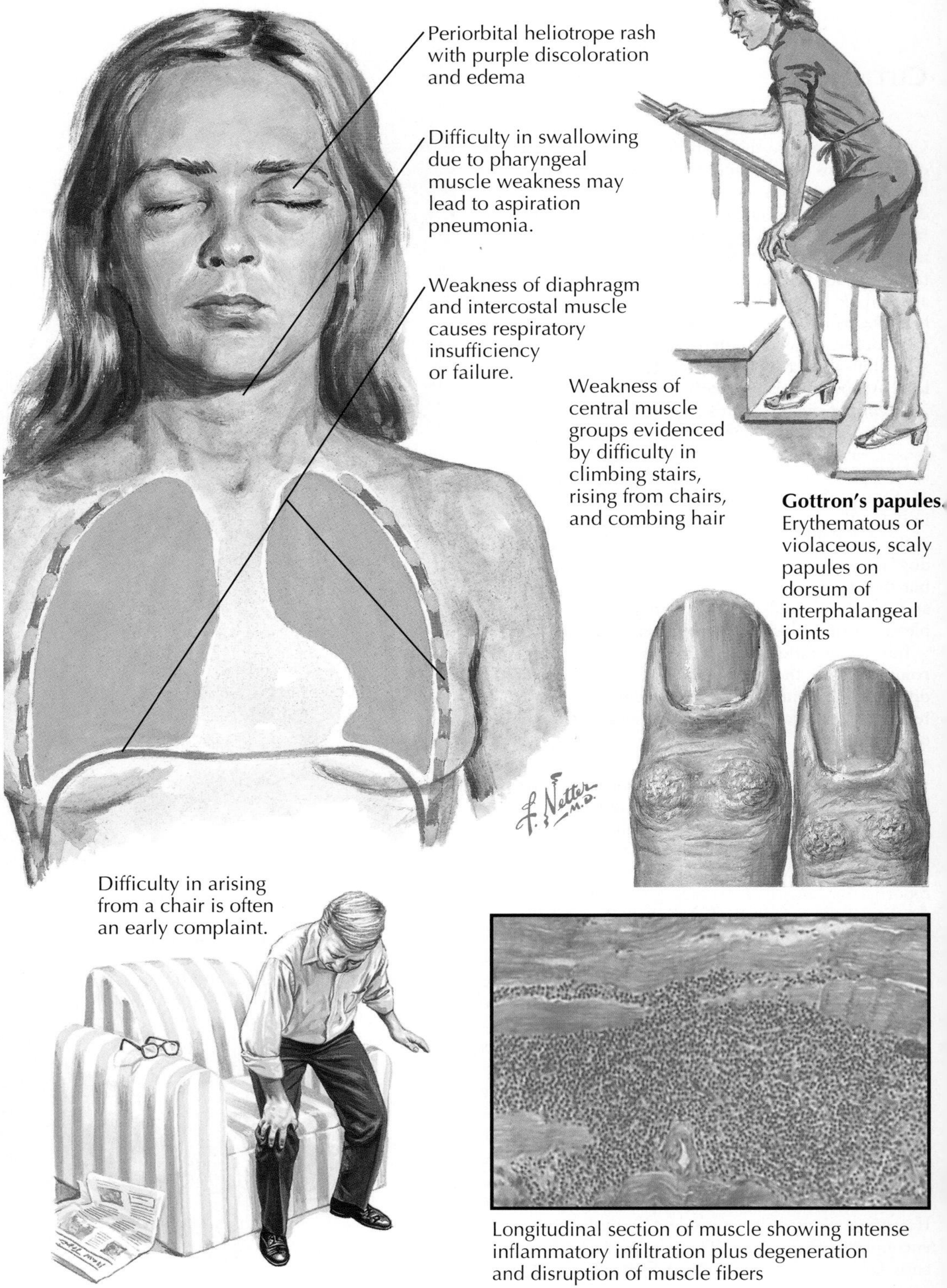

Periorbital heliotrope rash with purple discoloration and edema

Difficulty in swallowing due to pharyngeal muscle weakness may lead to aspiration pneumonia.

Weakness of diaphragm and intercostal muscle causes respiratory insufficiency or failure.

Weakness of central muscle groups evidenced by difficulty in climbing stairs, rising from chairs, and combing hair

Gottron's papules. Erythematous or violaceous, scaly papules on dorsum of interphalangeal joints

Difficulty in arising from a chair is often an early complaint.

Longitudinal section of muscle showing intense inflammatory infiltration plus degeneration and disruption of muscle fibers

Patients with dermatomyositis also complain of photosensitivity and notice a flare of their skin disease with ultraviolet light exposure. Children with dermatomyositis are much more prone to develop calcinosis cutis than their adult counterparts, and approximately 50% of all children with dermatomyositis will develop this feature. Calcinosis cutis manifests as tender dermal nodules or as calcifications along the muscle fascia.

Leukocytoclastic vasculitis also is seen much more frequently in juvenile dermatomyositis than in the adult form.

Dermatomyositis is a multisystem disorder. Diagnostic criteria have been established by the American College of Rheumatology. They are based on the presence of clinical, laboratory, and histological findings. Not all patients have all aspects of the disease, and

Plate 4-20

Rashes

DERMATOMYOSITIS (Continued)

the diagnosis is based on the number of the criteria fulfilled.

Inflammation of the proximal muscle groups has been well described. Patients often complain of difficulty in standing from a sitting position or in raising their hands above their heads. Patients have elevated serum concentrations of creatinine kinase, aldolase, and lactate dehydrogenase. This is indicative of muscle inflammation and breakdown. An electromyogram (EMG) can be used to evaluate the weakness and to differentiate a nerve origin from a muscle origin. A muscle biopsy, most commonly of the deltoid muscle, shows active inflammation on histological examination.

This disease can rarely manifest with severe, diffuse interstitial pulmonary fibrosis. Patients with pulmonary fibrosis most often test positive for the anti-Jo1 antibody. Anti-Jo1 antibodies have been found to be targeted against the histidyl–transfer RNA synthetase protein. Overall, it is an uncommon finding except in dermatomyositis patients with pulmonary disease. More than 75% of patients with dermatomyositis test positive for antinuclear antibodies (ANA). Those with malignancy-associated dermatomyositis typically do not develop pulmonary fibrosis, and those with pulmonary fibrosis do not develop a malignancy.

The malignancy most commonly associated with dermatomyositis is ovarian cancer. Many other malignancies have been seen in association with dermatomyositis, including breast, lung, lymphoma, and gastric cancers. Malignancy is seen before the onset of the rash in about one third of the cases, concurrently with the rash in one third, and within 2 years after diagnosis of the dermatomyositis in one third. After the diagnosis of dermatomyositis, it is imperative to search for an underlying malignancy and to perform age-appropriate cancer screening. Childhood dermatomyositis is rarely associated with an underlying malignancy.

Pathogenesis: The exact etiology of dermatomyositis is unknown. It has been theorized to occur secondary to abnormalities in the humoral immune system. The precise mechanism is under intense research.

Histology: Histological examination of a skin biopsy specimen shows an interface lymphocytic dermatitis. Hydropic change is seen scattered along the basilar cell layer. The epidermis has varying degrees of atrophy. A superficial and deep periadnexal lymphocytic infiltrate is common. The presence of dermal mucin in abundance is another histological clue to the diagnosis. A muscle biopsy often shows atrophy of the involved muscle with a dense lymphocytic infiltrate.

Treatment: There is no known cure for dermatomyositis, although some cases spontaneously remit. Cases associated with an underlying malignancy have been shown to go into full remission with cure of the underlying cancer. Relapse of dermatomyositis in these patients should prompt the clinician to search for a recurrence of their malignancy. Initial treatment is usually with prednisone, which acts as a nonspecific immunosuppressant. The addition of a steroid-sparing agent is almost always needed to avoid the long-term side effects of prednisone. Some patients require a smaller dose of prednisone along with a steroid-sparing

agent to keep the disease at bay. Many steroid-sparing agents have been used, including hydroxychloroquine, quinacrine, cyclosporine, intravenous immunoglobulin (IVIG), azathioprine, and methotrexate, all with variable success. Combination therapy is the norm.

The use of sun protection and sunscreen cannot be overemphasized. Topical corticosteroids help relieve

the itching and decrease some of the redness. The treatment of juvenile dermatomyositis is similar. It is believed to have a better prognosis, because few cases are associated with an underlying cancer. It is thought that early treatment of juvenile dermatomyositis decreases the risk of developing severe calcinosis cutis during the course of the disease.

CUTANEOUS AND LABORATORY FINDINGS IN DERMATOMYOSITIS

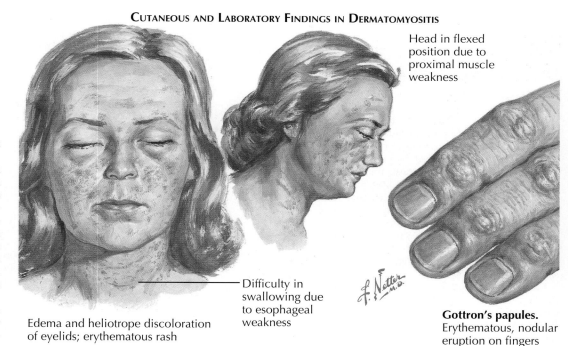

Head in flexed position due to proximal muscle weakness

Difficulty in swallowing due to esophageal weakness

Edema and heliotrope discoloration of eyelids; erythematous rash

Gottron's papules. Erythematous, nodular eruption on fingers

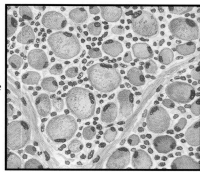

Atrophy of muscle fibers and lymphocyte infiltration (muscle biopsy)

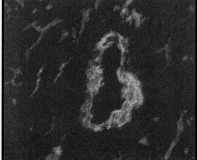

Immunoglobulin deposition in blood vessel of muscle (immunofluorescence)

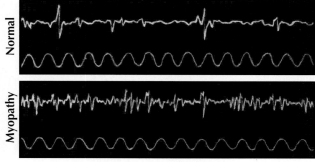

Normal

Myopathy

Electromyogram shows fibrillations

Laboratory findings

1. Nonspecific hypergammaglobulinemia; low incidence of antinuclear antibodies and rheumatoid factor

2. Elevated serum enzymes. creatine phosphokinase (CPK), aldolase, and aspartate amine transferase (AST, SGOT)

3. Elevated urinary creatine and myoglobulin levels

Plate 4-21

Integumentary System

DISSEMINATED INTRAVASCULAR COAGULATION

Disseminated intravascular coagulation (DIC) is a serious, life-threatening condition of the blood clotting system that can be caused by myriad insults to the body. It has a grave prognosis unless caught and treated early in the course of disease. Skin manifestations occur early and continue to progress unless the patient recovers. The skin lesions may lead to gangrene and secondary infection, further worsening the prognosis. DIC is seen as an end-stage process, caused by the consumption of blood clotting factors, that results in uncontrolled clotting and bleeding occurring simultaneously.

Clinical Findings: DIC occurs in males and females with equal incidence and has no racial or ethnic predilection. DIC has a wide range of cutaneous findings. Patients are often gravely ill and hospitalized in a critical care setting. A small subset of patients with early DIC present with cutaneous findings. The remainder of patients are first diagnosed with DIC and eventually develop cutaneous manifestations. The initial cutaneous clinical appearance is that of small petechiae that enlarge and coalesce into large macules and plaques of erythema. There may be a livedo reticularis pattern to the extremities. This fishnet-like appearance can be seen in other dermatological conditions. The petechiae quickly convert to purpuric plaques. Ulceration, necrosis, and blister formation are commonly seen in the areas of involvement. As the disease progresses, gangrene may develop in the affected areas as the blood flow to the skin is significantly decreased due to clotting of various components of the vascular system. Gangrene may lead to secondary infection. The finding of gangrene indicates a grave prognosis, and most of these patients do not survive. If DIC is treated aggressively and early, the survival rate is still only 40% to 50% at best.

DIC is considered to be a consumptive coagulopathy. The initial event that starts the reaction can be multifactorial. The most common causes of DIC are underlying malignancy (especially leukemia), severe traumatic events, sepsis, and obstetric complications. Each of these associated conditions has its own specific clinical setting. As DIC progresses, uncontrollable clotting and bleeding coexist, and patients often succumb to infection, thrombosis, or exsanguination. Thrombocytopenia is a common laboratory finding, as is an elevation of the bleeding time, prothrombin time (PT), and partial thromboplastin time (PTT). Fibrinogen is consumed, leading to an increase in fibrin degradation metabolites.

Pathogenesis: DIC may be subdivided into predominantly hemorrhagic and predominantly thrombotic types, although overlapping features of both occur in all cases. An inciting event such as trauma or infection initiates the clotting cascade in which the clotting factors are used up (or lost, in cases of severe bleeding) faster than they can be replaced. This sets off a cascade of events within the clotting system that results in consumption of all the factors used in clotting, leading to thrombosis and hemorrhage.

Histology: Examination of skin biopsies shows necrosis of the overlying epidermis and parts of the dermis. Thrombosis of the small veins and arterioles is seen, as

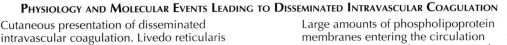

PHYSIOLOGY AND MOLECULAR EVENTS LEADING TO DISSEMINATED INTRAVASCULAR COAGULATION

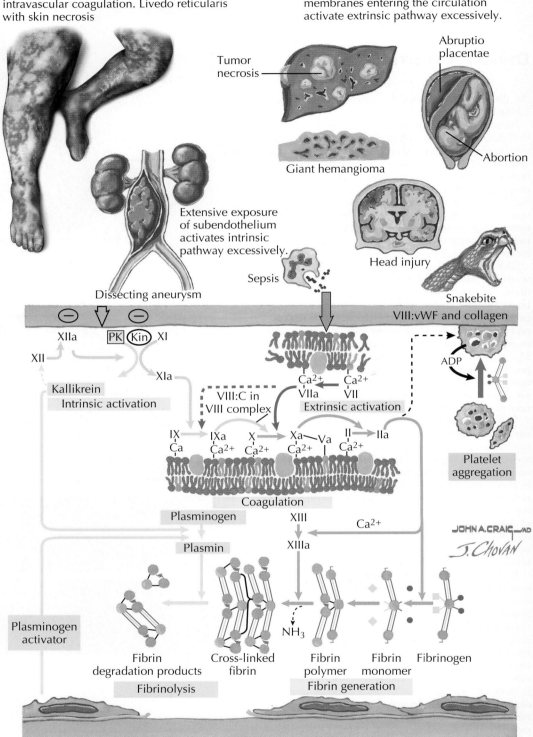

is widespread hemorrhage. In cases of sepsis-induced DIC, evidence of the causative organism may be found in the biopsy specimen.

Treatment: Treatment requires prompt recognition of the condition and immediate supportive care. Treatment of the underlying infection is a must, and in trauma-induced cases, bleeding must be stopped and coagulation factors replaced as they are lost. The main

component of therapy is treatment of the underlying cause that has precipitated the DIC event. The treatment of DIC is complicated and should be undertaken in a critical care setting. Many agents are used to help decrease thrombosis and replace lost clotting factors. A fine balance must be maintained between clotting and thrombosis. Patients with severe DIC have a poor prognosis.

Plate 4-22

Rashes

ELASTOSIS PERFORANS SERPIGINOSA

Elastosis perforans serpiginosa is classified as a perforating skin disorder. This rare cutaneous eruption is believed to be caused by an abnormal expulsion of fragmented elastic fibers from the dermis. The elastic fibers penetrate the surface of the epidermis and manifest as an unusual serpiginous eruption. It has been seen as an isolated finding but also can be seen in association with many underlying conditions, including Down syndrome, Ehlers-Danlos syndrome, and Marfan syndrome.

Clinical Findings: Elastosis perforans serpiginosa is a rare cutaneous perforating skin disease. It is much more commonly seen in the young adult population, and it has a significant male predominance, with a ratio of 4:1 to 5:1. The condition has been most often reported on the neck. The eruption typically begins as small red papules with an excoriated or slightly ulcerated surface. Initially, pruritus is the main symptom. Over time, the papules coalesce into serpiginous, "wandering" eruptions. They can be annular or semicircular. The rash runs a waxing and waning course, but most cases resolve spontaneously with or without therapy. Resolution on average occurs within 6 months, but cases lasting up to 5 years have been reported in the literature. Most cases are solitary in nature. Patients with underlying Down syndrome may have only one lesion or widespread cutaneous involvement. It has been estimated that up to 1% of patients with Down syndrome will develop evidence of this rash over the course of their lifetime. Approximately 33% of cases of elastosis perforans serpiginosa are associated with an underlying disorder (see box to *right*). An autosomal dominant pattern of inheritance has been described in a small number of cases, independent of any of the listed underlying conditions. The medication penicillamine has long been known to cause abnormalities of elastic fibers, and use of this medication has been shown to induce an eruption resembling elastosis perforans serpiginosa.

As the lesions progress, the epidermis ulcerates in pinpoint regions and the underlying fragmentized and abnormal elastic tissue extrudes. The areas may become more pruritic over time, and occasionally they are slightly tender. Most are asymptomatic. The appearance is most concerning for the patient and family members.

Histology: Abnormally fragmented eosinophilic elastic tissue can be appreciated on routine hematoxylin and eosin staining. Special elastic tissue stains can be used to better isolate and appreciate the elastic tissue. Examination of biopsy specimens shows an isolated area of acanthotic epidermis in which a passageway has formed. The passage begins in the superficial dermis and leads to the surface of the epidermis. This is filled with the abnormal elastic tissue, a few histiocytes, and an occasional giant cell. Early biopsies can show a cap of keratin overlying the passageway.

Pathogenesis: The cutaneous eruption is caused by the transepidermal extrusion of abnormally fragmented

Elastosis perforans serpiginosa. This unusual skin finding is often associated with Down syndrome, osteogenesis imperfecta, and Marfan syndrome. Isolated idiopathic cases may also occur.

Associations with Elastosis Perforans Serpiginosa
▶ Acrogeria
▶ Chronic renal failure
▶ Down syndrome
▶ Ehlers-Danlos syndrome
▶ Marfan syndrome
▶ Medications—penicillamine
▶ Osteogenesis imperfecta
▶ Pseudoxanthoma elasticum
▶ Rothmund-Thomson syndrome
▶ Scleroderma

Dense connective tissue

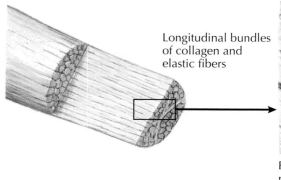

Longitudinal bundles of collagen and elastic fibers

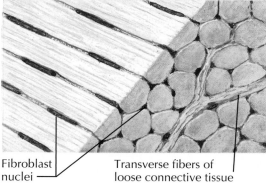

Fibroblast nuclei

Transverse fibers of loose connective tissue

elastic fibers. The reason for the abnormality in the elastic fibers has yet to be determined, except in those cases induced by penicillamine. Penicillamine has been shown to disrupt proper formation of elastic tissue. The abnormally formed fibers are then extruded from the dermis.

Treatment: Many therapies have been attempted, and their use is anecdotal at best. There have been no randomized, prospective, placebo-controlled trials for the treatment of this eruption. Many destructive modalities have been attempted with varying success. Cryotherapy has the most information to support its use, but ablative carbon dioxide lasers have also been used with good results. No therapy is required, because these eruptions almost always spontaneously remit.

Plate 4-23

Integumentary System

ERUPTIVE XANTHOMAS

Abnormal accumulation of triglycerides in various tissues, including the skin, may lead to the cutaneous finding of eruptive xanthomas. The xanthomatous diseases are a diverse group of conditions with unique clinical, laboratory, and systemic findings. An abnormality in lipid and cholesterol metabolism is what links these conditions together. Fatty acids provide the body with more than 40% of its daily energy requirements. The majority of fatty acids are supplied directly by the normal diet. Proteins and carbohydrates, when present in excess, can be converted to triglycerides to be stored as a future energy source. This process makes up the remaining source of free fatty acids and triglycerides supplied to the body.

Normal metabolism of triglycerides occurs through complex biochemical pathways. Triglycerides are converted into free fatty acids, which are broken down into acetyl-coenzyme A (acetyl-CoA). Acetyl-CoA then enters the Krebs cycle to be oxidized and turned into adenosine triphosphate (ATP), one of the main forms of energy used in cellular processes.

Ingested triglycerides are broken down into free fatty acids in the lumen of the intestine by bile acids. The free fatty acids are then transported across the gut lining as chylomicrons. This process is very rapid and occurs within 6 hours after eating. The chylomicrons are absorbed by many tissues and are converted back into free fatty acids and glycerol by the enzyme lipoprotein lipase. The free fatty acids can be converted to acetyl-CoA, converted to triglyceride and stored as an energy source for later use, or used to make various phospholipids. The storage of triglycerides for future energy use is ideal, because it yields higher amounts of energy than either proteins or carbohydrates. Triglycerides can yield 9 kcal/g of energy, whereas proteins and carbohydrates produce about 4 kcal/g. This is an efficient means of storing energy. Abnormalities in the production, breakdown, or storage of triglycerides may lead to complications resulting in cutaneous and systemic findings.

Eruptive xanthomas are one of the cutaneous findings caused by an abnormality in lipid metabolism. They can be caused by various familial hyperlipoproteinemias (types I, III, and V), by medications, or as a complication of diabetes. The cutaneous findings are identical in all of these conditions. Eruptive xanthomas should not be confused with tuberoeruptive, tendinous, or planar xanthomas, because these conditions have different biochemical bases and other systemic features that are unique. Treatment of eruptive xanthomas requires a team approach including endocrinology, cardiology, and dermatology specialists.

Clinical Findings: Eruptive xanthomas, as the name implies, have a rapid eruptive onset (hours to a few days). The most common location to be involved is the buttocks, but these eruptions can be seen anywhere on the body, including the mucous membranes. They have a predilection for the extensor surfaces of the skin.

CONGENITAL HYPERLIPOPROTEINEMIA

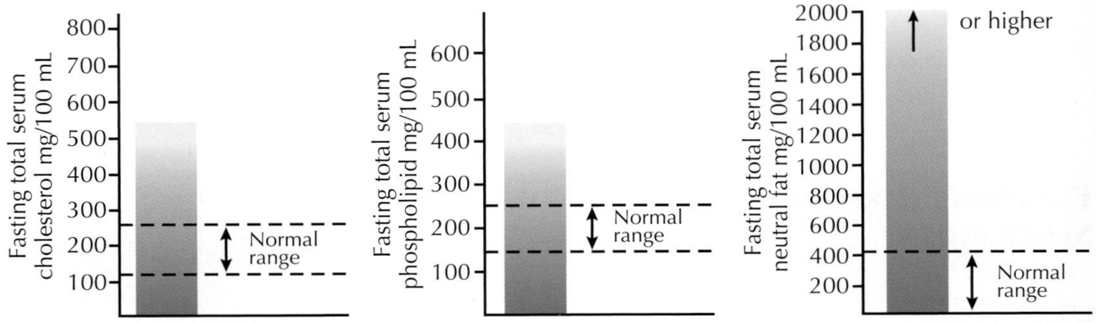

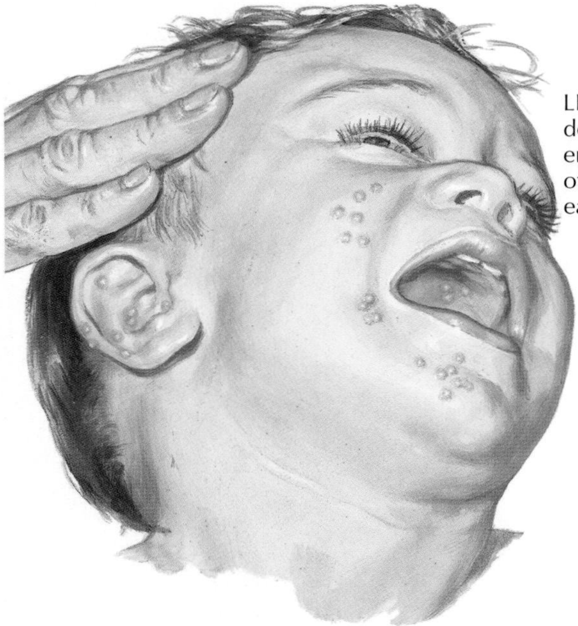

LPL or apo CII deficiency: eruptive xanthomas of cheek, chin, ear, and palate

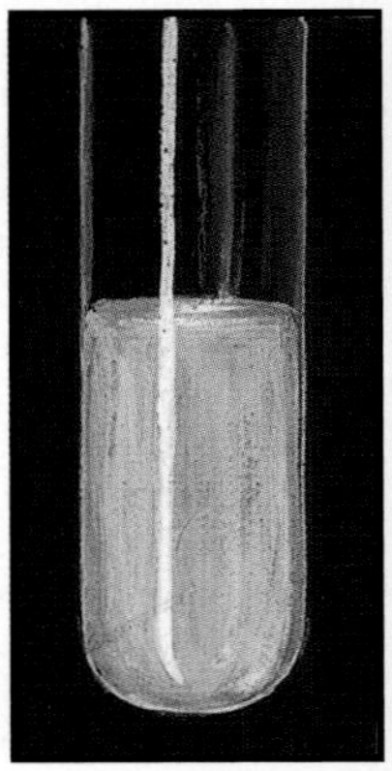

Creamy serum

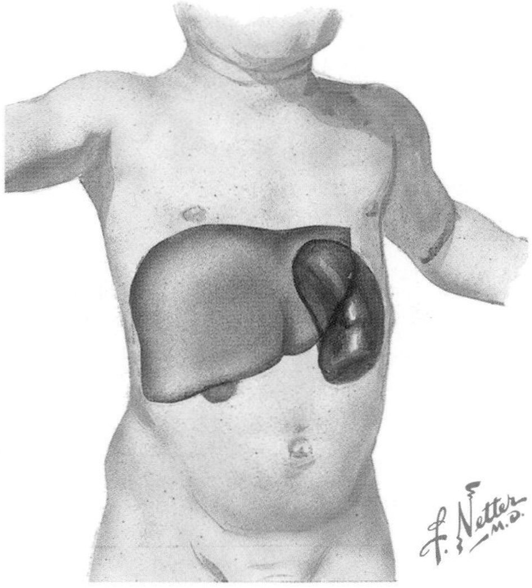

Hepatosplenomegaly

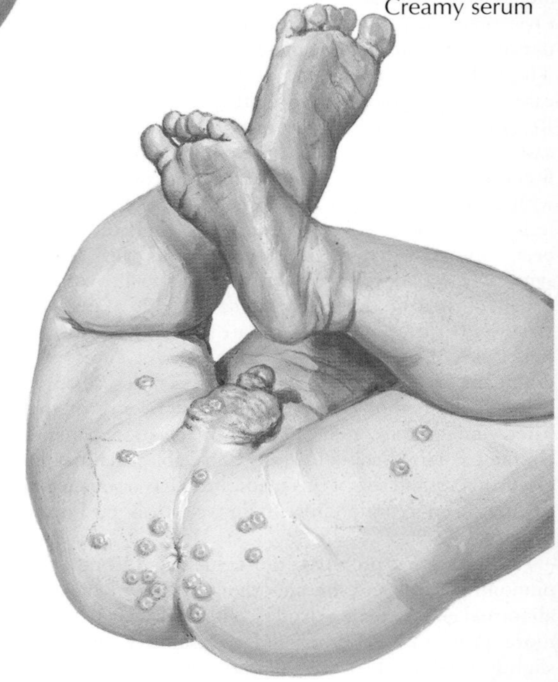

Umbilicated eruptive xanthomas of buttocks, thighs, and scrotum. Yellowish papules with some slight surrounding erythema

They appear as yellow to slightly red-orange, dome-shaped papules with an erythematous base. Patients often complain of mild pruritus, but occasionally they describe a painful sensation when the lesions are palpated. Eruptive xanthomas are rare in both children and adults, but they are more commonly seen in adulthood. There are no racial or sexual differences in incidence.

Patients diagnosed with eruptive xanthomas that are found to be caused by a deficiency in the enzyme

lipoprotein lipase are classified as having type I hyperlipoproteinemia. This is a rare form of hyperlipoproteinemia with onset in childhood. Systemic involvement is significant, with recurrent bouts of pancreatitis and hepatosplenomegaly. These patients have extremely elevated triglyceride and chylomicron levels but normal cholesterol levels. The eye may also be affected with lipemia retinalis. Lipemia retinalis can be seen only by means of a funduscopic examination. Vision is typically

Plate 4-24

Rashes

ACQUIRED HYPERLIPOPROTEINEMIA

ERUPTIVE XANTHOMAS
(Continued)

normal, and the patient is unaware of any eye abnormalities. The blood vessels within the eye have a creamy white color because of the excess lipid in the bloodstream. The arteries and veins are equally affected, and the only way to differentiate the two is by comparing the caliber of the vessel. The arterial light reflex is lost. The vessels appear flat, and the rest of the fundus is a uniform creamy color. Lipoprotein lipase enzyme activity can be measured, and this test is used to help diagnosis type I hyperlipoproteinemia. Eruptive xanthomas can also be seen as part of hyperlipoproteinemia type III (familial dysbetalipoproteinemia) and hyperlipoproteinemia type V. Type III has been found to be caused by a defect in the *APOE* gene, which encodes the apolipoprotein E protein. This protein is particularly important in clearing chylomicrons and intermediate-density lipoproteins.

Multiple medications have been implicated in the production of hypertriglyceridemia. They include isotretinoin, glucocorticoids, olanzapine, protease inhibitors (especially ritonavir), and indomethacin. Alcohol abuse can also be a cause of hypertriglyceridemia. Patients presenting with eruptive xanthomas who are taking any of these medications should have the medication discontinued or another substituted and should be reevaluated after treatment.

Diabetes is the most common cause of hypertriglyceridemia, and it probably is also the most common cause of eruptive xanthomas. Insulin is required for normal functioning of the lipoprotein lipase enzyme. Diabetic patients who are deficient in insulin have lower activity levels of lipoprotein lipase and increased levels of chylomicrons and triglycerides as a result.

On laboratory evaluation, the patient has triglyceride levels that are extremely elevated, in the range of 2000 mg/dL sometimes even surpassing the laboratory's ability to quantify it. If a sample of blood is centrifuged for a few minutes, the white to creamy-colored triglycerides will become evident and will take up a considerable amount of the specimen. On occasion, there are so many triglycerides present that the blood sample is a light creamy color even before centrifugation.

Histology: The histological findings from biopsies of early lesions of eruptive xanthomas can mimic those of granuloma annulare. Neutrophils can be evident during the formation of an eruptive xanthoma. The neutrophilic infiltrate lessens and disappears once the lesion has had time to establish itself. It is recommended that the biopsy specimen be taken from an established lesion (one that has been present for a day or two) so that more characteristic findings will be seen. Foam cells are present with a stippled cytoplasm. The number of foam cells is not as prominent as in tuberous or tendinous xanthomas. One unique finding is the presence of extracellular lipid, which is seen between bundles of collagen.

Pathogenesis: The varying conditions that can manifest with eruptive xanthomas all have unique ways of

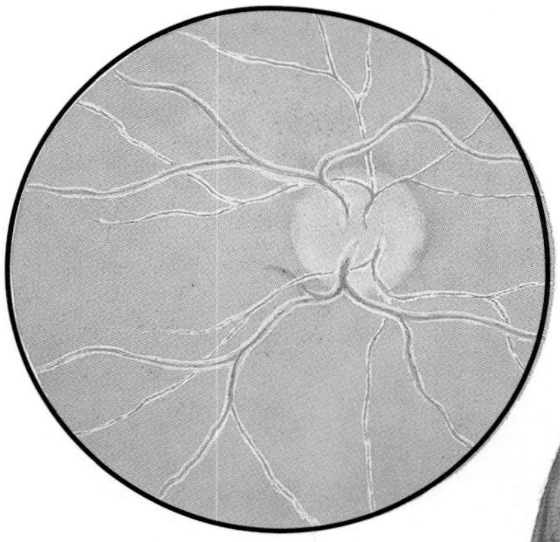

Hyperlipemia retinalis

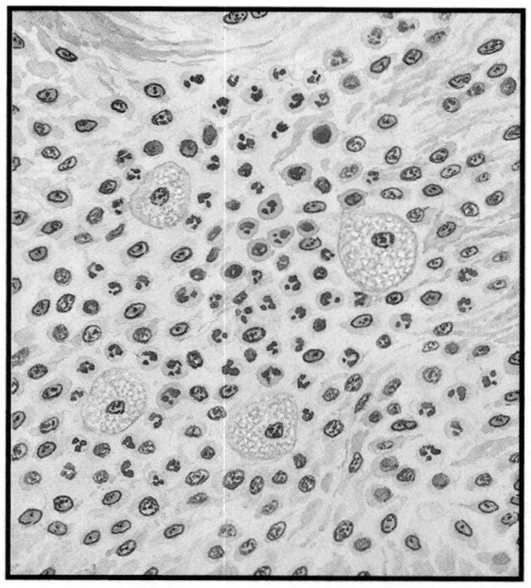

Hyperlipemic xanthomatous nodule (high magnification): few foam cells amid a mixed inflammatory infiltrate

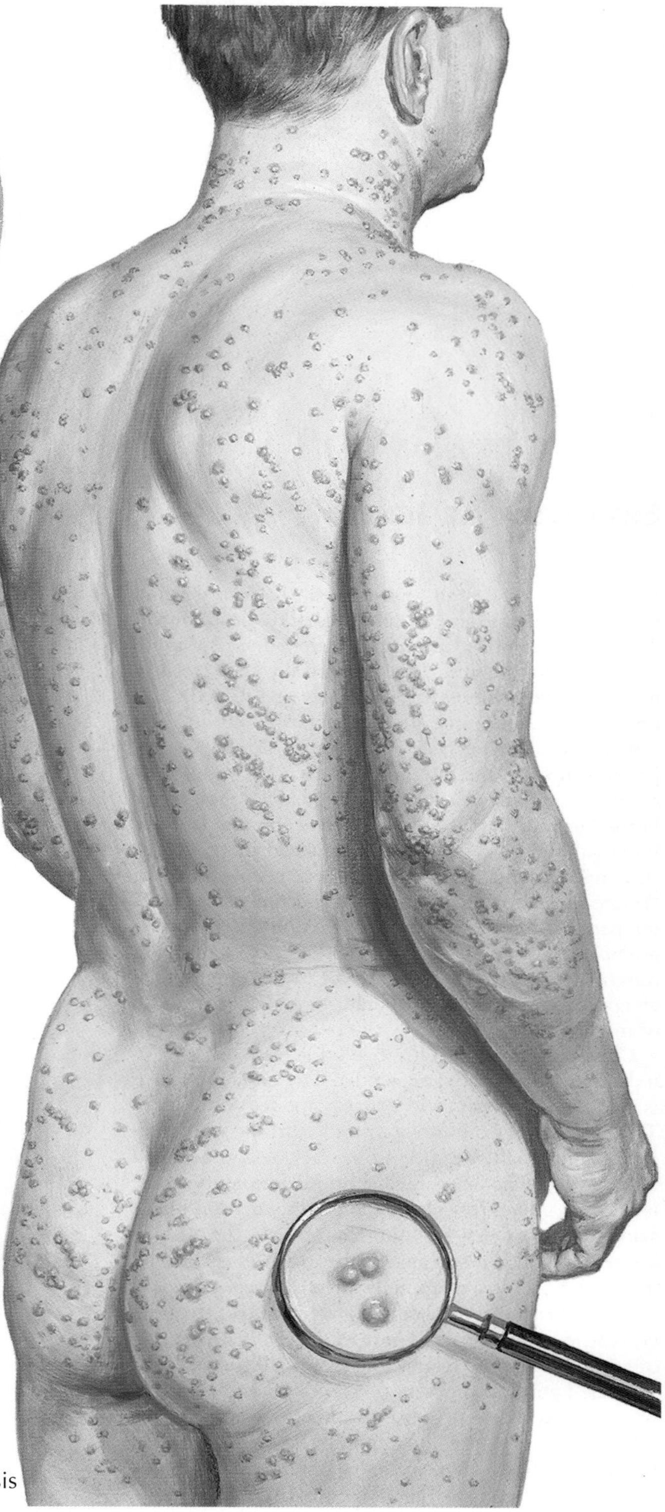

Eruptive xanthomatosis

causing hypertriglyceridemia. The final common pathway in the pathogenesis of eruptive xanthomas is the presence of significantly elevated triglyceride levels.

Treatment: The main goal of therapy is to return the triglyceride level back to a normal range. Medications that can cause hypertriglyceridemia need to be discontinued. Underlying diabetes needs to be treated aggressively to get better control of glucose metabolism

and insulin requirements. Those patients with familial causes need to institute dietary changes (to avoid medium-chain triglycerides), increase their activity level, and take triglyceride-lowering medications. These medications can be used for all causes of hypertriglyceridemia. The medications most commonly used to lower triglyceride levels are fenofibrate and gemfibrozil.

Plate 4-25

Integumentary System

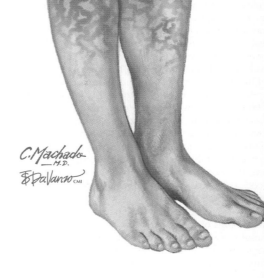

The abdomen, lower back, and legs are most frequently affected.

ERYTHEMA AB IGNE

Erythema ab igne is an unusual rash that can develop secondary to exposure to an exogenous heat source. The name is derived from the Latin phrase meaning "redness from the fire." It has a clinically characteristic pattern. The differential diagnosis is limited. For unknown reasons, not all persons exposed to heat sources develop the rash of erythema ab igne. Many patients develop the rash without even knowing of its existence. Reported causes have included hot water bottles, heating blankets, heaters, and computer laptops. Essentially any exogenous heat source can cause this reaction. Erythema ab igne has also been called the "roasted skin" or "toasted skin" syndrome. The exact temperature needed for the reaction to occur is unknown, and for some reason it does not occur from hot tub use, most likely because the causes of erythema ab igne are dry heat or temperatures higher than those of most hot tubs.

Clinical Findings: This condition can be seen in individuals of any race and gender. The initiating factor is an exogenous heat source that is applied to the skin. The heat source exposure is typically chronic and repetitive. Patients often notice a fine, lacy, red, reticulated macule or patch. Occasionally, no inflammatory phase is noticed, only a reticulated hyperpigmentation of the skin. Some patients do not realize that the rash is located on skin in direct approximation to a heat source. The lower back is a commonly affected area, secondary to the use of heating blankets or bottles to help treat chronic lower back pain. There have been many reports of erythema ab igne from exposures to all sorts of heat sources. Laptop computers can release a large amount of energy as infrared radiation; if someone is chronically using a laptop computer in direct approximation to their skin (e.g., anterior thighs), the rash of erythema ab igne may develop. The diagnosis is typically made by clinical examination and historical information. Patients often need to be asked whether they have been using a heating device or consistently using a laptop computer, because the correlation is not evident to them. The development of actinic keratosis or squamous cell carcinoma within the areas of erythema ab igne has rarely been reported.

Pathogenesis: Erythema ab igne is caused by the direct effects of heat on the skin. The temperature required has not been precisely defined, but the range of 43°C to 47°C seems to be most likely. In any case, there must be repeated exposure to subthermal burning

Also known as "toasted skin syndrome," erythema ab igne is caused by excessive heat transfer to the underlying skin. Hot water bottles and heating pads are most commonly implicated.

Common Etiologies of Erythema Ab Igne

▶ Heating blanket/pad
▶ Hot water bottles
▶ Localized heaters/radiators
▶ Laptop computers

temperatures. More frequent exposures and longer exposures seem to increase the risk of development of erythema ab igne. The exact mechanism by which the rash develops is unknown.

Histology: The skin may be slightly atrophic, and elastotic tissue is seen within the dermis. The rete ridges may be thinned. Some areas may show evidence of changes such as those seen in actinic keratosis. Vacuolar degeneration of the basal layer can be seen.

Treatment: The goal of therapy is to discover and remove the exogenous heat source. Once the heat source is removed, most of these rashes slowly fade away over months. Some of the hyperpigmented areas may persist, however. Use of emollient creams or Kligman's formulation has been reported. Kligman's formulation includes a retinoid, a steroid, and a skin-lightening cream. Laser therapy has also been used to decrease the pigmentary disturbance.

Plate 4-26

Rashes

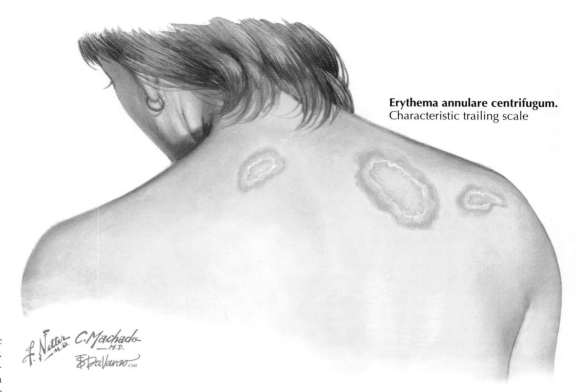

Erythema annulare centrifugum.
Characteristic trailing scale

ERYTHEMA ANNULARE CENTRIFUGUM

Erythema annulare centrifugum (EAC) is an idiopathic rash that is classified with the gyrate erythema family. It is believed to be a cutaneous reaction to many different antigenic stimuli, although no firm conclusion on the pathogenesis has been made. It has a characteristic clinical presentation that is easily recognized. The pathology of EAC is also characteristic and helps make the diagnosis by ruling out other conditions. EAC can be a marker of internal malignancy, but most cases, by far, are not associated with an underlying malignancy.

Clinical Findings: EAC often manifests insidiously. It has been reported to occur at any age and has no sexual or racial predilection. It has an unusual and peculiar morphology. The lesions start as small, pink papules that slowly expand. The patches of EAC are pink to red with a slowly expanding border. The peculiar and characteristic finding is the presence of a trailing scale. The leading edge of the rash advances and is followed by a few millimeters of fine trailing scale that continues to track the leading edge. As the rash expands outward, a central area of clearing forms. This central area is flesh colored. In tinea infections, in contrast, the scale represents the leading edge and travels in front of the expanding erythema. The main differential diagnosis is between erythema annulare centrifugum, tinea corporis, and mycosis fungoides. Potassium hydroxide (KOH) examination will rule out a dermatophyte, and a biopsy is required to differentiate EAC from mycosis fungoides.

The rash of EAC can be asymptomatic to severely pruritic. Most cases are mildly pruritic, but the most common complaint is of the unsightly appearance. The trunk is the body area most commonly involved, followed by the extremities. It is rarely seen on the face. Some areas may resolve at the same time that new areas are occurring.

Pathogenesis: The exact etiology of EAC is unknown. It is believed to be a reaction to many different antigenic stimuli. Research has suggested that EAC can be seen as a reaction pattern to an underlying tinea infection; this is thought to be a type IV hypersensitivity reaction. Many causes have been reported, including infections (fungal, bacterial, and viral) and medications, and EAC has been reported in association with many different underlying malignancies.

Histology: Biopsies of EAC lesions should be taken from the advancing border. EAC has a superficial

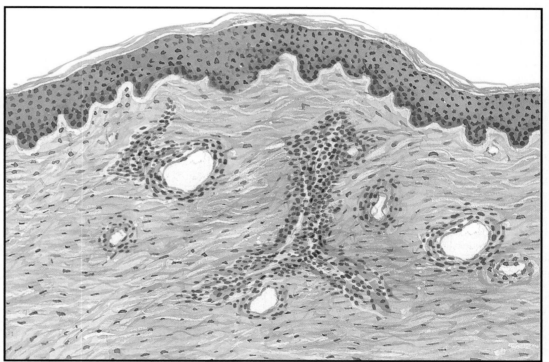

Histology of erythema annulare centrifugum will show tight perivascular infiltrates of lymphocytes often referred to as "coat sleeving" of the vessels.

and deep perivascular lymphocytic infiltrate. The infiltrate has a highly characteristic "coat sleeve" appearance around the vessels. The lymphocytic infiltrate is concentrated immediately around the vessels in the dermis, and the lymphocytes appear to be coating the vessel walls.

Treatment: EAC is almost always a self-limited process that spontaneously resolves. If an underlying infection is suspected, treatment and resolution of the infection has been shown to help resolve the rash of EAC. Malignancy-associated EAC is chronic in nature; it tends to resolve with treatment of the malignancy and to recur with relapses. Drug-induced EAC responds to discontinuation of the offending medication. Topical corticosteroids such as triamcinolone may be used to help decrease the erythema and pruritus.

Plate 4-27   Integumentary System

ERYTHEMA MULTIFORME, STEVENS-JOHNSON SYNDROME, AND TOXIC EPIDERMAL NECROLYSIS

ERYTHEMA MULTIFORME, STEVENS-JOHNSON SYNDROME, AND TOXIC EPIDERMAL NECROLYSIS

Erythema multiforme minor, erythema multiforme major, Stevens-Johnson syndrome (SJS), and toxic epidermal necrolysis are all classified as hypersensitivity reactions, with the most common initiating event being a medication or an infection. Some authors consider these to be completely distinct entities with specific etiologies. Until that is proven, a simple way of approaching these diseases is to consider them as representing a continuum with varying degrees of mucocutaneous involvement. Erythema multiforme minor is the most likely of all these conditions to be a unique entity, because it is more commonly caused by infection (e.g., herpes simplex virus, *Mycoplasma pneumoniae*). It is also more commonly seen in childhood. The other entities are much more likely to be initiated by medications. Almost all types of medications have been reported to cause these reactions, but a few classes account for most of these severe skin reactions. The classes of medications most commonly implicated are antibiotics (especially sulfa-based products), antiepileptics, allopurinol, and the nonsteroidal antiinflammatory drugs (NSAIDs).

Clinical Findings: There is no racial or ethnic predilection, and males and females are equally affected. For unknown reasons, patients with coexisting human immunodeficiency virus (HIV) infection are much more likely to develop a serious drug eruption than HIV-negative controls. The pathomechanism of this reaction is poorly understood.

Erythema multiforme minor is the most frequently seen of these eruptions. It is more common in children and young adults and can be caused by a myriad of infections and medications. Exposures to topical antigens such as urushiol in the poison ivy plant have also been reported to cause rashes resembling erythema multiforme minor. The most common cause that has been isolated is the herpes simplex virus. The rash of erythema multiforme minor can be seen in association with a coexisting herpesvirus infection or independent of the viral infection. Most episodes last for 2 to 3 weeks. A subset of patients have recurrent episodes. The rash appears acutely as a well-defined macule with a "target" appearance—a red center, a surrounding area of normal-appearing skin, and a rim of erythema that encircles the entire lesion. The peripheral rim is very well circumscribed and demarcated from the normal skin. Over a day, the macules may turn into edematous plaques. As time progresses, the center of the lesion becomes purple or dusky red. There may be only one area of involvement or hundreds in severe cases. Erythema multiforme minor affects the palms and soles; the target lesions in these areas can be very prominent and classic in appearance. The mucous membranes of the oral mucosa are involved in 20% of cases of erythema multiforme minor. Edematous pink-red plaques can be seen, as well as the more classic target lesions. If other mucous membranes are involved, the classification of erythema multiforme minor should not be used; the patient more likely has erythema multiforme major.

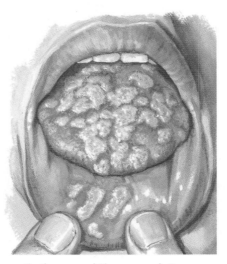

Erythema multiforme exudativum

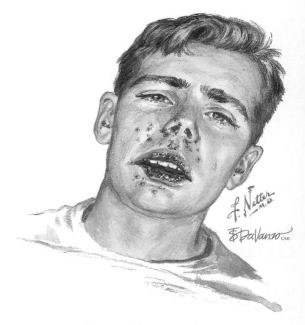

Stevens-Johnson syndrome

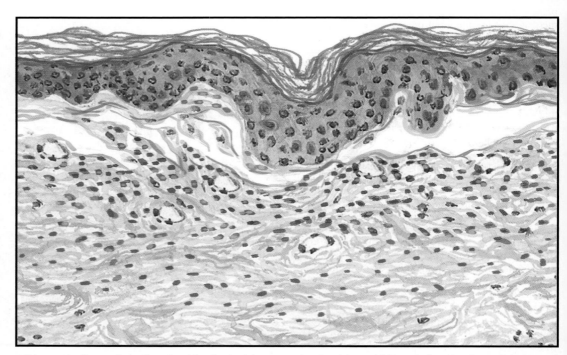

All have similar and overlapping histological features. A subepidermal blister is forming here due to necrosis of the overlying epidermis. There is a lymphocytic predominate perivascular infiltrate.

Most cases of erythema multiforme minor self-resolve, but they do have a tendency to recur.

Erythema multiforme major has been considered by many to be the same entity as SJS. This may be true, because the pathogenesis and clinical appearance can be similar. However, subtle differences exist and warrant classifying this condition independently. Both erythema multiforme major and SJS are most often induced by medications. The mucocutaneous surfaces are affected

to a significant degree. In severe cases, the mucosal membranes of the respiratory and gastrointestinal tract may also be affected. Erythema multiforme major and SJS typically begin with a nonspecific prodrome of fever and malaise. Fever is the most frequent nonmucocutaneous symptom. The rash begins insidiously as pink macules that quickly develop a dusky purple central region. The typical target-like lesion of erythema multiforme minor is usually absent in SJS but may be seen

Plate 4-28

Rashes

ERYTHEMA MULTIFORME, STEVENS-JOHNSON SYNDROME, AND TOXIC EPIDERMAL NECROLYSIS (Continued)

in erythema multiforme major. Erythema multiforme major is differentiated from erythema multiforme minor in that it affects a larger surface area and affects two mucous membranes.

In SJS, the dusky center of the lesion soon begins to blister, first as small vesicles and then coalescing into larger bullae. The extent and body surface area (BSA) of blistering is used to differentiate SJS from toxic epidermal necrolysis. Most authors consider blistering of 10% of the BSA and involvement of at least two mucosal surfaces to be definitive for SJS. Those cases with 10% to 30% BSA involvement have been termed *SJS–toxic epidermal necrolysis overlap*. Cases with greater than 30% BSA involvement are considered to represent toxic epidermal necrolysis. Light lateral pressure at the edge of a bulla or vesicle is an objective physical test that can be performed at the bedside. Spreading or an increase in size of the blister with pressure indicates separation of the epidermis from the underlying dermis and is termed *Nikolsky sign*.

Pathogenesis: Erythema multiforme major/SJS is believed to be a hypersensitivity reaction to certain medications. The insulting medication is thought to be metabolized into a recognizable antigen or to act as an antigen without metabolic degradation. Antibodies bind to the drug antigen and form antigen-antibody complexes that can deposit in the skin and other regions, causing an inflammatory cascade and the clinical findings.

Histology: The classic histological picture of erythema multiforme minor and major shows an acute inflammatory infiltrate along the dermal-epidermal junction. The stratum corneum is normal. There is an interface dermatitis with vacuolar degeneration of the basal cell layer. The interface dermatitis leads to necrosis and death of the basilar keratinocytes. If the necrosis spreads and coalesces, small areas of subepidermal blister formation may be seen. Erythema multiforme minor can share some features with fixed drug eruptions. In fixed drug eruptions melanophages are typically present, whereas this is not the case in erythema multiforme. Biopsy specimens of SJS and toxic epidermal necrolysis show more interface damage and blistering of the skin. The plane of separation is in the subepidermal space.

Treatment: Therapy for erythema multiforme minor and erythema multiforme major requires supportive care. The skin lesions typically self-resolve with minimal to no sequelae. Topical corticosteroids may help decrease the time to healing and decrease symptoms of pruritus. Recurrent episodes of erythema multiforme due to herpesvirus infection can be treated with chronic daily use of an antiviral agent such as acyclovir. This decreases the recurrence of herpes simplex infection and the resulting erythema multiforme reaction. Oral lesions can be treated with topical analgesics; the use of oral steroids is reserved for severe cases.

SJS can be a life-threatening condition and can progress to toxic epidermal necrolysis. For both SJS and toxic epidermal necrolysis, the cause of the reaction should be identified and withdrawn, and infections should be treated appropriately. These patients require aggressive supportive care, including wound care and

DRUG ERUPTIONS

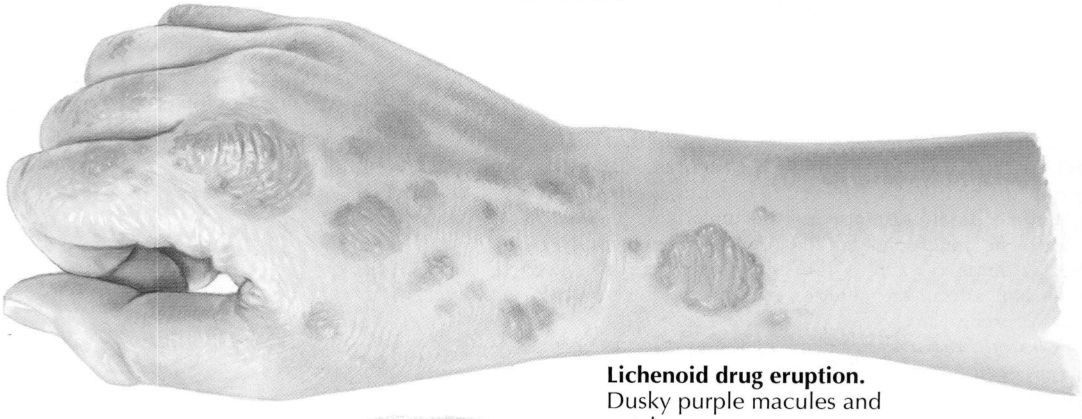

Lichenoid drug eruption. Dusky purple macules and patches

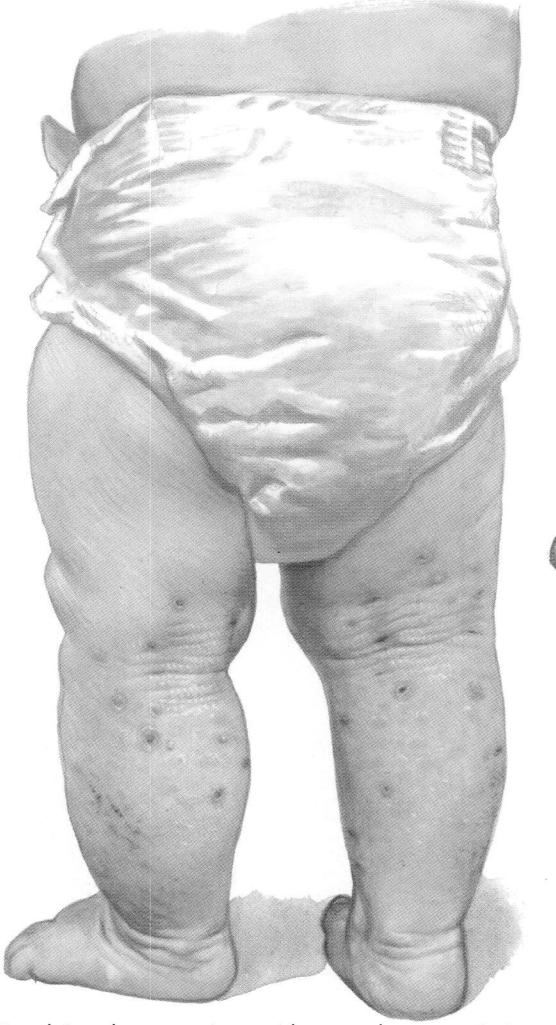

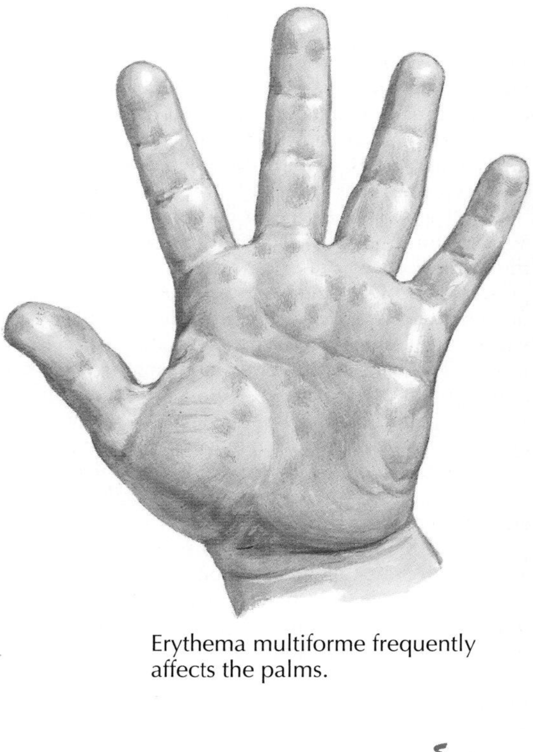

Erythema multiforme frequently affects the palms.

Resolving drug eruptions with secondary excoriations. Drug rashes typically start on the trunk and spread to the extremities.

fluid and electrolyte balancing. Most patients with severe involvement will benefit from the experience of a burn unit. SJS and toxic epidermal necrolysis can be treated similarly to burns, because the same technical issues are involved. There is no consensus on how to treat these two conditions with medications. The use of oral steroids early in the course of disease may help lessen the overall involvement, but steroids increase the risk of secondary infection and should not be used in

patients with infection-induced disease. If used late in the course of disease, they appear not to help and only increase risk of side effects. Intravenous immunoglobulin (IVIG) has been used to treat these conditions with varying success. If used early, it may modify the disease course; if used late, it is unlikely to be of any help. The amount of BSA involved with blistering is related to the prognosis. Those with greater BSA blistering tend to fare worse than those with smaller BSA involvement.

Plate 4-29

Integumentary System

ERYTHEMA NODOSUM

Erythema nodosum, an idiopathic form of panniculitis, is seen in association with a wide range of inflammatory and infectious diseases. Pregnancy and use of oral contraceptives are two of the most common associations. Erythema nodosum is believed to occur as a secondary phenomenon in response to the underlying disease state. The condition typically resolves spontaneously, but in some cases it is difficult to treat. Erythema nodosum affects the anterior part of the lower legs almost exclusively.

Clinical Findings: Erythema nodosum is most commonly seen in young adult women. There is no racial predilection. The skin findings in erythema nodosum have an insidious onset. Small, tender regions begin within the dermis and develop into firm, tender dermal nodules, with the anterior lower legs almost always involved. The rash typically affects both lower legs in synchronicity. The lesions can be multifocal or solitary in nature. Most patients have multiple areas of involvement, with varying sizes of the lesions. Involvement of other areas of the body has been reported but is exceedingly uncommon. In these dermal nodules, there is a slight red or purplish discoloration to the overlying normal-appearing epidermis. If ulcerations are present, one should consider another diagnosis, and a biopsy is warranted. Although almost all cases can be diagnosed on clinical grounds, skin biopsies are required for cases that are atypical in location or have unusual features such as ulcerations, surface change, palpable purpura, or other features inconsistent with classic erythema nodosum.

The diagnosis of erythema nodosum should lead to a search for a possible underlying association. One of the most frequent causes is use of oral contraceptive pills. If the rash is thought to be related to the use of oral contraceptives, they should be discontinued, after which the lesions of erythema nodosum typically resolve. Pregnancy is another major cause of erythema nodosum. The lesions may be difficult to treat during pregnancy, but they will spontaneously resolve after delivery. Erythema nodosum may also be seen in association with sarcoid. Löfgren's syndrome is the combination of fever, erythema nodosum, and bilateral hilar adenopathy that occurs as an acute form of sarcoid. In patients with no known reason for erythema nodosum, a standard chest radiograph should be considered to evaluate for sarcoid or the possibility of an underlying fungal or atypical infection. Valley fever (coccidioidomycosis), which is caused by the fungus *Coccidioides immitis*, has been linked with the development of erythema nodosum. Patients presenting with erythema nodosum who have lived in or traveled to an endemic area should be evaluated for this fungal infection. Streptococcal infection and tuberculosis are two other infections that should be considered. Erythema nodosum has also been reported to occur in the inflammatory bowel diseases and in Hodgkin's lymphoma.

Histology: Erythema nodosum is a primary septal panniculitis. The inflammation is isolated primarily to the fibrous septa that are present within the subcutaneous tissue. The fibrous septa are responsible for providing a framework for the adipose tissue. No vasculitis is seen, and its presence should make one reconsider the diagnosis. The overlying dermis has a superficial and deep perivascular lymphocytic infiltrate. A characteristic finding is that of Miescher's radial granulomas, which represent multiple histiocytes surrounding a central cleft. Multinucleated giant cells are also present within the septal infiltrate.

Erythema nodosum occurs in <5% of patients with inflammatory bowel disease. The anterior lower legs is the most frequent location.

One of the mainstays of therapy is leg elevation.

Main Forms of Panniculitis
Predominantly septal panniculitis
▶ Erythema nodosum
Predominantly lobular panniculitis
▶ Lipodermatosclerosis
▶ α_1-antitrypsin deficiency panniculitis
▶ Erythema induratum
▶ Sclerema neonatorum
▶ Traumatic panniculitis
▶ Pancreatic panniculitis

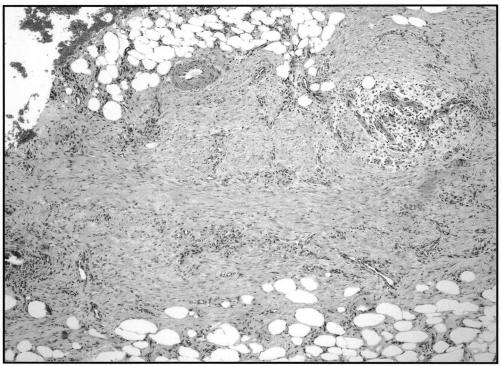

Erythema nodosum is a panniculitis that predominantly affects the septal portions of the adipose tissue. The septal tissue is expanded with a lymphocytic infiltrate.

Pathogenesis: The etiology of erythema nodosum is unknown, but it is thought to be a hypersensitivity reaction pattern to multiple unique stimuli. It is theorized that the antigenic stimulus causes the formation of antibody-antigen complexes that localize to the septal region of the adipose tissue.

Treatment: Treatment is primarily symptomatic. One must pursue the possibility of an underlying disorder. Erythema nodosum induced by medications or pregnancy resolves spontaneously once the medication is withdrawn or after delivery. Those cases associated with an underlying infection, malignancy, or inflammatory bowel disease may be longer lasting and may show a waxing and waning course. Topical corticosteroids, compression stockings, elevation, and nonsteroidal antiinflammatory agents are first-line therapies. Severe cases can be treated with a short course of prednisone. Supersaturated potassium iodide and colchicine have also been reported to be used successfully.

Plate 4-30

Rashes

FABRY DISEASE

Fabry disease (Anderson-Fabry disease) is a rare disease caused by a deficiency in the enzyme ceramide trihexosidase (α-galactosidase A). Fabry disease is also known by its alternative descriptive name, angiokeratoma corporis diffusum. It is inherited in an X-linked recessive pattern and is classified as a lysosomal storage disease. The defect in this enzyme causes a lack of proper metabolism of globotriaosylceramide (ceramide trihexoside) and accumulation of this lipid in various tissues throughout the body. Fabry disease affects the skin, kidneys, cardiovascular system, eye, and neurological system. There is no known cure, but advances in enzyme replacement therapy have shown promising results. Males are more severely affected; females can be affected to varying degrees or can act as carriers of the disease. Fabry disease has been estimated to occur in 1 of every 50,000 males. There is an increase in the mortality rate, with the average age at death for a man with classic Fabry disease being 40 years.

Clinical Findings: The clinical manifestations of Fabry disease have a slow onset during childhood; the average age at onset is 5 to 6 years. Acroparesthesias are the initial presenting symptoms in most children. Patients have severe pain in the hands and feet that is episodic in nature and can last from minutes to hours or, in extreme cases, days. The pain is often described as a burning sensation. Episodes of stress can induce the acroparesthesias. This is accompanied by bouts of hypohidrosis or, less commonly, anhidrosis. This inability to sweat properly may lead to heat exhaustion and heat intolerance. Patients also eventually develop varying degrees of hearing loss.

The cutaneous findings consist of numerous angiokeratomas in unusual locations. These fine, red, hyperkeratotic papules occur on the trunk and lower extremities and are almost always located between the umbilicus and the knees. The number of angiokeratomas continues to increase with time, eventually reaching hundreds to thousands. The mucous membranes may also be involved with angiokeratomas. Presentation of a child or a young adult with multiple angiokeratomas should prompt the clinician to consider the diagnosis of Fabry disease and to search for any other symptoms consistent with the disease. If the diagnosis of Fabry disease is made, patients should be referred to a specialty center that cares for these patients.

The most characteristic ocular finding is that of cornea verticillata. This is a whorl-like corneal opacity that can be observed only by slit-lamp examination. They do not impede vision.

With time, patients begin to develop progressive kidney disease. The earliest sign is often asymptomatic proteinuria. Continued kidney damage eventually leads to chronic renal failure and end-stage renal disease. Maltese cross–shaped deposits are often found in the urine sediment from patients with Fabry disease and represent lipid accumulations. Cardiovascular changes can be seen and lead to ischemic heart disease. Stroke and cerebral vascular disease are common and cause a significant amount of mortality in these patients.

The diagnosis of Fabry disease can be made by evaluating the plasma for α-galactosidase A activity. Males

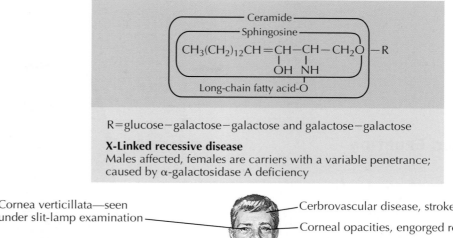

R=glucose−galactose−galactose and galactose−galactose

X-Linked recessive disease
Males affected, females are carriers with a variable penetrance; caused by α-galactosidase A deficiency

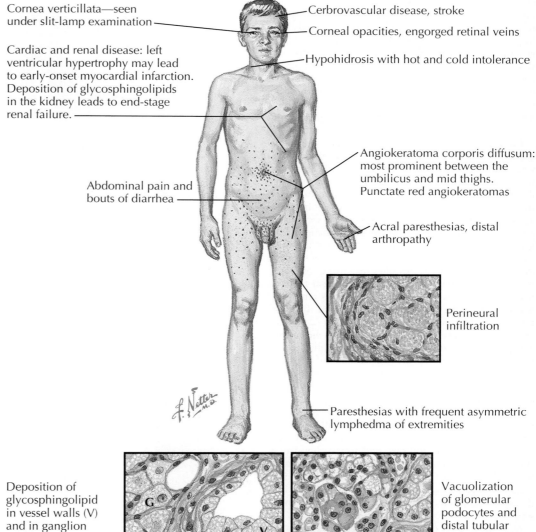

Cornea verticillata—seen under slit-lamp examination

Cardiac and renal disease: left ventricular hypertrophy may lead to early-onset myocardial infarction. Deposition of glycosphingolipids in the kidney leads to end-stage renal failure.

Abdominal pain and bouts of diarrhea

Cerbrovascular disease, stroke

Corneal opacities, engorged retinal veins

Hypohidrosis with hot and cold intolerance

Angiokeratoma corporis diffusum: most prominent between the umbilicus and mid thighs. Punctate red angiokeratomas

Acral paresthesias, distal arthropathy

Perineural infiltration

Paresthesias with frequent asymmetric lymphedma of extremities

Deposition of glycosphingolipid in vessel walls (V) and in ganglion cells (G)

Vacuolization of glomerular podocytes and distal tubular epithelial cells

with classic Fabry disease have less than 1% of proper enzyme activity. DNA gene sequencing can be performed to isolate the exact genetic defect. Genetic testing is the only reliable way to diagnosis females with the disease, because female carriers do have some plasma enzyme activity.

Treatment: Many medications can be used to treat the acroparesthesias, and they typically come from the antiseizure class of medications. Phenytoin and

gabapentin are used to help control the frequency and duration of the episodes. In the past, there were no specific therapies for Fabry disease. End-stage renal disease often required kidney transplantation. Enzyme replacement therapy has been available since 2003 and has begun to have an impact on morbidity in these patients. Long-term studies are needed to make any conclusions regarding their effects on mortality.

Plate 4-31

Integumentary System

FIXED DRUG ERUPTION

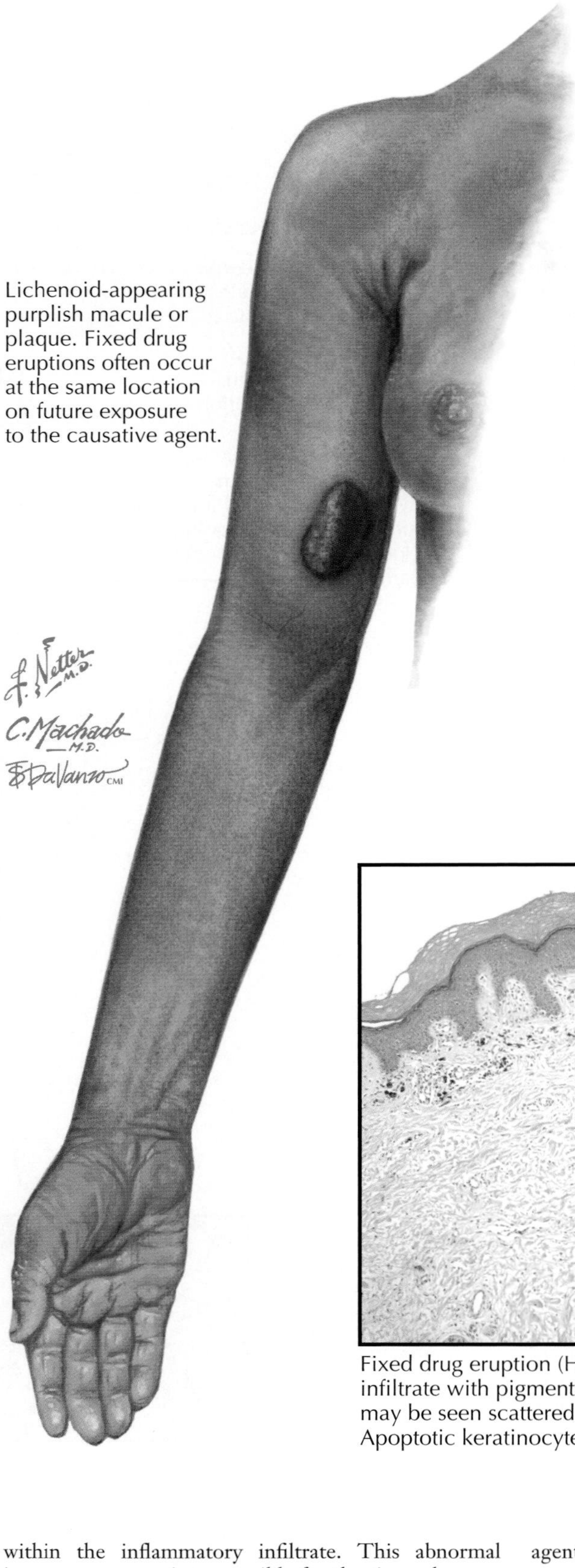

Fixed drug eruptions are responsible for up to 20% of all cutaneous drug eruptions. They can occur anywhere on the body and have been reported to occur in reaction to a long list of medications. There are a few medicines in particular that have been associated with fixed drug eruptions. One of the most frequent causes in the past was phenolphthalein contained in over-the-counter laxatives. After the numerous side effects from this medication were revealed, it was withdrawn from the market and is now of only historical significance. Fixed drug eruptions are unique in many ways, both clinically and histologically. The exact pathogenesis is unknown.

Clinical Findings: Clinically, fixed drug eruptions appear as oval to round, dusky red to purple macules with minimal surface change. Some cases have shown bullous-type reactions. The fixed drug eruption is unique in that it recurs in the same location time and time again as the patient is reexposed to the offending agent. Sometimes months may pass between exposures, and yet the reaction recurs in the same location. The glans penis, the oral mucosa, and the hands are the most commonly involved areas, although any area of the skin may be involved. Most cases show one area of reaction, but some have more than one. It is unusual to have more than five areas of involvement, but case reports of widespread involvement have been reported. In these cases, the differential diagnosis includes erythema multiforme. Another characteristic feature is the postinflammatory hyperpigmentation that occurs after resolution. This is caused by the vast amount of pigment incontinence that results from disruption of the dermal-epidermal junction. This hyperpigmentation can take months to years to resolve.

The list of medications that can cause fixed drug eruptions continues to grow. The most frequently reported culprits are the sulfa-based antibiotics, nonsteroidal antiinflammatory medications, and tetracycline-based antibiotics. Common over-the-counter medications have also been reported to cause fixed drug eruptions, including acetaminophen and herbal supplements. For this reason, a thorough history that includes both prescription and other medications is required.

Histology: Fixed drug eruptions are categorized in the lichenoid pattern of histological skin disease. These drug reactions show a prominent lichenoid infiltrate with lymphocytes. The infiltrate is associated with very noticeable vacuolar change of the basilar layer of the epidermis and prominent formation of necrotic keratinocytes (Civatte bodies). There is melanin incontinence within the dermis in all cases, and this can be used to differentiate fixed drug eruption from other lichenoid reactions. The bullae form within the subepidermal space in the bullous variant of fixed drug eruption. Rare variants of fixed drug eruption have been described that have included evidence of vasculitis. This form is exceedingly rare.

Pathogenesis: The etiology is unknown. Research has indicated that CD8+ T cells are the primary cell type

Lichenoid-appearing purplish macule or plaque. Fixed drug eruptions often occur at the same location on future exposure to the causative agent.

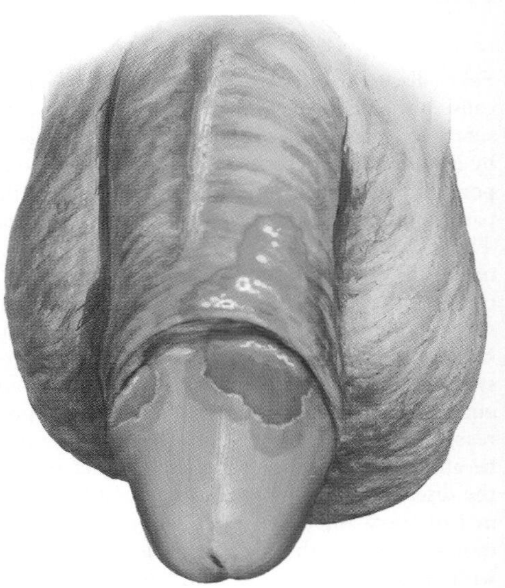

The glans penis is one of the most frequently involved areas in fixed drug eruptions.

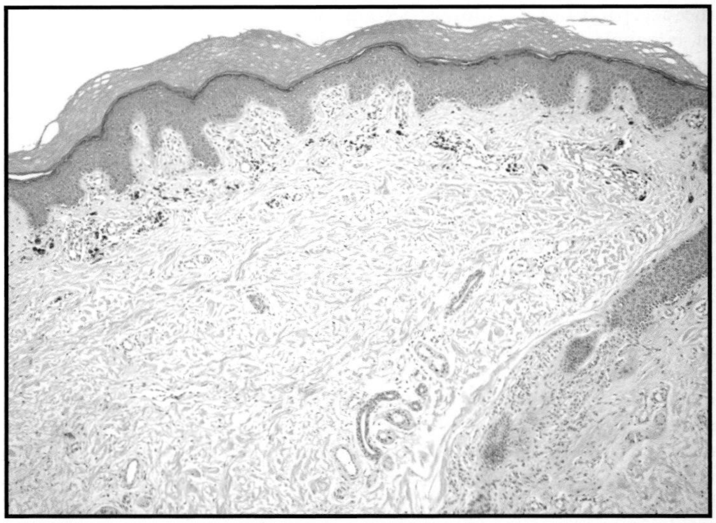

Fixed drug eruption (H&E stain) exhibiting a lymphocytic lichenoid infiltrate with pigmentary incontinence. Some vacuolar alteration may be seen scattered about the epidermal-dermal interface. Apoptotic keratinocytes can be variable in number.

within the inflammatory infiltrate. This abnormal immune response is responsible for the tissue damage. The precise interaction and mechanism by which certain medications react with the immune system of susceptible individuals to cause fixed drug eruptions has not been elucidated.

Treatment: The main point in therapy is making the correct diagnosis and removing the offending agent. Once this is done, the lesions heal within a month. Medium to potent topical corticosteroids can be used to help relieve pruritus and potentially speed healing. Fixed drug eruptions often leave an area of postinflammatory hyperpigmentation or hypopigmentation after the initial reaction has resolved. This pigmentary abnormality can last for months to years.

Plate 4-32

Rashes

GOUT

Gout is one of the crystal-induced arthropathies that is caused by precipitation of uric acid crystals in the joint spaces, kidneys, and cutaneous locations. It is divided into acute and chronic phases, which have different presentations and different treatments. The human body's immune reaction against the urate crystals causes more damage than the crystals themselves. Gout has been described for centuries and is clinically easily diagnosed. Medications, genetic predisposition, and dietary habits all contribute to cases of gout. There are other crystal-induced arthropathies that must be considered in the differential diagnosis of gout, the most common being calcium pyrophosphate crystals.

Clinical Findings: Gout is a disease predominantly found in the male population. Podagra is the classic presentation of an acute gouty attack. Descriptions of podagra have been published in the medical literature for centuries. It manifests as an acute monoarticular arthritis. The joint most commonly affected is the metatarsophalangeal articulation of the great toe. The clinical signs start as redness overlying the joint, swelling, warmth, and severe pain. Podagra has often been described as one of the most painful experiences a patient can perceive. A clue to the diagnosis is that the pain is often so severe that it appears to be out of proportion to the clinical picture. Patients complain of the slightest movement or touch; they are unable to wear shoes or bear weight on the foot; and they often have trouble with placement of a thin sheet over the affected joint. Acute attacks may be frequent, and the need for therapy is quite apparent. If no treatment is undertaken, an acute case of gout may last 7 days or longer. Any joint in the body can be affected by acute gout, but the great toe is by far the most common joint of involvement. Patients with acute gout have abnormal laboratory test results that can help in the diagnosis. An increased white blood cell count with a left shift is almost always seen. The markers of acute phase reactants are elevated, including the erythrocyte sedimentation rate (ESR), ferritin, and C-reactive protein.

The diagnosis can be made at the bedside by joint aspiration and microscopic evaluation. The affected joint is tapped with a fine-gauge needle and aspirated. The aspirate is then evaluated under polarized microscopy. Needle-like, elongated crystals of uric acid are seen freely within the synovial aspirate and also within the leukocytes of patients with gout. Radiographs of the affected joint do not show uric acid crystals and are likely to show only grossly abnormal soft tissue swelling. The serum uric acid level in acute gout can be normal, slightly elevated, or abnormally elevated; therefore, this test by itself is unreliable in making the diagnosis.

Chronic gout, which is seen as a sequela of multiple attacks of acute gout, leads to joint destruction and chronic arthritis. Patients with chronic gout may also

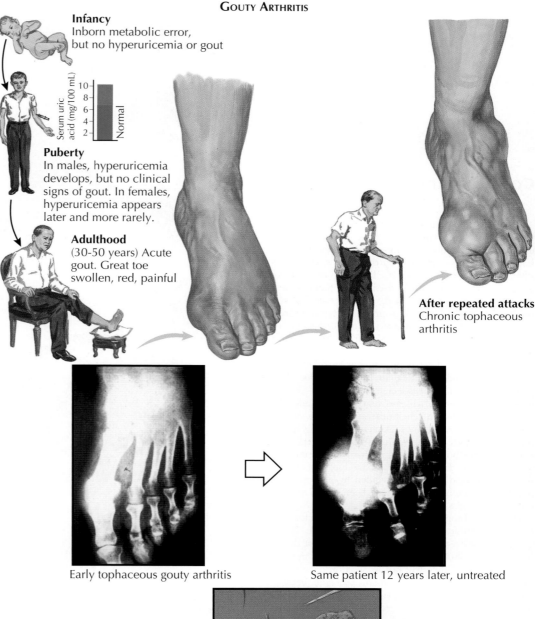

GOUTY ARTHRITIS

Infancy
Inborn metabolic error, but no hyperuricemia or gout

Puberty
In males, hyperuricemia develops, but no clinical signs of gout. In females, hyperuricemia appears later and more rarely.

Adulthood
(30-50 years) Acute gout. Great toe swollen, red, painful

After repeated attacks
Chronic tophaceous arthritis

Early tophaceous gouty arthritis

Same patient 12 years later, untreated

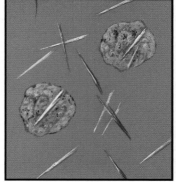

Free and phagocytized monosodium urate crystals in aspirated joint fluid seen on compensated polarized light microscopy

develop acute episodes of gout. Patients with chronic gout are predisposed to the development of tophaceous gout. This form of gout manifests as skin deposits of urate crystals. It can occur in any location and is most often located within the subcutaneous tissue. These tophi appear clinically as subcutaneous nodules, often overlying the extensor joints, particularly the elbows, Achilles tendons, and hands. For some reason, the ear is another area that is affected by tophi. The nodules of tophi may become thinned and partially translucent. The tophi may show an underlying yellowish appearance beneath the skin, and occasionally the clumping of crystals is appreciated just underneath the skin. With trauma, the nodules occasionally ulcerate, and crystals drain from the tophi. Saturnine gout is a specific form of gout that has been found to be caused by the consumption of homemade moonshine that is contaminated with lead.

Plate 4-33

Integumentary System

TOPHACEOUS GOUT

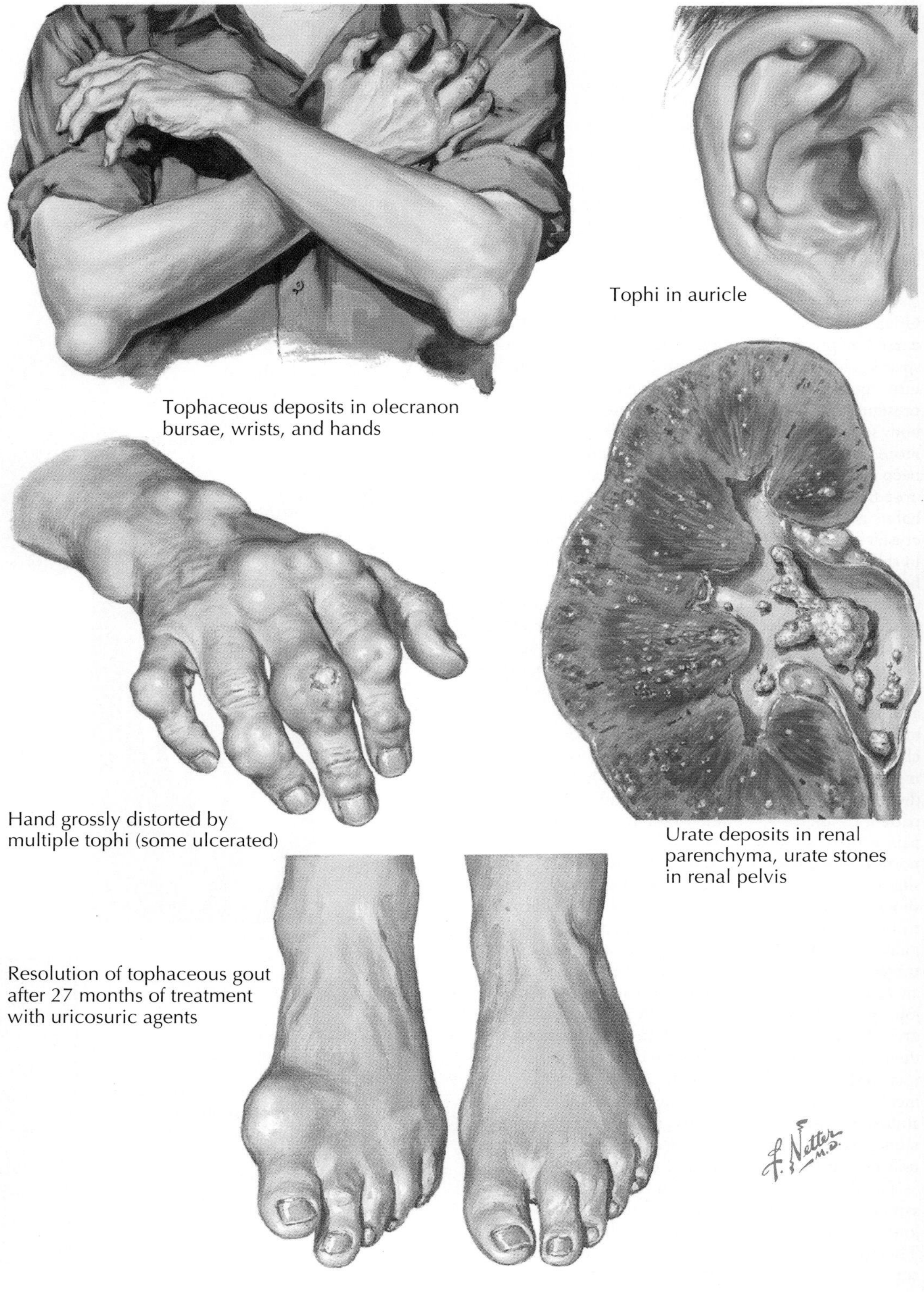

Tophi in auricle

Tophaceous deposits in olecranon bursae, wrists, and hands

GOUT (Continued)

Pathogenesis: Gout is caused by increased levels of uric acid resulting from a decrease in secretion, an increase in production, or an increase in dietary intake. Underexcretion of uric acid by the kidneys is responsible for most cases of gout. This can result from genetic causes or from use of medications that compete with the transport of uric acid, especially alcohol and the loop diuretics. Uric acid is produced under normal circumstances from the breakdown of purine nucleotides. Patients with the Lesch-Nyhan syndrome have a defect in the hypoxanthine-guanine phosphoribosyltransferase (HGPRT) enzyme, which is encoded by the gene *HPRT1* and is critical in the purine recycling pathway. This syndrome is seen in children and can lead to severe neurological disease that is confounded by severe gout. Certain chemotherapies cause severe immediate death of many leukocytes, resulting in the release of a high concentration of uric acid that can overwhelm the body's normal mechanisms of removal, leading to gout. Foods found to have high concentrations of uric acid should be avoided by patients with preexisting gout, because they have been shown to exacerbate the disease.

Histology: Biopsies of gout are rarely performed, because the clinical scenario is often diagnostic. When tissue of tophi is procured for biopsy, it is best that it be fixed in alcohol, because formalin dissolves the uric acid crystals, and they will not be seen on histological examination. The diagnosis can still be made, because the needle-shaped, clefted areas left by the dissolved crystals is characteristic. The crystals can be appreciated on alcohol-fixed tissue, and they appear needle shaped and birefringent under polarized light. The appearance of gout is much different from that of calcium pyrophosphate histologically, and there is usually no problem differentiating the two conditions. The crystals of pseudogout are rhomboid shaped and weakly birefringent.

Treatment: The therapeutic goal in acute gouty attacks is to control the patient's pain, and nonsteroidal antiinflammatory drugs (NSAIDs) have long been the medications of choice. Indomethacin also has been widely used for years. Aspirin should never be used in acute gout, because it can transiently increase uric acid levels when initiated. Colchicine is another medication that is used for the treatment of acute gouty attacks. Prednisone can be used to decrease the acute inflammation, pain, and swelling. Medications for the prophylactic treatment of gout are not used in acute episodes, because they may make an acute attack worse. They have also been shown to cause attacks of acute gout on rare occasions.

The most commonly used prophylactic medications to help prevent future acute attacks in patients with chronic gout are allopurinol and probenecid. Allopurinol is used exclusively for those patients who

Hand grossly distorted by multiple tophi (some ulcerated)

Urate deposits in renal parenchyma, urate stones in renal pelvis

Resolution of tophaceous gout after 27 months of treatment with uricosuric agents

overproduce uric acid, and probenecid is used for those whose kidneys underexcrete uric acid. Up to one third of patients started on allopurinol develop a cutaneous rash. If this happens, prompt discontinuation is wise, because allopurinol can lead to a severe drug hypersensitivity syndrome. Allopurinol works by inhibiting the purine breakdown enzyme, xanthine oxidase. This ultimately decreases the amount of uric acid produced from the breakdown of purine byproducts. Historically,

allopurinol was the first medication devised to inhibit a specific enzyme.

Tophi can be treated with the long-term use of allopurinol or probenecid. Over time, the goal is to mobilize the tissue uric acid and increase its excretion from the body. This can take years. Individual tophi have been surgically removed to help increase range of motion, if located around joints, or to improve cosmesis.

Plate 4-34

Rashes

GRAFT-VERSUS-HOST DISEASE

With the ever-increasing number of bone marrow transplantations and increasing survival rates of patients undergoing these procedures, graft-versus-host disease (GVHD) is becoming more prevalent. Two distinct clinical cutaneous forms exist, acute and chronic, each with its own manifestations and treatment options. Acute GVHD is often manifested by mucocutaneous eruptions that can range from a mild macular rash to life-threatening blistering of the skin. Chronic cutaneous GVHD is entirely different in clinical manifestation than its acute counterpart. The two forms are also seen during specific time frames: Acute GVHD is most likely to occur within the first 3 months after transplantation, whereas chronic GVHD occurs later, typically 4 months or longer after transplantation.

GVHD can be seen not only after bone marrow transplantation but in any immunosuppressed patient who has receives antigenically and immunologically viable cells from a donor. This may occur during organ transplantation or, rarely, during blood transfusion. The use of leuko-poor blood has helped decrease the chance of GVHD after blood transfusions.

Clinical Findings: Acute GVHD is a common complication after bone marrow transplantation. The incidence has been reported to be as high as 90%. The degree of involvement is variable. GVHD affects males and females equally, and there is no racial preference. Patients who develop acute GVHD typically begin having symptoms soon after their cell counts recover, usually 1 to 2 weeks after transplantation. Skin rashes that develop within the first week after transplantation are usually not from GVHD. The skin, upper and lower digestive tract, and liver are frequently involved, and these organ systems are evaluated to help make the diagnosis of GVHD. The rash of acute GVHD can range from a fine maculopapular rash to severe blistering of the skin that can resemble toxic epidermal necrolysis and can be life-threatening. It is difficult, if not impossible, to predict the development and course of acute GVHD. These patients are always taking multiple medications, and the differential diagnosis includes a drug rash. Histological evaluation of a skin biopsy cannot differentiate the two. The coexistence of mucositis, diarrhea, and elevated liver enzymes makes the diagnosis of acute GVHD more plausible. The constellation of all these symptoms leads one to make the diagnosis.

Chronic GVHD has entirely different clinical manifestations. This form of GVHD typically begins 3 to 6 months after transplantation. The skin is the organ system most commonly involved. Two distinct forms of chronic cutaneous GVHD occur, lichenoid and sclerodermatous. The lichenoid variant manifests as red papules, patches, and plaques. They can occur anywhere on the surface of the skin. There is a slight resemblance to lichen planus. The sclerodermatous variant is less common and manifests as thickened, firm skin with poikilodermatous changes. The surface of the skin is shiny, and the loss of adnexal structures is variable. This variant of chronic GVHD can be localized to a small area, or it can be generalized and may include the entire surface area of the skin. The amount of surface area involved is directly related to the morbidity the patient experiences.

Histology: Histological evaluation of skin biopsy specimens cannot differentiate acute GVHD from drug exanthems. Acute GVHD has been graded on a histological scale of 1 to 4. Grade 1 shows basal layer

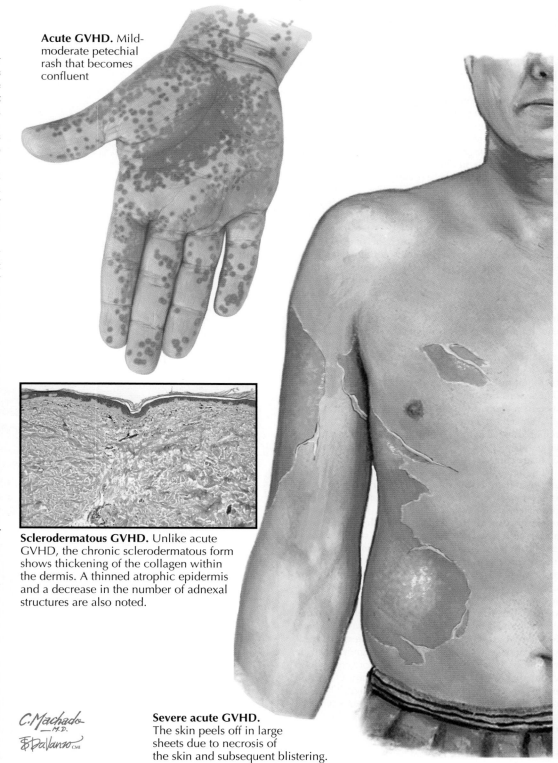

Acute GVHD. Mild-moderate petechial rash that becomes confluent

Sclerodermatous GVHD. Unlike acute GVHD, the chronic sclerodermatous form shows thickening of the collagen within the dermis. A thinned atrophic epidermis and a decrease in the number of adnexal structures are also noted.

C. Machado
— M.D.
B. DaVanzo CMI

Severe acute GVHD. The skin peels off in large sheets due to necrosis of the skin and subsequent blistering.

vacuolar and interface changes; grade 2 shows signs of keratinocyte death; grade 3 shows clefting within the subepidermal space; and grade 4 is full bulla formation with epidermal parting.

Lichenoid chronic GVHD shows a lichenoid dermatitis with a predominantly lymphocytic infiltrate. The sclerodermatous form of chronic GVHD shows abnormally thick dermal collagen, much like that seen in scleroderma.

Treatment: The treatment of acute GVHD is based on the clinical symptoms and the type of skin lesions.

Corticosteroids are commonly used in cases of GVHD, both acute and chronic. The acute form has also been treated with FK506 and cyclosporine. Many other immunosuppressants have been used.

Chronic GVHD is difficult to manage. There is no cure for GVHD, and treatment is directed at stabilizing and improving skin function and increasing the patient's functional capabilities. Phototherapy has been used successfully, as has extracorporeal photopheresis.

Plate 4-35

Integumentary System

GRANULOMA ANNULARE

Granuloma annulare is a commonly encountered rash. The etiology of this rash is unknown. There are various clinical presentations, including localized, generalized, subcutaneous, actinic, and perforating forms. The generalized version has been seen in association with diabetes. Most cases spontaneously resolve. Multiple treatment strategies exist.

Clinical Findings: Granuloma annulare is a rash that occurs commonly in children but can be seen in any age group. There is no race predilection, but it is twice as common in females as in males. The localized form of granuloma annulare typically starts insidiously as a small, flesh-colored to slightly yellow papule that expands centrifugally. Once the lesion gets to a certain size, its characteristic appearance becomes evident. Fully formed, the area appears as an annular plaque with minimal to no surface change. The plaque appears to have a raised rim around the edge, and the central portion of the lesion is almost normal in appearance. The peripheral rim is slightly yellow in color. The lesions can be entirely flesh colored. Patients experience minimal symptoms. Slight itching may be present. It is not uncommon to have multiple areas of involvement. The dorsal aspects of the feet and hands are common locations for this rash. Some patients relate that their rash is improved during the summer months. The lesions can range from small papules a few millimeters in diameter to larger plaques a few centimeters in diameter. If only small papules exist, a biopsy is required for diagnosis. The clinical appearance of the larger plaques is so characteristic that the diagnosis can be made clinically.

The generalized version of granuloma annulare consists of numerous widespread papules and small plaques. In most cases, there are no annulare-appearing plaques; the diagnosis is considered clinically, but a biopsy is required to confirm the diagnosis. This form occurs almost exclusively in adults and may be seen in association with diabetes. Patients with a diagnosis of generalized granuloma annulare should be screened for diabetes. The other variants of granuloma annulare are uncommonly encountered. They include the subcutaneous form, the perforating variant, and the actinic variant. The actinic variant may be considered a unique entity, termed *annular elastolytic giant cell granuloma.* Subcutaneous granuloma annulare manifests as deep-seated nodules within the dermis. A diagnosis is made via biopsy. This variant appears to be more common in children. The perforating variant is the rarest form and is the only variant to exhibit surface change. The areas of involvement develop small erosions. This is reported to occur most commonly on the dorsal surface of the hands.

Pathogenesis: The etiology is unknown. It has been theorized to represent an abnormal immune response to a foreign antigen such as a virus or bacteria. This has not been proven, and many other theories of pathogenesis exist. Ultimately, the collagen within the lesions is disrupted, and the resulting inflammatory response causes the clinical findings.

Histology: The histological findings in biopsy specimens of granuloma annulare are very specific. There are areas of necrobiotic collagen with a surrounding granulomatous infiltrate. The collagen is being destroyed centrally. A varying amount of mucin is present. The main histological differential diagnosis is between granuloma annulare and necrobiosis lipoidica. The inflammation in necrobiosis lipoidica is typically

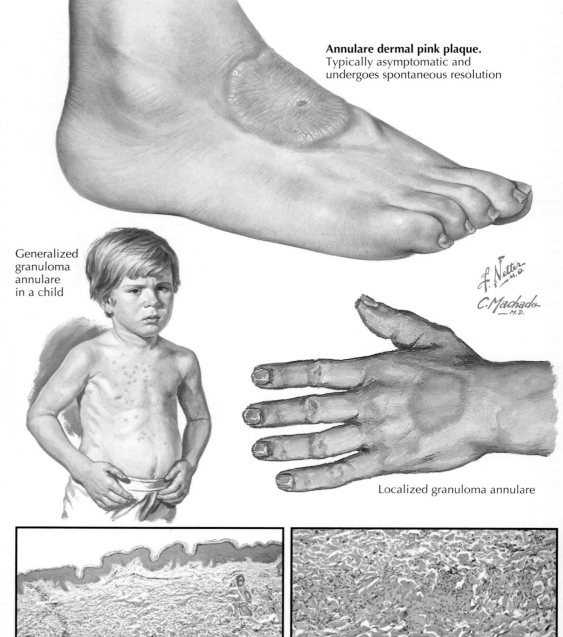

Annulare dermal pink plaque.
Typically asymptomatic and undergoes spontaneous resolution

Generalized granuloma annulare in a child

Localized granuloma annulare

Low power. Granulomatous inflammation throughout the specimen with necrobiotic collagen bundles

High power. Necrobiotic collagen within the granulomatous region

oriented across the entire biopsy specimen in a layered fashion. Histological variants of granuloma annulare exist, including interstitial granuloma annulare.

Treatment: Localized forms of granuloma annulare that are asymptomatic and not causing any distress to the patient can be left alone. Most cases resolve spontaneously over time with no residual scarring and no clinically noticeable abnormality. Topical corticosteroids may be used to try to decrease the inflammatory response. Intralesional corticosteroids can be used in some cases, but the risk of atrophy from the steroid injection must be considered. Generalized forms are not amenable to topical therapy. Phototherapy has been used successfully. Psoralen + ultraviolet A light (PUVA) therapy has had more success than ultraviolet B (UVB) light therapy, most likely because UVA light penetrates deeper into the dermis than UVB. Phototherapy with UVA_1 appears promising.

Plate 4-36

GRAVES' DISEASE AND PRETIBIAL MYXEDEMA

Graves' disease is the form of hyperthyroidism that is most often seen in the young adult population. It is an autoimmune disease that causes the thyroid gland to produce thyroid hormones. This results in the clinical manifestations.

Clinical Findings: Graves' disease is seen in females more frequently than males, in a ratio of approximately 7:1. Most patients have an insidious onset of symptoms. Heat intolerance and nervousness are two of the early and more common findings. Anxiety and emotional difficulties can be life altering. Patients often complain of difficulty sleeping. Constitutional symptoms can manifest as weight loss, increased appetite, increased sweating, and profound nervousness. Women may suffer from menstrual irregularities. Cardiac arrhythmias are common as the disease progresses. Hypertension and tachycardia can be two of the earliest cardiovascular signs of the disease. As the disease progresses, exophthalmos becomes prominent, a goiter can be seen or felt, and patients develop pretibial myxedema.

The exophthalmos may lead to intermittent double vision and a feeling of posterior ocular pressure. Photophobia can be a part of the disease, as can frequent tearing and a feeling of "sand" in the eyes that causes frequent tearing and pain. Goiter may be noticeable to the patient, and it may be appreciated initially because of difficulty buttoning one's collar. The goiter is diffuse in nature. The thyroid is easily palpable and is firm to the touch. On occasion, the astute clinician can auscultate a bruit over the thyroid gland; this represents the increased blood flow to the growing gland.

Pretibial myxedema is the most widely recognized skin finding in Graves' disease. It begins as small, indurated papules that coalesce into plaques on the anterior shin. The plaques indent easily when palpated and clinically act like lymphedema, causing a nonpitting edema. Pretibial myxedema can occur in other areas of the body, but this is a rare finding. The skin is typically warm to the touch and can have a velvety feel. Increased sweating is noticeable most often as warm, moist palms and soles, similar to what is observed in patients with hyperhidrosis. Clubbing of the fingers is seen in a small proportion of affected individuals. Facial flushing with an increase in sweating is also seen. Females may develop breast enlargement, and males may develop gynecomastia.

Laboratory testing is needed to help define the condition. Radioactive iodine uptake imaging shows a diffuse, symmetric uptake of iodine in the patient with Graves' disease. The pattern of uptake is very different from that seen in patients with a "hot" thyroid nodule, in which the radioactive signal is dramatically increased in the nodule. Thyroid antibody testing is very helpful in differentiating Graves' disease from other forms of thyrotoxicosis. Antithyroglobulin, antimicrosomal, and anti–thyroid-stimulating hormone (TSH) receptor antibodies can be evaluated.

Pathogenesis: Graves' disease is an idiopathic autoimmune disease that causes autoantibodies against the TSH receptor. The antibodies act as agonists to the receptor and cause non-stop activation of the TSH receptor on the thyroid. This leads to increased production of thyroid hormones, both triiodothyronine (T_3) and (T_4), by the thyroid. The increase in metabolic functioning of the thyroid leads to diffuse enlargement and goiter. The increased production of thyroid

hormones and their effects on target tissues lead to the clinical findings.

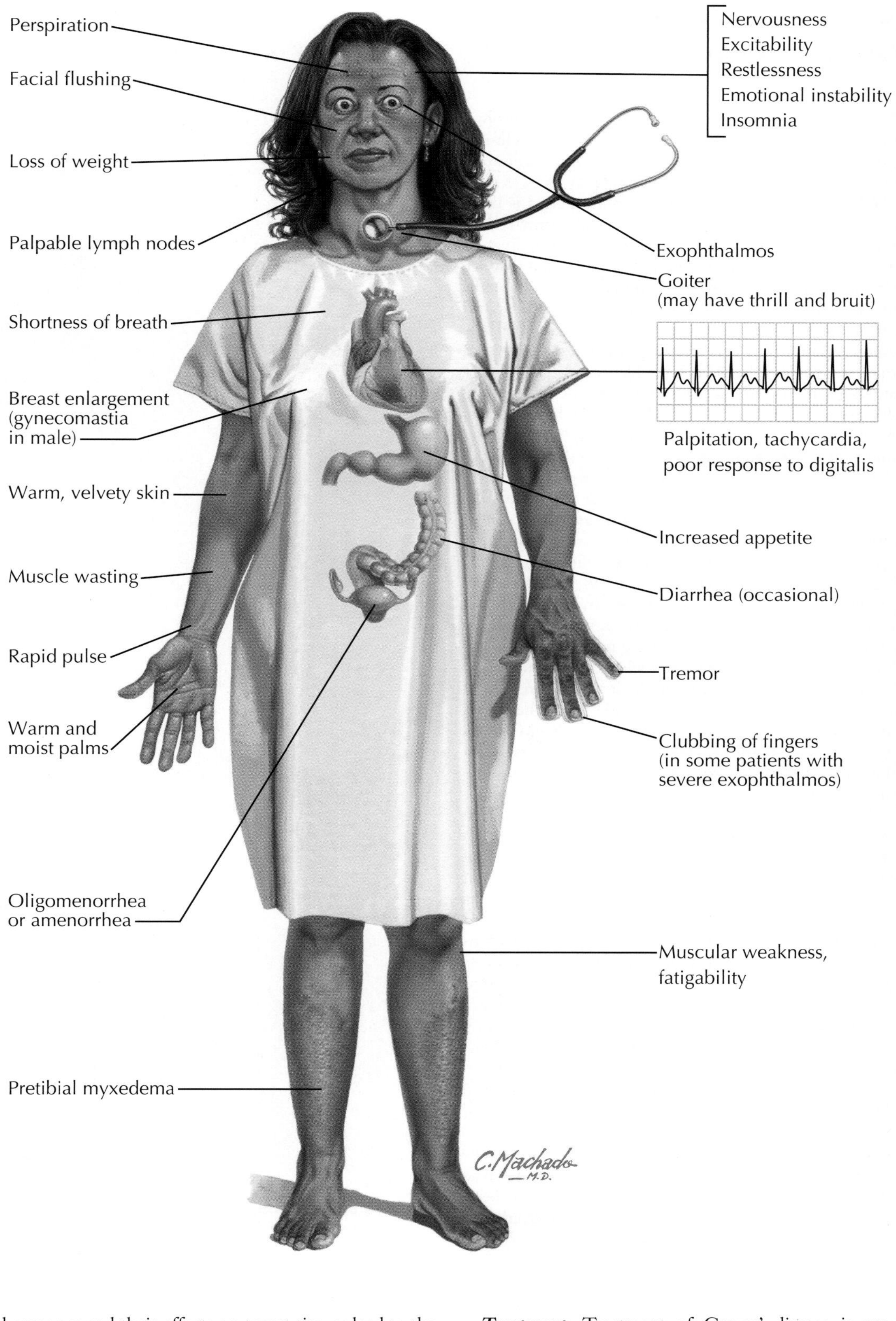

Histology: Biopsy specimens of the pretibial skin show large amounts of mucin deposits within the middle and lower dermis, between collagen bundles. The mucin is so thick that it causes the dermal collagen bundles to be splayed apart. Overlying hyperkeratosis can be appreciated. Biopsy specimens from clinically nonaffected skin may show some of the same histological findings but on a lesser scale.

Treatment: Treatment of Graves' disease is predicated on stopping the excessive thyroid hormone production. Ablation of the thyroid can be achieved with radiation therapy or surgical removal. Medications such as β-blockers are used to lessen the symptoms of the disease until it is rendered under control. Medical management of Graves' disease can be achieved with propylthiouracil or methimazole, both of which act to decrease thyroid hormone production.

Perspiration

Facial flushing

Loss of weight

Palpable lymph nodes

Shortness of breath

Breast enlargement (gynecomastia in male)

Warm, velvety skin

Muscle wasting

Rapid pulse

Warm and moist palms

Oligomenorrhea or amenorrhea

Pretibial myxedema

Nervousness
Excitability
Restlessness
Emotional instability
Insomnia

Exophthalmos

Goiter (may have thrill and bruit)

Palpitation, tachycardia, poor response to digitalis

Increased appetite

Diarrhea (occasional)

Tremor

Clubbing of fingers (in some patients with severe exophthalmos)

Muscular weakness, fatigability

C. Machado
—M.D.

Plate 4-37

Integumentary System

Hidradenitis Suppurativa (Acne Inversa)

Hidradenitis suppurativa (acne inversa) is a rare chronic, life-altering disease. It can be an isolated clinical finding, or it can be associated with cystic acne, dissecting cellulitis of the scalp, and pilonidal cysts.

Clinical Findings: Hidradenitis suppurativa is most commonly encountered in postpubertal women. The ratio of female-to-male involvement is approximately 4:1. This condition preferentially affects areas that are rich in apocrine glands and terminal hairs. The areas most commonly involved are the axillae, groin, and inframammary folds. It is rare in other areas. Hidradenitis suppurativa starts as tiny red papules or nodules that tend to be folliculocentric. The papules are tender and firm to palpation. At this point, the differential diagnosis includes an early folliculitis or furunculosis. As the disease progresses, the hard nodules become fluctuant and spontaneously drain to the surface of the skin. The nodules may coalesce into plaques with varying amounts of scarring. The longer the process has been going on, the more scarring is prevalent. Eventually, sinus tracts develop that interconnect multiple subcutaneous nodules with multiple cutaneous openings. Clinically, pressing on one of the nodules may produce drainage from a distant sinus tract. The disease is relentless, and new crops of lesions repeatedly develop. Pain is significant and is a main cause of morbidity. Obesity tends to be seen in association with hidradenitis suppurativa. Hidradenitis has been seen in association with Crohn's disease, and some believe that hidradenitis suppurativa is a cutaneous form of Crohn's disease. Long-standing disease has been associated with the development of squamous cell carcinoma. The tumors tend to be large at diagnosis

The drainage from the cutaneous nodules often requires extensive bandaging to keep clothing from getting soiled. The drainage has a malodorous, foul smell. The draining sinus tracts and nodules are often colonized with various bacteria, and cultures of the purulent drainage show growth of a number of different organisms, including *Staphylococcus aureus* and streptococcal species. However, this is not primarily an infectious disease. The bacteria in these cases are present secondary to the underlying inflammatory condition and the lack of normal cutaneous skin barrier function.

Pathogenesis: Hidradenitis suppurativa is an inflammatory disease with secondary bacterial superinfection and colonization. Routine culturing of the nodules and the drainage is often sterile. Hidradenitis is theorized to be caused by rupture of the mature follicular epithelium along areas of apocrine glands; hence, its propensity to occur in areas with high densities of apocrine glands. A hormonal control over the process has been theorized, given that it is more common in postpubertal women and in obese individuals. Once the hair follicle ruptures, an inflammatory cascade is set off and causes the resulting nodules, cysts, fistulas, and scarring. It appears to be a self-perpetuating process. The exact mechanism by which this occurs is unknown.

Histology: Chronic lesions show a dense, mixed inflammatory infiltrate with abscess and sinus tract formation. Varying amounts of fibrosis and scar tissue are present. Apocrine gland inflammation can be appreciated in a fair number of cases. The inflammation extends into the subcutaneous tissue.

Treatment: Therapy is often aimed at reducing inflammation and bacterial superinfection. There is no curative therapy, and most treatments have only

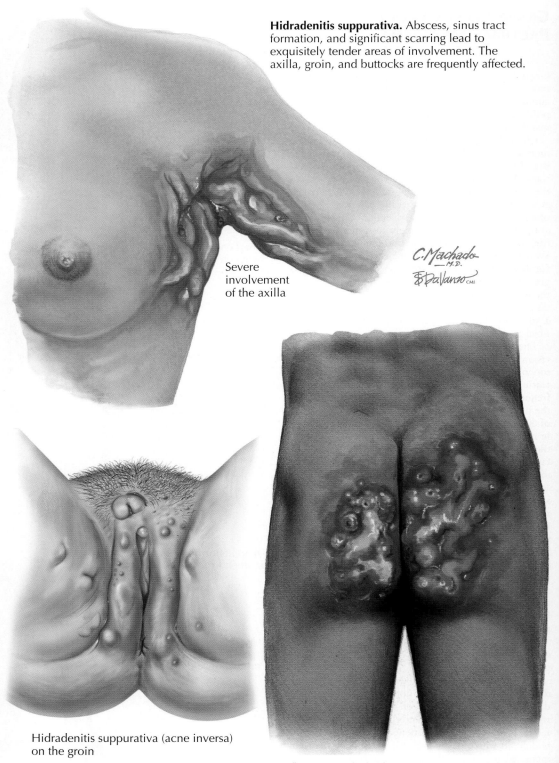

Hidradenitis suppurativa. Abscess, sinus tract formation, and significant scarring lead to exquisitely tender areas of involvement. The axilla, groin, and buttocks are frequently affected.

Severe involvement of the axilla

Hidradenitis suppurativa (acne inversa) on the groin

Severe inflammatory hidradenitis suppurativa of the buttocks

anecdotal reports of success. Topical clindamycin and other antibacterial products such as benzyl peroxide are often the first-line agents employed for mild disease. Oral antibiotics, typically in the tetracycline class, are often used because they have both antiinflammatory and antibacterial properties. Weight loss must be advocated. Other agents that have had limited success include isotretinoin, etanercept, and infliximab. Surgical options include wide local excisions to remove the affected tissue and repair with complex flap closure. Liposuction has also been tried in an attempt to remove the affected apocrine gland hair follicle unit. The only potential for cure is with a surgical approach. This approach seems to work best for axillary disease; groin and inframammary disease almost always recurs after surgery. It is also of the utmost importance to address patients' psychosocial needs, because this disease has a devastating toll on the patients it afflicts.

Plate 4-38

Rashes

IRRITANT CONTACT DERMATITIS

Irritant contact dermatitis is one of the most commonly encountered dermatoses in the dermatology clinic. Its true incidence is unknown. Irritant contact dermatitis can be caused by a multitude of factors, and the morphology of its appearance can be varied. One of the most common forms of irritant contact dermatitis is seen on the hands and is caused by occupational exposures to irritant chemicals or excessive hand washing.

Clinical Findings: Irritant contact dermatitis can occur at any age. Some studies show that women are more commonly affected. There is no racial predilection. There are many exposures that can eventually lead to the development of irritant contact dermatitis. The final clinical manifestations are similar despite the different instigating chemicals. Variations exist in the location of the dermatitis. The hallmark of irritant contact dermatitis is xerosis. Once the skin dries out to a certain point, it becomes inflamed. This leads to the clinical picture of dry pink or red patches. On the hands, painful fissures or splits may occur within the skin lines.

Diaper dermatitis in infants is one specific form of irritant contact dermatitis. The wet diaper rubbing against the child's buttocks and legs can cause skin irritation, red patches, and occasionally erosions. The child can become irritable with pruritus and is at higher risk for secondary bacterial infections.

Many chemicals are direct irritants to the skin, and injuries from these agents are occasionally seen in a dermatologist's office. Exposure of the skin to hydrochloric acid results in skin cell death, necrosis, and inflammation. This, in turn, leads to the development of red patches or plaques with varying amounts of erosion and ulceration. These patients often receive care in an occupational work setting or in the emergency room. The same can be said for exposure of the skin to strong basic chemicals such as sodium hydroxide. Basic chemicals can cause an irritant contact dermatitis that is directly related to the necrotic effect of the chemical on the skin surface.

One of the most common causes of irritant contact dermatitis is frequent hand washing. The use of soaps removes the natural oils and waxes that the skin produces as a way of physiologically keeping the skin from drying out. Once the removal of these oils outweighs their production, dryness begins to set in. If the skin is not given enough time to repair itself, the epidermis continues to dry out and becomes inflamed. Pink to red patches are evident, and, as the irritation continues, the dryness worsens until fissuring and cracking occur.

Ring dermatitis is another common form of irritant contact dermatitis. It is believed that soap residue builds up between the surface of the ring and the skin. This prolonged contact causes an irritant contact dermatitis underlying the ring. It can be misdiagnosed as an allergic contact dermatitis, and on initial presentation, these two forms of dermatitis cannot be differentiated. The main differential diagnosis is between an irritant and an allergic contact dermatitis. The two have similar clinical appearances and can be almost impossible to differentiate. Irritant contact dermatitis typically has an acute onset and a decrescendo resolution, unless there is repeated exposure to the irritant. Allergic contact dermatitis usually has a crescendo-decrescendo clinical course. These patterns can be helpful in differentiating the two conditions.

Pathogenesis: Exposure to an irritant chemical, whether an acid or a base, or repeated exposure to

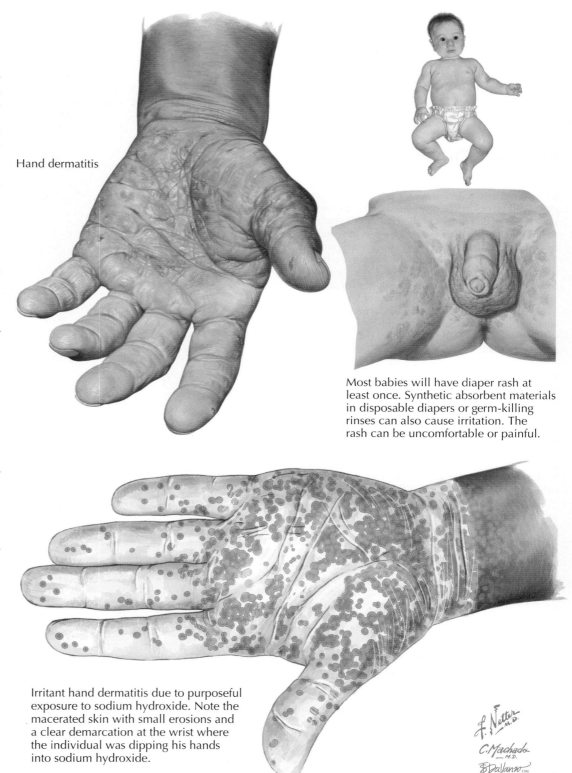

Hand dermatitis

Most babies will have diaper rash at least once. Synthetic absorbent materials in disposable diapers or germ-killing rinses can also cause irritation. The rash can be uncomfortable or painful.

Irritant hand dermatitis due to purposeful exposure to sodium hydroxide. Note the macerated skin with small erosions and a clear demarcation at the wrist where the individual was dipping his hands into sodium hydroxide.

soap and water leads to a similar inflammatory cascade. The damaged keratinocytes release myriad inflammatory cytokines. The intensity of the reaction is based on the concentration of the irritant and the exposure time. The recruitment of T cells occurs later in the time course of irritant contact dermatitis, when compared with allergic contact dermatitus.

Treatment: The goal of treatment is to remove the skin from exposure to the irritant. Barrier creams and

frequent diaper changes may be all that is needed to resolve irritant contact diaper dermatitis. Hand dermatitis can be treated with a combination of moisturizers, topical corticosteroids, and avoidance of frequent hand washing. If these changes can be accomplished, the prognosis is excellent. Workers with potential occupational exposures to irritant chemicals must be properly trained in handling them and given the correct protective gear to prevent exposure.

Plate 4-39

Integumentary System

KERATOSIS PILARIS

Keratosis pilaris is an extremely common dermatosis that in mild states can be considered a variant of normal skin. It is usually brought to the clinician's attention as an afterthought, or the clinician observes the condition and tells the patient about it for educational purposes. There are more severe forms of keratosis pilaris in which patients present to the dermatologist for therapy. Many distinct variants of keratosis pilaris exist, and they are named based on area of involvement.

Clinical Findings: Keratosis pilaris is one of the most common dermatoses and is thought by some to be a variant of normal. It is found in more than 40% of the adult population and in as many as 80% of children. There is no sex or race predilection. It typically begins soon after a child reaches 5 years of age. Most cases are asymptomatic and are of no concern to the patient or of only cosmetic concern. The upper lateral arms are the most common site of involvement. Small (1-2 mm), pink-to-red follicular hyperkeratotic papules are present to a varying extent. Some are so fine that they are noticeable only on palpation. Other cases are more widespread and can include the upper thighs, shoulders, and cheeks. Widespread cases tend to be more noticeable, and the small papules tend to be more inflammatory in nature.

This inflammatory form of keratosis pilaris is also called keratosis pilaris rubra. It is typically manifested by bright red, small, hyperkeratotic papules that may resemble pustules. They can be mistaken for acneiform lesions. A small scraping of the inflammatory lesion results in removal of a small keratin plug rather than the contents of an acneiform pustule. The location on the outer arms and upper thighs also helps to differentiate this condition from acne. Both keratosis pilaris and acne are extremely common, and they are frequently seen together in the same patient.

Ulerythema ophryogenes is a keratosis pilaris variant that manifests in early childhood. The lateral one third of the eyebrow is affected with minute, red keratotic papules. Hair loss of the lateral eyebrows is common. The rash may affect other parts of the face and may heal with tiny pitted scars. It is almost always seen along with keratosis pilaris. Over time, alopecia may develop in the affected regions, especially the lateral eyebrows.

Atrophoderma vermiculata is one of the rarest of the keratosis pilaris variants. It manifests as small, hyperkeratotic plugs on the cheeks that resolve and leave behind small, atrophic scars in a fine mesh-like pattern.

Erythromelanosis follicularis faciei et colli is similar in nature to atrophoderma vermiculata, but it lacks any evidence of scarring. This condition has been reported to occur most commonly in young men during the second and third decades of life. Postinflammatory hyperpigmentation is another unusual feature not seen with the other variants.

Keratosis follicularis spinulosa decalvans is probably the least common keratosis pilaris variant. It is inherited in a X-linked fashion and thus affects males. It is manifested by areas of skin thickening and follicular plugging

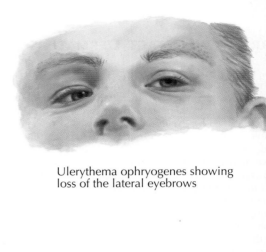

Ulerythema ophryogenes showing loss of the lateral eyebrows

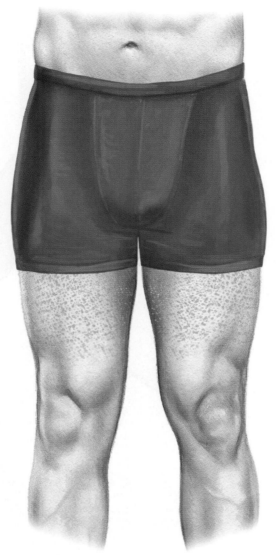

Keratosis pilaris of upper thighs. The upper arms and thighs are two commonly affected areas. Small 1- to 2-mm hyperkeratotic red papules

Keratosis Pilaris Variants

▶ Keratosis pilaris rubra
▶ Ulerythema ophryogenes (keratosis pilaris atrophicans faciei)
▶ Atrophoderma vermiculata (folliculitis ulerythematosa reticulata)
▶ Erythromelanosis follicularis faciei et colli
▶ Keratosis follicularis spinulosa decalvans

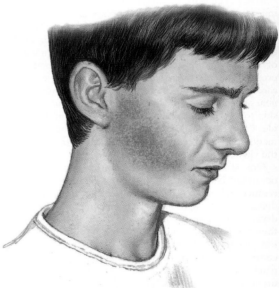

Keratosis pilaris atrophicans faciei. Perifollicular erythema is prominent, as are small regions of atrophic scarring.

along with areas of scarring alopecia. This condition may also affect the eyelashes. Corneal dystrophy and blepharitis can be seen.

Pathogenesis: The exact etiology of keratosis pilaris is unknown. It is believed to be caused by an abnormality in follicular keratinization of the infundibulum.

Histology: Keratosis pilaris is rarely biopsied. A keratin plug is the most prominent feature. The plug is typically 1 to 2 mm in diameter and may lie on top of a meager lymphocytic infiltrate.

Treatment: No therapy is required for most cases. A keratolytic moisturizer or humectant moisturizer works well. These include lactic acid– and salicylic acid–based moisturizers. After discontinuation, however, the rash of keratosis pilaris returns over a period of a few weeks to months. Many other therapies have been used. Vitamin A derivatives (e.g., tretinoin) are among the more commonly used prescription medications. The cream is applied daily and has been successful in removing the redness and hyperkeratosis.

Plate 4-40

Rashes

LANGERHANS CELL HISTIOCYTOSIS

Langerhans cell histiocytosis (LCH) is a rare disorder caused by the proliferation of Langerhans cells in various tissues. Historically, the disease was categorized based on the grouping of symptoms and organs affected, with names such as Letterer-Siwe disease and Hand-Schüller-Christian disease. Over the last decade, the classification of LCH has been standardized. The new classification does not remove the eponyms that have been used for years but rather categorizes the LCH into subgroups based on prognosis and amount of involvement. These histiocytoses are a heterogeneous group of diseases that may affect both the skin and various internal organs. The main pathological finding is the accumulation of pathological Langerhans cells within the affected tissue. The diagnosis is made on clinical, histological, laboratory, and radiographic findings. The newer classification of LCH is based on the number of organ systems involved. It includes the subtypes of restricted single-system LCH, extensive multisystem LCH, and single-system pulmonary LCH. The extensive multisystem form of LCH can be further divided into those cases with and without organ dysfunction. Prognosis and therapy depend on the organ systems involved and the number of systems implicated. Optimal therapy has yet to be determined.

Clinical Findings: LCH is a very rare condition that affects approximately 8 of every 1,000,000 people. There is a 2:1 male-to-female predilection, and all races are affected equally. Usually, the condition is first noticed in childhood, but adult-onset disease does occur. LCH isolated to the skin has one of the best prognoses of all of the forms of LCH. Most cases of LCH manifest first in the skin, even before the development of systemic findings; therefore, all patients with cutaneous LCH should be routinely screened for systemic diseases.

In infants, the typical presenting skin findings are those of a persistent papulosquamous eruption on the scalp that resembles cradle cap. On closer inspection, small petechiae are observed. These petechiae are very characteristic for LCH and can be easily overlooked. The scalp form is often misdiagnosed as seborrheic dermatitis early in infancy, and frequently it is not until the child is 3 to 6 months old and the rash has persisted that the diagnosis of LCH is entertained. The other common presentation in children is that of persistent diaper dermatitis. The rash has a unique predisposition to affect the groin folds and can be quite inflammatory and resistant to typical therapy for irritant contact dermatitis or diaper rash. The groin rash appears as red to yellowish-orange papules that coalesce into plaques. Ulcerations and erosions are common. Superinfection with bacteria often leads to an odor. Both of these forms are almost always considered to be another diagnosis before LCH is considered and a skin biopsy is done to prove the diagnosis. Other skin findings that can be observed by the astute clinician are adenopathy, ear inflammation and drainage from the external ear, and soft tissue swelling. The soft tissue swelling is seen only in those patients with underlying bony disorders. Gingival hypertrophy may also be seen, but it is often subtle. Infants may also have premature eruption of their teeth, which is most commonly noticed by the still breast-feeding mother.

Twenty percent of patients do not exhibit any cutaneous signs of disease and present solely with varying

PRESENTATION OF LANGERHANS CELL HISTIOCYTOSIS IN CHILDHOOD

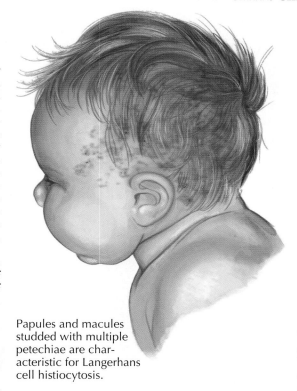

Papules and macules studded with multiple petechiae are characteristic for Langerhans cell histiocytosis.

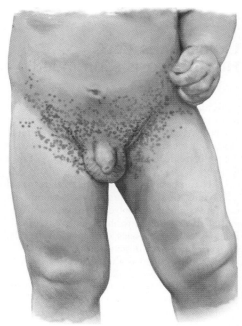

The diaper area is one of the more common areas of involvement with Langerhans cell histiocytosis. This disease should be in the differential diagnosis of diaper rash that does not respond to therapy for dermatitis, especially if petechiae are present.

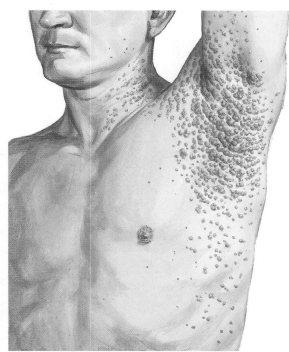

Disseminated Langerhans cell histiocytosis lesions in axilla and on neck and trunk

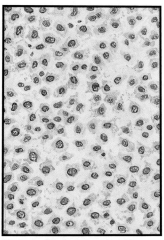

Sheets of Langerhans cell histiocytes with abundant pink cytoplasm and folded nuclei with prominent nuclear grooves

systemic complaints. The most common extracutaneous form of LCH, formerly designated eosinophilic granuloma, is now called single-system unifocal bone disease. Children present with a painless to slightly tender soft tissue swelling overlying the bony area of involvement, most commonly the calvarium. Palpation of the swelling reveals the fluctuant nature of the soft tissue distention, and in some cases the defect in the underlying bone can be felt. Plain radiographs can help delineate the extent of disease. If one area of bony involvement is found, a skeletal survey should be performed to evaluate for other silent bony lesions, which can occur in up to 15% of cases. The involved bone has a radiolucent appearance that is sharply demarcated from the surrounding bone. Bony involvement has been described to occur in almost every bone in the body. Most cases are inconsequential, but if the involvement affects a critical portion of the spine, the possibility of

Plate 4-41

Integumentary System

LANGERHANS CELL HISTIOCYTOSIS (Continued)

weakening of the joint and potential fracture could have life-threatening implications. The term "floating teeth" has been used to describe the finding of radiolucent aspects of the mandible that give the appearance that the teeth are floating without the support of the underlying bone.

LCH can be a life-threatening, progressive disease. The lymphatic system, lungs, hypothalamus, and pituitary are commonly involved. Lymphadenopathy in the region of skin or bony involvement is usually seen. Biopsies of lymph nodes can show involvement with Langerhans cells or dermatopathic changes.

Lung involvement is almost always a component of multisystem disease. Radiographs may be normal or may show cystic spaces or a nonspecific interstitial infiltrate. Pulmonary function testing may reveal a decrease in diffusion capacity and a decrease in forced expiratory volume. Lung abnormalities are very frequently seen in adults with LCH.

The pituitary stalk can also be affected in this disease. The eponym *Hans-Schüller-Christian disease* describes those patients with LCH who have the constellation of diabetes insipidus, lytic bony lesions, and exophthalmos. The involvement of the pituitary stalk leads to the diabetes insipidus. The lack of antidiuretic hormone causes the excretion of large amounts of dilute urine and increased thirst. The skull is the bony region most commonly involved.

Letterer-Siwe disease is the name given to the constellation of symptoms that include severe skin involvement, hepatosplenomegaly, anemia, and leukopenia. These patients have early onset of disease in infancy and have a poor prognosis because of the aggressiveness and extent of the disease load.

The diagnosis and prognosis of LCH depend on the number of organ systems involved and the extent of disease. Treatment likewise depends on these factors, and a multidisciplinary approach should be taken.

Pathogenesis: The exact etiology is unknown, and there is considerable ongoing research to determine whether this is a clonal malignant process or a reactive process. The Langerhans cells that are present within the areas of involvement have a different morphology from their normal counterparts. The affected Langerhans cells are round, without dendritic processes, and have been found to express different cell surface markers. The initiating factor or factors for these findings are as yet only theoretical. No gene defect has been described.

Histology: Histological findings from the skin and other involved tissues are only slightly different. The main pathology is found within the sheets of abnormal-appearing Langerhans cells. On microscopic evaluation, the cells have kidney bean–shaped nucleus and show varying amounts of epidermotropism. Immunohistochemical staining shows CD1a, S100 and CD207 positivity. On electron microscopy, the characteristic tennis racket–shaped Birbeck granules are seen.

Treatment: Therapy is determined by the extent and location of disease state. Mild, localized cutaneous single-system disease may be observed and watched carefully for the development of systemic involvement. Supportive care is given with topical antiinflammatory

EOSINOPHILIC GRANULOMA

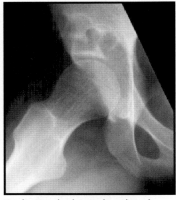

Radiograph shows loculated, bubble-like, radiolucent lesion in supraacetabular region of right ilium.

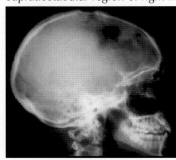

Variegated defects in flat bones of skull

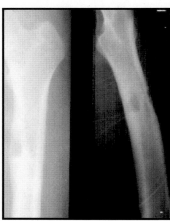

Anteroposterior and lateral views show typical marginated, radiolucent lesions in femoral shaft.

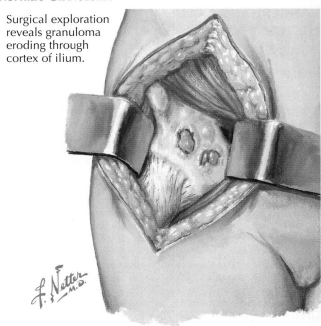

Surgical exploration reveals granuloma eroding through cortex of ilium.

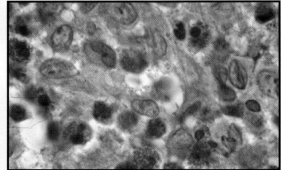

Section reveals pale-staining, foamy histiocytes interspersed with bilobed eosinophilis (H&E stain).

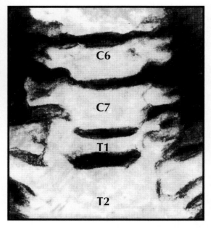

Marked narrowing of first thoracic vertebra that led to spinal cord injury in 13-year-old boy. Vertebra plana in young patients strongly suggests eosinophilic granuloma.

agents and antiinfectives to help treat and prevent possible infections, especially infections of the groin region in infants. A small percentage of patients experience spontaneous remission. Single bony lesions may also remit spontaneously.

Bony lesions have been treated with resection of the involved tissue, with curettage of the region, and with systemic steroid therapy. The use of steroids has been associated with recurrences after the drug is stopped.

Multisystem disease is treated in myriad manners, depending on the burden of disease, the systemic involvement, and the patient's symptoms. The disease can be difficult to treat, and systemic chemotherapies are the mainstay of treatment. Vinblastine- or etoposide-based regimens are most commonly used as first-line therapy. Some refractory disease has been treated with ablative chemotherapy and subsequent bone marrow transplantation.

Plate 4-42

Rashes

LEUKOCYTOCLASTIC VASCULITIS

Many forms of vasculitis can affect the skin, the most common one being leukocytoclastic vasculitis. Other forms of vasculitis known to affect the skin as well as other organ systems include Churg-Strauss vasculitis, Henoch-Schönlein purpura, Wegener's granulomatosis, polyarteritis nodosa, and urticarial vasculitis. Leukocytoclastic vasculitis is by far the most commonly encountered of the cutaneous vasculitides. The causes and pathomechanisms vary, and diagnosis and treatment depend on the results of the clinical and histological evaluations.

Clinical Findings: Leukocytoclastic vasculitis most commonly affects the lower extremity or dependent areas of the body. For example, this form of vasculitis is most commonly seen on the legs of ambulatory patients but on the back and buttocks of bedridden patients. The clinical hallmark of vasculitis is the presence of palpable purpura. The rash may start as small, pink, violaceous macules that rapidly develop into red or purple palpable papules; hence the term *palpable purpura*. Most of the lesions of palpable purpura are uniform in size, but they can range from minute to 1 cm or more in diameter. Patients are most likely to complain of mild itching or no symptoms at all, and the appearance of the rash is what brings them to see the clinician. Mild constitutional symptoms are often present, with mild fever, fatigue, and malaise most commonly reported. Skin-specific symptoms can range from mild pruritus to pain and tenderness to palpation.

The etiology of cutaneous leukocytoclastic vasculitis is heterogeneous. The three most common causes are infections, medications, and idiopathic causes. Almost every possible infection (bacterial, viral, parasitic, and fungal) has been reported to be an initiating factor for leukocytoclastic vasculitis. Medications are a common culprit and can easily be overlooked if a thorough history is not obtained. If the offending infection is treated properly or the offending medication is removed, the vasculitis resolves in approximately 1 month. The symptoms also cease, often faster than the rash resolves. Postinflammatory hyperpigmentation with some hemosiderin deposition often is a residual finding after the lesions have cleared. This resolves slowly over 6 to 12 months.

Pathogenesis: Leukocytoclastic vasculitis is a type III hypersensitivity reaction. Soluble antigens are believed to become complexed with antibodies. As these antigen-antibody complexes enlarge, they get trapped in the tiny vasculature of the dependent regions of the body. There, they can initiate the complement cascade and cause endothelial cell wall death, recruitment of neutrophils, and continued blood vessel destruction, leading to the typical cutaneous findings.

Histology: The pathology is centered on the blood venules in the dermis. A prominent neutrophilic infiltrate is present. Degeneration of the neutrophils is always seen, with nuclear dust; this is termed *leukocytoclasis*. Fibrinoid necrosis of the vessel walls is easily seen. Extravasated red blood cells are seen in the vicinity of the vasculitis. Thrombosis of affected vessel walls is a secondary finding and is not the primary pathology.

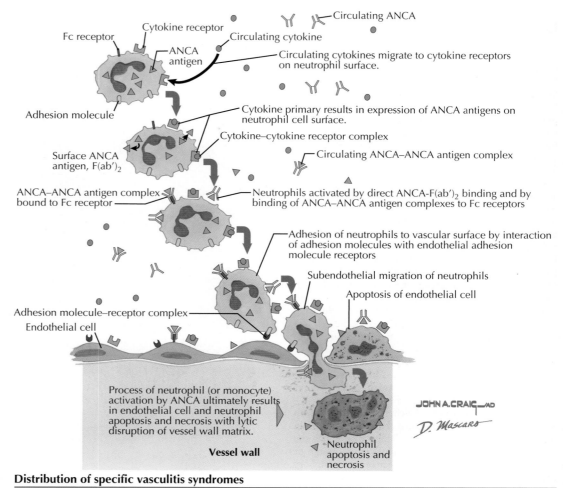

Process of neutrophil (or monocyte) activation by ANCA ultimately results in endothelial cell and neutrophil apoptosis and necrosis with lytic disruption of vessel wall matrix.

Distribution of specific vasculitis syndromes

Treatment: Therapy is based on the cause of the leukocytoclastic vasculitis. New offending medications should be withdrawn and replaced with substitutes of a different class. Infections need to be thoroughly treated. The use of topical high-potency corticosteroids is helpful in some cases, and oral steroids may be used in medication-induced leukocytoclastic vasculitis. In cases of infection-induced vasculitis, prednisone should be reserved until after the infection has been properly treated. Idiopathic vasculitis is treated with oral steroids, and often a search for an infection or other cause is undertaken. A thorough history and physical examination are needed, as well as some screening laboratory tests. Laboratory testing usually is not helpful unless the history or review of symptoms points in a particular direction. If patients are suffering from more than just very mild systemic symptoms, an evaluation should be done to rule out the more serious forms of vasculitis.

Plate 4-43

Integumentary System

LICHEN PLANUS

Lichen planus is a common inflammatory skin disease. It is unique in that it can affect the skin, the mucous membranes, the nails, and the epithelium of the hair follicles. Lichen planus most commonly affects the skin, but the other areas can be involved either solely or in conjunction with one another. Lichen planus that involves the skin has a tendency to spontaneously remit within 1 to 2 years after onset, whereas the oral version is almost always chronic in nature.

Clinical Findings: Lichen planus can affect people at any age, but it is much more common in adulthood. It has no gender or racial predilection. The rash classically has been described as flat-topped, polygonal, pruritic, purple papules. Frequently, a whitish, lacy scale, referred to as Wickham's striae, overlies the papules. Lichen planus is unusual in that the pruritus causes the patient to rub the area, rather than scratch. Lichen planus exhibits the Koebner phenomenon, and often areas of linear arrangement are seen secondary to trauma or rubbing. This is helpful when clinically examining a patient, because scratch marks and excoriations are rarely seen, whereas lichenification from repeated rubbing of the lesions is frequently seen. The rash has a tendency to be more prominent on flexural surfaces, especially of the wrists. The glans penis is another distinctive location in which lichen planus commonly occurs.

Many clinical variations of lichen planus have been described. An afflicted individual may have more than one morphology. Hypertrophic lichen planus has the appearance of thickened, scaly plaques with a rough or verrucal surface. There may be areas on the periphery that appear more classic in nature. This variant can be difficult to diagnosis clinically, and often a biopsy is required. It also can be difficult to treat effectively, and it runs a chronic course. Rarely, hypertrophic lichen planus has been reported to transform into malignant squamous cell carcinoma. Bullous lichen planus is an extremely uncommon variant that usually occurs on the lower extremities. The vesicle or bulla typically forms within the center of the lichen planus lesion.

Lichen planopilaris is the term given to describe lichen planus affecting the terminal hair follicles. This is most common on the scalp and leads to a scarring alopecia. The typical findings are small, erythematous patches surrounding each hair follicle. As the disease progresses, loss of hair follicles is observed, signifying that scarring is taking place. The central crown is the area most often affected. It is uncommon for the entire scalp to be affected. Once scarring has occurred, the hair loss is permanent. Lichen planopilaris runs a chronic waxing and waning clinical course.

Lichen planus may affect the mucous membranes of the oral cavity, the genital region, and the conjunctiva. These areas appear as glistening patches with lacy, white reticulations on the surface. Mucous membrane lichen planus has a higher tendency to ulcerate than the cutaneous form does. There have been reports of malignant transformation to squamous cell carcinoma. For this reason, long-term follow-up is required. Lichen planus may also affect the nail matrix and nail bed, leading to dystrophy and nail abnormalities. The most frequently seen nail abnormality is longitudinal ridging, but the most characteristic nail finding is pterygium formation.

Pathogenesis: Lichen planus appears to be mediated by an abnormal T-cell immune response. The T cells act locally on the keratinocytes to induce the clinical

findings. The exact pathomechanism has yet to be described.

Histology: The lesions show characteristic findings that include a dense lichenoid lymphocytic infiltrate along the dermal-epidermal border. Necrotic keratinocytes are frequently encountered within the hyperplastic epidermis and have been named Civatte bodies. Hypergranulosis is a prominent feature as is the "sawtooth" pattern of epidermal hyperplasia. The presence

of eosinophils should lead one to consider the diagnosis of a lichen planus–like drug eruption or lichenoid contact dermatitis.

Treatment: Isolated lesions can be treated with topical corticosteroids. Up to two thirds of skin lesions resolve spontaneously. Patients with widespread disease present a therapeutic challenge. Ultraviolet phototherapy, oral corticosteroids, and oral retinoids such as acitretin and isotretinoin have been used.

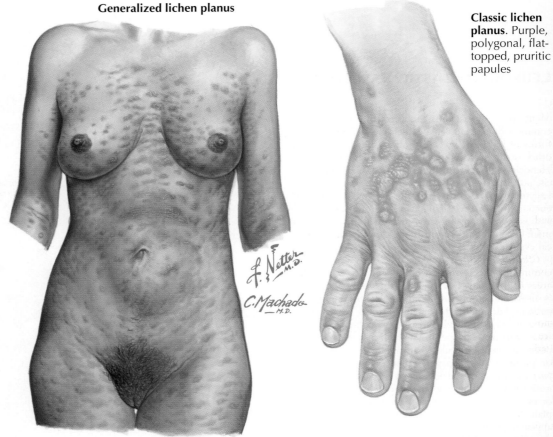

Generalized lichen planus

Classic lichen planus. Purple, polygonal, flat-topped, pruritic papules

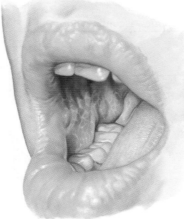
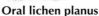

Oral lichen planus

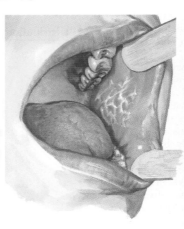

Wickham's striae. White reticulated patches on the buccal mucosa

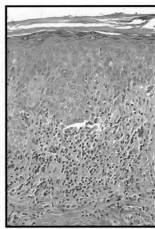

Histology of lichen planus. Lichenoid lymphocytic infiltrate with "saw-toothing" of the rete ridges, decreased granular cell layer, and a Max Joseph space at the dermal-epidermal junction.

Plate 4-44

Rashes

LICHEN SIMPLEX CHRONICUS

Lichen simplex chronicus is a commonly encountered chronic dermatosis that can be initiated by many events. Certain regions of the body are more prone to develop lichen simplex chronicus, such as the lower leg and ankle region and the posterior scalp, but it can occur anywhere. The initiating factor can be any skin insult that induces itching. The itch-scratch cycle is never broken, and the skin in the region being manipulated takes on a lichenified appearance. This is believed to be a localized skin condition that has no systemic associations or causes. Many therapies have been attempted with varying rates of success.

Clinical Findings: There is a slight female preponderance and no racial predilection. Most patients who present with lichen simplex chronicus do not relate an underlying insult that initiated the chronic itching. Some report a previous bug bite, trauma, or initiating rash such as allergic contact dermatitis caused by poison ivy. Involvement is localized to one region of the body, most often the ankle. Other commonly involved areas are the occipital scalp and the anogenital region. Patients report that they have a constant itching or burning sensation, and they respond to it by chronically rubbing or itching the area. Initially, a fine red patch with some excoriations is present. As the condition becomes chronic, the rash takes on the clinical appearance of lichen simplex chronicus. The skin becomes thickened and lichenified. There is an accentuation of the normal skin lines, and the region of involvement shows varying degrees of hyperpigmentation. Small excoriations and even small ulcerations may occur if the pruritus is severe and the patient cannot control the itching.

The cycle of pruritus and itching is perpetuated and can last for years to decades if untreated. Patients often relate that stressful events can initiate a flare of preexisting lichen simplex chronicus. They also commonly state that the itching is worse during the evening hours just before sleep. The main theory to explain this is that the cortex is not as busy processing information at that time, and other areas of the brain that are responsible for itching become activated or become disinhibited from cortical control. Even with treatment, some cases last for years. Patients typically become frustrated with therapy and are willing to pursue the help of other physicians or ancillary medical caregivers, such as acupuncturists. A fully developed area of lichen simplex chronicus is a well-defined lichenified plaque with excoriations and blood-tinged crust.

Pathogenesis: The exact pathomechanism of development of lichen simplex chronicus is unknown. Initiating events have been investigated, including insect bite reactions, underlying atopic diathesis, anxiety, stressful events, and other psychiatric conditions. Many patients have none of these factors, yet the clinical and pathological picture is identical.

Histology: The epidermis is acanthotic with elongation of the rete ridges. A varying amount of parakeratosis is present, with excoriations and superficial ulcerations observed in some cases. The collagen bundles within the papillary dermis show a vertical arrangement, parallel to the rete ridges. The rete ridges are irregular in elongation, unlike the regular pattern seen in psoriasis. A varying degree of epidermal spongiosis is seen, but no epidermotropism. The inflammatory infiltrate is composed primarily of lymphocytes.

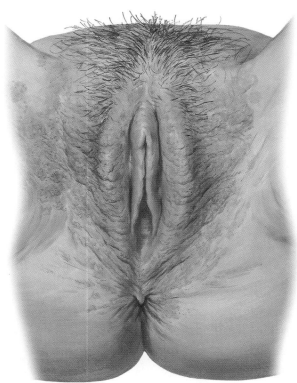

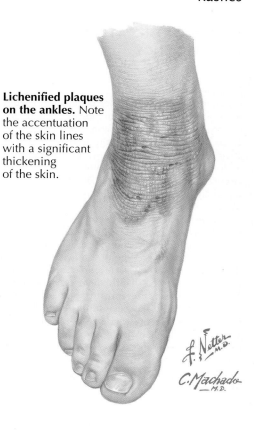

Lichenified plaques on the ankles. Note the accentuation of the skin lines with a significant thickening of the skin.

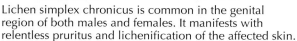

Lichen simplex chronicus is common in the genital region of both males and females. It manifests with relentless pruritus and lichenification of the affected skin.

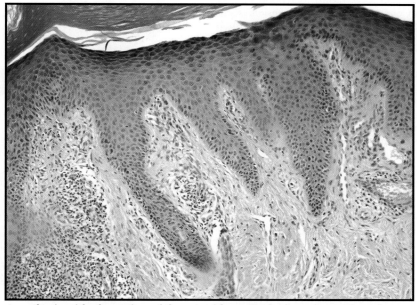

Acanthosis with elongation of the rete ridges. Patchy hyperkeratosis and parakeratosis. Vertically arranged collagen is present within the dermal papilla.

Treatment: Therapy is often directed at breaking the itch-scratch cycle. This is attempted with a combination of topical high-potency corticosteroids and oral antihistamines or gabapentin. The sedating antihistamines work better than the newer, nonsedating ones. Topical steroids may be used under occlusion for better penetration of the lichenified region. Intralesional injection with triamcinolone may be attempted. Capsaicin, which is derived from capsicum peppers, may be used. This agent works by depleting the superficial nerve endings of substance P, the neurotransmitter required for the itching sensation. Patients should be advised to trim their fingernails to help prevent trauma when they scratch. Behavioral modification may be attempted, but it is best accomplished by a professional psychiatrist or psychologist. Precipitating causes such as stress should be addressed. Patients often have remissions with frequent relapses.

Plate 4-45

Integumentary System

LOWER EXTREMITY VASCULAR INSUFFICIENCY

Vascular insufficiency of the lower extremity is a common finding in the older population. Factors that increase the risk of vascular disease include diabetes, obesity, smoking, hypertension, and hypercholesterolemia. Both the venous and the arterial systems may be affected, and the signs and symptoms are unique to each. The combination of venous and arterial insufficiency is commonly seen in older diabetic patients, especially those who smoke. Abnormalities of the lymphatic system may cause findings similar to those of venous insufficiency. Risk factors for lymphatic disease include prior surgeries (e.g., inguinal lymph node dissection), radiotherapy, and idiopathic lymphedema.

Clinical Findings: Venous insufficiency is a common disease that has no racial or ethnic predilection. It has been reported to be slightly more common in women. Venous insufficiency eventually leads to venous stasis and ulcerations. It has been estimated to be the cause of more than 50% of lower extremity ulcerations, with arterial insufficiency being the next most common cause, and neuropathic causes and lymphedema accounting for the remainder.

The first signs of venous insufficiency may be the development of varicose veins or smaller dilated reticular veins. As time progresses, venous stasis changes are seen, including dry, pink to red, eczematous patches with varying amounts of peripheral pitting edema. Red blood cells are extravasated into the dermis where, over time, they break down and form hemosiderin deposits, which appear as brown to reddish macules and patches. Continued venous hypertension, stasis, and swelling may eventually lead to a venous stasis ulcer. These ulcers are most commonly present on the medial malleolus region of the ankle but can occur almost anywhere on the lower extremity. They are usually nontender, but some can be exquisitely painful.

Arterial insufficiency is most often caused by atherosclerosis of the larger arteries of the lower extremity. Patients often have coexisting risk factors including older age, hypertension, smoking, diabetes, and hypercholesterolemia. Arterial ulcers are slightly more common in men, and there is no racial predilection. The clinical presenting signs are often dependent rubor, claudication, and rest pain. Physical examination confirms the absence of peripheral pulses in the dorsal pedal and posterior tibial arteries. At this point, the patient is at high risk for arterial ulcerations and subsequent gangrene. Surgical intervention is the only viable means of treatment.

Pathogenesis: Venous drainage of the lower extremity is accomplished via the superficial and deep systems of veins that are connected through horizontally arranged communicating vessels. These veins contain one-way bicuspid valves that prevent backflow and work with the action of muscle contraction to force the venous flow in a superior direction, eventually to empty into the inferior vena cava. The flow of venous blood toward the vena cava is the primary responsibility of the leg muscles, especially the calf muscle. Patients with sedentary lifestyles are at higher risk for venous insufficiency. During ambulation, the venous pressure normally decreases as the blood flow is increased toward the vena cava. If an abnormality exists and this does not occur, venous hypertension ensues. Congenital absence of the venous valves, incompetent valves, and a history of deep venous thrombosis are just three of the potential reasons for venous insufficiency. Once venous

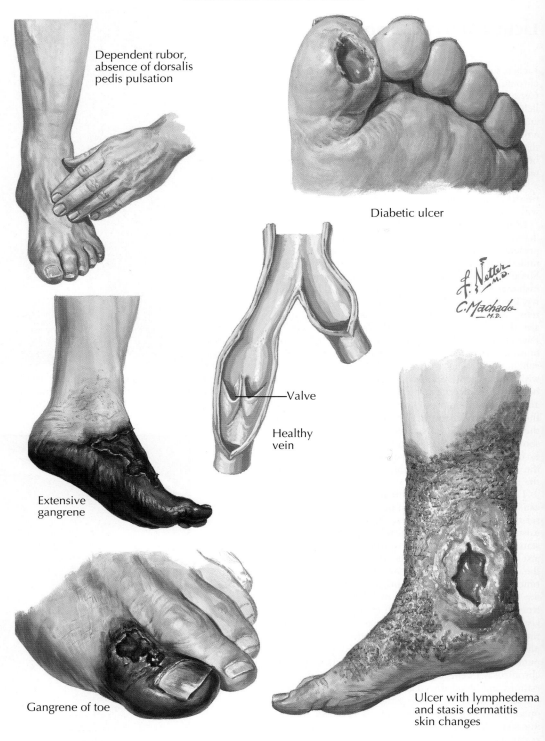

VASCULAR INSUFFICIENCY IN DIABETES

Dependent rubor, absence of dorsalis pedis pulsation

Diabetic ulcer

Valve

Healthy vein

Extensive gangrene

Gangrene of toe

Ulcer with lymphedema and stasis dermatitis skin changes

hypertension occurs, the patient is at risk for development of venous stasis and venous ulcerations.

Arterial insufficiency is caused by a slow narrowing of the arteries due to cholesterol plaque. This narrowing restricts the amount of blood flow to the tissue. Once the flow is decreased to less than the requirement needed for muscle and normal physiological functioning, symptoms arise.

Histology: Biopsies should not be performed in cases of arterial insufficiency, because they lead to ulcerations, infections, and, most likely, emergent surgery.

Histological evaluation of venous ulcerations shows a nonspecific ulcer, edema, proliferation of superficial dermal vessels, and extravasated red blood cells with a varying amount of hemosiderin deposition.

Treatment: Venous insufficiency is treated with a combination of compression and leg elevation. Losing weight and increasing the activity level may also help. Arterial insufficiency is best treated surgically with stent placement or arterial bypass of the narrowed artery. Pentoxifylline has also been used, with variable success, in early disease.

Plate 4-46

Rashes

MAST CELL DISEASE

Solitary mastocytoma with Darier's sign. Solitary mastocytomas almost always self-resolve. Darier's sign is elicited by rubbing the mastocytoma, causing urtication.

MAST CELL DISEASE

Mast cell disease is an uncommon condition that has many clinical variants and subtypes. It can be seen as a solitary finding, as in the solitary mastocytoma, or it can result in widespread cutaneous disease, as in urticaria pigmentosa. Most mast cell disease is caused by an abnormality in the *c-kit* gene *(KIT)*. There are many other forms of mast cell disease, most in the benign category; some affect the skin predominantly, and others are more systemic in nature. One systemic type is the rare mast cell leukemia. Other systemic forms have been reported, such as mast cell sarcoma, and carry a poor prognosis. It is important to recall that mast cells are derived from the bone marrow and share certain things in common with other hematopoietic cells. The World Health Organization (WHO) has developed a simplified classification system for mast cell disease (see box to *right*).

Clinical Findings: Solitary mastocytoma is one of the most common of all the mast cell disease types. It manifests in early childhood, often in the first few years of life. It appears as a yellowish to brownish macule, papule, or plaque. On rare occasions, a lesion develops a vesicle or bulla. Most lesions are asymptomatic until rubbed or scratched. When this takes place, a localized urticarial reaction occurs above the mastocytoma and extends into the surrounding skin. This sign, called Darier's sign, can be used in any of the cutaneous mast cell diseases to help make the diagnosis. These solitary mast cell collections almost always spontaneously resolve with no sequelae.

Urticaria pigmentosa is a more diffuse affliction of the skin with mast cells; it has been reported to be the most common variant of mast cell disease. From a few to hundreds of slightly hyperpigmented macules and plaques occur across the surface of the skin. Some develop into vesicles and bullae. This most commonly occurs in early childhood but has also been reported to occur in adulthood. Most children are diagnosed on the basis of the clinical presentation and demonstration of a positive Darier's sign. The condition typically runs a benign course in children, and most cases spontaneously remit over a few years and then disappear at about the time of puberty. Adult-onset urticaria pigmentosa is a more chronic disease that rarely remits. Special care should be taken to continually screen adult patients for the development of systemic mast cell involvement.

Telangiectasia macularis eruptiva perstans is a less commonly seen variant of mast cell disease. It occurs almost exclusively in the adult population. Patients often present with widespread telangiectases in unusual locations such as the back, chest, and abdomen. There can be a background erythema, and Darier's sign may

WHO Classification for Mast Cell Disease
▶ Cutaneous disease only (includes cutaneous mastocytoma, urticaria pigmentosa, and telangiectasia macularis eruptiva perstans) ▶ Indolent systemic disease ▶ Systemic mastocytosis with associated clonal non–mast cell hematological disease ▶ Aggressive systemic disease ▶ Mast cell leukemia ▶ Mast cell sarcoma ▶ Noncutaneous mastocytoma

C. Machado
—M.D.
B. DaVanzo CMI

Urticaria pigmentosa. This is the most common form of cutaneous mastocytosis. It can manifest with reddish-brown macules and papules and in severe cases with vesicles and bullae.

or may not be present. The most common symptom is pruritus. The appearance can be bothersome for some. It is most often limited to the skin, but the clinician should evaluate for systemic involvement.

Measurement of the serum tryptase level is the most accurate means of screening for systemic involvement with mastocytosis. Levels in the normal range indicate cutaneous disease only; levels greater than 20 ng/mL are indicative of systemic involvement, and further systemic workup is warranted. Urine histamine and histamine metabolites can also be assessed but seem to be less sensitive and less specific than the serum tryptase level. If systemic involvement is considered, further testing with a bone marrow biopsy may be indicated. Molecular genetic testing can be performed on the bone marrow sample to assess for the *KIT* gene mutation.

Plate 4-47

Integumentary System

MAST CELL DEGRANULATION BLOCKERS

MAST CELL DISEASE
(Continued)

Histology: The histological features depend on the form of mast cell disease. Most biopsy specimens show an excessive number of mast cells, typically surrounding the cutaneous vasculature. These mast cells are best appreciated with special staining techniques. The Leder (chloracetate esterase) stain, the Giemsa stain, and the toluidine blue stain are the most commonly used special stains to help highlight the cutaneous mast cells. CD117 immunostaining also stains mast cells.

Pathogenesis: Darier's sign is caused by direct release of histamine and other inflammatory mediators from the excessive collection of mast cells within the affected skin. On direct stimulation such as scratching or rubbing, the mast cells automatically release the contents of their granules. These granules contain histamine and other vasoactive substances that cause edema, redness, and pruritus.

Mast cell disease is caused by a mutation in the *KIT* gene. *KIT* is a protooncogene that encodes a protein called stem cell factor receptor (SCFR). SCFR is a transmembrane protein tyrosine kinase protein. This receptor is prominent in two skin cell types, mast cells and melanocytes. It is also present on a host of other primitive hematological cell types. Stem cell factor is also known by various other names, including KIT ligand, CD117, Steel factor, and mast cell growth factor. It is the molecule that binds to the transmembrane SCFR and acts to promote the reproduction of mast cells. The activating mutation of SCFR seen in mast cell disease causes an upregulation of signaling via this pathway and an uncontrolled proliferation of mast cells. The continuous activation of the stem cell factor allows for prolonged survival of mast cells, which also contributes to their increased number. Numerous mutations of *KIT* have been described, and it is believed that the different mutations play a role in the varied clinical expression of the disease. The most common mutation is a D816V mutation that is caused by replacement of the normal aspartic acid at the 816 position with a valine amino acid.

Treatment: Cutaneous mast cell disease in children is often self-limited and resolves spontaneously with time. Therapy with antihistamines may help decrease the pruritus and provide symptomatic relief until the condition resolves on its own. The most important aspect for children with cutaneous mast cell disease, especially urticaria pigmentosa, is to avoid agents or physical insults that may cause massive degranulation of mast cells. These triggers include medications such as anesthetics, narcotics, polymyxin B, and many others. Physical triggers include extremes of temperature, vigorous exercise, repeated rubbing of the involved skin,

Mast cell degranulation effects

J. Perkins
MS, MFA

A. Antigen reacts with antibody (IgE) on membrane of mast cells, which respond by secreting pharmacological mediators.

Vagus nerve

Mast cell degranulation blockers ⊖ →

Histamine

Mucous gland hypersecretion

SRS-A (slow-reacting substance of anaphylaxis)

Smooth muscle contraction

Increased capillary permeability and inflammatory reaction

ECF-A (eosinophil chemotactic factor of anaphylaxis)

Eosinophil attraction

B. End-organ (airway) response compounded by nonspecific reactions (ciliostasis, particle retention, and cell injury)

◄---- Prostaglandins ◄

? ◄----- Serotonin ◄

? ◄------- Kinins ◄

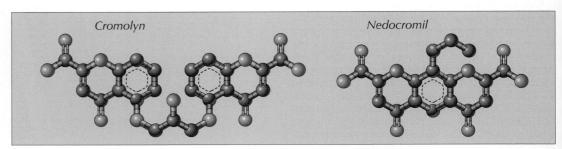

Cromolyn

Nedocromil

and many other stimuli that differ from individual to individual.

Antihistamines are the mainstay of therapy. The leukotriene inhibitors are also used as adjunctive therapy to the antihistamines. Cromolyn is a mast cell stabilizer that is not absorbed through the gastrointestinal tract. Its use is limited to treatment of coexisting diarrhea caused by mast cell disease of the gut. Telangiectasia macularis eruptiva perstans has been treated with the

585-nm pulsed dye laser to decrease the redness and telangiectases for cosmetic purposes. Some success has been achieved in treating systemic disease with the tyrosine kinase inhibitor, imatinib. Depending on the symptoms and the body systems involved, systemic chemotherapy may be warranted to decrease the mast cell load. These agents rarely put patients into long-term remission, and the response is transient. At this point, there is no cure for mast cell disease.

Plate 4-48

Rashes

MORPHEA

Morphea is a skin dermatosis that is idiopathic in nature. The most common form is solitary, but many clinical variants have been described, including linear, guttate, and generalized forms. A small subset of patients (<1%) progress to progressive systemic sclerosis. It is likely that many patients do not seek medical advice because the onset is insidious or the area of involvement is so small that it is hardly noticeable or bothersome.

Clinical Findings: Morphea is typically seen in young Caucasian females. The ratio of females to males has been estimated at 2:1. Morphea begins as a small erythematous macule. The lesion expands outward with a violaceous to red border. As it expands, the central portion becomes slightly hypopigmented and indurated in nature. The trunk is the most commonly involved region of the body. Most areas of involvement are asymptomatic to slightly pruritic. If the involved area crosses over a joint, there may be some loss of motion of the affected joint and pain with flexion and extension. The main differential diagnosis is between morphea and lichen sclerosis et atrophicus. Lichen sclerosis et atrophicus is typically more strikingly white in coloration and is less indurated.

Many variants of morphea have been described. Guttate morphea manifests with tiny, teardrop-shaped areas of hypopigmented macules with slight induration scattered about the trunk or extremities. The induration of guttate morphea is not nearly as prominent as that of localized morphea and may not be appreciable. These guttate lesions may be impossible to distinguish clinically from lichen sclerosis et atrophicus, and a biopsy is the only way to differentiate the two. Biopsies are not always conclusive, and the term *morphea–lichen sclerosis overlap* has been used to describe these lesions with features of both conditions. Generalized morphea is a rare variant with extensive involvement of the cutaneous surface. By definition, generalized morphea does not have systemic involvement, differentiating it from progressive systemic sclerosis. However, patients with generalized morphea may develop atrophy of the adipose and muscle tissues underlying the areas of involvement.

Linear morphea, also called linear scleroderma, is a unique cutaneous variant that is well described and has a distinctive appearance and potential underlying complications. It is commonly found along the length of the affected extremity. This form occurs most commonly in childhood. The affected skin may become bound down and cause limb length discrepancies as the child grows. Joint mobility is also a potential complication. Cortical hyperostosis of the long bones underneath the area of linear morphea has been well reported and is termed *melorheostosis.* There are subtypes of linear morphea that have been given the names *en coup de sabre* and *Parry-Romberg syndrome.*

En coup de sabre is a specific type of morphea that occurs along the forehead, as well as partially onto the cheek and into the scalp. It appears as a depressed linear furrow from the scalp vertically down the forehead. The appearance can be subtle or extremely noticeable and can cause significant cosmetic problems. Parry-Romberg syndrome is a name given to linear morphea that occurs vertically across the face, causing hemifacial atrophy. The underlying adipose tissue, muscle, and bone are involved, with significant disfigurement. Patients may have neurological involvement leading to seizures.

Pathogenesis: The pathogenesis of morphea is poorly understood. An unknown factor sets off this cutaneous reaction in which an excessive amount of collagen is produced locally by fibroblasts. Potential factors that may initiate the reaction are endothelial damage, certain *Borrelia burgdorferi* infections, and fibroblast abnormalities that lead to increased collagen production. *Borrelia*-induced morphea has yet to be described in the United States; it has been reported in Europe and Asia.

Histology: A punch biopsy specimen of morphea appears as a nicely formed cylinder. The dermis is expanded with excessive amounts of collagen. A slight inflammatory infiltrate is often seen along the dermal-subcutaneous border. Plasma cells are common.

Treatment: Therapy for localized morphea is not needed but can be attempted with topical corticosteroids, calcipotriene, and phototherapy. Linear morphea should be treated, because it has significant functional and cosmetic implications. Immunosuppressive agents such as methotrexate and prednisone have been the most thoroughly studied therapeutic agents.

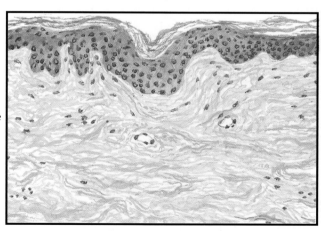

En coup de sabre. Rare form of localized morphea on the forehead and face. May be associated with the Parry-Romberg syndrome

Localized morphea. Atrophic plaques that are firm and nonflexible on palpation. Often surrounded by a violaceous or erythematous rim

Progressive systemic sclerosis (scleroderma). Typical skin changes in scleroderma: extensive collagen deposition and some epidermal atrophy

Plate 4-49

Integumentary System

MYXEDEMA

Myxedema is seen in patients with untreated severe hypothyroidism. This condition results from a total lack of thyroid hormone secretion and resultant deposition of mucopolysaccharides into the skin and other organs. Many skin and systemic findings are present in severe hypothyroidism. This is a condition seen in adults. The infantile form, called cretinism, is still found in parts of the world that do not routinely test newborn infants. If it is left untreated, mental retardation and various neurological deficits can occur. Adult myxedema is an uncommon clinical disease.

Clinical Findings: Patients usually develop severe hypothyroidism slowly. It can be caused by autoimmune thyroiditis, a thyroid tumor, a pituitary tumor or infarction, or hypothalamic disease. It can also be seen after treatment of hyperthyroidism with improper replacement of thyroid hormone. The onset of symptoms begins as mild, nondescript findings and advances to severe clinical disease as the lack of thyroid hormone worsens. Patients have many constitutional symptoms and always complain of fatigue, cold intolerance, and a generalized malaise. Constipation and weight gain are almost universal. Some patients develop a pericardial effusion and bradycardia. Neurological reflexes are blunted, and patients complain of slow mental reflexes.

The skin findings are specific to myxedema and can help one make the diagnosis. Patients develop diffuse, nonscarring alopecia. The hair is often dry and breaks easily. The lateral half of the eyebrows is shed. Fingernails become brittle and lift off the nail bed. The facial features appear lethargic. Periorbital edema is prominent. Dry skin is severe and can mimic ichthyosis vulgaris. The skin on the lips is thickened, as is the tongue. The tongue may enlarge to the point that the impression of the teeth is seen on its lateral edges. If the infiltrate of mucopolysaccharides is extreme, the scalp can become thickened and furrowed, taking on the appearance of cutis verticis gyrate. The skin may acquire a subtle yellow hue due to carotinemia; this is most likely to be observed on the glabrous skin.

Laboratory findings are diagnostic and necessary. A nonspecific mild anemia is seen, consistent with anemia of chronic disease. Hypercholesterolemia and hyponatremia are two of the nonspecific findings. Electrocardiography shows bradycardia and a prolonged PR interval. The results of various thyroid hormone tests are characteristic. An elevated level of thyroid-stimulating hormone (TSH) is confirmatory for a diagnosis of primary hypothyroidism. Thyroxine (T_4) levels are low and can be measured in various ways.

It is critical to differentiate adult generalized myxedema, as seen in hypothyroidism, from pretibial myxedema. Pretibial myxedema is a marker for hyperthyroidism, not hypothyroidism.

Pathogenesis: Thyroid hormone is required for multiple metabolic pathways to work properly, including the breakdown of glycosaminoglycans. When there is a decrease or a total lack of thyroid hormone, glycosaminoglycans cannot be properly metabolized, and they accumulate in the subcutaneous tissue, most prominently in the tissue of the face and scalp. This leads to the characteristic skin findings in myxedema.

Histology: Biopsy specimens of involved skin show mild deposition of mucin between collagen bundles

within the dermis. Hyaluronic acid makes up the majority of the mucin deposits. The alopecia is nonscarring.

Treatment: Prompt recognition and diagnosis of myxedema is required. It is a fatal condition if left untreated, and myxedema coma is precipitated by a total lack of thyroid hormone. Thyroid replacement with levothyroxine (synthetic T_4) is required.

Supportive care is necessary until the patient can be adequately stabilized. Determining the cause of the hypothyroidism is necessary to probe for thyroid cancer, pituitary problems, or other hypothalamic disease. Prompt recognition of the skin manifestations and referral to an endocrinologist can be life-saving. Once proper thyroid replacement has been achieved, the skin and hair findings slowly resolve over time.

Clinical manifestations

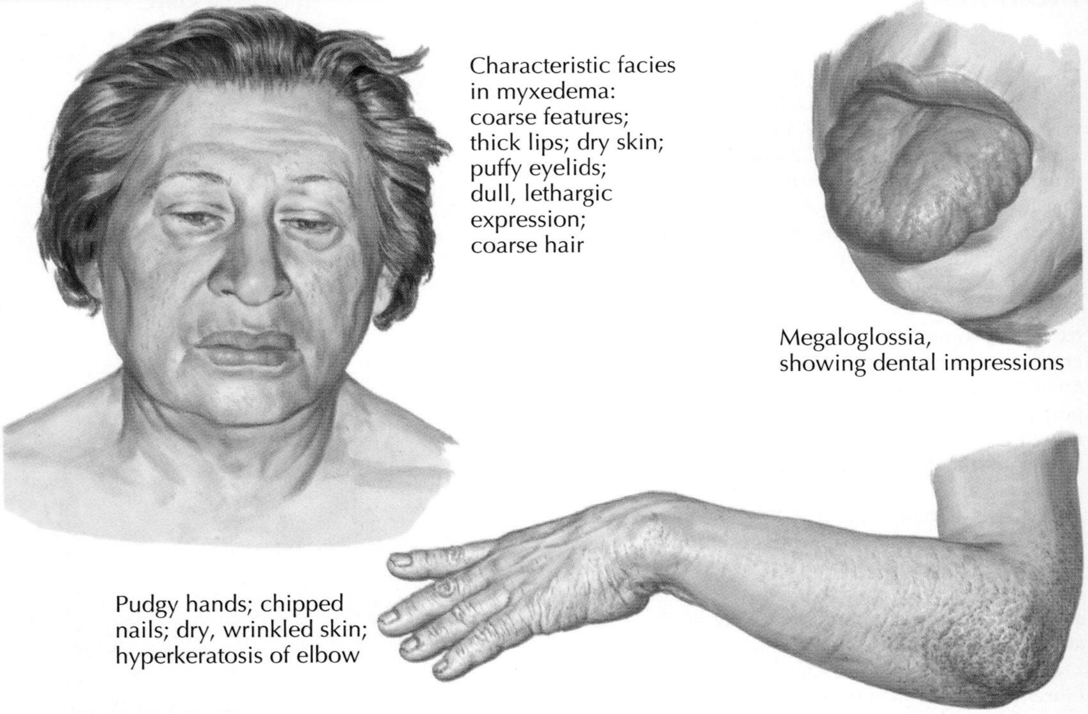

Characteristic facies in myxedema: coarse features; thick lips; dry skin; puffy eyelids; dull, lethargic expression; coarse hair

Megaloglossia, showing dental impressions

Pudgy hands; chipped nails; dry, wrinkled skin; hyperkeratosis of elbow

Hypothyroidism

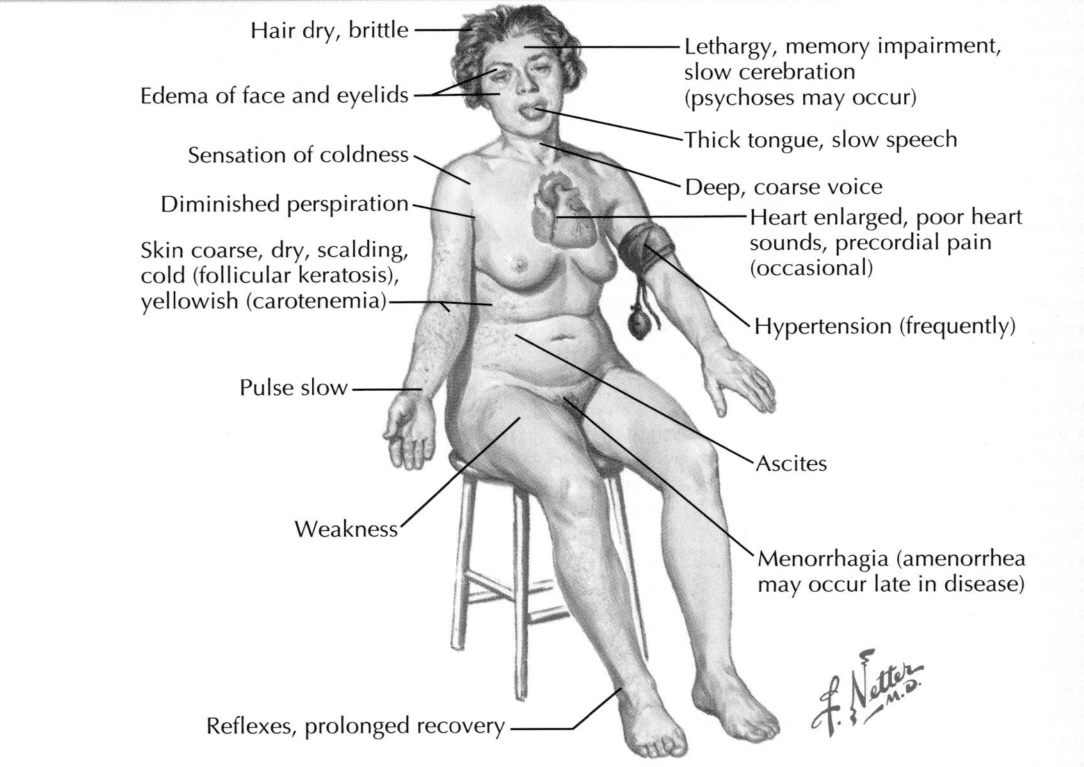

Hair dry, brittle

Lethargy, memory impairment, slow cerebration (psychoses may occur)

Edema of face and eyelids

Thick tongue, slow speech

Sensation of coldness

Deep, coarse voice

Diminished perspiration

Heart enlarged, poor heart sounds, precordial pain (occasional)

Skin coarse, dry, scalding, cold (follicular keratosis), yellowish (carotenemia)

Hypertension (frequently)

Pulse slow

Ascites

Weakness

Menorrhagia (amenorrhea may occur late in disease)

Reflexes, prolonged recovery

Plate 4-50

Rashes

NECROBIOSIS LIPOIDICA

Necrobiosis lipoidica is a rash that is frequently encountered in the dermatology clinic. It is most commonly seen in association with diabetes and is referred to as necrobiosis lipoidica diabeticorum. However, not all cases are seen in conjunction with diabetes mellitus, and the name *necrobiosis lipoidica* is a more inclusive designation. Patients who present with necrobiosis lipoidica should all be evaluated for underlying diabetes and screened periodically over their lifetime, because 60% to 80% will have or develop some form of glucose intolerance. Necrobiosis lipoidica has been reported to appear any place on the skin, but it is most frequently encountered on the anterior lower extremities. It has a characteristic clinical appearance, and the diagnosis can often be made on clinical grounds alone, without the use of a skin biopsy. The histologic findings are diagnostic of necrobiosis lipoidica. A punch or excisional biopsy is required for diagnosis, because a shave biopsy does not allow for proper histological evaluation of this condition.

Clinical Findings: There appears to be no sexual or racial predilection, and the disease is most commonly diagnosed in early adulthood. In most instances, necrobiosis lipoidica occurs on the anterior lower extremities. The rash typically begins as a tiny red papule that slowly expands outward and leaves behind a depressed, atrophic center with a slightly elevated rim. The borders are very distinct. They are slightly elevated and have a more inflammatory red appearance. They are well demarcated from the surrounding normal-appearing skin. The lesions have a broad range of sizes, from a few millimeters in some cases to affecting the entire aspect of the anterior lower legs. The plaques have a characteristic orange-brown coloration and significant atrophy. The underlying dermis appears to be thinned dramatically; the dermal and subcutaneous veins can easily be seen and appear to be popping out of the skin. When palpated, the center of the lesions feel as if there is no dermal tissue present at all. The difference between palpation of the normal skin and palpation of affected skin is striking.

A small percentage of patients experience ulcerations that can be slow and difficult to heal. Rarely, transformation of chronic ulcerative necrobiosis lipoidica into squamous cell carcinoma has been reported. This transformation is more likely to be a result of the chronic ulceration and inflammation than the underlying necrobiosis lipoidica. There are no other associations with necrobiosis lipoidica except for diabetes.

Pathogenesis: The pathomechanism of necrobiosis lipoidica is unknown. Theories have been suggested, but no good scientific evidence has pinpointed the cause.

Histology: The histology of necrobiosis lipoidica is characteristic. A punch or excisional biopsy is needed to ensure a full-thickness specimen. There is a "cake layering" appearance to the dermis, with necrobiotic collagen bundles within palisaded granulomas alternating with areas of histiocytes and multinucleated giant cells of both the foreign body and the Langhans type. The differential diagnosis histologically is between granuloma annulare and necrobiosis lipoidica. In necrobiosis lipoidica, the inflammatory infiltrate contains less mucin and more plasma cells. The inflammation in necrobiosis lipoidica also tends to extend into the subcutaneous adipose tissue.

Treatment: Treatment is typically initiated with the use of high-potency topical steroids. It may seem counterintuitive to treat an atrophic condition with topical

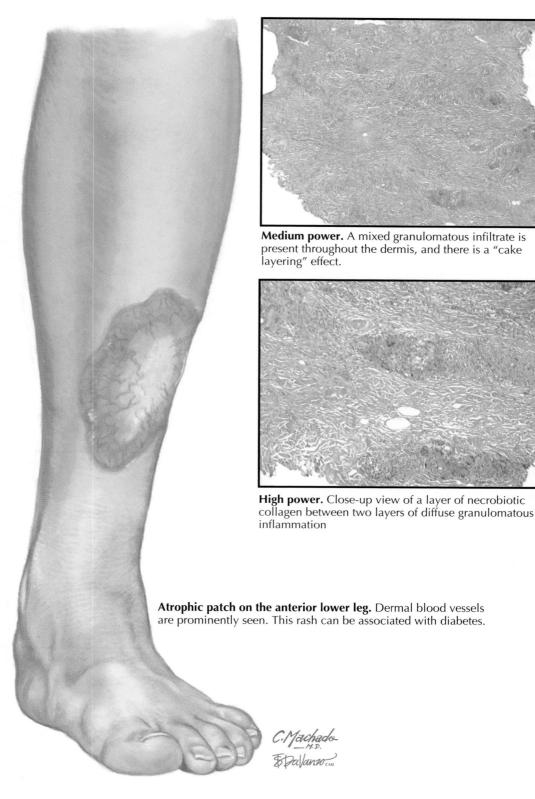

Medium power. A mixed granulomatous infiltrate is present throughout the dermis, and there is a "cake layering" effect.

High power. Close-up view of a layer of necrobiotic collagen between two layers of diffuse granulomatous inflammation

Atrophic patch on the anterior lower leg. Dermal blood vessels are prominently seen. This rash can be associated with diabetes.

corticosteroid creams, which can cause atrophy. In cases of necrobiosis lipoidica, however, the high-potency steroid agents do not lead to an increase in the atrophy. The steroid agents act to decrease and stop the inflammatory infiltrate from occurring and perpetuating itself. Intralesional injections of triamcinolone have also been successful. Many other agents have been anecdotally reported to be successful in treating this condition, although they have not been tried in standardized, placebo-controlled studies. Gaining control of the underlying diabetes does not seem to play a role in the outcome of the skin disease. Ulcerations should be treated with aggressive wound care, and compression garments should be worn if edema or venous insufficiency is present. Ulcers may take months to heal. Once the inflammation has been stopped, most people have residual atrophy that may be permanent or may improve slightly with time.

Plate 4-51

Integumentary System

NECROBIOTIC XANTHOGRANULOMA

Necrobiotic xanthogranuloma is a rare skin condition that is frequently associated with an underlying mono-clonal gammopathy. It was first described in the early 1980s. Since then, many cases have been reported that have confirmed this to be a distinct, albeit unusual and infrequently encountered, skin condition. The pathological findings of necrobiotic xanthogranuloma are distinctive and are required to make the diagnosis. Patients with this diagnosis need to be monitored routinely to watch for the development of a monoclonal gammopathy and the possibility of multiple myeloma.

Clinical Findings: So few cases of necrobiotic xanthogranuloma have been reported that no firm conclusion can be made on the epidemiology of the disease. However, it is a disease of older adulthood, with almost all cases occurring after the age of 50 years. The lesions have been reported to occur anywhere on the human body, but they are found most often on the forehead, cheeks, and temporal regions around the eyes. The periorbital region is almost always affected. Necrobiotic xanthogranulomas are typically yellowish to red papules and plaques. There may be intervening atrophy between the areas of involvement. The leading edge of the plaques may have a red or violaceous hue. Occasionally, nodules form. Secondary ulceration is frequently reported, as are telangiectases and dilated dermal vessels, which are most prominent in the regions of atrophy. The ulcerations take an extended period to resolve. Most patients are distraught by the appearance of the rash and complain of a mild pruritus, although many have no symptoms. The clinical differential diagnosis includes forms of planar xanthomas. A skin biopsy helps differentiate these conditions. This disease progresses over time and typically does not spontaneously remit.

Patients almost always complain of dry eyes or have objective findings of proptosis. In rare cases, necrobiotic xanthogranuloma affects the lacrimal gland and retrobulbar fat tissue.

Necrobiotic xanthogranuloma is associated with an immunoglobulin G-κ (IgG:κ) monoclonal gammopathy in most cases. The presence of a gammopathy should make the clinician seek the advice of a hematologist to perform a bone marrow biopsy to help evaluate for multiple myeloma. A small percentage of patients with this gammopathy have or will develop multiple myeloma. Other frequently abnormal laboratory tests in necrobiotic xanthogranuloma include an elevated erythrocyte sedimentation rate (ESR), a decreased level of complement C4, and leukopenia. Many other abnormalities have been described, providing more evidence that this is a systemic disease and not an isolated skin disease. Lesions of necrobiotic xanthogranuloma have also been described to occur in the upper respiratory system and in the heart.

Pathogenesis: The pathogenesis has been theorized to be an antibody response to a self-antigen, most likely a form of lipid. This is unproven, and the exact etiology is unknown.

Histology: The biopsy findings of necrobiotic xanthogranuloma are unique and characteristic. A punch biopsy or excisional biopsy should be performed to allow for adequate evaluation. On first glance, the entire dermis is filled with inflammatory cells. The inflammation is in the granulomatous category. A

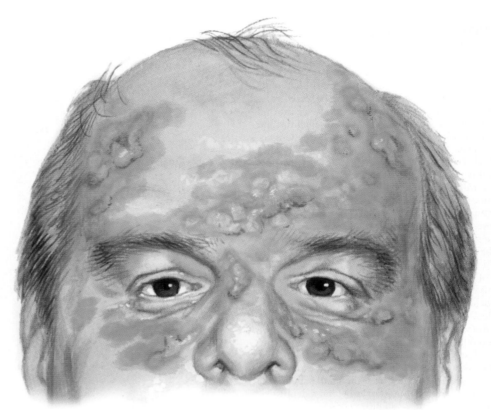

Patches and plaques on the face. Necrobiotic xanthogranuloma is most frequently encountered in a periocular location.

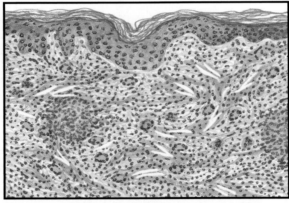

Low power. Diffuse dermal granulomatous infiltrate with giant cells

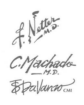

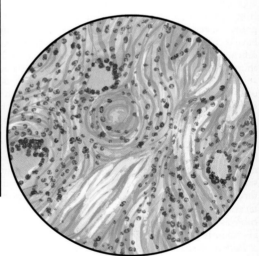

High power. The giant cells can be best appreciated on higher-power microscopy. The giant cells are predominantly the Touton type.

unique and characteristic finding, when seen, is that of cholesterol-filled, needle-shaped clefts within the granulomatous infiltrate. Giant cells, both the foreign body type and the Touton type, are commonly seen. The granulomatous infiltrate surrounds and envelops necrobiotic collagen tissue. There is usually an underlying, predominantly lobular panniculitis without vasculitis.

Treatment: Therapy is difficult. No randomized prospective studies have been performed on this rare condition, so only anecdotal therapies have been reported. Topical and oral steroids have been somewhat successful. Chemotherapeutic agents have been used with variable success, including the alkylating agents. Results have been varied, with some patients experiencing long-term remission. Patients all need to be screened for gammopathy and for the development of multiple myeloma. The presence of myeloma portends a worse prognosis.

Plate 4-52

Rashes

NEUTROPHILIC ECCRINE HIDRADENITIS

Neutrophilic eccrine hidradenitis is also known by other names, such as palmoplantar eccrine hidradenitis and idiopathic recurrent plantar hidradenitis. These names imply that it is seen only on the palms and soles. Neutrophilic eccrine hidradenitis is a more accepted term, because it includes all cases independent of location. This peculiar and uncommon rash can be seen anywhere on the body where eccrine glands are present. The palms and soles have a higher density of eccrine glands than other regions do, and this may be one reason why the disease is seen more frequently in this location. This condition has been frequently described in patients with leukemia who are undergoing chemotherapy. It has been reported to occur in other clinical settings, including human immunodeficiency virus infection, bacterial infections, other malignancies, and use of medications other than chemotherapeutics, as well as in patients with no other associations.

Clinical Findings: Clinically, neutrophilic eccrine hidradenitis manifests in a myriad of ways. It usually occurs in association with an underlying predisposing condition such as those listed previously. Patients develop the sudden onset of tender red papules and nodules with minimal to no ulceration. The papules blanch when pressed. The palms and soles are the areas most frequently involved, but this condition can occur anywhere on the body. The lesions may be asymptomatic, slightly tender, painful, or pruritic. The differential diagnosis includes hot foot syndrome, which is caused by pseudomonal bacterial infections. This condition typically affects the foot, and it can be associated with a folliculitis, such as hot tub folliculitis. Patients usually have a benign medical history and have had recent exposure to a hot tub or swimming pool.

Pathogenesis: Chemotherapy-induced neutrophilic eccrine hidradenitis is believed to occur secondary to accumulation of the chemotherapeutic agent within the eccrine glands to a level that is toxic to the secretory cells of the gland, resulting in cell necrosis. The neutrophilic inflammation is poorly understood. Only theories exist on the pathogenesis of non–chemotherapy-induced neutrophilic eccrine hidradenitis; the true pathogenesis is unknown.

Histology: The histological evaluation requires a punch biopsy or excisional biopsy to evaluate the

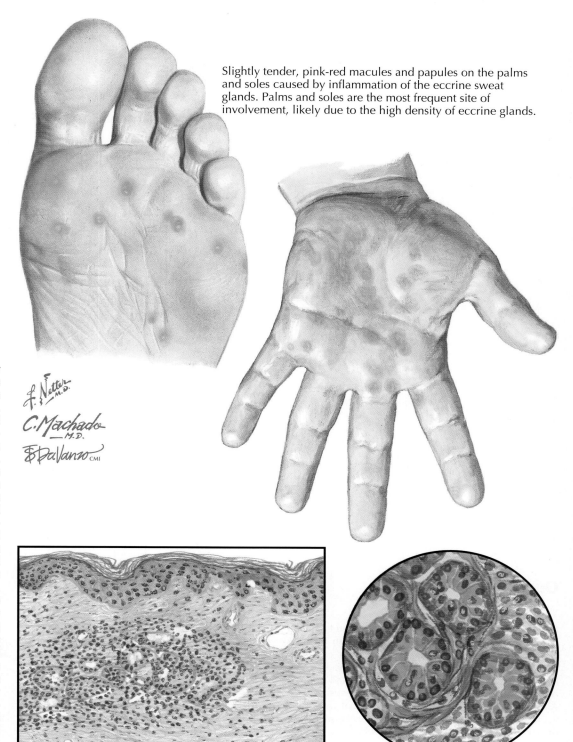

Slightly tender, pink-red macules and papules on the palms and soles caused by inflammation of the eccrine sweat glands. Palms and soles are the most frequent site of involvement, likely due to the high density of eccrine glands.

Low power. A neutrophilic infiltrate surrounds the dermal eccrine glands.

High power. Neutrophils infiltrating the eccrine ductal apparatus

eccrine glands. A shave biopsy is usually inadequate. There is a striking amount of neutrophilic inflammation in and around the eccrine apparatus. The eccrine glands show varying degrees of necrosis. No vasculitis is present.

Treatment: Treatment is supportive. Underlying infections need to be treated adequately. The main goals are pain control and prevention of secondary infection. If the patient's neutrophilic eccrine

hidradenitis is caused to a chemotherapeutic agent, a change in the chemotherapy regimen can be considered. If the patient's chemotherapy cannot be changed, topical corticosteroids and nonsteroidal antiinflammatory agents may be used. If this is unsuccessful, dapsone and colchicine may be considered because of their antineutrophilic effects. Oral steroids have been used with variable success. No placebo-controlled studies have been performed for this condition.

Plate 4-53

Integumentary System

METABOLIC PATHWAYS AND CUTANEOUS FINDINGS OF OCHRONOSIS

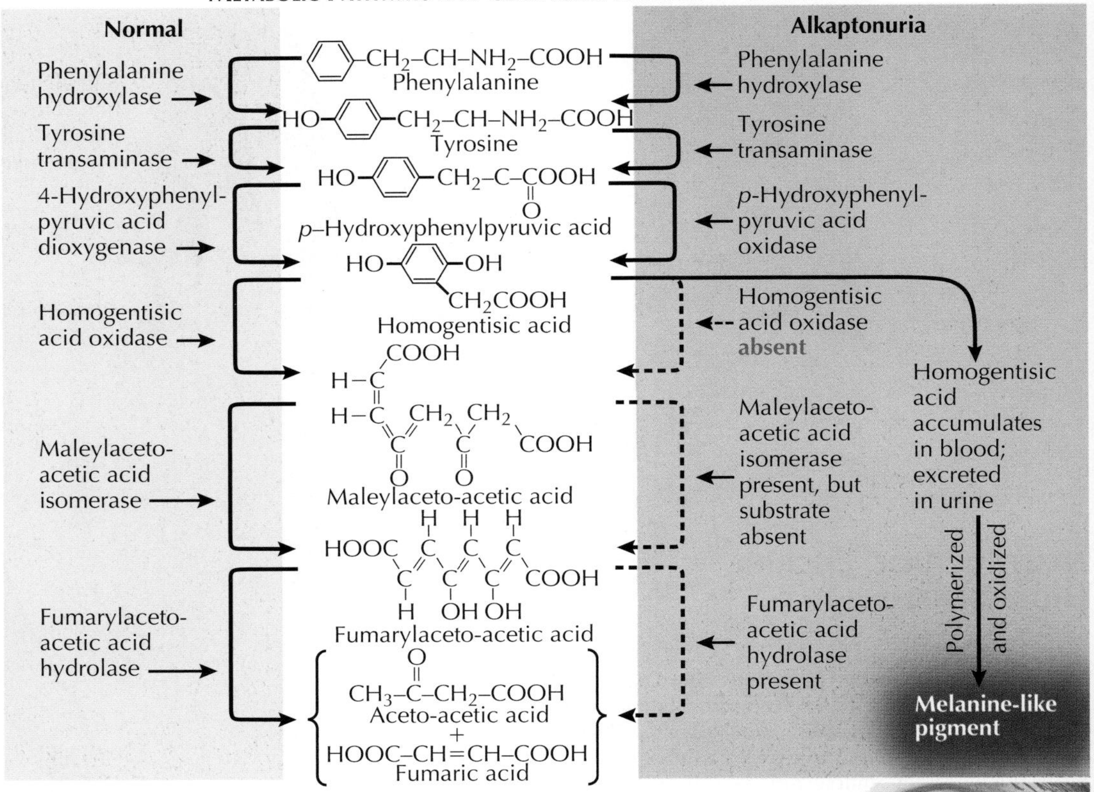

Normal | Alkaptonuria

Phenylalanine hydroxylase →

← Phenylalanine hydroxylase

CH_2–CH–NH_2–$COOH$
Phenylalanine

Tyrosine transaminase →

← Tyrosine transaminase

HO–CH_2–CH–NH_2–$COOH$
Tyrosine

4-Hydroxyphenyl-pyruvic acid dioxygenase →

← p-Hydroxyphenyl-pyruvic acid oxidase

HO–CH_2–C–$COOH$
O
p–Hydroxyphenylpyruvic acid

Homogentisic acid oxidase →

← Homogentisic acid oxidase absent

HO–OH
CH_2COOH
Homogentisic acid

Homogentisic acid accumulates in blood; excreted in urine

Maleylaceto-acetic acid isomerase →

← Maleylaceto-acetic acid isomerase present, but substrate absent

$COOH$
H–C
H–C CH_2 CH_2
C C $COOH$
O O
Maleylaceto-acetic acid

Polymerized and oxidized

Fumarylaceto-acetic acid hydrolase →

← Fumarylaceto-acetic acid hydrolase present

H H H
$HOOC$ C C C $COOH$
C C C
H OH OH
Fumarylaceto-acetic acid

Melanine-like pigment

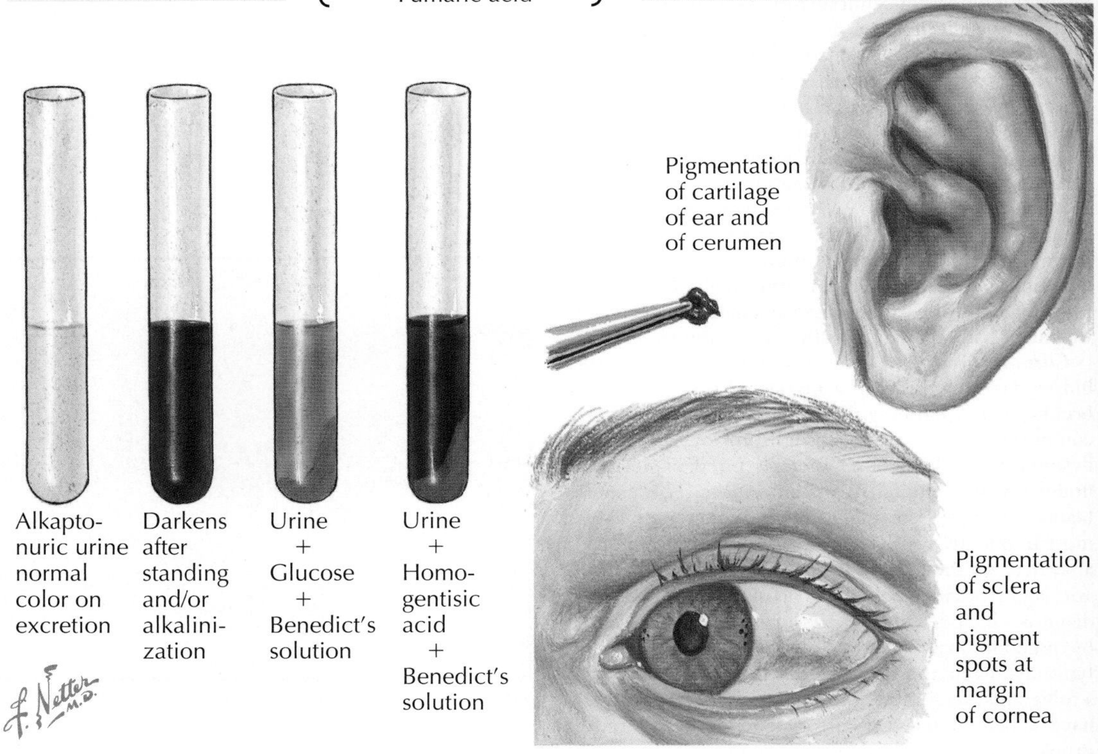

O
CH_3–C–CH_2–$COOH$
Aceto-acetic acid
+
$HOOC$–CH=CH–$COOH$
Fumaric acid

Alkapto-nuric urine normal color on excretion

Darkens after standing and/or alkalini-zation

Urine + Glucose + Benedict's solution

Urine + Homo-gentisic acid + Benedict's solution

Pigmentation of cartilage of ear and of cerumen

Pigmentation of sclera and pigment spots at margin of cornea

OCHRONOSIS

Ochronosis is the name given to the later clinical findings of alkaptonuria. Alkaptonuria is caused by an inborn error of metabolism resulting from a defect or deficiency of the enzyme homogentisic acid oxidase. A complete lack of the enzyme in the kidneys and liver is responsible for the buildup of the homogentisic acid. Alkaptonuria is transmitted in an autosomal recessive manner. Homogentisic acid oxidase is responsible for the metabolism of homogentisic acid, which is a breakdown product of the amino acids phenylalanine and tyrosine. This enzyme metabolizes homogentisic acid into maleylaceto-acetic acid, which is eventually converted to fumaric acid and aceto-acetic acid. When, as in alkaptonuria, the homogentisic acid oxidase enzyme is deficient, homogentisic acid accumulates in the blood and is excreted in the urine. The disease has a slow, insidious onset, and patients often present initially in young adulthood.

Clinical Findings: The first clinical sign is that of dark urine found in an affected baby's diaper, which often causes concerned parents to seek medical advice. If left to stand for a few minutes, the urine turns dark black because of the oxidative effects of the atmosphere. The urine can be alkalinized with a strong basic solution such as sodium hydroxide; addition of the basic solution to a sample of urine promptly turns it dark black. Benedict's reagent can also be used to test the urine of patients with alkaptonuria; when it is added, the supernatant turns dark black, and this finding is diagnostic of alkaptonuria.

As the homogentisic acid accumulates in these patients, it eventually begins depositing in skin and cartilage tissue, for which it has an affinity, becoming visibly noticeable in the fourth decade of life. The sclera is one of the first areas to be noticeably involved. A subtle brown discoloration begin to form on the lateral aspect of the sclera and continues to darken over the lifetime of the patient. The ear cartilage becomes dark brown to almost bluish due to the accumulation of the homogentisic acid. The cerumen is dark black, and evaluation of the ear may also show a darkening of the

Plate 4-54

Rashes

SYSTEMIC FINDINGS OF OCHRONOSIS

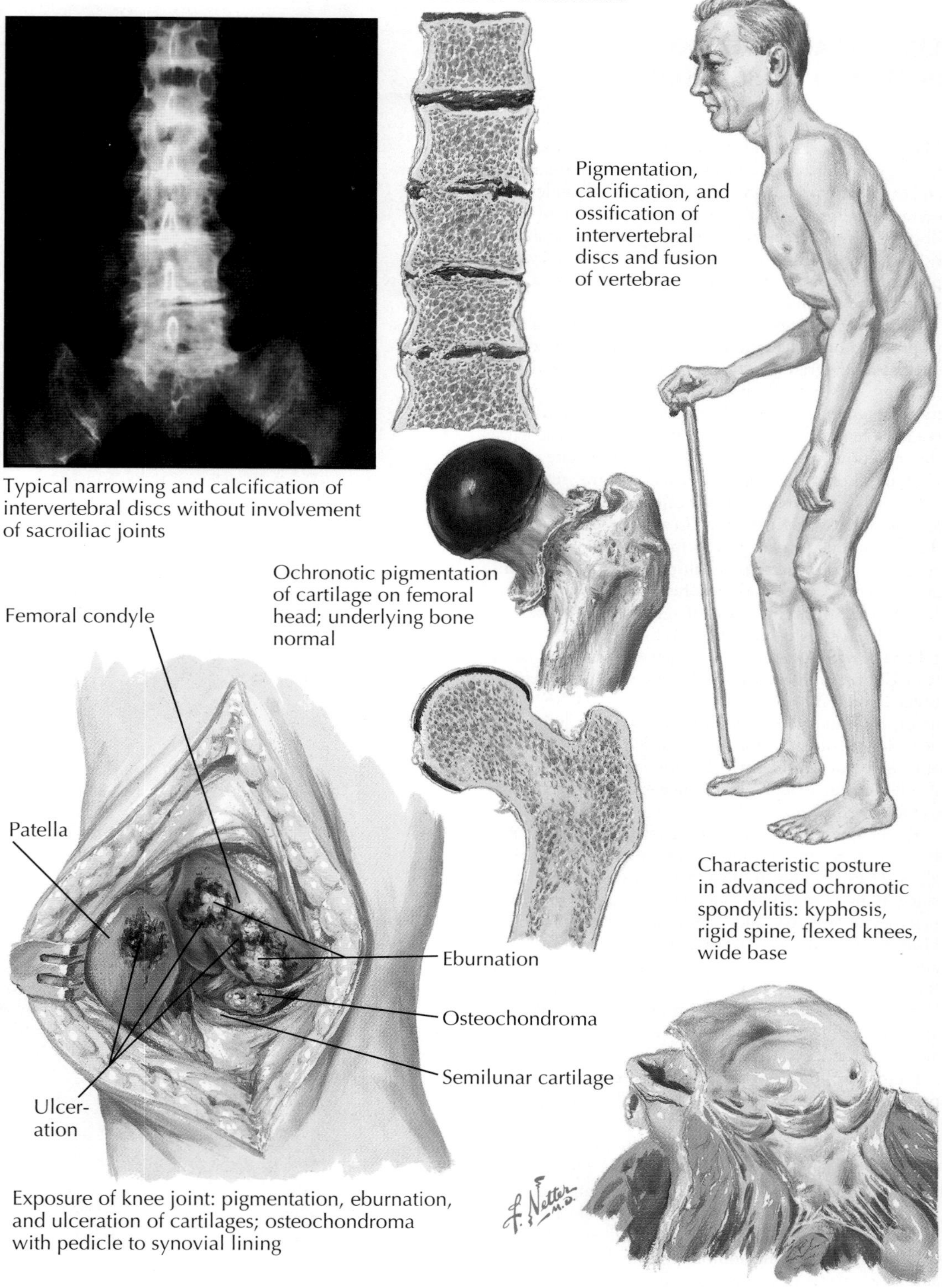

Typical narrowing and calcification of intervertebral discs without involvement of sacroiliac joints

Pigmentation, calcification, and ossification of intervertebral discs and fusion of vertebrae

Ochronotic pigmentation of cartilage on femoral head; underlying bone normal

Characteristic posture in advanced ochronotic spondylitis: kyphosis, rigid spine, flexed knees, wide base

Femoral condyle

Patella

Eburnation

Osteochondroma

Semilunar cartilage

Ulceration

Exposure of knee joint: pigmentation, eburnation, and ulceration of cartilages; osteochondroma with pedicle to synovial lining

Pigmentation of endocardium

OCHRONOSIS (Continued)

tympanic membrane and the stapes, incus, and malleus bones of the inner ear. The patient may suffer from tinnitus.

With time, the skin in various regions begins to become hyperpigmented. This occurs first and foremost in the areas with a high concentration of sweat glands. The axillae and the groin are noticeably affected. The excessive homogentisic acid is secreted in the sweat, and the pigment discolors the surrounding skin. The cheeks are also prominently affected.

The most disabling aspect of this disease is the deposition of homogentisic acid in the fibrocartilage and hyaline cartilage. This leads to severe degenerative joint disease at an early age. The pigment alters the cartilage and makes it brittle and friable. The cartilage begins to fragment and disintegrate and can get embedded in the synovial tissue, causing synovial polyps. The intervertebral disks become severely pigmented and begin to calcify because of the massive destruction of the cartilage. The disks are destroyed, causing a severe reduction in the patient's height, as well as chronic pain and rigidity of the spine. Eventually, the heart, prostate, aorta, and kidneys all show evidence of ochronosis.

Pathogenesis: Ochronosis is the result of an autosomal recessive inherited disorder that causes the affected patient to be deficient in the enzyme homogentisic acid oxidase. This deficiency, over time, leads

to the accumulation of homogentisic acid in various tissues throughout the body and the subsequent clinical manifestations.

Histology: The findings on skin biopsy are pathognomonic for ochronosis. Large ochre bodies are found within the dermis. These are obvious on low-power microscopy and can be used to confirm the diagnosis.

Treatment: No known cure is available, and there is no effective therapy. Physical therapy and joint

replacement increase flexibility and range of motion and help to decrease morbidity. Some researchers advocate a diet low in phenylalanine and tyrosine, although the success of this approach is anecdotal at best. The National Institutes of Health is currently studying an inhibitor of the enzyme 4-hydroxyphenylpyruvic acid dioxygenase, which would decrease the production of homogentisic acid and theoretically help to decrease joint destruction.

Plate 4-55

Integumentary System

ORAL MANIFESTATIONS IN BLOOD DYSCRASIAS

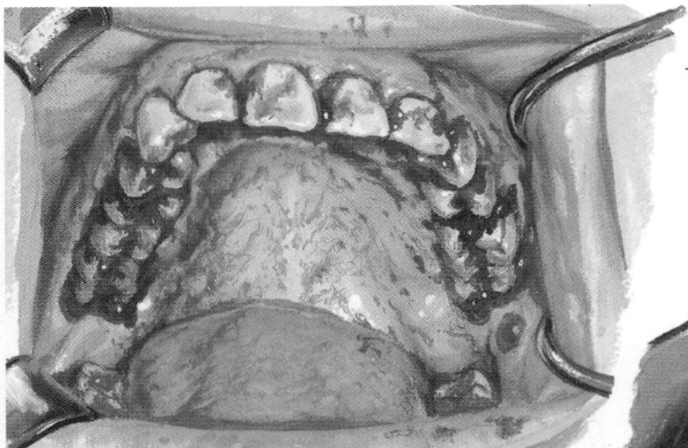

Many systemic hematological diseases have cutaneous findings as well as oral mucosal findings that are unique and can be the presenting clinical sign of the underlying disease. Awareness of the oral manifestations of these disorders is of paramount importance. Oral manifestations of blood dyscrasias can be seen in agranulocytosis, pernicious anemia, leukemia, polycythemia vera, and thrombotic thrombocytopenic purpura (TTP).

Clinical Findings: Agranulocytosis has been shown to produce oral ulcerations and erosions. Many different causes of agranulocytosis may result in these clinical findings. Medication-induced agranulocytosis is the most frequent cause of a decreased absolute neutrophil count of less than 500/μL. Many medications can cause this reaction, including dapsone, methotrexate, and a host of chemotherapeutic agents. A rare autosomal recessively inherited disease called infantile genetic agranulocytosis or Kostmann disease has been described. These patients present in the first months of life with recurrent oral ulcerations, multiple bacterial infections, and severely depressed absolute neutrophil counts. Death is the norm by 1 year of age unless the disease is correctly diagnosed and treated. Successful therapy is achieved with granulocyte colony-stimulating factor (G-CSF) or, in more advanced cases, with bone marrow transplantation. Even with successful G-CSF treatment, patients still develop oral ulcerations and severe periodontal disease. This is caused by the lack of an antimicrobial peptide, which allows certain bacteria to proliferate unabated. The species most frequently found is *Actinobacillus actinomycetes comitans.*

Pernicious anemia is caused by a deficiency of vitamin B_{12}. This deficiency is most commonly seen in individuals with an inability to absorb vitamin B_{12} or in strict vegetarians. Pernicious anemia can manifest with a macrocytic anemia and neurological complications. Hunter's glossitis is a form of atrophic glossitis that affects the tongue, leading to atrophy of the tongue filiform and fungiform papillae. The tongue takes on a beefy red appearance with a smooth surface. Varying amounts of glossodynia and decreased ability to taste are also found.

Gingival infiltration with leukemic cells may be the presenting sign of an acute leukemia, and gingival bleeding is the most frequent oral manifestation of leukemia. Oral ulcerations are commonly associated with the gingival leukemic hypertrophy. The gums appear red and swollen, with varying degrees of gingivitis. The gums may grossly enlarge to cover the majority of the teeth. This form of leukemic infiltration is seen almost exclusively in acute myelomonocytic leukemia (M4) and acute monocytic leukemia (M5). It is estimated to occur in two thirds of patients with M5 disease and in 20% of those with M4 disease. Other forms of leukemia have been implicated in causing gingival enlargement to a much lesser degree.

Polycythemia vera (previously termed *polycythemia rubra vera*) is caused by excessive production of red blood cells, which results in abnormally high hemoglobin and hematocrit values. The majority of cases are complicated by thrombosis. Most of these patients have a mutation in the *JAK2* gene, which encodes a Janus family tyrosine kinase protein. The ability to test for these mutations has made diagnosis much easier. Oral manifestations are limited to the tongue and gingival

Thrombocytopenic purpura, diffuse bleeding

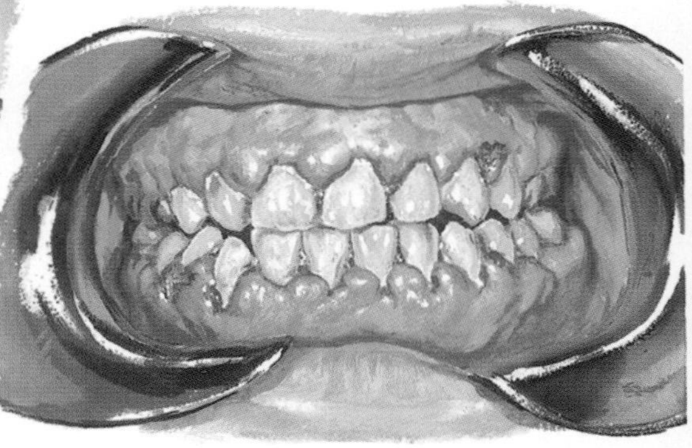

Leukemia (chronic), gingival infiltration

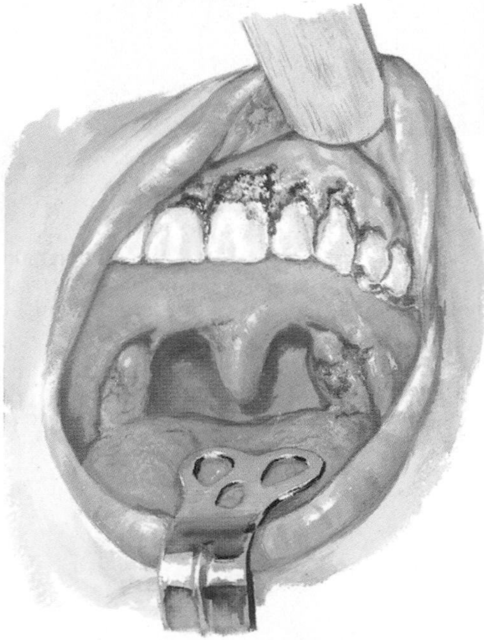

Agranulocytosis, multiple oral ulcers

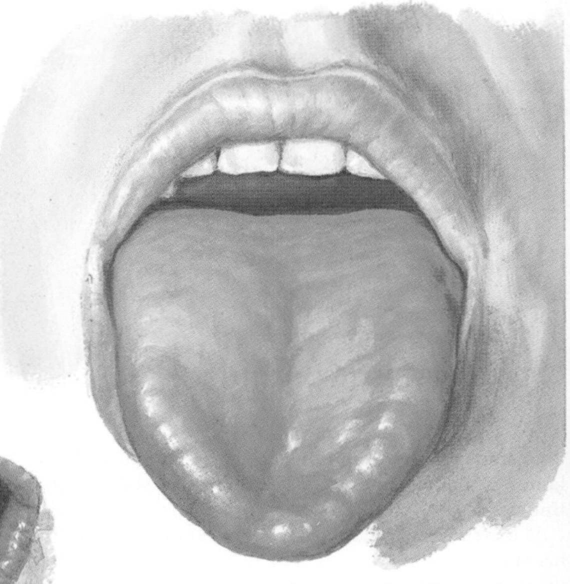

Pernicious anemia, smooth red tongue

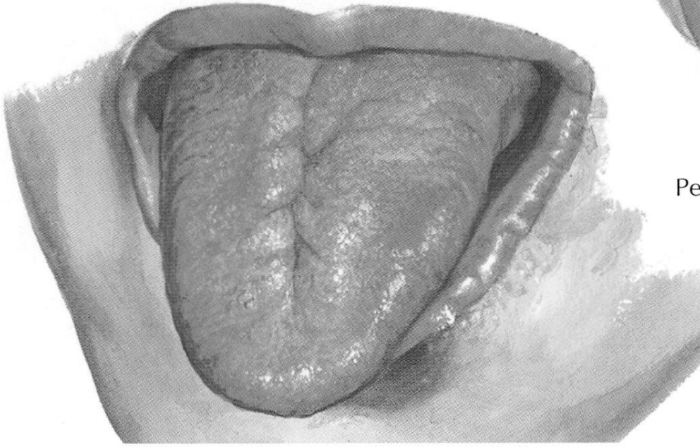

Polycythemia vera, beefy red tongue

mucosa. The tongue may become slightly enlarged, smooth, and hyperemic. Bleeding from the gingival mucosa can also be seen. The disease is manifested by many other systemic signs and symptoms.

TTP is a rare, life-threatening disease that can develop rapidly. It is manifested by the formation of microthrombi throughout the small vasculature. This causes multisystem organ failure and rapid death if not promptly treated. Most cases have been found to be

caused by a hereditary defect in the *ADAMTS13* gene or by decreased platelet levels caused by medications or autoimmunity. *ADAMTS13* is a gene that encodes a plasma metalloprotease, which is important in regulating von Willebrand factor function. Oral manifestations of the disease include widespread petechiae and ecchymosis of the tongue, gingival, labial, and buccal mucosa. Petechial hemorrhages of the gums may appear later in the course of the disease.

Plate 4-56

Rashes

PHYTOPHOTODERMATITIS

Phytophotodermatitis is a specific form of phototoxic or photoirritant contact dermatitis. The offending agent is a plant species from one of a few specific families. This form of dermatitis has an insidious onset and is typically preceded by little to no inflammation. This can make the diagnosis difficult for the clinician. Recognition of the key clinical features and the species of plant involved help make the diagnosis.

Clinical Findings: Phytophotodermatitis is caused by certain species of plants that come into contact with the skin. Lone contact with skin is not enough to cause the inflammatory reaction and subsequent postinflammatory hyperpigmentation: After exposure to the plant material, there is a time frame during which the exposed area must be introduced to ultraviolet radiation. It is the plant oils and resins in combination with the correct ultraviolet source that leads to the characteristic rash.

The most typical clinical scenario encountered is one in which the patient comes into contact with a plant that contains a psoralen compound. One of the most frequently reported causes is the juice of a lime *(Citrus aurantifolia).* This plant is categorized within the Rutaceae family. The Rutaceae family is the most widespread family of plants that have been described to cause these types of reactions, with the lime being by far the most common offender.

Patients often describe the use of a lime in a mixed drink while vacationing on the beach. The lime juice contacts the skin, and when the skin is exposed to a specific threshold of ultraviolet light, the reaction develops. Most often, patients do not complain of any acute symptoms. If the reaction is severe, burning occurs acutely and the diagnosis is relatively straightforward. However, most reactions are subtle and do not appear for a few days to weeks. Patients typically return home from vacation and notice a subtle hyperpigmentation around the mouth or scattered on the body where they have splashed or consciously applied the juice from a lime during sun bathing. The hyperpigmentation may last for months to years. On rare occasions, a severe acute reaction occurs with red plaque and vesicle formation.

The many families of plants capable of initiating this type of reaction all contain the chemical psoralen. Psoralen is a potent photosensitizer that is used clinically. Once purified, it can be given orally in the form of psoralen + ultraviolet A light (PUVA) therapy or painted on for topical PUVA therapy. It is especially helpful for treating refractory hand and foot dermatoses.

The areas of involvement are typically asymptomatic and do not show any overt inflammatory features. They appear as hyperpigmented, irregularly shaped macules on the skin. These spontaneously remit over a few months. Many plants are capable of producing the reaction.

Pathogenesis: Almost all of the plants responsible for phytophotodermatitis come from four specific families: Umbelliferae, Rutaceae, Moraceae, and Leguminosae. These plants all contain potent photosensitizers in varying concentrations. The chemicals responsible for photosensitization are the furocoumarins; more specifically, the psoralens are by far the most important of the photosensitizer chemicals. On contact, the psoralen penetrates the skin. Subsequent exposure to ultraviolet A light in the spectrum of 320 to 400 nm causes pyrimidine dimers to form within the DNA strands, which act

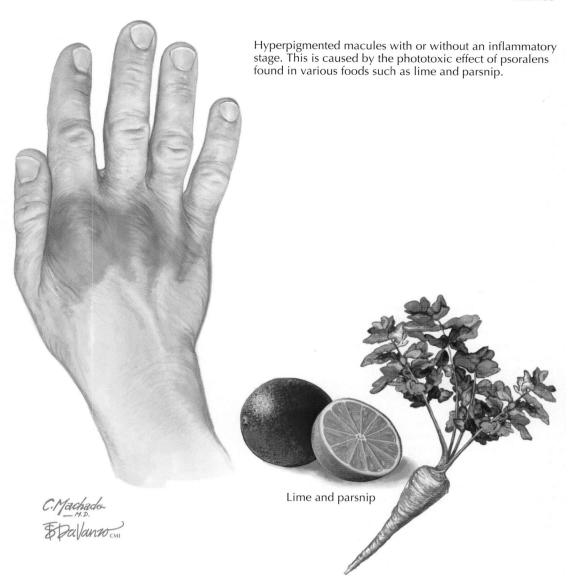

Hyperpigmented macules with or without an inflammatory stage. This is caused by the phototoxic effect of psoralens found in various foods such as lime and parsnip.

Lime and parsnip

The lime is the most frequent cause of this reaction. Bartenders and beach vacationers who drink beverages with a slice of lime are commonly afflicted.

Families of Plants Known to Cause Phytophotodermatitis and Some Representative Species	
Umbelliferae ▶ Dill–*Anethum graveolens* ▶ Parsley–*Petroselinum crispum* ▶ Parsnip–*Heracleum sphondylium* ▶ Giant hogweed–*Heracleum mantegazzianium* **Moraceae** ▶ Fig–*Ficus carica*	**Rutaceae** ▶ Rue–*Cneoridium dumosum* ▶ Lemon–*Citrus limon* ▶ Lime–*Citrus aurantifolia* ▶ Orange–*Citrus sinensis* **Leguminosae** ▶ Scurf pea–*Psoralea corylifolia*

to interrupt DNA synthesis. The psoralen and ultraviolet light also can cause hyperpigmentation (tanning).

Histology: The pathological features are dependent on the timing of the biopsy. An acutely inflamed lesion shows a superficial perivascular lymphocytic infiltrate and dermal edema with apoptotic keratinocytes within the epidermis. Late lesions show melanophages within the dermis.

Treatment: Acute areas of involvement can be treated with topical corticosteroid creams. The main issue in management is dealing with the prolonged postinflammatory hyperpigmentation. No therapy has been shown to be helpful, but almost all reactions resolve slowly over time. Care should be taken not to perform a treatment that might lead to a worse cosmetic outcome.

Plate 4-57

Integumentary System

PIGMENTED PURPURA

The pigmented purpuras are a group of idiopathic rashes that can occur at any age. They are grouped together because of their similar clinical and histological presentations. They are believed to be caused not by vasculitis but by inflammation of the small cutaneous capillaries, which produces a capillaritis. The rash is typically of no clinical significance to the patient, but it can cause significant cosmetic concern, and the purpuras need to be differentiated from other conditions that can cause similar rashes. The five rashes that make up the pigmented purpuric family of rashes are Schamberg's disease, eczematous pigmented purpura of Doucas and Kapetanakis, pigmented purpura of Gougerot and Blum, lichen aureus, and Majocchi's disease (annular telangiectatic pigmented purpura).

Clinical Findings: These entities are grouped together for many reasons. They are believed by some to be slightly different manifestations of the same disease state, and the histopathology of all the variants is strikingly similar. The pigmented purpuric dermatoses are benign and are not associated with any underlying abnormality. They can occur at any age. They are almost entirely asymptomatic in nature. The true incidence of these conditions is unknown, because they are often not reported. They are believed to occur very commonly.

Schamberg's disease is the most frequently encountered of the pigmented purpuric eruptions. It almost universally begins on the lower extremities. It manifests as tiny (1-mm) cayenne pepper–like petechial macules of the skin. Over time, a brownish-red hyperpigmented background forms secondary to the extravasation of red blood cells and their subsequent breakdown within the skin to release hemosiderin. The lesions are nonblanching and nonpalpable. The rash may spread proximally up the lower extremity but rarely affects other areas of the body. Most patients are referred to the dermatologist to rule out vasculitis, which is easily done by not finding any evidence of palpable purpura. The rash is almost always entirely asymptomatic, and patients frequently complain only of the appearance. If one sees widespread petechia, a platelet count should be performed to look for thrombocytopenia. If the platelet count is normal, a skin biopsy of the upper extremity or truncal area of involvement should be performed to evaluate for the very rare form of pigmented purpuric mycosis fungoides.

Eczematoid pigmented purpura of Doucas and Kapetanakis is a rare variant that manifests with petechiae and hyperpigmentation but is also associated with an overlying eczematous eruption. This form is typically pruritic and can show secondary excoriations.

Pigmented purpura of Gougerot and Blum is also known as lichenoid pigmented purpura. Small, light pink to purple papules form on the lower extremities. They can be mistaken initially for lichen planus. Biopsies of these papules show a lichenoid infiltrate. This pigmented purpura can be distinguished from Schamberg's disease in that the skin findings are palpable. There is no true palpable purpura.

Lichen aureus can be seen at any age and manifests with the presence of multiple tiny, golden-colored macules that coalesce into a large macule or patch. Lichen aureus can occur anywhere on the body and is solitary in nature.

The involved regions in Majocchi's disease show annular patches with petechiae and hyperpigmentation

Lichen aureus. Golden-colored macules and patches are characteristic of lichen aureus. This is one of the variants of pigmented purpura.

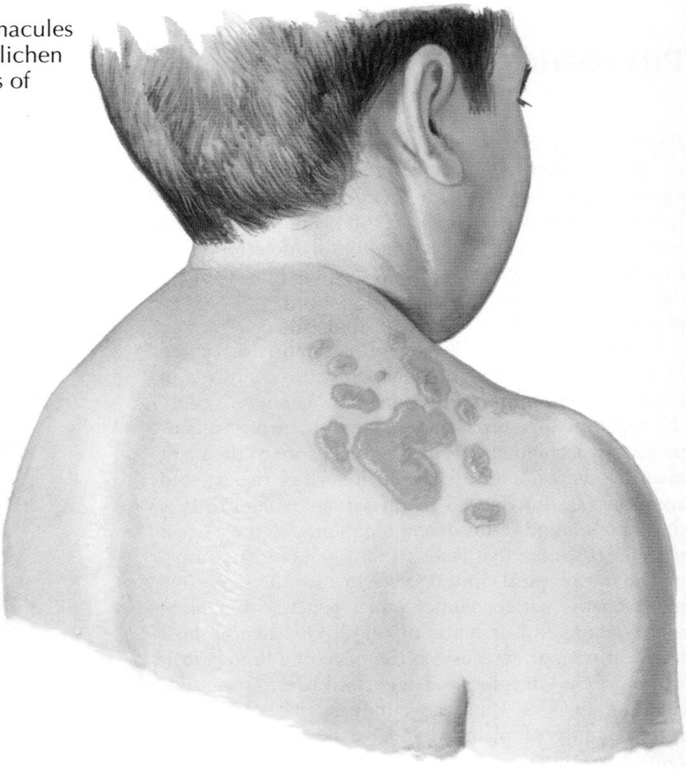

Schamberg's disease. Cayenne pepper–like petechiae. This asymptomatic idiopathic rash is almost exclusively seen on the lower legs.

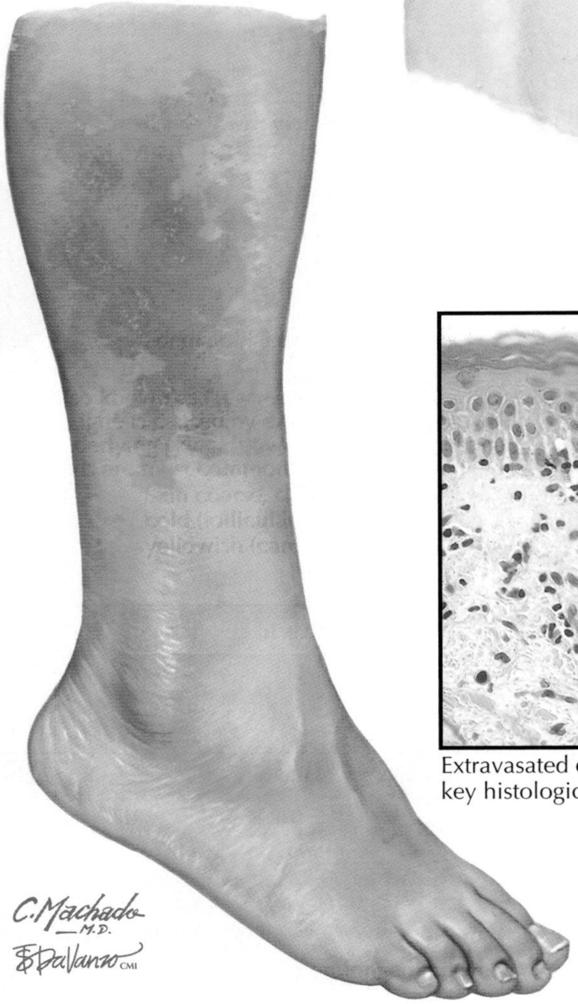

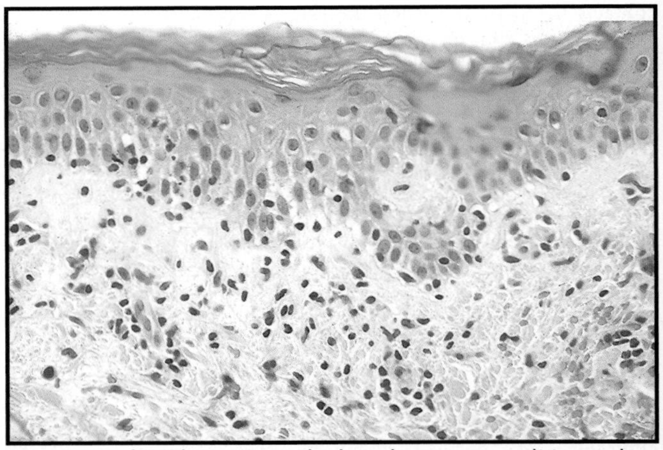

Extravasated erythrocytes and a lymphocytic vasculitis are the key histological features.

from hemosiderin deposition. This is a rare form of pigmented purpura that typically starts on the legs and spreads slowly over time.

Pathogenesis: The pigmented purpuric dermatoses are believed to be caused by capillaritis. The exact etiology is unknown.

Histology: The histological findings are similar across all variants. Extravasation of red blood cells is prominent. The extravasation is seen in the vicinity of the

capillaritis. The infiltrate is predominantly lymphocytic. The presence of hemosiderin is more easily seen in chronic lesions.

Treatment: There is no agreed-upon standard therapy, and withholding therapy is a frequently used option. Anecdotally, topical corticosteroids may be tried for a few weeks. Oral vitamin C and bioflavonoids have been reported to be successful, again mostly in anecdotal reports.

Plate 4-58

Rashes

PITYRIASIS ROSEA

Pityriasis rosea is a common idiopathic rash with a characteristic onset and distribution. It is a self-limited rash that spontaneously resolves within a few months. A few distinct clinical variants have been described. The main goal in treatment is to differentiate pityriasis rosea from other rashes that can have a similar clinical picture.

Clinical Findings: Pityriasis rosea is a common rash of young adults and children. It has no racial predilection. It is most often seen during the spring and fall months. Clustering of cases has been reported. A small but significant subset of patients have had a preceding upper respiratory tract infection. This has led some to search for a viral cause of the rash, although none have been found. The rash of pityriasis rosea can have a varying morphology, but it most commonly begins with a herald patch. The herald patch, or mother patch, is the first noticeable skin lesion. It typically precedes the entire outbreak of pityriasis rosea by a few days. The herald patch is a 2- to 4-cm, pink-red patch with fine adherent scale that commonly occurs on the trunk. After a few days, smaller, oval-shaped patches 0.5 to 1 cm in diameter begin appearing on the trunk and extremities. The rash follows the skin tension lines and has a peculiar "fir tree" pattern. This pattern mimics the down-sloping branches of a fir tree. The rash typically spares the face and glabrous skin.

Patients may complain of mild to moderate pruritus, but most are asymptomatic. The main differential diagnosis includes guttate psoriasis and, in cases that affect the palms and soles, secondary syphilis. Pityriasis rosea is a self-limited, spontaneously resolving rash. It typically does not last longer than 2 to 3 months. Guttate psoriasis usually begins after a streptococcal infection and does not exhibit a herald patch. The teardrop-shaped patches of guttate psoriasis also do not follow the skin tension lines, and this fact can be used to differentiate the two. Tinea corporis is almost always in the differential diagnosis of any rash that has a patch-type morphology and fine surface scale. Tinea corporis can be easily diagnosed with a microscopic evaluation of a small scraping of the skin. Widespread tinea is almost always associated with onychomycosis, and it is more commonly seen in patients who are taking chronic immunosuppressive agents or using topical steroids. These traits can be used to help differentiate the two conditions. The rash of secondary syphilis is the great mimicker. Any patient who has pityriasis rosea that affects the palms and or soles should be tested for syphilis.

A few unique variants of pityriasis rosea exist. One is papular pityriasis rosea. This form more commonly affects school-aged children with Fitzpatrick type IV, V, or VI skin. This version tends to be a bit more widespread and more pruritic. Instead of small, oval-shaped patches, this variant consists of small (0.5 cm) papules that have a small amount of surface scale. It runs the same benign course, with self-resolution after a few weeks to months. On healing, postinflammatory hyperpigmentation or hypopigmentation may result and may persist for several months.

Histology: A superficial and deep lymphocytic and histiocytic infiltrate is seen surrounding the vessels of

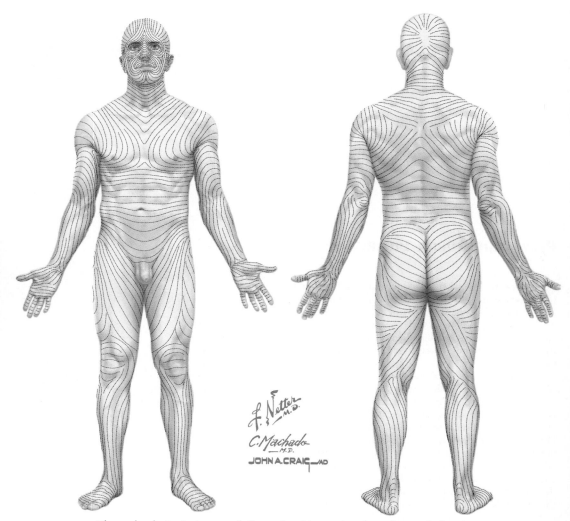

The rash of pityriasis rosea follows the skin tension lines (Langer's lines).

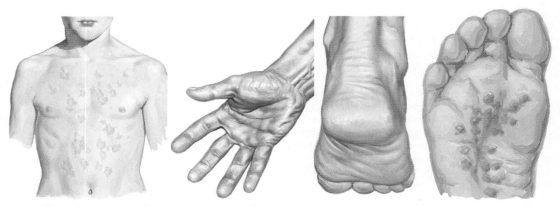

Generalized thin oval patches are distributed on the trunk following the skin tension lines.

The palms and soles are typically unaffected in pityriasis rosea. If they are affected, an RPR must be obtained to rule out secondary syphillis.

Secondary syphillis affecting the sole

the dermis. Varying amounts of extravasated red blood cells are appreciated within the upper dermis. The stratum corneum shows varying degrees of acanthosis and parakeratosis.

Pathogenesis: Many attempts to isolate a viral or a bacterial element in patients with pityriasis rosea have been met with frustration. To date, no infectious cause has been determined. The true nature and cause of pityriasis rosea remain elusive.

Treatment: No therapy is needed. Most cases are asymptomatic and mild. Pruritus can be treated with oral antihistamines and adjunctive topical steroids. The use of oral erythromycin, twice a day for 2 weeks, was shown to decrease the duration of the rash. Ultraviolet therapy is very helpful in treating the rash and pruritus. If there is any consideration for syphilis in the history or the physical examination, a rapid plasma reagin (RPR) blood test should be performed.

Plate 4-59   Integumentary System

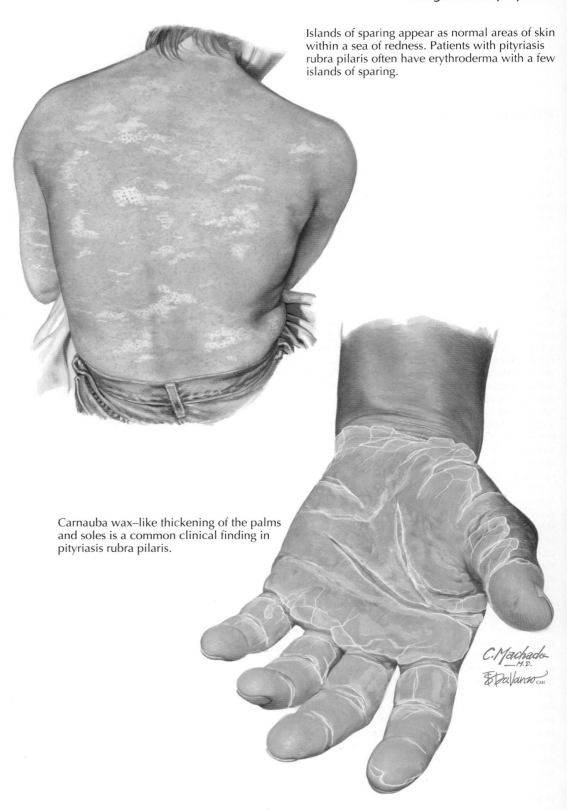

Islands of sparing appear as normal areas of skin within a sea of redness. Patients with pityriasis rubra pilaris often have erythroderma with a few islands of sparing.

Carnauba wax–like thickening of the palms and soles is a common clinical finding in pityriasis rubra pilaris.

PITYRIASIS RUBRA PILARIS

Pityriasis rubra pilaris (PRP) is an idiopathic rash that has many cutaneous manifestations. It is an uncommon entity that often manifests with near-erythroderma. There are several clinical variations of the condition, and it has a characteristic histological pattern, although this pattern is not always seen on microscopic examination.

Clinical Findings: PRP has a unique bimodal age of distribution, with an early onset of disease in the first 5 years of life and adult onset in the sixth decade. There is no gender or racial predilection. PRP tends to run a chronic course. It starts insidiously with small follicular, keratotic, pink to red papules. These papules have been described as "nutmeg grater" papules. The papules coalesce into larger patches and plaques. Eventually, large surface areas are involved, with a near-erythroderma. Characteristic islands of sparing occur within the erythrodermic background. These islands of completely normal skin are usually small, a few centimeters in diameter, but they can be much larger. The islands typically have an angulated shape, and they are rarely perfectly round or oval. The palms and soles become thickened and yellowish. This is highly characteristic of PRP and is called "carnauba wax–like" palms and soles. Fissuring is very common within the keratoderma and can be a source of pain and a site for secondary infection.

PRP has historically been separated into five subtypes: classic adult, classic juvenile, atypical adult, atypical juvenile, and a circumscribed or localized form. The classic adult and classic juvenile forms were described earlier. They typically run a chronic clinical course, with most cases spontaneously resolving a few years after onset. Paraneoplastic variants of PRP have been described. Onset of the malignancy precedes the rash of PRP, and the patients seem to improve with treatment of the underlying tumor. This is a very rare clinical scenario. Patients with human immunodeficiency virus infection seem to be at a higher risk for developing PRP.

The differential diagnosis of classic forms of PRP includes psoriasis, drug rash, and cutaneous T-cell lymphoma. Skin biopsy and clinical pathological correlation help the clinician make a firm diagnosis.

Pathogenesis: The etiology is undetermined. Theories on the formation of PRP have centered on abnormal metabolism of vitamin A or an abnormal immune response to a foreign antigen. These theories have not been thoroughly studied or proven. The report of a familial form of PRP may shed some light on the etiology.

Histology: The pathognomonic histological finding in PRP is the appearance of alternating layers of parakeratosis and orthokeratosis, both in a vertical and a horizontal direction, lending the appearance of a chess board. This pattern is not always present, and sometimes it can be seen only with close inspection.

Treatment: Therapy for PRP is difficult. Many agents have been used with varying degrees of success. Topical corticosteroid wet wraps, oral retinoids, and ultraviolet therapy have long been used as first-line agents. The retinoids are considered first-line therapy, and both isotretinoin and acitretin have been used. Other immunosuppressants have been used, including methotrexate, azathioprine, and the newer anti–tumor necrosis factor inhibitors. No randomized, placebo-controlled trials have been performed to date.

Plate 4-60

Rashes

POLYARTERITIS NODOSA

Polyarteritis nodosa is a rare chronic form of vasculitis of the medium to small vessels with significant cutaneous and systemic manifestations. It is a rare condition, with an estimated incidence of 5 per 1,000,000 persons. The symptoms depend on the organ system involved and the extent of vasculitis. Uniquely and for unknown reasons, the respiratory system is spared. Polyarteritis nodosa has been found in some cases to be a chronic, non–life-threatening disease that affects only the skin. More often, it is a multisystem disease, with the skin being affected along with other organ systems. Many other organ system may be involved, and the skin features may be the presenting sign of the disease. Excisional skin biopsies of cutaneous lesions of polyarteritis nodosa show the characteristic necrotizing vasculitis of medium vessels within the deep reticular dermis. The cutaneous diagnosis of polyarteritis nodosa should alert the clinician to the possibility of systemic disease, and appropriate testing should be undertaken to evaluate for widespread disease. Most cases of polyarteritis nodosa are idiopathic, but this condition can be seen in association with viral infections, malignancy, or autoimmune disease. Coinfection with the hepatitis B virus is the most classic and most frequent association with polyarteritis nodosa.

Clinical Findings: The primary cutaneous manifestation of polyarteritis nodosa is palpable purpura. The cutaneous findings tend to be spread over wide areas of the body and are not found entirely in dependent regions, as is the case with leukocytoclastic vasculitis. Deeper, tender dermal nodules may form. These nodules usually follow the course of an underlying artery. The patient may develop livedo reticularis of the extremities, and secondary ulcerations may form as the vasculitis progresses and causes necrosis of the overlying skin. The diagnosis of the type of vasculitis is difficult to make from clinical examination alone. Tissue sampling is needed to determine the type of vessel affected by the inflammatory vasculitis. Polyarteritis nodosa has also been shown to have nonspecific findings, such as red macules and papules, that mimic drug eruptions or viral infections. If the only organ system involved is the integumentary system, the prognosis is good, and the disease typically follows a chronic, treatable course.

Once the diagnosis of cutaneous polyarteritis nodosa has been made, a systemic evaluation must be undertaken to pursue potential life-threatening involvement. If other organ systems are involved, the patient will need to undergo systemic therapy, and a multidisciplinary approach is required. The sensory nerves are almost always affected by mononeuritis multiplex. This leads to a peripheral neuropathy, and it is cited as the most common extracutaneous finding in polyarteritis nodosa. The kidneys, heart, and gastrointestinal tract are also routinely affected, and any of these can lead to life-threatening complications. Renal artery aneurysms can form along the branches of the renal artery and can become thrombosed. This leads to wedge-shaped infarcts in the kidney with varying amounts of kidney function loss. Gastrointestinal arterial infarcts can also cause bowel ischemia and symptoms of an acute abdomen. The central nervous system and the musculoskeletal system are also frequently affected.

Pathogenesis: The pathomechanisms that incite polyarteritis nodosa are poorly understood. Hepatitis-induced polyarteritis is believed to be partially caused by viral disruption of arterial endothelial cells as a result of circulating antigen-antibody complexes.

Polyarteritis nodosa with characteristic multisystem involvement

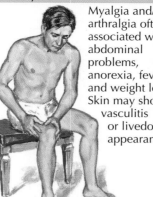

Myalgia and/or arthralgia often associated with abdominal problems, anorexia, fever, and weight loss. Skin may show vasculitis or livedoid appearance.

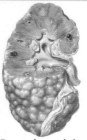

Coarsely nodular, irregularly scarred kidney. Cut section reveals organizing infarcts and thrombosed aneuysms in corticomedullary region.

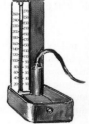

Hypertension common

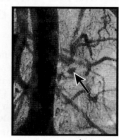

Angiogram showing microaneurysm of small mesenteric artery

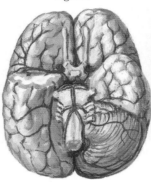

CNS involvement may cause headache, ocular disorders, convulsions, aphasia, hemiplegia, and cerebellar signs.

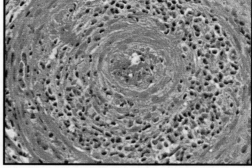

Inflammatory cell infiltration and fibrinoid necrosis of walls of small arteries lead to infarction in various organs or tissues.

Mononeuritis multiplex with polyarteritis nodosa

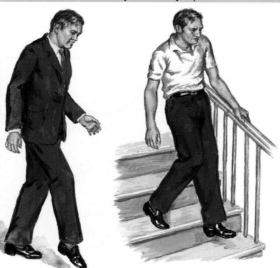

Sudden occurrence of foot drop while walking (peroneal nerve)

Sudden buckling of knee while going downstairs (femoral nerve)

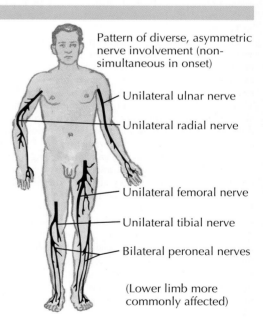

Pattern of diverse, asymmetric nerve involvement (non-simultaneous in onset)

Unilateral ulnar nerve

Unilateral radial nerve

Unilateral femoral nerve

Unilateral tibial nerve

Bilateral peroneal nerves

(Lower limb more commonly affected)

Histology: Necrotizing vasculitis of medium and small arteries in the deep reticular dermis is the hallmark of polyarteritis nodosa. The inflammatory infiltrate is predominantly made up of neutrophils with an admixture of other leukocytes. Fibrinoid necrosis is prominent, and intraluminal clotting is often seen. Depending on the type of skin lesion biopsied, varying amounts of skin necrosis are seen. This is most commonly observed in areas of infarcted skin and ulceration.

Treatment: The first-line therapy is with oral corticosteroids. The use of steroid-sparing agents early in the course of the disease may help decrease steroid-induced side effects. Cyclophosphamide is the major steroid-sparing agent used. Therapy for polyarteritis nodosa induced by hepatitis B virus infection is targeted at the replicating viral particles.

Plate 4-61

Integumentary System

PRURITIC URTICARIAL PAPULES AND PLAQUES OF PREGNANCY

Pruritic urticarial papules and plaques of pregnancy (PUPPP), also known as polymorphous eruption of pregnancy (PEP), is the most common dermatosis associated with pregnancy. The name describes the variable appearance that the rash can take. Idiopathic in nature, it is seen most commonly during an expectant mother's first pregnancy. It has been shown to have no bearing on pregnancy outcome or on the fetus or newborn. It is diagnosed on clinical grounds and rarely biopsied. There are no associated laboratory abnormalities. The classic history and variable morphology of the rash are characteristic.

Clinical Findings: PUPPP occurs during the late third trimester of pregnancy or has its onset soon after delivery. The rash almost always begins within the striae distensae of the abdomen. Small urticarial papules and plaques begin to form within the striae. They are extremely pruritic and cause significant discomfort. As the name implies, the rash can have a polymorphous nature. Papules, plaques, macules, and even small vesicles have been described. The rash may spread from the abdomen to other regions of the body. PUPPP has been described to occur more commonly during the first pregnancy with a male fetus. The reasons for this are unknown. The rash spontaneously remits after delivery, in most cases within 2 to 4 weeks. Those patients with onset after delivery typically have a shorter course, with 1 week of severe itching followed by remission soon afterward. PUPPP typically does not recur in subsequent pregnancies. PUPPP also does not flare when birth control medications are started, as does herpes gestationis.

The main differential diagnosis is between PUPPP and prurigo gestationis. Prurigo gestationis has no primary lesions and manifests as diffuse itching with excoriations. Liver function enzymes may be elevated in this condition. Prurigo gestationis is associated with an increased risk for prematurity. Scabies infection can also be highly pruritic and can be considered in the differential diagnosis. Scabies is easily diagnosed with a scraping and microscopic evaluation of a burrow. Scabies can have its onset at any time during a pregnancy, and urticarial papules and plaques within striae are not typically seen. If they are seen, they are not as numerous or uniform in appearance as the lesions of PUPPP. Herpes gestationis, also known as pemphigoid gestationis or bullous pemphigoid of pregnancy, is the most severe of all the pregnancy-associated rashes. It can begin as urticarial red plaques on the abdomen and then spread to other regions. Compared with PUPPP, it tends to occur earlier in the pregnancy. The biggest differentiating point is that the rash of herpes gestationis will begin to blister: Small vesicles form and quickly coalesce into larger bullae. Bullae are never seen in PUPPP. Herpes gestationis is caused by maternal antibody formation against hemidesmosomal antigens. Titer levels can be measured, and the most commonly found antibody is against the 180-kd bullous pemphigoid antigen (BP180). There is a risk of prematurity and low birth weight with this rash. Oral corticosteroids are often needed to keep herpes gestationis under control. The rash remits after delivery but tends to recur during subsequent pregnancies, and it can flare when an affected patient starts taking birth control medications.

Pathogenesis: The etiology is unknown. PUPPP is most commonly seen in first pregnancies and possibly

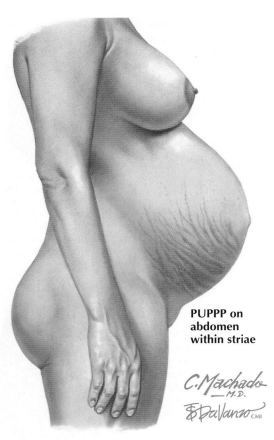

PUPPP on abdomen within striae

C. Machado M.D.
B. DaVanzo CMI

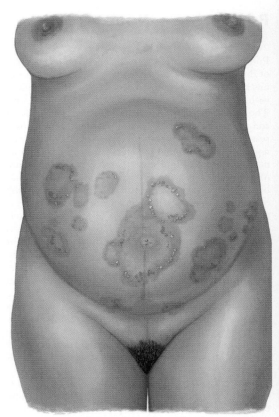

Herpes gestationis. Also known as bullous pemphigoid of pregnancy. Pruritic bullae develop on a background of erythematous or urticarial-appearing skin.

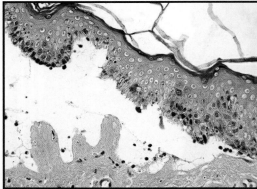

Herpes gestationis (pemphigoid gestationis) (H&E stain). Prominent subepidermal bulla formation is seen along the specimen. Separation is caused by antibodies against the BP180 protein, which leads to bulla formation.

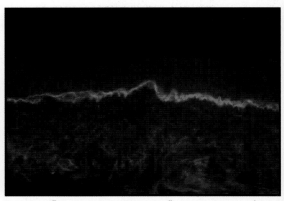

Immunofluorescence. Immunofluorescence studies show linear staining of C3 along the basement membrane zone in herpes gestationis.

is more common in multiple-birth pregnancies. The exact roles played by skin distention, hormonal changes, and interactions with the immune system in the pathogenesis of PUPPP are being studied.

Histology: Histological findings of PUPPP biopsy specimens are nonspecific; there is a superficial and deep perivascular lymphocytic infiltrate. Occasional eosinophils are seen, with some dermal edema.

Treatment: The main treatment for PUPPP is to give supportive care and to try to suppress the itching symptoms. There are no ill effects on the fetus, and expectant mothers can be given topical medium- or high-potency corticosteroids to help decrease the itching. Occasionally, antihistamines such as diphenhydramine are also needed to control the itching.

Plate 4-62

Rashes

PSEUDOXANTHOMA ELASTICUM

Pseudoxanthoma elasticum is a rare genetic disorder with both cutaneous and systemic findings. It is inherited in an autosomal recessive manner. This disease is caused by a defect in an adenosine triphosphate (ATP)-binding protein that is found in many tissues, including the skin, eye, gastrointestinal tract, and cardiovascular systems. The cutaneous findings often precede the appearance of the systemic findings. Recognition of the cutaneous findings can help lessen the risk of systemic complications. A multidisciplinary approach to the care of these patients is required. The skin findings have no bearing on mortality.

Clinical Findings: Pseudoxanthoma elasticum manifests in late childhood or early adulthood. The cutaneous findings are almost always the first sign of the disease. The skin on the neck is most commonly affected early and most severely. There is a "plucked chicken" appearance to the skin. Small yellow papules are studded within the involved region, and over time they coalesce into larger, symmetric plaques. The intervening skin has a dull appearance with a fine pebbly texture. The neck is by far the area most noticeably affected, but other regions may become involved, including the intertriginous regions. A rare generalized cutaneous form has been reported. The mucous membranes may also become involved with tiny yellow papules. As time progresses, the skin may become loose, appearing to hang from the body, and this can be a significant cosmetic concern to the patient. The areas of cutaneous involvement are essentially asymptomatic. On occasion, mild pruritus is reported. A nonspecific skin finding that is seen with increased frequency in pseudoxanthoma elasticum is elastosis perforans serpiginosa. This perforating disorder has been described to occur in many different clinical settings, and it is caused by the transepidermal elimination of damaged elastic tissue. The reason this occurs in pseudoxanthoma elasticum is unknown.

It is important to diagnosis this disease at a young age so that some of the severe systemic complications can be prevented. The globe is affected in pseudoxanthoma elasticum. The first sign is a yellowish discoloration of the retina. Later in life, cracks or ruptures in Bruch's membrane can be seen on funduscopic examination; these are termed *angioid streaks*. Angioid streaks have a later age at onset than the cutaneous findings do. Abnormalities of the elastic fibers in Bruch's membrane are responsible for their formation. Angioid streaks can be seen in many disorders of connective tissue and are not specific for pseudoxanthoma elasticum. Retinal hemorrhage and resultant visual field loss is the most severe ophthalmological complication.

Cardiovascular and gastrointestinal manifestations arise because of the abnormal calcification of elastic tissue within blood vessel walls. Gastrointestinal hemorrhage may occur and may be life-threatening. Angina and hypertension may occur from involvement of the coronary and renal arteries, respectively.

Histology: Findings on skin biopsies are very characteristic and show abnormal fractured, calcified elastic tissue within the dermis. The findings can be accentuated with special staining methods to highlight the calcified elastic fibers. However, the diagnosis can be made easily on routine hematoxylin and eosin staining.

Pathogenesis: Pseudoxanthoma elasticum is inherited in an autosomal recessive fashion and is caused by a defect in the *ABCC6* gene. This gene is responsible for encoding the multidrug resistance–associated protein 6

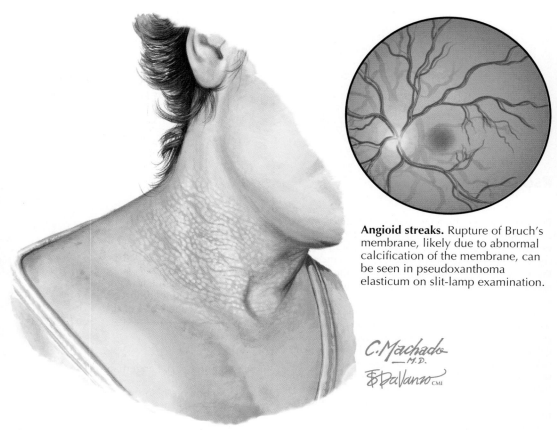

Angioid streaks. Rupture of Bruch's membrane, likely due to abnormal calcification of the membrane, can be seen in pseudoxanthoma elasticum on slit-lamp examination.

C. Machado
—*M.D.*
B DaVanzo CMI

The neck is often the first area of skin involvement. Often clinically noted to have the appearance of "plucked chicken skin"

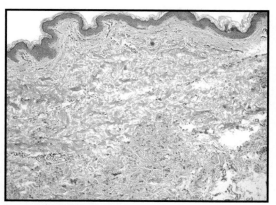

Low power (H&E). Fragmented and calcified elastic fibers appear as basophilic clumps within the middle to lower dermis. This is highly characteristic for pseudoxanthoma elasticum.

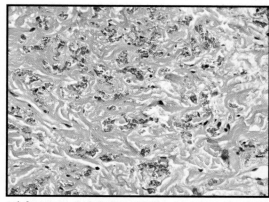

High power (H&E). Basophilic clumping of calcified elastic fibers that have become fragmented is well appreciated in this highpower view. The abnormality in the elastic fibers leads to the various clinical manifestations of the disease.

(MRP6), which is also known as ATP-binding cassette transporter 6 (ABCC6). This protein is found within the liver and kidneys and is expressed at low levels in the tissues that are affected by this disease. It has been proposed that the defect causes a metabolic abnormality, possibly resulting in a buildup of a metabolite that damages to the elastic fibers in the affected tissue.

Treatment: Therapy is directed at preventive care. Routine cardiovascular and ophthalmological examinations can help keep hypertension and early signs of retinal disease in check. Retinal hemorrhages need to be treated acutely by an ophthalmologist. Routine examinations for blood in the stool and routine gastrointestinal examinations are warranted to screen for gastrointestinal bleeding, which is the main cause of morbidity and mortality in these patients. Patients should be encouraged to stay within a healthy weight range and not to smoke. Most patients live a normal life span.

Plate 4-63

Integumentary System

HISTOPATHOLOGICAL FEATURES AND TYPICAL DISTRIBUTION OF PSORIASIS

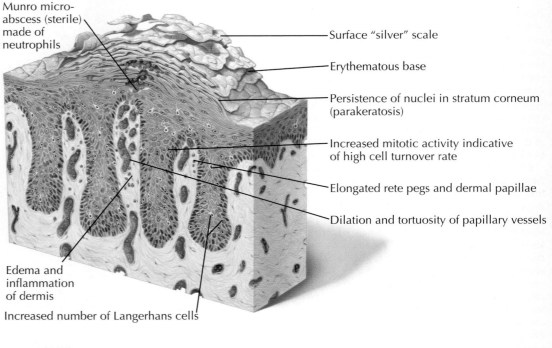

Munro micro-abscess (sterile) made of neutrophils

Surface "silver" scale

Erythematous base

Persistence of nuclei in stratum corneum (parakeratosis)

Increased mitotic activity indicative of high cell turnover rate

Elongated rete pegs and dermal papillae

Dilation and tortuosity of papillary vessels

Edema and inflammation of dermis

Increased number of Langerhans cells

PSORIASIS

Psoriasis is an autoimmune disease that affects 1% to 2% of the U.S. population. There is a large regional variation in the incidence of psoriasis. Scandinavian countries have a much higher incidence than the rest of the world, and the Native American population has one of the lowest rates of psoriasis. Much has been learned about the pathogenesis of psoriasis, and dramatic advances in therapy have helped many patients. Psoriasis is grouped with the other papulosquamous skin diseases. It can cause not only skin disease but also joint disease. The total effect that psoriasis has on patients cannot be judged solely on the basis of skin involvement, because the disease has been shown to have profound psychological and social effects as well. There is no known cure for psoriasis, but research is moving forward, and new therapies are being developed.

Clinical Findings: Psoriasis is a papulosquamous skin disease that can affect people at any age of life. There is no gender predilection. Approximately 40% of affected individuals have a family history of psoriasis. Most patients with early age at onset tend to have a more severe course of disease. Psoriasis often starts with silvery, ostraceous, scaly patches and plaques with a predilection for the knees, elbows, and scalp. The term *ostraceous scale* refers to the oyster shell–like appearance of the hyperkeratotic scale that is oriented in a concave manner. The term *rupioid scale* is used to describe the psoriatic plaques that appear to mimic the cone shape of limpet shells. A characteristic clinical finding is that of Woronoff's ring, the peripheral rim of blanching seen around the early psoriatic plaques. Auspitz's sign is another characteristic clinical sign used to differentiate psoriasis from other rashes. It refers to the pinpoint bleeding that occurs after the upper scale has been removed from a psoriatic plaque. Woronoff's sign is specific to psoriasis and most likely is caused by localized vasoconstriction surrounding the area of the lesion, which has an increased blood flow. There is a striking symmetry to the rash. Psoriasis can have various skin morphologies. There are many well-recognized clinical variants with distinctive clinical findings.

Psoriasis vulgaris is the most common form of psoriasis encountered. It manifests with symmetrically located, silvery, scaly patches and plaques on the scalp, knees, elbows, and lower back. Patients can have a small amount of body surface area involvement, or they can have widespread disease approaching near-erythroderma. The face is usually spared from patches and plaques of psoriasis. Patients with a higher body surface area of involvement tend to have a higher risk for development of psoriatic arthritis and psoriatic nail disease. All patients with psoriasis exhibit the Koebner phenomenon. Koebnerization of psoriasis occurs when a previously normal area of skin is traumatized and psoriatic plaques develop within the traumatized skin.

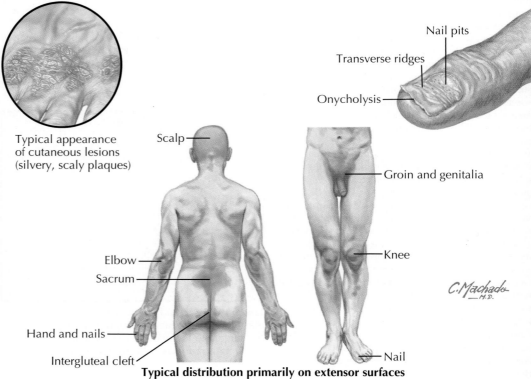

Typical appearance of cutaneous lesions (silvery, scaly plaques)

Nail pits

Transverse ridges

Onycholysis

Scalp

Groin and genitalia

Elbow

Sacrum

Knee

Hand and nails

Intergluteal cleft

Nail

Typical distribution primarily on extensor surfaces

Inverse psoriasis is a well-recognized clinical variant that manifests in intertriginous areas of the groin, gluteal cleft, axillae, and umbilicus. The patches tend not to be as thick as in the other forms, and the scale is fine. This is due to their location in occluded areas, which have an increased amount of moisture and help to keep the scale to a minimum. The patches can be bright red and are often misdiagnosed as a cutaneous

Candida infection. Inverse psoriasis is also symmetric in nature and can present therapeutic challenges.

Guttate psoriasis is a variant of psoriasis that can occur after an infection, most notably a streptococcal bacterial infection. The guttate lesions develop soon after or during the infection and appear as tiny teardrop-shaped patches with fine adherent scale. The word *guttate* means "droplet," and the lesions of guttate

Plate 4-64

Rashes

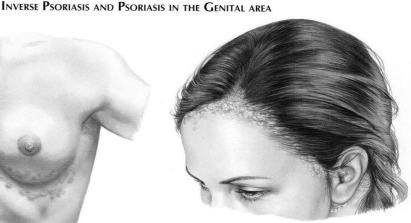

INVERSE PSORIASIS AND PSORIASIS IN THE GENITAL AREA

PSORIASIS (Continued)

psoriasis appear as tiny droplets of psoriatic patches found generalized over the skin, as if areas of psoriasis had developed within sprinkled water droplets. Children with guttate psoriasis may have only one isolated episode after a streptococcal infection and no evidence of psoriasis thereafter. Adults with guttate psoriasis, on the other hand, almost always develop psoriasis vulgaris at some later point.

Scalp psoriasis is a unique variant that occurs only on the scalp. Patients complain of thick, scaly patches that itch and can cause a dramatic amount of seborrhea. Most patients who present with localized scalp psoriasis eventually develop areas of psoriasis elsewhere on their bodies.

Pustular psoriasis is a rare and distinctive form. It can occur in patients with a preexisting history of psoriasis, or it can be the initial presenting morphology. The diagnosis is straightforward in a patient with a long-standing history of psoriasis who develops a pustular flare. The most common reason for this is the rapid withdrawal of systemic corticosteroids, for example, when a patient with psoriasis is prescribed methyl-prednisolone for some unrelated condition, such as allergic contact dermatitis due to poison ivy. The rapid decrease in the dose of the corticosteroid can induce a pustular flare. The patches of psoriases develop pinpoint (1-2 mm) pustules that can coalesce into superficial pools of pus. These patients are often ill appearing and can have associated hypocalcemia. Patients presenting with pustular psoriasis without a preexisting history of psoriasis pose a difficult diagnostic problem at first. The differential diagnosis is among psoriasis, a pustular drug eruption, and Sneddon-Wilkinson disease. A skin biopsy and clinical follow-up will eventually make the diagnosis clear.

Nail psoriasis is most often associated with severe psoriasis vulgaris and psoriatic arthritis. It can occasionally be a solitary finding. Oil spots, onycholysis, nail pitting, and variable amounts of nail thickening can be present. Nail disease is refractory to most topical therapies, and often systemic therapy is required to get a good clinical response. Nail psoriasis is a marker for psoriatic arthritis, and patients with nail psoriasis are at a higher risk for development of psoriatic arthritis.

Palmar and plantar psoriasis is another of the less commonly seen clinical variants. It can manifest on the palms and soles as red, scaly patches and plaques or as patches studded with a variable amount of small pustules. This variant of psoriasis is more commonly found in females, and smoking has been shown to make the clinical course worse.

Psoriatic erythroderma is a rare variant that is seen as a sequela of steroid withdrawal or of other, undefined triggers. It manifests with near-total redness of the skin. The redness is caused by massive vasodilatation of the cutaneous vasculature, which can lead to high-output cardiac failure. These patients are universally treated in the inpatient setting.

Psoriatic arthritis can manifest in association with psoriatic skin disease or as arthritis with nail

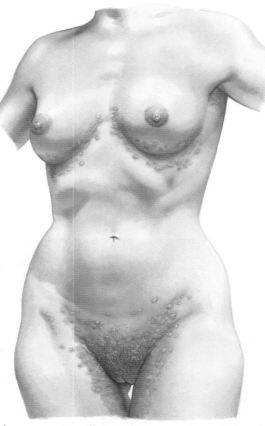

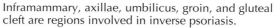

Inframammary, axillae, umbilicus, groin, and gluteal cleft are regions involved in inverse psoriasis.

Thick, adherent, silvery, scaly patches and plaques on scalp

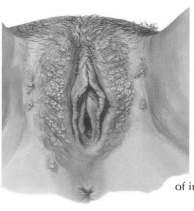

Typical appearance of intertriginous lesion

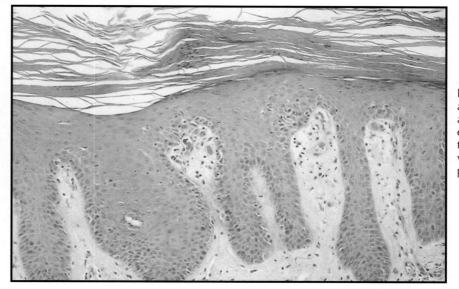

Regularly spaced and shaped acanthosis of the epidermis, with telangiectatic vessels in the papillary dermis

findings. Patients typically present with an asymmetric oligoarticular arthritis, a symmetric polyarticular arthritis, distal interphalangeal–predominant disease, spinal spondylitis, or arthritis mutilans. Arthritis mutilans is the rarest form of psoriatic arthritis, but it is life altering and can lead to a devastating loss of function. Psoriatic arthritis is considered to be a seronegative form of inflammatory arthritis.

Pathogenesis: Psoriasis is an autoimmune disease caused by an abnormality within the cells of the immune system. There is a genetic susceptibility, and the human leukocyte antigen (HLA) Cw6 locus is the most commonly found (but not the only) susceptibility factor in patients who develop psoriasis. The success of therapy with cyclosporine, a medication that dramatically decreases T-cell function, was one of the first

Plate 4-65

Integumentary System

PSORIATIC ARTHRITIS

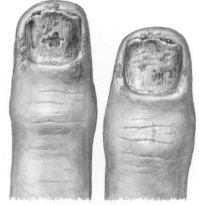

Pitting, discoloration, and erosion of fingernails with fusiform swelling of distal interphalangeal joints

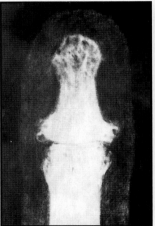
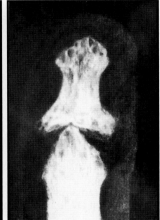

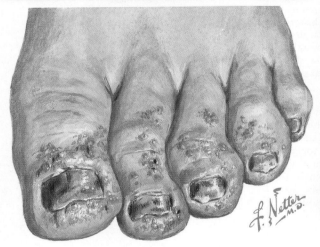

Toes with sausage-like swelling, skin lesions, and nail changes

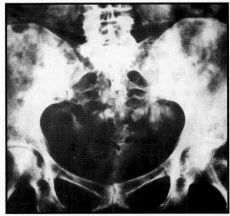

Psoriatic patches on dorsum of hand with swelling and distortion of many interphalangeal joints and shortening of fingers due to loss of bone mass

Radiographic changes in distal interphalangeal joint. *Left,* In early stages, bone erosions are seen at joint margins. *Right,* In late stages, further loss of bone mass produces "pencil point in cup" appearance.

Radiograph of sacroiliac joints shows thin cartilage with irregular surface and condensation of adjacent bone in sacrum and ilia.

PSORIASIS (Continued)

clues to the pathogenesis of psoriasis. Psoriatic patients given this medicine almost always have rapid clinical improvement.

T-cell lymphocytes and dermal dendritic cells are the most likely precursor cells to be the cause of psoriasis; they are both found in increased numbers in psoriatic plaques. CD8+ T cells are the predominant lymphocyte found within the epidermis; they contain the cutaneous lymphocyte antigen (CLA) antigen on their cell surface. The CLA antigen is important because it directs these cells into the skin. Many subsets of dermal dendritic cells have been found within psoriatic plaques. Dendritic cells have been shown to be potent stimulators of T cells, and they are believed to be required to propagate the inflammatory reaction. These two cell types interact with each other and change the local cytokine profile into one that is proinflammatory and provides a milieu that is required for the development of the clinical findings of psoriasis. What is still unknown is the initial stimulus that sets off this cascade of events and how it is propagated and perpetuated.

Histology: Histological examination of biopsy specimens of psoriasis vulgaris show regular psoriasiform hyperplasia of the epidermis. Multiple normal-appearing mitotic figures are seen within keratinocytes. Neutrophils are prominent within the stratum corneum and within the lumen of the papillary dermal blood vessels. Mounds of parakeratosis are seen in the stratum corneum and contain many neutrophils. The papillary dermis shows a proliferation of ectatic capillary vessels with a perivascular infiltrate made up of lymphocytes, Langerhans cells, and histiocytes. Collections of neutrophils within the stratum corneum are called Munro microabscesses. Kogoj microabscesses are similar collections of neutrophils within the stratum spinosum. There is a decrease in the thickness of the granular cell layer. With time, some of the tips of the rete ridges coalesce and form thickened ends.

Pustular psoriasis shows varying amounts of intraepidermal pustules; acanthosis and psoriasiform hyperplasia are not prominent. Again, there are multiple dilated capillary blood vessels in the papillary dermis.

Treatment: There is no cure for psoriasis. Treatment should be based on the amount and location of the psoriatic plaques and consideration of the psychological well-being of the affected individual. Small areas in discrete locations can be treated with topical corticosteroids, anthralin, tar compounds, or vitamin D or A analogues or left alone without therapy. Ultraviolet therapy with natural sunlight, narrow-band ultraviolet B light (UVB), or psoralen + ultraviolet A light (PUVA) has been used with great success. Often, combinations of therapies are implemented.

As the body surface area of involvement increases or the psychological well-being of the individual is affected such that systemic therapy is warranted, many agents are available to treat the psoriasis. Phototherapy with narrow-band UVB or PUVA has been used for decades

with excellent results. In the long term, these therapies increase the patient's risk of developing skin cancers, and lifelong dermatologic follow-up is required.

Oral systemic agents are also used for moderate to severe psoriasis. Methotrexate taken on a weekly basis has been used for years. Oral cyclosporine has been used with great success for erythrodermic and pustular psoriasis. Its use is limited to 6 to 12 months because of nephrotoxicity. Many biological agents have become

available over the last decade. These medications are given by subcutaneous, intramuscular, or intravenous injection. They include etanercept, alefacept, adalimumab, infliximab, and ustekinumab. All of these agents have had excellent response rates. They are all considered to be immunosuppressive, and patients taking these medications need close clinical follow-up, because they are at increased risk for infections and possibly for systemic cancers, such as lymphoma, after years of use.

Plate 4-66

Rashes

RADIATION DERMATITIS

With the ever-increasing use of adjunctive radiotherapy for a plethora of indications in the treatment of cancer, radiation dermatitis has been increasing in incidence. There are acute and chronic forms of radiation dermatitis, and their development is based on the total dose of radiation given. The skin is particularly sensitive to radiation damage, and it responds to the radiation in various ways. In the 1950s, the use of radiation to treat common skin conditions such as acne, tinea, and many common dermatoses was widespread. It was not until a better understanding of the long-term effects of radiation was achieved that this practice was discontinued. Localized or widespread radiotherapy is still used for some skin conditions, but it is most commonly reserved to treat malignancies such as tumor-stage mycosis fungoides or as an adjunctive therapy for melanoma, squamous cell carcinoma, Merkel cell carcinoma, or, uncommonly, unresectable basal cell carcinoma. External-beam radiotherapy can cause other complications depending on the location to which it is applied. Irradiation of the head and neck region often produces xerostomia and mucositis. Dysphagia is also a possibility. If care is not taken to protect the globe, vision alteration or blindness may occur.

The method by which the radiation dose is given (fractionated, hyperfractionated, or accelerated hyperfractionated) is less critical in the development of radiation dermatitis than the total dose or the coexisting use of chemotherapy. Chemotherapy in combination with radiotherapy increases the chance of radiation dermatitis dramatically.

Clinical Findings: Radiation dermatitis can be divided into an acute form and a chronic form. The acute form begins within weeks after the radiation therapy has started. There is a graded scale of acuity from grade I to grade IV. Almost all patients undergoing radiotherapy develop some symptoms of grade I radiation dermatitis. Grade I is defined as a slight erythema of the skin overlying the radiation site associated with xerosis of the skin. Grade II manifests with more inflammatory red patches and edema. Grade III shows evidence of bright erythema, edema, and desquamation of the epidermis. Grade IV, the most severe form of acute radiation dermatitis, manifests as full-thickness skin necrosis, erythema, and ulcerations. This is the least common form of acute radiation dermatitis but the most severe, and it requires immediate management.

Chronic radiation dermatitis is commonly seen many months to years after exposure to radiation. Poikilodermatous skin changes are most prominent, and there is a thickening and hardness to the exposed skin. Poikiloderma manifests as telangiectases, atrophy, and hyperpigmentation and hypopigmentation. Hair loss is common, as is the loss of all appendageal structures such as eccrine glands and apocrine glands. The hair loss is permanent.

Treatment: Therapy for acute radiation dermatitis is grade dependent. There is no acceptable or reliable prophylactic method to prevent radiation dermatitis. Grade I acute dermatitis is treated with moisturizers, and the use of a low-potency cortisone cream can be considered. Grade II or III acute dermatitis should be treated with moisturizing creams such as zinc oxide paste. Strict sun protection is required. Medium-potency corticosteroids may be used, and care should be taken to avoid superinfection. If a cutaneous infection is suspected, culture and use of appropriate antibiotics is required. Grade IV dermatitis requires treatment by a team of wound care specialists adept at treating burns.

Chronic radiation dermatitis, in and of itself, does not require therapy unless the patient experiences severe tightness or hardness of the skin. In anecdotal reports, pentoxifylline has been successful in softening the areas of chronic radiation dermatitis. Topical moisturizers may help with the dryness. The most critical aspect is routine inspection of the area of chronic radiation dermatitis for the development of skin cancers, most commonly basal cell carcinoma and squamous cell carcinoma.

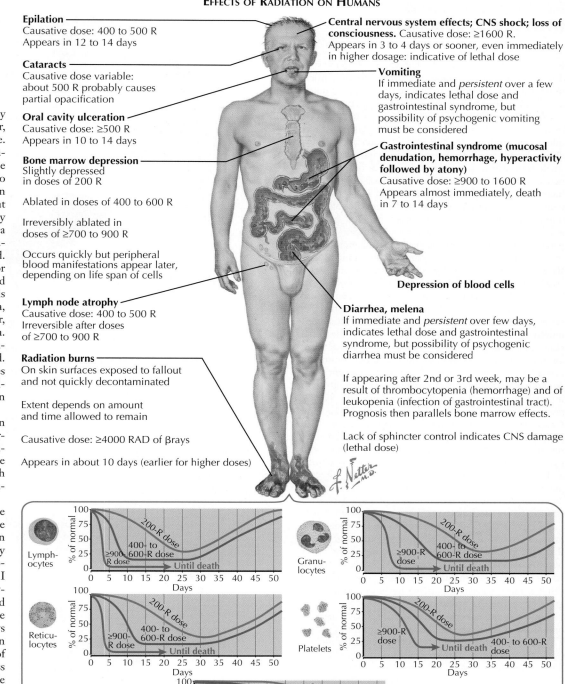

EFFECTS OF RADIATION ON HUMANS

Epilation
Causative dose: 400 to 500 R
Appears in 12 to 14 days

Cataracts
Causative dose variable: about 500 R probably causes partial opacification

Oral cavity ulceration
Causative dose: ≥500 R
Appears in 10 to 14 days

Bone marrow depression
Slightly depressed in doses of 200 R

Ablated in doses of 400 to 600 R

Irreversibly ablated in doses of ≥700 to 900 R

Occurs quickly but peripheral blood manifestations appear later, depending on life span of cells

Lymph node atrophy
Causative dose: 400 to 500 R
Irreversible after doses of ≥700 to 900 R

Radiation burns
On skin surfaces exposed to fallout and not quickly decontaminated

Extent depends on amount and time allowed to remain

Causative dose: ≥4000 RAD of βrays

Appears in about 10 days (earlier for higher doses)

Central nervous system effects; CNS shock; loss of consciousness. Causative dose: ≥1600 R. Appears in 3 to 4 days or sooner, even immediately in higher dosage: indicative of lethal dose

Vomiting
If immediate and *persistent* over a few days, indicates lethal dose and gastrointestinal syndrome, but possibility of psychogenic vomiting must be considered

Gastrointestinal syndrome (mucosal denudation, hemorrhage, hyperactivity followed by atony)
Causative dose: ≥900 to 1600 R
Appears almost immediately, death in 7 to 14 days

Depression of blood cells

Diarrhea, melena
If immediate and *persistent* over few days, indicates lethal dose and gastrointestinal syndrome, but possibility of psychogenic diarrhea must be considered

If appearing after 2nd or 3rd week, may be a result of thrombocytopenia (hemorrhage) and of leukopenia (infection of gastrointestinal tract). Prognosis then parallels bone marrow effects.

Lack of sphincter control indicates CNS damage (lethal dose)

Plate 4-67

Integumentary System

REACTIVE ARTHRITIS (REITER'S SYNDROME)

Reactive arthritis (formerly known as Reiter's syndrome) comprises a unique constellation of clinical findings. The syndrome is believed to be precipitated by an infectious agent, often shigella or chlamydia.

Clinical Findings: Reactive arthritis usually affects men in the third to fifth decades of life. The most frequent skin findings are balanitis circinata and keratoderma blennorrhagica. Balanitis circinata manifests as small psoriasiform, pink-to-red patches on the glans penis. It can appear identical to psoriasis. Keratoderma blennorrhagicum is less common than balanitis circinata. It occurs on the soles and palms, with the soles predominating. Small papulosquamous papules, patches, and plaques occur on the glabrous skin. Small, juicy papules and pustules can be scattered throughout the involved skin; the clinical appearance can mimic psoriasis. Some scholars think that reactive arthritis and psoriasis are one in the same, but other clinical findings of reactive arthritis make the two worthy of differentiation.

The unique clinical hallmarks that separate reactive arthritis from psoriasis are the triad of urethritis, conjunctivitis, and arthritis. Urethritis typically is the initial clinical finding. It often begins a few days to 1 week after an infection. The infective agent that most commonly precipitates this syndrome is *Chlamydia trachomatis*. Gastrointestinal bacterial infections have also been shown to initiate the reaction, including infections with *Shigella flexneri*, *Salmonella* species, *Yersinia enterocolitica*, and *Campylobacter jejuni*. Dysuria, urinary frequency, and pyuria can be the presenting findings. Women with severe urethritis can develop cervicitis, cystitis, and pyelonephritis. Men are prone to development of cystitis and prostatitis. A few days to weeks later, the affected patient develops conjunctivitis and arthritis. The conjunctiva is red and injected with a weeping exudate. Iritis and uveitis are rarely seen manifestations but can occur.

Reactive arthritis is considered to be a seronegative form of arthritis. It is typically polyarticular and affects the large joints such as the knees and hips. The joints become swollen, red, and tender. Movement can be restricted because of pain. Most cases spontaneously resolve, but a subset of patients develop chronic progressive destructive arthritis.

Some patients develop nondescript small, discrete oral ulcers that can appear the same as aphthous ulcers. They can be nontender, and this feature can be helpful in differentiating them from other forms of oral ulcers. These ulcers spontaneously resolve in most cases. Laboratory testing show seronegativity. Testing for both the rheumatoid factor and antinuclear antibodies (ANA) is negative. The sedimentation rate is often extremely elevated. Patients frequently carry the human leukocyte antigen (HLA)-B27 marker. This is a marker that has been found to occur with a higher than expected frequency in patients with ankylosing spondylitis and reactive arthritis. However, most patients who test positive for the HLA-B27 marker never develop either of these conditions. There is no blood test that can make the diagnosis of reactive arthritis. Radiographs can be helpful in assessing joint inflammation and joint destruction. The diagnosis of reactive arthritis is made on clinical grounds. Most patients do not exhibit all of the findings mentioned, and the diagnosis is based on the number of clinical findings and the length of time the patient has had them. The American College of Rheumatology has published complicated criteria to help make the diagnosis.

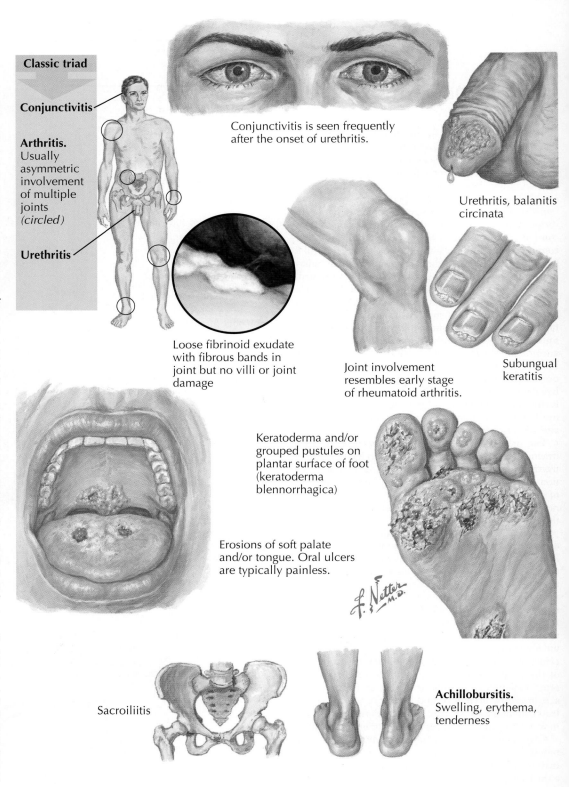

Classic triad

Conjunctivitis

Arthritis. Usually asymmetric involvement of multiple joints *(circled)*

Urethritis

Conjunctivitis is seen frequently after the onset of urethritis.

Urethritis, balanitis circinata

Subungual keratitis

Joint involvement resembles early stage of rheumatoid arthritis.

Loose fibrinoid exudate with fibrous bands in joint but no villi or joint damage

Keratoderma and/or grouped pustules on plantar surface of foot (keratoderma blennorrhagica)

Erosions of soft palate and/or tongue. Oral ulcers are typically painless.

Sacroiliitis

Achillobursitis. Swelling, erythema, tenderness

Pathogenesis: The leading theory is that an infection in a susceptible individual sets off this immunological reaction. HLA-B27 seems to be a marker that is frequently positive in patients with reactive arthritis, but only a small subset of HLA-B27–positive patients develop the disease. The exact pathomechanism is unknown. Possibly, a bacterial antigen causes epitope spreading and initiates the autoimmune reaction.

Histology: The pathological findings are nondiagnostic and appear identical to those of psoriasis. Psoriasiform hyperplasia of the epidermis is prominent, along with neutrophils. Increased numbers of blood vessels are seen in the dermis.

Treatment: Any underlying infection must be sought and appropriately treated with the correct antibiotic therapy. Nonsteroidal antiinflammatory drugs are used to treat the arthritis. An ophthalmologist should be consulted to evaluate the globe. Corticosteroid eye drops are frequently used. Topical steroids can be used to treat the skin manifestations. Many patients experience a spontaneous remission in a few months.

Plate 4-68

Rashes

ROSACEA

Rosacea is an extremely common chronic dermatosis. This inflammatory dermatosis is associated with many triggers or initiating factors that can cause a flare of the inflammatory response. There are various forms, including erythematotelangiectatic, papular pustular, ocular, and phymatous varieties and rosacea fulminans. The erythematotelangiectatic form is the most common. Rosacea fulminans is the least common but by far the most severe form.

Clinical Findings: Rosacea is most often seen in Caucasians, especially those of northern European heritage. There is a slight overall female predominance. The phymatous form occurs almost exclusively in men. The peak age at onset has been estimated to be in the third to fourth decades of life. Most patients start with a subtle redness to their cheeks and nose. The forehead and ears are less commonly affected. Most patients notice a trigger or inciting factor that makes their skin flush. Triggers include alcohol, hot spicy foods, hot liquids (e.g., coffee, tea), and exposure to extremes of temperature. Patients can have any, all, or none of the typical triggers. On exposure to a trigger, patients often experience a warmth to the skin and flushing of the areas involved by rosacea.

The diagnosis is typically straightforward and is made on clinical grounds; however, the differential diagnosis in some cases can include other causes of flushing and lupus erythematosus. The butterfly rash of lupus erythematosus can look very similar, and occasionally a skin biopsy is required to help differentiate the two. This is unusual, because the systemic manifestations of lupus are not seen in rosacea. This scenario is most common when a patient with known lupus erythematous presents with a facial rash and the underlying lupus must be differentiated from co-existing rosacea as the cause.

Other common forms of rosacea are the papular pustular and ocular forms. Patients with the papular pustular form typically start off with the erythematotelangiectatic form and progress to this form over time. Not every case of erthematotelangiectatic rosacea progresses, however. Patients begin to develop crops of inflammatory papules and pustules, predominantly on the nose and cheeks. The forehead and chin can also be involved. The appearance can be hard to differentiate from acne, but these patients typically have triggers, some flushing, and a later age at onset. The back and chest are not involved by rosacea. Patients with ocular rosacea present with conjunctivitis and blepharitis. These are manifested clinically by redness of the conjunctiva and a feeling of "sand" in one's eye. It can be a solitary finding, but it is more commonly seen in conjunction with skin disease.

Phymatous rosacea is caused by massive overgrowth of sebaceous glands with edema and enlargement of the structures affected. This is most common on the nose of men, in which cases it is called rhinophyma. The appearance of the nose can become distorted, leading to a red, edematous, bulbous deformity with accentuated follicular openings.

Rosacea fulminans is a rare variant that can have an acute onset of severe papules, pustules, nodules, and cyst formation.

Pathogenesis: The etiology of rosacea is unknown. Subtypes are most likely a heterogeneous group of similar-appearing disease states.

Histology: The findings on skin biopsy in rosacea depend on the form that is biopsied. The erthematotelangiectatic form typically shows a few dilated blood vessels and dermatoheliosis. A sparse, superficial

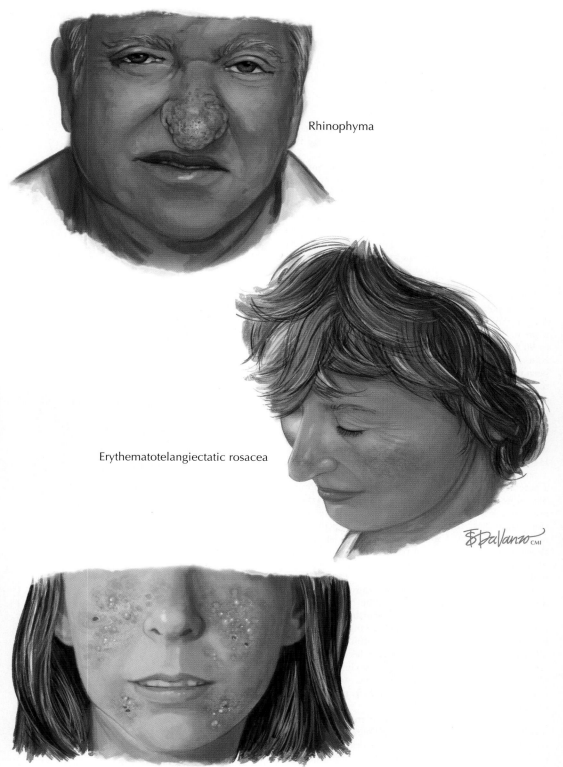

Rhinophyma

Erythematotelangiectatic rosacea

Rosacea Fulminans

lymphocytic infiltrate may surround adnexal structures. Papular rosacea shows perifollicular abscesses. An interesting finding with unknown relevance is that of multiple demodex mites within the hair follicle passage. A granulomatous form of rosacea can be seen histologically.

Treatment: Sun protection and sunscreen use are important for all patients with rosacea, especially the erthematotelangiectatic form. The use of topical and oral antibiotics (e.g., topical metronidazole, sulfacetamide, oral tetracyclines) has long been the mainstay of therapy. Topical azelaic acid has also been helpful. Avoidance of triggers is helpful in some individuals. Use of the 585-nm pulsed dye laser has led to excellent results in treating the underlying redness from telangiectatic blood vessels. Isotretinoin has been used in severe cases, including rosacea fulminans. Rhinophyma is typically treated with a surgical approach to debulk the extra tissue and reshape the nose.

Plate 4-69

Integumentary System

SARCOID

Sarcoid, or sarcoidosis, is a relatively common condition that can affect many organ systems. There is a wide spectrum of disease activity, from localized skin disease to widespread involvement of the integumentary, pulmonary, cardiac, renal, gastrointestinal, ophthalmic, endocrine, neurological, and lymphatic systems. However, most cases are mild in nature and can be controlled with proper care. Although an infectious etiology has often been theorized, no conclusive evidence has been established. This idiopathic condition can produce multiple skin findings. The skin findings should cause the attending physician to look for systemic involvement.

Clinical Findings: Sarcoidosis can occur in any ethnic population, but it is seen at a higher rate in African Americans. It also has a higher incidence in women. The usual age at onset is before 40 years. Up to 90% of patients with sarcoid have a benign clinical course with no increased mortality. Sarcoidosis has been reported to occur in a familial form, which has led researchers to look for specific genetic defects that could explain the disease. However, sarcoid remains an idiopathic multisystem disease. There are many distinct clinical expressions of the disease that are common enough that they have been named, including Löfgren's syndrome, lupus pernio, Darier-Roussy sarcoid, Heerfordt syndrome, and Mikulicz syndrome.

Sarcoid can affect the skin in a multitude of ways. There are both specific and nonspecific skin findings. The most common nonspecific skin finding is erythema nodosum. Erythema nodosum affects the lower anterior extremities. It manifests as tender subcutaneous nodules or plaques. Examination of biopsy specimens shows a nonspecific form of panniculitis. The etiology of erythema nodosum in patients with sarcoid is poorly understood.

The lesions of sarcoid that occur within the integumentary system are quite varied. The most common specific skin lesion is a slightly brownish to red-brown papule, plaque, or nodule with varying amounts of hyperpigmentation. Sarcoid is a mimicker of many other conditions, especially in its skin lesions. Macular lesions, ulcerations, subcutaneous nodules, annular plaques, ichthyosiform erythroderma, and alopecia have all been described as potential presentations of sarcoid.

The extracutaneous organ system most commonly involved is the pulmonary system. There is a relatively straightforward classification that describes the stages of pulmonary sarcoid based on radiographic findings. The higher the radiographic stage, the more severe the disease. Isolated bilateral hilar adenopathy is the most common pulmonary finding, and it is the basis for stage I radiographic disease. These patients are most commonly asymptomatic, and the adenopathy is found on routine radiographic testing. Any findings of pulmonary sarcoid should prompt referral of the affected individual to a pulmonologist for pulmonary function testing.

Löfgren's syndrome is defined by the acute onset of erythema nodosum, almost exclusively in young adult women; it is seen in association with fever, bilateral hilar adenopathy, and uveitis. Other, nonspecific constitutional signs are often present. The

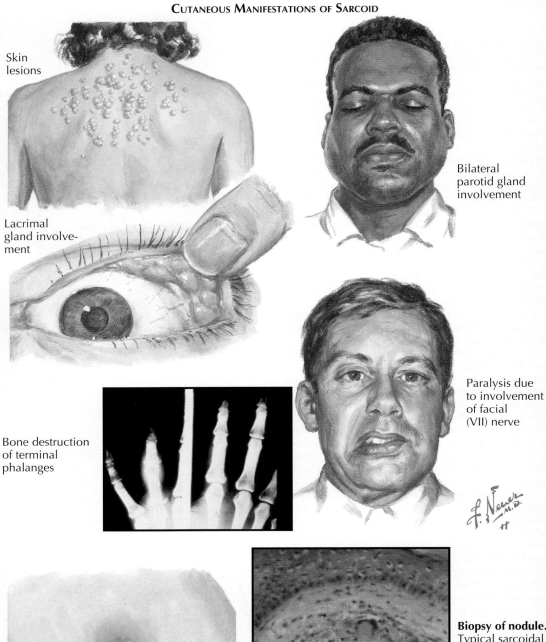

CUTANEOUS MANIFESTATIONS OF SARCOID

Skin lesions

Lacrimal gland involvement

Bilateral parotid gland involvement

Bone destruction of terminal phalanges

Paralysis due to involvement of facial (VII) nerve

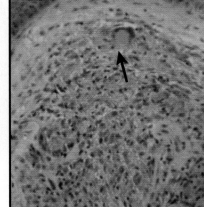

Positive Kveim test. Intracutaneous injection of saline suspension of human sarcoidal spleen or lymph nodes causes appearance of erythematous nodule in 2 to 6 weeks.

Biopsy of nodule. Typical sarcoidal granuloma (dense infiltration with macrophages, epithelioid cells, and occasional multinucleated giant cells [*arrow*])

erythrocyte sedimentation rate is uniformly elevated. For some unknown reason, this syndrome is most commonly seen in young Caucasian women. This form of sarcoidosis typically resolves spontaneously within 2 to 3 years.

Lupus pernio is the name given to the clinical findings of specific cutaneous sarcoid involvement of the

nose and the rest of the face. This form of sarcoid is quite resistant to therapy, runs a more prolonged course, and is often difficult to treat. The skin findings are typically shiny brown-red plaques, papules, and nodules overlying the nose and other regions of the face. The involvement can become so severe as to cause disfigurement of the nose by shiny red-brown papules

Plate 4-70

Rashes

SARCOID (Continued)

and plaques. Lupus pernio has nothing to do with the autoimmune disease lupus. Lupus pernio can be very difficult to treat, and systemic immune suppression is often required.

Subcutaneous sarcoidosis, also called Darier-Roussy sarcoid, is an uncommon condition that manifests as subcutaneous plaques of varying size. This is a rare finding in patients with sarcoid. It manifests as slightly tender, dermal nodules with an overlying hyperpigmentation or normal-appearing skin. A biopsy specimen taken from one of the subcutaneous nodules shows the typical findings of sarcoid.

Heerfordt syndrome is an extremely rare version of sarcoidosis that manifests more commonly in young adult men than in women. It is manifested by fever, parotid gland hypertrophy, and lacrimal gland enlargement in association with facial nerve palsy and uveitis. Neurological involvement with sarcoidosis may cause papilledema and cerebrospinal fluid pleocytosis, indicating an inflammatory reaction pattern. Meningism can occur with headache, spinal stiffness, and photophobia.

Mikulicz syndrome is not specific to sarcoid. It is manifested by bilateral enlargement of various glands, including the parotid, submandibular, and lacrimal glands. The tonsillar tissue may also be involved. Fever is common, as is the subsequent development of dry eyes and mouth due to the widespread, often painless, inflammation of the affected glands. It has been seen with uveitis and is considered by some as a variant of Sjögren's syndrome.

Diagnostic testing to confirm sarcoid includes, most importantly, a tissue biopsy. Tissue sampling is diagnostic and should lead the physician to search for other organ systems involved with sarcoidosis. Laboratory testing may show elevated levels of serum calcium and angiotensin-converting enzyme. Chest radiographs can identify a spectrum of disease that is staged by certain criteria. Patients uniquely show a decreased ability to mount a delayed-type hypersensitivity reaction. This may be manifested by an inability to react to intradermally placed antigens such as tuberculin or candida and is termed *anergy*. Sarcoid patients in the past were frequently found to have a positive Kveim test. This test is no longer clinically performed because of the danger of transmitting a bloodborne pathogen. The test was performed by interdermal placement of a small amount of a suspension of human spleen and lymph node that had been affected by sarcoid, similar to the placement of a purified protein derivative (PPD) test for tuberculosis. This test was found to be positive in more than 85% of patients with sarcoid.

Mortality is uncommon but may occur secondary to severe cardiac, renal, or pulmonary involvement.

Pathogenesis: The exact etiology of sarcoidosis is unknown. For years, scientists have been looking at the potential causative link between sarcoid and an infectious agent, usually an atypical mycobacterial agent. However, no conclusive evidence has been reported to indicate that sarcoid is caused by an infectious disease.

Histology: The classic finding of multiple, noncaseating epithelioid granulomas with a sparse surrounding inflammatory infiltrate is the hallmark of sarcoidosis.

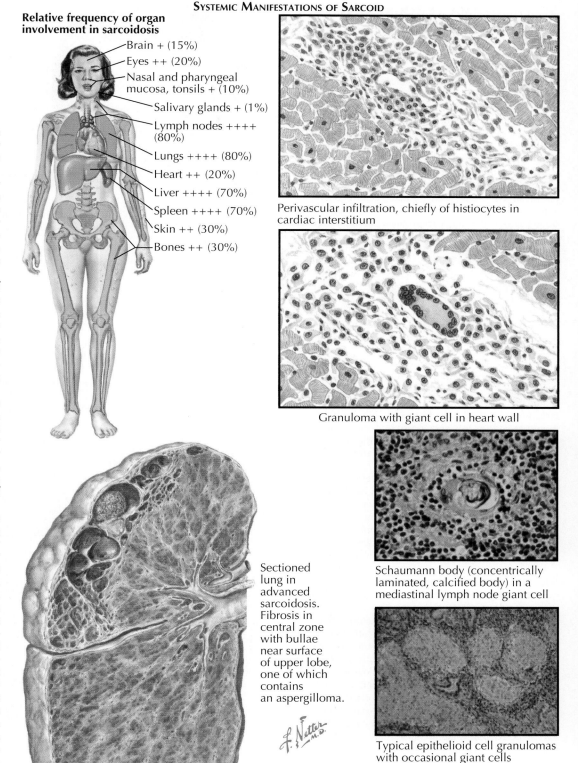

SYSTEMIC MANIFESTATIONS OF SARCOID

Relative frequency of organ involvement in sarcoidosis

Brain + (15%)
Eyes ++ (20%)
Nasal and pharyngeal mucosa, tonsils + (10%)
Salivary glands + (1%)
Lymph nodes ++++ (80%)
Lungs ++++ (80%)
Heart ++ (20%)
Liver ++++ (70%)
Spleen ++++ (70%)
Skin ++ (30%)
Bones ++ (30%)

Perivascular infiltration, chiefly of histiocytes in cardiac interstitium

Granuloma with giant cell in heart wall

Sectioned lung in advanced sarcoidosis. Fibrosis in central zone with bullae near surface of upper lobe, one of which contains an aspergilloma.

Schaumann body (concentrically laminated, calcified body) in a mediastinal lymph node giant cell

Typical epithelioid cell granulomas with occasional giant cells

The granulomatous findings are consistent across all of the various tissues affected by sarcoid. Many nonspecific histological findings can also be seen, but not on a consistent basis; these include Schaumann bodies and asteroid bodies.

Treatment: The treatment for sarcoid has been consistent over time and includes nonspecific immunosuppression, most commonly with oral corticosteroids such as prednisone. Isolated cutaneous findings may be treated with topical corticosteroids or intralesional steroid injections. Methotrexate is a steroid-sparing agent that is used for difficult-to-control disease and for lupus pernio. The anti–tumor necrosis factor medications, infliximab and adalimumab, have been used with some success. The use of hydroxychloroquine has also been advocated for treatment of cutaneous sarcoid.

Plate 4-71

Integumentary System

SCLERODERMA (PROGRESSIVE SYSTEMIC SCLEROSIS)

Scleroderma, or progressive systemic sclerosis, is an idiopathic, life-threatening connective tissue disease that involves many organ systems. There is often an insidious onset of diffuse skin thickening, sclerodactyly, Raynaud's phenomenon, capillary nail fold loops, and tightening of the skin around the orifice of the mouth. As the name implies, this is a progressive disease with significant morbidity and mortality.

Clinical Findings: Progressive systemic sclerosis is an unrelenting connective tissue disease that predominantly affects young adult women. African Americans appear to be slightly more affected than Caucasians. It occurs across all ethnic backgrounds. Skin findings are variable from patient to patient, but all have a persistent and relentless sclerosis of the skin. It begins insidiously, and slowly the skin begins to thicken and harden, causing the underlying dermis to become firm to palpation. The progressive sclerosis causes digital tip ulceration as the peripheral distal blood vessels begin to thrombose. The hair shafts in the affected skin disappear at a slow and steady, almost unnoticeable rate. This is caused by crowding out of the hair follicles by the excessive production of dermal collagen.

As the dermal sclerosis progresses, skin tightness is noticed, and the patient may become aware of difficulty with movement of the fingers. The tightness around the mouth is manifested by an increase in the furrowing circumventing the oral orifice and inability to open the mouth as wide as was once possible. Patients may lose the ability to make facial expressions as the skin tightens and hardens in place. Patients may be left in an expressionless state.

The skin overlying the sclerosis develops hyperpigmentation and hypopigmentation; this has been given the name "salt-and-pepper discoloration." The capillary loops around the nail folds become enlarged and engorged and are visible without magnification. These dilated capillary loops occur in up to three quarters of all patients with progressive systemic sclerosis.

Sclerodactyly is the term given to the progressive thickness and associated tightness of the digits. It is caused by the overabundance of collagen production within the dermis.

Progressive systemic sclerosis is a multisystem disorder that not only affects the skin but also causes significant, life-threatening damage to internal organs. The esophagus is affected early, and patients complain of dysphagia and an inability to swallow food easily. Aspiration of food and liquids is common and often leads to aspiration pneumonia. Pulmonary fibrosis is a leading cause of morbidity and mortality. Patients complain of shortness of breath and a cough. Pulmonary hypertension is almost universally seen. Conduction defects can develop in the cardiovascular system, and thickening of the myocardial wall may cause a constrictive cardiomyopathy. The kidneys are also involved, and a subset of patients develop renal failure and hypertension.

Pathogenesis: The initiating factor that causes the fibroblast to make ever-increasing amounts of collagen in an unregulated manner is unknown. Many possible targets are being explored as potential causes of progressive systemic sclerosis, including fibroblasts, endothelial cells, various environmental antigens, and internal defects within T cells.

Histology: The histological findings in the skin are characteristic. Punch biopsy specimens are very square

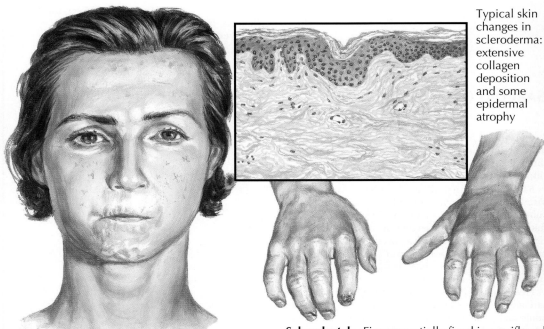

Typical skin changes in scleroderma: extensive collagen deposition and some epidermal atrophy

Characteristics. Thickening, tightening, and rigidity of facial skin, with small, constricted mouth and narrow lips, in atrophic phase of scleroderma

Sclerodactyly. Fingers partially fixed in semiflexed position; terminal phalanges atrophied; fingertips pointed and ulcerated

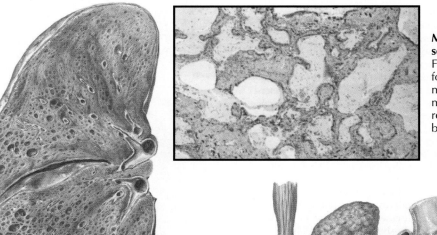

Microscopic section of lung. Fibrosis with formation of microcysts, many of which represent dilated bronchioles.

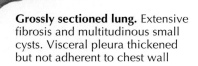

Grossly sectioned lung. Extensive fibrosis and multitudinous small cysts. Visceral pleura thickened but not adherent to chest wall

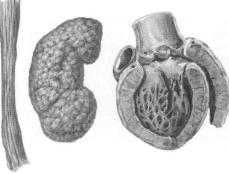

Esophagus, kidneys, heart, skin, and other organs, as well as joints, may also be affected.

on gross evaluation because of the increased amount of dermal collagen. Microscopic evaluation shows an increased amount of collagen that replaces everything including the adnexal structures and subcutaneous fat. The extensive collagen is so vast that it can appear as an amorphous eosinophilic mass with nothing between the collagen bundles. A sparse inflammatory infiltrate is present at the interface of the collagen and underlying remaining tissue. Plasma cells may be prominent.

Treatment: Treatment for this skin disease is difficult. Pruritus can be controlled with antihistamines and topical corticosteroids. Ultraviolet phototherapy has been used. The deeper-penetrating ultraviolet A (UVA) rays work best. This is often administered in the form of psoralen + UVA (PUVA) therapy. Systemic corticosteroids and nonsteroidal immunosuppressant therapy are the main treatment strategies for this disease. Progressive systemic sclerosis requires a multidisciplinary approach to achieve the best therapeutic results.

Plate 4-72

Rashes

SEBORRHEIC DERMATITIS

Seborrheic dermatitis is a commonly encountered rash with a bimodal age distribution. There is an infantile and an adult form. The two forms do not resemble each other clinically and are distinct in appearance. The infantile form has also been named "cradle cap" because of its prominent location on the scalp. The adult form has been found in association with many underlying conditions, although it is most commonly seen as an isolated skin finding.

Clinical Findings: The infantile form of seborrheic dermatitis manifests in the first weeks of life and lasts a few months at most. It affects males and females equally, and there is no racial predilection. The most usual location of involvement is the scalp. Most cases are mild and do not cause the parents to seek the advice of a medical professional. These mild cases manifest with a fine scale that may be slightly greasy or adherent. The child is unaware of the dermatosis, and it resolves spontaneously. Rarely, an infant develops greasy yellow, scaly patches and even plaques across the entire scalp (cradle cap). The dermatitis may become more inflamed, and weeping from the patches or plaques may ensue. The infant may try to scratch at the areas, indicating that pruritus is present. In these severe cases, weeping patches and plaques may also be seen in the groin and axillary folds. Only in the most exceptional of cases does the rash disseminate, but it has the ability to affect any region of the body.

The adult version is chronic in nature and affects a higher percentage of people than does the infantile form. Because of its chronicity, patients often seek medical advice. There is also quite a bit of clinical variability in adult seborrheic dermatitis. The face is the most commonly involved site, with a predilection for the nasolabial fold, eyebrows, ears, and scalp. It has a strikingly similarity to patches in other locations on the skin. Most cases are mild and consist of greasy yellow to slightly red, scaly patches. The scalp involvement is similar in appearance. Seborrheic dermatitis has a propensity to affect the areas of the skin that have a high density of sebaceous glands. On occasion, patients have not only facial involvement but signs of involvement on areas of the upper chest and back.

Many conditions have been associated with the adult form of seborrheic dermatitis, including Parkinson's disease and other chronic neurological disorders. Adult onset of severe seborrheic dermatitis has been reported to occur with a higher incidence in patients with underlying human immunodeficiency virus (HIV) infection. HIV-associated seborrheic dermatitis tends to be widespread, with severe facial involvement. Patients who present with severe seborrheic dermatitis should be assessed for HIV risk factors.

Pathogenesis: The exact pathogenesis is unknown. Seborrheic dermatitis is believed to be caused by an interaction of various components of the skin, including the production of sebum, with the normal skin immune system response to the fungus, *Malassezia furfur*. The role that each of these factors plays in the formation of seborrheic dermatitis is not completely understood.

Histology: Seborrheic dermatitis is almost never biopsied to confirm the diagnosis. Classic biopsy specimens show parakeratosis overlying a slightly spongiotic epidermis with a mild lymphocytic perivascular infiltrate in the dermis. Spores of fungus can be seen lying on the surface of the epidermis.

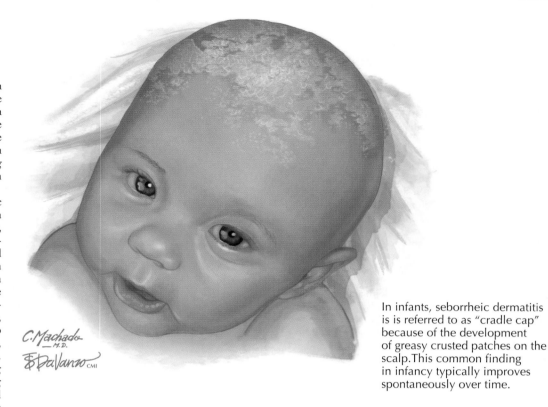

In infants, seborrheic dermatitis is is referred to as "cradle cap" because of the development of greasy crusted patches on the scalp. This common finding in infancy typically improves spontaneously over time.

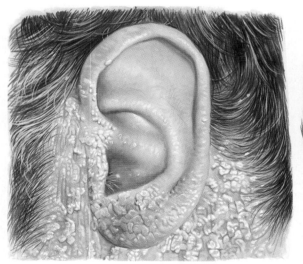

Severe seborrheic dermatitis may be associated with human immunodeficiency virus (HIV) infection.

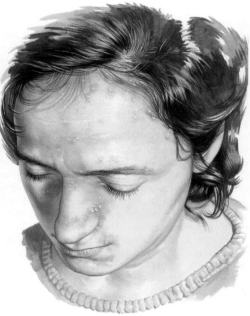

Seborrheic dermatitis in adults frequently manifests with greasy yellow, scaly patches in the scalp, ears, and eyebrows and along the nasolabial fold.

Treatment: Most cases of infantile seborrheic dermatitis can be ignored or treated with nothing more than daily baths and a bland emollient. More involved cases can be treated with more frequent shampooing of the scalp and the use of a mild topical corticosteroid. The use of ketoconazole cream has also been advocated in some cases.

Because of its chronic nature, adult seborrheic dermatitis is treated with topical ketoconazole as a first-line therapy. The other azole antifungal agents are just as effective. The addition of a weak topical corticosteroid used intermittently can also lead to excellent results. The scalp is most commonly treated with a ketoconazole-based shampoo or a tar- or selenium-based shampoo. There is no cure for seborrheic dermatitis, but most therapeutic regimens, if adhered to, lead to an excellent clinical response.

Plate 4-73

Integumentary System

SKIN MANIFESTATIONS OF INFLAMMATORY BOWEL DISEASE

Crohn's disease and ulcerative colitis are two common autoimmune gastrointestinal disorders with many cutaneous findings. Most patients do not have the cutaneous findings, but a small proportion of the population with inflammatory bowel disease develop one of the cutaneous manifestations, which include pyoderma gangrenosum, aphthous ulcerations, oral candidiasis, erythema nodosum, metastatic Crohn's disease, iritis, and conjunctivitis. Arthritis, although not a skin manifestation, can produce red, tender swelling around an afflicted joint space.

Clinical Findings: Ulcerative colitis and Crohn's disease are more commonly seen in the Caucasian population. Crohn's disease is slightly more common in women, and ulcerative colitis affects men and women equally. Up to 20% of individuals with inflammatory bowel disease have a family history of the condition. Ulcerative colitis affects the large intestine, whereas Crohn's disease has been shown to affect any part of the gastrointestinal tract.

Skin manifestations occur in 5% to 10% of those affected by inflammatory bowel disease. The most common skin finding is erythema nodosum. Erythema nodosum manifests as tender dermal nodules predominantly on the shin region. They typically are symmetric in location. There are many associations with erythema nodosum in addition to inflammatory bowel disease, including pregnancy, use of birth control medications, sarcoidosis, deep fungal infections such as coccidiomycosis, and an idiopathic form. The etiology and pathogenesis are unknown. Erythema nodosum can occur in areas other than the pretibial region, but this is uncommon.

Pyoderma gangrenosum is one of the most severe skin manifestations of inflammatory bowel disease. It can manifest as a small, red papule or pustule that can rapidly expand to form a large ulceration with a violaceous undermined rim. The ulcer may form in a cribriform pattern. The skin involved develops small cribriform ulcerations centrally that expand outward and coalesce into one large ulcer. These ulcers are extremely tender and cause significant morbidity. Pyoderma gangrenosum can also be seen as an idiopathic finding or in association with an underlying malignancy, typically in the lymphoproliferative group of malignancies. It has been estimated that approximately 1% of patients with inflammatory bowel disease will develop pyoderma gangrenosum.

Aphthous ulcers can occur anywhere within the oral mucosa. They are shallow ulcerations with a white fibrinous base. They are quite tender and can cause patients to avoid eating because of the severe discomfort. Oral candidiasis is typically an iatrogenic manifestation of inflammatory bowel disease. Most patients are prescribed systemic steroids to treat their underlying disease, and this predisposes them to the development of *Candida* infections, both oral and vaginal.

Arthritis is seen in approximately 10% of patients with inflammatory bowel disease and is considered to be in the seronegative classification of inflammatory arthropathies.

Metastatic Crohn's disease is unique to Crohn's. It represents the spread of the granulomatous disease onto the skin. It most commonly occurs in areas with close approximation to the gastrointestinal tract, such as the perianal and perioral regions. It manifests as tender,

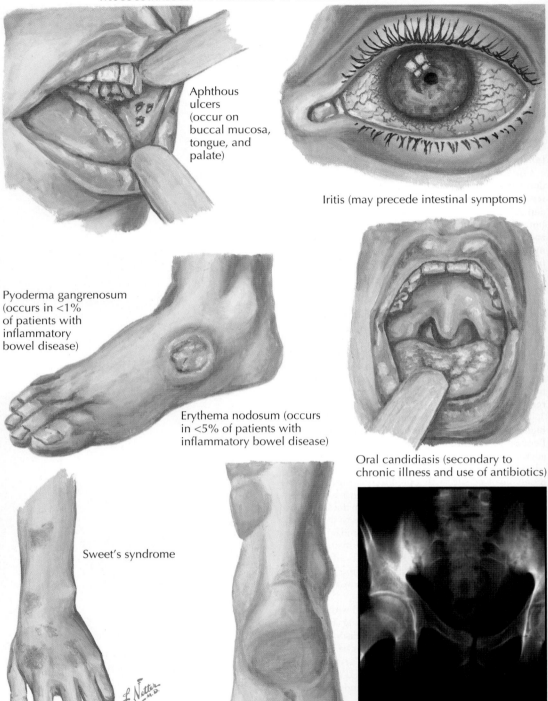

MUCOCUTANEOUS MANIFESTATIONS OF INFLAMMATORY BOWEL DISEASE

Aphthous ulcers (occur on buccal mucosa, tongue, and palate)

Iritis (may precede intestinal symptoms)

Pyoderma gangrenosum (occurs in <1% of patients with inflammatory bowel disease)

Erythema nodosum (occurs in <5% of patients with inflammatory bowel disease)

Oral candidiasis (secondary to chronic illness and use of antibiotics)

Sweet's syndrome

JOHN A. CRAIG—AD

Arthritis (occurs in <10% of patients with inflammatory bowel disease)

draining papules and nodules. A peculiar variant has been described to occur along the inguinal creases. It appears as fissures or ulcerations that can penetrate deeply into the dermis and even the subcutaneous fat tissue. It has been described as slit-like or knife-like linear ulcerations. Isolated genital swelling is another unusual presentation of metastatic Crohn's disease. Metastatic Crohn's disease has been described in many other cutaneous locations. This form of cutaneous disease can be difficult to treat.

Other rare skin findings that have been seen in association with inflammatory bowel disease are skin fistulas, vasculitis including polyarteritis nodosa, urticaria, Sweet's syndrome, epidermolysis bullosa acquisita, and psoriasis.

Pathogenesis: The pathogenesis of these cutaneous manifestations of inflammatory bowel disease is unknown. They are theorized to be caused by an autoimmune mechanism of defective cell-mediated immunity. Metastatic Crohn's disease is believed to be caused

Plate 4-74

Rashes

SKIN MANIFESTATIONS OF INFLAMMATORY BOWEL DISEASE (Continued)

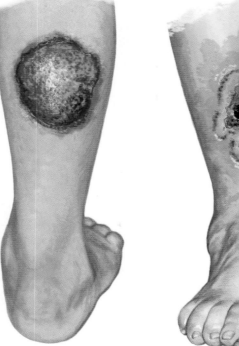

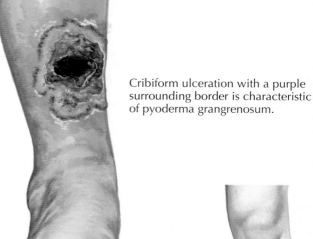

Cribiform ulceration with a purple surrounding border is characteristic of pyoderma grangrenosum.

when the inflammatory bowel disease recognizes the skin as gut tissue and develops the same granulomatous process within the cutaneous structures.

Histology: Pyoderma gangrenosum shows non-specific ulceration when biopsied. The findings are nondiagnostic, and the diagnosis is one of exclusion. The presence of multiple neutrophils leads one to look for cutaneous infection, and appropriate tissue cultures should be performed and found negative before a diagnosis of pyoderma gangrenosum is made. The appearance of pyoderma gangrenosum histologically is highly dependent on the time and type of lesion biopsied. Early lesions show a follicle-centered neutrophilic infiltrate with a dermal abscess. As the lesions progress, ulceration is seen with a predominant neutrophilic infiltrate. The ulcers are often very deep and enter the subcutaneous tissue. Changes of vasculitis can often be seen, but they are believed to be caused by the overlying ulceration; the vasculitis is not thought to be the predominant pathological process.

Biopsy specimens of erythema nodosum shows a septal panniculitis. The fibrous septa are inflamed with a mixed inflammatory infiltrate with heavy lymphocyte predominance. Giant cells are frequently seen within the widened septal tissue. A unique finding is that of Miescher's radial granuloma formation, in which multiple histiocytes are arranged flanking a small area. They are organized circumferentially around a central slit-like space. The reason for this finding is unknown. Erythema nodosum is the most common form of septal panniculitis.

Aphthous ulcerations, if biopsied, show small ulcerations or erosions of the mucosa. The predominant cell type found within the infiltrate is the neutrophil. These findings are nonspecific.

Oral candidiasis should be diagnosed without a skin biopsy. A scraping of the white oral plaques shows an easily removed, whitish, sticky tissue. A microscopic examination shows candidal elements. Examination of the biopsy specimen shows the candidal organisms on the surface of the mucosa, with an underlying mixed inflammatory infiltrate.

Metastatic Crohn's disease is a unique phenomenon. It is histologically described as noncaseating granulomas. These granulomas are identical to the bowel granulomas. The skin granulomas are centered in the dermis but can be seen around blood vessels and into the adipose tissue.

Treatment: Therapy is aimed at controlling the underlying bowel disease. If it is well controlled, the skin manifestations typically follow in line. Conversely, if the bowel disease is poorly controlled, one can expect the skin disease to be poorly controlled as well. It is useful to use the skin manifestations as a sign of active bowel disease. If a patient who has been in a long remission suddenly develops pyoderma gangrenosum, it is highly plausible that the bowel disease has become active once more. Ulcerative colitis can be cured by colectomy. Crohn's disease cannot be cured by colectomy because it affects the entire gastrointestinal tract. Oral or intravenous immunosuppressive medications are used to treat both these conditions. Oral prednisone, sulfasalazine, azathioprine, methotrexate, mycophenolate mofetil, and intravenous infliximab have shown excellent results in patients with these chronic diseases. They also have the added benefit of helping

Older lesion of pyoderma gangrenosum with granulation tissue present. The rolled borders are not as prominent as in acute lesions.

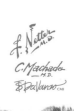

Erythema nodosum manifesting as tender dermal nodules

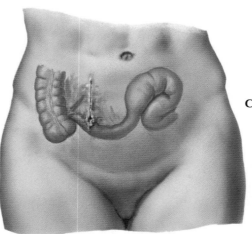

External fistula (via appendectomy incision)

Crohn's disease

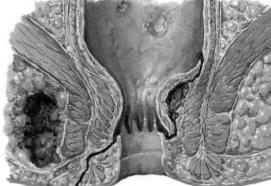

Perianal fistulae and/or abscesses

the skin disease. Cyclosporine and prednisone have shown excellent results in treating pyoderma gangrenosum. Intralesional triamcinolone can be attempted on small, early lesions of pyoderma gangrenosum.

Oral aphthous ulcers can be treated with topically applied steroid gels or ointments compounded in dental paste formula to increase adherence to the mucosa. Topical anesthetics are commonly used.

Erythema nodosum can be treated with compression stockings, topical potent steroids, and oral steroids in severe cases. Intralesional injection of triamcinolone is also effective. Metastatic Crohn's disease is difficult to treat and requires systemic immunosuppressive agents such as azathioprine, prednisone, or infliximab. It is best treated by a multidisciplinary approach.

Plate 4-75

Integumentary System

STASIS DERMATITIS

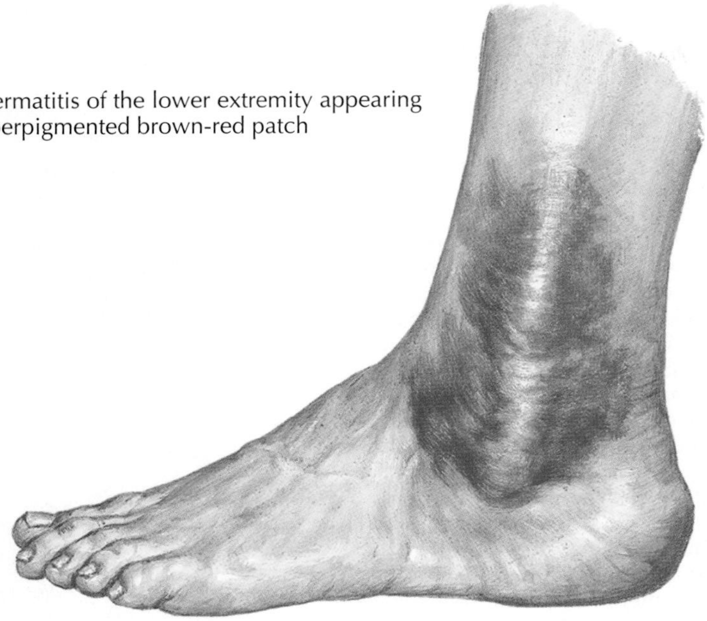

Stasis dermatitis is a common chronic dermatosis that is seen almost exclusively on the lower extremities. The inflammation can lead to chronic discoloration, ulceration, and infection. Underlying systemic disease such as congestive heart failure and renal failure can predispose to stasis dermatitis. Any condition that can cause edema of the lower extremities has the potential to cause stasis dermatitis.

Clinical Findings: Stasis dermatitis is a chronic inflammatory skin disease that indicates underlying insufficiency of the venous return system. It is most commonly seen in the older population, and there is no gender or racial predilection. Most often, congestive heart failure is the associated disease causing the edema. Many other conditions of venous insufficiency can also be causative, including varicose veins and postsurgical complications, such as after a saphenous vein harvest for coronary artery bypass surgery or an inguinal lymph node dissection.

Stasis dermatitis is a skin manifestation of a wide range of underlying venous diseases. The lower extremities account for more than 99% of cases of stasis dermatitis, and the diagnosis in other areas of the body should be questioned. The legs tend to have a range of edema, from the very mild amount that accumulates at the end of a long day of standing to severe chronic edema that is always present. Red-brown patches, some with a light yellow discoloration, typically begin around the medial malleolus. As the condition progresses, the patches begin to spread and can encompass the entire lower extremity, although much more commonly they are found at knee level or just below knee level. There can be complete confluence of the dermatitis around the affected limb, or it can affect only part of the leg.

The rash is almost always symmetric, and it is not uncommonly misdiagnosed as bilateral lower extremity cellulitis. The rash is typically pruritic, and the itching can be so severe as to cause excoriations and small ulcerations. Depending on the severity, weeping vesicular patches and plaques can form. A rare bulla can also be seen in some cases, and one must consider bullous pemphigoid in the differential diagnosis. Varicose veins are often present on examination, or there may be a history of bypass surgery. If left untreated, venous stasis can lead to venous ulcerations, which have been described as slightly painful ulcerations on the lateral malleolus. The ulcerations can occur anywhere on the leg and in some cases are very tender. Peripheral pulses are intact, and this physical examination finding helps to rule out arterial insufficiency. If the ulcerations and edema are not controlled, the ulcerations will continue to expand and can become secondarily infected; if they become deep enough, they can lead to underlying osteomyelitis or cellulitis. These neglected cases can end in loss of the affected portion of the limb if medical therapies do not successfully clear the infection and ulcerations.

Pathogenesis: Increased pressure within the venous system of the lower extremity causes extravasation of serum and blood into the surrounding dermis and subcutaneous tissue. As the edema in the lower extremity worsens, the skin begins to develop signs of chronic inflammation mediated by the abnormal location of fluid.

Histology: Biopsies are not routinely performed in stasis dermatitis, and the diagnosis is almost always

Stasis dermatitis of the lower extremity appearing as a hyperpigmented brown-red patch

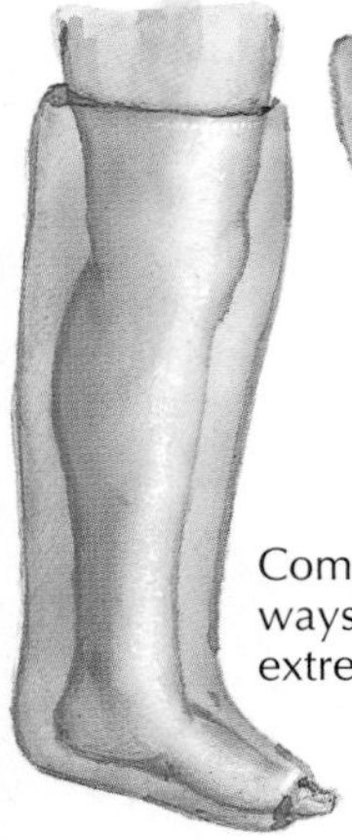

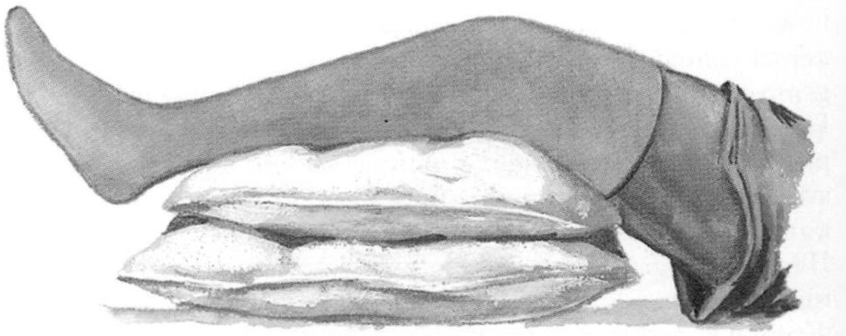

Compression dressings or stockings are one of the best ways to keep fluid from accumulating in the lower extremities. Leg elevation is a mainstay of therapy.

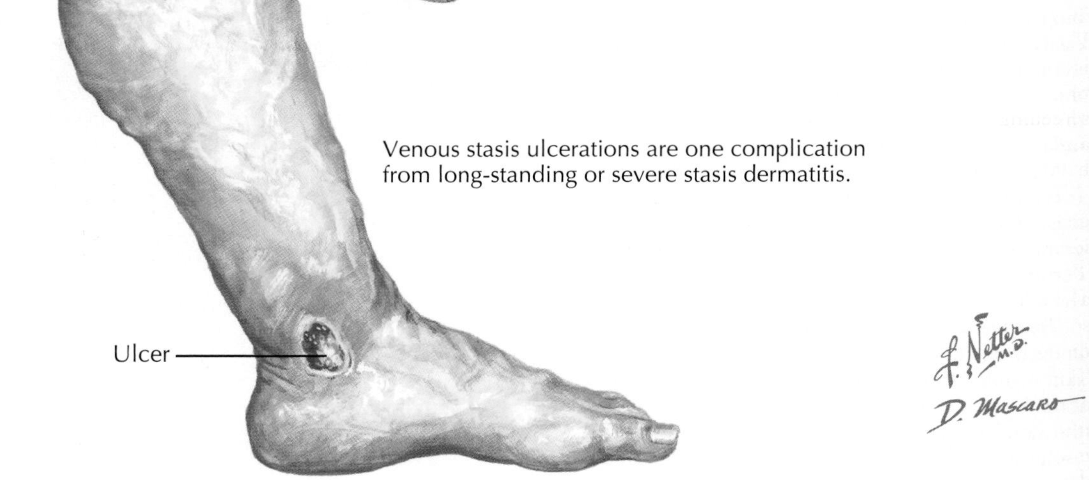

Venous stasis ulcerations are one complication from long-standing or severe stasis dermatitis.

Ulcer

made clinically. Histological examination shows an increase in small vessels, extravasation of red blood cells, and hemosiderin deposition in the dermis. The epidermis shows varying amounts of spongiotic dermatitis.

Treatment: The rash can be treated symptomatically with topical corticosteroids and emollients. The main goal of therapy is to restore the proper venous flow.

Depending on the underlying reason for the stasis dermatitis, this may or may not be possible. If it is not possible, the mainstay of therapy is the use of compression stockings or wraps. However, the compliance rate is low because of difficulty putting them on and discomfort. Those patients who are able to use the compression gear and topical corticosteroids usually have a good prognosis.

Plate 4-76

Rashes

URTICARIA

Urticaria is a commonly encountered skin condition with a multitude of causes. There are primary and secondary forms of urticaria. Most secondary causes are acute in nature and can be explained by an underlying disease state, medication, or food. Urticaria can be a manifestation of many disease states, such as Muckle-Wells syndrome. Urticaria can also be a secondary sequela of an underlying malignancy, acute or chronic infection, genetic disease, and rheumatologic disease. It can also be seen as an acute reaction in a patient with anaphylaxis.

Primary urticaria can be divided into subsets of disease. The most common type is chronic idiopathic urticaria. Other forms of primary urticaria include the physical urticarias. There are many forms of physical urticaria, and the astute clinician can perform provocative testing to determine the type. There is no known cure for urticaria, but most cases of primary urticaria spontaneously resolve within 2 to 3 years.

Clinical Findings: Primary idiopathic urticaria is one of the most frequently encountered forms of urticaria. If no underlying cause is found and the urticaria lasts longer than 6 weeks, it is given the designation *chronic idiopathic urticaria*. This form of urticaria comes and goes at will with no provocative or remitting factors. Lesions appear as evanescent, pink to red, edematous plaques or hives. They can occur anywhere on the body and can cause much distress to the patient because of their appearance and because of the severe pruritus. Patients are particularly distressed when the hives affect the face and eyelids, causing periorbital and periocular swelling. Patients with chronic urticaria usually undergo a battery of laboratory and allergy tests. A complete blood count, metabolic panel, chest radiograph, and measurements of thyroid-stimulating hormone and antithyroid should be performed, as well as testing for various infectious diseases if the medical history warrants. Testing for hepatitis B, hepatitis C, and HIV infection can be done in the appropriate clinical setting. Patients with a travel history often undergo stool examinations for ova and parasites. A full physical examination is warranted, together with age-appropriate cancer screening. Most patients with chronic urticaria have no appreciable cause for their hives and are diagnosed as having chronic idiopathic urticaria.

The physical urticarias are a group of conditions that cause hives; they represent a unique form of chronic idiopathic urticaria in that there is a precipitating factor. There are many types of physical urticaria, including aquagenic and cholinergic forms and cold-, pressure-, solar-, and vibratory-induced urticaria. These forms are diagnosed based on the results of provocative testing. The clinical history often leads to the diagnosis and the appropriate testing regimen. As an example, a patient may develop hives only under tight-fitting socks. This is typical for pressure-induced urticaria. If the patient develops hives on appropriate provocative testing, the diagnosis is made.

Pathogenesis: The pathogenesis of urticaria is poorly understood. Mast cells play a critical role. A stimulus causes mast cells to release histamine, which acts on the local vasculature to increase vascular permeability. The increased permeability causes localized swelling. Some forms of urticaria, such as those seen in anaphylaxis, are caused by a type I hypersensitivity reaction. Other forms of secondary urticaria may be caused by specific immunoglobulin E (IgE) antibodies that interact with mast cells.

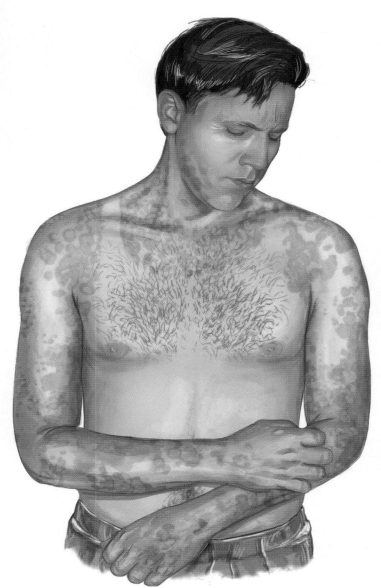

Solar Urticaria: Note the areas affected are those only exposed to the sun in this sleeveless shirt wearing man.

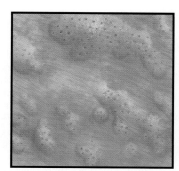

Urticaria: Pink edematous plaques with follicular accentuation caused by the dermal edema.

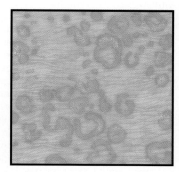

Annular and serpiginous urticaria: This is a less commonly seen variant of urticaria.

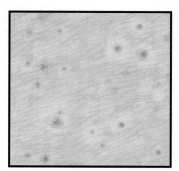

Cholinergic urticaria: This form of urticaria can be induced by increasing the body temperature through exercise or submersion in a warm bath.

Many medications have been shown to cause mast cell degranulation without an IgE-mediated pathway. The most common of these are the opiates and anesthetic agents. Chemical transmitters other than histamine also play a role in urticaria; they include the leukotrienes, serotonin, and various kinins.

Histology: The histological findings in urticaria are bland. The specimen typically shows a superficial perivascular lymphocytic infiltrate with some dermal edema. The epidermis is normal.

Treatment: Treatment of chronic idiopathic urticaria is based on symptom relief. Antihistamines are the first-line therapy and can be used in combination. The lack of response can be frustrating for both patient and physician. Physical urticarias are treated in the same manner, with emphasis on avoidance. Patients who can avoid exposure to the physical stimulus responsible for the urticaria have been shown to have a better clinical outcome.

Plate 4-77

Integumentary System

VITILIGO

Vitiligo is a common acquired skin disease with multiple clinical variants. Vitiligo occurs because of loss of function or complete loss of melanocytes within the epidermis and follicular epithelium. There are many theories as to its development, but it is believed to be an autoimmune skin disease. Vitiligo may be seen in association with other autoimmune conditions. Patients afflicted with vitiligo can be psychologically affected by the disease.

Clinical Findings: Approximately 1% of the population is affected by vitiligo. It has been reported to occur at any age, but it is most common in the teenage years and the early twenties. There is no sex or racial predilection. A small percentage of cases are familial in nature. The exact inheritance pattern and the reason for this configuration are unknown. Many clinical variants of vitiligo exist. All forms have varying degrees of involvement of the skin. When melanin is no longer produced, patients are left with depigmented macules. These macules appear as stark white areas of skin, which can be a few millimeters to many centimeters in diameter. The areas of involvement have a well-defined border region. Hair within the areas of depigmented skin may also be depigmented. With time, the loss of pigment in the hair becomes more prominent. Hair depigmentation within the regions of vitiligo is not universal, and normal-appearing pigmented hair may grow within such an area. Most commonly, no inflammation is seen, and the areas are completely asymptomatic in nature.

Patients with Fitzpatrick type I skin are less obviously affected than those with Fitzpatrick type VI skin. The areas of vitiligo will not tan after sun exposure. Sun exposure typically makes the difference between affected and nonaffected skin more noticeable, because it increases melanin production in the unaffected skin, resulting in a darkening or tanning of the skin around the vitiliginous region. The areas of vitiligo are prone to easy burning and must be protected.

Various clinical variants or classifications of vitiligo exist, including localized, generalized, linear, trichrome, and blaschkoid variants. The generalized form can cause near-universal involvement of the skin, with a only few tiny islands of normal-appearing skin remaining within the areas of vitiliginous skin. Linear areas of involvement are rare and typically affect a limb. Blaschkoid vitiligo follows the embryological Blaschko lines.

Histology: There is no inflammation, and hematoxylin and eosin staining of the biopsy specimen may appear normal unless compared with a biopsy specimen from unaffected skin. When this is done, the lack of melanin production and melanocytes is appreciated. Special staining to accentuate melanocytes can make them much more visible.

Pathogenesis: The exact cause of vitiligo has yet to be determined. The leading theory on its development is the autoimmune theory. An unknown trigger causes the immune system to begin destroying melanocytes. The immune system recognizes melanocytes as somehow abnormal and causes their destruction. The autoimmune theory also may explain why vitiligo is seen clustered with diabetes, thyroid disease, and other autoimmune conditions.

Treatment: Patients with vitiligo should be screened for underlying autoimmune conditions such as diabetes and thyroid disease. The treatment of these conditions has not been shown to help the vitiligo. No therapy is needed. For those patients who seek treatment, many therapies are available, mostly on an anecdotal basis. Potent topical corticosteroids and topical

Vitiligo affecting both skin and hair

Localized burning within the areas of vitiligo secondary to phototherapy is a potential side effect

Symmetric vitiligo

Various clinical presentations of vitiligo

immunomodulators such as tacrolimus and pimecrolimus have been used. Phototherapy with narrowband ultraviolet B light (UVB) and with psoralen + ultraviolet A light (PUVA) has been used successfully. The risk of burning is very high in the affected regions, and care should be used when starting this treatment. Small areas have been treated successfully with surgical techniques involving autotransplantation of skin from unaffected regions. If the therapy works, melanocyte rejuvenation typically occurs in a speckled pattern

centered on the hair follicles. The hair follicle is believed to be a reservoir of melanocytes for repopulation of areas that are devoid of their normal complement of melanocytes.

Rarely, complete depigmentation is undertaken, for those who are so severely affected that only a few islands of normal-appearing skin remain, to allow for a uniform skin tone. Monobenzylether of hydroquinone is used to eliminate any remaining melanocytes and depigment the skin.

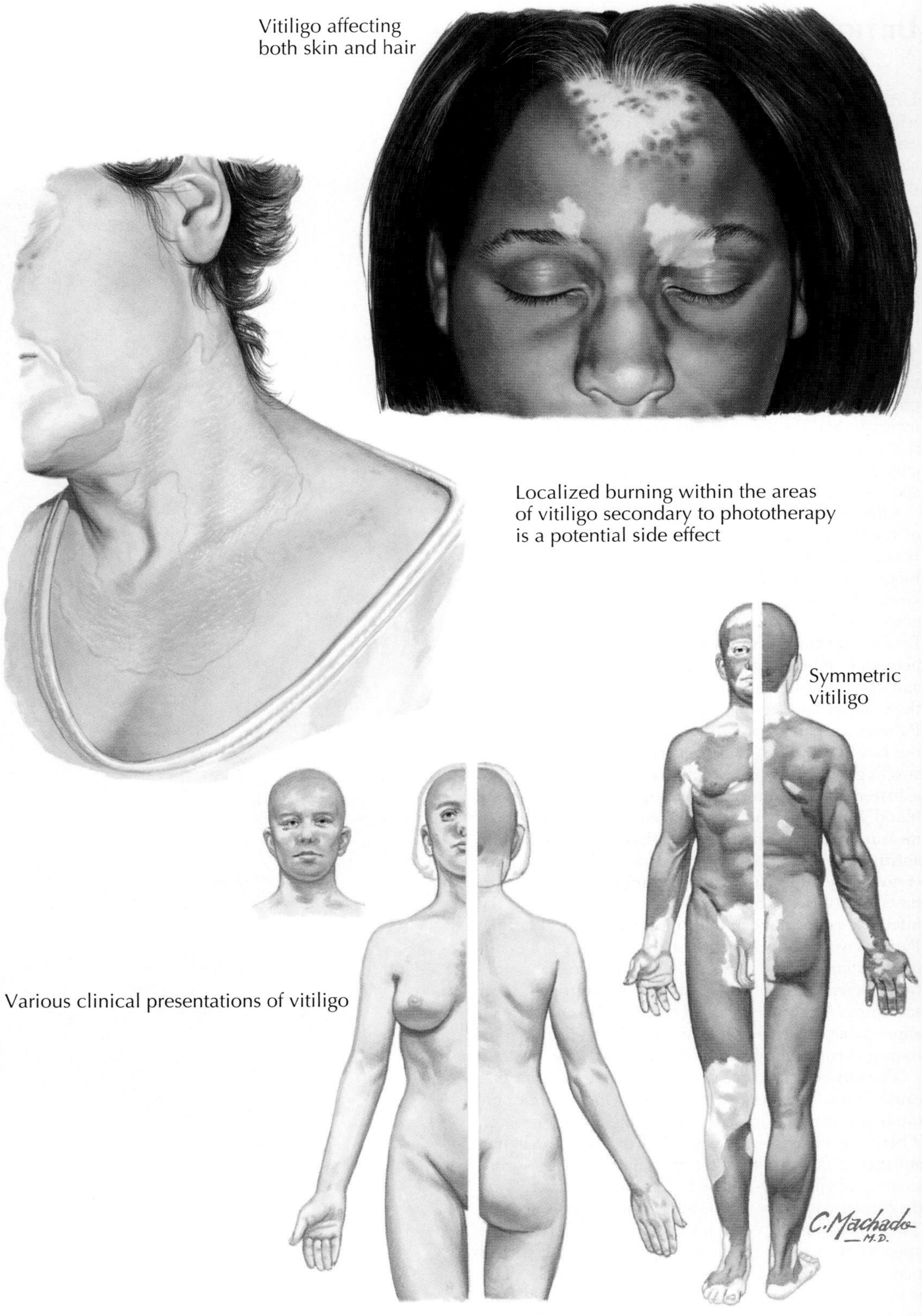

AUTOIMMUNE BLISTERING DISEASES

Plate 5-1

Integumentary System

BASEMENT MEMBRANE ZONE AND HEMIDESMOSOME

Basement membrane zone

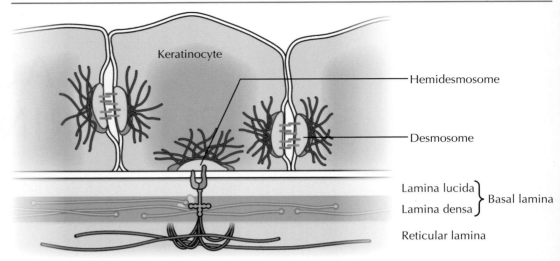

BASEMENT MEMBRANE ZONE, HEMIDESMOSOME, AND DESMOSOME

BASEMENT MEMBRANE ZONE

The basement membrane zone (BMZ) of the epidermis is a beautiful and complex structure and a marvel of biological engineering. The zone acts to attach the overlying epidermis to the underlying stromal tissue, in this case the papillary dermis, which is made predominantly of collagen bundles. A plethora of unique and specialized proteins play critical roles in the proper functioning of the BMZ. Any defect or abnormal antibody that can cause disruption of the normal architecture can result in fracturing of the BMZ and blister formation.

The BMZ can be appreciated on routine hematoxylin and eosin (H&E) staining as an eosinophilic band below the basilar keratinocytes. The components of the BMZ are produced in two locations: the epidermal keratinocyte and the dermal fibroblast. These cells act to produce the required proteins in the correct ratio to maintain a functional basement membrane. The basement membrane's most important function is to keep the epidermis firmly attached to the underlying dermis. This is necessary for life. This specialized structure also acts to encourage migration of cells and repair of the epidermal-dermal barrier after trauma. Many other critical processes and physiological roles depend on the proper functioning of the BMZ, including permeability of water and other chemical substrates, proteins, and cellular elements. The BMZ is a highly organized structure that is consistent from person to person.

The structure of the BMZ can be subdivided into individual compartments for study, with the understanding that the entire unit functions as one. These are the epidermal basilar cell cytoskeleton, hemidesmosome, lamina lucida, lamina densa, and sublamina papillary dermis. Each of these components is made up of unique proteins that act in harmony to preserve the functional role of the BMZ. The basilar keratinocytes contain intracellular cytoskeleton components made of keratin intermediate filaments, predominantly keratin 5 and keratin 14. The keratin intermediate filaments are interwoven into the hemidesmosomal plaque to firmly adhere the basilar cell to the hemidesmosome.

The keratin intermediate filaments interact with bullous pemphigoid antigen 1 (BP230) and plectin. These two proteins are the main components of the hemidesmosomal plaque. Plectin and BP230 are bound tightly together. Plectin and bullous pemphigoid antibody 1 also bind to the integrin class of proteins and to bullous pemphigoid antigen 2 (BP180). Integrins and BP180 are transcellular proteins that bind to the intracellular molecules, plectin and BP230; they also extend out from the basilar keratinocyte and interact with the laminin 5 and collagen IV molecules in the lamina lucida and lamina densa.

The lamina lucida is so named because of its translucent appearance on electron microscopy. In comparison, the lamina densa is an electron-dense region that lies just below the lamina lucida. The lamina lucida is

Hemidesmosome

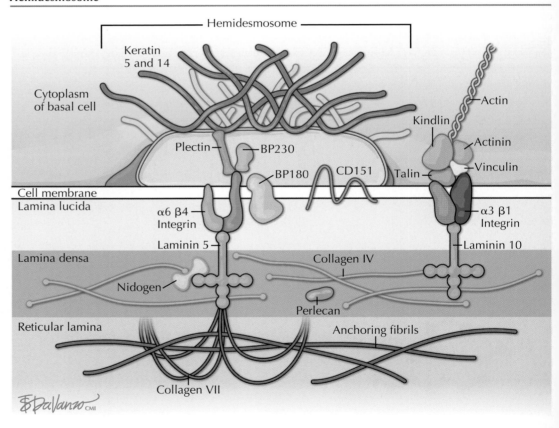

composed of the transversing parts of the integrin and BP180 proteins. These two molecules attach to the laminin class of proteins in the lamina densa. The lamina lucida is considered to be the weakest part of the BMZ, and it is the blister plane in suction blisters, junctional epidermolysis bullosa, and salt-split skin. The lamina densa is composed of a latticework of type IV collagen. Type IV collagen is found only in the

lamina densa. It is unique in that it retains its globular regions on either end. These form attachments to other type IV collagen molecules to create the lattice. Collagen type IV binds strongly to a dumbbell-shaped protein named *nidogen*. This nidogen protein is critical in attaching the laminin proteins in the lamina densa. Nidogen locks the type IV collagen to the laminins, which are bound to the overlying integrin and BP180.

Plate 5-2

Autoimmune Blistering Diseases

BASEMENT MEMBRANE ZONE, HEMIDESMOSOME, AND DESMOSOME (Continued)

The laminin proteins appear as inverted crosses and serve to attach the aforementioned proteins to the papillary dermis that underlies the lamina densa by interacting with type VII collagen. Type VII collagen, which is made up of three identical alpha chains, is also known as the anchoring fibril. These fibrils interweave among the type I and type II collagens of the papillary dermis and attach either end to the laminin proteins in the lamina densa, thus firmly anchoring the entire overlying epidermis and BMZ to the papillary dermal collagen.

Many blistering diseases are caused by genetic abnormalities in the BMZ proteins; these are classified as the epidermolysis bullosa group of blistering diseases. Each of these diseases is unique due to different protein defects that lead to the various phenotypes. Autoimmune blistering diseases of the pemphigoid class target the BMZ and its components, including the hemidesmosome. Autoimmune diseases in the pemphigus class of diseases target the desmosome.

HEMIDESMOSOME

The hemidesmosome is one of the main components of the BMZ. Its purpose is to attach the basilar layer keratinocytes to the underlying stroma—that is, the papillary dermis. The hemidesmosome is made up of many unique and highly integrated groups of protein-to-protein connections. The main proteins in the hemidesmosomal plaque are the bullous pemphigoid antigens BP180 and BP230, integrin, plectin, and laminin. Their interactions and how they connect the keratinocyte cytoskeleton to the underlying collagen have already been described. Antibodies directed against the components of the hemidesmosome can be seen in the pemphigoid group of disease states.

DESMOSOME

The desmosome provides the major connection between one keratinocyte and another. It is the most complex of the keratinocyte connection points, which also include tight junctions, adherens junctions, and gap junctions. Desmosomes are present on all keratinocytes from the stratum basalis through the stratum granulosum. Once they reach the stratum corneum, the desmosomes start to degrade and break apart as the corneocytes are desquamated off the surface of the skin. The main purpose of desmosomes is to connect the actin cytoskeleton of one keratinocyte to that of the adjacent keratinocyte. They achieve this goal through a series of highly coordinated protein connections. The main proteins that allow for the connection between adjacent cells and the strength of the connection are the cadherin proteins, desmoglein and desmocollin. These are calcium-dependent adhesion molecules. Desmoglein and desmocollin are transmembrane proteins.

A desmocollin protein from one keratinocyte interacts with a desmoglein protein from the adjacent keratinocyte in a one-to-one ratio. There is more than one type of desmogleins and desmocollins, but they all interact similarly. Some of the subtypes are expressed at slightly different rates in various locations such as mucous membranes and the different levels of the epidermis. Each desmoglein or desmocollin molecule is anchored within the keratinocyte to plakoglobin, which in turn is bound to a group of proteins named *desmoplakins*. The desmoplakin proteins ultimately connect with the intercellular actin cytoskeleton.

The pemphigus group of diseases are autoimmune blistering diseases caused by the formation of autoantibodies against desmoglein and, in some cases, also against desmocollin. These autoantibodies interrupt the cell-to-cell adhesion process, resulting in superficial blistering of the skin and mucous membranes.

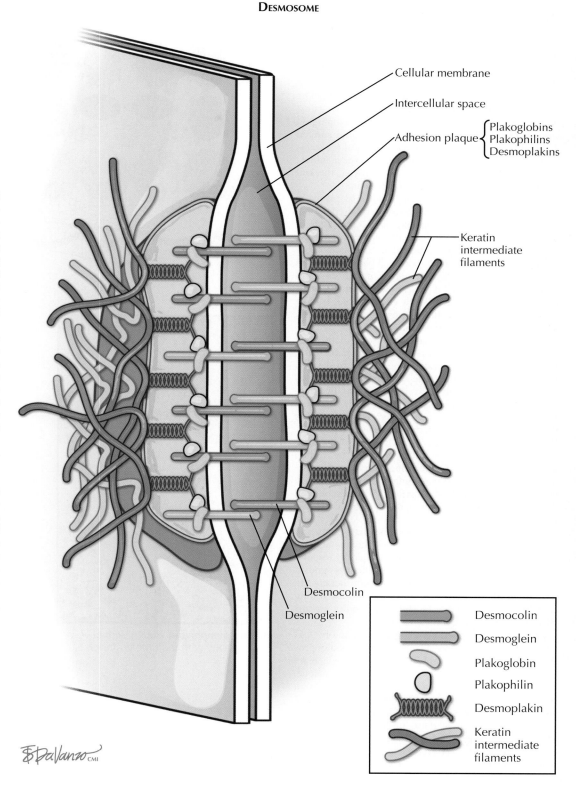

DESMOSOME

Cellular membrane

Intercellular space

Adhesion plaque { Plakoglobins
Plakophilins
Desmoplakins

Keratin intermediate filaments

Desmocolin

Desmoglein

	Desmocolin
	Desmoglein
	Plakoglobin
	Plakophilin
	Desmoplakin
	Keratin intermediate filaments

Plate 5-3

Integumentary System

BULLOUS PEMPHIGOID

Bullous pemphigoid is the most frequently encountered of all the autoimmune blistering diseases. It has a characteristic clinical course and appearance. The pathomechanism has been described in detail. The cause is the formation of autoantibodies directed against two hemidesmosomal proteins, bullous pemphigoid antigen 180 (BP180) and bullous pemphigoid antigen 230 (BP230). These two proteins are critical for stabilization of the hemidesmosomal plaque. If the hemidesmosomal plaque is interrupted or destroyed, the end result is subepidermal blistering of the skin.

Clinical Findings: The hemidesmosomal plaque is the main anchoring system of the dermal-epidermal junction. It is a complex apparatus with a multitude of proteins that interact to bind the epidermis to the underlying dermis. If it is interrupted, the pemphigoid complex of diseases may occur. These conditions include bullous pemphigoid, herpes gestationis, and cicatricial pemphigoid. Of these, bullous pemphigoid is the disease state most frequently encountered. It most commonly occurs in the fifth to seventh decades of life, with no race or sex predilection.

Clinically, patients often have a prodrome of intensely pruritic patches and plaques on the trunk, particularly the abdomen. Soon thereafter, they begin to develop large, tense bullae. The bullae can range from 1 cm to 10 cm in diameter, with an average of 2 cm. The blisters are tense to palpation and are not easily ruptured. If they do rupture, a fine, clear to slightly yellow serous fluid drains, and the underlying dermis is exposed. Reepithelialization is fairly rapid. Patients have continuous formation of new bullae, followed by healing and then repetition of the blistering pattern, until treatment is obtained. Scarring is minimal unless secondary infection has occurred. Most patients with pemphigoid do not have oral involvement, in direct contrast to those with the pemphigus class of diseases.

Bullous pemphigoid can spontaneously remit and relapse over time. Most patients seek therapy and are treated with a host of agents. Patients typically respond well to therapy and overall have an excellent prognosis. Secondary infections and side effects from therapy can lead to morbidity and mortality. Laboratory testing reveals immunoglobulin G (IgG) antibodies against BP180 or BP230 or both.

Pathogenesis: Bullous pemphigoid is caused by IgG autoantibody production. The two autoantibodies produced attack the BP180 and BP230 proteins, which are integral components of the hemidesmosomal plaque. BP180 is a transmembrane protein, and BP230 is an intracellular protein that lies within the keratinocyte and binds to BP180 and keratin filaments. The reason for the development of these antibodies is unknown. Once they have formed, they attach to the hemidesmosomal proteins. This activates a plethora of pathogenic mechanisms that act to induce separation of the epidermis from the dermis. Critical in the pathogenesis is activation of the complement cascade by the IgG antibodies. Complement activation may lead to further recruitment of inflammatory cells, which can be activated and thereafter release cytokines and enzymes that perpetuate the response.

Histology: Routine hematoxylin and eosin staining reveals a cell-poor subepidermal blister with scattered eosinophils. The histological differential diagnosis can be between bullous pemphigoid and epidermolysis bullosa acquisita (EBA). Immunofluorescence staining can be used to help differentiate the two. IgG and

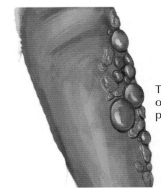

Autoantibody-mediated blisters: location of cleavage plane

→ PF (Dsg 1)

→ PV (Dsg 3)

BP (BP180, BP230)
→ CP, HG, LABD

→ EBA (Col VII), LABD

BP, bullous pemphigoid; Col VII, type VII collagen; CP, cicatricial pemphigoid; Dsg 1, desmoglein 1; Dsg 3, desmoglein 3; EBA, epidermolysis bullosa acquisita; HG, herpes gestationis; PF, pemphigus foliaceous; PV, pemphigus vulgaris; LABD, linear immunoglobulin A bullous dermatosis

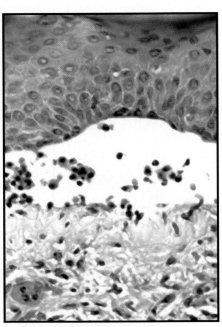

Bullous pemphigoid. Subepidermal blister cavity with multiple eosinophils

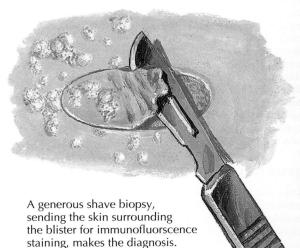

Tense bullae of bullous pemphigoid

A generous shave biopsy, sending the skin surrounding the blister for immunofluorscence staining, makes the diagnosis.

complement C3 localize to the basement membrane zone and appear as a linear band. The salt-split skin technique can also be used to differentiate the two diseases. This is achieved by incubating skin in a 1M NaCl solution to split the skin through the lamina lucida. When immunofluorescence staining is used on salt-split skin, the immunoreactants localize to the blister roof in bullous pemphigoid and to the dermal base in EBA.

Treatment: The severity of bullous pemphigoid varies. Therapy needs to be tailored to the individual. Many patients are older and have comorbidities that must be taken into account. Mild, localized disease can be treated with high-potency topical steroids. Severe disease is treated initially with oral steroids, and then the patient is transitioned to a steroid-sparing agent. The medications that have been routinely used include mycophenolate mofetil, azathioprine, and the combination of tetracycline and nicotinamide. Newer agents such as intravenous immunoglobulin (IVIG) have been used for severe refractory disease.

Plate 5-4

Autoimmune Blistering Diseases

MUCOUS MEMBRANE PEMPHIGOID

Mucous membrane pemphigoid goes by other names, including cicatricial pemphigoid, Brunsting-Perry pemphigoid, ocular pemphigoid, and benign mucous membrane pemphigoid. The last name should not be used because this is a chronic progressive, disabling disease with severe morbidity and mortality. The term *cicatricial* inherently states that the disease is associated with scarring, but this is not always the case. Hence, one patient without scarring may be referred to as having ocular pemphigoid and another with scarring may be said to have cicatricial ocular pemphigoid. Almost all patients will have some form of scarring, albeit very mild in some cases, if monitored for a long enough period. In reality, these are names given to a heterogeneous group of autoimmune blistering diseases that express a unique phenotype and have been shown to have small variances in the basement membrane zone autoantibodies they produce.

Clinical Findings: Mucous membrane pemphigoid can be seen in any racial group and affects females more often than males, in a 2 : 1 ratio. It is a disease of older persons and is most commonly seen in the seventh and eighth decades of life. Mucous membrane pemphigoid is a severe, chronic autoimmune blistering disease with grave consequences. It is a major cause of morbidity and mortality, and therapy can be difficult. Up to one quarter of these patients have eye involvement, which can lead to decreased vision and blindness. Mucous membrane disease is typically the initial sign: Patients present with painful erosions in the nasal passages, oropharynx, genitalia, and pulmonary tree. Patients complain of pain and difficulty eating secondary to severe discomfort. Erosions are the most common clinical findings, but vesicles and bullae may also be seen. Pulmonary and esophageal involvement may lead to strictures that result in difficulty with breathing or eating. Weight loss typically ensues, as does malaise and fatigue.

The skin can also be affected, leading to blister formation that heals with scarring and milia. If blisters develop on the scalp, they heal with a scarring alopecia. This form of the disease has been given the name *Brunsting-Perry pemphigoid*. This term is typically reserved for only those cases involving the scalp and skin that do not affect the mucous membranes.

Ocular pemphigoid is a chronic symmetric disease. The initial symptoms are inflamed conjunctiva, discomfort, pain, and increased tear production. Scarring soon develops and forms fibrous adhesions between the palpebral and bulbar conjunctivae. This scarring is termed *symblepharon*. The scaring is progressive, and it may cause the eyeball to become frozen in place. Entropion is common, and as it progresses, the eyelashes turn inward (trichiasis) and are forced against the cornea, which causes severe pain, irritation, and corneal ulceration. Patients cannot entirely close their eyelids because of the severe scarring. The damaged cornea undergoes keratinization, leading to opacity of the cornea and blindness.

Histology: Subepidermal blistering that heals with scar formation is the hallmark of this disease. The blistering takes place just below the keratinocyte, within in the lamina lucida. Immunohistochemical staining with collagen type IV shows that the blister plane is above the level of the lamina densa. The immunostaining and routine hematoxylin and eosin staining show a picture very similar to that of bullous pemphigoid. Linear immunoglobulin G and complement C3

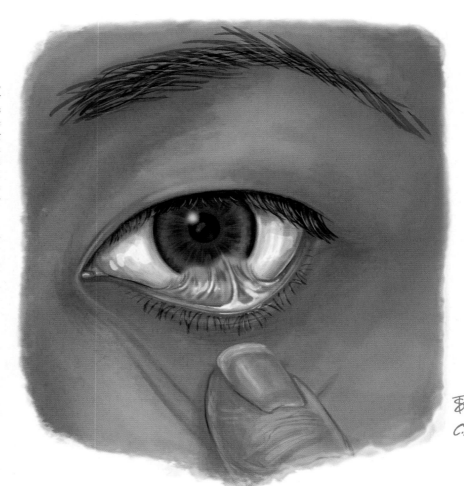

Ocular cicatricial pemphigoid. Scarring can become so severe as to cause vision loss. Symblepharon is commonly seen.

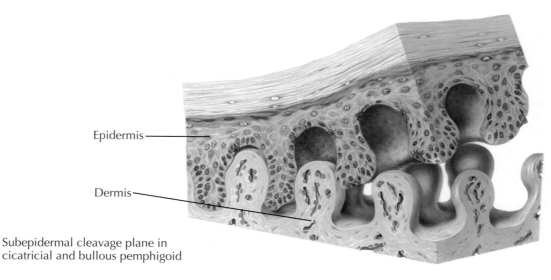

Epidermis

Dermis

Subepidermal cleavage plane in cicatricial and bullous pemphigoid

immunofluorescent staining is present along the basement membrane zone.

Pathogenesis: Autoantibody formation against proteins of the basement membrane zone has been linked to cicatricial pemphigoid. Many different antibodies against these proteins exist, including antibodies against the laminins, bullous pemphigoid antigens 180 and 230, and many other proteins as yet unclassified. The heterogeneity in antibody production likely accounts for the varying clinical phenotypes that are expressed.

Treatment: Prednisone is the drug used to treat the disease initially. After the disease is under some control, the addition of a steroid-sparring immunosuppressant should be attempted. Commonly used medications include azathioprine, methotrexate, mycophenolate mofetil, and cyclophosphamide. Dapsone and sulfapyridine, a similar medication that can be used in place of dapsone, have had some success treating this disease. Intravenous immunoglobulin (IVIG) has been used with success in refractory cases.

Plate 5-5

Integumentary System

DERMATITIS HERPETIFORMIS

Dermatitis herpetiformis is a unique chronic blistering disease that can be seen in isolation or in conjunction with celiac sprue. Dermatitis herpetiformis is the cutaneous manifestation of underlying gluten sensitivity. Patients with a genetic predisposition seem to be at risk for development of immunoglobulin A (IgA) autoantibodies that cross-react with gluten proteins and specific components of the skin and gastrointestinal tract. Dermatitis herpetiformis is always associated with small-bowel disease, and in some cases celiac sprue coexists. Patients with dermatitis herpetiformis are at increased risk for development of lymphoma of the gastrointestinal tract, potentially caused by the chronic inflammation and stimulation of the gastrointestinal-associated lymphatic tissue. Following a gluten-free diet cures the disease in both the skin and gastrointestinal locations.

Clinical Findings: Dermatitis herpetiformis is most frequently seen in the fourth and fifth decades of life, with a higher prevalence in the female Caucasian population. The reason for this preference may be that dermatitis herpetiformis has associations with the human leukocyte antigen (HLA) DQ2 and DQ8 haplotypes. Dermatitis herpetiformis manifests as a symmetric vesicular eruption, which is often preceded by a burning sensation or pruritus. The extensor surfaces of the elbows, knees, and lower back, as well as the scalp, may be involved. The vesicles are fragile and break easily. Erosions and excoriations are frequently seen. Diarrhea can be a recurrent complaint, secondary to involvement of the small bowel. Patients frequently report a flare of the rash and abdominal pain and diarrhea after eating certain foods.

Laboratory testing is frequently performed. High levels of IgA anti–tissue transglutaminase (anti-tTG) antibody and antiendomysial antibodies (EMAs) are commonly found and are highly specific for dermatitis herpetiformis. In cases of suspected sprue, an upper endoscopy can be performed, with a biopsy of the small bowel to evaluate for the characteristic villous atrophy.

Pathogenesis: Dermatitis herpetiformis is an autoimmune blistering disease that is caused by the development of specific antibodies, notably anti-tTG and EMAs. Tissue transglutaminase (tTG) is very similar to epidermal transglutaminase, and it is believed that the anti-tTG antibodies attack both proteins. This disruption of the epidermal transglutaminase is thought to be responsible for the blistering skin findings. Once the antibodies attach to the epidermal transglutaminase protein, the complement cascade and various cytotoxic cellular events are activated. The anti-EMA test is the most specific of the antibody tests for dermatitis herpetiformis.

Histology: Early lesions of dermatitis herpetiformis show subepidermal clefting with a neutrophil-rich infiltrate in the papillary dermis. As the lesions progress, subepidermal blistering becomes prominent, and the papillary dermis is filled with neutrophils. The histological findings of dermatitis herpetiformis can be difficult to differentiate from those of linear IgA bullous dermatosis on routine hematoxylin and eosin staining. Direct immunofluorescence is required to differentiate the two diseases. The direct immunofluorescence staining pattern in dermatitis herpetiformis is that of a speckled arrangement of IgA within the papillary dermis. In linear IgA bullous disease, as the name implies, a linear pattern along the basement membrane zone is seen.

Treatment: The treatment of dermatitis herpetiformis is twofold. The first aspect of therapy is to control

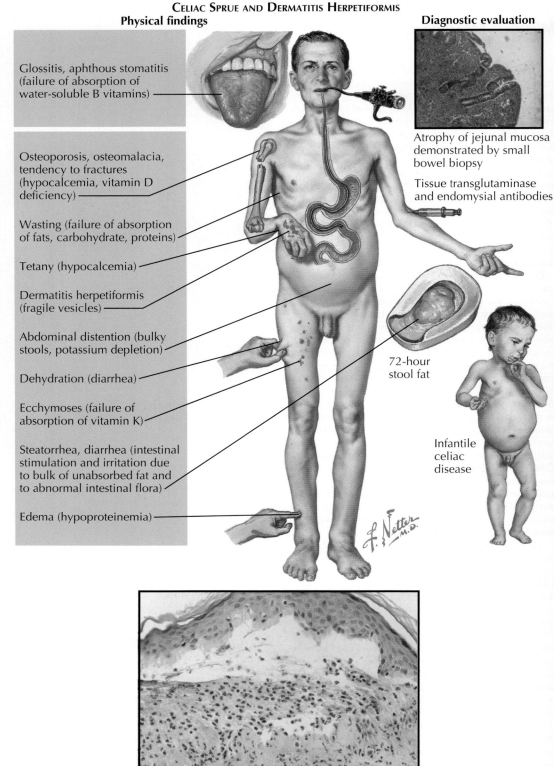

CELIAC SPRUE AND DERMATITIS HERPETIFORMIS

Physical findings

Glossitis, aphthous stomatitis (failure of absorption of water-soluble B vitamins)

Osteoporosis, osteomalacia, tendency to fractures (hypocalcemia, vitamin D deficiency)

Wasting (failure of absorption of fats, carbohydrate, proteins)

Tetany (hypocalcemia)

Dermatitis herpetiformis (fragile vesicles)

Abdominal distention (bulky stools, potassium depletion)

Dehydration (diarrhea)

Ecchymoses (failure of absorption of vitamin K)

Steatorrhea, diarrhea (intestinal stimulation and irritation due to bulk of unabsorbed fat and to abnormal intestinal flora)

Edema (hypoproteinemia)

Diagnostic evaluation

Atrophy of jejunal mucosa demonstrated by small bowel biopsy

Tissue transglutaminase and endomysial antibodies

72-hour stool fat

Infantile celiac disease

Neutrophilic infiltrate underlying a subepidermal blister

the itching and blistering. This can be rapidly achieved with dapsone or sulfapyridine. The response to these two medications is remarkably quick, with most patients noticing near-resolution of their symptoms within 1 day. In cases of suspected dermatitis herpetiformis that has not been confirmed histologically, dapsone can be used as a therapeutic test: If the patient sees a rapid response after the first day of dapsone therapy, the diagnosis is most certainly dermatitis herpetiformis. Dapsone or alternative medications can treat the blistering and pruritus, but they do not decrease the long-term risk of small-bowel lymphoma. The only means of decreasing and removing the risk of lymphoma is to have the patient adhere to a strict gluten-free diet. This requires nutritional education. If patients are able to entirely avoid gluten-containing products, not only will the rash resolve, but the gastrointestinal abnormalities will resolve, and the risk of lymphoma will return to that of the general population.

Plate 5-6

Autoimmune Blistering Diseases

EPIDERMOLYSIS BULLOSA ACQUISITA

Epidermolysis bullosa acquisita (EBA) is a rare chronic autoimmune blistering disease that is caused by auto-antibodies against type VII collagen. EBA has many features in common with the dominantly inherited form of the blistering disease, dystrophic epidermolysis bullosa (DEB). DEB is caused by a genetic defect in collagen VII that leads to a reduced amount or total lack of this type of collagen. Collagen VII serves as the anchoring fibrils that attach the epidermis via a series of protein connections to the dermis. Any defect in the production of collagen VII or abnormal destruction of this protein leads to blistering of the skin. EBA has been shown to be associated with a number of underlying systemic diseases, including inflammatory bowel disease, leukemia, and other autoimmune diseases.

Clinical Findings: EBA is an extremely rare disease that affects 1 in 2,000,000 to 3,000,000 people. It is almost always seen in the adult population, with the peak incidence in the fifth decade of life. A small number of cases of children affected by EBA have been reported. There is no race or sex predilection. EBA manifests with blister formation or with fragile skin and erosions from slight trauma. This can have a similar clinical appearance to porphyria cutanea tarda (PCT). The blistering is most frequently located in regions that experience mechanical friction or trauma. The dorsal surfaces of the hands are almost always involved, and patients complain of skin fragility and blister formation after slight trauma. The blisters heal slowly with scarring, and on close inspection, milia are found in the region of the healed blister. The mucous membranes are frequently involved, and oral disease can lead to weight loss. Other clinical variants of EBA have been described, and they typically mimic the clinical appearance of other autoimmune blistering diseases. For this reason, the only method to correctly diagnosis any blistering disease is by correlation of clinical and pathological findings.

Pathogenesis: EBA is caused by the production of autoantibodies directed against type VII collagen. The noncollagenous portions of type VII collagen are the most antigenic sections. Type VII collagen is the main component of the anchoring fibrils found within the dermis. The antibodies that have been found are in the immunoglobulin G subclass. They activate complement, which results in inflammation and destruction of the anchoring fibrils, eventually leading to fractures within the dermal-epidermal junction and, ultimately, to blistering. The etiology of antibody formation is not fully understood.

Histology: Biopsy specimens of EBA show a cell-poor subepidermal blister. The amount of inflammation is often minimal, but in some subtypes of the disease a lymphocytic infiltrate can be appreciated. The histological differential diagnosis includes bullous pemphigoid, and only with immunostaining can one decisively make the correct diagnosis. With immunohistochemical staining for collagen IV, the main component of the lamina densa, the blistering can be localized to the plane above the lamina densa in bullous pemphigoid or below the lamina densa in EBA. The salt-split skin method has also been used to split skin through the lamina lucida by incubating the skin specimen in 1M NaCl. Immunofluorescence staining of the split skin shows staining below the split in EBA and above the split in bullous pemphigoid.

Formation and composition of collagen

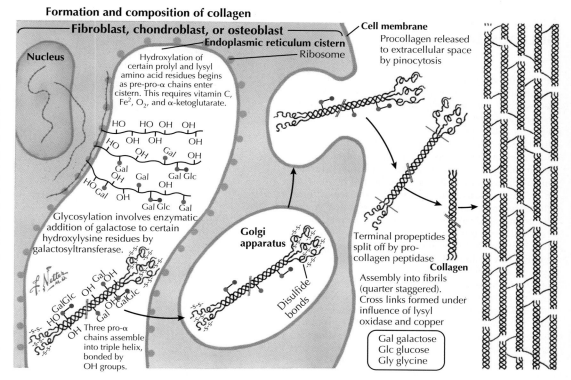

Three pro-α chains assemble into triple helix, bonded by OH groups.

Structure of α chains

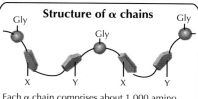

Each α chain comprises about 1,000 amino acids. Every third amino acid in chain is glycine, smallest of amino acids. Glycine has no side chains, which thus permits tight coil. X and Y here indicate other amino acids (X often proline; Y often hydroxyproline). Proline and hydroxy-proline, respectively, constitute about 10% and 25% of total amino acids in each α chain.

Types of collagen
(based on a chain composition of fibrils)

Type I
$\alpha 1(I)$
$\alpha 2$

Two α1(I) chains and one α2 chain = $(\alpha 1[I])_2 \, \alpha 2$; in bone, tendon, ligament, fascia, skin, artery, uterus

Type II
$\alpha 1(II)$

Three α1(II) chains = $(\alpha 1[II])_3$; in articular cartilage

Type III $(\alpha 1[III])_3$; in skin, artery, uterus, GI tract. Type IV $(\alpha 1[IV])_3$; in basement membranes, lens capsule. Type V $(\alpha B)_3$ or $(\alpha B)_2 \, \alpha A$; in basement membranes, other tissues. At least 12 different collagen molecules identified.

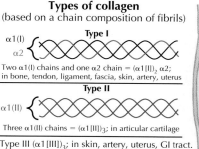

Type I in Bone, Tendon, Ligament, Skin

Type II in Articular cartilage and cartilaginous part of growth plate

Types of Collagen and Main Locations

Type	Location	Type	Location
Type I	Dermis, other tissue (most common form)	Type XII*	Dermis around hair follicles
Type II	Hyaline cartilage	Type XIII	Cell-to-cell adhesion
Type III	Skin and vascular tissue, fetal dermis	Type XIV*	Dermis, cornea
Type IV	Lamina densa of basement membrane zone	Type XV	Basement membrane zone
Type V	Found in association with type I collagen	Type XVI*	Dermis, cartilage
Type VI	Cartilage, dermis	Type XVII	Bullous pemphigoid antigen 180
Type VII	Anchoring fibrils	Type XVIII	Basement membrane zone
Type VIII	Vascular tissue, eye	Type XIX*	Basement membrane zone
Type IX*	Articular cartilage	Type XX *	Unknown
Type X	Cartilage	Type XXI*	Extracellular vascular wall matrix
Type XI	Cartilage		
*FACIT collagen, fibril-associated collagens with interrupted triple helices.			

Treatment: Therapy is difficult. Treatment of any underlying autoimmune disease or malignancy may help keep the blistering disease under control. Even with therapy, EBA tends to run a chronic waxing and waning course with frequent flares. Immunosuppressive agents have been used in EBA with varying success. Azathioprine, methotrexate, prednisone, intravenous immunoglobulin (IVIG), rituximab, mycophenolate mofetil, and cyclophosphamide have all been used.

Dapsone and colchicine have had anecdotal reports of success as well.

Supportive care is critical. Protection of the skin from trauma can help decrease blister formation. Early detection of infection and intervention to treat superinfection are critical. Even with all the current treatment strategies that have been attempted for EBA, the disease tends not to go into remission and remains chronic in nature.

Plate 5-7

Integumentary System

LINEAR IMMUNOGLOBULIN A BULLOUS DERMATOSIS

Linear immunoglobulin A (IgA) bullous dermatosis is an infrequently encountered autoimmune blistering disease that was originally described in 1979. This disease has a characteristic immunofluorescence staining pattern that is used to differentiate it from other blistering diseases such as dermatitis herpetiformis. As the name implies, linear IgA is deposited along the length of the dermal-epidermal junction. Chronic bullous disease of childhood is considered by most to be the same disease, although there are a few clinical differences in age at onset and associations that can be used to justify separating them into two distinct, albeit very similar, entities. Most cases of chronic bullous dermatosis of childhood are idiopathic, whereas most cases of linear IgA bullous dermatosis are drug induced and occur in an older population.

Clinical Findings: Linear IgA bullous dermatosis is rare and is estimated to occur in 1 of every 2,000,000 people. There is no race or sex predilection. It occurs most frequently in the adult population. The blistering disease has an insidious onset with small vesicles that may mimic dermatitis herpetiformis. The blisters are pruritic and do not have the same burning sensation as occurs in dermatitis herpetiformis, nor is there any relationship to dietary intake. The bullae in linear IgA bullous dermatosis are characteristically arranged in a "string of sausages" configuration. Each bulla is elongated and tapers to an end, with a small area of intervening normal-appearing skin before the tapering beginning of a new bulla. This string can be linear or annular in orientation. The blisters are tense and eventually rupture and heal with minimal scarring. Mucous membrane involvement is frequently seen and can resemble that of mucous membrane pemphigoid.

Chronic bullous disease of childhood manifests in early childhood (4-5 years of age). The blistering is similar to that of linear Ig bullous dermatitis, and the histological findings are identical. Blistering in chronic bullous disease of childhood is more often localized to the abdomen and lower extremities but may occur anywhere on the skin; it also commonly affects mucous membranes. Chronic bullous disease of childhood is most often idiopathic, whereas linear IgA bullous dermatosis can also be seen in association with underlying medications, malignancies, or other autoimmune conditions. Many medications have been implicated in causing linear IgA bullous dermatosis, with vancomycin being the most common by far.

Histology: The immunofluorescence staining pattern is characteristic and shows linear IgA all along the basement membrane zone. This is highly specific and sensitive for the diagnosis of linear IgA bullous dermatosis and chronic bullous disease of childhood. Routine hematoxylin and eosin staining shows a subepidermal blister with an underlying neutrophilic infiltrate. This can be impossible to distinguish from dermatitis herpetiformis or bullous lupus, so immunostaining is required.

Pathogenesis: The exact target antigen in linear IgA bullous dermatosis is unknown. It is speculated that the IgA antibodies are directed against a small region of bullous pemphigoid antigen 180 (BP180). Other possible antigens exist and have been localized to the lamina lucida and lamina densa regions of the basement membrane. The reason for formation of these antibodies and how certain medications induce them are unknown. Once present, the antibodies target the basement membrane zone and cause inflammation by

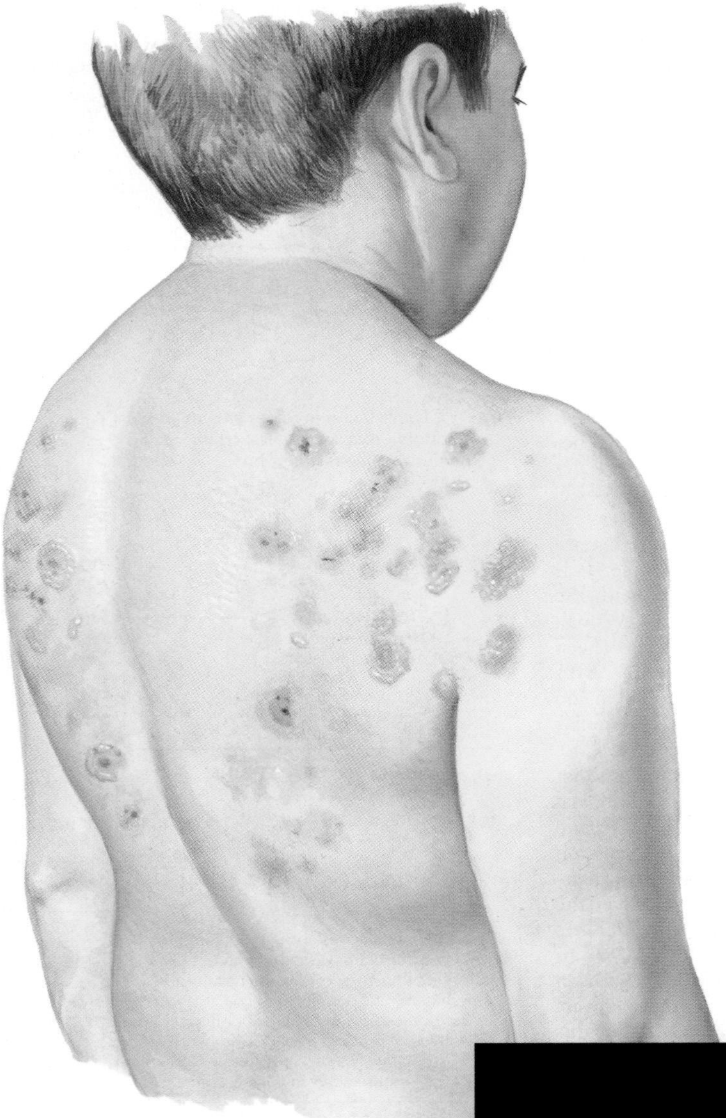

Characteristic bullae of linear IgA disease, or chronic bullous disease of childhood. They are configured in an annular manner with small areas of intervening normal skin.

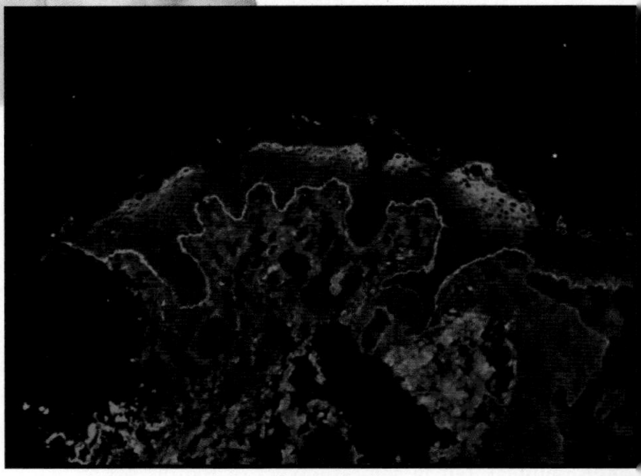

Linear deposition of IgA along the basement membrane zone

various mechanisms, ultimately leading to disruption of the dermal-epidermal junction and blistering.

Treatment: The first line of therapy is dapsone. Patients respond quickly to this medication. Low doses of dapsone are usually all that is needed. Alternative substitutes for dapsone include sulfapyridine and colchicine. Oral prednisone can be helpful initially, but because of the long-term side effects, patients should be transitioned to one of the other medications mentioned. Drug-induced variants of this blistering disease are best treated by recognizing the common culprits and removing them immediately. Over a period of a few weeks, most patients who have discontinued the offending medication return to a normal state. If the disease is found to be associated with an underlying malignancy or other autoimmune condition, therapy with dapsone is warranted. Treatment of the underlying condition should also be undertaken. If the malignancy or the associated disease is put into remission, there is a good possibility that the blistering disease will remit as well.

Plate 5-8

Autoimmune Blistering Diseases

PARANEOPLASTIC PEMPHIGUS

Paraneoplastic pemphigus was not described until the early 1990s. It is a rare subset of the pemphigus family of diseases that is associated with the synchronous occurrence of a systemic neoplastic process. The neoplastic disease may precede the diagnosis of paraneoplastic pemphigus. This disease has been differentiated from other forms of pemphigus by its unique antibody profile and staining patterns. Most cases have occurred secondary to hematological malignancy, but solid tumors have also been with paraneoplastic pemphigus.

Clinical Findings: Paraneoplastic pemphigus is most likely to occur in the older population, usually during the seventh or eighth decade of life. It has also been reported to occur in young children with neoplastic disease. There is no sex or race predilection. Most patients develop paraneoplastic pemphigus after the diagnosis of an internal malignancy or at the same time as their diagnosis.

The oral mucosa is almost always the first mucocutaneous surface to be affected. Severe erosions and ulcerations occur throughout the oropharynx. This leads to significant pain and difficulty eating. Patients avoid eating because of the severe, unremitting pain. Weight loss and blistering, in combination with the underlying malignancy, result in a severe, life-threatening illness. The hallmark of this disease is the severe oral mucous membrane involvement. In fact, if the patient does not have oral involvement, the diagnosis of paraneoplastic pemphigus should be reevaluated, and the patient most likely has another form of pemphigus. Soon after the onset of oral disease, the patient's skin begins to break out in vesicles and flaccid bullae. These blisters are identical to those seen in pemphigus vulgaris. Histologically, there are some subtle differences in immunofluorescence.

The bullae can spread, and large surface areas of skin may become involved. Other clinical morphologies of skin disease have been described, including an erythema multiforme–like eruption, a pemphigoid-like eruption, and a lichenoid eruption that can mimic both graft-versus-host disease and lichen planus. These variants are infrequently seen. The combination of paraneoplastic pemphigus and an underlying malignancy has led to poor outcomes; this condition is refractory and very difficult to treat. The diagnosis is made by consistent clinical features in a patient with an underlying malignancy who also has serum autoantibodies against certain proteins, most frequently the plakin family of proteins.

Pathogenesis: Paraneoplastic pemphigus is caused by circulating autoantibodies directed against various intercellular keratinocyte proteins. The most commonly found antibodies are directed against the plakin

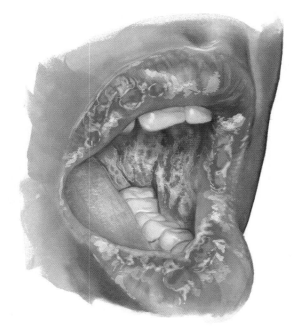

Severe involvement of the oral mucosa is the hallmark of paraneoplastic pemphigus.

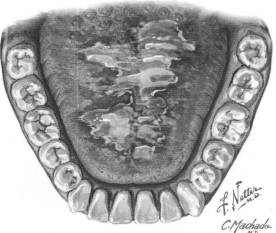

Diffuse erosions on the tongue

Antibodies Found in Paraneoplastic Pemphigus
Bullous pemphigoid antigen II
Bullous pemphigoid antigen I
Desmoglein 1
Desmoglein 3
Desmoplakin 1
Desmoplakin 2
Envoplakin
Periplakin
Plectin

Associations with Paraneoplastic Pemphigus
Hematologic malignancies (85% of cases)
Non-Hodgkin's lymphoma
Hodgkin's lymphoma
Chronic lymphocytic leukemia
Lymph node hyperplasia
Castleman's disease
Solid tumors (15% of cases)
Thymoma
Sarcomas—predominantly retroperitoneal location
Adenocarcinoma
Breast
Pancreas
Lung
Prostate
Colon
Squamous cell carcinoma
Oral cavity
Melanoma

family of proteins, which include envoplakin and periplakin. Many other autoantibodies have also been found. It is theorized that the underlying neoplasm stimulates the cellular and humoral immune systems to form these autoantibodies. The exact mechanism by which the tumor causes this to occur is unclear.

Histology: Acantholysis is the main histological feature on routine staining. Varying amounts of keratinocyte necrosis are also appreciated. The blister forms within the intraepidermal space. Routine staining cannot differentiate among the various members of the pemphigus family of diseases. Direct immunofluorescence staining in these diseases shows a fishnet staining pattern caused by intercellular hemidesmosomal keratinocyte staining. Paraneoplastic pemphigus is much more likely than any of the other pemphigus diseases to have a positive indirect immunofluorescence staining pattern when rat bladder epithelium is used, whereas the pattern when monkey esophagus epithelium is used

is routinely negative. The opposite pattern is seen with most other types of pemphigus. The unique histological and immunofluorescence staining patterns seen in paraneoplastic pemphigus can lead one to the diagnosis. Immunoblotting may also be done.

Treatment: Therapy needs to be directed at the underlying neoplastic process. The overall outcome is extremely poor. The 2-year survival rate has been estimated at 10%. Supportive care to prevent superinfection of the skin is imperative. Immunosuppressants are used to help decrease the blistering, but they may have deleterious effects on the underlying neoplasm. If the underlying neoplasm can be cured, there is a better chance that this disease will go into remission, although this does not always happen. Corticosteroids, azathioprine, intravenous immunoglobulin (IVIG), rituximab, plasmapheresis, bone marrow transplantation, and a host of other therapies have been attempted with limited success.

Plate 5-9

Integumentary System

PEMPHIGUS FOLIACEUS

Pemphigus foliaceus is a chronic autoimmune blistering disease. Pemphigus foliaceus can be seen in an isolated form or as an endemic form called *fogo selvagem*. These diseases are caused by autoantibody production against desmosomal proteins. The endemic form of the disease is seen in small regions in the jungles of South America, predominantly in Brazil. Pemphigus foliaceus is closely related to pemphigus vulgaris, and in some cases the clinical picture and antibody profile can shift from one disease to the other, leading to difficulty in classification.

Clinical Findings: Pemphigus foliaceus is a rare disease that most frequently affects patients who are about 50 years of age. There is no sex or race predilection. Blistering of the skin is prominent and can affect large body surface areas. The blisters tend to be more superficial than those of pemphigus vulgaris. The blisters are rarely found intact because of their superficial and fragile nature. Mucous membranes are rarely affected, because the mucocutaneous surfaces do not contain high concentrations of the desmoglein 1 protein. Patients exhibit a positive Nikolsky's sign. This sign is positive when exertion of pressure (rubbing) induces a blister or erosion on nonaffected skin.

Fogo selvagem (Portuguese for "wild fire") affects a younger population, occurring in patients approximately 25 years of age. It is believed to be transmitted by the bite of the black fly or the mosquito in patients who are susceptible to the disease. It has been postulated that the bite begins a cascade of immune system antibody production, resulting in formation of the pathogenic antibodies against desmoglein 1. The infectious agent transmitted by the flies has not been discovered. A fair percentage of patients have a family member who is also affected, and this provides some clinical evidence for a genetic predisposition to the disease. The disease exhibits photosensitivity in the ultraviolet B range.

Indirect immunofluorescence testing of the patient's serum shows autoantibodies against desmoglein 1.

Histology: The histological findings of pemphigus foliaceus and its endemic form, fogo selvagem, are identical. Intraepidermal blistering is caused by acantholysis. The acantholysis is most prominent in the upper epidermis, usually starting in the granular cell layer and above. Typically, a mixed inflammatory infiltrate is seen within the dermis. Varying amounts of crust and superficial bacteria are seen in areas of chronic erosion. Immunofluorescence staining shows a fishnet pattern of intercellular staining with immunoglobulin G and complement.

Pathogenesis: Abnormal antibody production is directed against the desmoglein 1 protein, which is a critical component of the desmosomal attachment between adjacent keratinocytes. Desmogleins are calcium-dependent adhesion proteins known as cadherins. As the autoantibodies attach to the desmoglein protein and are deposited within the epidermis, they activate complement. Complement activation, along with the cytotoxic effects of lymphocytes, leads to acantholysis of keratinocytes and the eventual blistering of the epidermis. The hemidesmosome is unaffected, and the basilar layer of keratinocytes stays attached to the basement membrane zone.

Treatment: Because mucous membrane involvement is almost nonexistent and the blistering is more superficial, the course of pemphigus foliaceus is typically less severe than that of pemphigus vulgaris; however, this is not always the case. Therapy is directed toward decreasing the antibody formation. Immunosuppressants are

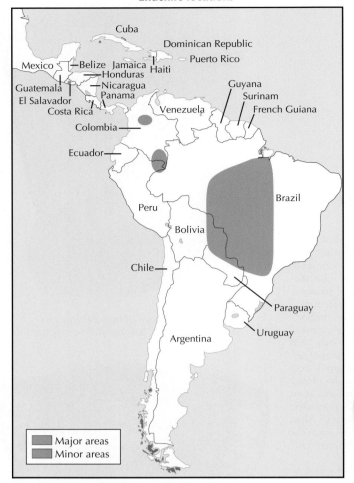

Endemic locations

Cuba
Dominican Republic
Mexico — Belize Jamaica Haiti — Puerto Rico
Honduras
Guatemala — Nicaragua Guyana
El Salvador Panama Surinam
Costa Rica Venezuela French Guiana
Colombia —
Ecuador —
Brazil
Peru
Bolivia
Chile —
Paraguay
Uruguay
Argentina

☐ Major areas
☐ Minor areas

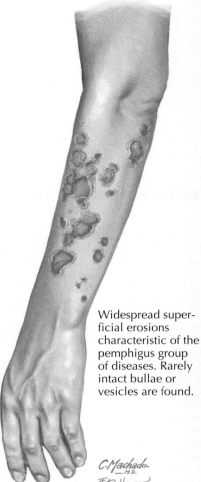

Widespread superficial erosions characteristic of the pemphigus group of diseases. Rarely intact bullae or vesicles are found.

C. Machado M.D.
B. Palanzo CMI

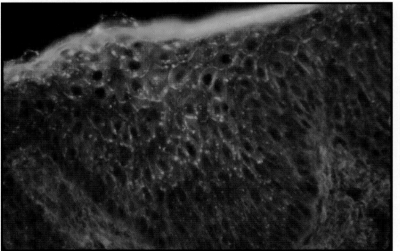

Direct immunofluorescence showing uniform staining between keratinocytes in the dermis. The antibody is directed against the desmoglein 1 protein.

the mainstay of therapy, and combinations are occasionally required to get the disease under control. Oral corticosteroids are typically the first medications used, along with a steroid-sparing agent. Azathioprine, mycophenolate mofetil, cyclophosphamide, and rituximab have all been used with varying success. Intravenous immunoglobulin (IVIG) has also been used. Use of the non-immunosuppressive agents, tetracycline and nicotinamide, has shown variable success. The same can be said of hydroxychloroquine. The treatment of pemphigus foliaceus requires chronic therapy, because this is a chronically relapsing and remitting disease. Supportive care is required to avoid excessive trauma and friction to the skin, which can induce blistering. Bacterial superinfection needs to be treated promptly.

Therapy for fogo selvagem is similar in many respects. The use of mosquito and fly control measures may be of help in the endemic regions, because these insects are believed to be the vectors of transmission to susceptible humans.

Plate 5-10

Autoimmune Blistering Diseases

PEMPHIGUS VULGARIS

Pemphigus vulgaris is the prototypical acantholytic autoimmune blistering disease. It is one of the most serious of all blistering diseases. Blister formation in this subset of skin diseases occurs secondary to intraepidermal acantholysis. The desmosomal plaque is the target of the autoantibodies found in this disease.

Clinical Findings: The mean age at onset is approximately 55 years. Patients present with rapid onset of vesicles and bullae that rupture easily. The flaccid bullae are rarely found intact. The disease often begins within the oral cavity, and the oral lesions can either precede the skin disease or occur independently of skin manifestations. Vesicles and bullae are almost never seen in the oral cavity, because the blisters in pemphigus are superficial and rupture almost immediately after they are formed. The oral erosions are excruciatingly painful and are frequently misdiagnosed as a herpes simplex infection. Often, it is not until the erosions become chronic that the diagnosis of pemphigus is entertained. Patients eventually avoid eating because of the pain, and they often complain of weight loss, fatigue, and malaise.

If skin lesions are also present, the diagnosis can be made with more confidence based on the clinical findings. However, one must perform a biopsy to rule out the other pemphigus variants. Paraneoplastic pemphigus always starts in the mouth and tends to be much more severe and refractory to therapy than pemphigus vulgaris. This diagnosis should be considered in a patient who has a coexisting malignancy and treatment-refractory disease. Immunoblotting is a specific test to look for the exact autoantibody present in paraneoplastic pemphigus; it can be performed in highly specialized laboratories. In pemphigus vulgaris, indirect immunofluorescence almost always shows a high titer against desmoglein 3. The antibody titer correlates with the disease activity, and titers have been monitored to assess the treatment of the disease. Pruritus is uncommon in patients with pemphigus; the overwhelming complaint is skin pain. If left untreated, the disease is progressive and carries a mortality rate of 60% to 65%.

The skin blisters of pemphigus vulgaris rupture early in the course of their formation. The remaining erosions can become quite large, however. Weeping of serous fluid is present, and bleeding from the erosions can also be seen. Secondary superinfection is common and may cause an increase in autoantibody production.

Pathogenesis: Pemphigus vulgaris is a chronic autoimmune blistering disease in which autoantibodies are directed against the desmosomal plaque. The desmosomal plaque is the most crucial element that holds adjacent keratinocytes in place and juxtaposed to one another. There are other intercellular connections between keratinocytes, including gap junctions, adherens junctions, and tight junctions. The desmosomal

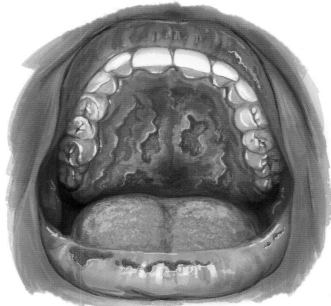

Oral erosions can be the first mucocutaneous sign of the disease pemphigus vulgaris.

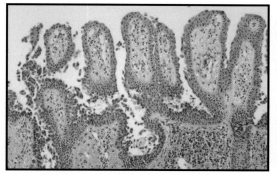

Blister formation via acantholysis is the hallmark histological finding in pemphigus vulgaris.

Tombstoning

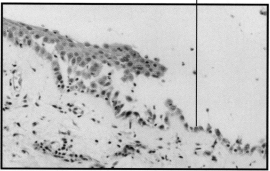

Pemphigus vulgaris. Severe acantholysis with "tombstoning" along the basement membrane zone (BMZ). This is caused by uninvolved hemidesmosomes, which adhere the basilar keratinocytes to the BMZ.

plaque is composed of various proteins that act to connect the intracellular actin cytoskeleton of one keratinocyte to that of another; these include various desmoglein, desmocollin, desmoplakin, plakophilin, and plakoglobin proteins. The central portion of the desmosome contains the proteins desmoglein and desmocollin. They are responsible for the tight binding of adjacent keratinocytes. There are many members in each of the desmoglein and desmocollin families.

Autoantibodies to the desmoglein family of proteins, specifically desmoglein 3, are responsible for the formation of pemphigus vulgaris. Antibodies against desmoglein 1 have also been found in patients with pemphigus vulgaris and pemphigus foliaceous.

Histology: Skin biopsies of pemphigus vulgaris shows intraepidermal blister formation. The blisters are formed by acantholysis, and keratinocytes appear to be free floating within the blister cavity. "Tombstoning" may be present. This is the designation given to the

basilar keratinocytes that stay attached to the basement membrane zone by their unaffected hemidesmosomes. The basilar keratinocytes appear to be standing up in a row, mimicking tombstones. Immunofluorescence show immunoglobulin G staining in a fishnet pattern throughout the epidermis. Each intercellular connection between keratinocytes is highlighted.

Treatment: Appropriate therapy needs to be instituted as soon as the diagnosis is made. High-dose oral or intravenous corticosteroids have been the mainstay of therapy. However, patients need to be transitioned to a steroid-sparing agent. Many immunosuppressive medications have been used to treat pemphigus vulgaris. The more common ones are azathioprine, mycophenolate mofetil, cyclophosphamide, and the newer agents, intravenous immunoglobulin (IVIG) and rituximab. Morbidity and mortality have been dramatically reduced since the introduction of steroids and steroid-sparing agents.

INFECTIOUS DISEASES

Plate 6-1

Integumentary System

ACTINOMYCOSIS

Many species of the bacterial genus *Actinomyces* are able to cause disease in humans. The infection tends to run a chronic course that leads to suppurative granulomatous abscesses in the skin. The diagnosis may be suspected if there is clinical evidence of painful draining of suppurative material and histological evidence of granuloma formation. The exact diagnosis is based on tissue culture or culture of the suppurative material. The disease is progressive if appropriate therapy is not instituted. The organisms responsible for these infections are normally found within the oral cavity and are commensal organisms. They can also be found throughout the gastrointestinal tract.

Clinical Findings: Males are much more likely to develop this infection than females, with an estimated ratio of 3:1. Most patients are between 30 and 50 years of age. Predisposing factors include poor dental hygiene. The infection is believed to be endogenous in origin. It is a rare infection in the United States. There are several clinical pictures of actinomycosis. The most common form seen is the cervicofacial subtype, which accounts for more than 50% of cases. It is related to oral trauma, such as recent dental work. The area that has been traumatized provides a portal of entry for the bacteria, and there is a progressive induration of the underlying tissue. With time, the firm swelling begins to break through the skin and to drain through multiple cutaneous fistulas. Pain can be intense and is relieved as the fistulas spontaneously drain. The designation "lumpy jaw" signifies the induration and fistula formation seen in patients with actinomycosis cervicofacial disease.

The next most prevalent form of the disease is the pulmonary form. This is believed to be caused by aspiration of the causative bacteria. Patients often complain of hemoptysis and low-grade fever. Chest radiographs can show features similar to those of tuberculosis infections. Any lobe of the lung may be involved, but the right lower lobe is most frequently affected because the infection is caused by aspiration. If the disease goes unrecognized, sinus tracts eventually form through the lung lining, muscle, and skin to the thoracic cutaneous wall. Skin abscess and a draining sinus in this location should lead one to look for pulmonary involvement, including the development of empyema. Abdominal forms of the disease are believed to occur after trauma to the bowel. This has been reported most frequently after appendectomy, and for unknown reasons the bacteria localize to that area. The last form of the disease is the disseminated form, which is rare and can occur after any form of the disease that is not appropriately treated. Any organ system may be involved.

Histology: Biopsy specimens show a suppurative granulomatous reaction pattern. Neutrophils, histiocytes, and lymphocytes make up the majority of the inflammatory infiltrate. Basophilic granules (sulfur granules) are surrounded by a predominantly neutrophilic infiltrate.

Anaerobic culture of the purulent material or a portion of the tissue is critical for proper identification of the responsible organism and ultimately for choosing the appropriate therapy. Material should be sent anaerobically immediately to the laboratory. Yellow to white sulfur granules form as the culture material grows. Evaluation of the sulfur granules with the use of an oil immersion microscope shows the filamentous bacteria.

Pathogenesis: Actinomycosis is caused by one of the gram-positive filamentous bacteria of the *Actinomyces* genus: *A. israelii, A. turicensis, A. lingnae, A. gravenitzii,*

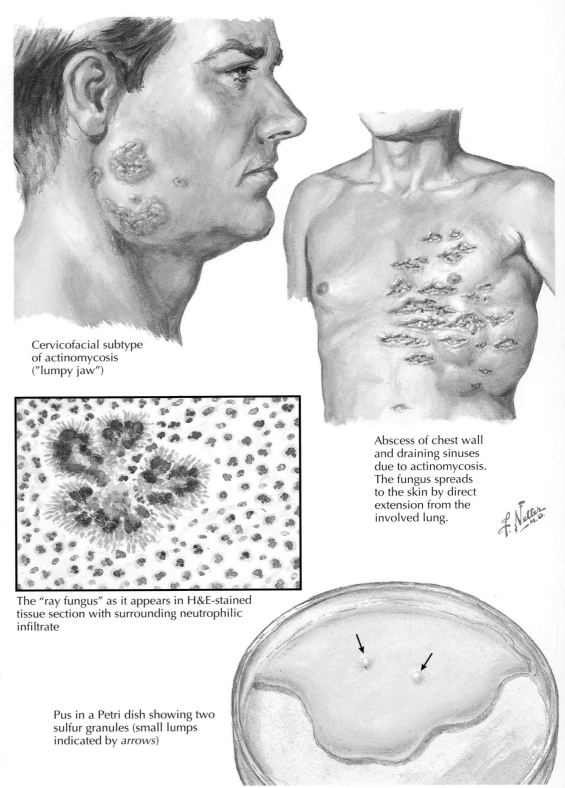

Cervicofacial subtype of actinomycosis ("lumpy jaw")

Abscess of chest wall and draining sinuses due to actinomycosis. The fungus spreads to the skin by direct extension from the involved lung.

The "ray fungus" as it appears in H&E-stained tissue section with surrounding neutrophilic infiltrate

Pus in a Petri dish showing two sulfur granules (small lumps indicated by *arrows*)

A. meyeri, A. naeslundii, A. radingae, A. europaeus, A. viscosus, A. neuii, or *A. odontolyticus. A. israelii* is the organism most frequently observed to cause disease. These are anaerobic, acid-fast bacteria that have a filamentous morphology with varying amounts of branching. The definitive diagnosis is made by culture of the organism.

Treatment: The drug of choice to treat this bacterial infection is penicillin. Therapy needs to be maintained for months to be certain of complete cure. If the infection is treated promptly, almost all patients have a full and complete recovery. Patients who are allergic to penicillin can be treated with any of the tetracycline-based antibiotics.

Plate 6-2

Infectious Diseases

BLASTOMYCOSIS

Blastomycosis is a fungal infection that is found predominantly in North America. This disease is also known as North American blastomycosis or Gilchrist's disease. However, because it has also been reported in Central and South America, the preferred name of this disease is blastomycosis. It is endemic in the areas of the United States and Canada that border the Great Lakes, the Saint Lawrence Riverway, and the Mississippi River Valley. Most cases have been reported from Wisconsin and Ontario. The infection is common in other mammals such as dogs. Most cases are isolated and sporadic in nature; however, outbreaks of the infection have occurred in which many people who came into contact with the same environmental source were infected.

Clinical Findings: The organism is first inhaled into the lungs, where it quickly reverts to its yeast state. Most infections are controlled by the local immune response, and minimal to no symptoms occur. The disease most frequently stays localized within the pulmonary system. It can, however, spread to any other organ system in an immunosuppressed host. After the conidia (spores) are inhaled, the most frequent symptoms are coughing, fever, pleurisy, weight loss, malaise, arthralgias, and hemoptysis. The symptoms may initially mimic those of an influenza infection. Approximately half of the patients with symptomatic disease have only pulmonary findings; the other half have both pulmonary and other organ system findings.

Cutaneous findings are nonspecific and have been classified as verrucous or ulcerative. The verrucous lesions can range from small papules and plaques to large nodules with sinus tract formation. The central face and nose are common locations of involvement. Ulcerated lesions can occur anywhere and are associated with underlying abscess formation and drainage. The skin lesions can mimic those of skin cancers, and biopsy is required to make the appropriate diagnosis.

Histology: Biopsies of blastomycosis show pseudoepitheliomatous hyperplasia of the epidermis. Within the dermis is a granulomatous infiltrate of predominantly noncaseating granulomas. Neutrophils are prominent. The yeast can be appreciated on routine hematoxylin and eosin staining. They appear as oval cells with a thick, refractory wall. Often, broad-based budding is noted. This form of solitary broad-based budding is specific for *Blastomyces dermatitidis*. Other special stains can be used to better highlight the fungus, including the periodic acid–Schiff and silver stains.

The best means of diagnosing this fungal infection is by culture on Sabouraud's media. The mold begins to grow quickly and forms white to gray, waxy colonies. Special DNA probes can be used to quickly identify the fungus growing in the medium.

Pathogenesis: Blastomycosis is directly caused by infection with the dimorphic fungus, *B. dermatitidis*. This organism inhabits soil and vegetation in its mold or mycelial form. When the environment that contains the fungus is disrupted, the spores of this fungus may gain entry into a human (or other mammal) by direct inoculation or by inhalation. Once the fungus has entered the human body, the increase in temperature causes it to convert to its yeast form. The yeast form is not contagious, and the human acts as a host for reproduction but is unable to transmit the disease to any other human. The normal host is able to contain the inhaled spores within alveolar macrophages and

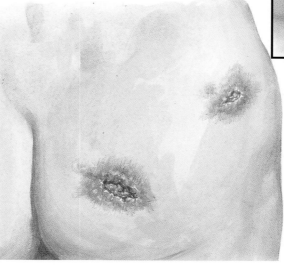

Verrucous ulcerated plaques and nodules

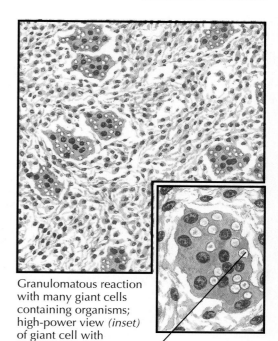

Very high-power view of a budding and a nonbudding organism

Broad-based budding is characteristic of blastomycosis.

Granulomatous reaction with many giant cells containing organisms; high-power view *(inset)* of giant cell with organisms

Organism with thick, refractory cell wall

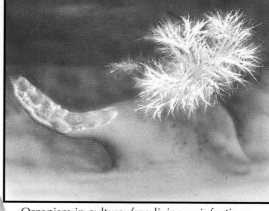

Organism in culture: free-living or infectious phase of *Blastomyces dermatitidis*. Sabouraud's dextrose agar medium

granulomas in the lung, but the yeast form of the fungus is much more resistant to killing by natural host responses. If the host is immunocompromised, the fungus may disseminate to other organs, particularly the cutaneous surface. Dissemination occurs via vascular spread of the yeast organisms.

Treatment: Prompt treatment with amphotericin B is the therapy of choice for those with disseminated or severe disease or any evidence of immunosuppression. Milder cases can be treated with prolonged courses of the azole antifungal agents; amphotericin B is used if the disease fails to respond to this treatment. Fluconazole and itraconazole are the two antifungal agents most frequently used, although other options are available. Before antifungal therapy was available, more than 80% of cases were fatal.

Plate 6-3

Integumentary System

CHANCROID

Chancroid is a sexually transmitted disease caused by *Haemophilus ducreyi*. Infection with this bacterium is one of the most common causes of acute genital ulcerations in the world. Although it is most frequently encountered in Africa and Asia, it can be seen worldwide. Infection with this agent is frequently associated with other sexually transmitted diseases. *H. ducreyi* infection has been shown to increase the likelihood of contracting the human immunodeficiency virus (HIV) after exposure. Although specialized serology testing is being developed, the diagnosis is based on the clinical scenario and culture results.

Clinical Findings: *H. ducreyi* is transmitted via sexual contact, and the first sign of the disease is the formation of a papule at the site of inoculation. The papule occurs, on average, 3 to 5 days after exposure. The papule, which is often surrounded by a red halo, quickly turns into a vesiculopustule and then a painful ulceration. The ulcer is nonindurated and has undermined edges with a well-demarcated boundary. If left untreated, the ulcerations can become enormous and serpentine in appearance. The base of the ulcer has a gray appearance with granulation tissue present. The infection is associated with massive inguinal adenitis, termed *buboes*, in about 50% of cases. The disease is transmitted by unprotected sexual intercourse with an infected individual. Women may develop subclinical undetected disease, in which case they can act as carriers for transmission. This is likely the reason that sexual intercourse with female prostitutes increases one's chance of developing disease. Active disease is much more frequently encountered in males, in a 4:1 ratio.

Pathogenesis: *H. ducreyi* is a gram-negative coccobacillus. The organism is transmitted from one human host to another by intimate physical contact. The bacterium requires a break in the integrity of the epidermis to gain entrance to the body. It then multiples locally and forms the initial papule, which soon becomes a pustule teeming with bacteria. Once the papulopustule ulcerates, the bacterial load is high and allows for further transmission. It has been shown that the bacteria can be shed from nonulcerated lesions. The formation of ulcerations on epidermis that opposes the original ulcer has been termed a "kissing ulcer" and is caused by direct autoinoculation of the bacteria. The bacteria cannot live long outside its human host, and this characteristic can make it difficult to properly culture. Many virulence factors have been detected, including the cell surface lipooligosaccharide protein. The bacteria grow on chocolate agar culture medium.

Histology: A skin biopsy from the edge of the ulcer may be helpful in diagnosis. There are three zones of inflammation from superficial to deep. Zone 1 is the necrotic superficial tissue. The second zone is the largest and consists of a proliferation of freshly made blood vessels. The last zone is a deep layer consisting of an inflammatory infiltrate with many plasma cells. Detection of the bacteria is difficult on tissue biopsies unless the bacterial load is tremendous. If a high burden of bacteria is present, they may be seen on microscopy lined up in a "school of fish" pattern. This is rarely

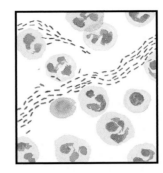

Soft chancre of chancroid with surrounding redness

Haemophilus ducreyi in a "school of fish" pattern with surrounding neutrophils

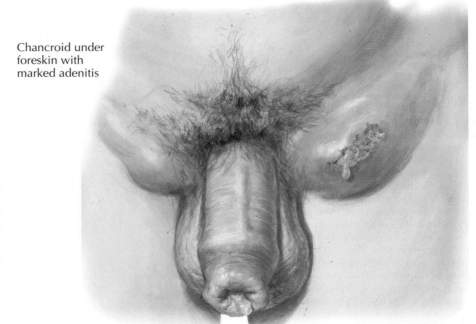

Chancroid under foreskin with marked adenitis

Swollen lymph nodes (buboes) can spontaneously drain to the skin surface.

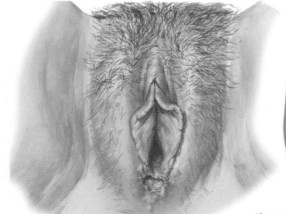

Chancroid ulcerations show a well-demarcated border and a gray discolored base.

observed in skin biopsy specimens. Culturing of the bacteria is the best means to firmly make the diagnosis.

Treatment: Treatment can be accomplished with azithromycin, erythromycin, or ceftriaxone. The clinician should also consider treating empirically for other sexually transmitted diseases, because they tend to congregate together. This is especially true of gonorrhea, which is often a coinfection with *H. ducreyi*. For some reason, the disease is more difficult to treat in patients who have a coexisting HIV infection. This may be because HIV-positive patients have a lowered cell-mediated immunity, and an intact cell-mediated immune system is needed to treat *H. ducreyi* infection. Surgical incision and drainage of fluctuant nodules should be considered as an adjunct to oral antibiotics. Drainage decreases the bacterial load and potentially makes antibiotic therapy more effective.

Plate 6-4

Infectious Diseases

COCCIDIOIDOMYCOSIS

Coccidioidomycosis, or valley fever, is endemic in the southwestern United States. Patients who breathe in spores (arthroconidia) from the fungus *Coccidioides immitis* may become infected. Most patients do not develop active disease; instead, their exposure is confirmed by the presence of a positive delayed hypersensitivity test to the fungus. Primary cutaneous coccidioidomycosis is a rare entity caused by inoculation of the fungus directly into the skin. By far the most common form of cutaneous coccidioidomycosis is caused by dissemination to the skin from a primary pulmonary infection.

Clinical Findings: This infection has a slightly increased incidence in African Americans. The Filipino population appears to be at greatest risk for developing severe disease. Males and females are equally affected. Most individuals who inhale the spores do not develop active disease. Rather, the fungus lies dormant or trapped within pulmonary granulomas. About one third of patients who are exposed to the fungus develop an acute pneumonitis. Fever, cough, malaise, and pleurisy are the main symptoms. The pneumonitis may be severe enough to bring the patient to the clinic to seek therapy, but many cases are mild and patients routinely dismiss them as the common cold. Reactivation later in life may occur secondary to acquired immunosuppression, pregnancy, or older age.

Cutaneous findings in coccidioidomycosis have a variable morphology. Papules, plaques, and nodules are the most frequent forms of disseminated coccidioidomycosis. These skin lesions have a predilection to affect the face, and in particular the nasolabial skin fold. Multiple draining cutaneous abscesses with fistula and sinus formation can occur in late untreated disease. Chronic ulcerations have also been reported to be a manifestation of cutaneous disease.

Nonspecific skin findings attributed to fungal infection with *C. immitis* are well recognized. The best reported and most clearly associated finding is erythema nodosum. Erythema nodosum is a reaction that occurs in many internal and cutaneous disease states. Almost any deep fungal infection can induce erythema nodosum. Patients who have a history of travel to an endemic area should be screened for this fungal disease. Rarely, erythema multiforme and Sweet's syndrome have been reported in association with coccidioidomycosis.

Pulmonary disease is almost always present and should be thoroughly searched for in patients presenting with cutaneous coccidioidomycosis. Chest radiographs may show many findings, including cavitary lesions, hilar adenopathy, pneumonitis, pleural effusions, and lobar disease.

The only method to make a diagnosis is with an appropriate tissue culture that shows growth of the causative fungus. The clinical examination and history are not as sensitive or specific as culture of the fungus. If one has a high index of suspicion for this disease, treatment should be instituted and then adjusted after the culture results become available.

Histology: Punch biopsy or excisional biopsy specimens show a diffuse granulomatous inflammatory infiltrate. Pseudocarcinomatous epithelial hyperplasia often overlies the granulomatous infiltrate. Within the granulomatous portion of the dermal infiltrate are the characteristic spherules that contain endospores. The spherules are thick walled and can readily be seen on specimens routinely stained with hematoxylin and eosin stain. The spherule can be highlighted with the use of a silver stain.

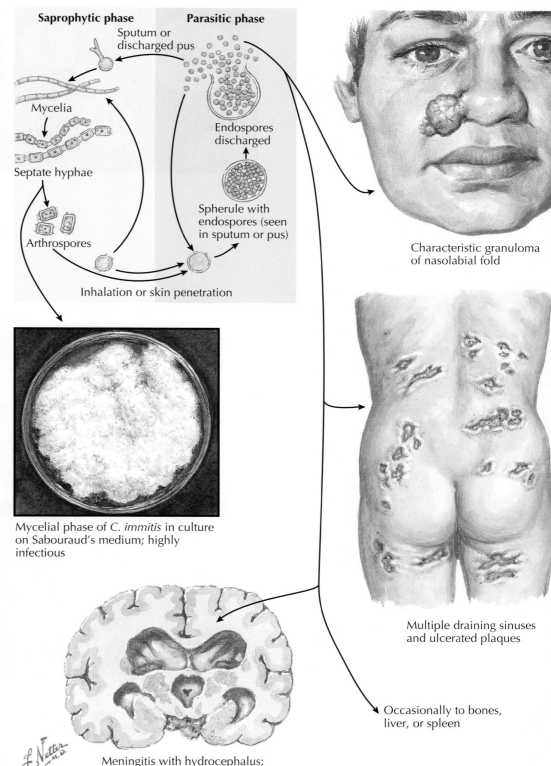

Characteristic granuloma of nasolabial fold

Mycelial phase of *C. immitis* in culture on Sabouraud's medium; highly infectious

Multiple draining sinuses and ulcerated plaques

Occasionally to bones, liver, or spleen

Meningitis with hydrocephalus; uncommon but often fatal

Pathogenesis: Coccidioidomycosis is caused by the soil-dwelling fungus, *C. immitis*. Endemic to the southwestern United States, Central America, and parts of South America, this fungus is found in the environment in its mycelial or mold phase. It produces white, light, and fluffy arthrospores. These arthrospores are highly infectious. Once inhaled, this dimorphic fungus turns into its yeast form. The yeast form is made of thick-walled spherules with multiple, centrally located endospores that can be released from the host by coughing or by drainage of an abscess. The resulting endospore readily converts back to its mycelial phase and can infect another host.

Treatment: The azole antifungals fluconazole and itraconazole are first-line therapies for coccidioidomycosis. Treatment typically lasts 6 to 12 months; prolonged therapy may be required in some cases. Severe, life-threatening cases and those refractory to azole antifungal medications are usually treated with amphotericin B. Adjunctive surgical treatment can be used to debride abscesses and remove isolated pulmonary disease.

Plate 6-5

Integumentary System

CRYPTOCOCCOSIS

Cryptococcosis is an opportunistic fungal infection caused by *Cryptococcus neoformans* or, less frequently, by *Cryptococcus gattii*. It is seen primarily in immunosuppressed patients such as patients taking chronic immunosuppressive medications and those with the acquired immunodeficiency syndrome (AIDS). A diagnosis of cryptococcosis in a patient with human immunodeficiency virus (HIV) infection is considered to be an AIDS-defining illness.

It is primarily a lung disease, but dissemination to the skin and to the central nervous system (CNS) are well described. Cryptococcosis has a higher tendency to affect the CNS than the other opportunistic fungi do. Primary cutaneous cryptococcosis is a rarely seen condition that is caused by direct inoculation of the yeast into the skin.

Clinical Findings: A variety of infectious outcomes can occur after exposure to this encapsulated yeast. Immunocompetent hosts typically do not show any signs or symptoms. On occasion, the fungus can be found colonizing the oropharynx and upper airway; this has been shown to be transient and appears to cause no harm. Most of the population in North America show serological evidence of exposure. If a colonized patient subsequently becomes immunosuppressed, the dormant fungus may cause disease. Cryptococcosis is ubiquitous in North America, and patients routinely come in contact with the fungus. Immunosuppressed patients who contact the fungus during routine outdoor environmental exposure may become infected. The fungus can be found in soil and is frequently found in bird droppings, especially those of pigeons. The fungus gains entry via inhalation. Once in the lung tissue, it is able to grow and reproduce. The host may develop signs of lung inflammation including cough, hemoptysis, pain, pleurisy, and pneumonia. The fungus eventually disseminates through the bloodstream to infect various tissues.

The skin is affected in up to 25% of patients with disseminated disease, especially those patients with AIDS. The lesions can appear as small white papules with a central dell that mimic molluscum contagiosum. The most commonly described morphology of cutaneous cryptococcosis is that of a red macule that can be large and can imitate cellulitis. Many other cutaneous morphologies have been described in the literature. Cutaneous nodules with underlying abscess formation and overlying ulcerations are not uncommon. Clinical suspicion should lead the physician to perform an incisional or punch biopsy for histological evaluation and microbiological culture to ascertain the diagnosis.

Pathogenesis: *C. neoformans* and *C. gattii* are opportunistic yeasts that are encapsulated. The capsule is critical in that it helps the fungus avoid host defenses. Various serotypes of the species exist. The host inhales the organism or accidentally becomes inoculated through a penetrating skin wound. The yeast can overcome the host's cell-mediated immunity if the immune system is compromised. This can lead to fungal abscess and hematogenous spread of the fungus. *Cryptococcus* is a unique fungus that has a neurotrophic behavior and often causes CNS disease.

Histology: The histological features are somewhat dependent on the immune status of the patient. In severely immunosuppressed patients, the biopsy specimen often shows a gelatinous appearance with numerous yeast cells and a mixed inflammatory infiltrate.

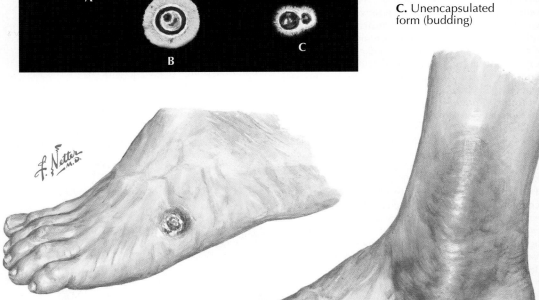

India ink preparation showing *C. neoformans*. No hyphae are seen.

A. Budding organism with thick capsule

B. Nonbudding organisms

C. Unencapsulated form (budding)

Skin lesions on foot and ankle. *Above,* Molluscum-like lesion. *Right,* Diffuse lesion involving lateral aspect of limb mimicking cellulitis.

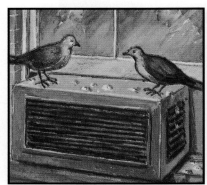
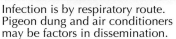

Infection is by respiratory route. Pigeon dung and air conditioners may be factors in dissemination.

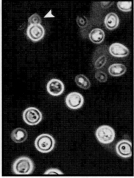

India ink preparation showing budding and capsule

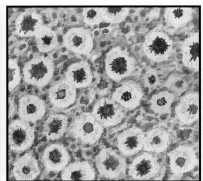

Accumulation of encapsulated cryptococci in subarachnoid space (PAS or methenamine-silver stain)

Immunocompetent patients are more likely to have a granulomatous infiltrate with few yeast organisms and a vigorous host granulomatous response. The yeast capsule can be stained with Alcian blue, India ink, or mucicarmine. Periodic acid–Schiff stain can be used to demarcate the central portion of the yeast.

Cultures of the fungus reveal fast-growing, off-white, mucoid colonies. The fungus is unique in that it can grow at varying temperatures, including the routine culture temperature of 24°C to 25°C and body temperature of 37°C. Microscopic examination reveals round, budding, encapsulated yeasts without hyphae. *C. neoformans* has unique biochemical features, such as its inability to ferment sugars, that allow mycologists to study and differentiate this organism from other fungi and from other cryptococcal species.

Treatment: Patients with a diagnosis of cutaneous cryptococcosis need to be evaluated for CNS involvement, because the therapy is very different. If a spinal fluid analysis shows evidence of fungal involvement, the treatment of choice is amphotericin B with or without flucytosine. If no nervous system involvement is present, long-term use of itraconazole or fluconazole can be prescribed. Cutaneous abscesses should be incised and drained to decrease the fungal load. Treatment considerations should also include the immune status of the patient and appropriate screening and testing for HIV infection.

Plate 6-6

Infectious Diseases

CUTANEOUS LARVA MIGRANS

Parasitic Diseases
Necatoriasis and Ancylostomiasis

Cutaneous larva migrans is a tropically acquired skin disease caused by the aimless wandering of a nematode larva. This disease has also been termed "creeping eruption" because of the slow, methodical movement underneath the skin, which subsequently manifests with the classic cutaneous findings. The most frequent cause of cutaneous larva migrans is the larva of *Ancylostoma braziliense* or *Ancylostoma caninum*. The cutaneous findings are similar among the various species that can cause disease. Treatments are effective for this condition, which causes more psychological than physical harm. Establishment of the specific larva responsible for the disease is not routinely attempted, nor is it practical or cost effective.

Clinical Findings: The larvae gain entrance into the epidermis through tiny abrasions, cuts, or any disruption of the normal epidermal layer. The larvae are frequently obtained during a barefoot walk on a contaminated beach or from a similar environment. Travelers to Central and South America often acquire the larvae on the beach while lying on or playing in the sand. The initial entry of the larvae goes entirely unnoticed. It is not until days to weeks later that the human host begins to develop cutaneous signs of the disease. The first evidence is a pink to red, edematous eruption that begins to take on a serpiginous course. The involved skin appears as red, squiggly lines. If only one larva is present, only one serpiginous line will be present. The line meanders and slowly elongates over days to weeks until the patient seeks medical advice. Patients who are infected with multiple parasites have multiple serpiginous areas of involvement, with some in a criss-crossing pattern. Pruritus is universal, but pain is infrequent. The lesions are typically elevated but can become vesicular in nature.

Pathogenesis: Cutaneous larva migrans is caused by penetration of the epidermis by one of the various larvae known to cause disease. The larvae are derived from eggs that are laid in the intestines of an infected animal, such as a dog, and then released in the stool. When the animal defecates, the eggs are readily passed into the soil, where they hatch into larvae. The human is an incidental or dead-end host, because the larva is unable to replicate or complete its life cycle in humans. This is very much different than infections with the gastrointestinal parasites *Ancylostoma duodenale* and *Necator americanus*, which require the human host to replicate. The larvae wander around the epidermis, unable to penetrate the basement membrane zone and therefore unable to enter the dermis. If the condition is left untreated, the larvae die in the skin within a few months. The larvae have been shown to secrete enzymes that help them travel throughout the epidermis, but they lack an enzyme to penetrate the dermal-epidermal junction.

Histology: The histopathology is nonspecific unless the actual larva is biopsied. This is highly unlikely, because the larva is typically an estimated 2 to 3 cm ahead of the leading edge of the serpiginous rash, and most biopsies are taken from the serpiginous region. The biopsy specimen shows a lymphocytic dermal infiltrate with eosinophils. Occasionally, a space is seen within the spongiotic epidermis, which indicates the area through which the larva passed.

Treatment: The mainstays of treatment are the anthelmintic agents. Albendazole and ivermectin are

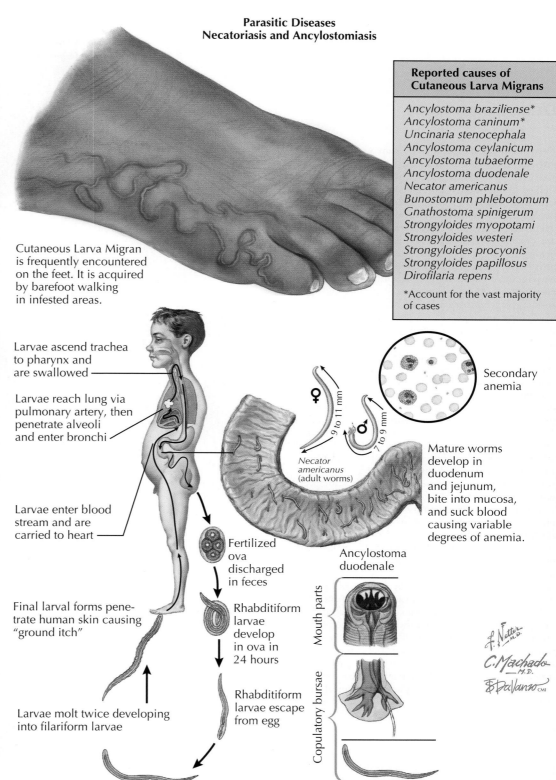

Cutaneous Larva Migran is frequently encountered on the feet. It is acquired by barefoot walking in infested areas.

Reported causes of Cutaneous Larva Migrans

Ancylostoma braziliense*
Ancylostoma caninum*
Uncinaria stenocephala
Ancylostoma ceylanicum
Ancylostoma tubaeforme
Ancylostoma duodenale
Necator americanus
Bunostomum phlebotomum
Gnathostoma spinigerum
Strongyloides myopotami
Strongyloides westeri
Strongyloides procyonis
Strongyloides papillosus
Dirofilaria repens

*Account for the vast majority of cases

Larvae ascend trachea to pharynx and are swallowed

Larvae reach lung via pulmonary artery, then penetrate alveoli and enter bronchi

Larvae enter blood stream and are carried to heart

Final larval forms penetrate human skin causing "ground itch"

Larvae molt twice developing into filariform larvae

Fertilized ova discharged in feces

Rhabditiform larvae develop in ova in 24 hours

Rhabditiform larvae escape from egg

Secondary anemia

♀ 9 to 11 mm   ♂ 7 to 9 mm

Necator americanus (adult worms)

Mature worms develop in duodenum and jejunum, bite into mucosa, and suck blood causing variable degrees of anemia.

Ancylostoma duodenale

Mouth parts

Copulatory bursae

the most frequently used medications. Oral ivermectin is well tolerated and works equally as well as the others. Ivermectin binds to glutamate-gated chloride channels in the parasites, allowing free passage of chloride and eventually death of the cell. Thiabendazole and albendazole work by inhibiting microtubule polymerization in the parasite, ultimately leading to its death. Thiabendazole and albendazole can cause severe gastrointestinal side effects, and they are best used topically. A pharmacist can compound these agents into a topical solution to apply to the affected area. Other therapies that have been attempted include cold therapy with topical liquid nitrogen, which is no longer advocated. The larvae have been shown to survive at subfreezing temperatures, and because one cannot predict with high certainty the location of the larva, a large area of skin must be treated with liquid nitrogen for the treatment to be effective.

Plate 6-7   Integumentary System

TINEA FACIEI AND TINEA CORPORIS

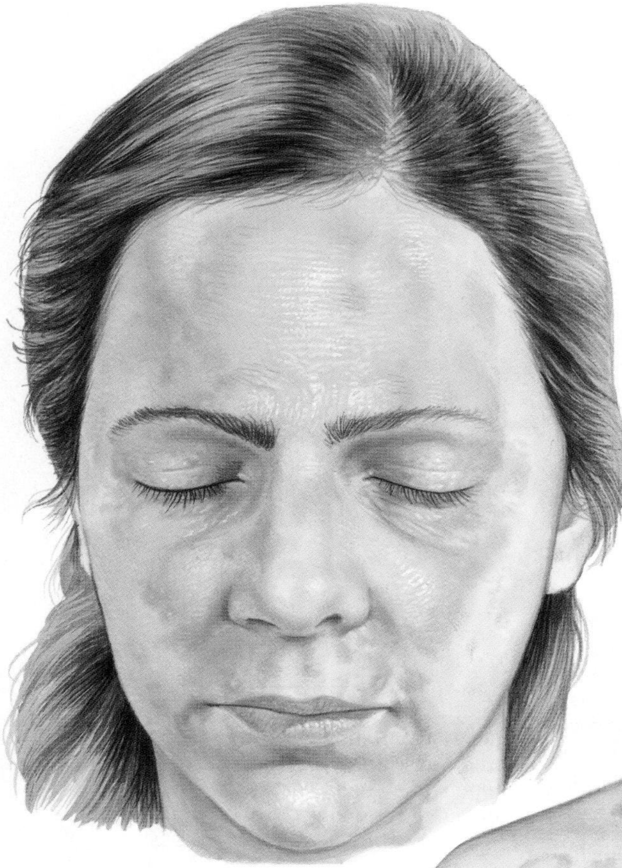

DERMATOPHYTOSES

Dermatophytes are classified in many ways by mycologists and physicians. One of the simplest classification systems is based on the natural living conditions of the studied fungi. Fungi can be classified as zoophilic (affecting mammals only), anthropophilic (affecting predominantly humans with little transference to other mammals), or geophilic (predominantly soil fungi that are capable of affecting mammals under the correct living conditions). This classification is widely used by physicians, because more complicated categorizations have minimal impact on the overall therapy and prognosis. Most of these infections are treated with topical antifungal agents that can be purchased over the counter, which have very high success rates. Fungal infections of the hair shaft and nails require systemic therapy for the highest efficacy of treatment. Topical antifungal agents do not penetrate the deeper layers of the stratum corneum, the nail plate, or the hair shaft, and in these cases systemic antifungals are required for therapy.

Clinical Findings: Superficial fungal infections have been around for millennia and have been reported in the literature under various names and descriptions. Most of the terms used for these infections are based on the location of the disease. An individual may be affected by more than one of these types concurrently. Immunocompetent individuals are less likely than those who are immunosuppressed to develop widespread disease.

Tinea corporis (ringworm) is a superficial dermatophyte infection of the skin of the trunk or extremities. It begins as a small red macule or papule and, over time, spreads out in an annular or polycyclic nature. The primary morphology of tinea infections is the scaly patch with a leading trail of scale. On close examination, one can observe a random amount of hair loss within the affected area. Most cases are mild and affect only one or two areas, but some can be widespread and can be associated with other forms of tinea such as tinea unguium. If tinea corporis is left untreated, the fungus will continue to spread out from the center of each lesion; lesions can merge into very large patches that may envelop almost the entire trunk or extremity.

Tinea faciei, as the name implies, occurs on the face. It appears as annular patches with a leading edge of scale. The scale is easily scraped off. In adult men, the term *tinea faciei* is used to describe disease in regions of the face other than terminal hair–bearing skin, such as the beard and scalp. The lesions may converge into polycyclic patches and are typically pruritic. This form of superficial fungal infection.is commonly seen in children. Sleeping in the same bed as pets may increase the risk of exposure to the causative fungus and the chance of acquiring any of the superficial fungal infections. *Trichophyton tonsurans* is the most likely etiological agent in North America.

Tinea barbae is a fungal infection in the beard region of postpubertal men. This infection often affects the skin as well as the hair follicles, and it can appear as red patches with follicle-based pustules. Many fungal species have been shown to cause this condition, with the zoophilic agents being more commonly responsible. *Trichophyton verrucosum* has been frequently reported,

Tinea faciei. Annular patches occur in a diffuse pattern. Extensive disease may be caused by topical corticosteroid use.

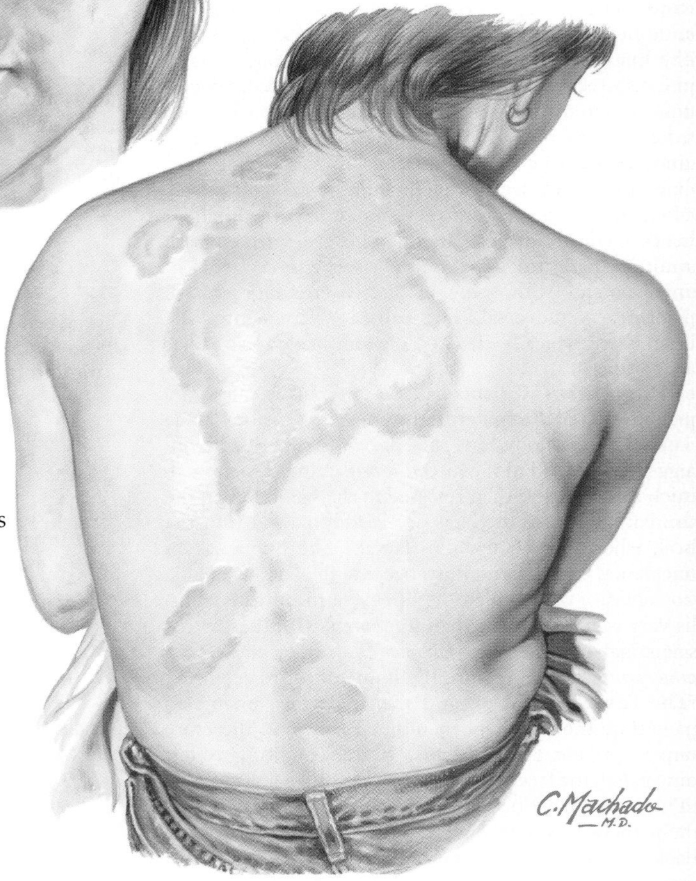

Tinea corporis. Annular scaly patches with a leading edge of scale

along with other *Trichophyton* species. The infection may form boggy, crusted plaques identical to a kerion of the scalp. If the lesions are plaque-like and affect the hair follicles, systemic therapy is needed.

Tinea cruris (jock itch) is one of the most easily recognized and prevalent forms of superficial fungal infections. The fungus prefers to live in dark, moist regions of the skin that stay at body temperature. The

groin a perfect location for fungal infections. The disease is often very pruritic, and this is what gives it the vernacular name, "jock itch." It is seen frequently in athletes but is by no means limited to them. *Trichophyton rubrum* and *Epidermophyton floccosum* are the most commonly reported etiological agents.

Tinea pedis (athlete's foot) is probably the superficial fungal infection that is best known to members of the

Plate 6-8

Infectious Diseases

DERMATOPHYTOSES (Continued)

general public, because of personal involvement or that of someone they know. This fungal infection is seen in two predominant types, the interdigital type and the moccasin type. The interdigital subtype forms macerated, red patches in the toe web spaces. The areas can become pruritic and can lead to onychomycosis. Moccasin-type tinea pedis involves the entire foot and is the less common of the two types. *T. rubrum* is the most frequent isolate in these cases.

Tinea manuum, also most frequently caused by *T. rubrum*, predominantly affects one hand only. It is commonly seen in association with bilateral tinea pedis and therefore has been called "one hand two feet disease." The reason that it affects only one hand is unknown. The most frequent complaint is itching and the appearance of the red annular patches.

Majocchi's granuloma is a form of fungal folliculitis caused by one of the dermatophyte species. It is universally seen in patients who have been treated with corticosteroids for a presumed form of dermatitis. As the patient continues to apply the steroid cream to the patch of fungal infection, the redness spreads, and pustules may form within the affected region. The pustules are based on a hair follicle, and the hair may be absent or easily pulled from the region with minimal or no discomfort. Removal of the hair and use of a potassium hydroxide (KOH) preparation allows the fungus to be seen. This form of folliculitis must be treated with a systemic agent, because the topical antifungals do not penetrate deep enough into the depths of the hair follicle or into the hair shaft, as would be required to treat an endothrix fungus. Fungal species are designated as endothrix or ectothrix species based on their ability to penetrate the hair shaft epithelium.

Tinea capitis is seen almost exclusively in children and is most commonly caused by *T. tonsurans*. This infection begins as a small, pruritic patch in the scalp that slowly expands outward. Hair loss is prominent because the fungus invades the hair shaft and can cause the hair to break. A frequent clinical sign is "black dot" tinea. This is the clinical finding of tiny, broken-off hairs that appear as black dots just at the level of the scalp. Posterior occipital adenopathy is always seen in cases of tinea capitis, and its absence should make one reconsider the diagnosis. If a child presents with a scaly patch in the scalp and associated hair loss, it should be treated as tinea capitis until proven otherwise. A KOH examination of the hair or of a scalp scraping often, but not always, shows evidence of a dermatophyte. A fungal culture can be used in these cases to confirm the diagnosis if the KOH examination is negative. The culture sample is easily obtained by rubbing the scaly patch with a toothbrush and collecting the scale that is removed in a sterile container. The cultures are grown in the laboratory on dermatophyte test medium (DTM), and growth is often seen in 2 to 4 weeks. Tinea capitis requires at least 6 weeks of systemic oral therapy to clear, and all the patients' pets, especially cats, should be evaluated by a veterinarian for evidence of disease.

A kerion is a boggy plaque found on occasion in tinea capitis that results from a massive immune inflammatory response to the causative fungal agent. The fungi most likely to cause this reaction are in the zoophilic

TINEA CRURIS AND TINEA CAPITIS

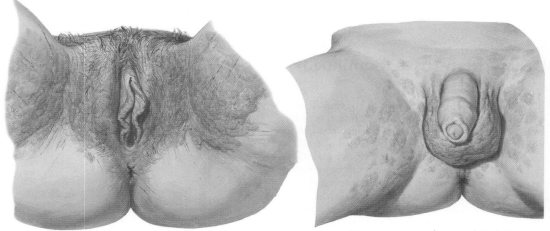

Tinea cruris (female)

Tinea cruris (male), "jock itch," a very common infecton in males

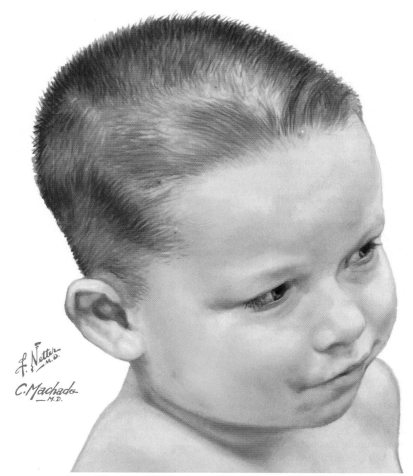

Tinea capitis. Scaly patches with associated alopecia

class. The kerion often appears as a large, inflamed, boggy-feeling plaque with alopecia. Serous drainage and crusting are also present. These plaques are very tender to palpation, and children complain of pain even when the lesions are not manipulated. Alopecia overlies the plaque, and if it is severe, a kerion can lead to permanent scarring alopecia. Posterior occipital and cervical adenopathy is present and tender to palpation. The kerion often become impetiginized with

bacteria, especially *Staphylococcus* species. Treatment is based on the use of systemic oral antifungals in association with an oral corticosteroid to decrease the massive inflammatory response. Any bacterial coinfections must be treated at the same time. Scarring alopecia may be permanent and may lead to morbidity for the child.

Tinea unguium, or onychomycosis, is clinically recognized by thick, dystrophic, crumbling nails. One or

Plate 6-9   Integumentary System

TINEA PEDIS AND TINEA UNGUIUM

Tinea pedis

The two most common forms of tinea pedis are interdigital and moccasin.

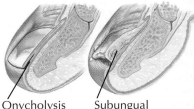

Area typically affected by interdigital tinea pedis

Area typically affected by the moccasin form of tinea pedis

Moccasin form of tinea pedis

DERMATOPHYTOSES (Continued)

all the nails on a foot or hand may be involved. Toenail infection is much more common than infection of the fingernails. Most patients start with tinea pedis, after which the fungus spreads to infect the nail plate. This results in thickening and yellowing of the nail. Over time, the nail becomes thickened with subungual debris that is easily removed with a blunt instrument such as a curette. The nail may become onycholytic and fall off the nail bed. Patients are most frequently asymptomatic, but some complain of discomfort and difficulty clipping their nails. Diabetic patients and those with peripheral vascular disease are at risk for bacterial cellulitis. The dystrophic nails serve as a nidus for infection with various bacteria. Nail disease requires the use of systemic oral medications to get the best therapeutic response. Topical agents have shown some benefit, but only for very mild nail involvement. A deep green discoloration under the nail is an indication of *Pseudomonas* nail colonization. The bacteria make a bright green pigment that is easily visible. Soaks in acetic acid (vinegar) diluted 1:4 in water are effective in clearing up the secondary *Pseudomonas*.

Dermatophytid reactions can occur with any dermatophyte infection. They are infrequently seen. They manifest as monomorphic, pink-red, scattered papules. They are typically pruritic and are most commonly seen in patients with a tinea capitis or kerion infection. Another manifestation of dermatophytid reactions is a deep vesicular reaction on the palms or soles. This can closely mimic dyshidrotic dermatitis. Treatment of the underlying fungal infection clears the dermatophytid reaction. Topical or oral corticosteroids may be used for relief until the fungal infection is cured.

The easiest, most sensitive, and most specific means of diagnosing the infection is by KOH examination. A scraping of the leading edge of the rash is taken and placed on a slide; KOH is added, and the preparation is heated for a few seconds. It is then viewed under a microscope for the characteristic branching and septated fungi of a dermatophyte. This method does not allow speciation of the fungus, which requires growth of cultures on fungal growth media. Each fungus has characteristic growth requirements and appears slightly different on microscopic evaluation of the cultured colonies.

Histology: Tinea corporis infections are rarely biopsied. When they are, one sees on close inspection fungal hyphae within the stratus corneum. Hyphae can be demonstrated with various staining methods. Neutrophils are the predominant cell type seen in the stratum corneum.

Pathogenesis: Dermatophyte infections are predominantly caused by three fungal genera: *Trichophyton*, *Microsporum*, and *Epidermophyton*. Multiple species within each of the first two genera have cutaneous effects; *Epidermophyton floccosum* is the only known species in the last genus to cause skin disease. Other genera have been implicated, but 99% of dermatophyte infections are caused by these three genera of fungi.

Treatment: Topical antifungal agents are the mainstay of treatment for tinea corporis, pedis, manuum, and cruris. Terbinafine is a topical fungicidal agent that has excellent efficacy against dermatophytes. The

Tinea unguium

Proximal subungual onychomycosis (PSO) Proximal white subungual onychomycosis (PWSO) Fungus infection reaches the nail plate via the cuticle, eponychium, or ventral face of the proximal nail fold.

Superficial white onychomycosis (SWO) The fungus infects the dorsal surface of the nail.

PSO secondary to paronychia Fungus from the lateral and/or proximal nail folds reaches the nail plate through the injured cuticle.

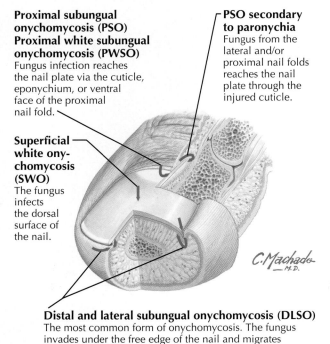

C. Machado M.D.

Distal and lateral subungual onychomycosis (DLSO) The most common form of onychomycosis. The fungus invades under the free edge of the nail and migrates proximally to involve the nail bed.

Onychomycosis. Classification by portals of entry

Oncholysis, subungual hyperkeratosis, splitting, crumbling and yellow longitudinal spikes are clinical features of distal and lateral subungual onychomycosis.

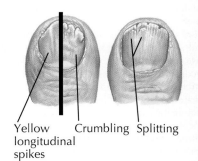

Onycholysis (detachment of the nail from its bed)

Subungual hyperkeratosis

Yellow longitudinal spikes

Crumbling

Splitting

topical azoles are used equally as often and also show excellent therapeutic results. Twice-daily treatment for 2 to 4 weeks usually is an effective treatment course. The importance of cleaning and drying the involved skin thoroughly cannot be understated. The fungi do not like to live in dry environments, and these simple steps can help treat and prevent the disease. Immunosuppressed individuals with widespread disease are candidates for oral antifungal agents.

Tinea capitis, tinea barbae, Majocchi's granuloma, and onychomycosis all require oral systemic treatment. Topical antifungals are ineffective in these cases because they do not penetrate deeply into the hair shaft or into the nail plate. Topical antifungals may be used in conjunction with the oral agents. The two most commonly prescribed oral antifungals are terbinafine and griseofulvin. The azole antifungal agents have also been used with excellent efficacy rates.

Plate 6-10

Infectious Diseases

LESIONS OF HERPES SIMPLEX

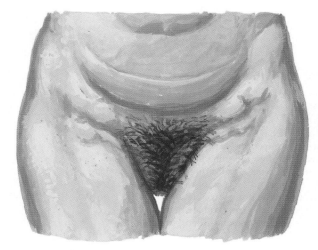

Regional tender lymphadenopathy is commonly seen in genital herpes.

HERPES SIMPLEX VIRUS

Herpes simplex virus type 1 (HSV1) and type 2 (HSV2) are the two viruses that are responsible for the production of both mucocutaneous and systemic disease. Mucocutaneous disease is overwhelmingly more common than systemic disease such as HSV encephalitis. HSV infections are ubiquitous in humans, and almost all adults develop antibodies against one of these viruses. Most infections are subclinical or so mild that they are never recognized by the patient. HSV infections are predominantly oral or genital. The virus becomes latent in local nerves and can be reactivated to produce future outbreaks. Currently, there are eight known herpesviruses that infect humans, including HSV1 and HSV2. HSV infections can cause severe, life-threatening central nervous system (CNS) disease in immunocompromised patients and in neonates. Many unique cutaneous forms of HSV have been described with their own clinical characteristics.

Clinical Findings: HSV can be spread from infected to uninfected individuals by close contact (e.g., kissing, sexual contact). The virus is shed from the infected host both when active lesions are present and when no clinical evidence of disease can be seen. It is believed that subclinical shedding of the virus is responsible for a great deal of transmission. HSV can cause oral labial disease (gingivostomatitis or herpes labialis) or genital disease, the main mucocutaneous forms of the disease. Most cases of oral labial disease are caused by HSV1, and genital disease is caused predominantly by HSV2. This is not always the case, and one can no longer assume the viral type from the clinical location of disease. HSV infections in other areas are becoming more common, and recurrent bouts of disease on the buttocks is one of the most frequently seen presentations.

The initial HSV infection can be subclinical, mild, or severe. Subsequent reactivation of the virus typically never approaches the severity seen in the initial primary infection. The exception occurs with immunosuppressed patients, in whom a widespread or chronic localized version of the infection may occur. Primary infection manifests with severe, painful mucocutaneous blistering and erosions. Primary oral labial herpes can lead to weight loss, fever, gingivitis, and pain. This is most commonly seen in children and is associated with tender cervical adenopathy. The infection spontaneously resolves within 2 to 3 weeks. If treated, the disease may be slightly decreased in length and severity, but this is highly dependent on the timing of diagnosis and initiation of therapy.

Herpes labialis is the term given to recurrent episodes of oral labial herpes. The episodes are milder than the primary infection and often start with a prodrome. Most patients complain of a tingling or painful sensation hours to a day before the appearance of herpes labialis. Patients can use this knowledge to their advantage and begin antiviral therapy at the first indication of recurrence to decrease the severity of the episode or abort it all together. Herpes labialis, also known as a cold sore, appears as a vesicle or bulla that quickly breaks down and forms an erosion and crusted papule or plaque. The lesions last for a few days to 1 week and can cause significant psychological issues.

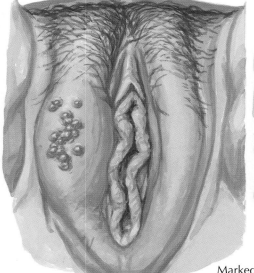

Grouped vesiculopustules on a tender red base

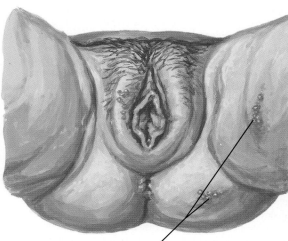

Marked edema and vesicle formation in primary herpes

Autoinoculation lesions

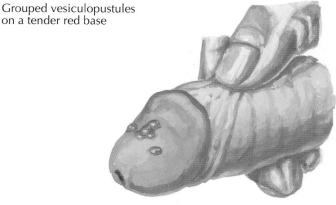

Primary HSV disease is almost always more severe than reactivation of HSV.

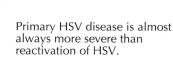

JOHN A. CRAIG—MD

Herpes infection of the genital region is spread by sexual contact and is one of the most common of all sexually transmitted diseases. Initial episodes of genital herpes infection manifest with fever, adenopathy, and painful ulcerations and blistering of the affected region. The primary episode is always more severe than subsequent reactivations of the virus. The ulcerations are grouped vesiculopustules on an erythematous base. They are extremely tender and easily rupture to form shallow ulcerations that appear "punched out" with an overlying serous crust. The cervix is often involved, and scarring can occur. Genital herpes infection almost universally causes dysuria and inguinal adenopathy that is tender.

Plate 6-11

Integumentary System

LESIONS OF HERPES SIMPLEX (CONTINUED)

HERPES SIMPLEX VIRUS
(Continued)

Recurrent episodes of genital herpes produce a milder version of the primary infection. The systemic constitutional symptoms are often absent, but the grouped vesicles and ulcers can cause excruciating pain and social stigma. The frequency and severity of recurrent episodes in an individual patient are variable and impossible to predict. A generalization can be made that those who have more severe primary infections tend to have more relentless recurrences.

Herpetic whitlow is the name given to a specific form of infection that is most commonly seen in medical laboratory workers and health care providers. It occurs from accidental inoculation of the herpesvirus into the skin. The finger is the area most commonly involved, because of accidental needle sticks. A painful primary viral infection may occur at the site of inoculation.

Eczema herpeticum, Kaposi's varicelliform eruption, is often encountered in a young child with severe atopic dermatitis who is exposed to the herpesvirus. Because of the widespread skin disease, the virus is able to infect a large surface area of the body. This results in extensive skin involvement with multiple vesicles and punched-out ulcerations.

The transmission of HSV from mother to child during the birthing process is of significant concern, and mothers with active HSV disease at the time of delivery most likely should undergo cesarean section to help decrease the risk of transmission. Neonatal HSV infection is a life-threatening disease. The neonate may have widespread multiorgan disease, with CNS involvement being the major cause of morbidity and mortality. Temporal lobe involvement can lead to seizures, encephalitis, and death. The skin is always infected, and this is a clue for the clinician to search for other organ system involvement, especially involvement of the CNS and the eye. Ocular infection can lead to severe corneal scarring and blindness.

HSV encephalitis is a life-threatening disease that causes a necrotizing encephalitis. Patients complain of an acute onset of fever and headache, with rapidly evolving seizures and focal neurological deficits. Without treatment, coma and death occur in three quarters of affected patients. The temporal lobes and insula are almost always affected. Prompt recognition and therapy have decreased the mortality rate to 1 in 4.

A Tzanck preparation is a long-used bedside procedure that takes only a few minutes to perform and is positive in cases of HSV1, HSV2, or varicella-zoster virus (VZV) infection. The procedure does not differentiate among the three viruses. However, HSV infection can be distinguished from varicella clinically. The procedure is done by unroofing a vesicle and scraping its base with a no. 15 blade scalpel. The scrapings are placed on a glass slide and allowed to air dry for 1 to 2 minutes. A blue stain such as Giemsa or toluidine blue is applied for 60 seconds and then gently rinsed off. The slide is dried, mineral oil is applied, and the preparation is covered with a microscope cover slip. It is then ready to be viewed. Multinucleated giant cells are readily seen throughout the sample, confirming the viral etiology of the blister.

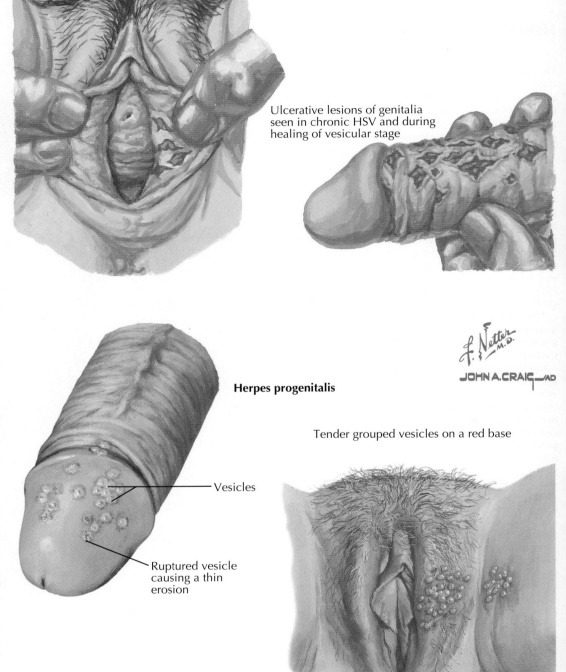

Ulcerative lesions of genitalia seen in chronic HSV and during healing of vesicular stage

Herpes progenitalis

Tender grouped vesicles on a red base

Vesicles

Ruptured vesicle causing a thin erosion

Herpes genitalis. Regional adenoopathy is often appreciate

Rapid immunostaining is available and can be used with high sensitivity and specificity to diagnose and differentiate the various herpesvirus types. This form of direct fluorescent antibody (DFA) testing is similar to the Tzanck preparation. As in the Tzanck preparation, scrapings of the blister base are placed on a glass microscope slide. The slide is stained with antibodies corresponding to the various herpesviruses. The sample is viewed under fluorescent microscopy, and a positive sample fluoresces with one of the specific viral stains. This test takes 1 to 2 hours to perform.

Viral tissue cultures can also be performed to differentiate the HSV types, but the results can take days to 1 week to obtain. This is the most sensitive and specific test for the infection.

Histology: Examination of a biopsy specimen of a blister shows ballooning degeneration of the epidermal keratinocytes. This degeneration forms the blister

Plate 6-12

Infectious Diseases

HERPES SIMPLEX VIRUS
(Continued)

cavity. There is a mixed inflammatory infiltrate around the superficial and deep dermal vascular plexus. Multinucleated giant cells are found at the base of the blister pocket. The skin biopsy findings are unable to differentiate HSV1 from HSV2 or from VZV infection.

Pathogenesis: HSV1 and HSV2 are double-stranded DNA viruses encased within a lipid envelope. Along with VZV, they are classified in the subfamily Alphaherpesvirinae. The five other human herpesviruses are classified slightly differently. The virus attaches to the host cells via specialized glycoproteins expressed on its lipid envelope. The lipid envelope then fuses with the host cell, allowing the virus to gain entry into the cytoplasm. Many glycoproteins are responsible for this attachment and fixation and the entrance into the host cell. The HSV capsid, which is an icosahedron-shaped structure, migrates from the cytoplasm to the nucleus of the cell. The viral capsid attaches to the nuclear membrane through the interaction of various membrane proteins and is capable of transferring its DNA into the cell nucleus.

Once the HSV DNA has gained entrance into the nucleus, it can become latent and quiescent or can actively replicate new virus particles. When they are actively replicating, the HSV particles often have a cytotoxic effect on the affected cell after viral replication has occurred; this ensures the production of viral progeny and their release from the host cell. HSV is capable of hijacking the host cell's replication protein apparatus. HSV uses the host cell DNA polymerase to replicate its DNA and uses the cellular machinery to produce proteins required for viral replication. The virus carries various DNA genes that can be expressed early during the course of infection or later when the virus is ready to produce progeny. The early gene products are important for replication and regulation of the viral DNA genes. The late gene products encode the viral capsid. Once the viral elements have been produced in sufficient quantity and in the proper ratio, the viral particles spontaneously converge to produce a capsid, which encapsulates the viral DNA. This occurs within the host cell nucleus. The virus then passes through the nuclear membrane and the cytoplasmic membrane, acquiring its lipid bilayer. At this point, the virus is free to infect another host.

Alternatively, after it enters the cell's nucleus, the virus may become latent. This is particularly the case in neural tissue. The viral DNA inserts itself into the host DNA, where it lies dormant and hidden from expression until reactivation occurs at some later time. It accomplishes this by specialized folding of the DNA and histone complex so as not to allow for viral gene expression. When the virus is reactivated and ready to produce viral particles, this mechanism of latency is somehow deactivated, allowing for viral reproduction.

Treatment: Therapy and its efficacy are highly dependent on the timing of administration. Antiviral medications work by inhibiting viral synthesis, and they work best when used early in the course of disease. Primary infections should all be treated with one of the antiviral agents in the acyclovir family. These closely

HERPES SIMPLEX VIRUS ENCEPHALITIS

Possible route of transmission in HSV encephalitis

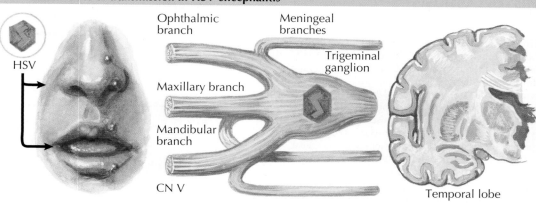

Ophthalmic branch · Meningeal branches · Trigeminal ganglion · Maxillary branch · Mandibular branch · CN V · Temporal lobe · HSV

Primary infection
Virus enters via cutaneous or mucosal surfaces to infect sensory or autonomic nerve endings with transport to cell bodies in ganglia.

Latent phase
Virus replicates in ganglia before establishing latent phase.

Reactivation (lytic phase)
Reactivation of HSV in trigeminal ganglion can result in spread to brain (temporal lobe) via meningeal branches of cranial nerve V.

Clinical features of HSV encephalitis

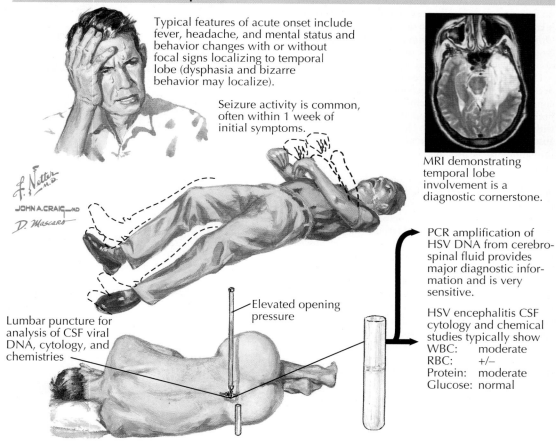

Typical features of acute onset include fever, headache, and mental status and behavior changes with or without focal signs localizing to temporal lobe (dysphasia and bizarre behavior may localize).

Seizure activity is common, often within 1 week of initial symptoms.

MRI demonstrating temporal lobe involvement is a diagnostic cornerstone.

Lumbar puncture for analysis of CSF viral DNA, cytology, and chemistries

Elevated opening pressure

PCR amplification of HSV DNA from cerebrospinal fluid provides major diagnostic information and is very sensitive.

HSV encephalitis CSF cytology and chemical studies typically show
WBC: moderate
RBC: +/−
Protein: moderate
Glucose: normal

related medications include acyclovir, famciclovir, valacyclovir, and topical penciclovir. Recurrent episodes of the disease can be treated at the time of outbreak or with a chronic daily suppressive regimen. Widespread eczema herpeticum, CNS infection, or infection in an immunosuppressed patient is probably best treated with intravenous antiviral medication. The acyclovir family of medications are converted to their active form by viral-specific thymidine kinase. After conversion, this

metabolite is a potent inhibitor of viral DNA polymerization. These medications are highly specific for the viral enzymes and have an excellent side effect profile. Acyclovir-resistant HSV has become well recognized and is best treated with foscarnet. Foscarnet does not require modulation by thymidine kinase to become an active inhibitor of HSV replication, thereby bypassing the HSV resistance mechanism. No medication to date has shown activity against latent viral infection.

Plate 6-13

Integumentary System

HISTOPLASMOSIS

Histoplasmosis is endemic in the Ohio River Valley but exists throughout North America and is also seen in Central and South America. It is a primary pulmonary disease, with the skin being secondarily involved in disseminated disease; however, isolated cutaneous disease can result from direct inoculation. The disease is typically seen in immunocompromised patients. Patients typically breathe in the infective spores, which lodge in the pulmonary tree. Most infections are subclinical.

Clinical Findings: The disease is seen primarily in immunocompromised patients. Other risk factors include occupations that increase the patient's contact with bat or bird droppings in an endemic region. The fungus is not found within bird droppings, but the droppings provide the perfect environment for the fungus to grow and reproduce. Patients inhale the spores into the lungs. Most have no symptoms. Some have mild flu-like symptoms that go undiagnosed or misdiagnosed as an upper respiratory infection. The primary infection heals, and the lungs may have visible findings on chest radiography. Variable radiographic findings are seen. Small, symmetrically located areas of hilar miliary calcification are the most common finding. Other lung findings can mimic those of tuberculosis, lung cancer, or metastatic cancer. Bilateral hilar adenopathy may be seen, as may lobar pneumonia.

Dissemination of the disease to other organs can occur in the immunocompromised host. The skin is commonly affected in disseminated disease. The skin findings often appear as papules, plaques, or nodules with varying degrees of ulceration. Subcutaneous abscess formation may occur, and fistulas and sinus tract formation may be prominent. Surrounding redness may give the appearance of cellulitis. Adenopathy in the draining lymph nodes is commonly appreciated. The diagnosis is dependent on the histological findings and the culture results.

Histology: Skin biopsy specimens show pseudocarcinomatous hyperplasia of the epidermis with an underlying granulomatous infiltrate. Ulceration and abscess formation are not uncommon with widespread necrosis. The yeast-like organisms can be appreciated in the cytoplasm of histiocytes. This is one of the few infections in which one sees phagocytized histiocytes. The yeast structures are round to oval, and there may be a clear region surrounding the yeast cell. Yeast organisms are also appreciated within the dermis, between and within the inflammatory infiltrate. They can be highlighted by use of special histology stains such as the periodic acid–Schiff stain or the Grocott silver stain.

The fungus is best cultured on Sabouraud's media. The fungus in its mycelial phase grows slowly. It appears as a brown, fluffy fungus on culture.

Pathogenesis: *Histoplasma capsulatum* is a dimorphic fungus that is responsible for a wide range of infections including pulmonary, pericardial, and cutaneous diseases. The fungus is ubiquitous in nature and is found in soil, where it lives as a saprophyte. Spores from the mycelial phase of the fungus are inhaled or inoculated directly into the skin. Once they have entered the body, the change in temperature causes transformation of the spores into the yeast form of *H. capsulatum*. Most infections go unnoticed, and most of the others induce a subclinical scenario or a mild, flu-like illness. Most cases are self-contained, and the only evidence of disease is the formation of granulomas within the lungs and a positive skin delayed-hypersensitivity test. If a

Ulcerating plaque of tongue due to histoplasmosis. Lesion may be identical in appearance to carcinoma of tongue.

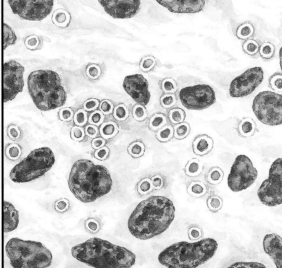

Mycelial or free-living phase of *H. capsulatum* as it exists in nature or in culture

Spores of mycelial phase of *H. capsulatum*. Inhalation of these is the source of infection.

Dimorphic fungus. *H. capsulatum* in tissue

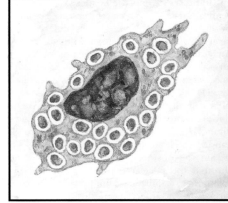

H. capsulatum in a macrophage, termed a *phagocytized histiocyte*. In this yeast or tissue phase, the organism is not transmissible from person to person.

preexposed or newly exposed patient becomes immunosuppressed, the patient is at risk for disease reactivation and serious sequelae.

Treatment: Most cases of primary pulmonary disease go undiagnosed, and the patient's immune system contains the fungus. In those patients with mild pulmonary symptoms who are not immunocompromised, therapies can be withheld, because most cases resolve spontaneously. Patients who have more severe disease or are

immunocompromised should be started on therapy with one of the three most efficacious and best-studied medications: fluconazole, itraconazole, or amphotericin B. Treatment may be prolonged. Patients who are found to have the acquired immunodeficiency syndrome benefit from directed therapy against the human immunodeficiency virus. Patients taking chronic immunosuppressants should have their medications discontinued or decreased, if possible.

Plate 6-14

Infectious Diseases

LEPROSY (HANSEN'S DISEASE)

Leprosy is a chronic multisystem disease with cutaneous findings that is caused by the bacteria, *Mycobacterium leprae*. It also goes by the name *Hansen's disease*. Gerhard Hansen was the Norwegian physician who first described *M. leprae* as the cause of leprosy in 1873. Leprosy is most prevalent in regions of Africa, Southeast Asia, and South America, and it can be seen in isolated regions of North America.

Clinical Findings: Cutaneous findings often begin as a solitary hypopigmented macule. The area of involvement often has a loss of sensation and temperature discrimination. This initial phase has been termed *indeterminate* leprosy. At this point, it is unknown what type of overall immune response the host will mount. After a period of time, if the host's cell-mediated immune response is able to keep the bacteria in check, the patient develops tuberculoid leprosy or paucibacillary leprosy. Tuberculoid leprosy manifests with one to three patches or plaques. The border tends to be raised, with a central depression. Adnexal structures, such as hair, are lost, and the lesions are often hypopigmented. This form of leprosy tends to affect the peripheral nerves (e.g., median nerve, ulnar nerve). Palpation of the involved nerve demonstrates enlargement and irregularly spaced nodules. Nerve involvement leads to impairment of the innervated skin and muscle.

Those patients who do not mount a strong cell-mediated immune reaction develop lepromatous leprosy or multibacillary leprosy. Up to hundreds of hypopigmented patches and plaques may be present. Hair loss may occur in the affected skin and along the eyelashes and eyebrows. This form of leprosy can affect many nerves in a widespread region, leading to neuropathy. There are varying degrees of cell-mediated immune response, and the disease is classified by the Ridley-Jopling system.

Pathogenesis: *M. leprae* is an acid-fast mycobacterium that is found in environments where the temperature averages approximately 29°C. Most likely, the bacterium is inhaled and subsequently invades the skin and other tissues by hematogenous spread. This bacterium is classified as an obligate intracellular organism. It survives within histiocytes, in which it is protected from host defense systems. Infected individuals with a poor immune response develop lepromatous leprosy, whereas those with an excellent response develop tuberculoid leprosy. Several genes are being evaluated as potential susceptibility markers, because it appears that the organism is not highly contagious. It is estimated that only 5% of those exposed eventually develop disease. This bacterium is highly unusual in that it can infect peripheral nerves. The bacterium expresses a protein, phenolic glycolipid 1 (PGL-1), that has the ability to bind to peripheral nerve cells. This allows initial entry into the host and provides the bacteria with a place to replicate. Many other tissue types can be infected.

Histology: The skin biopsy can be extremely helpful in confirming or making the diagnosis of leprosy. The biopsy findings are highly dependent on the type of leprosy the patient develops. Biopsies of paucibacillary leprosy show a granulomatous infiltrate with few bacteria present. The bacteria can be sparsely located, and the tissue must be stained with a modified acid-fast stain (Fite method) to appreciate the small, red, rod-shaped bacteria. These can be seen only with an oil-immersion objective.

In multibacillary leprosy, the infiltrate is a mixed dermal infiltrate with an overlying Grenz zone. The

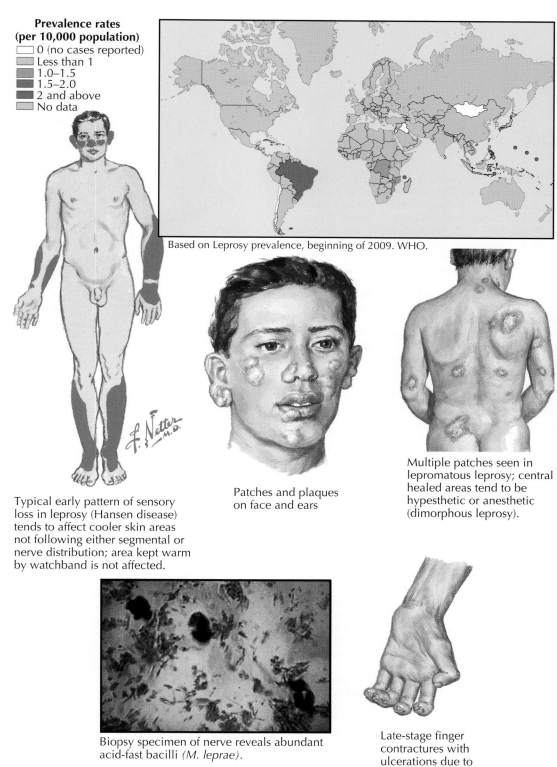

Prevalence rates (per 10,000 population)
- 0 (no cases reported)
- Less than 1
- 1.0–1.5
- 1.5–2.0
- 2 and above
- No data

Based on Leprosy prevalence, beginning of 2009. WHO.

Typical early pattern of sensory loss in leprosy (Hansen disease) tends to affect cooler skin areas not following either segmental or nerve distribution; area kept warm by watchband is not affected.

Patches and plaques on face and ears

Multiple patches seen in lepromatous leprosy; central healed areas tend to be hypesthetic or anesthetic (dimorphous leprosy).

Biopsy specimen of nerve reveals abundant acid-fast bacilli *(M. leprae)*.

Late-stage finger contractures with ulcerations due to sensory loss

dermal infiltrate is made up of plasma cells, lymphocytes, and foamy histiocytes. The histiocytes, when observed under oil immersion, show numerous bacteria. Bacteria are also seen scattered throughout the dermis.

Treatment: Guidelines for the treatment of leprosy have been established by the World Health Organization (WHO), and one should always refer to the most recent information when treating this disease.

Treatment is based on the bacillary load. Paucibacillary disease can be treated with a regimen of rifampin, minocycline, ofloxacin, and dapsone. The treatment schedule varies during the course of therapy, which is 6 months long, and following the protocol is extremely important. Multibacillary disease requires longer therapy and uses a combination of dapsone, clofazimine, and rifampin.

Plate 6-15   Integumentary System

LICE

Lice are nonflying insects that live off the blood meal from a human host. They have been human pathogens for thousands of years and continue to cause millions of cases of disease annually. Three variants of the louse exist: the head louse, the body louse, and the pubic louse. For the most part, lice cause localized skin disease from the biting they do to secure their blood meal. However, some lice have been known to transmit other diseases to humans. The most important infectious agents transmitted by body lice are the bacteria that cause epidemic typhus, relapsing fever, and trench fever. These infections are uncommon in the United States and North America but are still seen, and one should be aware of their causes and vectors.

Clinical Findings: Lice are capable of infesting any human, independent of age, sex, or race. Body lice are seen more frequently in patients of low socioeconomic status and especially in homeless individuals. Underlying mental health issues in this subset may also predispose one to conditions that are opportune for infestation. Pubic lice, or "crabs," is a sexually transmitted disease that is seen in younger adults more frequently than in other age groups; however, it has been reported to occur in people all ages.

Pediculosis capitis (head lice infestation) is probably the most common louse infestation in North America and Europe. The louse, *Pediculus humanus capitis*, preferentially locates to the scalp and lives between the hair shafts. These lice are transmitted by close contact and from fomites such as combs, pillows, and head rests. Patients complain of severe itching on the scalp and neck. On inspection, small (1-2 mm), red, excoriated papules are seen. Evidence of scratching becomes prominent as time goes on without a diagnosis. The diagnosis is confirmed by finding a louse, which is typically 2 to 4 mm long and light brown in color. On occasion, the abdomen of the louse can appear red, which is the case directly after a blood meal. These insects are not particularly fast moving, nor can they fly or jump; as a result, they are easy to capture and identify. Egg sacks (nits) are firmly adhered to the hair. This is in contrast to the common hair cast, which can easily be moved up and down the hair shaft with minimal effort. The nits are laid in close proximity to the scalp, usually within 0.5 mm. The nits hatch within 2 weeks. Therefore, nits found more than 2 cm from the scalp are often nonviable, and the larva has already emerged from the nit. Persistent infections can lead to bacterial superinfection and pyoderma with cervical adenopathy.

Pediculosis pubis (pubic lice infestation) is a commonly acquired sexually transmitted disease. The pubic louse, *Phthirus pubis*, is structurally different from the body or head louse and can easily be distinguished. Patients complain of itching and often note pinpoint drops of blood in their undergarments. This is caused by small amounts of bleeding after the pubic lice feed. These lice have specialized arms that allow them to climb around the entire human body, and they may be seen at any location. They have a tendency to affect the

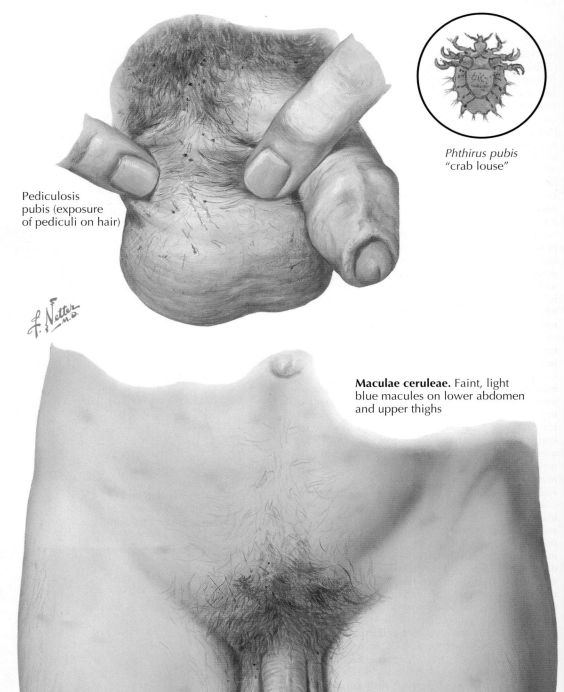

Pediculosis pubis (exposure of pediculi on hair)

Phthirus pubis "crab louse"

Maculae ceruleae. Faint, light blue macules on lower abdomen and upper thighs

eyelashes and eyebrows. This is important to look for clinically, to appropriately treat all affected regions.

Pediculosis corporis (body lice infestation) is commonly seen in homeless individuals and in those with poor hygiene. Historically, body lice have been associated with epidemics during times of war, because close contact for extended periods leads to easy transfer from one host to another. The body louse, *Pediculus humanus corporis*, is indistinguishable from the head louse on inspection with the naked eye. Entomologists trained in differentiating the species are capable of discerning the two. Body lice live on the clothing and leave it to feast on human blood. Patients present with multiple pruritic, red to pink, excoriated papules anywhere on the body. On inspection of the skin, one typically will not find lice. It is only with close inspection of the clothing or bedding material that the infestation becomes apparent. Hundreds to thousands of lice may

Plate 6-16

Infectious Diseases

LICE (Continued)

be present on the clothing, particularly in small hiding spaces such as the seams. Along with the lice, many eggs and larvae may be seen.

The body louse has been shown to be a carrier of the bacterial agents that cause relapsing fever, trench fever, and epidemic typhus: *Borrelia recurrentis*, *Bartonella quintana*, and *Rickettsia prowazekii*, respectively. The louse carries the bacteria within its gut.

B. recurrentis is responsible for causing the disease relapsing fever. It is transmitted from one human to another when the fecal material of a human body louse gains entry into the bloodstream. This bacterium is unique in that it can rearrange its surface proteins. This is believed to be the reason for the relapsing and recurrent fevers: The host immune system reacts in a periodic manner to the changing surface of the bacteria.

B. quintana is a bacterium that is transmitted through the feces of the louse. After a louse defecates on a patient's skin and the patient scratches, the stool and the bacteria are implanted into the skin, which causes infection. Also, the louse often bites after defecating and causes skin trauma that transfers the bacteria into the skin. *B. quintana* is the etiologic agent of trench fever, bacillary angiomatosis, and peliosis and has also been shown to cause endocarditis. *B. quintana* infections are most commonly seen in patients who are infected with the human immunodeficiency virus and in homeless individuals.

R. prowazekii is an obligate intracellular parasite that is transmitted to humans through the feces of the human body louse. The natural environmental reservoir for this bacterium is the flying squirrel (*Glaucomys volans*). The infected louse feeds on the human, and the fecal material that contains the *R. prowazekii* bacteria is deposited into the fresh wound, allowing for infectious transfer. This infection is most frequently seen during times of war, when individuals are in close contact with one another for significant periods. Signs and symptoms of epidemic typhus include fever, rash, pain, delirium, and other constitutional symptoms.

Pathogenesis: *P. humanus capitis* affects humans and has a high propensity to infest the scalp. These lice live on the host and periodically take a blood meal from the scalp or neck area. In patients with very long hair, the blood meal may be taken from the back or any area of skin that is in contact with the hair. The lice are able to reproduce rapidly. The females, which are a bit larger than the males, lay eggs that hatch and develop into adults capable of reproducing within 4 weeks.

Histology: The histological findings on skin biopsy are similar among all forms of louse bites. Histological evaluation cannot differentiate a louse bite from any other insect bite with certainty. Skin biopsies are rarely performed in these cases, because the diagnosis is made clinically. Biopsy specimens show a nonspecific, mixed superficial and deep inflammatory infiltrate with eosinophils. This may suggest a bite reaction. Unlike tick bites or scabies, in which occasionally tick parts or scabies mites are seen in a biopsy specimen, a biopsy from a patient with a lice infestation will never show mouth parts or other elements of the louse.

CLINICAL FINDINGS AND MANAGEMENT OF LICE

Clinical findings

Intense itching in pubic area (often nocturnal) is a hallmark of parasitic infection, and excoriations are common.

Bluish skin discolorations (maculae ceruleae) are often seen with *Phthirus pubis* infestations.

Secondary infection of excoriations or bites may yield impetiginized lesions.

Examination of pubic area and pubic hair may reveal ova and parasites.

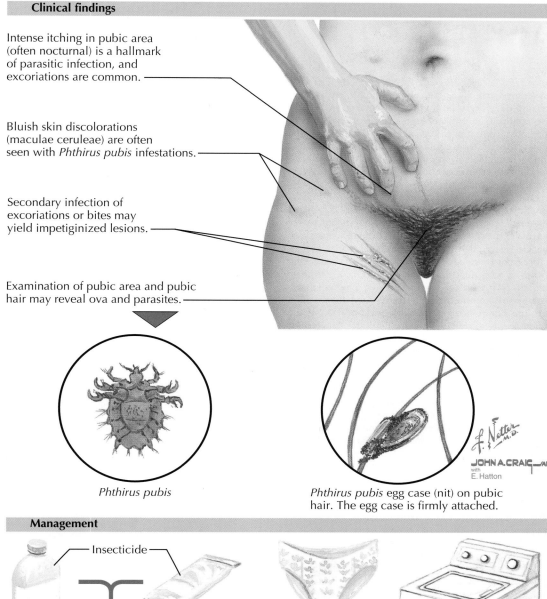

Phthirus pubis

Phthirus pubis egg case (nit) on pubic hair. The egg case is firmly attached.

Management

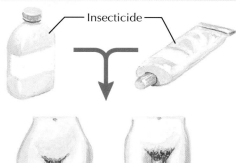
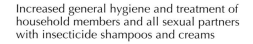

Insecticide

Increased general hygiene and treatment of household members and all sexual partners with insecticide shampoos and creams

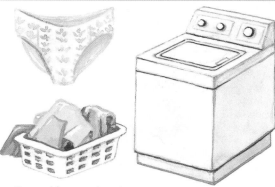

General house cleaning with emphasis on disinfection and laundering of underclothing and bedding

Treatment: Therapeutic agents to treat lice are similar among all species of human lice. The most commonly used therapies are based on permethrin; when used appropriately, they show good cure rates. These treatments should be used in conjunction with an agent that helps remove the nits from the hair shafts, and physical removal with a lice hair comb is a must. Therapy should be repeated on a weekly basis. Bedding and clothing need to be disinfected. The use of lindane has decreased because of its potential neurotoxicity. Malathion and oral ivermectin show excellent efficacy. Oral ivermectin needs to be repeated in 1 week, because it does not kill the developing larvae within the nits.

Therapy for body lice also requires complete disinfection of the household or living areas. Overtly infested clothing should be thrown away. Professional fumigation should be considered.

Plate 6-17

Integumentary System

LYME DISEASE

Lyme disease is a tickborne infection caused by the spirochete bacteria, *Borrelia burgdorferi*. The deer tick, *Ixodes scapularis*, is the main tick responsible for transmitting the disease to humans. Discovered in 1975 in the Connecticut town of Lyme, this disease has become the most common tickborne disease in the United States. Most cases are reported in the spring, summer, and early fall, correlating with tick activity. The disease not only affects humans but has been reported to affect dogs, horses, and cattle.

Clinical Findings: Erythema migrans is the characteristic cutaneous rash of Lyme disease. Erythema migrans typically manifests as a solitary "bull's-eye" macule at the site of the tick bite. There is a central red macule surrounded by nonaffected skin, which is then entirely surrounded by an expanding erythema that blends in with the normal skin. The rash of erythema migrans is larger than 2 cm in diameter. The rash manifests soon after the tick has transmitted the bacteria into the skin. Occasionally, the central portion of the lesion forms a vesicle or bulla. Solitary skin lesions are the most frequent skin manifestation, but one can also encounter early disseminated Lyme disease. This results in multiple areas of skin involvement. The numerous skin lesions are smaller than the original lesion, lighter in color, and not as fully developed as bull's-eye lesions. This early dissemination of *B. burgdorferi* occurs in one quarter of infected individuals. Most patients also exhibit constitutional symptoms at the time of diagnosis, including headache, fever, and malaise.

Erythema migrans occurs in approximately 75% of those infected with the spirochete. Individuals who do not exhibit the rash and those who go without treatment are likely to develop chronic disease, which manifests in many ways. Lyme arthritis is one of the most frequent manifestations of chronic Lyme disease; it is typically oligoarticular in presentation. Another of the more frequently seen manifestations is Bell's palsy, which is caused by involvement of the central nervous system. The cardiovascular, nervous, musculoskeletal, and hematological systems may all be involved in chronic Lyme disease.

Histology: Skin biopsies of erythema migrans show a lymphocytic superficial and deep dermal infiltrate. Numerous plasma cells may be seen in conjunction with eosinophils. Spirochetes are seen in fewer than half of specimens. The pathological findings of erythema migrans are used to help confirm the clinical findings. However, one should not wait for the pathology report to treat a patient with clinical evidence of Lyme disease.

Pathogenesis: *B. burgdorferi* is a spirochete that is transmitted to humans via the bite of the deer tick (*I. scapularis*). The white-tailed deer and the white-footed mouse are the two reservoirs for *B. burgdorferi*. These two animals are typically unaffected by the bacteria. The larval, nymph, or adult form of the *I. scapularis* tick takes a blood meal from one of these reservoirs and acquires the bacteria. The spirochete causes the tick no harm and can survive in the gut of the tick for prolonged periods. The tick can then transmit the bacteria to an incidental host such as a human. Transmission of the bacteria is increased the longer the tick is attached to the host. It is generally believed that a tick must be attached for 24 hours to transmit the bacteria.

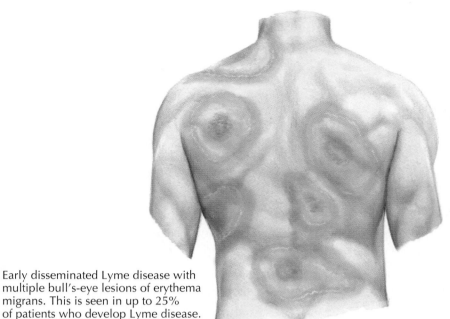

Early disseminated Lyme disease with multiple bull's-eye lesions of erythema migrans. This is seen in up to 25% of patients who develop Lyme disease.

Lyme disease is spread by a bite from an *Ixodes scapularis* tick that is infected with *Borrelia burgdorferi*.

Bell's Palsy: Common Manifestation of Chronic Lyme Disease

Hyperacusis	Left peripheral VII facial weakness	Left central VII facial weakness
	Attempt to close eye results in the eyeball rolling superiorly, exposing sclera (Bell's phenomenon), but no closure of the lid per se.	

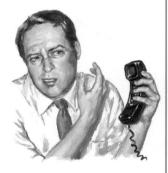

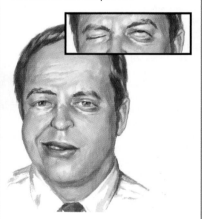

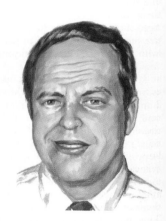

This may be an early or initial symptom of a peripheral VII nerve palsy: patient holds phone away from ear because of painful sensitivity to sound. Loss of taste also may occur on affected side.

Patient is unable to wrinkle forehead; eyelid droops very slightly; cannot show teeth at all on affected side in attempt to smile; and lower lip droops slightly.

Patient has an incomplete sm with very subtle flattening of affected nasolabial fold and relative preservation of brow and forehead movement.

Treatment: Treatment of erythema migrans consists of a 3-week course of doxycycline. The therapy is highly effective and has an excellent safety profile. Amoxicillin can be used for patients who cannot take doxycycline and for young children. Central nervous system involvement requires intravenous therapy with ceftriaxone or penicillin. Prevention is critically important. Permethrin-based insect repellants are effective at repelling deer ticks. Clothing impregnated with permethrin can be purchased for those who spend time outdoors in endemic areas.

After being in a wooded region, people should check their skin for the presence of ticks and remove them immediately, because the transmission of the spirochete requires approximately 24 hours of attachment. This inspection method works for adult ticks, but the larvae and nymphs are too small to see routinely and are almost always overlooked.

Plate 6-18

Infectious Diseases

Lymphogranuloma Venereum

Lymphogranuloma venereum (LGV) is a sexually transmitted disease (STD) that is produced by infection with *Chlamydia trachomatis* serotypes L1, L2, and L3. The disease progresses through three distinct phases of transmission. This bacterial disease was once limited to tropical regions, but with the ease of worldwide travel, it can now be seen globally. The skin manifestations are found predominantly in the groin and genital region. This disease is often seen in conjunction with other STDs, and screening for other STDs should be done routinely in patients diagnosed with LGV.

C. trachomatis has also been shown to be responsible for many infectious complications, including pneumonia, urogenital infections, conjunctivitis, and trachoma. Trachoma, which often starts as conjunctivitis, results in chronic intense inflammation of the bulbar and eyelid conjunctiva that causes scarring and eventually blindness if left untreated. Trachoma and conjunctival disease are caused by the A, B and C serotypes of *C. trachomatis*.

Clinical Findings: LGV is a rare disease in the United States and Europe but should be considered in the differential diagnosis of all anogenital ulcerations. The disease is seen more frequently in patients with a low socioeconomic status and in those with multiple sexual partners. LGV is passed from one individual to another via sexual intercourse. After a short incubation period (a few days to a few weeks), a painless papule forms and ultimately ulcerates. The ulcer is small (≤1 cm in diameter) and without induration. This ulceration is often described as painless, but it causes the patient irritation and discomfort with pressure and manipulation. This primary stage of the disease spontaneously resolves without therapy. The ulcer heals, leaving only a slight scar.

The secondary stage of disease begins with inguinal adenopathy. The inguinal lymph nodes become enlarged and painful. Initial involvement occurs within 2 to 3 weeks after healing of the ulcer and typically results in discrete, painful lymph nodes on each side of the inguinal crease. The lymph nodes coalesce over time and mat together into a large mass of tissue called buboes. If both sides of Poupart's ligament are involved, this can lead to a characteristic clinical finding named the *groove sign*. This name denotes the massive adenopathy on each side of Poupart's ligament; the groove is the area overlying the ligament with no adenopathy. The massive adenopathy may become necrotic, and suppurative lymph nodes are frequently seen. Sinus tracts from the adenopathy to the surface of the skin form and drain. This second stage is associated with fever and constitutional symptoms.

The third stage or late stage of LGV is less frequently seen and consists of scarring and fibrosis as well as elephantiasis of the genitals. If the primary and secondary diseases have affected the rectum, rectal fissures and strictures may be present, leading to chronic pain. Rectal disease is most frequently encountered in the male homosexual population.

Pathogenesis: *C. trachomatis* is a gram-negative obligate intracellular bacterium. It is unique in that it has no ability, or only limited ability, to produce its own adenosine triphosphate (ATP) energy source. This inability to create a steady source of energy forces the bacterium to reside within a host cell. The infectious form of the bacterium, called the elementary body, gains entry into a host cell. Within the cell, it forms a larger, actively reproducing reticulate body. The reticulate body undergoes binary fission to produce progeny

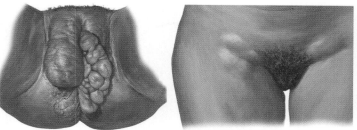

Lymphogranuloma venereum causing chronic lymphedema *(left)* and inguinal adenopathy *(right)*

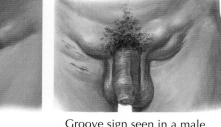

Groove sign seen in a male patient wih lymphogranuloma venereum caused by massive adenopathy on either side of Poupart ligament

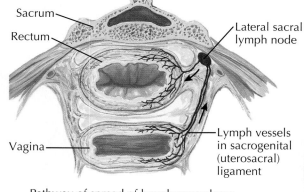

Sacrum

Rectum

Lateral sacral lymph node

Vagina

Lymph vessels in sacrogenital (uterosacral) ligament

Pathway of spread of lymphogranuloma (lymphopathia) venereum from upper vagina and/or cervix uteri to rectum via lymph vessels

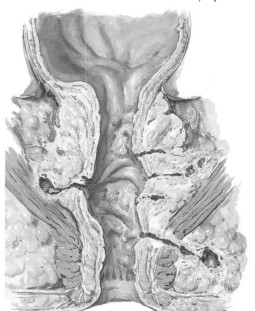

Stricture of rectum with multiple blind sinuses; strictures cause chronic pain and are a significant source of morbidity

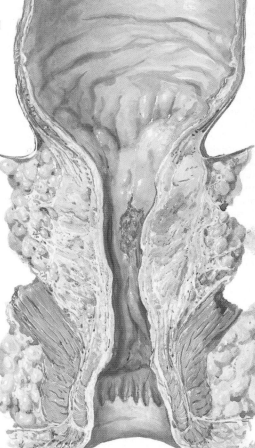

Long tubular stricture of rectum

(elementary bodies), which are then released from the cell to infect other cells or hosts.

Histology: A skin biopsy of a primary ulcer of LGV shows epithelial necrosis with a mixed, nonspecific inflammatory infiltrate. There are no pathognomonic histological findings in LGV. A tissue culture (McCoy cell culture) is the only reliable means of diagnosis. The finding of iodine-staining, glycogen-containing inclusion bodies is sensitive and specific for the presence of

C. trachomatis. Various serological tests are available, but they cannot reliably differentiate between past and present disease.

Treatment: The routine application of erythromycin to the eyes of newborns has dramatically decreased the risk of trachoma. LGV is treated with oral antibiotics in the tetracycline or erythromycin class. All sexual partners should also be treated, even if they do not exhibit overt signs of disease.

Plate 6-19   Integumentary System

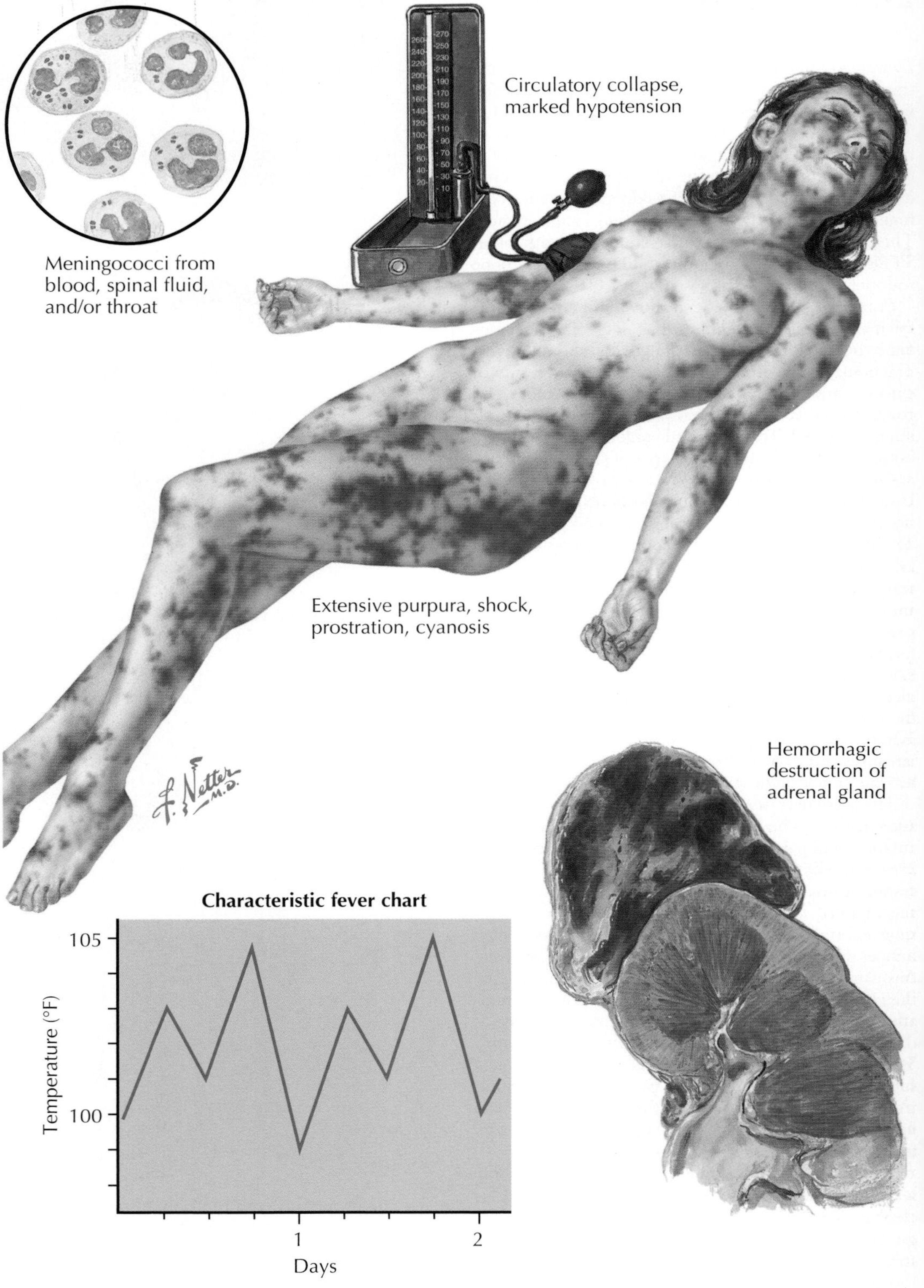

MENINGOCOCCEMIA

Meningococcemia can cause a wide range of clinical diseases, of which neisserial meningitis is the most severe and life-threatening. The bacteria, *Neisseria meningitidis*, is capable of causing septicemia, pneumonia, and meningitis. These are all relentless diseases that are universally fatal if not promptly treated. The bacteria has been known to cause severe disseminated intravascular coagulation (DIC) and the Waterhouse-Friderichsen syndrome. The latter syndrome, also known as acute adrenocortical insufficiency, is directly caused by hemorrhagic destruction of both adrenal glands. This syndrome can result from a wide range of conditions, including infections, and *N. meningitidis* is one of the more frequent infectious causes.

Clinical Findings: Children younger than 1 year of age are those most likely to develop disease from *N. meningitidis* infection. Boys are more apt to develop this infection than girls, and there is no race predilection. One risk factor appears to be the presence of a smoker in the household. It is theorized that the secondhand smoke damages the child's respiratory epithelium just enough to allow the bacteria to penetrate the mucous membranes and enter the bloodstream. Other risk factors include a deficiency of the complement components C5, C6, C7, and C8. Asplenia also increases one's risk, because the spleen is extremely important in removing encapsulated bacteria from the bloodstream. Chronic immunosuppression increases the risk, as does living in crowded conditions. This is why military barracks and college dormitories are often sources of outbreaks.

Patients who develop meningitis have fever, headache, vomiting, stiff neck, and meningeal physical signs, including Kernig's sign and Brudzinski's sign. Kernig's sign is positive when placing a patient's hips and knees in 90-degree flexion and extending the knee joint elicits pain. Brudzinski's sign is more sensitive for meningitis and is positive when flexing of the patient's neck causes flexion of the hips and knees. These signs have long been used to help diagnosis meningitis clinically. As the disease progresses, seizures or coma may occur.

Cutaneous findings include palpable purpura, ecchymosis, widespread macular purpura, and necrosis of the skin with secondary vesiculopustules. The purpura can be angulated with an irregular border. Centrally within the purpuric region, there is often a dusky gray discoloration of the skin. Patients often complain of skin pain. Necrosis may progress to cause gangrene of the digits or distal extremities. In severe cases, entire limbs can become gangrenous. If DIC sets in, the clinical skin findings of DIC may be seen on top of the initial skin findings. The presence of DIC is a poor prognostic indicator.

Fulminant meningococcal septicemia may lead to hemorrhagic necrosis of the adrenal glands; this is termed the Waterhouse-Friderichsen syndrome. It leads ultimately to acute adrenal dysfunction. This

ACUTE ADRENAL INSUFFICIENCY (WATERHOUSE-FRIDERICHSEN SYNDROME)

Meningococci from blood, spinal fluid, and/or throat

Circulatory collapse, marked hypotension

Extensive purpura, shock, prostration, cyanosis

Hemorrhagic destruction of adrenal gland

Characteristic fever chart

syndrome is seen in fewer than 5% of patients with *N. meningitidis* septicemia, but it occurs in more than 50% of the fatal cases. Patients present with skin findings of widespread purpura and cyanosis. They have signs and symptoms of hemodynamic collapse, hypotension, acute renal failure, and a biphasic fever. The skin findings are caused by small-vessel embolization or endothelial destruction from the septicemia. Blood extravasates through the damaged endothelial walls and produces massive purpura. The more extensive the cutaneous purpura in meningococcal septicemia, the higher the incidence of Waterhouse-Friderichsen syndrome.

Laboratory testing can be used to diagnosis the disease, but one should not wait for the results to begin therapy if there is a high clinical suspicion of

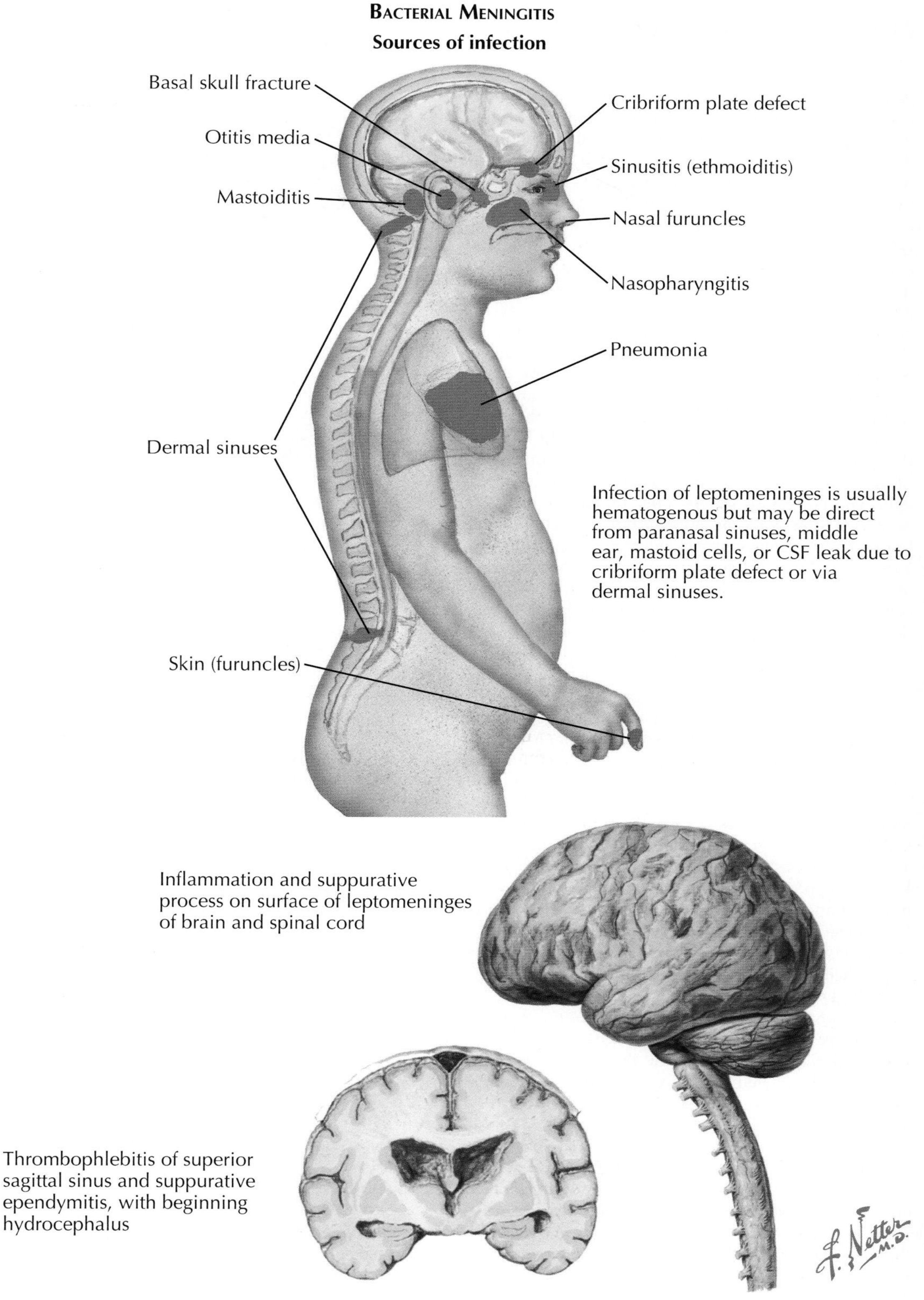

Plate 6-20

Infectious Diseases

MENINGOCOCCEMIA (Continued)

N. meningitidis infection. Culture of *N. meningitidis* from blood, cerebral spinal fluid (CSF), or tissue is diagnostic. The gram-negative diplococcal bacteria grows on the chocolate agar plate and appears as small, round, moist, gray colonies. Gram staining of CSF shows intracellular gram-negative diplococcal bacteria. This bacteria also grows well on the Thayer-Martin agar plate. The bacteria is oxidase positive and is able to acidify certain sugars. These laboratory data can be used to help differentiate *N. meningitidis* from other bacteria. CSF samples can be used for polymerase chain reaction (PCR) testing for the bacteria, but this is not routinely done in these cases. All cases of *N. meningitidis* infection should be reported to state and national health organizations.

Pathogenesis: Meningococcal infections, including septicemia and meningitis, are caused by the gram-negative bacteria, *N. meningitidis*. This is a diplococcal bacterium that requires an iron source for survival. Because of this unique metabolic requirement, humans are the only known host. The meningococcus bacteria can be found as a transient colonizer in the oropharynx of up to 10% of sampled individuals. These carriers express no sequelae but serve as a potential reservoir for meningococcal disease. The organisms are spread by close contact and sharing of saliva. If the bacteria is able to reproduce to such an extent as to cause bacteremia, it then becomes a potential pathogen. Bacteremia can quickly lead to septicemia (meningococcemia). This is a severe, life-threatening disease that can kill quickly. Meningeal involvement leads to neisserial meningitis. The bacteria exhibit a neurotrophic behavior and attack the lining of the central nervous system.

At least 13 serotypes of *N. meningitidis* are known, 9 of which have been conclusively shown to cause human disease. Currently, a vaccine is available that protects against the serotypes that most frequently cause disease: serotypes A, C, Y, and W-135. The remaining five serotypes can affect any individual regardless of vaccination status. The bacteria expresses a toxin (lipooligosaccharide) on its surface that causes many of the systemic symptoms of disease. *N. meningitidis* is an encapsulated bacteria, and this helps protect it from the host's immune system.

Histology: Most skin biopsy specimens show evidence of vasculitis with neutrophils, fibrinoid necrosis, and extravasated red blood cells. Organisms can be appreciated on tissue Gram stains. Embolism of capillaries and small venules is often seen, and necrosis and ulceration can be secondary findings.

Treatment: Treatment requires prompt recognition of symptoms and immediate intravenous antibiotic therapy. Any close contacts of the patient should be screened for evidence of disease and given prophylactic oral therapy to decrease the potential of an epidemic. The main intravenous antibiotic of choice is

ceftriaxone, followed by penicillin or by chloramphenicol in penicillin-allergic patients. Patients with Waterhouse-Friderichsen syndrome need adrenal gland replacement therapy.

Contacts should be treated with ciprofloxacin, rifampin, or ceftriaxone. This prophylactic therapy, as well as intravenous therapy, should be started immediately if clinical suspicion is high enough; delaying therapy for even a few hours to wait for laboratory

confirmation can be the difference between life and death.

Immunization is helping to keep the disease incidence low, and guidelines have been established for which high-risk groups should get the vaccine and when. Although the vaccine protects against only 4 of the 13 serotypes of *N. meningitidis*, it has the potential to decrease the incidence of this disease and save many lives.

BACTERIAL MENINGITIS
Sources of infection

Basal skull fracture
Otitis media
Mastoiditis
Dermal sinuses
Skin (furuncles)
Cribriform plate defect
Sinusitis (ethmoiditis)
Nasal furuncles
Nasopharyngitis
Pneumonia

Infection of leptomeninges is usually hematogenous but may be direct from paranasal sinuses, middle ear, mastoid cells, or CSF leak due to cribriform plate defect or via dermal sinuses.

Inflammation and suppurative process on surface of leptomeninges of brain and spinal cord

Thrombophlebitis of superior sagittal sinus and suppurative ependymitis, with beginning hydrocephalus

Plate 6-21

Integumentary System

Molluscum Contagiosum

As its name implies, molluscum contagiosum is a highly contagious viral infection that has little morbidity. This infection is most commonly encountered in children. The diagnosis is made on clinical grounds after inspection of the characteristic skin findings. When seen in the genital region of adults, molluscum contagiosum is considered to be a sexually transmitted disease. This infection rarely occurs in immunocompetent adults outside sexual transmission. In adults with no clear evidence of transmission, an evaluation for an immunosuppressed state should be undertaken. Patients taking chronic immunosuppressive medications and those with the acquired immunodeficiency syndrome are more prone to infection with molluscum contagiosum.

Clinical Findings: Young children are often affected by this common viral infection. Children pass the virus from one to another through close contact. The incubation period is 2 to 4 weeks. The characteristic finding is of small (3-5 mm), dome-shaped papules with a central dell. The coloration can be pink to slightly whitish. Solitary lesions may be appreciated, but clusters of lesions are often encountered. They may appear on any part of the body. Slight pruritus may accompany the lesions, but otherwise there are no symptoms. Molluscum lesions have a tendency to become inflamed. When this occurs, they can become tender. Inflamed lesions are bright red and can bleed if the child scratches or traumatizes them. The more inflamed a lesion becomes, the more likely it is to leave scarring. Scarring can also occur if the lesion becomes secondarily infected. Most noninflamed lesions spontaneously resolve within 6 months.

Young and older adults who present with molluscum contagiosum in the genital region are believed to have acquired the infection through sexual contact. The number of lesions in these cases tends to be increased, and the lesions tend to be localized to the groin. These also spontaneously resolve over time with no therapy. Immunosuppressed individuals, especially those with human immunodeficiency virus (HIV) infection, have a high incidence of molluscum contagiosum viral infections. These infections tend to be widespread and can be larger than the typical version acquired in childhood.

Pathogenesis: Molluscum contagiosum is caused by an enveloped, large, double-stranded DNA poxvirus, of which there are four unique types. Humans are the only known species to be infected by this virus. The virus has been designated molluscum contagiosum virus (MCV), and the four types MCV1 through MCV4. The virus is spread by close physical contact, and transmission on fomites has also been established. The virus attaches to the glycosaminoglycans on the surface of the targeted cell. The viral DNA gains entry into the cell cytoplasm, where it replicates itself. The virus carries with it a viral RNA polymerase, which acts to transcribe the viral genes, as well as a viral DNA polymerase for replication of its DNA. Early and late proteins are produced. The early proteins are generally for viral replication, and the late proteins are for production of the structural shell of the virus. These processes all occur within the cytoplasm of the infected cell. Once the virus has replicated, the infected cell typically dies, and the brick-shaped viral particles are released.

Histology: Skin biopsies of molluscum contagiosum are very characteristic, and the infection is easily diagnosed histologically. However, biopsies usually are not obtained because the disease is diagnosed clinically. The virally infected cells have molluscum bodies. The molluscum bodies change from small, eosinophilic

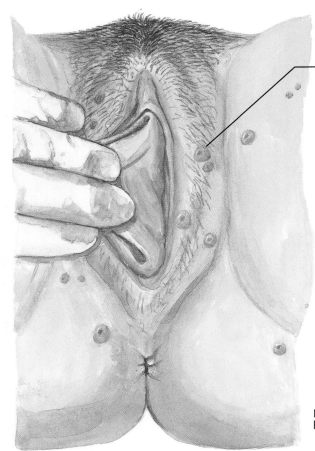

Scattered distribution of molluscum lesions over perineum, buttocks, and thighs. Lesions spread by physical contact and autoinoculation. The disease can be sexually transmitted in adults.

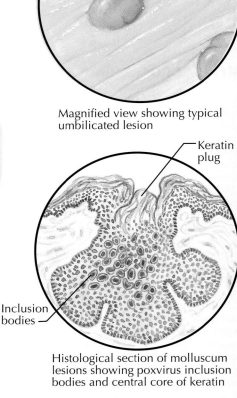

Magnified view showing typical umbilicated lesion

Histological section of molluscum lesions showing poxvirus inclusion bodies and central core of keratin

Local eradication of lesions can be obtained with desiccation, cryotherapy, laser ablation, chemical cautery, or curettage.

Application of liquid nitrogen to lesion using cotton swab

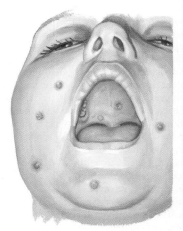

Molluscum contagiosum is commonly encountered in children.

cytoplasmic bodies in the stratum basalis into larger basophilic bodies in the outer epidermis. As they enlarge, they often compress the nucleus of the infected cell. These intracytoplasmic inclusion bodies have been termed *Henderson-Patterson bodies*.

Treatment: Often in children, a watch-and-wait approach is the best therapy, because most cases resolve spontaneously. Many destructive methods are available. Liquid nitrogen cryotherapy is highly effective, but most children have difficulty tolerating the pain it can

cause. Many other therapies have been used, including tretinoin cream, salicylic acid, curette, cantharidin, and imiquimod. Patients who are immunosuppressed can be treated with any of these modalities. Attempts to decrease immunosuppressive medications should be coordinated through the patient's transplant surgeon or primary care physician. Patients with widespread molluscum contagiosum and coexisting HIV infection have benefited from highly active antiretroviral therapy (HAART).

Plate 6-22

Infectious Diseases

PARACOCCIDIOIDOMYCOSIS

Paracoccidioidomycosis, also known as South American blastomycosis, is a disease that is seen almost exclusively in regions of Central and South America. It is caused by the dimorphic fungus, *Paracoccidioides brasiliensis*. Most infections are acquired by direct inhalation of the chlamydospores. The fungus is found in the environment in the mycelial or mold phase; it converts to the yeast phase at body temperature. Brazil has the highest incidence of paracoccidioidomycosis. Primary lung infection may lead to disseminated disease, with the skin being secondarily infected. Direct inoculation into the skin causes primary cutaneous disease.

Clinical Findings: This fungal infection is more common in men than in women, for reasons poorly understood. It may be that men are more likely to have occupational exposures (most commonly, farming). A protective effect of estrogen also has been hypothesized. There is no race predilection. Immunocompetent hosts who are exposed to the fungus are likely to develop a subclinical infection. Then, either the fungus becomes walled off in the form of granulomas within the lung or the patient goes on to develop clinical disease. Serological testing may show evidence of past exposure in healthy subjects with no clinical findings. Some hosts have a constellation of flu-like symptoms that include malaise, weight loss, fatigue, fever, pneumonitis, and pleurisy. Progressive pulmonary lesions may occur regardless of immune status, but they are more severe in patients who are immunosuppressed.

Bilateral pulmonary infiltrates are seen on chest radiography and are similar to the radiographic findings of tuberculosis. The infiltrates often form consolidated areas with cavitations that heal with emphysematous changes. Almost all cases of paracoccidioidomycosis affect the lung. Once established, the fungus is able to disseminate to the skin, draining lymph nodes, adrenal glands, central nervous system, peritoneum, and gastrointestinal tract.

Skin lesions in paracoccidioidomycosis come in two distinct varieties. Disseminated disease is the more frequently encountered subtype. The lesions are predominantly on the head and neck, especially around the oral and nasal passages. The oral mucosal membranes and tongue are involved. Nasal and pharyngeal ulcerations are so frequently encountered that they have been given a name, *Aguiar-Pupo stomatitis*. The mucosal lesions are often peppered with pinpoint hemorrhagic areas. The skin findings may include papules, nodules, or fungating plaques. Ulceration is almost universal, and patients complain of pain and swelling. Cervical lymph nodes are enlarged. The infected lymph nodes often form sinus tracts to the skin and drain spontaneously.

The second form of cutaneous paracoccidioidomycosis is caused by direct inoculation of the fungus. The fungal elements are normally found in the soil, and piercing of the skin with a contaminated object can lead to primary cutaneous paracoccidioidomycosis. These lesions appear as papules or draining tender nodules with or without overlying ulceration. Some may spontaneously resolve, but most slowly enlarge.

Histology: Skin biopsy specimens show pseudocarcinomatous hyperplasia of the epidermis with varying degrees of ulceration and abscess formation. There is a mixed inflammatory infiltrate. Suppurative granulomatous inflammation is seen within the underlying dermis. The fungus can be seen on routine hematoxylin and eosin staining with close inspection. The cells of the yeast phase are thick walled and refractile. They can be

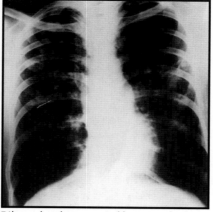

Bilateral pulmonary infiltrates, which closely resemble tuberculosis. Pulmonary lesions may range from minimal to very extensive.

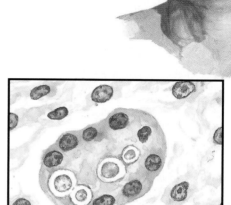

Plaques on lips, nose, and tongue with cervical lymphadenopathy

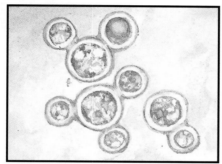

Yeast phase of *P. brasiliensis* in fresh unstained sputum prepared with 10% NaOH, showing double walls with single and multiple budding

Several double-contoured yeast-phase cells with single buds in a giant cell from a skin lesion

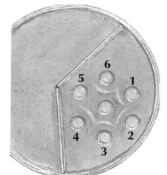

Precipitin test. Antigen in central well; serum from five different patients in peripheral wells showing precipitin bands. Wells *4* and *5* are from the same patient before and after treatment, evidencing response.

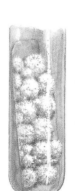

Mycelial colonies of *P. brasiliensis* grown on Sabouraud's medium at room temperature. Downy appearance is caused by filamentous hyphae with intercalate or terminal chlamydospores.

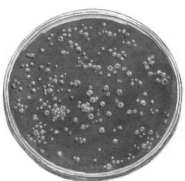

Colonies of yeast form of *P. brasiliensis* grown on blood agar at 37°C

seen in the shape of a "mariner's wheel," which is highly characteristic and specific for *P. brasiliensis*. The fungus can be highlighted with a multitude of special staining methods, including periodic acid–Schiff and sliver stains. The fungus is easily cultured on Sabouraud's medium and shows fluffy white colonies.

Pathogenesis: The fungus *P. brasiliensis* has unusual living requirements, and its growth in the environment is dependent on the soil pH, the altitude, and a consistent temperature. Alterations in the optimal growing conditions decrease the survivability of the organism.

The host response to this fungus depends on an intact Th1 helper T-cell response.

Treatment: Treatment with itraconazole has had great success and has drastically altered the prognosis of this disease. As with all systemic fungal infections, treatment courses last for months to a year. Historically, sulfonamides were used. If left untreated, this disease has a significant mortality rate. Ketoconazole and fluconazole have also been used successfully, and amphotericin B is now reserved for the most severe cases and for those that fail to respond to azole or sulfonamide therapy.

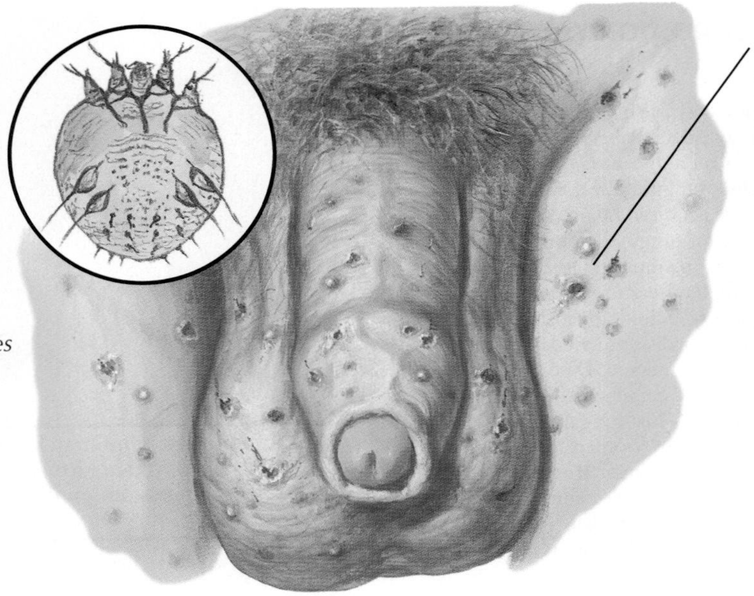

Plate 6-23

Integumentary System

SCABIES

Human infection with the parasite *Sarcoptes scabiei* var *hominis* causes scabies. Humans are the only known host, and the parasite is transferred from one person to another by close physical contact.

Clinical Findings: Scabies mites can affect any human. Men and women are equally affected, and there is no race predilection. The rash of scabies is highly pruritic. Patients often scratch in front of the examining physician and cannot stop themselves from doing so. Patients often state that it is the worst itching sensation they have ever experienced. The itching sensation is worse in the evening, especially when one is trying to sleep. Cutaneous findings are variable. Burrows are the hallmark of scabies and are pathognomonic for the disease.

Burrows consist of a fine, 0.5- to 1.0-mm-wide, 0.5- to 1.5-cm-long area of undulating or serpentine regions with a tiny black speck at one end. This tiny black speck is the scabies mite that is burrowing along the skin. If one were to scrape the area of the burrow where the mite is located and examine the scraping under the microscope, a mite would surely be seen. The mite may also be seen in association with eggs and scybala (mite feces). Any of these findings confirms the diagnosis. Burrows are most commonly appreciated along the sides of the fingers and the wrists.

The palms are commonly affected with tiny (1 mm) patches within the skin lines. They are intensely pruritic and are associated with excoriations. Scabies mites avoid the areas of the body that contain numerous sebaceous glands and for this reason are almost never seen on the face of anyone past the age of puberty. They may be found on the face of infants and children, who have not yet formed mature sebaceous glands. Scabies also has a propensity to affect the genitalia. The scrotum is almost always affected in cases that are more than a few weeks old. Very few rashes cause papules or nodules on the scrotum, and the presence of itchy nodules on the scrotum should be considered a sign of scabies until proven otherwise.

Crusted or Norwegian scabies is a rare form of scabies seen in immunosuppressed individuals. The crusted lesions represent the actions of hundreds to thousands of scabies mites. Patients are often covered from head to toe and are extremely pruritic. A scraping shows the presence of numerous mites. Individuals with crusted scabies should be treated with a multimodal approach.

Scabies can cause outbreaks in long-term care facilities. These outbreaks can affect many individuals within the facility and are difficult to eradicate.

Histology: Skin biopsies are rarely performed. If a biopsy were to be done, one would see a mixed inflammatory infiltrate in the dermis with many eosinophils. This is a nonspecific finding and can be the result of any bug bite reaction. If the actual mite is biopsied, scabies parts will be present within the epidermis.

Pathogenesis: *S. scabiei* is spread from one human to another by close physical contact. The mite burrows into the epidermis but is unable to penetrate the basement membrane zone. Its presence sets off a massive inflammatory response. The female mites lay eggs as they burrow through the skin. Each egg hatches within 2 to

3 days and releases a larva. The larvae quickly grow and form nymphs and then mature adult mites. This process occurs within 1 week's time. The mites have a life span of 2 months. The female mite can lay 3 eggs per day.

Treatment: Permethrin is currently the drug of choice to treat scabies. It should be applied overnight and repeated in 1 week, because it is pediculicidal but not ovacidal. The second application makes sure that

Scabies (*Sarcoptes scabiei* in *circle*)

Inflammatory excoriated papules (note penile involvement). Involvement of genitalia, umbilicus, and finger webs is characteristic for scabies.

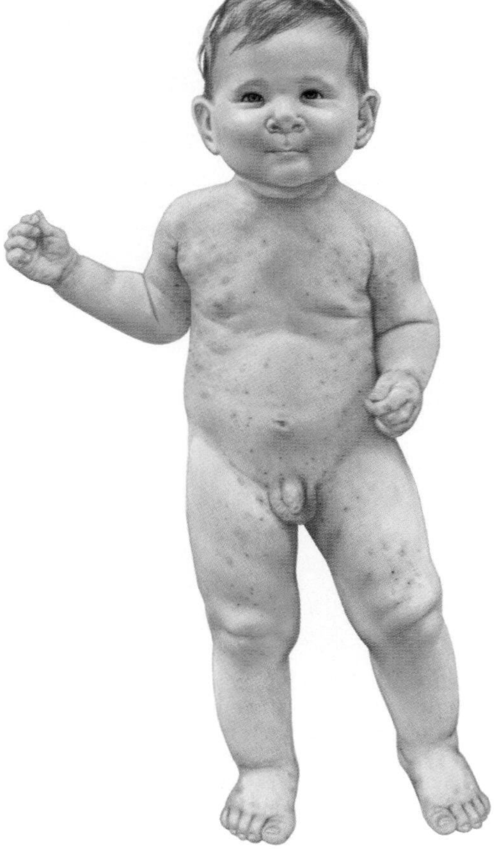

Child with scabies, ventral view

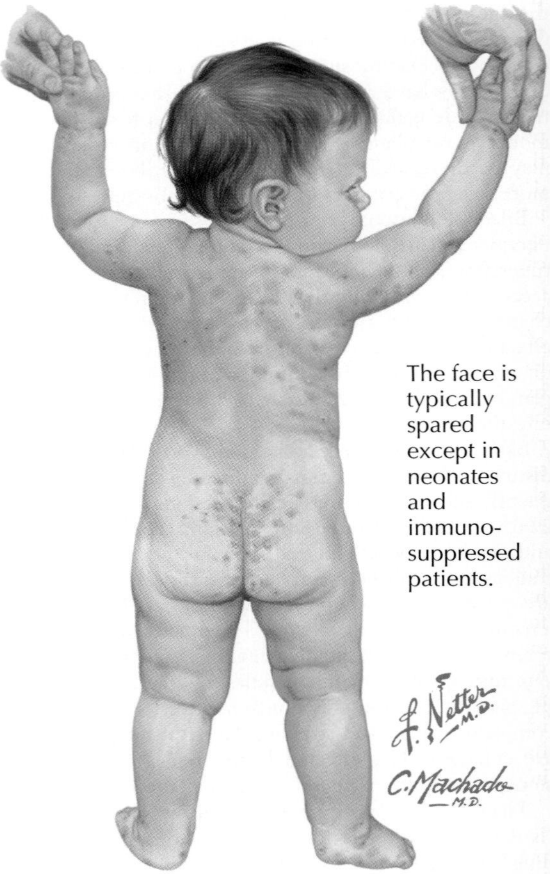

Child with scabies, dorsal view

The face is typically spared except in neonates and immunosuppressed patients.

any recently hatched mites are killed before they can reach reproductive age. Colloidal sulfur may be used on pregnant women. It is efficacious and safe but has a terrible odor. Outbreaks in long-term care facilities are often treated with oral ivermectin, which has shown good efficacy. Lindane has fallen out of favor because of its potential neurotoxicity. The use of malathion is advocated if permethrin fails.

Plate 6-24

Infectious Diseases

SPOROTRICHOSIS

Sporothrix schenckii is an environmental fungus that is capable of causing human disease after direct inoculation into the skin. Inoculation is the cause of cutaneous sporotrichosis, which is considered to be a subcutaneous mycosis. Unusual cases of inhalation sporotrichosis have been described in the literature, as have cases of central nervous system disease. These cases occur almost exclusively in immunosuppressed hosts. Sporotrichosis has classically been associated with inoculation after the prick from a rose plant. This is well reported; the fungus can be isolated from rose plants but is also found on many other plants and in soil environments.

Clinical Findings: Gardeners, florists, and outdoor enthusiasts are at highest risk for infection from *S. schenckii*. These activities and occupations increase the likelihood of contact with the soil fungus. The fungus lives in the environment, and humans become infected by direct implantation of the fungus into the skin. Common methods of inoculation are the prick of a thorn or an injury contaminated with soil or plant material. Within a few days after entry into the skin, a papule and then a pustule form at the site of inoculation. Patients may initially be given an antibiotic in the belief that they have a bacterial infection. Often, it is not until the pustule ulcerates and develops into a larger plaque that the diagnosis is suspected or considered. Once this has occurred, the fungus enters the local lymphatics and proceeds to migrate proximally. As the fungus travels through the lymphatic system, it periodically causes draining sinus tracts to the surface, which appear as papules or nodules. This characteristic lymphangitic spread, also called sporotrichoid spread, is seen in most cases of cutaneous sporotrichosis.

Although a few other infections can manifest with lymphangitic spread, its presence along with a history of trauma suggests an infection with sporotrichosis. If lymphangitic spread is present, a skin biopsy and fungal, bacterial, and atypical mycobacterium cultures should be performed. Less commonly, solitary plaques of sporotrichosis occur without any evidence of sporotrichoid spread. The disease manifests as solitary, nonhealing, slowly enlarging plaques with various amounts of ulceration and drainage.

Pathogenesis: *S. schenckii* is a dimorphic soil fungus found throughout the environment. *S. schenckii* causes human infection by direct implantation of the mold form of the fungus into the skin. Once the fungus has entered the human body, it transforms into its yeast form in response to the stable temperature. Most infections stay localized in the skin. In rare cases of severe immunosuppression, *S. schenckii* becomes disseminated; this occurs most frequently in association with human immunodeficiency virus infection.

Histology: Findings from skin biopsy specimens of sporotrichosis are not diagnostic in many cases. The presence of a granulomatous infiltrate is often the main histological feature. The periodic acid–Schiff (PAS) stain and Gomori's methenamine silver (GMS) stain are two excellent stains that highlight the fungus and allow the pathologist to more readily appreciate the few cigar-shaped fungal elements that are present within the dense inflammation. Multiple fungal organisms are rarely seen; they are observed most frequently in patients with an underlying immunodeficiency.

S. schenckii is best cultured on Sabouraud's media at room temperature. In these conditions, a white to brown colony of mold forms readily. As time elapses, the fungus forms a brown pigment that turns the entire colony brown to black. Because of its dimorphic nature,

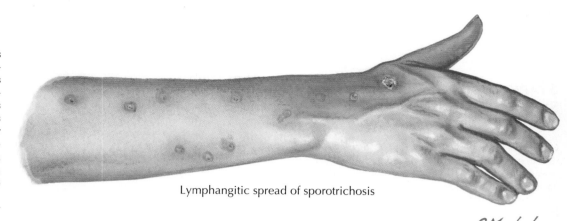

Lymphangitic spread of sporotrichosis

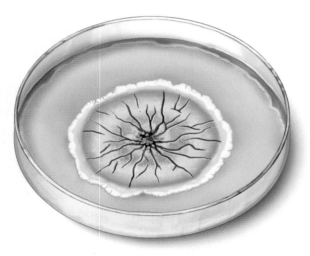

Sporothrix schenckii on Sabouraud plate

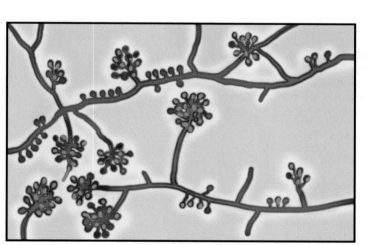

Structural growth pattern of *Sporothrix schenckii*

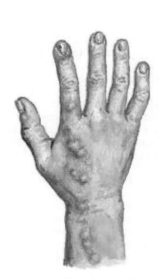

Begins as small nodule and spreads to hand, wrist, and forearm (even systemically). This and other mycotic infections are diagnosed with biopsy and culture.

S. schenckii can be grown at 37°C, although it grows much more slowly at that temperature.

Treatment: Saturated solution of potassium iodide (SSKI) has been used for decades to treat cutaneous infections with *S. schenckii*. This medication has an unknown mechanism of action in treating fungal infections, but it is believed to interrupt protein synthesis of the fungus and to boost local host immune function. The treatment of choice is one of the azole antifungal medications. Itraconazole has been the most widely studied and used antifungal and is the preferred agent. All the azole antifungal agents inhibit the fungal cytochrome P450 enzyme 14-α-sterol-demethylase (CYP51A1). This inhibition prevents the fungus from producing ergosterol, a vital cell membrane component. Patients with pulmonary or central nervous system involvement or disseminated disease should be treated with amphotericin B.

Plate 6-25   Integumentary System

STAPHYLOCOCCUS AUREUS SKIN INFECTIONS

Cutaneous infection with *Staphylococcus aureus* can manifest in many ways. With the emergence of methicillin-resistant *S. aureus* (MRSA), these cutaneous infections have once again been given the attention they deserve. Most cases of MRSA are community acquired, and they have entirely different sensitivity patterns than those of hospital-acquired MRSA infections. These cutaneous infections are increasing in incidence. They not only cause significant skin disease but have the potential to become systemic and cause septicemia, pneumonia, osteomyelitis, and other internal infections. *S. aureus* is a transient colonizer of the skin and nasopharynx. This bacteria has shown a remarkable ability to develop and acquire antibacterial resistance mechanisms. *S. aureus* and MRSA are major hospital-acquired *S. aureus* infections, and now community-acquired MRSA has become just as important. MRSA accounts for more than 50% of hospital-acquired *S. aureus* infections.

The emergence of community-acquired MRSA has led to an increase in the number of serious *S. aureus* infections. These community-acquired strains have been shown to cause an increased incidence of skin furuncles and abscesses as well as severe pneumonia. Most of these infections occur in young, previously healthy individuals.

Clinical Findings: *S. aureus* and MRSA can cause a wide range of cutaneous infections. The most superficial of all infections that this bacteria causes is impetigo. Impetigo is often seen in children and in people with preexisting skin diseases, which increase the likelihood of cutaneous infections. The two most common causes of impetigo are *S. aureus* and *Streptococcus pyogenes* or group A streptococcus. The disease often manifests on the face. Regardless of the location, the infection appears as small, superficial, honey-colored crusts with some weeping of yellow, clear serum. There is a bullous variant, and it manifests with superficial blisters that easily rupture. The disease is contagious and can be spread among children. Typically, topical therapy yields excellent results, and oral therapy can be avoided. If one were to biopsy a lesion of impetigo, a superficial infectious process would be seen in the stratum corneum. Neutrophils and bacterial elements would be found within the stratum corneum.

Infection of the hair follicle shaft, termed *folliculitis*, can occur with a wide variety of bacterial infections, including both *S. aureus* and streptococcal species. Many other forms of folliculitis have been described with other etiologic agents. Hot tub folliculitis is caused by *Pseudomonas aeruginosa*, which grows in improperly disinfected hot tubs. Gram-negative folliculitis can be seen in patients receiving long-term antibiotic therapy for acne and other conditions. Regardless of the bacterial agent, the appearance of folliculitis is the same. A small (1-3 mm) pustule is present and surrounds a hair follicle. The pustule is easily broken and can be slightly itchy to slightly painful. The hair can easily be removed from the pustule with minimal effort. The pustule is surrounded by a millimeter or two of erythema, which in turn is surrounded by a blanched region extending out another few millimeters. Typically, entire regions of the body are affected, such as the legs or buttocks.

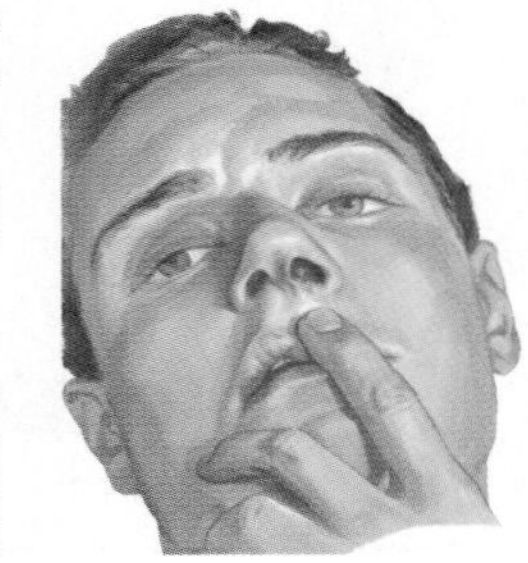

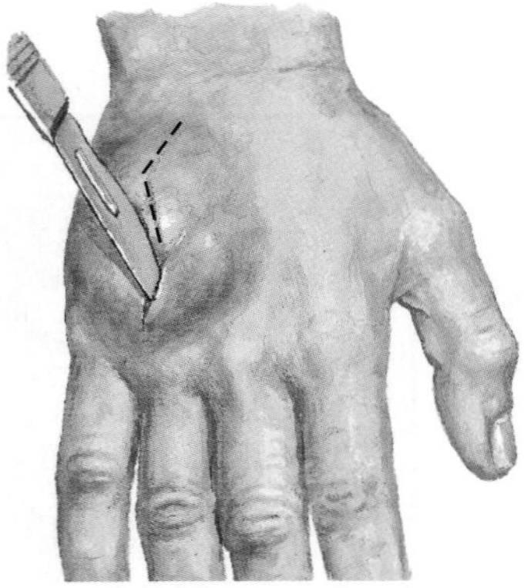

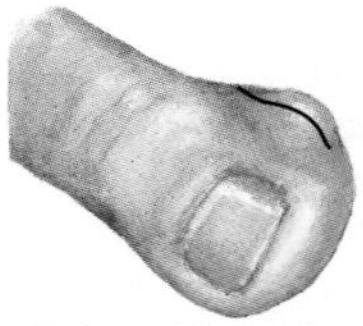

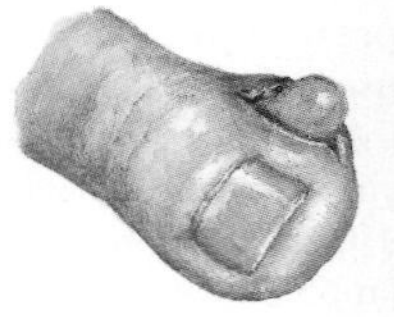

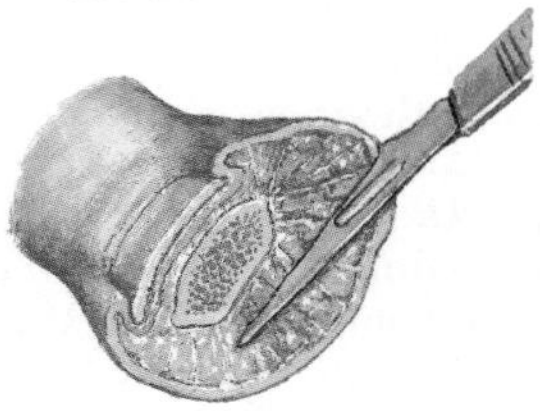

TYPES OF SKIN INFECTIONS
Cross section of the skin showing layers and types of infection

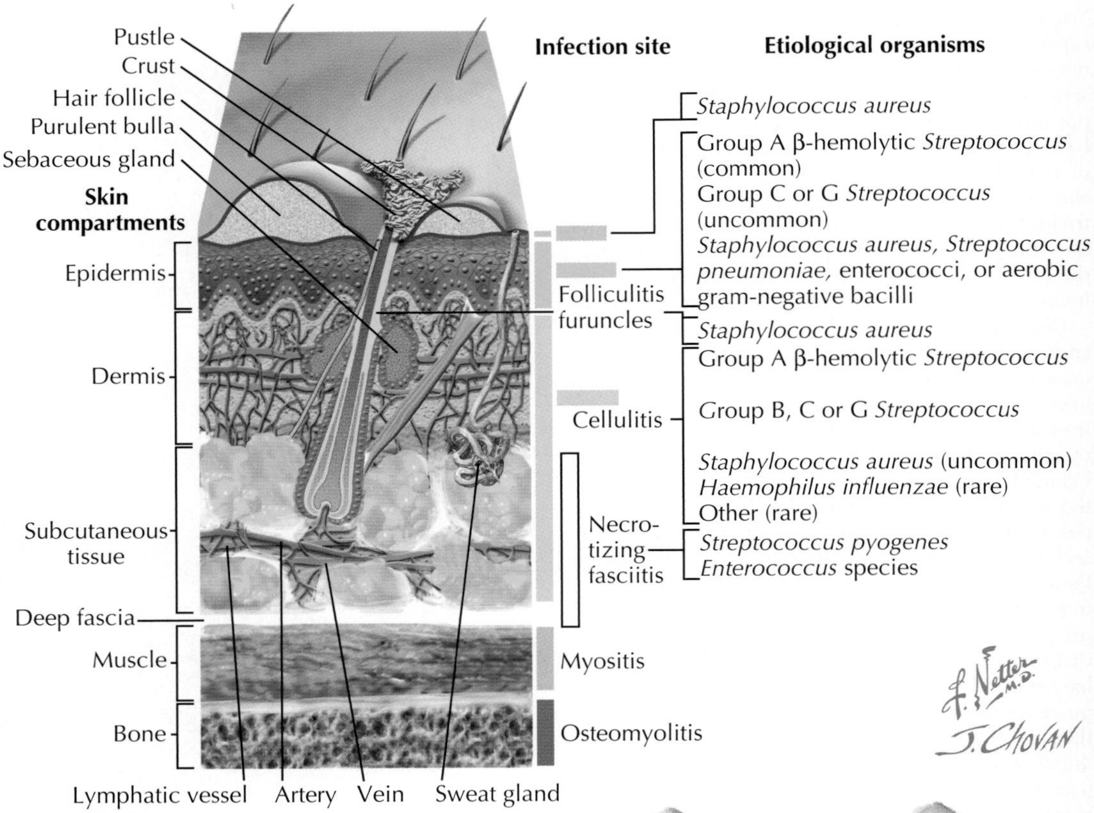

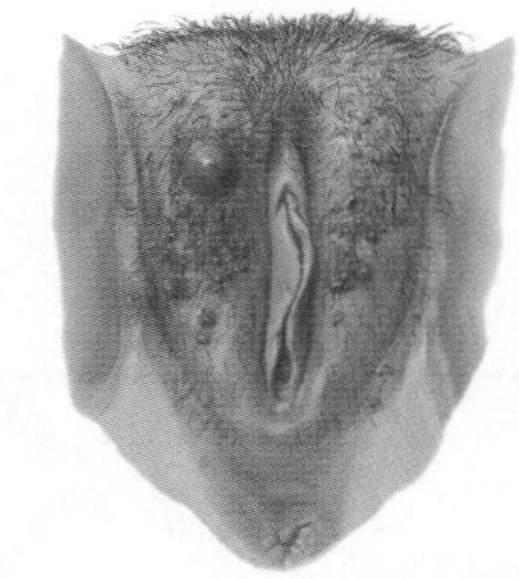

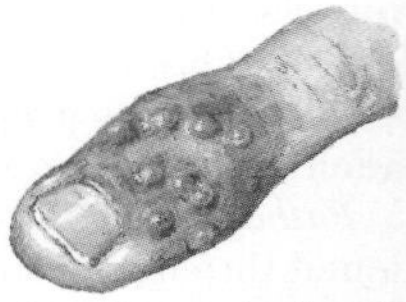

Folliculitis can lead to furuncles (boils) or carbuncles (large furuncles). However, most furuncles do not develop from a preexisting folliculitis. The furuncle is a deep-seated, red, inflamed, tender nodule. Furuncles can occur in any location and are commonly found within the nostril. The nostril is a location that *S. aureus* is known to colonize. Furuncles may become quite large and spontaneously drain to the surface. Before the drainage occurs, one can often appreciate the presence of a pustule developing within the central portion of the furuncle. Carbuncles appear to result from the coalescence of multiple furuncles. They can be large and can have multiple draining sinus tracts to the surface of the epidermis. Multiple pustules may precede the drainage. Pain and localized adenopathy are hallmarks of both furuncles and carbuncles.

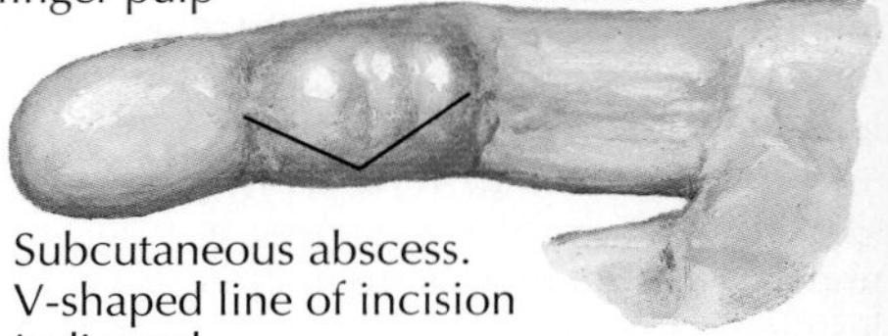

Plate 6-26

Infectious Diseases

STAPHYLOCOCCUS AUREUS SKIN INFECTIONS (Continued)

Cellulitis develops from a bacterial infection within the dermis or the subcutaneous fat of the skin. The most frequent location is on the lower extremities. It occurs more commonly in people with diabetes, trauma to the skin, poor vascular circulation, or immunosuppression. Cellulitis starts as a small, pink-to-red macule that slowly expands and can encompass large portions of the skin. This is associated with edema and pain. The condition is almost always unilateral. The pain can be severe. Tender adenopathy of regional lymph nodes is present. Fever and systemic symptoms are almost always present. The redness is able to travel many centimeters a day. The presence of red lines is more indicative of a lymphadenitis than a cellulitis, but these conditions can coexist. Erysipelas is a more superficial form of cellulitis that occurs in the upper dermis. It manifests clinically as a well-demarcated, edematous red macule that is tender to the touch. The lower extremities and the face are common areas of involvement.

Toxic shock syndrome (TSS) is the name given to the development of fever, hypotension, and near-erythroderma. The rash can appear as widespread, red, blanching macules. If appropriately treated, the rash causes desquamation of the skin and return to normal within a few weeks. TSS was initially reported after the use of superabsorbent tampons, which were left in place for the entire menstrual cycle. These tampons are no longer available. The superabsorbent tampons provided an environment conducive to the rapid growth of *S. aureus*. Toxins produced by the bacteria are responsible for the symptoms. TSS can occur after any *S. aureus* infection but is much more likely with an abscess. The toxins act as superantigens and activate T cells without the normal immune system processing. This can lead to massive activation of the immune system.

Pathogenesis: *S. aureus* is a gram-positive bacteria that is found throughout the environment and can be a colonizer of humans. It is most likely to be found colonizing the nares, the toe web spaces, and the umbilicus. The bacteria grows in grape-like clusters on blood agar cultures. *S. aureus* is one of the most common bacterial causes of human infection.

Histology: The histological findings are based on the form of infection biopsied. The common underlying theme is a neutrophilic infiltrate that can be present throughout the biopsy specimen. Bacteria are present and can be highlighted on tissue Gram staining. The inflammation in impetigo is often limited to the epidermis, with bacteria and neutrophils present within the stratum corneum. Superficial blistering may occur within the granular cell layer in bullous impetigo. Folliculitis shows edema and a neutrophilic infiltrate in and around the hair follicle. Furuncles, carbuncles, and abscess show a massive dermal infiltrate with neutrophils and bacterial debris.

The pathology of cellulitis is more subtle, with neutrophils around blood vessels. Bacteria can be difficult to see or to culture from skin biopsies of cellulitis. Most cases of cellulitis are not biopsied. TSS shows a superficial and deep mixed inflammatory infiltrate. No bacteria are seen, because the rash is toxin mediated.

Treatment: Impetigo can be treated with topical therapy against *S. aureus* and streptococcal species.

TOXIC SHOCK SYNDROME

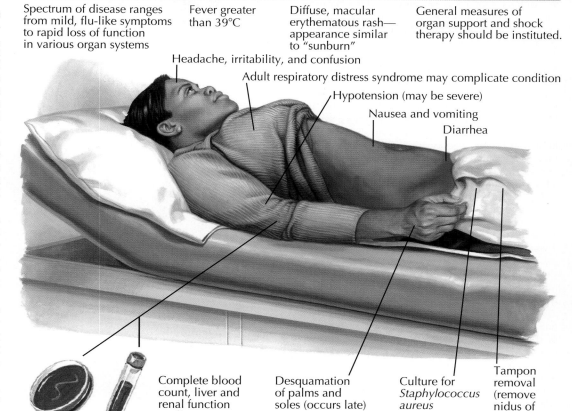

Etiology and pathogenesis

Often associated with superabsorbent tampon use

Staphylococcal exotoxins (TSS1), enterotoxins (A,B,C)

Vaginal colonization by *Staphylococcus aureus* with exotoxin production

Conditions required for development of toxic shock syndrome:
1. Bacterial colonization
2. Exotoxin production
3. Entry portal for toxin

Early phase manifests with flu-like symptoms, fever, rash, and hypotension

C. Machado M.D.
JOHN A. CRAIG AD

Clinical features of toxic shock syndrome

Spectrum of disease ranges from mild, flu-like symptoms to rapid loss of function in various organ systems

Fever greater than 39°C

Diffuse, macular erythematous rash—appearance similar to "sunburn"

General measures of organ support and shock therapy should be instituted.

Headache, irritability, and confusion

Adult respiratory distress syndrome may complicate condition

Hypotension (may be severe)

Nausea and vomiting

Diarrhea

Complete blood count, liver and renal function studies

Desquamation of palms and soles (occurs late)

Culture for *Staphylococcus aureus*

Tampon removal (remove nidus of infection)

Mupirocin is one such topical agent that is highly effective. The other forms of infection need to be treated with oral antibiotics. Cephalexin or dicloxacillin is a good first choice. In areas with high rates of community-acquired MRSA, one should consider covering for this agent with a sulfa-based medication or a tetracycline derivative in adults. Culturing of the bacterial agent should be done in all cases to select the most effective medication.

Severe cases of cellulitis and all cases of TSS should be treated in the hospital in the appropriate setting. Intravenous antibiotics are always used, and vancomycin is the initial choice until the strain of *S. aureus* is isolated and sensitivities are assessed. Once the sensitivities of the bacteria have been determined, the antibiotic treatment can be tailored to the individual patient. Patients with TSS often require intensive care with pressure support and respiratory support.

Plate 6-27

Integumentary System

SYPHILIS

Syphilis has been well described in the literature since the late 1400s. The history behind the discovery and treatment of the disease is a story of perseverance and the willpower of many scientists working separately and together to help treat one the most deadly diseases of their time. Philip Ricord, a French scientist, is given credit for describing the three stages of syphilis and differentiating it from other diseases such as gonorrhea. The infectious organism, *Treponema pallidum*, was described in 1905 by Fritz Schaudinn, a German zoologist, and Erich Hoffman, a German dermatologist. Soon after this discovery, the German scientist Paul Ehrlich developed the first specific therapy for syphilis. The oral medication he and his team discovered was initially called 606, because it was the 606th compound they had attempted to use to treat the disease. This organoarsenic molecule was soon renamed salvarsan. This medication is highly effective against *T. pallidum*.

T. pallidum is classified as a spirochete. Spirochetes are gram-negative bacteria that have a winding or coiled linear body. There are three subspecies of *T. pallidum*; the one responsible for syphilis is named *Treponema pallidum pallidum*. The other subspecies of *T. pallidum* cause endemic syphilis or bejel, pinta, and yaws. Syphilis is a highly infectious disease that is transmitted via sexual contact or vertically from an infected mother to her unborn child. Syphilis has been recognized to progress through three stages: primary, secondary, and tertiary. Not all cases progress through all of the stages, and only about one third of untreated cases eventually progress to tertiary syphilis. The secondary and tertiary phases are interrupted by a latent phase of variable length.

Clinical Findings: Both historically and today, most cases of syphilis have been transmitted via sexually intercourse. The disease is often seen in conjunction with other sexually transmitted diseases (STDs), especially human immunodeficiency virus (HIV) infection. The two infections may actually facilitate each other's infectious potential. There is no race or sex predilection; the organism is able to infect any host with whom it comes in contact. The initial infection in most cases results in clinical findings in the genital region.

Primary syphilis is marked by a nonpainful ulceration that begins as a red papule and ulcerates over a period of a few days to weeks. The average time to onset of the ulcer is 3 to 4 weeks after exposure, but it can occur 3 to 4 months later. This primary ulcer, called a

chancre, is firm to palpation. The ulcer can be found anywhere on the genitalia, including the labia, vaginal introitus, and mons in females and the glans, foreskin, and penile shaft in males. Lesions on the foreskin of males often show the Dory flop sign. This occurs when one grasps the area of the prepuce containing the ulcer and slowly retracts the proximal edge; after a critical angle has been achieved, the entire ulcer flops over.

This occurs because the ulcer is firm and does not bow under pressure. If left untreated, these ulcers self-resolve within 1 to 3 weeks. After this occurs, the bacteria hematogenously disseminate to other organ systems.

The timing of secondary syphilis is variable: It can occur immediately after primary syphilis or up to 6 months after the chancre of primary syphilis has healed.

SYPHILIS OF GENITALIA

Chancre with inguinal adenopathy
1° syphillis

Condylomata lata
2° syphillis

Chancre of coronal sulcus; nontender ulcer

Chancre of glans: firm rubbery, nontender ulcer

Multiple chancres (shaft and meatus)

Penoscrotal chancre with inguinal adenopathy

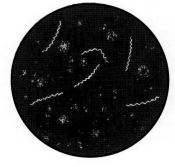
Spirochetes under darkfield examination

Plate 6-28

Infectious Diseases

SYPHILIS OF ORAL CAVITY

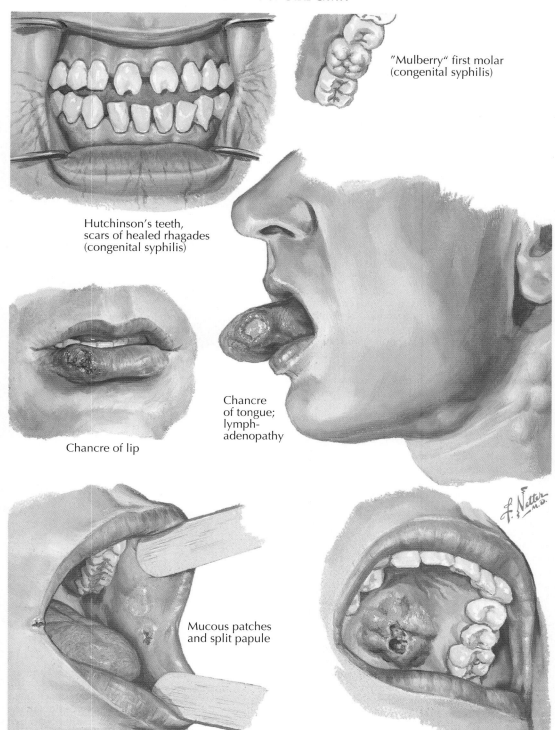

"Mulberry" first molar (congenital syphilis)

Hutchinson's teeth, scars of healed rhagades (congenital syphilis)

Chancre of lip

Chancre of tongue; lymphadenopathy

Mucous patches and split papule

Gumma of palate; tendency to perforation

SYPHILIS (Continued)

The average time frame is approximately 6 weeks after healing of the primary ulcer. Without treatment, most if not all patients experience symptoms and skin lesions of secondary syphilis. Patients universally complain of constitutional symptoms such as malaise, fever, chills, fatigue, and weight loss. Cutaneous findings can be multifaceted. The most prevalent skin finding is that of skin-colored to red to slightly hyperpigmented papules and patches. The palms and soles are characteristically involved, and this is a clue that the diagnosis of syphilis should be entertained.

Condylomata lata is the name given to the moist plaques that develop in the groin region from secondary syphilis. These lesions contain numerous *T. pallidum* organisms. Adenopathy is almost always present. Some rare findings of secondary syphilis include ulcers in the mouth, which can mimic aphthous ulcerations, and a nonscarring alopecia. The alopecia has been described as having a "moth-eaten" appearance. This is in reference to the random arrangements of patches of alopecia. All the lesions of secondary syphilis contain the bacteria, and samples can be taken and directly observed under darkfield microscopy. The organisms are seen as mobile spirochetes with a spiral configuration. Patients with secondary syphilis may have early central nervous system (CNS) involvement and may complain of headaches and other meningeal signs. Approximately 3 to 4 months after the first signs and symptoms of secondary syphilis appear, they spontaneously resolve. This is the beginning of the latent phase, which is a phase of wide variability. Some patients never develop tertiary syphilis, and approximately 1 in 5 develop a recurrence of secondary syphilis.

Tertiary syphilis follows the latent phase of syphilis in 30% to 40% of untreated individuals. The average time from initial development to tertiary syphilis is approximately 4 years. Tertiary syphilis can affect the skin, bone, and mucous membranes. The characteristic skin finding is the gumma. Gummas appear frequently as individual lesions, although a multitude of gummas may occur at the same time. The gumma starts as a papule and then evolves into a nodule, which ulcerates over the course of a few days to weeks. The ulceration is caused by significant necrosis of the involved tissue. This leads to deep ulcers with well-defined borders. The surface of the ulcer may be covered with gelatinous exudates. Another form of tertiary syphilis is the nodular syphilid skin lesion. These lesions are red to red-brown nodules that slowly enlarge and can

develop various configurations, including serpiginous and annular formations. These lesions rarely, if ever, ulcerate.

Unique forms of syphilis that do not fit neatly into one of the categories already described include neurosyphilis, congenital syphilis, and late syphilis. Involvement of the CNS by *T. pallidum* is termed neurosyphilis. Neurosyphilis can occur during any of the numerous forms and stages of syphilis. It is caused by direct

infection of the CNS by the spirochete. Most patients with syphilis exhibit no signs of CNS involvement, even when the bacteria can be isolated from the CNS. However, almost all of these cases of asymptomatic neurosyphilis eventually progress to symptomatic clinical illness. Some of the common symptoms of neurosyphilis are headache, hearing difficulty, neck stiffness, and muscle weakness. As the disease progresses untreated, patients develop seizures, delirium,

Plate 6-29

Integumentary System

SYPHILIS IN PREGNANCY

SYPHILIS (Continued)

and tabes dorsalis. Tabes dorsalis results from degeneration of the posterior columns of the spinal cord. The posterior columns are critical for proper sensation, and patients with tabes dorsalis develop gait disorders, diminished reflexes, proprioception abnormalities, pain, paresthesias, and a host of other neurological symptoms. If neurosyphilis remains untreated, the patient dies of the disease. Therefore, any patient who exhibits signs or symptoms of neurosyphilis should undergo a spinal tap to evaluate the cerebrospinal fluid for involvement with *T. pallidum*.

Congenital syphilis occurs as the result of vertical transmission from an infected mother to her unborn fetus. Up to one third of infected neonates die of the disease. In neonates who survive, the disease manifests in many ways. Neonates may present with macerated erosions associated with cachexia and failure to thrive. "Snuffles" is the term used to describe the chronic runny nose with a bloody purulent discharge. Rhagades are one of the most common signs seen in congenital syphilis; they appear as scarring around the mouth and eyes. Many bony abnormalities have been reported, including a saddle-nose deformity, the Higoumenakis sign (medial clavicular thickening), saber shins, and Clutton's joints. Teeth abnormalities include Hutchinson's teeth (notched incisors) and, less frequently, mulberry molars.

Histology: Skin biopsies of syphilis that are evaluated with routine hematoxylin and eosin (H&E) staining show varying features depending on the stage and form of disease being biopsied. A universal finding in all forms is the presence of numerous plasma cells within the inflammatory infiltrate. Ulceration, granulomas, and vasculitis are often encountered. The spirochetes cannot be appreciated with routine H&E staining; special staining techniques are required. The Steiner stain and the Warthin-Starry stain are the two most commonly used stains. Immunohistochemical stains can also be used, and they have been shown to be highly sensitive and specific.

Pathogenesis: Syphilis is caused by the spirochete, *T. pallidum pallidum*. This bacteria is highly infective and is predominantly spread by sexual contact and by transmission from an infected mother to her unborn child.

Treatment: The *T. pallidum* organism has very little antibiotic resistance, and the therapy of choice is still penicillin. A single intramuscular dose of 2.4 million IU of benzathine penicillin G is recommended, and some now recommend a follow-up dose—the same as the initial dose—at 1 or 2 weeks. Patients who develop neurosyphilis need to be treated with intravenous

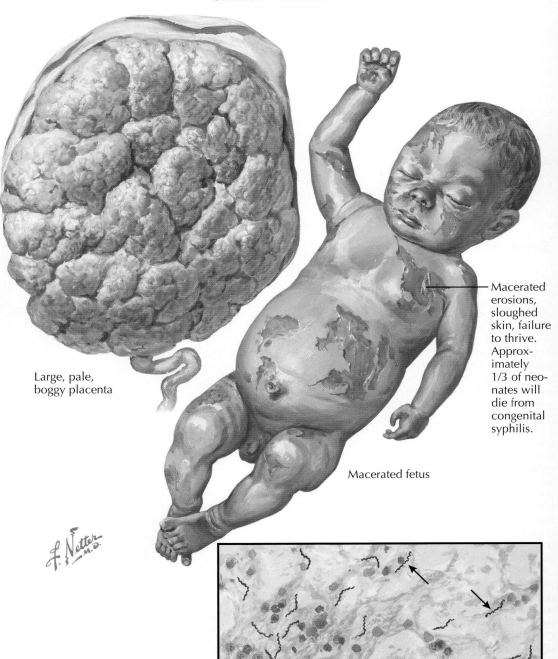

Large, pale, boggy placenta

Macerated fetus

Macerated erosions, sloughed skin, failure to thrive. Approximately 1/3 of neonates will die from congenital syphilis.

Spirochetes in fetal tissue (Levaditi stain). *T. pallidum*

penicillin for at least 2 weeks. Most patients who are treated for syphilis develop the Jarisch-Herxheimer reaction. This reaction is the result of the decimation of the *T. pallidum* organisms due to therapy with penicillin. As the scores of bacteria are killed, the dead spirochetes induce an inflammatory reaction. This reaction may manifest as fever, chills, fatigue, malaise, and rashes of varying morphology. It can often make

the rash of secondary syphilis appear worse for a period of time. This reaction is not specific to *T. pallidum* and has been reported with other infectious agents. It is critical to follow patients long enough after therapy ensure adequate treatment as measured by titers on rapid plasma reagin (RPR) or venereal disease research laboratory (VDRL) testing. All patients with syphillis should be tested for HIV.

Plate 6-30

Infectious Diseases

VARICELLA

The varicella-zoster virus (VZV) causes two discrete clinical infections: chickenpox (varicella) and herpes zoster (shingles). Although chickenpox was once a universal infection of childhood, the incidence of this disease has plummeted since the advent of the chickenpox vaccine. VZV belongs to the herpesvirus family and is primarily a respiratory disease with skin manifestations.

Clinical Findings: The disease is seen predominantly in children and young adults. Disease in adults tends to be more severe. Varicella is caused by inhalation of the highly infectious viral particle from an infected contact. The virus replicates within the pulmonary epithelium and then disseminates via the bloodstream to the skin and mucous membranes. Most children do not have severe pulmonary symptoms. A prodrome of headache, fever, cough, and malaise may precede the development of the rash by a few days.

The rash of varicella is characteristic and is present in almost 100% of those infected. It begins as a small, erythematous macule or papule that vesiculates. After vesiculation, the lesion may form a small vesiculopustule and then quickly rupture and form a thin, crusted erosion. The resulting vesicle has a central depression or dell, and it is localized over a red base. This gives rise to the classic description of a "dew drop on a rose petal." The rash is more common on the trunk and on the head and neck, and it often is less severe when found on the extremities. A characteristic finding is an enanthem. The mucous membranes of the mouth are frequently involved with pinpoint vesicles with a surrounding red halo. A clinical clue to the diagnosis is the finding of lesions of multiple morphologies occurring at the same time. Most cases of varicella are self-resolving and heal with minimal to no scarring. Scarring can be significant if the vesicles or crusts become secondarily infected. Children are considered infectious from 1 to 2 days before the rash breaks out until the last vesicle crusts over. The diagnosis of chickenpox is made clinically. A Tzanck test, direct immunofluorescence, or viral culture can be used in nonclassic cases to confirm the diagnosis.

Adults who develop primary varicella infection are at risk for severe pulmonary complications and severe skin disease with a dramatically increased risk for scarring. Adults who are exposed to VZV for the first time are more likely to develop pneumonia and encephalitis. Children who develop pneumonia during an infection with chickenpox have most likely acquired a secondary bacterial pneumonia.

Since the universal adoption in the United States of routine childhood vaccination against varicella in 1995, the incidence of varicella has precipitously dropped. The VZV vaccine is a live attenuated vaccine that is highly effective in achieving protective titer levels. Those individuals who develop chickenpox after vaccination have an attenuated course that is manifested by a few vesicles and more macules. This atypical variant of chickenpox is often misdiagnosed, or it may be so mild that the parents do not seek medical care.

Histology: A skin biopsy of a vesicle shows an intraepidermal blister that forms via ballooning degeneration of the keratinocytes. There is a perivascular lymphocytic infiltrate in the dermis. Multinucleated giant cells can be seen at the base of the blister.

Pathogenesis: Varicella (chickenpox) is caused by VZV. This is a double-stranded DNA virus with a lipid capsule. It is spread from human to human via the respiratory route. Once inhaled, the highly infectious

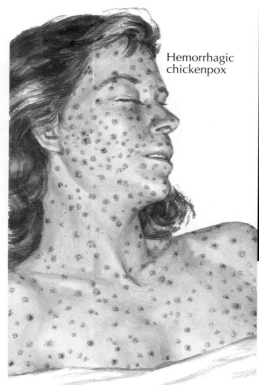
Hemorrhagic chickenpox

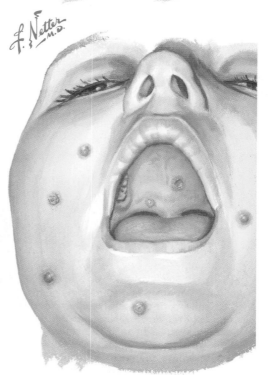
Chickenpox in child; "dew drops on a rose petal"

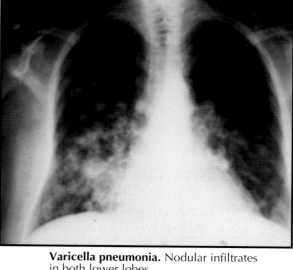
Varicella pneumonia. Nodular infiltrates in both lower lobes

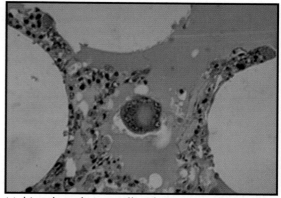
Multinucleated giant cell with massive edema of the alveolus

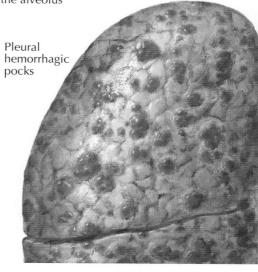
Pleural hemorrhagic pocks

virus invades endothelial cells in the respiratory tract. The virus quickly disseminates to the lymphatic tissue and then to other organ systems. This virus is neurotrophic and can lie dormant in the dorsal root ganglion, with the potential to reactivate much later in the form of shingles.

Treatment: Most childhood infections require no specific therapy other than supportive care and treatment of secondary bacterial infection. Immunocompromised individuals, including pregnant women, should be treated with an antiviral medication such as acyclovir. Neonates are also at high risk for serious disease and need to be treated. The vaccine provides long-term effectiveness that has been shown to last for decades. More time is needed to firmly establish the need for and timing of any booster vaccinations.

Plate 6-31

Integumentary System

CLINICAL PRESENTATION OF HERPES ZOSTER

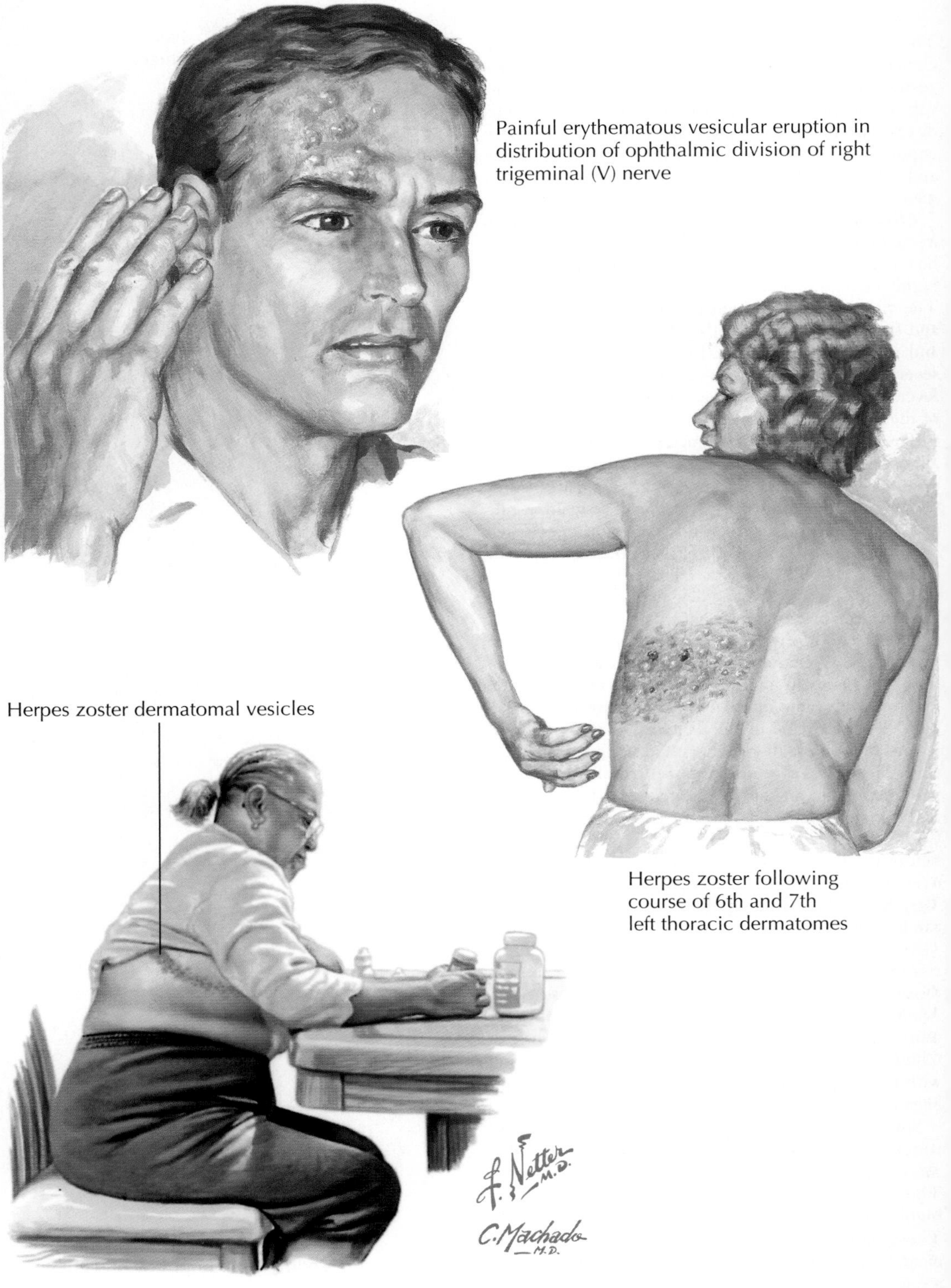

HERPES ZOSTER (SHINGLES)

The varicella zoster virus (VZV) is responsible for causing varicella (chickenpox) as well as herpes zoster (shingles). Herpes zoster is caused by reactivation of dormant VZV. Only hosts who have previously been infected with VZV can develop herpes zoster. The incidence of herpes zoster is sure to decrease in the future, because the zoster vaccine has good efficacy in increasing immunity against the virus. The live attenuated vaccine is currently recommended for those individuals 60 years of age and older who fulfill the criteria for receiving a live vaccine. This age was chosen because the incidence of herpes zoster increases after age 60, possibly related to a waning immune response and antibody titer remaining from the patient's original VZV infection. Whether the VZV vaccine protects against herpes zoster will take years to determine. The United States introduced widespread childhood immunization against VZV in 1995, and none of these children have yet reached the age of 60. Whether future booster vaccinations or VZV revaccination will be required is yet to be determined.

Clinical Findings: Herpes zoster is caused by reactivation of VZV, as acquired previously, that has been lying dormant in the dorsal root ganglia of the spinal cord or the ganglia of the cranial nerves. Patients are typically older individuals. The incidence increases with each decade of life and peaks at about 75 years of age. Herpes zoster is infrequently encountered in children. Men and women are equally affected. The initial symptom typically is a vague pain, tingling, or itching sensation. This may precede the rash by 1 or 2 days. Constitutional symptoms are commonly seen in older patients. After this prodrome, the characteristic vesicular rash develops in a dermatomal distribution. The location most frequently affected is the thoracic spine region; however, the trigeminal nerve is the most frequently involved nerve. The vesicles spread out to involve almost the entire dermatome of the nerve that has been infected. The rash does not cross the midline, and this is a clue to the diagnosis. Bilateral herpes zoster is very rare and is seen more frequently in immunosuppressed individuals.

The rash is exquisitely tender and can lead to significant sleep disturbances and significant morbidity. With healing, which usually occurs within 1 to 2 weeks, scarring is common. Pain typically dissipates over time, but a small subset of individuals, usually older than 50 years of age, develop postherpetic neuralgia. Postherpetic neuralgia can be a life-altering condition of abnormal sensation within the region affected by the herpes zoster outbreak. Patients often describe pain and paresthesias. Clothing or bedding rubbing against the skin can cause severe discomfort and pain. Postherpetic neuralgia can last for weeks to months or even years and can be devastating.

Painful erythematous vesicular eruption in distribution of ophthalmic division of right trigeminal (V) nerve

Herpes zoster dermatomal vesicles

Herpes zoster following course of 6th and 7th left thoracic dermatomes

Although the thoracic dorsal ganglia, taken as a whole, are responsible for the most cases of herpes zoster, the trigeminal nerve is the most frequently involved single nerve. The severity of the infection depends on the branch or branches involved. Herpes zoster infections on the face are typically more severe than those on the trunk or extremities. Infections on the face can affect the eye and ear and can lead to blindness or to hearing loss in severe cases. If the vesicles of herpes zoster affect the tip of the nose, the eye is likely to be involved. The nasociliary branch of the ophthalmic division of the trigeminal nerve innervates the nasal tip, and involvement of this region indicates that the infection is within the ophthalmic nerve. This involvement of the nasal tip with subsequent involvement of the globe is termed *Hutchinson's sign*. VZV infection of the eye is a medical emergency, and the patient must be evaluated by an ophthalmologist as soon as possible.

Plate 6-32

Infectious Diseases

HERPES ZOSTER (SHINGLES)
(Continued)

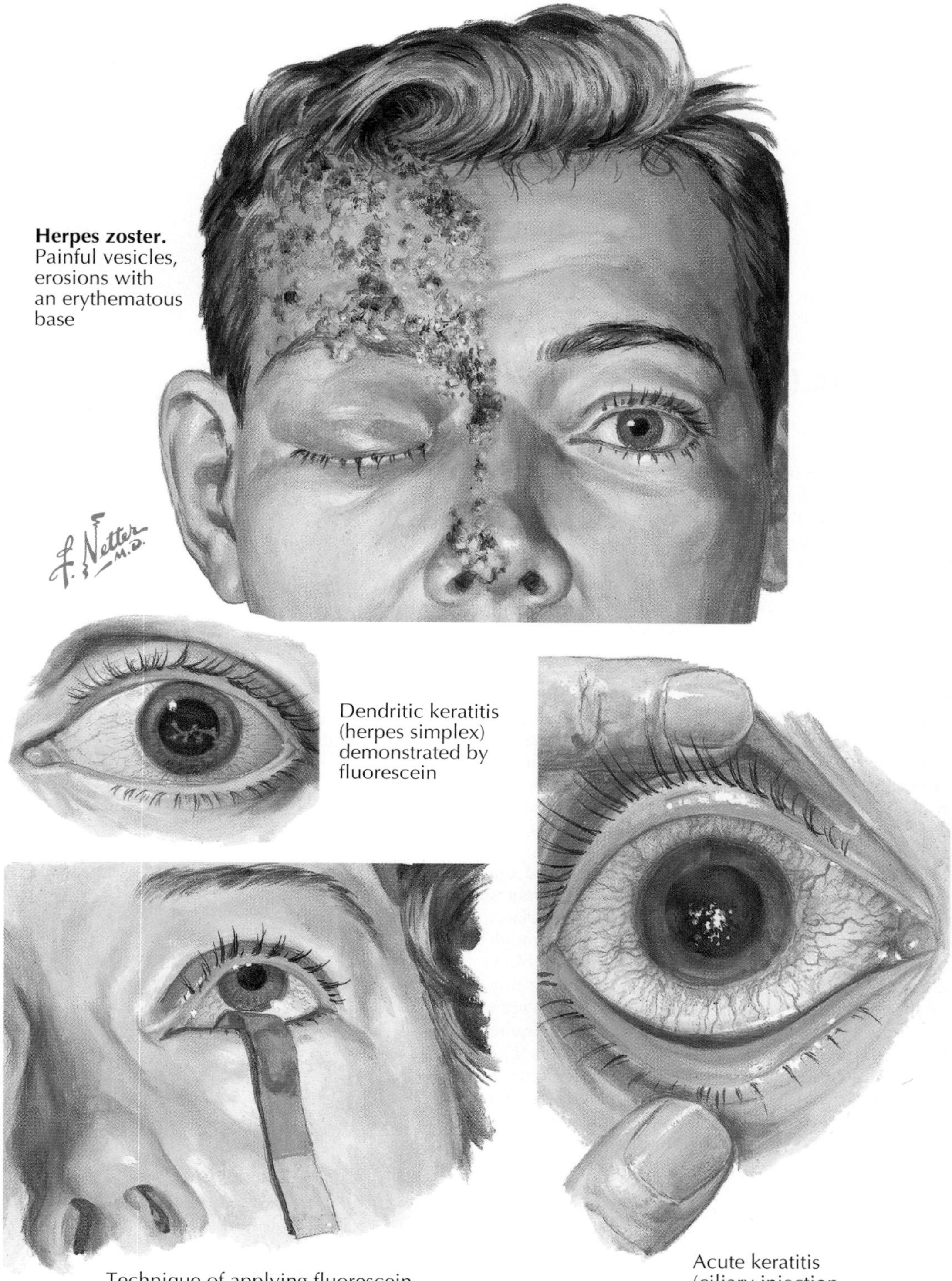

Simultaneous involvement of the facial and vestibular nerves is not infrequent and has been termed the Ramsay Hunt syndrome. These two nerves originate in close proximity to each other, and reactivation of VZV within the geniculate ganglion may involve both these nerves. This can lead to hearing loss and motor nerve loss due to involvement of the vestibular and the facial nerve, respectively. The ear and the anterior tongue develop the vesiculation seen in routine VZV infections. The motor loss may mimic Bell's palsy, and hearing loss may be permanent. Other cranial nerves have been reported to be affected in Ramsay Hunt syndrome, but the seventh and eighth nerves are those most frequently affected by far.

Scarring may be a severe sequela of this infection, and it can be made worse by bacterial superinfection. The presence of any honey-colored crusting or expanding erythema outside the dermatome should suggest the possibility of secondary impetigo or cellulitis. Prompt recognition and therapy are required to help prevent serious, disfiguring scarring.

The diagnosis is made clinically, and the Tzanck test can confirm the diagnosis. The presence of multinucleated giant cells on a Tzanck preparation taken from a vesicular rash in a dermatomal distribution confirms the diagnosis. Viral culture can be performed, but is not cost-effective. Direct immunofluorescent antibody testing (DFA) is a rapid method to determine the viral cause, but it is expensive and is rarely needed in these cases.

Histology: Skin biopsies are not needed for diagnosis of this infection. If one were to biopsy a vesicle, ballooning degeneration of the keratinocytes would be present. This ballooning degeneration leads to the vesiculation and bulla formation. Multinucleated giant cells can be seen at the base of the blister. A mixed dermal inflammatory infiltrate is present.

Pathogenesis: Any individual previously infected with VZV in the form of chickenpox is predisposed to develop herpes zoster later in life. Most cases occur with advancing age, as cell-mediated immunity tends to wane with time. The virus remains latent in the nerve ganglia until it reactivates. The ability to reactivate and the exact signal for reactivation are unknown. Once the virus reactivates, it begins to replicate and to cause necrosis of the affected nerve cells. The virus travels along the cutaneous sensory nerves and eventually affects the skin that is innervated by the nerve root where the virus became reactivated.

Treatment: Treatment with antiviral medications from the acyclovir family should be instituted immediately. The sooner therapy is started, the better is the chance of decreasing the length of disease. Therapy may also decrease the incidence of postherpetic neuralgia. The use of oral corticosteroids in conjunction with the antiviral medication has been advocated to help

VARICELLA ZOSTER WITH KERATITIS

Herpes zoster. Painful vesicles, erosions with an erythematous base

Dendritic keratitis (herpes simplex) demonstrated by fluorescein

Technique of applying fluorescein strip in previously anesthetized eye

Acute keratitis (ciliary injection, irregular corneal surface)

decrease the risk of postherpetic neuralgia, but large studies have thus far shown inconclusive data to support this approach. The therapy has the best chance of changing the course of the disease if given within the first 72 hours after the onset of disease symptoms.

A live attenuated zoster vaccine for the prevention of herpes zoster is being given to patients older than 60 years of age. This vaccine has been shown to boost natural immunity against VZV and to decrease the number of cases of herpes zoster and the frequency of postherpetic neuralgia in those who do develop herpes zoster after vaccination. As with all live vaccines, its use in immunosuppressed patients is contraindicated.

Currently, the treatment of postherpetic neuralgia is not optimal. Amitriptyline, gabapentin, lidocaine patches, pregabalin, anticonvulsants, and opioids are all used with varying success.

Plate 6-33

Integumentary System

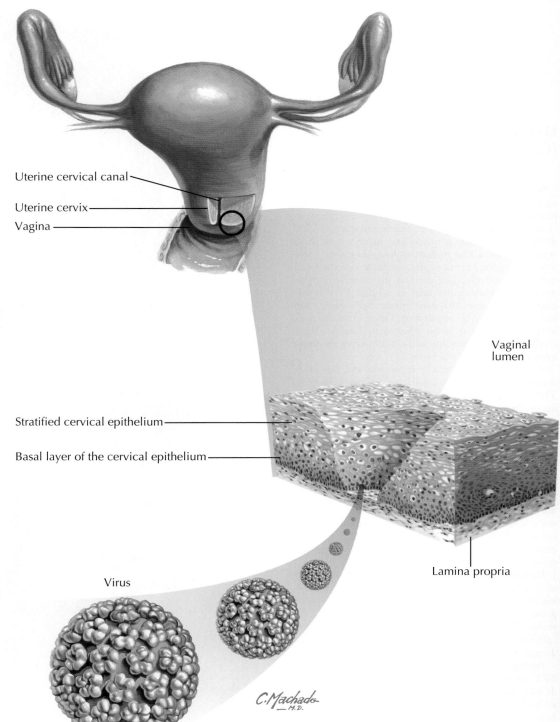

HUMAN PAPILLOMAVIRUS (HPV) INFECTION

Uterine cervical canal

Uterine cervix

Vagina

Vaginal lumen

Stratified cervical epithelium

Basal layer of the cervical epithelium

Lamina propria

Virus

C. Machado
—M.D.

VERRUCAE (WARTS)

Verrucae are one of the most frequently encountered viral infections in humans. They are capable of causing disease in any individual, but severe infections seem to be more likely in those who are immunocompromised. Warts can affect any cutaneous surface, and unique wart subtypes are more prone to cause disease in different clinical locations. By far the most important aspect of infection with the human papillomavirus (HPV) is the ability of the virus to cause malignant transformation. This malignant potential is specific to certain subtypes and is especially a concern in women, who are at risk for cervical cancer. Most cases of cervical cancer can be traced to prior infection with certain HPV strains. In June 2006, the U.S. Food and Drug Administration approved the use of a prophylactic HPV vaccine in prepubertal girls. The vaccine is a recombinant quadrivalent vaccine against HPV types 6, 11, 16, and 18. Types 16 and 18 are believed to have been responsible for up to 70% of cervical cancers.

Clinical Findings: Verruca vulgaris, also called the common wart, is the most prevalent wart that infects the human. It can be located on any cutaneous surface. These warts often appear as small papules with a rough surface studded with pinpoint, dark purple to black dots. These dots represent the thromboses of the tiny capillaries within the wart. Most warts are between 5 mm and 1 cm in diameter, but some can become quite large and encompass much larger areas of the skin. The coalescence of multiple warts into one larger wart is called mosaic warts. These are most commonly seen on the plantar aspect of the foot. Verruca vulgaris can come in many sizes and shapes. Most lesions spontaneously resolve within a few years. A good rule of thumb is that 50% of verrucae will disappear spontaneously in 2 years. Many distinctive clinical forms of warts exist.

The filiform wart is represented by a small verrucal papule with finger-like projections extruding from the base of the papule. The projections are typically 1 to 2 mm thick and 4 to 7 mm long. They are commonly found on the face. The flat wart is frequently encountered and manifests as a 3- to 5-mm, flat papule with a slight pink to red to purple coloration. Flat warts are frequently seen on the legs of women and in the beard region of men, and they can be arranged in a linear pattern if the warts are spread during the act of shaving. Flat warts have been found to be highly associated with HPV types 3 and 10.

Plantar warts (myrmecia) are seen on the plantar aspect of the foot and are caused for the most part by HPV types 1, 2, and 4. They are deep-seated papules and plaques that may coalesce into large mosaic warts.

The warts are well defined and characteristically interrupt the skin lines. This is in contrast to a callus, in which the skin lines are retained, and this sign can be used to differentiate the two conditions. Plantar warts can cause pain and discomfort if they are located in areas of pressure such as the heels or across the skin underlying the metatarsal heads. Palmar warts are very similar to plantar warts and have the same clinical appearance.

Subungual and periungual warts, a subclassification of palmar/plantar warts, are found around and under the nail apparatus. These warts can cause nail dystrophy and pain on grasping of objects. They tend to affect more than one finger and can be more difficult to treat than the common wart. Long-standing periungual or subungual warts that have a changing morphology should be biopsied to rule out malignant transformation into a squamous cell carcinoma. This is not

Plate 6-34

Infectious Diseases

CONDYLOMATA ACUMINATA (GENITAL WARTS)

In females
"Cauliflower"-appearing plaques

VERRUCAE (WARTS) (Continued)

infrequently encountered, and a high clinical suspicion
should be used when investigating these types of warts.

Ring warts are seen after various treatments of
common warts, most frequently after liquid nitrogen
therapy. The central portion of the wart resolves,
leaving a ring-shaped or donut-shaped wart with central
clearing. These warts can become larger than the wart
originally treated.

Condylomata acuminata (genital warts) are often
considered to be the most common form of sexually
transmitted disease in the United States. These warts
typically begin as small, flesh-colored to slightly hyperpigmented macules and papules. As they grow, they take
on an exophytic growth pattern and have often been
compared with the appearance of cauliflower. The
warts may stay small and localized, or they may grow to
enormous size, leading to difficulty with urination and
sexual intercourse. Females with cervical genital warts
are asymptomatic and may not realize they are infected.
Routine gynecological examinations and Papanicolaou
smears are the only reliable way to diagnosis cervical
warts. Diagnosis is extremely important, because cervical warts are the number one cause of cervical cancer.

Histology: Skin biopsies of wart tissue show the
pathognomonic cell called the koilocyte. This cell,
when present, is highly specific and sensitive for HPV
infection. It is a keratinocyte with a basophilic small
nucleus and a surrounding clear halo. There are few to
no keratohyalin granules in the koilocyte. Other findings include varying amounts of hyperkeratosis, acanthosis, and striking papillomatosis.

Pathogenesis: Warts are caused by infection with
HPV, of which more than 150 subtypes are known to
cause human disease. They are small viruses with no
lipid envelope, and they can stay viable for long periods.
HPV has a double-stranded, circular DNA. A variety
of subtypes are able to affect different regions of the
body. HPV is capable of infecting human epithelium,
including the keratinized skin and the mucous membranes. It gains entry through slightly abraded skin or
mucous membranes. The virus does not actively infect
the outer stratum corneum but rather the stratum
basalis cells. Like most viruses, HPV can produce early
and late gene products. The early genes encode various
proteins necessary for replication. These early gene
products also play a role in malignant transformation
of the infected cell. The exact mechanism is not completely understood. The late genes produce capsid proteins. At least eight early genes are present, and two late
genes are included in the viral DNA.

Treatment: Common warts can be treated in a
number of ways. Approximately 50% of the lesions

Cervical HPV infection
is the leading cause of
cervical cancer.

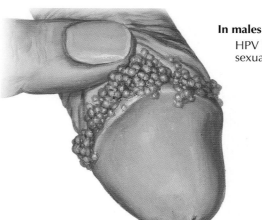

In males
HPV is one of the most common
sexually transmitted diseases.

spontaneously resolve. The others may or may not
respond to therapy. This lack of universal treatment
response is frustrating to patient and physician alike.
Many destructive therapies are available, including
liquid nitrogen cryotherapy, salicylic acid, trichloracetic
acid, cantharidin, podophyllin, and bleomycin. Immunotherapy can be used to induce an immunological
response; these options include imiquimod, interferon,
squaric acid, and Candida skin test antigen. No single

therapy appears to work better than any other, and
patients often need to undergo a variety of treatments
until they find one that works.

Genital warts should be treated with imiquimod or
one of the destructive methods to decrease the risk of
transmission. Women who are sexually active should
undergo routine gynecological screening. The advent
of the HPV vaccine may lead to a decreased incidence
of genital warts and cervical cancer.

HAIR AND NAIL DISEASES

Plate 7-1

Integumentary System

ALOPECIA AREATA

Alopecia areata is an autoimmune disease that causes discrete circular or oval areas of nonscarring alopecia. This form of alopecia has several clinical variants, including alopecia totalis, alopecia universalis, and an ophiasis pattern. Therapy is often difficult. The disease can have profound psychological impact, especially in young patients. It is critical to address this issue, because the effects on the patient's psychological well-being are often more severe than the actual hair loss.

Clinical Findings: Alopecia areata can affect individuals of any age but is most frequently seen in children and young adults. It is estimated to affect 1% of the population. Both sexes are equally affected, and there is no race predilection. The first sign is hair loss in one specific area of the scalp. The hairs fall out in large numbers, especially when pulled. The patches of hair loss typically have an oval or circular pattern. There may be one or more than a dozen areas of involvement. The scalp hair is the most commonly affected region. The affected scalp is smooth without evidence of scarring or follicular dropout. Small, stubby hairs may be present at follicular openings and have been termed "exclamation point hairs." All hair regions may be involved, including the eyebrows, eyelashes, and beard.

Alopecia areata has an unpredictable, waxing and waning course. Areas may begin to grow back as new patches form. It is not uncommon for a patient to have one solitary episode with spontaneous resolution and no future episodes. Some patients develop patches of alopecia intermittently over their lifetime. Complete loss of the scalp hair caused by alopecia areata is termed *alopecia totalis.* The rarest variant is alopecia universalis, which causes loss of all hair in all locations. These two forms of alopecia areata are very difficult to treat. Patients with both alopecia totalis and alopecia universalis need psychological assessment, because the loss of hair has severe social and self-esteem consequences. Patients often benefit from consultation with a professional psychologist or psychiatrist. Alopecia areata support groups can be extremely helpful.

The ophiasis pattern of alopecia areata is less commonly seen. It involves the parietal scalp dorsally to the occiput bilaterally. The diagnosis is typically made on clinical grounds. A skin biopsy is rarely needed. The hair pull test is a diagnostic test that can be performed at the bedside. It is positive when more than three hairs are pulled out in and around the patch of alopecia areata. If the hair is actively shedding, this test should be performed only once, because the number of hairs removed is large and can be very upsetting to the patient. The hair that regrows is often lacking in pigment and appears white or gray. Over time, these white hairs are replaced with pigmented hairs as the hair pigmentation machinery begins to work again.

Histology: Skin biopsies of the scalp of an affected area show a dense lymphocytic infiltrate surrounding all the hair bulbs in what has been termed a "swarm of bees" pattern. There are increased numbers of catagen and telogen hairs. The epidermis is normal.

Pathogenesis: Alopecia areata is believed to be an autoimmune inflammatory disease of T cells that, for unknown reasons, attacks certain hair follicles. It may be seen in association with other autoimmune diseases

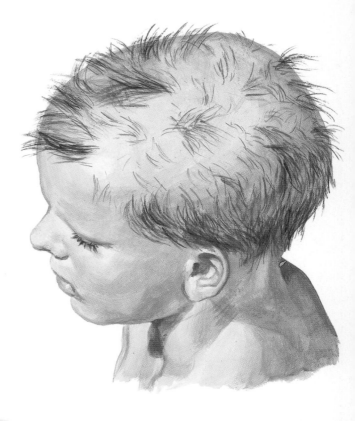

Alopecia areata approaching the alopecia totalis stage. This patient has lost almost all of her scalp hair.

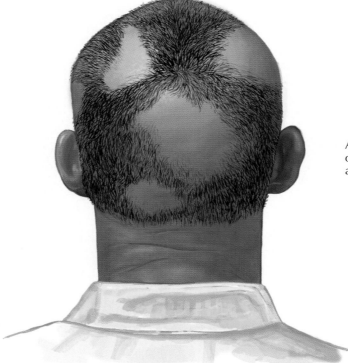

Alopecia areata with the characteristic oval and circular areas of nonscarring alopecia

such as autoimmune thyroid disease. It is believed to be polygenic in nature.

Treatment: Treatment consists of proper assessment of the patient and how the disease is affecting the patient's life in general. Some individuals tolerate the condition without adverse psychological effects; for them, the best treatment is a watch-and-wait approach. Others with mild disease may have severe self-esteem issues and should be offered therapy. However, no therapy has been shown to be uniformly effective, and most have only anecdotal reports of efficacy. Topical retinoids and corticosteroids are used, as well as intralesional steroid injections if the areas are small enough. Contact sensitization with squaric acid has had equivocal results. Oral steroids should be avoided, because the long-term side effects do not warrant their use.

Plate 7-2

Hair and Nail Diseases

ANDROGENIC ALOPECIA

Androgenic alopecia, also known as male pattern baldness or female pattern hair loss, is a major form of hair loss. The age at onset is variable and likely has a genetic determination. Some men lose their entire scalp hair, resulting in baldness. Baldness is rare in women, because their hair loss manifests as varying grades of thinning.

Clinical Findings: There are variable degrees of male pattern hair loss. The Hamilton-Norwood scale has been used to grade the degree of hair loss. Grade I is manifested by receding frontal hair. Grade VII is near-total loss of the scalp hair with some sparing of the inferior occiput. The age at onset of androgenic alopecia in men can be any time from puberty into adulthood. Most men older than 50 years of age exhibit some form of androgenic hair loss. The Caucasian population is much more prone to developing androgenic alopecia than the African American or Asian population.

Female pattern hair loss can be more difficult to treat because of the importance society places on appearance and the psychological effects that hair loss can have on women. Most women do not go bald, but some develop severe thinning of the vertex. A characteristic finding in androgenic female pattern hair loss is preservation of the frontal hair line. This form of hair loss is seen more commonly in the postmenopausal population.

Histology: Evaluation of a 4-mm punch biopsy specimen by the horizontal method is the best technique to evaluate hair loss. In androgenic alopecia, the follicles are normal in number, but they show evidence of miniaturization. Vellus hairs are increased in number. Whereas the normal scalp has been shown to have a vellus-to-telogen hair ratio of 1:7, the ratio in androgenic alopecia is 1:3.5. The hair shaft diameters of the terminal hairs are inconstant, which corresponds to the miniaturization affect.

Pathogenesis: Androgenic alopecia has been shown to follow an autosomal dominant pattern of inheritance. It is believed to result from an abnormal response of the hair follicle to androgens (i.e., dihydrotestosterone). This androgen has been shown to cause miniaturization of the terminal hairs over successive hair cycles. As the hair follicles miniaturize, they become smaller with a thinner caliber. This causes less scalp coverage, which manifests as hair thinning. The actual hair follicles are not scarred or lost. Inhibition of the production of dihydrotestosterone from its precursor, testosterone, is one therapeutic tactic.

Treatment: Therapy for male pattern baldness includes use of the topical agent minoxidil 5%, applied twice daily, with or without the oral 5α-reductase inhibitor, finasteride. 5α-Reductase is the enzyme responsible for converting free testosterone into dihydrotestosterone. Both these agents have been shown in multiple randomized studies to decrease the rate of hair loss and increase the hair shaft diameter. These medications are well tolerated and have minimal side effects. Patients with prostate cancer should avoid the use of finasteride unless approved by their oncologist. The only option at present for women with androgenic alopecia is topical minoxidil 2%. This has been shown to decrease the rate of hair loss.

Most patients who use minoxidil experience a slowing of hair loss, and some see increased growth. It is critical to treat early in the course of disease to maximize the effects of the medication. Topical minoxidil may cause excessive hair growth on the forehead and temples if it is applied in these regions. This can be disconcerting for patients, and they need to be educated on the proper application of the medication.

Hair transplantation techniques continue to improve. The goal of surgery is to leave a natural-appearing hair pattern. This is best accomplished with minigrafts of 1 to 2 follicles at a time. A strip of the patient's hair is removed from the occipital scalp, and each individual hair is dissected out. The separated hair follicles are then tediously inserted into the desired areas. Patients can have an excellent result, and the transplanted hair appear to be resistant to the effects of dihydrotestosterone.

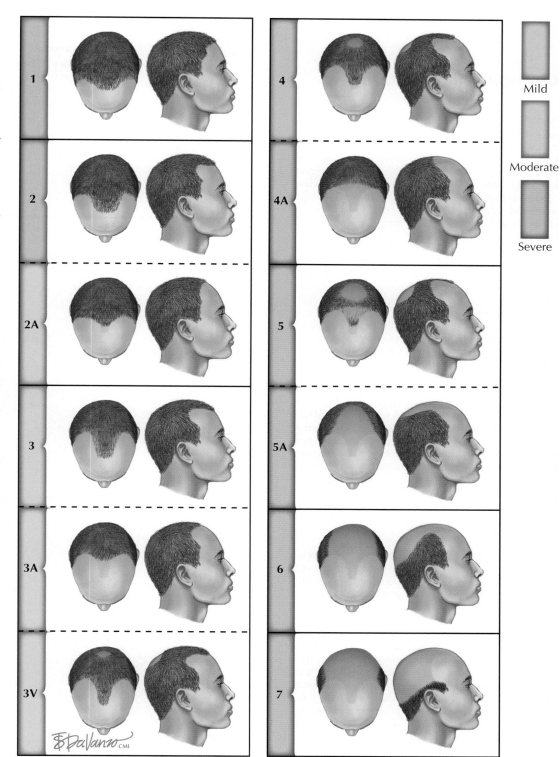

Plate 7-3

Integumentary System

COMMON FINGERNAIL DISORDERS

COMMON NAIL DISORDERS

Nail disorders are frequently encountered in the clinical setting. They can occur secondary to an underlying systemic disorder or as a primary disease of the nail unit. The nail unit consists of the nail matrix, bed, and plate and the proximal and lateral nail folds. Disorders of the nail plate and nail bed can manifest in a variety of ways. Systemic disease can manifest through changes in the nail unit. Beau's lines and Mees' lines of the nail are two nail findings seen in systemic disease. Beau's lines are caused by a nonspecific halting of the nail matrix growth pattern, and Mees' lines are specific for heavy metal toxicity. Dilation of the capillaries of the proximal nail fold or cuticular erythema can be a sign of connective tissue disease. The complete skin examination should also include an examination of the nails, because they offer insight into the patient's health.

One of the most serious nail unit disorders is melanoma of the nail matrix. Melanoma may manifest as a linear, pigmented band along the length of the nail. As time progresses, the proximal nail fold and hyponychium may also become pigmented and involved with melanoma. The finding of pigment on the proximal nail fold has been termed *Hutchinson's sign*. This sign is not seen in subungual hematomas. All new pigmented nail streaks should be evaluated and a biopsy considered. The biopsy requires nail plate removal and retraction of the proximal nail fold. The biopsy of a pigmented nail streak is performed within the nail matrix. Biopsies of the nail matrix may lead to a thinner nail or to chronic nail dystrophy due to disruption of the matrix. Subungual melanoma tends to be diagnosed late, because these tumors are easily overlooked or passed off as a subungual hematoma. It is critically important to differentiate the two.

Subungual hematomas are frequently encountered. Most are caused by direct trauma to the nail plate and nail bed, which causes bleeding between the plate and bed. Acute hematomas can be very painful. Most acute subungual hematomas are on the fingers and are caused by a crush injury or by a direct blow to the nail plate. As the blood accumulates under the nail plate, the pressure created can cause excruciating pain. This can be easily treated by nail trephination. A small-gauge hole is bored into the overlying nail plate with a hot, thin metal object or small drill. Once the nail plate has been punctured, the blood that has accumulated under the nail freely flows out of the newly formed channel, and near-immediate pain relief is achieved. Most traumatic injuries to the nail unit do not cause these very painful hematomas but rather cause small amounts of blood to accumulate under the nail plate. Pain is absent or minimal. Most people remember some trauma to the nail, but others do not. This form of subungual hematoma can involve small portions of the nail or the entire nail. There is often a blue, purple, and red discoloration of the underlying nail. Occasionally, the nail plate has a black appearance and is easily confused with subungual melanoma. The history can be misleading in these cases, because many patients with and without melanoma remember some form of trauma to the nail that might lead the clinician to pass the lesion off as a subungual hematoma. If any doubt about the diagnosis

Acute paronychia. Tender red nail fold, commonly caused by *Staphylococcus aureus*

Mees' lines. Mees' lines on fingernails and hyperpigmentation of the soles are characteristic of arsenic poisoning.

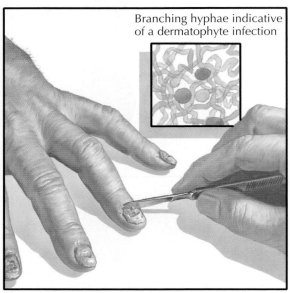

Branching hyphae indicative of a dermatophyte infection

Onychomycosis of the fingernails. A KOH preparation is done by scraping the crumbling nail plate and examining it under the microscope.

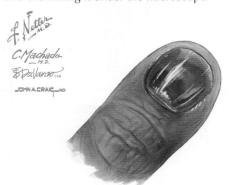

Subungal hematoma from trauma

Psoriatic arthritis with nail involvement. Sausage-shaped digits, psoriatic skin plaques and nail changes

Nail pits

Transverse ridges

Onycholysis

Psoriatic nail changes

exists, a nail biopsy should be considered. The nail plate is removed, and a subungual hematoma is easily distinguished from a tumor. Most subungual hematomas slowly grow outward toward the distal free edge of the nail. As the nail grows, its most proximal portion appears normal. The entire subungual hematoma eventually grows out and is shed or clipped off once it passes the hyponychium.

Onychocryptosis (ingrown nail) is almost universally seen in the great toenail. It is caused by burrowing of the lateral portion of the nail plate into the lateral nail fold. As the nail punctures the lateral nail fold, it sets off an inflammatory reaction that causes edema, redness, pain, and occasionally purulent drainage. Secondary infection is common. Ambulation may become difficult because the pain forces the patient to avoid pressure.

Plate 7-4

Hair and Nail Diseases

COMMON NAIL DISORDERS
(Continued)

The exact etiology of onychocryptosis is not entirely known, but it is believed to be caused, or at least made more likely, by improper trimming or removal of the lateral portion of the nail. If the nail plate is cut at varying angles or torn from its bed by picking, this may allow for the lateral free edge of the nail plate to enter into the lateral nail fold. Tight-fitting shoes have also been implicated as increasing the likelihood of developing ingrown nails. This condition is seen more frequently in young men, but it can be seen in all age groups. The fingernails are rarely affected. Treatment consists of lateral nail plate removal with or without a lateral nail matrixectomy. After proper anesthesia, a nail plate elevator is used to free the involved portion of the nail. A nail splitter is then used to remove the lateral third of the nail. The freed nail is grasped with a nail puller, and the nail is removed with a gentle, back-and-forth rocking motion. The portion of the nail that is removed from under the lateral nail fold is often larger than expected. Recurrent ingrown nails usually should be treated with nail matrixectomy. This destroys the lateral third of the nail matrix, eliminating the ability to form that portion of the nail and removing the potential nidus from causing further problems in the future. Application of phenol to the nail matrix after nail plate avulsion is one of the best methods for destroying the nail matrix. Bilateral nail fold involvement on the same toe is not infrequently encountered, and the entire nail can be removed in these cases. Onychocryptosis is not a primary infection of the nail unit, and any infection is believed to be secondary to the massive inflammatory response. This is in stark contrast to an acute paronychia.

Paronychia is a nail fold infection with either a bacterial agent (as in acute paronychia) or a fungal agent (in chronic paronychia). Acute paronychia manifests with redness and tenderness of the nail fold. The redness and edema continue to expand, causing pain and eventually purulent drainage. Removal of the cuticle or nail fold trauma may lead to an increased risk for this infection. *Staphylococcus aureus* and *Streptococcus* species are the most frequent etiological agents. Chronic paronychia typically is less inflammatory and manifests with redness and edema around the nail folds. Many digits may be involved. At presentation, patients typically report that they have been having difficulty for longer than 6 to 8 weeks. Tenderness is much less significant than in acute paronychia. Chronic paronychia is usually caused by a fungal infection of the nail fold with *Candida albicans*. Individuals who work in occupations in which their hands are constantly exposed to water are at higher risk for chronic paronychia. Therapy includes topical antifungal and antiinflammatory agents.

A felon is often confused with acute paronychia, but it is a soft tissue infection of the fingertip pulp. It may arise secondary to an acute paronychia. The clinical findings are those of a swollen, red, painful finger pad. The treatment is surgical incision and drainage together with oral antibiotics to cover *S. aureus* and *Streptococcus* species.

Onychomycosis is seen frequently in individuals of all ages, and its prevalence increases with age. Patients

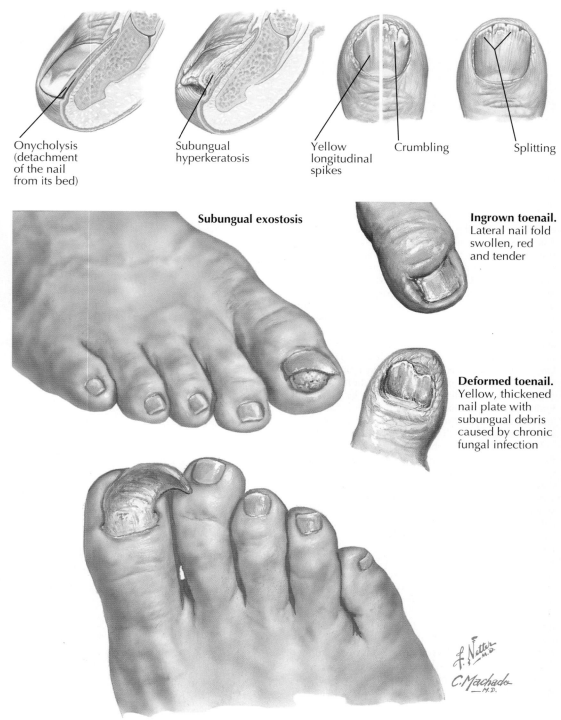

Onycholysis (detachment of the nail from its bed)

Subungual hyperkeratosis

Yellow longitudinal spikes

Crumbling

Splitting

Subungual exostosis

Ingrown toenail. Lateral nail fold swollen, red and tender

Deformed toenail. Yellow, thickened nail plate with subungual debris caused by chronic fungal infection

Onychogryphosis. "Ram's horn" nail. Nail plate is thick and curved.

can present with different variants of onychomycosis. The most frequent type is the distal and lateral subungual onychomycosis. Other variants include white superficial onychomycosis and proximal subungual onychomycosis. *Trichophyton rubrum* is the most frequent cause of all except white superficial onychomycosis, which is caused most often by *Trichophyton mentagrophytes*. Superficial white onychomycosis manifests with a fine, white, crumbling surface to the nail.

When it is curetted off, the white areas of fungal involvement are found to affect only the outermost portion of the nail plate. The material is a combination of fungal elements and nail keratin. Therapy includes curetting the white involved portion of the nail and applying a topical antifungal agent for at least 1 month.

Distal and lateral subungual onychomycosis manifests with thickened, yellow, dystrophic appearing nails with subungual debris. There are varying amounts of

Plate 7-5

Integumentary System

Onychogryphosis

COMMON NAIL DISORDERS
(Continued)

onycholysis (nail plate lifting off the nail bed). One nail may be solitarily involved but it is more common for several nails to be involved and for the surrounding skin to be involved with tinea manuum or tinea unguium. Fungal nail infections are much more frequently seen on the toenails than on the fingernails. The nails can become painful, especially with ambulation. Occasionally, the entire nail is shed as a result of significant onycholysis, and the nail that regrows will again be involved with onychomycosis. The thick and dystrophic nails may become a passage for bacterial invasion of the body. This is especially true in patients with diabetes. Bacteria can gain entrance into the skin and soft tissue via the abnormal barrier between nail and nail fold, and this can lead to paronychia, felon, and the most serious complication, cellulitis. Distal and lateral subungual onychomycosis almost always needs to be treated with an oral antifungal medication for any chance of a cure. Topical agents may be helpful in limited nail disease, but their use is typically limited to an adjunctive role. Oral azole antifungals, griseofulvin, and terbinafine have all been used, with similar results.

Psoriasis can affect the nails in many ways. Nail involvement appears more frequently in patients with severe disease and in those with psoriatic arthritis. The nails can show oil spots, pitting, ridging, onycholysis, and onychauxis (subungual hyperkeratosis). The oil spots are represented by a brownish to yellowish discoloration under the nail plate and associated onycholysis. The discoloration is caused by deposition of various glycoproteins into the nail plate. Nail pitting can be seen in other conditions besides psoriasis, such as alopecia areata; it is caused by parakeratosis of the proximal nail matrix, which is responsible for producing the dorsal nail plate. Ridging and onychauxis is caused by the excessive hyperkeratosis of the nail bed, which is directly caused by psoriasis. Therapy for psoriatic nails can involve intralesional steroid injections or use of systemic agents to decrease the abnormal immune response that is driving the psoriasis.

Onychogryphosis ("ram's horn" nail deformity) manifests with an unusually thickened and curved nail that takes the shape of a ram's horn.

A plethora of nail changes may be seen in response to systemic disease. Beau's lines are horizontal notches along the nails that may be caused by any major stressful event. The stressful event typically is induced by prolonged hospitalization, which causes temporary inadequate production of the nail bed by the nail matrix. It is entirely corrected spontaneously as the individual improves. Mees' lines are induced by heavy metal toxicity, most commonly from arsenic exposure. They appear as a single, white horizontal band across each nail. Mees' lines have also been reported in cases of malnutrition. Terry's nails is the name given to nail changes seen in congestive heart failure and cirrhosis of the liver: More than two thirds of the proximal nail

Correct Incorrect
Pedicure

Ingrowing tissue

Infected ingrowing tissue

Cotton pledget under nail

Removal of one third of nail bed

Nail avulsed
Distal nail bed
Skin flap
Proximal nail bed removed
Note the proximity of the nail bed to the underlying bone.

Suture of skin flap

plate and bed appear dull white with loss of the lunula. Half-and-half nails, also called Lindsay's nails, are seen in patients with chronic renal failure. The proximal half of the nail is normal appearing, whereas the distal half has a brown discoloration. Yellow nail syndrome manifests with all 20 nails having a yellowish discoloration and increased thickness of the nail plate. This syndrome is almost always seen in association with a pleural effusion, often secondary to a lung-based malignancy.

Koilonychia is one of the most easily recognized deformities of the nail; it is caused by iron deficiency. The nail plate develops a spoon-shaped, concave surface. Splinter hemorrhages may be a sign of bacterial endocarditis. Clubbing, which is defined as loss of Lovibond's angle, is typically caused by chronic lung disease. The nail unit can manifest disease in many ways, and awareness of the various nail signs can help the clinician diagnose and treat these conditions.

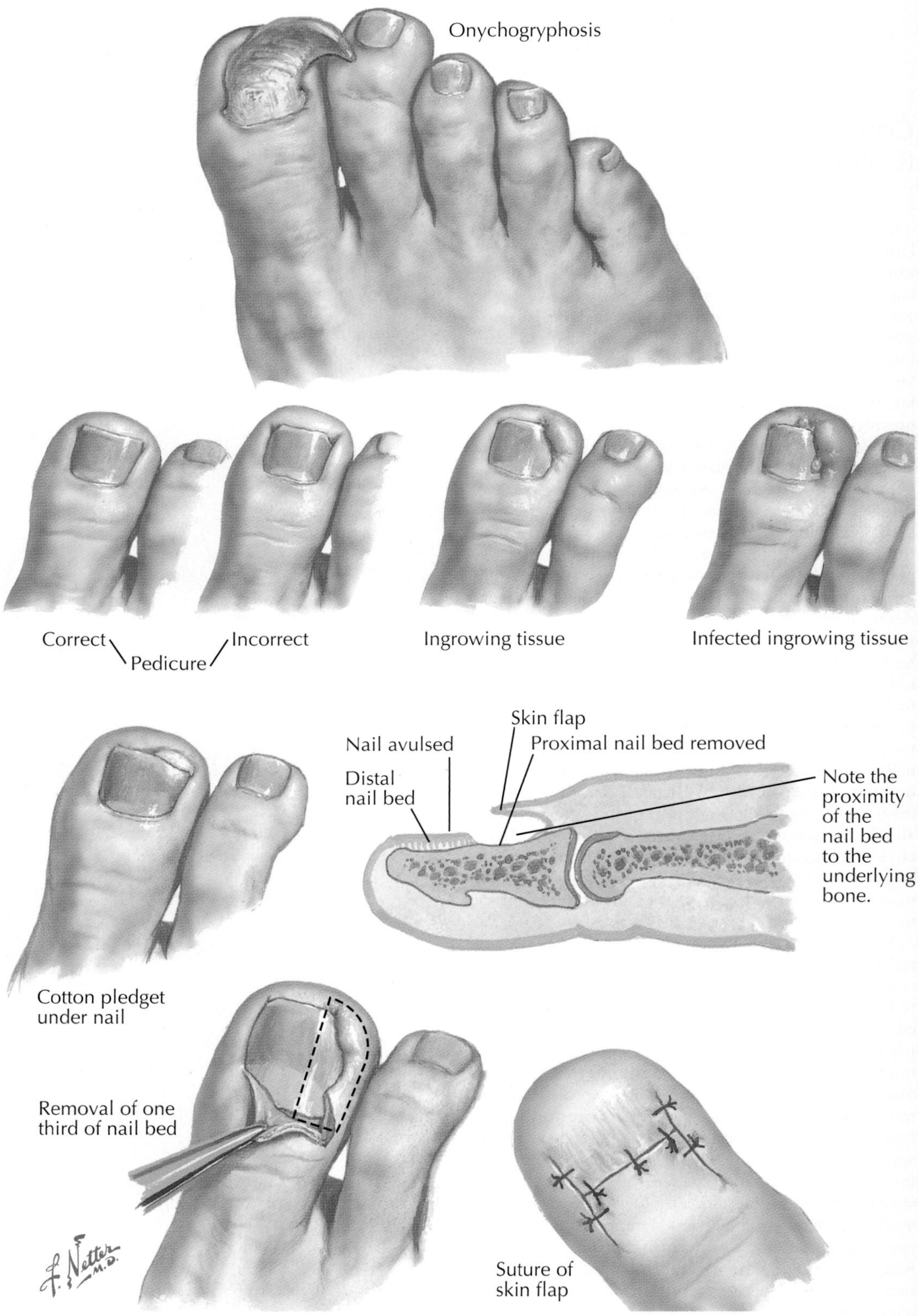

Plate 7-6

Hair and Nail Diseases

HAIR SHAFT ABNORMALITIES

There are a wide variety of hair shaft abnormalities. Most are nonspecific clinical findings that can be seen in a multitude of underlying conditions, as well as in the normal individual. Trichoptilosis, known by the lay term "split ends," is probably the most common hair shaft abnormality in humans. It is nonspecific and is not associated with any particular underlying syndrome. Trichoptilosis is believed to be caused by excessive trauma to the distal hair shaft. Trichorrhexis nodosa is another hair shaft abnormality that can be seen in individuals with no underlying disease state. A few highly specific hair abnormalities are indicative of particular disorders; for example, pili trianguli et canaliculi and trichorrhexis invaginata are seen only in uncombable hair syndrome and Netherton syndrome, respectively. The astute clinician uses knowledge of hair shaft abnormalities to help form a differential diagnosis and in some cases to confirm a diagnosis.

Pili torti is also known as "twisted hair" or "corkscrew hair." The hair twists on its axis in a corkscrew pattern. This twisting leads to increased pressure on the hair shaft, which results in early breakage and short, brittle hair. The involvement is almost exclusively on the scalp. Pili torti is nonspecific and can be found in a number of genetic skin conditions, including Björnstad syndrome, Menkes syndrome, and Crandall syndrome. It can also be seen as a primary hair disease with no underlying associations.

Monilethrix is a highly specific hair shaft abnormality. The hair has a beaded or undulating appearance, with nodes interspaced at regular intervals by abnormally thin hair. It is inherited in an autosomal dominant fashion and is caused by a mutation in the hair basic keratin 6 gene (HB6), which is officially known as keratin 86 (KRT86). The hair is fragile and breaks in the thinned internode regions. The internode regions are devoid of pigment, and this feature is used to discriminate this condition from pseudo-monilethrix. There is no known therapy. Many afflicted individuals improve after puberty. It is almost never associated with systemic disease.

Trichorrhexis nodosa is a completely nonspecific finding that may be seen in healthy individuals. This hair shaft abnormality has been described as "broomstick hair" because of the appearance of the distal end of the broken hair, which resembles the bristles of a broom. Trichorrhexis nodosa is the most frequent reason for hair breakage. Trauma to the hair is causative. This trauma can be self-induced by rubbing or twisting, which results in fracturing of the hair and the appearance of trichorrhexis nodosa. This finding on microscopic examination can be helpful in evaluating hair loss secondary to trichotillomania or chemical-induced alopecia.

Pili trianguli et canaliculus, also termed "spun glass hair," is the diagnostic finding in uncombable hair syndrome. This rare and highly unusual syndrome is associated with no underlying ill effects on the afflicted individuals. The hair is uncontrollable and impossible to comb straight. This effect is related to the abnormal triangular shape of the hair shaft as well as changes in the direction of the hair, which occur at uneven intervals. The condition is inherited in an autosomal dominant pattern and is believed to be the result of an abnormal inner root sheath. No therapy is needed, and most children with this condition spontaneously improve over time. The hair shafts appear almost triangular under electron microscopy.

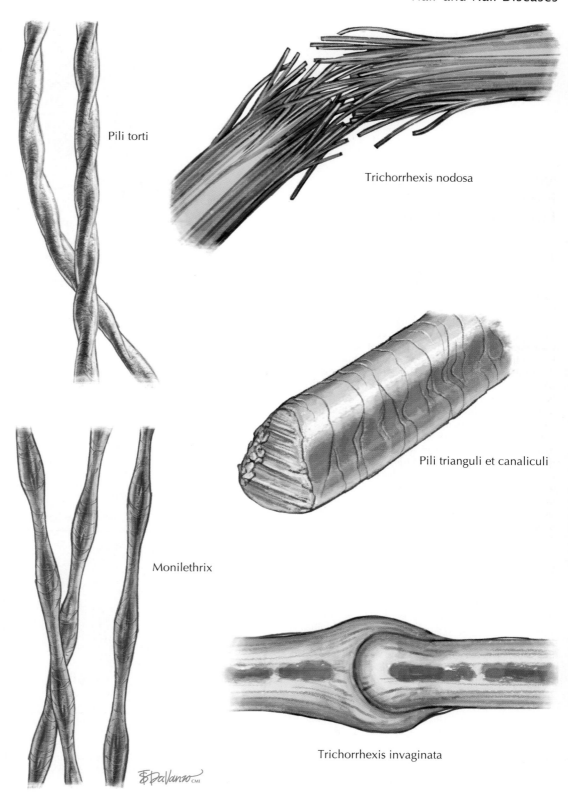

Pili torti

Trichorrhexis nodosa

Pili trianguli et canaliculi

Monilethrix

Trichorrhexis invaginata

Trichorrhexis invaginata is seen only in patients with the autosomal recessive Netherton syndrome. This hair shaft abnormality has been termed "bamboo hair" because of its resemblance to the growth rings of a bamboo plant. Another descriptive term is "ball and socket hair," because it appears that the distal portion of the hair invaginates into the proximal hair cortex. The hair is brittle and breaks easily, leading to alopecia. The eyebrow hair is the best place to look for trichorrhexis invaginata. Netherton syndrome is a multisystem disease caused by a mutation in the SPINK5 gene that is associated with erythroderma, alopecia, and elevated levels of immunoglobulin E. Ichthyosis linearis circumflexa is the name for the migratory, irregular, serpiginous patches and plaques with a double-edged scale that are seen only in Netherton syndrome. The SPINK5 gene encodes the serine protease inhibitor, Kazal type 5 protein, which is important in epithelial desquamation.

Plate 7-7   Integumentary System

NORMAL STRUCTURE AND FUNCTION OF THE HAIR FOLLICLE APPARATUS

The pilosebaceous unit is a complex apparatus that comprises a hair shaft and its follicle, sebaceous glands, arrector pili muscle, and, in some regions of the body, apocrine glands. Hair is a complex structure that is made of many different keratin proteins linked by disulfide bonds between neighboring cysteine amino acid molecules. The keratin molecules come in acidic and basic forms. An acidic keratin fiber localizes with a basic keratin fiber and cross-links via disulfide bonds.

The exact function of hair is unknown, but it is theorized to act as an insulator for heat retention and has been postulated to be important to attract a mate. No matter what the function, humans can live a normal life without the presence of hair with no ill effects.

Hair comes in a variety of colors. The amount of melanin or pheomelanin in the hair shaft determines the exact color of the hair. With time, the production of hair pigment decreases, and the hair becomes dull gray or white. This process is unpredictable in a given individual, and even those within the same family may show striking differences in hair color change. As people age, the scalp hair usually tends to thin. This is considered to be a normal physiological process.

There are two main types of hair in the adult. Terminal hair is thick hair that is present on the scalp, axilla, and groin and in the beard region in men. Vellus hair is the fine, thin, lightly pigmented hair that can be found in most areas of the body where terminal hair is not present. No hair is present on the lips, palms, soles, glans, or labia minora. Lanugo hair is present during fetal development and is predominantly seen in premature infants. This type of hair is shed in utero and replaced with vellus hair before delivery. Reversion of vellus hair and terminal hair back to lanugo hair is a sign of anorexia nervosa. Lanugo hair has a soft, fluffy white appearance.

The hair cycle is an extremely complex and highly coordinated process. The anagen phase is the growth phase. The anagen phase of the typical adult scalp hair lasts approximately 2 years. This growth phase is followed by the catagen phase, which is a short (2 week) transition period during which the hair follicle transforms from a growing, functioning hair into a club hair. This is followed by the telogen phase, which lasts approximately 2 months and ends with shedding of the club hair. Anagen hairs have a floppy, pigmented end that is easily distinguished from the telogen hair. Telogen hair is termed *club hair* because of its depigmented bulb at the proximal end. Catagen hairs are almost impossible to identify because they appear somewhere in the spectrum between anagen and telogen hair. The length of the anagen phase is responsible for the overall length of the hair: The longer the anagen phase, the longer the hair can grow. This

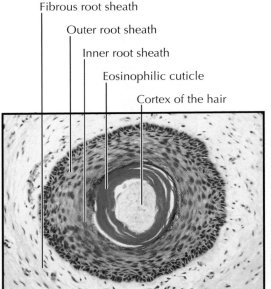

Pilosebaceous unit

Epidermis
Hair shaft
Hair cortex
Hair medulla
Dermal papilla

Sebaceous gland and its duct
Arrector pili muscle
Hair cuticle
Huxley layer } Inner root sheath
Henle layer
Outer root sheath
Hair bulb

Schematic diagram of a pilosebaceous unit and innervation of skin

Hair
Sebaceous gland
Hair follicle
Dermis
Hair bulb
Papilla

Fibrous root sheath
Outer root sheath
Inner root sheath
Eosinophilic cuticle
Cortex of the hair

Hair follicle
Sebaceous duct
Sebaceous gland
External root sheath
Dermis
Arrector pili muscle
Epidermis

Light micrograph of a hair and its follicle near the epidermis in transverse section*

Light micrograph of thin skin close to the epidermis*

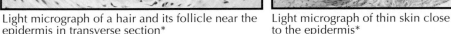

*Micrographs reprinted with permission from Ovalle W, Nahirney P. Netter's Essential Histology. Philadelphia: Saunders; 2008.

process is preprogrammed and is different for all hair types on the body. The normal scalp can shed up to 100 hairs per day. The hair follicle is remarkably capable of regeneration after the hair has entered into telogen phase. An unknown signal causes the hair follicle stem cells, which are located in the bulge region, to differentiate and begin producing another hair, restarting the anagen phase. The bulge region is an area found in approximation to the insertion of the arrector pili muscle into the hair follicle.

Histological examination of a cross section of a terminal hair shaft reveals a complex architecture. The hair is made up of various concentric layers. The innermost layer is the medulla, which is pigmented. The next layer is the cortex, followed by the cuticle, the inner root sheath (Huxley's and Henley's layers), and the outer root sheath. The outer root sheath seamlessly blends into the epidermis. The hair follicle undergoes trichohyalin keratinization, which is different from the keratohyalin keratinization of the epidermis.

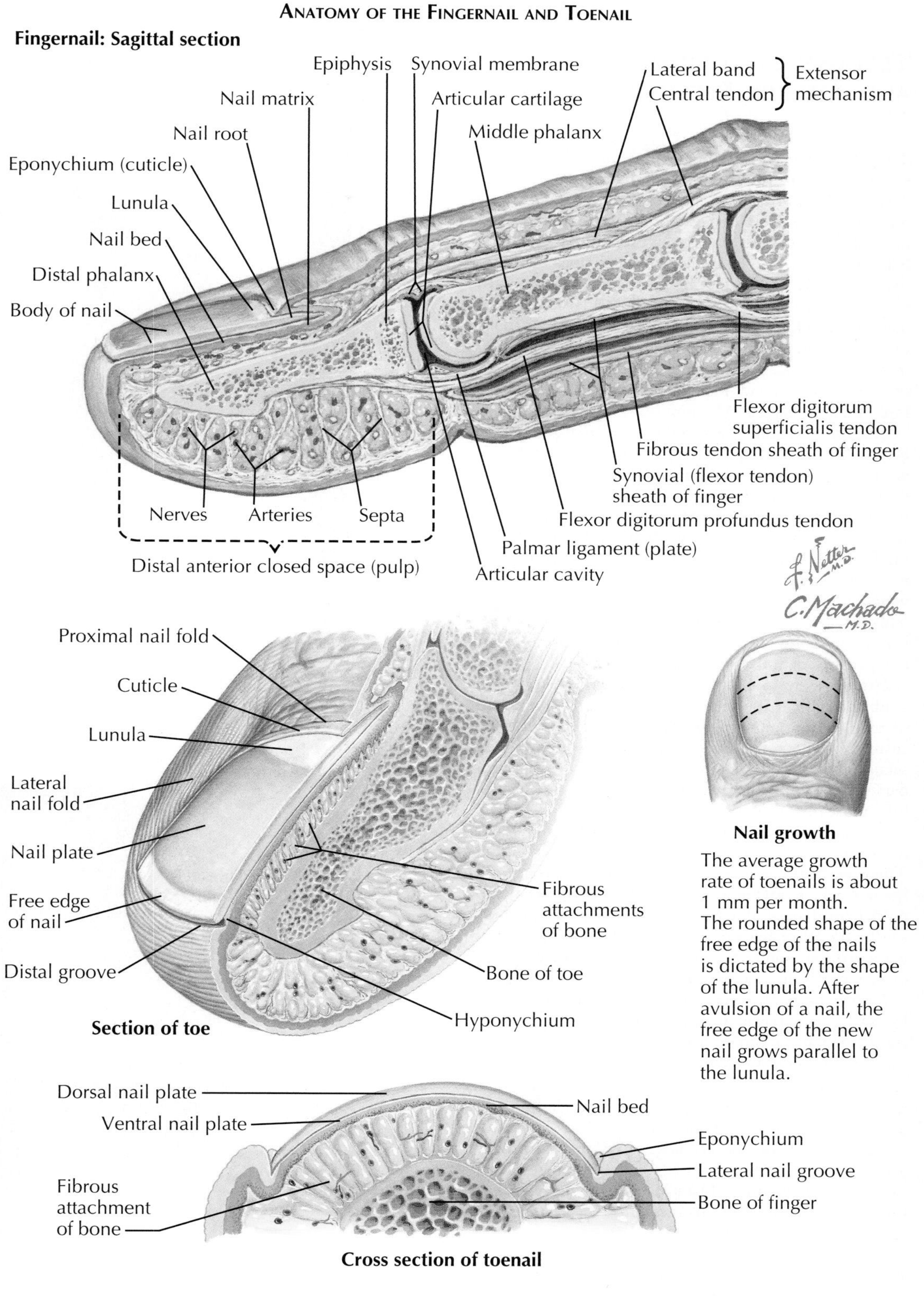

Plate 7-8

Hair and Nail Diseases

ANATOMY OF THE FINGERNAIL AND TOENAIL

Fingernail: Sagittal section

Epiphysis Synovial membrane
Nail matrix
Nail root
Eponychium (cuticle)
Lunula
Nail bed
Distal phalanx
Body of nail

Articular cartilage
Middle phalanx
Lateral band ⎫ Extensor
Central tendon ⎬ mechanism

Flexor digitorum superficialis tendon
Fibrous tendon sheath of finger
Synovial (flexor tendon) sheath of finger
Flexor digitorum profundus tendon
Palmar ligament (plate)
Articular cavity

Nerves   Arteries   Septa

Distal anterior closed space (pulp)

NORMAL STRUCTURE AND FUNCTION OF THE NAIL UNIT

The human nail is composed of a specialized form of keratin. All 20 nails have the same chemical makeup; the only difference is in the size of the nail. The nail unit is made up of highly specialized structures. The nail matrix is the portion of the nail unit that is responsible for production of the nail plate. The matrix lies a few millimeters behind the proximal nail fold, which ends as the cuticle (eponychium), and extends under the nail bed. Under the proximal nail bed, the nail matrix can often be appreciated as a half-circle termed the lunula. The color of the lunula is often creamy white with a hint of pink. Any damage to the nail matrix can potentially cause a temporary or permanent nail dystrophy.

The distal nail matrix is responsible for producing the ventral portion of the nail plate. The proximal nail matrix is responsible for producing the dorsal surface of the nail plate. The nail plate is made of keratin protein and is the hard portion of the nail. It is theorized to be protective to the underlying nail matrix and distal phalanx, as well as being helpful with grasping and dexterity of the fingertips. The nail plate is firmly attached to the underlying nail bed via tiny, vertically arranged interdigitations. These tiny undulations help lock the nail plate into the nail bed below. The nail plate is an avascular structure, and the underlying nail bed is highly vascular.

The nail bed is attached to the epidermis via the proximal nail fold and the cuticle, as well as the lateral nail folds on either side of the nail. Damage to the cuticle, whether by accident or during manicures or pedicures, can increase the risk of bacterial or fungal infection within the nail or the skin of the nail folds. This can lead to acute or chronic paronychia or onychomycosis. Improper trimming of the lateral aspects of the nail plate may lead to an ingrown toenail (onychocryptosis). The distal nail plate is attached to the underling epidermis by the hyponychium. Damage to this portion of the nail unit may allow for bacterial or fungal infections to take hold under or within the nail plate.

The nails grow continuously throughout a person's lifespan. Fingernails grow on average 3 mm per month, and toenails grow a bit more slowly, on average 1 mm per month. However, these growth rates are highly variable among individuals. Both hair keratin and skin keratin types have been described to comprise the various portions of the nail unit. The hair keratin Ha1 and the skin keratins K5, K6, K16, and K17 make up the majority of the keratin types found in the adult nail. Other keratins have been identified during development of the nail.

Primary and secondary nail disorders are commonly encountered. Primary nail disorders include onychomycosis, onychocryptosis, onychoschizia (horizontal

Section of toe

Proximal nail fold
Cuticle
Lunula
Lateral nail fold
Nail plate
Free edge of nail
Distal groove

Fibrous attachments of bone
Bone of toe
Hyponychium

Nail growth

The average growth rate of toenails is about 1 mm per month. The rounded shape of the free edge of the nails is dictated by the shape of the lunula. After avulsion of a nail, the free edge of the new nail grows parallel to the lunula.

Cross section of toenail

Dorsal nail plate
Ventral nail plate
Fibrous attachment of bone

Nail bed
Eponychium
Lateral nail groove
Bone of finger

splitting), onychogryphotic nail ("ram's horn" nail), leukonychia, median nail dystrophy, and onycholysis. These disorders are most often seen in isolation, with no underlying systemic abnormalities. Secondary nail disorders are seen in the presence of an underlying systemic disease; examples include koilonychia (caused by iron deficiency), nail plate pitting (many conditions including psoriasis and alopecia areata), pterygium

formation (lichen planus), longitudinal red and white streaks and distal V-shaped nicking (Darier's disease), clubbing (pulmonary disease), and yellow nail syndrome (pleural effusion and lymphedema). All skin examinations should include evaluation of the nails, because many systemic diseases can manifest with nail findings, and these clinical signs may be the first signs of underlying disease.

Plate 7-9

Integumentary System

TELOGEN EFFLUVIUM AND ANAGEN EFFLUVIUM

Telogen effluvium and anagen effluvium are commonly encountered forms of nonscarring hair loss.

Clinical Findings: Telogen effluvium is a form of nonscarring alopecia that can result in dramatic thinning of the scalp hair but rarely causes total hair loss. It has been found to be induced by a number of stressors that cause the anagen hairs to abruptly turn into telogen hairs. This results in an abnormal number of hairs in the telogen phase and an increase in hair shedding. The hair loss can be profound and disconcerting to the patient. Causes include childbirth, major illness or stress, surgery, and medications. The hair loss is less rapid than in anagen effluvium.

Anagen effluvium is a specific form of alopecia that is typically induced by chemotherapeutic agents. Alkylating agents such as busulfan and cisplatin and the antitumor antibiotics (bleomycin and actinomycin D) are frequently responsible. Other agents have been implicated, including the antimetabolites, topoisomerase inhibitors, and vinca alkaloids. The anagen phase hair is particularly sensitive to these chemotherapy agents, which inhibit proliferation of rapidly dividing cells. This form of hair loss is easier to diagnosis, because a history of taking one of the implicated chemotherapeutic agents is critical in making the diagnosis.

Histology: Scalp biopsies are one of the best ways of confirming the diagnosis. The standard procedure is to obtain a 4-mm punch biopsy from the affected region. Instead of the routine vertical sectioning, horizontal sectioning is performed. Punch biopsies have been standarized to 4 mm. The presence of scarring, the form of inflammation, and the ratio of anagen to telogen hairs are evaluated. In telogen effluvium, a normal number of hairs are present without evidence of miniaturization. The ratio of telogen to anagen hairs is increased from the normal 5 to 10 telogen hairs per 100 anagen hairs to more than 20 per 100. Biopsies of anagen effluvium show a normal ratio of anagen to telogen hairs, but the anagen hairs exhibit some evidence of abnormality, either broken shafts or apoptosis of the hair.

Pathogenesis: Telogen effluvium can almost always be traced to a recent illness, surgery, iron deficiency, child bearing, or other major stressor in the patient's life. Many medications have been reported to induce telogen effluvium, and the clinician should evaluate all medications taken. Dietary habits, especially crash dieting and anorexia nervosa, may lead to telogen effluvium. The hair follicles are not scarred and eventually grow back after the stressors have been resolved. Because the beginning of hair loss may be delayed after the stressful event, by 3 to 4 months on average, the patient may not realize the relationship.

Treatment: The treatment of telogen effluvium consists of determining the etiology and educating the patient. It is important to rule out an underlying disorder (e.g., iron deficiency, hypothyroidism) that may be triggering the hair loss. Once this has been accomplished, patients need to be educated and reassured that telogen effluvium almost always resolves within 6 to 8 months, and they may expect full regrowth. Supplemental vitamins and topical minoxidil have not been vigorously tested as therapies for telogen effluvium, and their use cannot be scientifically advocated. Referral to a psychological counselor may be appropriate in situations such as eating disorders.

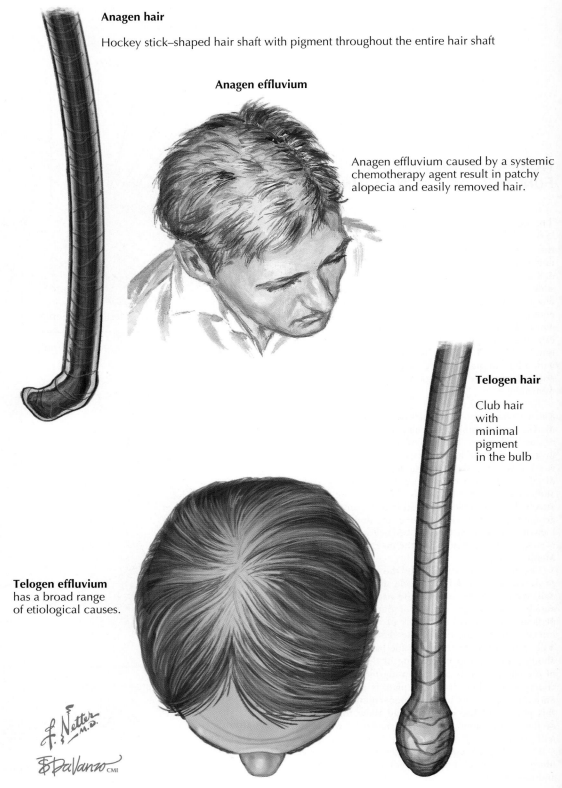

Anagen hair

Hockey stick–shaped hair shaft with pigment throughout the entire hair shaft

Anagen effluvium

Anagen effluvium caused by a systemic chemotherapy agent result in patchy alopecia and easily removed hair.

Telogen hair

Club hair with minimal pigment in the bulb

Telogen effluvium has a broad range of etiological causes.

Anagen effluvium is related to the use of chemotherapeutic agents to treat systemic cancer. The therapy should not be stopped because of this side effect. After therapy has been completed, most patients regrow their hair. Patients have reported many changes in the color, texture, and curling of their newly grown hair. These changes have not been fully explained. Topical minoxidil may shorten the duration of anagen effluvium, but its prophylactic use has not been helpful in preventing it. More studies are needed to confirm these findings. At this point, education and reassurance are the most important therapeutic considerations. Most patients will regrow their hair, and for the few that do not, other options exist. The use of hair pieces has been expanded for many medically related forms of alopecia.

Plate 7-10

Hair and Nail Diseases

TRICHOTILLOMANIA

Trichotillomania is defined as the compulsive act of deliberate hair plucking, pulling, or twisting that causes hair breakage. There has been a push to rename this condition *trichotill* to remove the negative connotation of "mania" from the diagnosis. Two subgroups of patients with trichotillomania exist. The first is a younger population of mostly elementary school–aged children, and the second is the adult population. The younger the patient is at the time of diagnosis, the better the overall prognosis for a cure.

Clinical Findings: Patients present with bizarre configurations of hair loss. This is often the first clue to the diagnosis. On close inspection, the hairs are often broken off close to the surface of the skin. A white 3 × 5 inch card can help as a background to appreciate the damage to the hairs. Many broken hairs of varying lengths are present. Hair shafts may show a twisting morphology. If the patient is evaluated soon after the hair pulling has been performed, pinpoint amounts of hemorrhage may be appreciated at the follicular openings. Microscopic examination of the ends of the hairs may show fracturing of the hair shaft and trichorrhexis nodosa. Most patients are not aware of the actions that are causing their hair loss. It is imperative to not be judgmental during patient visits, and the importance of developing a good rapport cannot be overestimated. One useful request that can be asked of patients is, "Show me how you manipulate your hair." Often patients unconsciously start to twist or tug at their hair. It is important to educate the parents to observe their child for any evidence of hair manipulation. After this form of education, the parents often become aware of the manipulation. It is important for them not to scold the child when this is taking place but rather to try to distract the child with positive reinforcement. Almost all children eventually outgrow the condition, and their hair then returns to normal.

Adults with trichotillomania have a much more chronic course. They typically have no insight into their condition. They commonly go from one doctor to another seeking therapy. In adults, biopsies are critically important to obtain objective diagnostic information. Referral to a psychologist or psychiatrist should be strongly considered for adult patients with trichotillomania.

Histology: Histopathological evaluation show a non-inflammatory, nonscarring alopecia. Characteristic to this diagnosis is the presence of trichomalacia, which is seen as follicular damage within the hair follicle. Varying degrees of follicular red blood cell extravasation are appreciated. Melanin pigment casts within the hair follicle are commonly seen. Overall, the number of hair shafts is normal. The performance of a scalp biopsy is advocated by many to give the patient or family objective information about the diagnosis.

Pathogenesis: Trichotillomania is a self-induced form of hair loss that is caused by intentional twisting, plucking, pulling or other forms of direct damage to the hair shaft. This can be a conscious or an unconscious behavior. Most cases involve some form of emotional disturbance, and one must be cognizant of this when addressing the patient and family.

Treatment: Trichotillomania may be considered in the spectrum of obsessive-compulsive disorders. Most children eventually abandon the actions that have caused their hair loss. Most cases in children are precipitated by emotional stress, and they tend to improve as that stress resolves. Positive reinforcement can be

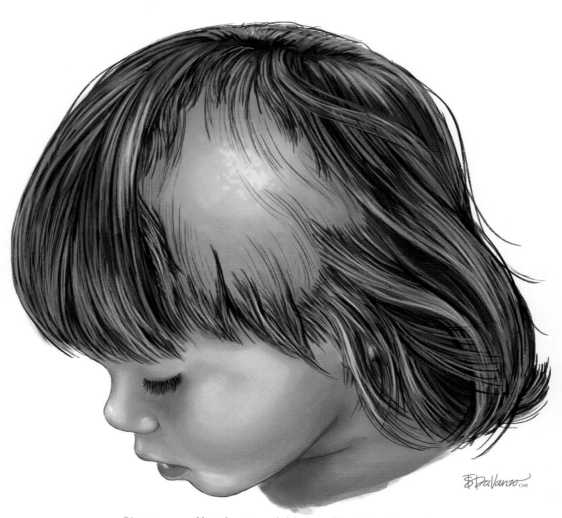

Bizarre area of hair loss in a child caused by trichotillomania

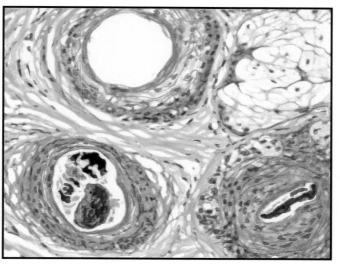

Trichomalacia is one of the histological hallmarks of trichotillomania.

a means to help the child become aware of the hair manipulation. Negative punishment tends to be ineffective. In some cases, a child psychologist or psychiatrist can be extraordinarily helpful in treating these patients.

Adults with trichotillomania have an entirely different clinical course. Most cases are chronic, and most patients never develop insight into their disease. Underlying psychological conditions may be at the root of the issue, and cognitive therapy in the care of a psychiatrist or psychologist may be instrumental in helping these patients. The use of medications traditionally prescribed for obsessive-compulsive disorders may be warranted in the adult patient.

NUTRITIONAL AND METABOLIC DISEASES

Plate 8-1   Integumentary System

BERIBERI

Beriberi is a nutritional deficiency state that is caused directly by a lack of thiamine (vitamin B₁) in one's diet or by a lack of proper absorption of the vitamin. A rare form of acquired thiamine deficiency occurs after the ingestion of thiaminase, an enzyme that cleaves thiamine into a nonfunctional state. These cases are exceedingly rare and are considered to occur after an accidental poisonous ingestion of a source high in thiaminase. Thiamine deficiency is a rare occurrence in most of the world but is still seen in people whose food supply is based primarily on polished rice. The other major cause of the disease is alcoholism. Alcoholics who obtain most of their caloric intake from alcohol may be deficient in a multitude of B vitamins including thiamine. Thiamine deficiency may be seen in neonates and infants who are breast feeding from mothers with borderline thiamine deficiency. The principal food sources of thiamine are fresh meats, liver, whole wheat bread, and vegetables. Nonpolished brown rice is also a good source of thiamine. Thiamine is absorbed in the gastrointestinal tract in the proximal jejunum.

Thiamine deficiency has been reported in cases of short gut syndrome and after bariatric surgery in which large parts of the jejunum are bypassed and absorption of thiamine is dramatically decreased. Most of these cases were complicated by the fact that patients were not following their prescribed diets. Beriberi has also been reported in patients with human immunodeficiency virus infection and in some people taking long-term furosemide therapy without adequate thiamine intake. Furosemide has been shown to increase the rate of excretion of thiamine from the kidneys.

Thiamine is a water-soluble vitamin that is critical in the formation of the energy storage molecule, adenosine triphosphate (ATP). Thiamine is crucial for the proper functioning of both glycolysis and the Krebs cycle. The U.S. Nutrition Board of the Institute of Medicine, National Academy of Sciences, has designated 1.2 mg/day of thiamine as the normal recommended daily intake for men and 1.1 mg/day for women.

Clinical Findings: The disease is most frequently seen in Asia, where polished rice is one of the main food sources. Alcoholics are at very high risk for development of this vitamin deficiency. There is no race or gender predilection, and it can occur in all people. The clinical findings in beriberi are highly variable and are dependent on the level of deficiency and the patient's underlying comorbidities. The organ systems most commonly involved are the central nervous system (CNS) and the muscular system. Two major forms of beriberi occur, although there is much overlap. Dry beriberi is a form of the disease in which the CNS symptoms predominate. Wet beriberi is the form in which the predominant symptoms are salt retention and congestive heart failure. Infantile beriberi is rare but is manifested by a combination of dry and wet beriberi with severe CNS depression, heart failure, and sudden death.

The first signs and symptoms of dry beriberi are typically those of a peripheral neuropathy and of muscle disease involving both skeletal and smooth muscle. Dry beriberi typically manifests with increasing fatigability, muscle weakness, paresthesias, a decrease in deep tendon reflexes, and loss of sensation. As the disease

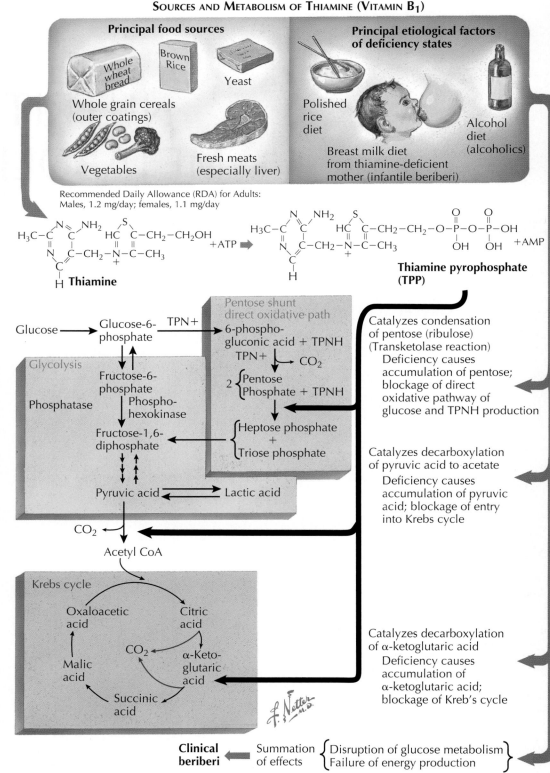

SOURCES AND METABOLISM OF THIAMINE (VITAMIN B₁)

progresses, patients may develop a foot or wrist drop (flaccid paralysis). The lower extremity is typically affected before the upper. Loss of muscle mass may be prominent. Elevated levels of creatinine phosphokinase are seen, as well as a creatinuria. Weakness is profound.

Wet beriberi predominantly affects the muscle tissue, particularly the cardiac system. The end stage is

high-output cardiac failure; without treatment, death follows. Beriberi rarely causes death if the diagnosis is made and proper treatment is instituted before end-stage heart failure sets in. Patients with wet beriberi experience a decrease in diastolic blood pressure and minimal change in systolic pressure, resulting in an overall increase in the pulse pressure. Tachycardia is prominent. As heart failure develops, pulmonary

Plate 8-2

Nutritional and Metabolic Diseases

BERIBERI (Continued)

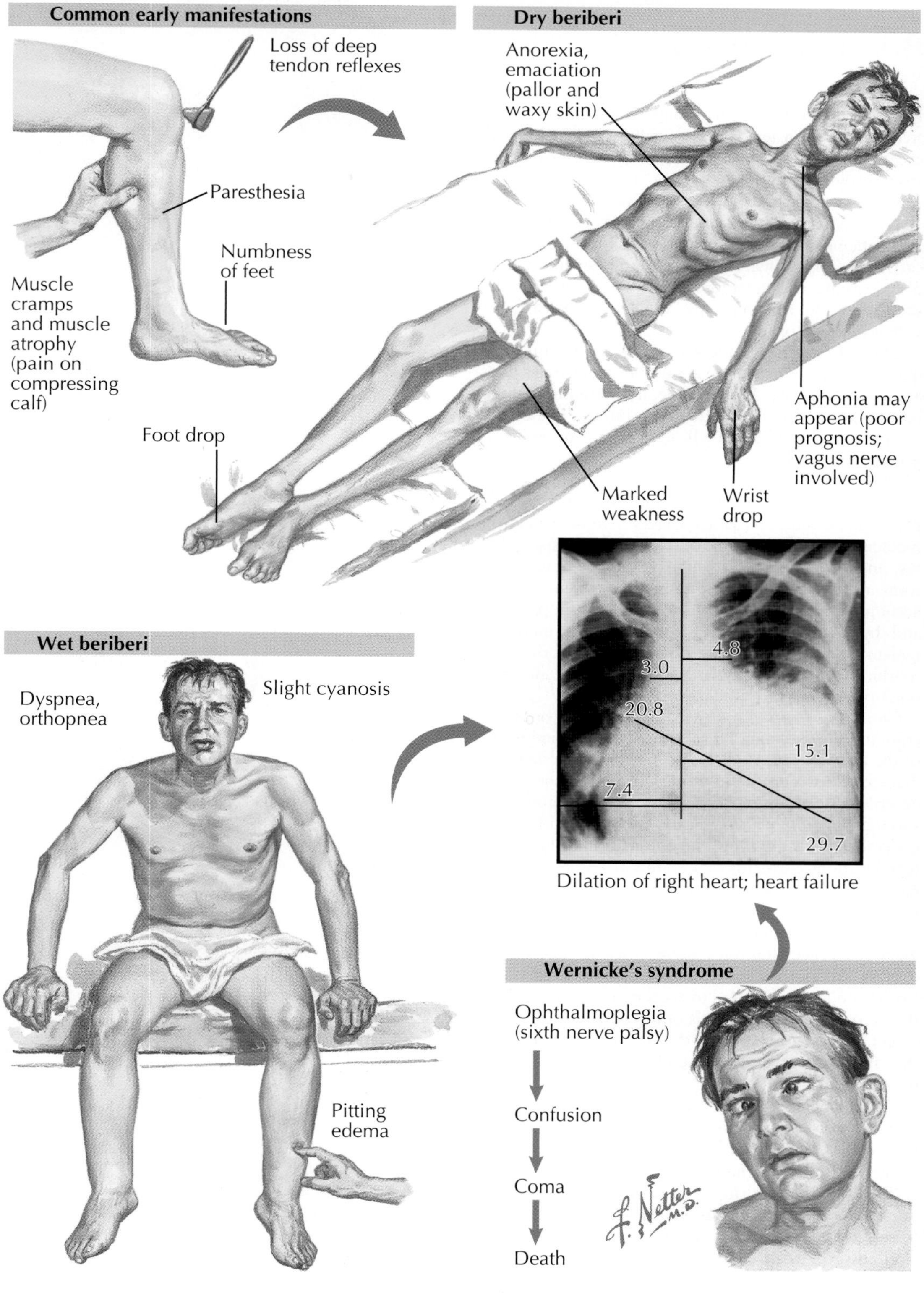

edema and fluid retention occur, causing dependent edema and difficulty breathing. Cyanosis may occur from poor oxygenation. Laboratory testing shows an increased QT interval on electrocardiography and increased serum levels of lactic acid, pyruvate, and α-ketoglutarate. Chest radiography shows an enlarged heart with dilation of the right side and pulmonary congestion, edema, or both.

The skin findings of beriberi are not specific, but when seen in conjunction with the rest of the clinical picture, they can definitely help make the diagnosis. The cutaneous findings of wet beriberi consist of cyanosis of the skin with variable amounts of peripheral edema. The skin has a waxy appearance and feel. Cutaneous pallor is prominent and, along with the cyanosis, gives the patient an ill appearance. Pallor is a common skin finding in dry beriberi as well. Patients may also present with accidental traumatic injuries to their extremities related to lack of sensation from the peripheral neuropathy. Hair loss has been reported, but most believe that this is secondary to a combination of niacin and thiamine deficiency.

The excretion of thiamine via the kidneys is markedly decreased in beriberi. Normally, 70 to 150 µg of thiamine is excreted per gram of creatinine. In beriberi, that level can drop to zero.

Histology: Biopsy specimens of the skin in patients with beriberi are of no clinical usefulness. A skin biopsy from an area of cyanosis or pallor shows normal skin. A biopsy from one of the waxy areas may show variable mild degrees of acanthosis and parakeratosis. A muscle biopsy shows vacuolization and hyalinization of the muscle fibers. An inflammatory process may be present that can cause varying degrees of necrosis of the muscle. The muscle fibers may show diffuse or focal fiber necrosis. These changes are most prominent in the cardiac muscle. In patients who develop Wernicke's syndrome, postmortem examinations of the brain have revealed small hemorrhages within the hypothalamus and upper brainstem. Peripheral nerve tissue shows noninflammatory degeneration of the neurons with atrophy and chromatolysis. This can occur in the neurons of the peripheral nervous system and the CNS.

Pathogenesis: All forms of beriberi are caused by a nutritional deficiency of thiamine. Thiamine is a critical vitamin that is needed for carbohydrate metabolism. Thiamine is the precursor for thiamine pyrophosphate (TPP). It is converted to TPP by the addition of one ATP molecule. TPP is needed as a cofactor for the proper function of many metabolic pathways. TPP helps transfer an aldehyde group from a donor to a beneficiary chemical structure. Three major energy-producing pathways are modulated by TPP: glycolysis, the Krebs cycle, and the pentose shunt (hexose monophosphate shunt). The hexose monophosphate shunt is important in producing other cofactors that play important biochemical roles for donation of hydrogen. The overall chemical state that occurs in patients with thiamine deficiency is a lack of ability to produce sufficient quantities of cellular ATP. This lack of the main source of energy for the cell results in the clinical findings. The nervous tissue and muscle tissue are particularly prone to damage from failure to produce sufficient ATP.

It has been estimated that 3 to 6 weeks of a thiamine-free diet in an average human is sufficient to cause development of the initial signs and symptoms of beriberi.

Treatment: Therapy consists of supplementation of the patient's diet with 50 mg/day intramuscularly of thiamine until the symptoms resolve. Treatment should also include other B-complex vitamins, because many patients who are deficient in one B vitamin also have low levels of the others. A nutritionist should be consulted to educate the patient on the need for a proper diet and how to achieve this. Alcoholics are prone to recurrence of beriberi and should be encouraged to participate in alcohol abstinence programs and to take a daily multivitamin supplement. The symptoms rapidly reverse on replacement of thiamine.

CLINICAL MANIFESTATIONS OF DRY AND WET BERIBERI

Common early manifestations
- Loss of deep tendon reflexes
- Paresthesia
- Numbness of feet
- Muscle cramps and muscle atrophy (pain on compressing calf)
- Foot drop

Dry beriberi
- Anorexia, emaciation (pallor and waxy skin)
- Aphonia may appear (poor prognosis; vagus nerve involved)
- Marked weakness
- Wrist drop

Wet beriberi
- Dyspnea, orthopnea
- Slight cyanosis
- Pitting edema

3.0   4.8
20.8
7.4   15.1
29.7

Dilation of right heart; heart failure

Wernicke's syndrome
- Ophthalmoplegia (sixth nerve palsy)
- Confusion
- Coma
- Death

Plate 8-3

Integumentary System

HEMOCHROMATOSIS

Hemochromatosis is a fairly common autosomal recessive genetic disorder of iron metabolism that leads to excessive iron absorption and eventually iron overload. Iron progressively accumulates in various tissues throughout the body, with the liver most severely affected. Most cases are caused by a genetic mutation in the hemochromatosis gene, *HFE*. This mutation is carried by approximately 10% of the population. The disease signs and symptoms typically do not appear until after child-bearing age, usually in the sixth or seventh decade of life.

Clinical Findings: Caucasian males are the most frequently affected, and there is variability of carrier rates among populations. For example, in Ireland the rate of homozygosity for the C282Y mutation in *HFE* is 1 in 85 individuals. The overall incidence worldwide is probably about 1 in 350.

The clinical manifestations of hemochromatosis patients who are homozygous for the mutated *HFE* gene can be quite variable. Classic hemochromatosis includes three main components: liver cirrhosis, diabetes, and generalized skin pigmentation. These symptoms are caused, respectively, by a persistent chronic accumulation of iron in the liver and in the pancreas and by iron deposition in the skin with increased melanin production. Cirrhosis is the main cause of morbidity and mortality, and it dramatically increases one's risk for hepatocellular carcinoma.

Cutaneous findings include a generalized bronze discoloration of the skin. This diffuse pigmentation is one of the first signs of the disease. This finding, along with diabetes, has led to the name "bronze diabetes" to describe the condition. Nails can be brittle and show varying degrees of koilonychia. There is widespread generalized hair thinning and loss, affecting all terminal hair locations. Arthritis is a common finding in these patients and can also be seen in asymptomatic heterozygous carriers of the disease.

Histology: Histology of the skin is not useful for diagnosis. Liver biopsies show varying degrees of damage on a spectrum from fibrosis to cirrhosis. The Prussian blue stain is used to accentuate the iron within the hepatocytes and the cells of the biliary tract. There is less iron accumulation in the Kupffer cells, which is the direct opposite of the findings in states of iron overload.

Pathogenesis: The *HFE* gene is located on the short arm of chromosome 6 and is mutated in this autosomal recessive genetic disorder of iron metabolism. The most frequently encountered genetic mutation is the C282Y mutation. Normal iron regulation is dependent on absorption of iron from dietary sources and normal losses. Regulatory mechanisms allow for equalization of iron absorption to balance the iron losses in normal physiological states. The defect in *HFE* leads to abnormal regulation of cellular uptake of iron as well as a loss of regulation of ferritin levels. The result of the excessive iron deposition is an increase in free radical oxygen species and their destructive interactions with various tissues. In the liver, this leads to fibrosis and eventually cirrhosis.

Treatment: Therapy requires removal of the excessive iron. This is best accomplished by routine scheduled phlebotomy. Phlebotomy decreases the amount of iron stores and is used to attempt to prevent the progression to cirrhosis. Prevention of cirrhosis is the single best predictor of morbidity and mortality in these patients. The goal in most patients is to keep the hemoglobin in the range of 12 g/dL. Other methods to remove excessive iron include erythrocytapheresis and iron chelation therapy. Erythrocytapheresis is a method by which predominantly red blood cells are removed from the blood while the serum, white blood cells, and platelets are returned to the patient's bloodstream. Iron chelation therapy with intravenous deferoxamine has been helpful for patients who cannot tolerate blood removal procedures. Methods to try to decrease the absorption of iron from the gastrointestinal tract can also be attempted. These treatments have shown the best results if implemented before evidence of cirrhosis is present. The importance of genetic counseling cannot be overemphasized.

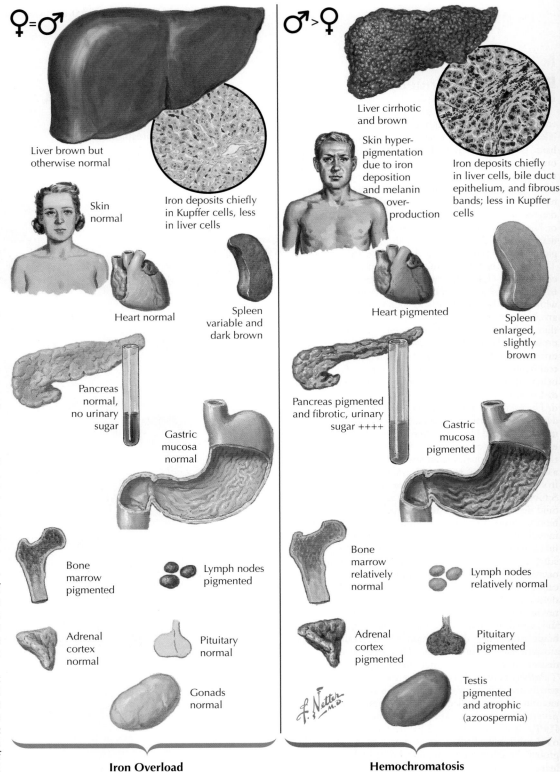

Liver brown but otherwise normal

Skin normal

Iron deposits chiefly in Kupffer cells, less in liver cells

Heart normal

Spleen variable and dark brown

Pancreas normal, no urinary sugar

Gastric mucosa normal

Bone marrow pigmented

Lymph nodes pigmented

Adrenal cortex normal

Pituitary normal

Gonads normal

Iron Overload

Liver cirrhotic and brown

Skin hyper-pigmentation due to iron deposition and melanin over-production

Iron deposits chiefly in liver cells, bile duct epithelium, and fibrous bands; less in Kupffer cells

Heart pigmented

Spleen enlarged, slightly brown

Pancreas pigmented and fibrotic, urinary sugar ++++

Gastric mucosa pigmented

Bone marrow relatively normal

Lymph nodes relatively normal

Adrenal cortex pigmented

Pituitary pigmented

Testis pigmented and atrophic (azoospermia)

Hemochromatosis

Plate 8-4

Nutritional and Metabolic Diseases

METABOLIC DISEASES: NIEMANN-PICK DISEASE, VON GIERKE DISEASE, AND GALACTOSEMIA

There are a plethora of metabolic diseases that can have various cutaneous skin findings. These conditions, on the whole, are uncommon and are rarely encountered by the practitioner except in a tertiary referral center. However, knowledge of these uncommon diseases is important, because prompt recognition and diagnosis can lead to proper referrals and a better outcome for all involved. Three such metabolic disorders are Niemann-Pick disease, von Gierke disease, and galactosemia.

Niemann-Pick disease is a heterogenous group of conditions resulting from inability to properly metabolize sphingomyelin. There are three clinical variants, which have been designated types A, B, and C. They are all inherited in an autosomal recessive pattern, with the highest prevalence in people of Ashkenazi Jewish descent. Most cases are fatal in early childhood. Mental delay is profound. The disease results in massive hepatosplenomegaly caused by the excessive accumulation of sphingomyelin in various tissues. Niemann-Pick disease is caused by an abnormal lysosomal lipid enzyme degradation system, and it is therefore considered to be a lysosomal storage disease. Sphingomyelin is degraded into ceramide by the action of the enzyme sphingomyelinase. Type A and type B disease are similar in that the *ASM* gene, which encodes the acid sphingomyelinase enzyme, is mutated. This mutation leads to an inability of the lysosomes to metabolize sphingomyelin. Sphingomyelin accumulates in the liver and spleen. Severe neurological disorders occur in type A disease, but not in type B, and this is the only factor differentiating the two. Patients present in infancy or early childhood. Skin findings include xanthomas and a waxy skin surface. Retinal examination reveals a cherry-red spot on the fovea. Niemann-Pick type C disease, which is caused by a mutation in the *NPC1* or the *NPC2* gene, does not involve any cutaneous findings. The cells are unable to normally process endocytosed cholesterol. Treatments are limited, with stem cell transplantation having been used with some efficacy.

von Gierke disease, also known as glycogen storage disease type I, can be subdivided into types Ia and Ib. These autosomal recessive diseases are caused, respectively, by defects in the enzymes glucose-6-phosphatase and glucose-6-phosphatase translocase. These defects prevent normal gluconeogenesis from glycogen stores. Patients develop profound hypoglycemia during periods of fasting because they are unable to break down glucose-6-phosphate into glucose within the liver. This leads to a fatty liver and increased glycogen storage. Glucose-6-phosphate is shunted into glycolysis, which results in increased lactate production.

Cutaneous findings in von Gierke disease include extensor xanthomas on the knees and elbows. Patients have a peculiar facies that has been described as a "doll-like face." This has been shown to be caused by an increased amount of fatty tissue deposited in the cheeks. Patients have frequent nose bleeds and severe gingivitis along with oral ulcerations. During periods of hypoglycemia, cyanosis may be very noticeable, and it may lead eventually to hypoxic brain injury. These patients are also at higher risk for skin infections due to an abnormal

neutrophilic response to gram-positive bacteria. Treatment is based on a diet of 60% to 70% carbohydrates to avoid episodes of hypoglycemia.

Galactosemia is a rare autosomal recessive disorder that results from a defect in the enzyme galactose-1-phosphate uridyltransferase. It is caused by a mutation of the *GALT* gene on the short arm of chromosome 9. This mutation results in an increase of galactose-1-phosphate in various tissues. Nervous tissue, the lens, and the liver are areas of massive accumulation. This

leads to the sequelae of the disease, predominantly mental delay, cataracts, and liver disease. The main cutaneous findings are jaundice secondary to liver disease and cutaneous signs of coagulopathy such as petechiae and hemorrhage. Cataracts are a well-known sign of galactosemia and are directly caused by the accumulation of galactitol in the lens, which results in edema and eventual cataract formation. Therapy requires the strict avoidance of galactose and lactose in the diet.

SELECTED METABOLIC DISEASES WITH SKIN FINDINGS

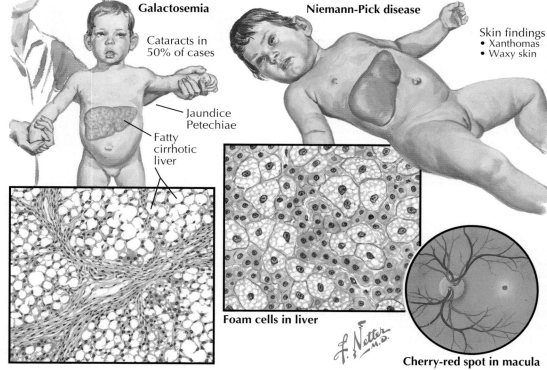

von Gierke disease

Skin findings
• Extensor xanthomas
• "Doll-like facies"
• Intermittent cyanosis

Liver section. Stained with hematoxylin-eosin large cells with fine vacuoles

Intracellular glycogen. Stained with Best's carmine technique

Galactosemia

Cataracts in 50% of cases

Jaundice
Petechiae
Fatty cirrhotic liver

Foam cells in liver

Niemann-Pick disease

Skin findings
• Xanthomas
• Waxy skin

Cherry-red spot in macula

Plate 8-5

Integumentary System

PELLAGRA

Pellagra is caused by inadequate dietary intake of niacin (nicotinic acid, vitamin B₃) or its precursor amino acid, tryptophan. It has also been discovered to occur on occasion in patients with carcinoid syndrome. In this syndrome, tryptophan is used entirely to produce serotonin, and there is none left to produce niacin. Pellagra was first identified as a unique disease in the early 1700s by a Spanish physician, Gaspar Casal, who observed it in Spanish peasants who ate diets almost entirely made of corn and corn-based foodstuffs. He named the disease "Asturian leprosy" after the region of Spain he was studying. An Italian physician, Francesco Frapoli, who studied the disease in endemic regions of northern Italy, later named it pellagra.

Pellagra has been dominant in regions of the world that rely heavily on corn as the main dietary staple. In the early twentieth century, the southern United States was inundated with cases of pellagra. Joseph Goldberger, a physician and epidemiologist studying the disease, discovered that pellagra was caused directly by a deficiency of vitamin B. He was unable at that time to isolate the specific B vitamin, but he has been given credit for discovering the cause of pellagra.

Clinical Findings: Pellagra can affect any individual regardless of race or gender. The incidence in the North America and Europe is low, and cases are mainly caused by abnormal diets and alcoholism. The disease can still be seen in endemic regions of the world where corn is the main food source. The clinical cutaneous hallmark of pellagra is a severe dermatitis. The dermatitis is photosensitive, and exposure to the sun often brings out the rash or exacerbates it. Patients often present initially after having spent many hours outdoors on an early spring day. The dermatitis is symmetric and is manifested by eczematous patches and thin plaques that tend to be tender to the touch. There is a fine line of demarcation between abnormal and normal skin. The head, neck, and arms are the most involved regions because of their higher level of sun exposure. The dermatitis along the anterior neck and upper thorax has been termed Casal necklace. This is represented by weeping pink and red patches and plaques in a distribution like that of a necklace touching the skin circumferentially around the neck. Because of its photosensitive nature, the dermatitis of pellagra often spares the skin directly behind the ears and beneath the chin. The nose, forehead, and cheeks are prime regions of involvement. Non–sun-exposed areas can also be involved, and the intertriginous regions are almost universally affected, including the perineum, axillae, and inframammary skin folds. The reason for the propensity to affect these non–sun-exposed regions is poorly understood but may be related to chronic friction that induces the dermatitis. In the areas of involvement, small vesiculations may occur because of separation of the epidermis from the dermis.

As time progresses, the dermatitis begins to desquamate. This process begins in the central portions of the dermatitis and spreads outward in a centrifugal manner. As the skin desquamates, it leaves behind red, eroded patches and plaques. Chronic involvement leaves permanent scarring and abnormal hyperpigmentation or hypopigmentation of the area. The epidermis over bony prominences (e.g., ulnar head) shows marked hyperkeratosis.

Mucous membrane involvement is common in all vitamin deficiency states, and pellagra is no exception. Angular cheilitis and a red, shiny, edematous tongue

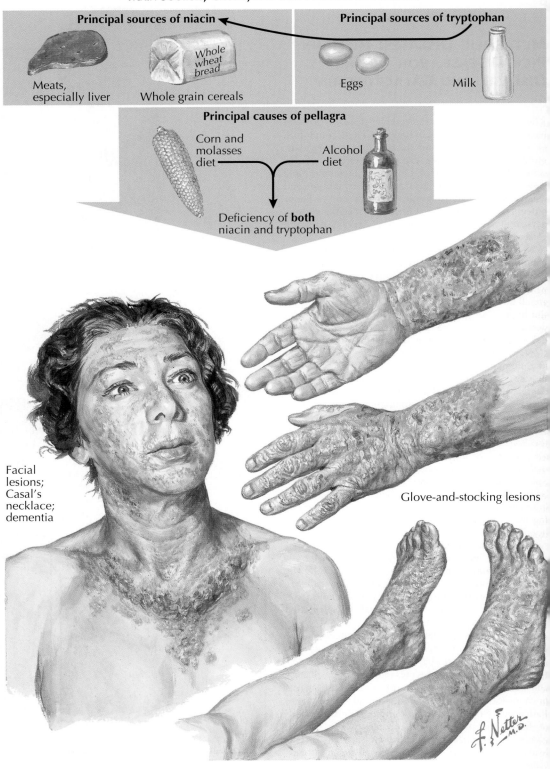

MAIN SOURCES, CAUSES, AND SKIN FINDINGS OF PELLAGRA

Principal sources of niacin

Meats, especially liver

Whole grain cereals

Whole wheat bread

Principal sources of tryptophan

Eggs

Milk

Principal causes of pellagra

Corn and molasses diet

Alcohol diet

Deficiency of **both** niacin and tryptophan

Facial lesions; Casal's necklace; dementia

Glove-and-stocking lesions

with atrophied papillae are seen routinely in patients with pellagra. The oral and gastrointestinal mucous membranes may be involved. Oral ulcerations are frequently seen. Patients routinely complain of a sore mouth and difficulty swallowing; these symptoms can lead to further lack of proper nutrition, exacerbating and compounding the disease.

Diarrhea is commonplace and is caused by the effect of niacin deficiency on the gastrointestinal tract. The diarrhea is watery and further complicates the patient's nutritional status and electrolyte and fluid balances. Blood and purulence may be present in the watery diarrhea as a result of ulceration and abscess formation. Ulcerations can be seen throughout the gastrointestinal

Plate 8-6

Nutritional and Metabolic Diseases

PELLAGRA (Continued)

tract, as can cystic dilation of the mucous glands. The colon may show small submucosal abscesses.

Subtle neurological findings precede full-blown encephalopathy in pellagra. These clinical findings include poor concentration, headaches, and apathy. Dementia eventually sets in as the disease causes a diffuse encephalopathy. The encephalopathy may mimic psychiatric disease, especially depression with suicidal tendency. Other well-defined symptoms include confusion, hallucination, delirium, insomnia, tremor, seizures, and extrapyramidal rigidity. The entire central nervous system is involved in severe pellagra. Cortical nerve cells show degeneration. The Betz cells show chromatolytic changes with displacement of the nucleus toward the cell wall. There is an increased amount of adipose in the nerve cells as well as an increase in the lipofuscin pigment within the cytoplasm of these cortical cells. The posterior columns may undergo demyelination, leading to tremor, gait disturbance, and movement difficulties. Chromatolysis has been shown to occur in the pontine nuclei, spinal cord nuclei, and multiple cranial nerve nuclei. As the encephalopathy progresses, disorientation and delirium take over, and the patient eventually slips into a coma. Death may shortly ensue unless the disease is diagnosed and treated appropriately. These unique clinical findings seen in pellagra can be simplified in the oft-quoted mnemonic, "4 D's": dermatitis, diarrhea, dementia, and death.

The diagnosis is typically made on clinical grounds, and laboratory analysis is used for confirmation. One should always consider other vitamin deficiencies when evaluating a patient with pellagra. The 24-hour urine secretion of N-methyl nicotinamide is normally in the range of 5 to 15 mg/day; in patients with pellagra, it is less than 1.5 mg/day. Measurement of this metabolite serves as an easy, noninvasive test to confirm the deficiency of niacin. Serum niacin levels can be measured directly, although they are not as accurate as the urinary excretion levels.

Histology: The skin biopsy findings are nonspecific and show epidermal pallor with a mixed inflammatory infiltrate that is predominantly composed of lymphocytes in a perivascular location. Occasional areas of inflammatory vesiculation within the epidermis may be seen.

Pathogenesis: Niacin is an essential vitamin that is found in many food sources, including whole grain breads and meats. Patients whose diet is deficient in niacin are seen in regions of the world where corn is the main food source. Various levels of niacin deficiency occur. This disease can also be seen in alcoholics who do not maintain a balanced diet and receive almost all their caloric intake from alcoholic products. Patients who develop pellagra also have a diet deficient in tryptophan. Major sources of tryptophan include eggs and milk. Tryptophan is a precursor of niacin and can be converted to niacin. Niacin is required for the proper production of nicotinamide adenine dinucleotide (NAD) and nicotinamide adenine dinucleotide phosphate (NADP), important coenzymes for many biochemical reactions. Both molecules are capable of acquiring two electrons and acting as reducing agents in various reduction-oxidation (redox) reactions. When a deficiency of niacin occurs, many biochemical reactions throughout the human body cannot be properly performed, and the clinical manifestations occur.

Carcinoid syndrome is a rare cause of pellagra. Carcinoid is a syndrome of excessive secretion of serotonin.

MUCOSAL AND CENTRAL NERVOUS SYSTEM MANIFESTATIONS OF PELLAGRA

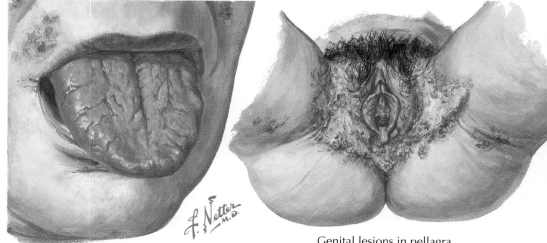

Pellagra tongue

Genital lesions in pellagra

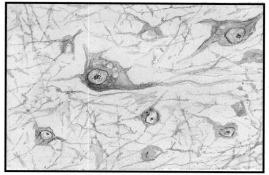

Degeneration of cells of cerebral cortex

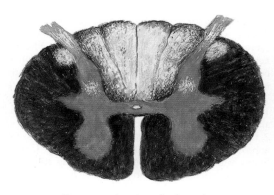

Degeneration in spinal cord

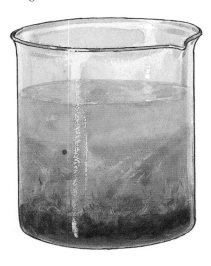

Aqueous stool in diarrhea of pellagra

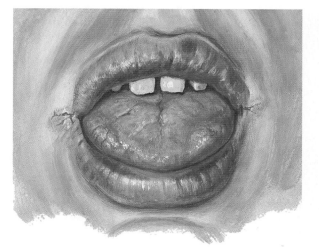

Glossitis and angular cheilitis are commonly seen in pellagra.

Tryptophan is the precursor for serotonin as well as niacin, and in this syndrome all tryptophan is shunted to make serotonin at the expense of tryptophan. This results in decreased production of niacin and, potentially, the clinical symptoms of pellagra.

Treatment: Pellagra rapidly responds to supplementation with niacin. Niacin is given orally every 6 hours until the patient responds. If a patient does not respond,

a coexisting vitamin deficiency should be sought. If possible, a nutritionist should be consulted to advise the patient on proper dietary intake. Alcoholics, who can be deficient in many B vitamins, are often treated with multiple B vitamins. Patients with carcinoid syndrome need to take supplemental niacin to avoid pellagra symptoms, but the goal of therapy is to treat the underlying tumor.

Plate 8-7

Integumentary System

NORMAL AND ABNORMAL METABOLISM OF PHENYLALANINE

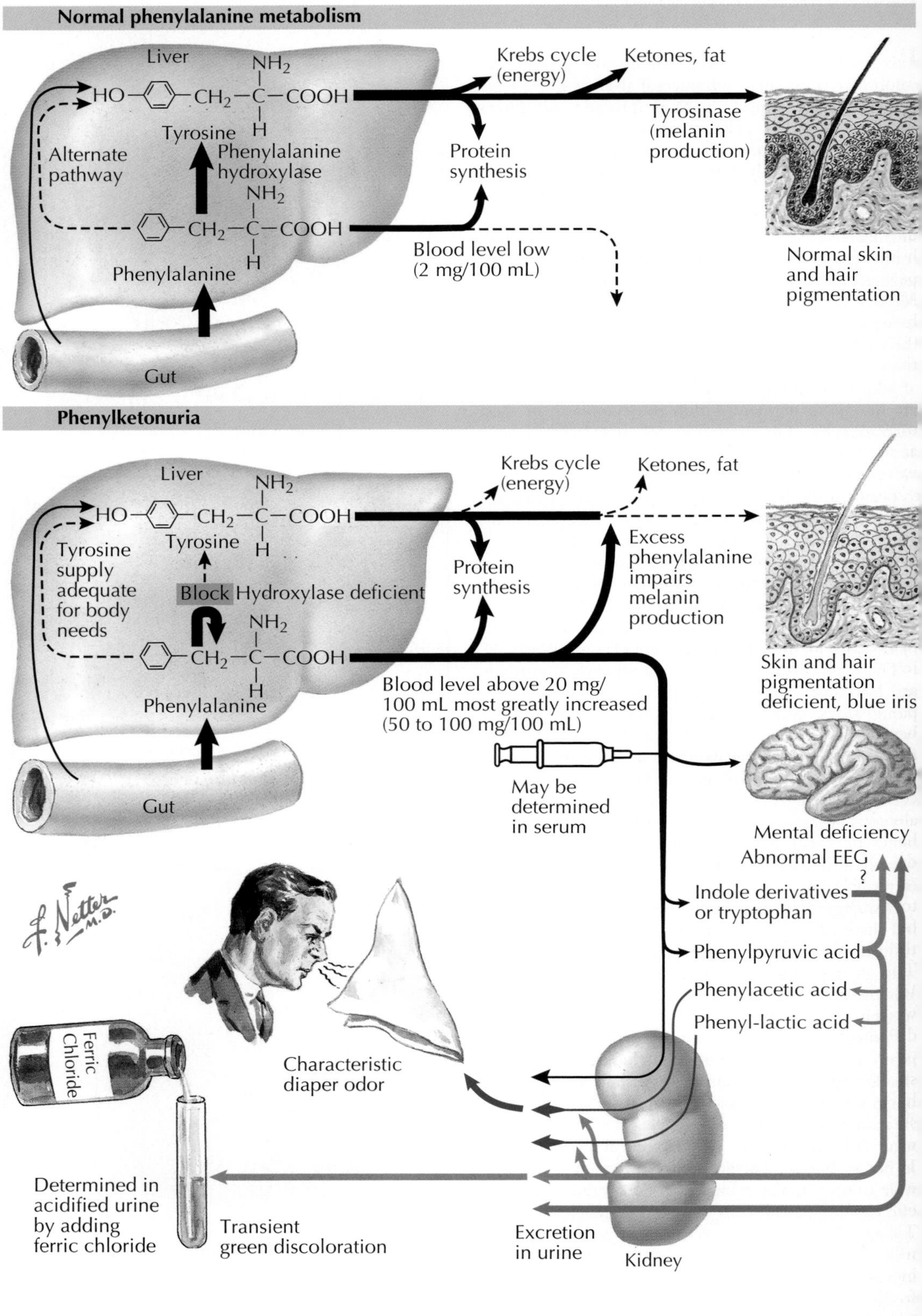

PHENYLKETONURIA

Phenylalanine is an essential amino acid that serves as a substrate for many different biochemical pathways. Two end products that use phenylalanine as their precursors are melanin and epinephrine. Under normal physiological and biochemical environments, any excess amount of phenylalanine is converted into tyrosine by the liver and used for a host of biochemical processes including protein synthesis. In patients with phenylketonuria, the enzyme in the liver that converts phenylalanine into tyrosine is completely absent. This inborn error of metabolism is one of the most thoroughly researched disease states. With early detection and therapy, the severe sequelae of phenylketonuria can be avoided. Screening is performed soon after birth for all children in the United States and in most of the world. Children born in regions with poor medical infrastructure and no testing are at risk for the disease. Once the disease symptoms have appeared, therapy usually cannot reverse the damage that has been done. Phenylketonuria is inherited in an autosomal recessive manner, but many genotypes have been described, and many mutations in the responsible gene have been reported. The defect is located on the long arm of chromosome 12, where the *PAH* gene encodes the protein, phenylalanine hydroxylase.

Clinical Findings: Phenylketonuria occurs in approximately 1 of every 10,000 births in the United States, with the Caucasian population being at highest risk. Worldwide, the Turkish population has the highest rate, 1 per 2500 newborns. Both genders are affected equally. Infants appear normal at birth. The small load of phenylalanine that is derived from the maternal source in utero is typically not high enough to cause any symptoms or signs of phenylketonuria. Soon after birth, the first symptoms appear as the neonate, lacking the PAH enzyme, rapidly begins to accumulate phenylalanine in serum and tissues. Other biochemical pathways are enacted to try to rid the body of the excess phenylalanine, but these make matters worse. The degradation metabolites that are produced from various deamination and oxidation metabolic modification reactions can cause end-organ damage. Phenyl-lactic acid, phenylpyruvic acid, and phenylacetic acid are the main byproducts. Because of these byproducts, the urine takes on a characteristic "mousy" odor.

Affected neonates have blond hair and a generalized hypopigmentation. Children with darker-skinned parents often have a lighter skin tone and lighter hair and eye coloration than either parent. Most have blue eyes. Evidence of early-onset dermatitis that may appear as atopic dermatitis is often present. Other skin changes that have been described include sclerodermoid changes of the trunk and upper thighs.

The most dreaded sequela of phenylketonuria is the profound brain damage that can occur secondary to the elevated levels of phenylalanine. The neonatal brain is easily damaged by excessive levels of this amino acid. Global brain damage is caused by phenylalanine, and the damage is typically irreversible. This is the reason that screening tests are performed on neonates. Mental retardation, seizures, and tremors are common effects of phenylketonuria. Seizures can be of the grand mal or petit mal type and occur in infancy or childhood. The seizures are reversible once a low-phenylalanine diet is undertaken. The electroencephalogram (EEG) of all

Normal phenylalanine metabolism

Phenylketonuria

infants and children with phenylketonuria shows abnormal results. As the child grows, the mental deficiencies begin to become more apparent. Physical growth and physical maturation are unaffected. Children tend to be hyperactive and are prone to develop self-mutilating rituals such as biting themselves or banging their heads violently against walls or floors. Tremors may be the only other neurological finding observed.

Laboratory testing shows elevated levels of phenylalanine in the serum. Normal levels are between 1 and 2 mg/dL, and those with untreated phenylketonuria have levels greater than 20 mg/dL. Phenylpyruvic acid typically is not present in the urine in appreciable amounts in the normal physiological state. In patients with phenylketonuria, urine levels are elevated. The addition of ferric chloride to the urine causes

Plate 8-8

Nutritional and Metabolic Diseases

PHENYLKETONURIA (Continued)

acidification of the urine, and a transient green discoloration is produced.

All neonates should be tested for phenylketonuria within the first day or two of life as part of routine metabolic screening. This test can be followed up in 7 days if the initial test was performed within the first 24 hours of life or if the initial test was positive. Testing is performed by the Guthrie inhibition assay or by the McCamon-Robins fluorometric test. These tests are highly accurate; levels greater than the normal value of 0.5 mg/dL are considered suspicious, and levels greater than 2 to 4 mg/dL are diagnostic.

Histology: Findings on skin biopsy are nondiagnostic and are rarely helpful in this disease. Biopsy specimens of the hypopigmented skin appear normal. Those from areas of dermatitis show a nonspecific, spongiotic dermatitis with a lymphocytic infiltrate.

Pathogenesis: Phenylketonuria is an autosomal recessive disorder of the metabolism of phenylalanine. It is caused by a genetic defect in the long arm of chromosome 12, which results in a nonfunctional phenylalanine hydroxylase enzyme. Phenylalanine and its metabolites, via other metabolic pathways, lead to the clinical signs and symptoms. Excessive phenylalanine causes skin and hair hypopigmentation by direct inhibition of the tyrosinase enzyme, which decreases the amount of melanin and other molecules that are dependent on this enzyme pathway. Once the phenylalanine levels have dropped below the threshold of tyrosinase inhibition, enzyme function returns to normal and the pigmentary abnormalities resolve. Phenylalanine is directly toxic to brain cells, resulting in severe central nervous system (CNS) abnormalities. Numerous mutations of the *PAH* gene have been reported, making in utero diagnosis very difficult.

Treatment: The most important aspect of therapy is to maintain a low-phenylalanine diet. The goal should be to continue this diet lifelong, because a subset of those who stop the diet early develop CNS disease. This is especially true for women of child-bearing age. Women with deficiencies of phenylalanine hydroxylase who become pregnant can cause irreversible brain damage to their offspring if they do not control their phenylalanine level. These women should stay on a strict phenylalanine-free diet and be managed by a high-risk obstetrics team. Phenylalanine serum levels should be tested routinely to make sure the gravid mother keeps her serum phenylalanine level below 5 to 10 mg/dL. Women who are considering getting pregnant should go on a low-phenylalanine diet before conception and should be under the care of an obstetrician. The diet is a prepared amino acid mixture. Strict elimination of foods high in phenylalanine is required, including meat, eggs, fish, milk, breads, and many other foodstuffs. The diet can be very difficult to follow for even the most dedicated of individuals. The artificial sweetener aspartame must also be avoided, because it is made up of aspartate and phenylalanine.

Approximately 50% of cases of phenylketonuria respond to the medication tetrahydrobiopterin (BH4, sapropterin). BH4 has been found to help metabolize excess phenylalanine, and its starting dose and maintenance dose are based on patient weight and response to Therapy. Levels of phenylalanine must be measured over a few weeks to months to determine the

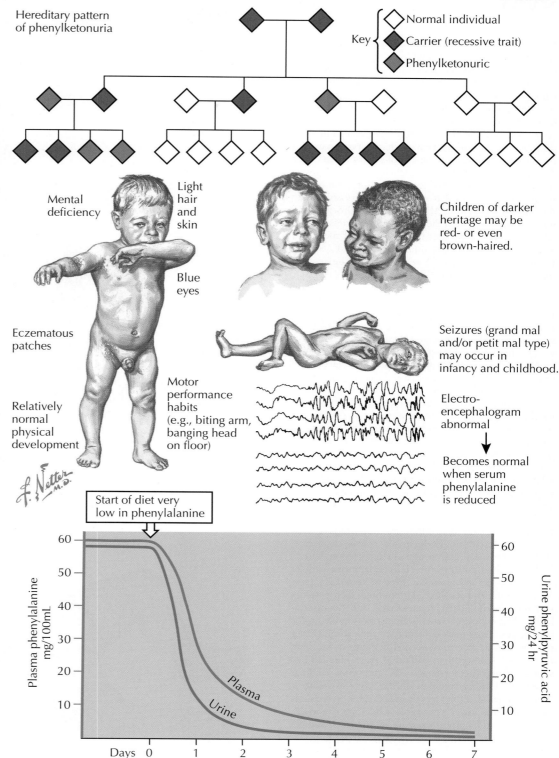

CLINICAL MANIFESTATIONS, HEREDITARY PATTERNS, AND EFFECTS OF PLASMA AND URINARY LEVELS IN PHENYLKETONURIA

Hereditary pattern of phenylketonuria

Key:
Normal individual
Carrier (recessive trait)
Phenylketonuric

Mental deficiency
Light hair and skin
Blue eyes
Children of darker heritage may be red- or even brown-haired.
Eczematous patches
Relatively normal physical development
Motor performance habits (e.g., biting arm, banging head on floor)
Seizures (grand mal and/or petit mal type) may occur in infancy and childhood.
Electro-encephalogram abnormal
Becomes normal when serum phenylalanine is reduced

Start of diet very low in phenylalanine

Plasma phenylalanine mg/100mL
Urine phenylpyruvic acid mg/24 hr
Plasma
Urine
Days 0 1 2 3 4 5 6 7

effectiveness of the medication. Those patients who are helped may potentially be able to increase the amount of protein in their diet.

During therapy, the skin disease, including discoloration of the hair and skin as well as dermatitis, disappears. The abnormal EEG pattern reverts to normal, and the patient's urine returns to normal. Mental performance may always lag, and permanent damage may be sustained early in the course of the disease. Only mild behavioral improvements have been reported. Those children who were diagnosed before the onset of any abnormal symptoms and are maintained on a low-phenylalanine diet do not develop any of the sequelae of the disease.

Plate 8-9

Integumentary System

SCURVY

Scurvy is a well-known nutritional disease that results from a lack of the water-soluble vitamin, ascorbic acid (vitamin C). Scurvy has a well-documented history. It was first recognized in the fourteenth century in sailors who spent long amounts of time at sea. The symptoms were recognized as being related to a lack of fresh foods, especially citrus products. In 1753, James Lind, a British surgeon aboard the HMS Salisbury, performed the first documented clinical trial proving that scurvy was caused by a lack of citrus fruit in the diet of sailors. After Lind's discovery, citrus fruits were included in ships' provisions, and the incidence of scurvy in sailors plummeted. It was not until 1928 that ascorbic acid was isolated by the Hungarian chemist, Albert von Szent-Grörgyi, who was eventually awarded the Nobel Prize for this discovery. Scurvy is still present in some areas of the world due to inadequate dietary intake of vitamin C. Scurvy is uncommon in North America but can be seen in individuals with abnormal diets.

Clinical Findings: Scurvy is a disease that can affect a wide range of organ systems. The skin and mucous membranes are always involved and may display the initial symptoms of the disease. Recognition of these symptoms is critical in diagnosing the disease and preventing long-term illness. Scurvy is a rare disease in regions of the world with access to proper dietary intake of vitamin C. In North America and Europe, most cases are the result of abnormal dieting, psychiatric illness, or alcoholism. Prompt recognition of the cutaneous manifestations can lead to treatment and cure of the disease. Scurvy has an insidious onset with nonspecific constitutional symptoms such as generalized weakness, malaise, muscle and joint aches, and easy fatigability with shortness of breath. These symptoms may be related to the macrocytic anemia that is frequently seen in patients with scurvy and is believed to be caused by a coexisting folic acid deficiency.

The first clinical findings are often in the mucous membranes and the skin. There are a multitude of cutaneous manifestations. Early in the course of disease, skin becomes dry and rough, in association with a dulling of the skin tone. Small, hyperkeratotic papules may be noticed and resemble those of keratosis pilaris. More specific and sensitive skin findings then develop, including perifollicular hemorrhage and "corkscrew hairs." The corkscrew hairs are most noticeable on the extremities. Swan-neck deformity of the extremity hair may also occur due to abnormal bending of the hair; this is less common than corkscrew hair. The nail bed shows splinter hemorrhages. All cutaneous findings appear to be more common on the lower extremities. This is believed to be a result of increased hydrostatic pressure in the lower extremities while one is upright, which leads to increased pressure on the small venules in the follicular locations, resulting in the perifollicular hemorrhages. These findings are also observed in areas of pressure directly on the skin, such as around the waist line. The Rumpel-Leede sign is positive: When a blood pressure cuff is inflated for 1 minute to a value that is greater than the diastolic pressure but less than the systolic pressure, numerous petechial hemorrhages occur distal to and underneath the blood pressure cuff. This test is a sign of capillary fragility induced by increased hydrostatic pressure.

The mucous membranes may show the first sign of the disease. The main finding is edematous, bleeding gums. As the disease progresses, the gums become friable and peel away from the teeth. The teeth may

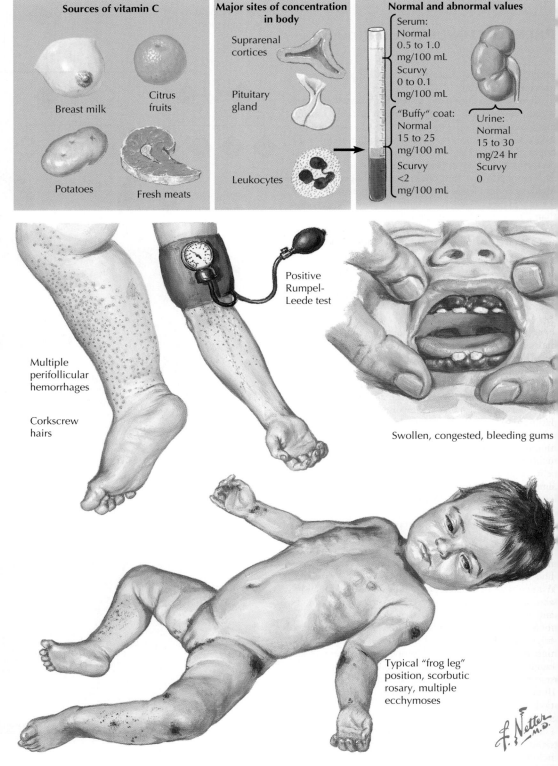

DIETARY SOURCES OF VITAMIN C AND CLASSIC CUTANEOUS MANIFESTATIONS OF SCURVY

Sources of vitamin C

Breast milk

Citrus fruits

Potatoes

Fresh meats

Major sites of concentration in body

Suprarenal cortices

Pituitary gland

Leukocytes

Normal and abnormal values

Serum:
Normal
0.5 to 1.0 mg/100 mL
Scurvy
0 to 0.1 mg/100 mL

"Buffy" coat:
Normal
15 to 25 mg/100 mL
Scurvy
<2 mg/100 mL

Urine:
Normal
15 to 30 mg/24 hr
Scurvy
0

Multiple perifollicular hemorrhages

Corkscrew hairs

Positive Rumpel-Leede test

Swollen, congested, bleeding gums

Typical "frog leg" position, scorbutic rosary, multiple ecchymoses

develop dental calculi at the base. This may result in loose teeth and pain. Teeth eventually become disrupted from their attachments and fall out.

Compared with scurvy in adults, congenital scurvy and scurvy during early childhood have unique manifestations related to bony development. Vitamin C is critically important for the development of collagen and cartilage, and abnormalities at a young age result in a variety of bony deformities. *Scorbutic rosary* is a term given to the prominence of the costochondral junctions. Infants with scurvy develop "frog legs" due to subperiosteal hemorrhage. This form of hemorrhage is painful and the infant naturally relaxes the lower limbs in this pattern to relieve the pain. Healing of the subperiosteal hemorrhage often involves abnormal calcification of the region and the formation of a more club-shaped bone

Plate 8-10

Nutritional and Metabolic Diseases

SCURVY (Continued)

BONY AND SKIN ABNORMALITIES OF SCURVY

This can lead to difficulty with movement. Radiographs of the long bones reveal the classic white line of Frankel, which represents the abnormal calcification of the cartilage within the epiphysial-diaphysial juncture. The periosteum appears ballooned out due to the presence of subperiosteal hemorrhage. Over time, the hemorrhagic areas become partially or completed calcified.

Infants with scurvy may also develop severe ecchymosis around the eye and in the retrobulbar space, which, when severe, can result in proptosis. Child abuse may be considered in the differential diagnosis.

Breast milk contains adequate amounts of vitamin C, so infantile scurvy is more likely to occur in children who are not breast fed and are given a diet devoid of vitamin C.

Pathogenesis: Vitamin C is an essential vitamin that is acquired through dietary intake. Humans lack the enzyme L-gluconolactone oxidase, which is required for the synthesis of L-ascorbic acid from its precursor, glucose. Dietary sources of vitamin C include fruits, vegetables, and fresh meats. Citrus fruits are the main source of dietary vitamin C. All human tissues contain vitamin C, with the adrenal glands and pituitary glands having the highest concentrations. Leukocytes contain appreciable amounts of vitamin C, and the buffy coat level is helpful in diagnosis. The clinical manifestations of scurvy do not appear until the buffy coat concentration has fallen to less than 4 mg/100 mL or the serum level to less than 20 μmol/L. The normal buffy coat concentration is in the range of 15 to 25 mg/100 mL, and that of the serum is 40 to 120 μmol/L. The kidney has an extraordinary ability to adjust its vitamin C reabsorption and secretion based on serum levels. In scurvy, the kidney salvages all available vitamin C, and the urine concentration is 0 mg/24 hours.

Vitamin C is required as a cofactor for various enzyme functions. Vitamin C supplies electrons to enzymatic reactions. If these are absent, the enzymes are unable to properly produce their intended end product, and the manifestations of scurvy begin to develop. One of the most important functions of vitamin C is to serve as a cofactor, along with ferrous iron (Fe^{++}), for the enzymes prolyl hydroxylase and lysyl hydroxylase. These enzymes are responsible, respectively, for hydroxylation of the proline and lysine amino acid residues in collagen. If the proper ratio of proline and lysine hydroxylation is not present, the collagen molecule is unable to form a proper triple helix, and its function is compromised. Defective collagen production is the main deficiency responsible for the cutaneous signs of scurvy, because collagen is the major structural protein in blood vessel walls and in the dermis. Vitamin C is also responsible for electron donation in other enzymatic reactions, including those that synthesize tyrosine, dopamine, and carnitine.

Histology: Histology is not required for the diagnosis. Biopsy of a petechial lesion shows perifollicular red blood cell extravasation and a minimal lymphocytic inflammatory infiltrate. If the specimen includes the area around a hair follicle, close inspection will reveal a coiled or corkscrew appearance to the hair follicle. It should be remembered that patients with scurvy have impaired wound healing: After biopsy without proper therapy, the freshly incised skin may take weeks to months to heal, and large ecchymoses typically develop around the biopsy site.

Treatment: Therapy requires the replacement of vitamin C at a dosage of 300 to 500 mg daily until the symptoms resolve. Then start the recommended daily

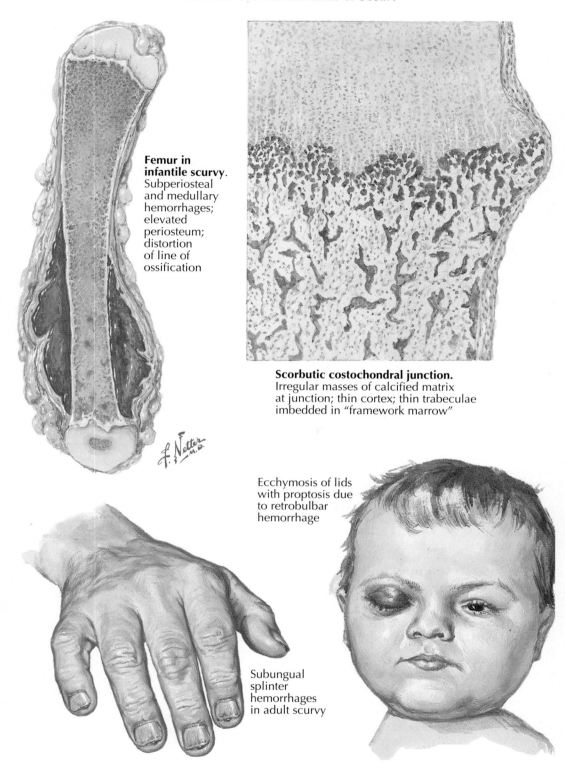

Femur in infantile scurvy. Subperiosteal and medullary hemorrhages; elevated periosteum; distortion of line of ossification

Scorbutic costochondral junction. Irregular masses of calcified matrix at junction; thin cortex; thin trabeculae imbedded in "framework marrow"

Ecchymosis of lids with proptosis due to retrobulbar hemorrhage

Subungual splinter hemorrhages in adult scurvy

allowance. Patients show rapid improvement. The root cause must be determined, and if the patient does not respond to therapy, serum levels should be rechecked. If they are still low, noncompliance with therapy should be considered. Often, patients with scurvy have an underlying alcoholism, eating disorder, or psychiatric illness that, if not properly addressed, will continue to occur. Patients should see a nutritionist, who can best educate them on the need for a balanced diet and which foods are high in vitamin C. Alcoholics need to be referred to experts who are adept at treating this common problem. Supplementation with the daily recommended amounts can be continued for life, because any excess vitamin C is not stored in the body but excreted by the kidneys. Supplementation ensures the avoidance of further episodes of scurvy.

Plate 8-11   Integumentary System

VITAMIN A DEFICIENCY

Vitamin A deficiency, also known as phrynoderma, is a multisystem disorder caused by a deficiency of vitamin A, either from lack of intake or from a decrease in normal absorption. Vitamin A is a fat-soluble essential vitamin that is stored in the fatty tissue and liver. Humans require a nutritional source for this vitamin. Foods high in vitamin A include all yellow vegetables (including carrots), green leafy vegetables, liver, milk, eggs, tomatoes, and fish oils. Many other food staples contain vitamin A. Hippocrates may have been the first to describe vitamin A deficiency and a therapy for it. However, it was not until the early twentieth century that scientists recognized the different forms of vitamin A and its carotene precursors.

Clinical Findings: Night blindness is one of the earliest findings in vitamin A deficiency. Vitamin A is crucially important for proper functioning of the retinal rods, through production of rhodopsin. Rhodopsin is the primary rod pigment that makes visual adaption in the dark possible. Xerophthalmia (dry eyes) often precedes the night blindness and is typically the first sign of vitamin A deficiency, although this sign is neither sensitive or specific. As the deficiency progresses, the xerophthalmia may result in corneal dryness, abrasions, ulceration, and keratomalacia, which leads to blindness. Bitot's spots can be seen on the lateral conjunctiva of the eye. These are highly specific for vitamin A deficiency and appear as stuck-on foamy white papules and plaques that cannot be removed by swabbing. Bitot's spots are caused by abnormal keratinization of the conjunctival epithelium. It is estimated that vitamin A deficiency is one of the leading causes of vision loss worldwide. Growth impairment in children can be caused by vitamin A deficiency.

Phrynoderma is the name given to the skin findings in vitamin A deficiency. *Phrynoderma* literally means "toad-like" skin, and it is manifested by hyperkeratotic follicle-based papules. The skin is dry and rough. Patients with vitamin A deficiency may also have cheilitis and glossitis. These latter two conditions are nonspecific and can be seen in a variety of vitamin deficiencies.

Hypervitaminosis A can result from excessive vitamin A supplementation. It manifests as dry skin, hair loss, joint aches, bone pain, and headaches. Vitamin A can cause birth defects when taken in high doses during pregnancy.

Pathogenesis: Vitamin A deficiency in the United States is most frequently caused by strange dietary habits that avoid foods rich in vitamin A. Other conditions may predispose individuals to this deficiency, including cystic fibrosis, because of the difficulty in absorption of fat-soluble vitamins. Short gut syndrome that occurs after bariatric surgery may also lead to vitamin A deficiency. Proper production of bile acids and pancreatic enzymes is required for absorption of vitamin A. Severe liver disease may result in functional vitamin A deficiency, because the liver is required to convert carotene into vitamin A.

Vitamin A is found in foods predominantly as retinol or β-carotene. Vitamin A is critical for nuclear signaling, through binding to its nuclear receptors, the retinoic acid receptors (RARs) and the retinoid X receptors (RXRs). Once this binding occurs, the resulting complexes can affect the transcription of various gene products. The vitamin is responsible for maturation and proliferation of epithelial cells.

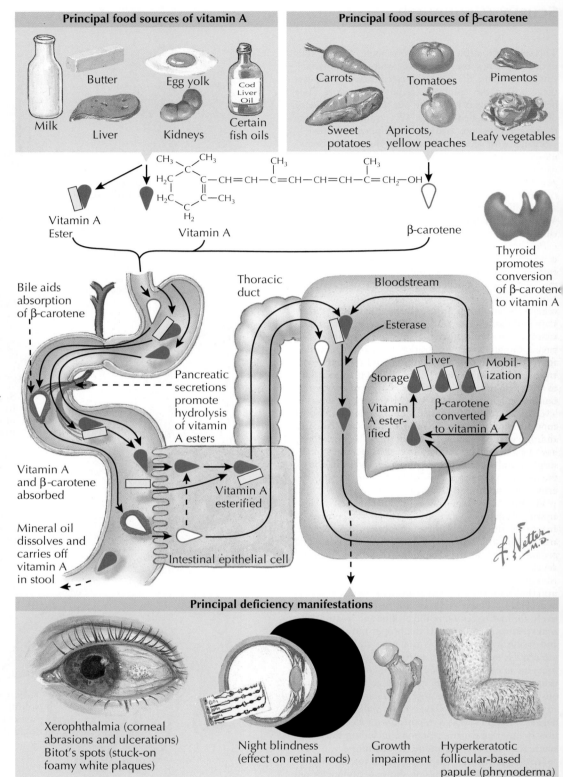

Principal food sources of vitamin A

Milk | Butter | Egg yolk | Cod Liver Oil
Liver | Kidneys | Certain fish oils

Principal food sources of β-carotene

Carrots | Tomatoes | Pimentos
Sweet potatoes | Apricots, yellow peaches | Leafy vegetables

Vitamin A Ester | Vitamin A | β-carotene

Thyroid promotes conversion of β-carotene to vitamin A

Bile aids absorption of β-carotene

Thoracic duct | Bloodstream

Esterase

Pancreatic secretions promote hydrolysis of vitamin A esters

Liver
Storage | Mobilization

Vitamin A esterified | β-carotene converted to vitamin A

Vitamin A and β-carotene absorbed

Vitamin A esterified

Mineral oil dissolves and carries off vitamin A in stool

Intestinal epithelial cell

Principal deficiency manifestations

Xerophthalmia (corneal abrasions and ulcerations) Bitot's spots (stuck-on foamy white plaques)

Night blindness (effect on retinal rods)

Growth impairment

Hyperkeratotic follicular-based papule (phrynoderma)

Histology: Cutaneous biopsies are nonspecific but may suggest a nutritional deficiency. There is pallor of the upper epidermis. Hyperkeratotic plugs are seen in follicles, with minimal to no inflammatory infiltrate.

Treatment: Treatment requires replacement of vitamin A and probably other essential vitamins in the patient's diet. The eye changes may be permanent, but the cutaneous findings respond well. Loss of only night vision has been shown to respond to therapy in some cases. Once blindness occurs, however, the only hope for vision is with corneal transplantation. Most cases in North America and Europe are caused by poor absorption due to an underlying cause, and the advice of a nutritionist who is an expert in malabsorption is indicated. These patients may require long-term replacement and monitoring of their vitamin A levels.

Plate 8-12

Nutritional and Metabolic Diseases

POTENTIAL CLINICAL CONSEQUENCES OF WARFARIN USE

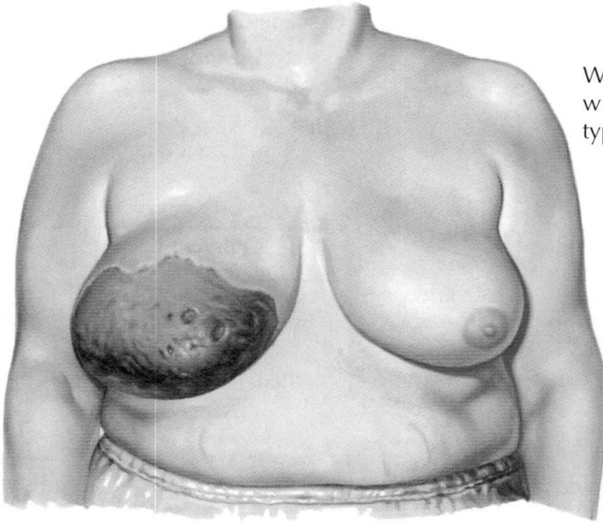

Warfarin-induced skin necrosis manifesting with purple hemorrhagic bullae and ulceration, typically over fatty tissue

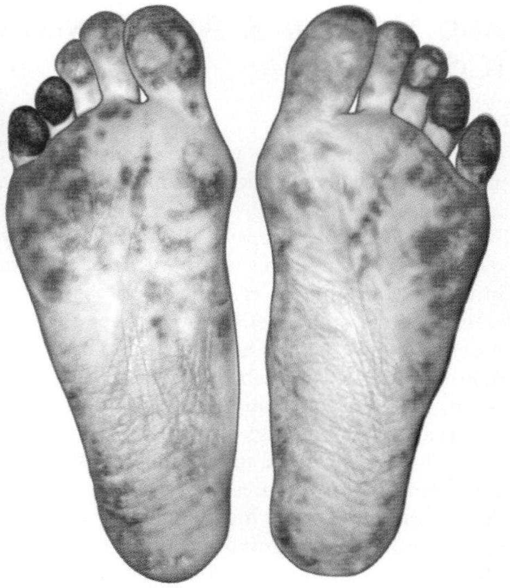

VITAMIN K DEFICIENCY AND VITAMIN K ANTAGONISTS

Vitamin K is an essential nutrient that is required as a cofactor for the production of a handful of coagulation cascade proteins. It is a fat-soluble vitamin that is efficiently stored in the human body. Vitamin K deficiency is rare and is typically seen only transiently in neonates and infants during the first 6 months of life. Affected neonates may show abnormally prolonged bleeding after minor trauma. Patients may have an elevated prothrombin time (PT) and decreased serum levels of vitamin K and coagulation factors. Therapy consists of replacement of vitamin K to normal levels and a search for any possible underlying cause, such as liver or gastrointestinal disease. Neonatal and infantile vitamin K deficiency is most likely caused by maternal breast milk insufficiency of vitamin K.

Vitamin K deficiency is rarely seen in adults, because most diets contain enough vitamin K for normal physiological functioning. Adult patients with liver disease and malabsorption states are at highest risk for the development of vitamin K deficiency. Vitamin K may be found in two natural forms: vitamin K_1 (phylloquinone) and vitamin K_2 (menaquinone). K_1 is found in plants, and K_2 is produced by various bacteria that make up the normal flora of the gastrointestinal tract. Antibiotics may cause a decrease in the bacterial production of vitamin K_2, resulting in a lack of vitamin K available for absorption. This is typically not a clinical issue unless the patient is taking a vitamin K antagonist such as warfarin. Vitamin K is absorbed in the distal jejunum and ileum via passive diffusion across the cell membrane. The majority of vitamin K is stored normally in the liver. There, the vitamin is converted to its active state, hydroxyquinone. An efficient vitamin K salvage pathway normally prevents an individual from becoming deficient in the vitamin. The enzyme vitamin K epoxide reductase is responsible for converting the inactive epoxiquinone to the active hydroxyquinone form of vitamin K.

Warfarin is a synthetic analogue of vitamin K and is the main vitamin K antagonist. It is indicated for use as an anticoagulant in the treatment of a number of conditions, including atrial fibrillation and deep venous thrombosis, and after heart valve replacement surgery. Warfarin acts by inhibiting the enzymes that are responsible for carboxylation of glutamate residues and epoxide reductase. This both decreases the available clotting factors and induces vitamin K deficiency, leading to added reduction of available clotting factors.

Clinical Findings: Vitamin K antagonists have been shown to cause a specific type of cutaneous eruption known as warfarin necrosis, which occurs in approximately 0.05% of patients taking the medication. Warfarin necrosis affects the areas of the body that have increased body fat, such as the breasts, the abdominal pannus, and the thighs. The feet are also particularly prone to development of warfarin necrosis. The skin

Purple toe syndrome associated with vitamin K antagonist therapy

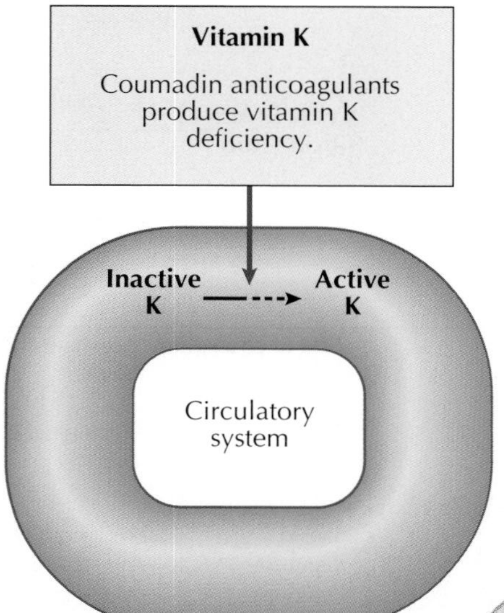

Vitamin K
Coumadin anticoagulants produce vitamin K deficiency.

Inactive K → Active K

Circulatory system

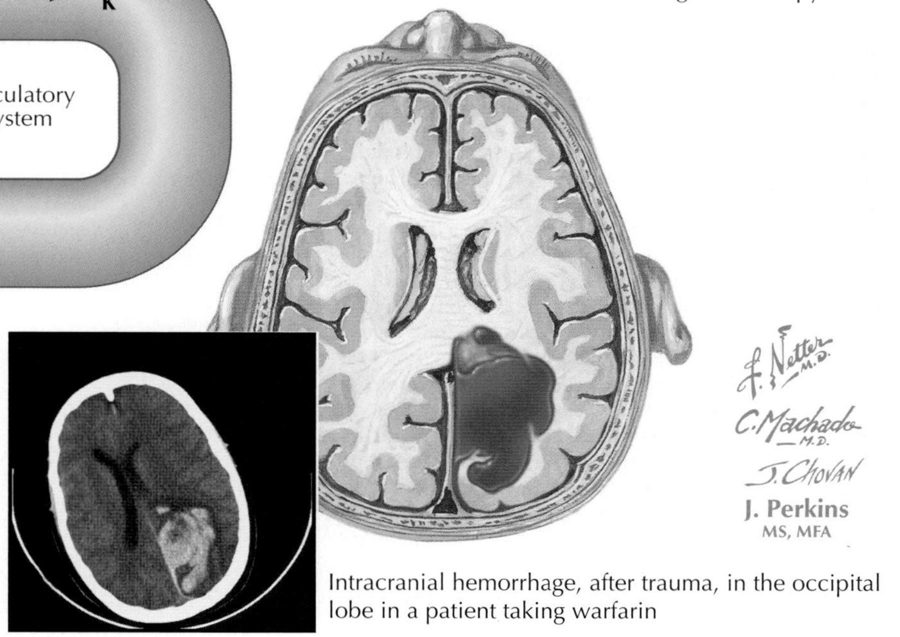

Intracranial hemorrhage, after trauma, in the occipital lobe in a patient taking warfarin

initially develops small, red to violaceous petechiae and macules preceded by paresthesias. These regions become erythematous and purple (ecchymoses) with intense edematous skin. The lesions eventually ulcerate or form hemorrhagic bullae. The hemorrhagic bullae desquamate, leaving deep ulcers. Painful cutaneous ulcers may occur, with some extending into the subcutaneous tissue, including muscle. Most ulcers appear

within 5 to 7 days after the initiation of warfarin therapy. Secondary infection may be a cause of significant morbidity. The affected areas continue to undergo necrosis unless the warfarin is withheld and the patient is treated with a different class of anticoagulant. The feet and lower extremities may have a reticulated, purplish discoloration called "purple toe syndrome." This cutaneous drug reaction can be eliminated or at least drastically

Plate 8-13

Integumentary System

ANTICOAGULATION EFFECTS ON THE CLOTTING CASCADE

Cascade of clotting factors and sites of action of heparin and warfarin

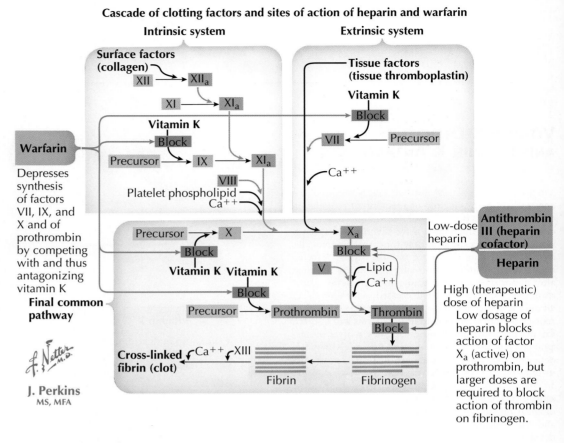

VITAMIN K DEFICIENCY AND VITAMIN K ANTAGONISTS (Continued)

decreased if the patient is pretreated with heparin or another equivalent anticoagulant before warfarin is initiated.

Histology: Skin biopsies from areas of warfarin necrosis show an ulcer with a mixed inflammatory infiltrate. Thrombosis is seen within the small vessels (venules and capillaries) of the cutaneous vasculature. Arterial involvement is absent. Minimal to no inflammatory infiltrate is present. Red blood cell extravasation is prominent. The main histopathological finding is microthrombi. Findings of inflammation, a neutrophilic infiltrate, arterial involvement, a strong lymphocytic infiltrate, or the presence of bacteria in or around vessels mitigate against the diagnosis of warfarin necrosis. Bacteria will be present on the surface of the ulcer and are believed to be a secondary phenomenon.

Pathogenesis: Vitamin K is needed for the modification of many coagulation cascade proteins, including protein C, protein S, factor II (prothrombin), factor VII, factor IX, and factor X. Factors II, VII, IX, and X are critical in forming a clot and are produced in the liver as inactive precursors. Preactivation of these clotting factors requires the action of vitamin K carboxylation on glutamate amino acid residues. Once preactivated, the clotting factors are available for full activation and clot formation when exposed to calcium and phospholipids on the surface of platelets.

Inhibition of these clotting factors by vitamin K antagonists leads to anticoagulation. Warfarin works by inhibiting the carboxylation of glutamate. On the other hand, protein C and protein S are responsible for turning off the clotting cascade and play a natural regulatory role in normal coagulation. When these proteins are inhibited, the clotting cascade may proceed unimpeded, allowing for excessive clotting. Protein C and protein S have shorter half-lives than factors II, VII, IX, and X. Therefore, when individuals are treated initially with warfarin, the levels of protein C and protein S are depleted before the other factors, leading to a prothrombic state. This initial prothrombic state is responsible for the clinical signs and symptoms of microvasculature blood clotting and skin necrosis. The clotting takes place in areas of increased adipose tissue because of the sluggish flow of blood through the fine vasculature in these regions. For this reason, most patients are given heparin or a similar anticoagulant until the full effect of warfarin on all clotting factors has occurred.

Therapy: Treatment of warfarin necrosis requires discontinuation of warfarin and initiation of heparin anticoagulation and supportive care with fresh-frozen plasma and vitamin K replace the lost protein C and protein S. Surgical debridement may be required, and one should be vigilant for any signs or symptoms of secondary infection. Therapy consists of proper

replacement of vitamin K and supportive care. Menadione is a synthetic form vitamin K that can be given therapeutically.

Vitamin K deficiency in neonates and infants is diagnosed by an isolated elevation in the prothrombin time. The levels of the vitamin K–dependent clotting cofactors can each be measured, and vitamin K replacement

should be administered to those who are deficient. Breast milk is not a strong source of vitamin K, and if the mother had previous children with vitamin K deficiency, the newborn should be given supplemental vitamin K. The best method for supplementation has yet to be determined, but it can be achieved with a one-time intramuscular injection or with oral replacement.

Element	Site of absorption	Mechanism
Ca^{++}	Duodenum and jejunum	Active
Fe^{++}	Duodenum and jejunum	Facilitated diffusion
Water-soluble vitamins		
Vitamin C	Ileum	Na^{+}-coupled/2° active
Thiamin (B_1)	Jejunum	Na^{+}-coupled/2° active
Riboflavin (B_2)	Jejunum	Na^{+}-coupled/2° active
Biotin	Jejunum	Na^{+}-coupled/2° active
Vitamin B_{12}	Ileum	Facilitated diffusion
Pyridoxine (B_6)	Jejunum and ileum	Passive diffusion
Fat-soluble vitamins		
Vitamin A	Jejunum and ileum	Passive diffusion
Vitamin D	Jejunum and ileum	Passive diffusion
Vitamin E	Jejunum and ileum	Passive diffusion
Vitamin K	Jejunum and ileum	Passive diffusion

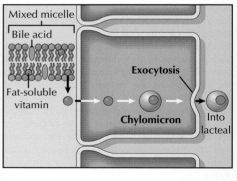

Plate 8-14

Nutritional and Metabolic Diseases

WILSON'S DISEASE

Wilson's disease, also known as hepatolenticular degeneration, is a disorder caused by a defect in copper metabolism. The disease is rare, with a worldwide incidence of approximately 1 in 18,000. It is an autosomal recessive condition that is caused by a defect in the *ATP7B* gene, which is located on the long arm of chromosome 13. The product of this gene is responsible for the proper transport of copper. The main clinical findings relate to nervous system involvement and liver disease. Wilson's disease has a variable phenotype depending on the specific genetic mutation. Cutaneous disease and ophthalmological disease are frequently seen.

Clinical Findings: Wilson's disease equally affects males and females, and its incidence varies among populations. The usual age at onset is in the first 2 decades of life. Liver disease and central nervous system (CNS) disease are often the first signs. Patients may present with unexplained hepatomegaly, cirrhosis, and end-stage liver disease. The CNS findings can manifest in various patterns. Mild to severe psychiatric symptoms of depression and mood lability are common; the manifestations in some patients may approach the diagnosis of schizophrenia. Impaired cognition and memory are frequently seen and may lead to early dementia. Extra-pyramidal features are always present and include tremor and rigidity. The tremor has been described as a "wing-beating" tremor of the shoulder girdle. Brady-kinesia is invariably a part of the disease. Ataxia and chorea, along with dysfunction of normal motor coordination, are evident as time progresses.

The cutaneous findings, when present in conjunction with liver and CNS disease, can make the diagnosis. Patients have varying amounts of pretibial hyperpigmentation, the cause of which is poorly understood. Rarely, patients present with a blue discoloration to the lunula of the nail. The most pathognomonic sign is the presence of Kayser-Fleischer rings on the cornea. A Kayser-Fleischer ring is a yellow to orange-brown ring around the iris. It represents an abnormal accumulation of copper in Descemet's membrane of the cornea. A slit-lamp examination is required to appreciate this clinical finding, which is unique to Wilson's disease.

Laboratory testing is required to confirm the diagnosis. A hallmark is a decreased ceruloplasmin level. The actual ceruloplasmin protein is not defective in any manner. Urinary copper excretion is elevated to more than 100 μg/day.

Pathogenesis: The *ATP7B* gene is mutated in Wilson's disease, and this leads to the systemic and cutaneous manifestations of the disease. The *ATP7B* gene encodes the P-type adenosine triphosphatase (ATPase) that serves as a metal-binding and metal-carrying protein. This P-type ATPase is primarily responsible for the transport of copper. When it is defective, copper builds up to abnormal levels in the liver, in the CNS, and to a lesser extent, in the cornea. Many different mutations have been discovered in the *ATP7B* gene and are responsible for the different phenotypes seen. Homozygous patients and compound heterozygotes have completely different phenotypes with some overlapping features. Certain mutations lead to liver and CNS disease or to a predominance of one over the other. The large number of mutations and the large size of the gene make it difficult to analyze. The prevalence of the different genetic mutations varies among populations.

Histology: Skin biopsies are not helpful in the diagnosis. Biopsies of the liver show varying degrees of portal inflammation and fibrosis with eventual

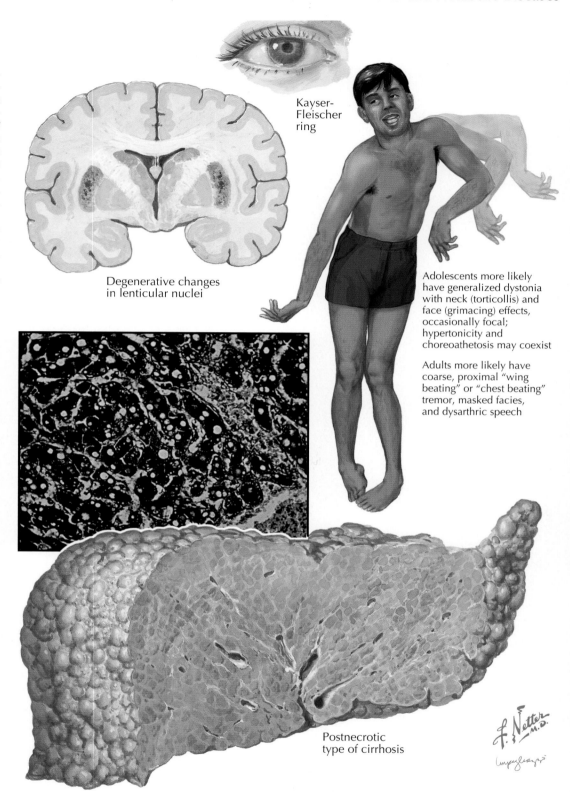

Kayser-Fleischer ring

Degenerative changes in lenticular nuclei

Adolescents more likely have generalized dystonia with neck (torticollis) and face (grimacing) effects, occasionally focal; hypertonicity and choreoathetosis may coexist

Adults more likely have coarse, proximal "wing beating" or "chest beating" tremor, masked facies, and dysarthric speech

Postnecrotic type of cirrhosis

cirrhosis. Hydropic degeneration of individual hepatocytes is seen to a varying degree, depending on the timing of the biopsy. Special staining methods can highlight the elevated copper within the hepatocytes.

Treatment: The only cure for the disease is liver transplantation. This procedure is becoming more common and has led to excellent therapeutic responses. The transplanted normal liver produces adequate levels of the P-type ATPase to bring the copper levels to

normal. CNS symptoms, if present at the time of transplantation, typically persist with minimal improvement over time. While awaiting liver transplantation, patients are usually treated with a combination of a low-copper diet, oral zinc supplementation, and D-penicillamine. Zinc competes with copper for absorption and decreases the amount of copper absorbed from the gastrointestinal tract. D-Penicillamine is a copper-chelating agent that helps to lower serum and tissue copper levels.

GENODERMATOSES AND SYNDROMES

Plate 9-1

Genodermatoses and Syndromes

ADDISON'S DISEASE

Addison's disease (chronic primary adrenocortical insufficiency) occurs when the adrenal gland has lost most of its functional capacity. Addison's disease can be caused by many different disease states that inhibit the functioning of the adrenal gland. The adrenal gland has a massive reserve capacity, and clinical manifestations of chronic adrenal insufficiency are not seen until the bilateral glands have lost at least 90% of their ability to produce adrenal hormones. Autoimmune destructive atrophy of the adrenal glands is the most common cause of Addison's disease. Infectious processes can cause destruction of the adrenal gland, with tuberculosis one of the more common causes of chronic adrenal gland insufficiency. Most cases of acute adrenal gland destruction are caused by bacteria (i.e., meningococcal disease).

Clinical Findings: Males and females are equally affected. The first symptoms are lethargy and generalized malaise. These symptoms may not be apparent until the affected patient undergoes a major stressful event, such as infection, which can lead to a prolonged disease course and a prolonged convalescence. Patients have excessive nervousness and may show emotional lability superimposed on periods of depression. Fatigue and weakness can be severe, to the point where even speaking causes fatigue. Weight loss and evidence of dehydration are present in most cases. Hypotension is frequently seen, and a small heart shadow is seen on chest radiography.

Cutaneous effects are always found in chronic primary adrenal insufficiency. Pigmentation is seen in many regions of the body and appears to occur in areas of friction, such as along the waist line and on elbows and knees. This is typically a generalized "bronze pigmentation," but it is accentuated in the groin, nipples, and scrotum. The palmar and plantar creases are accentuated. Hyperpigmentation may be prominent within previous scars. Vitiligo may be present in conjunction with autoimmune adrenal insufficiency. Increased pigmentation of hair is seen, but this may be subtle and may occur slowly. Pigmentary alterations of the gingival and labial mucosa may also be seen. Pigmentary anomalies are not seen in secondary adrenal insufficiency, which is caused by pituitary deficiency.

Body hair is dramatically decreased, with near loss of axillary and pubic hair. The hair loss is more pronounced in females, because males still produce androgens, primarily in the unaffected testes. Serum testing shows hyperkalemia and hyponatremia, with a low cortisol level. The diagnosis is confirmed by intravenously injecting a synthetic corticotropin and evaluating the adrenal gland's response by measuring cortisol levels after the injection. In patients with Addison's disease, the serum cortisol level is not increased by stimulation testing.

Histology: Skin biopsies are not helpful in making the diagnosis and are rarely performed. A normal number of melanocytes are present, with an increased amount of melanin pigment in the epidermis.

Pathogenesis: The adrenal glands are responsible for making cortisol, aldosterone, and the 17-ketosteroids. When the adrenal glands no longer are able to produce these molecules, Addison's disease sets in. In the presence of low circulating levels of cortisol, the pituitary responds by increasing production of adrenocorticotrophic hormone (ACTH, corticotropin) and melanocyte-stimulating hormone (MSH). ACTH and MSH are derived from the same precursor protein, pro-opiomelanocortin (POMC). The pigmentary anomalies

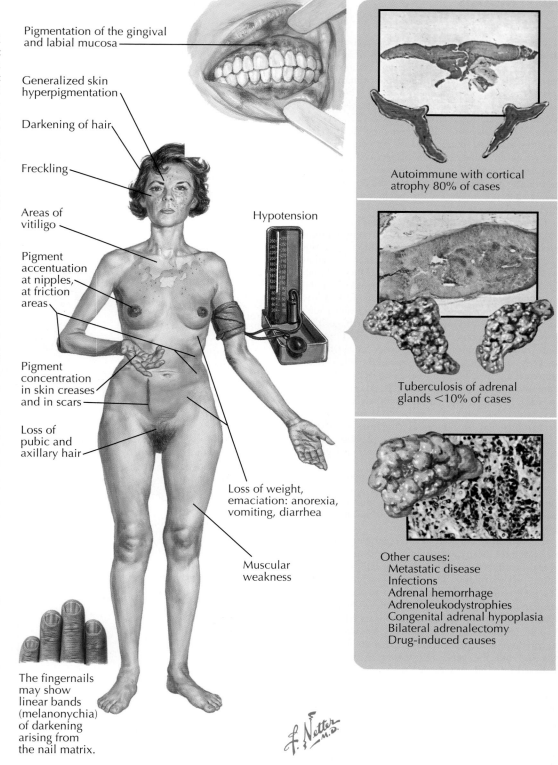

Pigmentation of the gingival and labial mucosa

Generalized skin hyperpigmentation

Darkening of hair

Freckling

Areas of vitiligo

Pigment accentuation at nipples, at friction areas

Pigment concentration in skin creases and in scars

Loss of pubic and axillary hair

Hypotension

Loss of weight, emaciation: anorexia, vomiting, diarrhea

Muscular weakness

The fingernails may show linear bands (melanonychia) of darkening arising from the nail matrix.

Autoimmune with cortical atrophy 80% of cases

Tuberculosis of adrenal glands <10% of cases

Other causes:
Metastatic disease
Infections
Adrenal hemorrhage
Adrenoleukodystrophies
Congenital adrenal hypoplasia
Bilateral adrenalectomy
Drug-induced causes

seen in Addison's disease are directly related to increased release of MSH. The increase in MSH causes pigment production by melanocytes in skin, hair, and mucous membranes. Pubic and axillary hair loss is related to the lack of 17-ketosteroids, whereas hypotension is caused by the lack of aldosterone. The lack of aldosterone causes a decreased blood volume and decreased serum sodium. The lack of cortisol production is responsible for weakness, fatigue, weight loss, and decreased mentation.

Addison's disease is seen frequently in association with other autoimmune endocrine disorders such as diabetes and autoimmune thyroiditis.

Treatment: Treatment requires the clearing of infection or treatment of the underlying cause of adrenal gland dysfunction. Supplemental hydrocortisone and fludrocortisone are used as replacement therapy for those with inadequate adrenal function. Hydrocortisone is used primarily to replace the missing cortisol, and fludrocortisone is used to replace aldosterone.

Plate 9-2											Integumentary System

AMYLOIDOSIS

The term *amyloidosis* refers to a heterogeneous group of diseases. Systemic and cutaneous forms of amyloidosis can occur and are caused by the deposition of one of many different amyloid proteins. The primary cutaneous forms are more frequently seen. They include nodular, lichen, and macular amyloidosis (also referred to as lichen or macular amyloidosis). The systemic form is a multisystem, life-threatening disorder that requires systemic therapy. Most systemic disease is caused by an abnormality in plasma cells; myeloma-associated amyloid is a distant second in incidence. In addition to amyloidosis of the skin, the central nervous system may be involved with amyloidosis, as it is in Alzheimer's disease.

Clinical Findings: Systemic amyloidosis is caused by abnormal production of amyloid AL protein (immunoglobulin light chains) and its deposition in various organ systems. These effects can be seen in patients with plasma cell dyscrasia or myeloma. Mucocutaneous findings are often part of systemic amyloidosis, and on occasion they are the initial presentation of the disease. The hallmark cutaneous finding is translucent papules and plaques with varying degrees of hemorrhage. These papules are composed of the abnormal AL protein. Soft, rubbery papules may also occur within the oral mucous membranes. Pinch purpura of the skin is almost universal and results from weakening of the superficial cutaneous vessels by deposition of the AL protein. Periorbital ecchymoses may circumferentially surround the eye, which has led to the term "raccoon eyes." The ecchymoses may be induced by coughing or by superficial trauma. The palms and soles may have a waxy appearance. The tongue is often strikingly enlarged due to amyloid deposits.

Deposition of the AL protein in close approximation to the dermal elastic fibers produces a rare finding termed amyloid elastosis. Clinically, this may mimic cutis laxa; the skin is easily distensible and lacks elastic recoil.

Deposition of amyloid in the renal glomeruli, liver, or heart muscle can cause significant end-organ damage. Renal insufficiency leading to renal failure is a major cause of morbidity and mortality. Hepatomegaly, leading to fibrosis and liver failure, may occur. Amyloid protein that is deposited in the muscle of the heart may lead to arrhythmias and congestive heart failure.

The primary cutaneous diseases known as lichen amyloidosis and macular amyloidosis are localized to the leg and the back, respectively. Most cases are believed to be directly caused by keratinocyte-derived amyloid protein. There are no systemic symptoms. Patients present with pruritic hyperpigmented macules and papules that may coalesce into plaques. Nodular primary cutaneous amyloidosis is caused by the local production of AL protein by plasma cells in the skin. This condition is extremely rare and may progress to systemic amyloidosis.

Pathogenesis: Systemic AL amyloidosis results from plasma cell dyscrasia or from myeloma-associated disease. It is directly caused by a proliferation of abnormal plasma cells. The plasma cells produce excessive amounts of immunoglobulin light chains, predominantly λ chains. The excessive amounts of AL protein are deposited within the walls of the cutaneous vasculature; this leads to weakening of the walls and is responsible for their easy rupture. The AL protein is deposited in many organ systems. Rarely, the plasma cells produce immunoglobulin heavy chains; this is termed AH protein.

Sites and manifestations of amyloid deposition that may occur in various combinations

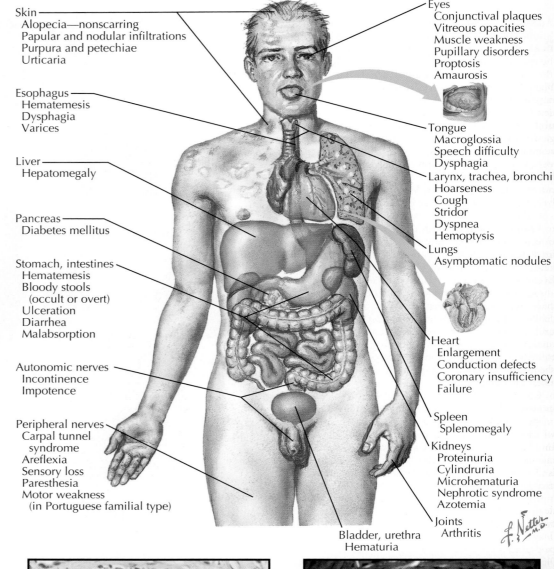

Skin
Alopecia—nonscarring
Papular and nodular infiltrations
Purpura and petechiae
Urticaria

Esophagus
Hematemesis
Dysphagia
Varices

Liver
Hepatomegaly

Pancreas
Diabetes mellitus

Stomach, intestines
Hematemesis
Bloody stools
(occult or overt)
Ulceration
Diarrhea
Malabsorption

Autonomic nerves
Incontinence
Impotence

Peripheral nerves
Carpal tunnel
syndrome
Areflexia
Sensory loss
Paresthesia
Motor weakness
(in Portuguese familial type)

Bladder, urethra
Hematuria

Eyes
Conjunctival plaques
Vitreous opacities
Muscle weakness
Pupillary disorders
Proptosis
Amaurosis

Tongue
Macroglossia
Speech difficulty
Dysphagia

Larynx, trachea, bronchi
Hoarseness
Cough
Stridor
Dyspnea
Hemoptysis

Lungs
Asymptomatic nodules

Heart
Enlargement
Conduction defects
Coronary insufficiency
Failure

Spleen
Splenomegaly

Kidneys
Proteinuria
Cylindruria
Microhematuria
Nephrotic syndrome
Azotemia

Joints
Arthritis

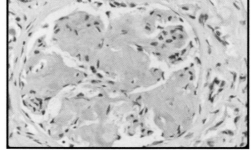

Extensive amyloid deposits in glomerulus of human kidney (Congo red and hematoxylin stain)

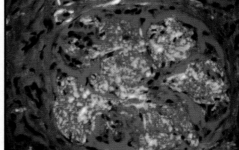

Same section, viewed under polarizing microscope, demonstrating green birefringence

Histology: Amyloidosis is a disease caused by the abnormal deposition of amorphous AL protein in the dermis and subcutaneous tissue. Biopsies of involved skin show eosinophilic deposits on routine staining. The amyloid protein is accentuated with special staining methods such as the Congo red stain. It shows an apple-green birefringence under polarized light microscopy and appears reddish under routine microscopy.

Treatment: Systemic amyloidosis is best treated with combination chemotherapy. Traditionally, prednisone and melphalan were the agents of choice. Newer proteosome inhibitors are currently used. Bone marrow transplantation is performed in certain cases.

Therapy for primary cutaneous amyloidosis is directed at symptomatic control. Topical corticosteroids and oral antihistamines are used to control itching. Varying results have been reported with ultraviolet phototherapy. No randomized, prospective studies of the treatment of primary cutaneous amyloid have been published.

Plate 9-3   Genodermatoses and Syndromes

BASAL CELL NEVUS SYNDROME

Basal cell nevus syndrome (BCNS), also known as nevoid basal cell carcinoma syndrome or Gorlin syndrome, is an uncommon autosomal dominant genodermatosis caused by mutations in the *patched-1 (PTCH1)* gene on chromosome 9. Approximately 40% of cases represent new, spontaneous mutations. Affected individuals are predisposed to the development of multiple basal cell carcinomas (BCCs), often in the hundreds over their lifetime. The diagnosis of this syndrome is based on a number of established criteria.

Clinical Findings: The incidence of BCNS is estimated to be 1 in 100,000 persons, and there is no race or sex predilection. It is inherited in an autosomal dominant fashion. Often, the first symptoms are painful keratogenic (odontogenic) jaw cysts. The early onset of BCCs often occurs before the age of 20 years.

Four of five BCNS patients have odontogenic jaw cysts on dental examination or dental radiographs. In children, the BCCs have been shown to mimic skin tags. Because skin tags are highly unusual in children, one should biopsy any skin tags seen in a young child to evaluate for BCC. About 90% of affected individuals show evidence of palmar pitting. This represents abnormal keratinization of the palmar skin. The lesions manifest as small (1-2 mm), pink to red, shallow defects in the glabrous skin of the palms or soles.

Medulloblastoma is uncommonly seen in patients with BCNS, occurring in only 1% to 2% of patients. Interestingly, 1% to 2% of children diagnosed with medulloblastoma are also diagnosed with BCNS. This is likely the most serious sequela of the syndrome and carries significant morbidity and mortality.

Diagnosis of BCNS is based on fulfillment of well-developed criteria. Two major criteria or one major and two minor criteria must be met to make the diagnosis. The six major criteria are (1) more than two BCCs; (2) palmar and plantar pitting; (3) odontogenic jaw cysts; (4) abnormalities of the ribs, including bifid or splayed ribs; (5) calcification of the falx cerebri; and (6) first-degree relative diagnosed with BCNS. The minor criteria are (1) congenital malformations (frontal bossing, hypertelorism, cleft palate, coloboma); (2) ovarian or cardiac fibromas; (3) macrocephaly; (4) skeletal abnormalities (scoliosis, syndactyly, Sprengel deformity of the scapula, pectus deformity); (5) medulloblastoma; and (6) other radiological abnormalities, including phalangeal lucencies in a flame shape and vertebral fusion.

Pathogenesis: BCNS is caused by to a defect in the *PTCH1* gene on the long arm of chromosome 9. This gene is responsible for encoding the sonic hedgehog receptor protein that is found on many cell membranes. In normal physiological states, the transmembrane protein encoded by *PTCH1* binds to the smoothened protein, turning off downstream cell signaling and ultimately decreasing cell proliferation. When the gene is mutated or when excessive sonic hedgehog protein is present, inhibition of the smoothened protein is removed, leading to uncontrolled cell signaling and a dramatically increased risk of cancer. Patients with BCNS are more sensitive to damage from ultraviolet light and radiation than normal controls.

Histology: BCC in the BCNS syndrome is histologically the same as any other BCC, and there are no distinguishing factors.

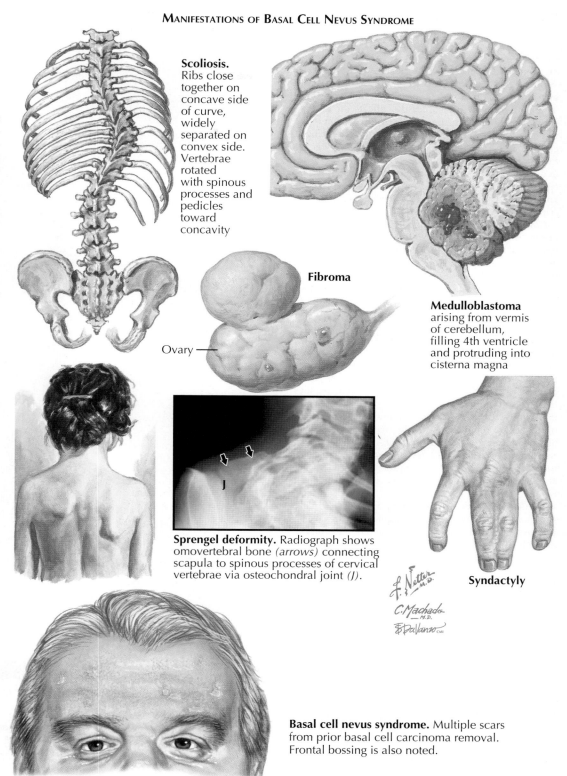

MANIFESTATIONS OF BASAL CELL NEVUS SYNDROME

Scoliosis. Ribs close together on concave side of curve, widely separated on convex side. Vertebrae rotated with spinous processes and pedicles toward concavity

Fibroma

Ovary

Medulloblastoma arising from vermis of cerebellum, filling 4th ventricle and protruding into cisterna magna

Sprengel deformity. Radiograph shows omovertebral bone *(arrows)* connecting scapula to spinous processes of cervical vertebrae via osteochondral joint *(J).*

Syndactyly

Basal cell nevus syndrome. Multiple scars from prior basal cell carcinoma removal. Frontal bossing is also noted.

Treatment: BCCs tend to be multiple. Routine skin examinations and prompt removal of basal cell skin cancers help decrease the size of scarring and disfigurement resulting from surgery. All patients need to be educated at an early age on avoiding excessive sun exposure, tanning, and unnecessary radiation exposure from medical testing, because all of these increase the likelihood of BCC development. Many ongoing research protocols are looking at oral agents to decrease the abnormal hedgehog signaling pathway; such studies may lead to medical options for these patients in the future. Jaw cysts are best removed surgically to relieve pain and discomfort. Medulloblastoma is a serious, life-threatening tumor most commonly seen in early childhood, before the age of 4 years. Surgical and chemotherapeutic options exist.

Plate 9-4

Integumentary System

CARNEY COMPLEX

Carney complex, also known as NAME syndrome (**n**evi, **a**trial myxomas, **m**yxoid neurofibromas, **e**phelides) or LAMB syndrome (**l**entigines, **a**trial myxomas, **m**ucocutaneous myxomas, **b**lue nevi), is an autosomal dominantly inherited disorder that affects the integumentary, endocrine, cardiovascular, and central nervous systems. This rare disorder is primarily caused by a genetic mutation in the tumor suppressor gene, *PRKAR1A*. Approximately 20% of patients have defects in an undescribed gene located at 2p16. Various genotypes and phenotypes exist, and the diagnosis is based on a complex list of major, supplemental, and minor criteria.

Clinical Findings: The phenotypic expression of the disease is variable, and research has shown the phenotype to be related to the underlying genotype of the disease. Cutaneous findings are often the first signs of the disease, and they are typically noticed in the first few months of life. Five prominent skin effects can be seen in isolation or, more commonly, in conjunction with one another. Multiple lentigines and common acquired nevi are the two most frequent skin findings. Multiple blue nevi are also seen. The blue nevi, lentigines, and nevi tend to group together on the head and neck region, lips, and sclerae. Mucocutaneous myxomas may be found at any location and appear as flesh-colored to slightly translucent, pedunculated papules that are soft and easily compressed. They vary widely in number, from a few to hundreds. Subcutaneous myxomas are often found on the margin of the tarsal plate and can have a slightly pink-red to somewhat translucent appearance. They are not as soft to the touch as the mucocutaneous myxomas. Ephelides are also found in abundance, primarily in the head and neck region.

Cardiac myxomas are the leading cause of morbidity and mortality, and each patient diagnosed with Carney complex needs routine echocardiography and follow-up with cardiology. Male patients should be screened for testicular tumors with physical and ultrasound evaluations. Pituitary adenomas may lead to a growth hormone–producing adenoma and subsequent evidence of acromegaly. Cushing's syndrome may result from excessive cortisol production by the adrenal glands. This is a multisystem disorder with great variation in potential organ system involvement. Carney complex is best treated and monitored with a multidisciplinary approach.

Pathogenesis: The *PRKAR1A* gene encodes a regulatory subunit of a protein kinase A. Protein kinase A belongs to a family of regulatory proteins that are dependent on cyclic adenosine monophosphate (cAMP) for proper functioning. Many different mutations in *PRKAR1A* have been discovered, including missense, frame-shift, and nonsense mutations, all leading to defects in the encoded protein. Because of the many unique mutations in this gene, researchers have been able to show that the type of genetic mutation correlates with the phenotype of the disease. As an example, mutations in the exon portions of the gene (compared with the intron portions) are much more likely to clinically express lentigines and cardiac myxomas.

Histology: Skin biopsies by themselves are not diagnostic, and the lentigines, myxomas, and blue nevi found in patients with this syndrome are not different histologically than those found outside the Carney complex. Testicular tumors usually show a Leydig cell or Sertoli cell tumor with various amounts of calcification. Histological findings on biopsy of the adrenal

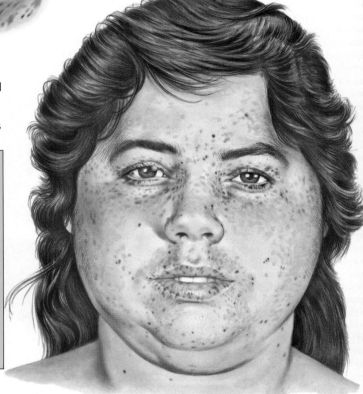

Mucocutaneous manifestations of Carney complex characterized by pigmented lentigines, blue nevi, myxomas, common acquired nevi, and subcutaneous myxomas

Additional features of Carney complex can include:

▶ Myxomas: cardiac atrium, mucocutaneous myxoma

▶ Testicular large-cell calcifying Sertoli cell tumors

▶ Growth hormone–secreting pituitary adenomas

▶ Psammomatous melanotic schwannomas (found along the sympathetic nerve chain)

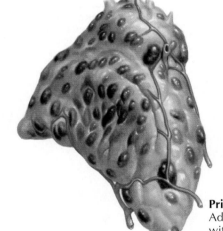

Primary pigmented nodular adrenocortical disease (PPNAD). Adrenal glands are usually of normal size and most are studded with black, brown, or red nodules. Most of the pigmented nodules are less than 4 mm in diameter and interspersed in the adjacent atrophic cortex.

gland characteristically show varying amounts of nodular pigmented regions; this has been termed primary *pigmented nodular adrenocortical disease (PPNAD)*. Adrenal disease may lead to increased production of cortisol and ultimately to the signs and symptoms of Cushing's syndrome. A unique tumor, almost always seen in conjunction with Carney complex, is the psammomatous melanotic schwannoma. These are not cutaneous tumors but are most likely to be found along the paraspinal sympathetic chain.

Treatment: Therapy for skin myxomas includes observation or excision of individual lesions. Lentigines and blue nevi can be removed for cosmetic purposes. Atrial myxomas are the leading cause of morbidity and mortality, and they require removal by cardiothoracic surgery. Patients need to be monitored by cardiology and endocrinology specialists for their entire lifetime. Routine screening evaluations of the heart, pituitary, adrenal gland, and testicles must be performed.

Plate 9-5

Genodermatoses and Syndromes

CUSHING'S SYNDROME AND CUSHING'S DISEASE

Cushing's syndrome is caused by excessive secretion of endogenous glucocorticoids or, more frequently, by intake of excessive exogenous glucocorticoids. The latter type is typically iatrogenic in nature. The excessive glucocorticoid levels lead to the many cutaneous and systemic signs and symptoms of Cushing's syndrome and Cushing's disease. Endogenous glucocorticoids are made and secreted by the adrenal glands, and benign adrenal adenomas are the most frequently implicated adrenal tumors causing Cushing's syndrome. Cushing's disease is caused by excessive secretion from the anterior pituitary of adrenocorticotropic hormone (ACTH, corticotropin) as the result of a basophilic or chromophobe adenoma. The increased amount of ACTH causes the adrenal glands to hypertrophy and boost their production of cortisol, eventually leading to a state of hypercortisolism. Excessive release of corticotropin-releasing hormone (CRH) from the paraventricular nucleus of the hypothalamus can also cause the syndrome. Any tumor that has the ability to produce ACTH also has the potential to cause Cushing's syndrome. The most frequently reported such tumor is the small cell tumor of the lung, which is able to produce many neuroendocrine hormones including ACTH in large amounts.

Clinical Findings: Cushing's disease is found more frequently in females than in males, and there is no race predilection. The most common age at onset of the disease is in the third to fourth decades of life. Cushing's syndrome, especially the exogenous form, can be seen at any age, and ACTH-secreting tumors typically manifest in the sixth to eighth decades of life, particularly if caused by small cell lung cancer.

Cutaneous findings in Cushing's syndrome and Cushing's disease are almost identical. The excessive cortisol levels affect the skin, including the underlying subcutaneous adipose tissue. Patients have an insidious onset of fat redistribution. This leads to thinning of the arms and legs and deposition of adipose tissue in the abdomen and posterior cervical fat pad ("buffalo hump"). The fat redistribution also causes the face to have a full appearance ("moon facies"). Supraclavicular fat pads are frequently appreciated on physical examination. Large, thick, purple-red striae are seen along the areas of fat redistribution on the abdomen and buttocks, as well as on the breasts in female patients. Striae are caused by an increase in fat and an increase in the catabolism of dermal elastic tissue. The catabolic effect of cortisol causes muscle wasting and the appearance of further thinning of the limbs. This also leads to weakness and easy fatigability. Cortisol directly causes thinning of the skin to the point that it appears translucent and almost paper-like. This thinning of the skin may impart a redness to the face (facial plethora) and other regions as the underlying vasculature becomes more noticeable. The skin is easily torn or bruised and shows poor wound healing ability.

Cortisol decreases elastic tissue within the cutaneous vasculature, leading to easy and exaggerated bruisability and prominent ecchymoses. The excessive cortisol may also lead to increases in acne papules, pustules, and nodules; in some cases, this is quite severe, with cysts, nodules, and scarring. A rare cutaneous finding is excessive facial lanugo hair. In Cushing's disease, the excessive production of ACTH is associated with an increase in the production of melanocyte-stimulating hormone

(MSH) and subsequent hyperpigmentation. This is not seen in untreated Cushing's syndrome.

Cushing's syndrome and Cushing's disease also manifest systemically with myriad symptoms. Excessive cortisol may lead to mood changes including depression, mania, and psychosis. Hypertension is common, and elevated blood sugar levels may occur and can be difficult to control. The skeletal system is always affected, and osteoporosis occurs early in the course of the disease; left untreated, this can lead to vertebral compression fractures and other bony fractures (e.g., femoral neck).

Treatment: Cushing's syndrome of exogenous origin requires removal of the responsible agent. In most cases, this is difficult, because these patients often

require the life-saving exogenous corticosteroids (e.g., after transplantation). In such cases, the practitioner should decrease the dose to the minimum possible or try to change to a different immunosuppressant. Cushing's syndrome caused by adrenal adenoma or bilateral adrenal hyperplasia requires surgical removal. After removal of both adrenal glands, the patient will need replacement therapy. If the syndrome is caused by abnormal secretion of ACTH from a malignant tumor such as a small cell carcinoma of the lung, the patient is best served by treating the underlying tumor. Cushing's disease is best treated by neurosurgical removal of the tumor, with consideration of postoperative radiotherapy.

CLINICAL FINDINGS OF CUSHING'S SYNDROME

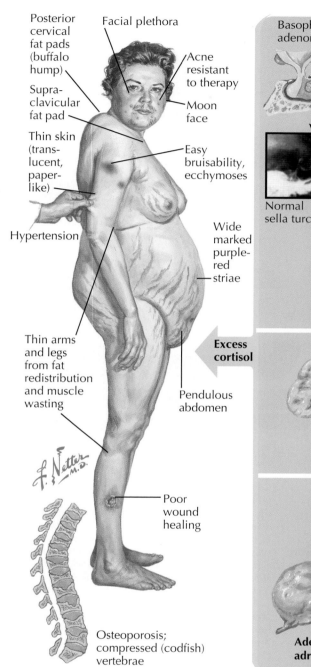

Posterior cervical fat pads (buffalo hump)

Facial plethora

Acne resistant to therapy

Supraclavicular fat pad

Moon face

Thin skin (translucent, paper-like)

Easy bruisability, ecchymoses

Hypertension

Wide marked purple-red striae

Thin arms and legs from fat redistribution and muscle wasting

Excess cortisol

Pendulous abdomen

Poor wound healing

Osteoporosis; compressed (codfish) vertebrae

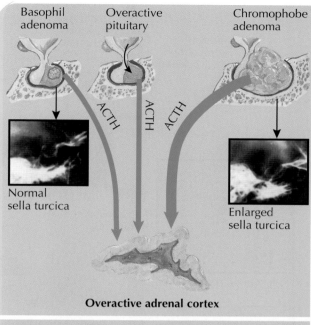

Basophil adenoma

Overactive pituitary

Chromophobe adenoma

ACTH

Normal sella turcica

Enlarged sella turcica

Overactive adrenal cortex

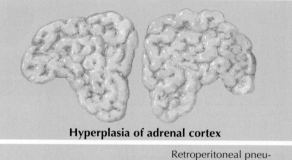

Hyperplasia of adrenal cortex

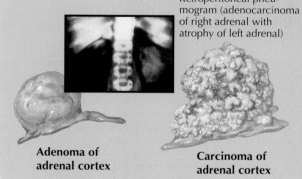

Adenoma of adrenal cortex

Retroperitoneal pneumogram (adenocarcinoma of right adrenal with atrophy of left adrenal)

Carcinoma of adrenal cortex

Plate 9-6   Integumentary System

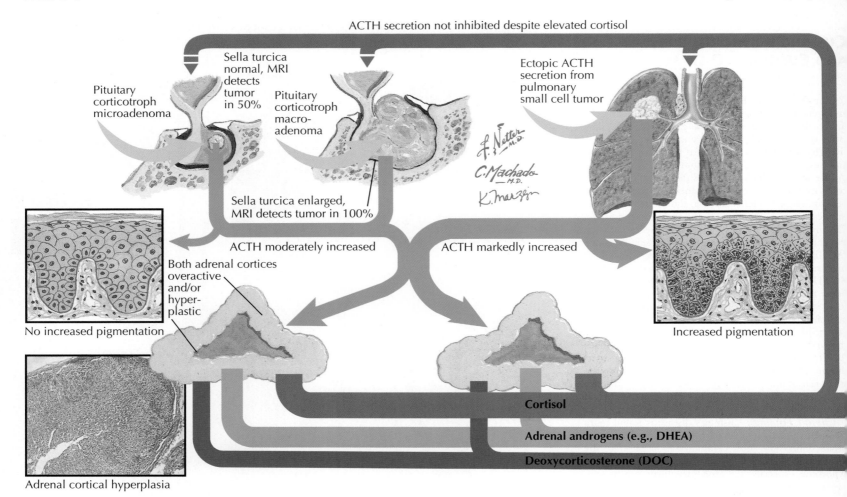

ACTH secretion not inhibited despite elevated cortisol

Pituitary corticotroph microadenoma

Sella turcica normal, MRI detects tumor in 50%

Pituitary corticotroph macro-adenoma

Ectopic ACTH secretion from pulmonary small cell tumor

Sella turcica enlarged, MRI detects tumor in 100%

ACTH moderately increased

ACTH markedly increased

Both adrenal cortices overactive and/or hyper-plastic

No increased pigmentation

Increased pigmentation

Adrenal cortical hyperplasia

Cortisol

Adrenal androgens (e.g., DHEA)

Deoxycorticosterone (DOC)

CUSHING'S SYNDROME: PATHOPHYSIOLOGY

Cushing's syndrome is directly caused by excessive amounts of glucocorticoids and their effects on numerous organ systems. Cortisol is strikingly elevated in all cases of Cushing's syndrome. In some cases, levels of 17-ketosteroids and aldosterone are slightly elevated, and this plays a role in the clinical manifestations of the disease. There are numerous disease states that can cause hypercortisolemia, including excessive secretion of adrenocorticotropic hormone (ACTH, corticotropin), adenoma and hyperplasia of the adrenal gland, carcinoma of the adrenal gland, primary pigmented nodular adrenocortical disease (PPNAD), and exogenous cortisol use. In all cases, it is the marked elevation of cortisol that ultimately is the cause of the disease.

Normally, ACTH is produced and regulated by the hypothalamic-pituitary-adrenal (HPA) axis. Corticotropin-releasing hormone (CRH) is the main hypothalamic regulator of pituitary ACTH production. CRH acts on the corticotroph cells of the anterior pituitary, causing them to secrete pro-opiomelanocortin (POMC), which is posttranslationally modified into ACTH. ACTH then acts on the adrenal glands to increase production of cortisol. Normally, cortisol and ACTH both act in a negative feedback loop to inhibit excessive secretion of CRH.

Excessive ACTH may be produced in several ways. Most often, it is produced from a basophilic adenoma of the anterior stalk of the pituitary gland. The term

Cushing's disease should be used in cases of anterior pituitary ACTH-secreting tumors. All other forms of the condition should be referred to as *Cushing's syndrome*. In basophilic adenomas of the pituitary, the size of the sella turcica can range from normal to dramatically enlarged. ACTH production is elevated and is not suppressed by the increase in the cortisol level. Bilateral adrenal hyperplasia is seen, because the ACTH acts to increase the production of cortisol by the adrenal glands.

ACTH is produced in the pituitary by posttranslational modification of the protein POMC. POMC is modified by various enzymes to produce ACTH, β-lipotropin, and melanocyte-stimulating hormone (MSH). ACTH is further broken down to produce MSH. β-lipotropin is broken down to produce β-endorphin. Cushing's disease is associated with a generalized skin hyperpigmentation caused by increased melanin production that is directly related to the effects of MSH on the cutaneous melanocytes. Hyperpigmentation of the skin is seen only in patients with an abnormally elevated ACTH secretion.

Excessive ACTH may also be produced from ectopic ACTH-producing tumors, most frequently bronchogenic small cell tumor. Most patients present with signs and symptoms of Cushing's syndrome before the underlying tumor is diagnosed. This form of Cushing's syndrome can be very difficult to differentiate from Cushing's disease in the early stages of each, and the clinician needs to be aware of the various pathophysiological mechanisms involved in excessive ACTH production. When faced with a patient with excessive ACTH production, the clinician must perform a thorough evaluation, including history, physical

examination, and laboratory and radiological testing, to determine the etiology.

Cortisol excess may also be seen in primary adrenal disease caused by benign bilateral adrenal hyperplasia, a cortisol-secreting adenoma, or, less likely, a carcinoma. In these cases, plasma ACTH levels are reduced to near zero, due to the effect of the negative feedback loop on the HPA axis. The uninvolved adrenal gland is typically atrophic. Exogenous steroid use can also lead to Cushing's syndrome. In those cases, the ACTH level is decreased and the adrenal glands are atrophic.

Regardless of the etiology of Cushing's disease or Cushing's syndrome, the clinical manifestations are caused almost entirely by excessive cortisol production in the zona fasciculata of the adrenal gland. Cortisol is a catabolic steroid and causes profound muscle weakness if allowed to persist. Adipose tissue redistribution is prominent. Central obesity is easily observed, with a thinning of the extremities. Supraclavicular and posterior cervical ("buffalo hump") fat pads are frequently encountered. Cortisol has negative effects on the connective tissue of the skin, leading to a decrease in collagen. This, in turn, leads to an increase in capillary fragility, easy bruising, ecchymoses, and a thin or translucent appearance to the skin. Prominent purple to red striae are seen as a result of the loss of normal connective tissue function within the skin. The striae are most prominent in areas of obesity and are made more noticeable by the central fat redistribution. Facial plethora is frequently seen and is likely caused by thinning of the skin and an underlying polycythemia. Excessive cortisol leads to increased blood glucose levels; this in turn can lead to poor wound healing and an increase in

Plate 9-6, *continued*

Genodermatoses and Syndromes

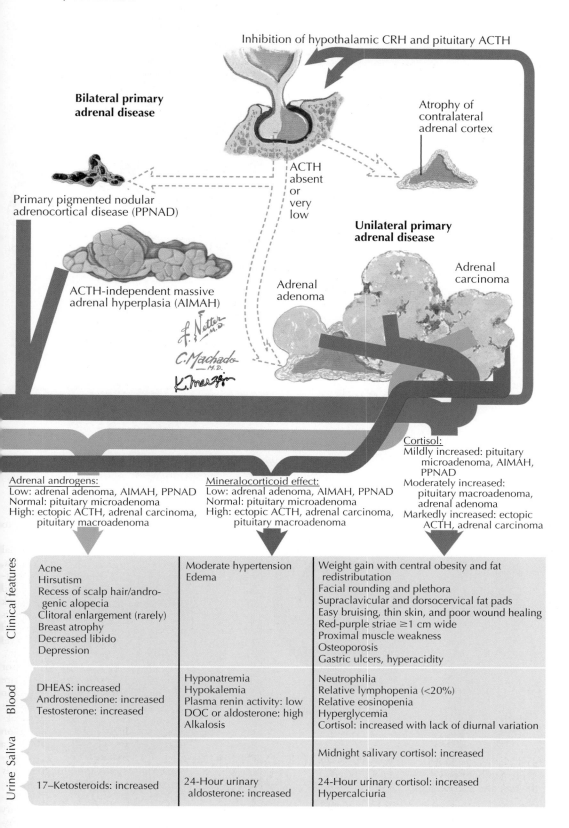

Inhibition of hypothalamic CRH and pituitary ACTH

Bilateral primary adrenal disease

Atrophy of contralateral adrenal cortex

ACTH absent or very low

Primary pigmented nodular adrenocortical disease (PPNAD)

Unilateral primary adrenal disease

ACTH-independent massive adrenal hyperplasia (AIMAH)

Adrenal adenoma

Adrenal carcinoma

Cortisol:
Mildly increased: pituitary microadenoma, AIMAH, PPNAD
Moderately increased: pituitary macroadenoma, adrenal adenoma
Markedly increased: ectopic ACTH, adrenal carcinoma

Adrenal androgens:
Low: adrenal adenoma, AIMAH, PPNAD
Normal: pituitary microadenoma
High: ectopic ACTH, adrenal carcinoma, pituitary macroadenoma

Mineralocorticoid effect:
Low: adrenal adenoma, AIMAH, PPNAD
Normal: pituitary microadenoma
High: ectopic ACTH, adrenal carcinoma, pituitary macroadenoma

	Clinical features		
Clinical features	Acne Hirsutism Recess of scalp hair/androgenic alopecia Clitoral enlargement (rarely) Breast atrophy Decreased libido Depression	Moderate hypertension Edema	Weight gain with central obesity and fat redistributation Facial rounding and plethora Supraclavicular and dorsocervical fat pads Easy bruising, thin skin, and poor wound healing Red-purple striae ≥1 cm wide Proximal muscle weakness Osteoporosis Gastric ulcers, hyperacidity
Blood	DHEAS: increased Androstenedione: increased Testosterone: increased	Hyponatremia Hypokalemia Plasma renin activity: low DOC or aldosterone: high Alkalosis	Neutrophilia Relative lymphopenia (<20%) Relative eosinopenia Hyperglycemia Cortisol: increased with lack of diurnal variation
Saliva			Midnight salivary cortisol: increased
Urine	17–Ketosteroids: increased	24-Hour urinary aldosterone: increased	24-Hour urinary cortisol: increased Hypercalciuria

CUSHING'S SYNDROME: PATHOPHYSIOLOGY (Continued)

infections. Hyperglycemia can lead to polyuria and polydipsia.

Most patients with elevated cortisol levels exhibit some degree of central nervous system involvement.

Fatigue, lethargy, emotional disturbance, depression, and occasionally psychosis are diagnosed in these patients. Excess cortisol can cause an increase in gastric acidity, leading to severe peptic ulcer disease. Patients with Cushing's syndrome are more likely to have severe recalcitrant peptic ulcer disease than the average peptic ulcer patient.

In some patients, levels of 17-ketosteroids and aldosterone are moderately elevated. This leads to acne,

which is often nodulocystic and recalcitrant to therapy. Hirsutism and premature or accelerated androgenetic alopecia may be seen. In rare cases, clitoral enlargement and breast atrophy are seen. A decrease in libido is extremely common. Excessive aldosterone may lead to hypertension, hyponatremia, and a metabolic hypokalemic alkalosis. The elevation of 17-ketosteroids and aldosterone is most frequently associated with adrenal carcinoma.

Plate 9-7   Integumentary System

DOWN SYNDROME

Down syndrome is a genetic disorder caused by trisomy of chromosome 21. Trisomy 21 occurs in approximately 1 of every 1000 births. Chromosome 21 is an acrocentric chromosome, and trisomy 21 is the most common form of chromosomal trisomy. Trisomy 21 most often occurs as the result of nondisjunction of meiosis, which leads to an extra copy of chromosome 21. Some patients with Down syndrome have a Robertsonian translocation to chromosome 14 or chromosome 22, which are two other acrocentric chromosomes. In these cases, the number of total chromosomes is normal at 46, but the extra chromosome 21 material is translocated to another chromosome. This, in effect, causes an extra chromosome 21. All or part of chromosome 21 may be translocated, leading to variations in phenotype. Mosaicism is a rare cause of trisomy 21 in partial cell lines, and the clinical phenotype depends on how early the genetic defect occurred during embryogenesis.

Clinical Findings: There is no race predilection in Down syndrome and only a slightly increased incidence in males. Down syndrome has been shown to increase in incidence with increasing maternal age. The estimated incidence increases to 1 in every 50 births for mothers who are 45 years of age. The clinical manifestations of Down syndrome are wide reaching and affect every organ system. Patients with Down syndrome have a decreased life span, although modern medicine continues to improve these patients' quality and quantity of life. Congenital heart disease is one of the most frequent problems and leads to a plethora of complications and increased morbidity and mortality. Endocardial cushion defects are the most frequently seen heart abnormality in Down syndrome. Central nervous system involvement leads to mental and physical delay. The incidence of childhood leukemia is increased in these patients, the most frequent type being acute megakaryoblastic leukemia.

The cutaneous findings in Down syndrome are vast. All patients with Down syndrome have cutaneous disease, but because of the variation in phenotype, not all have the same findings. Patients with Down syndrome are more likely to develop atopic dermatitis, which may be mild or severe. Generalized xerosis is universally found in Down syndrome. Patients may have an increase from the normal number of nuchal skin folds in infancy as well as a characteristic facies. Epicanthic folds and a flat-appearing face with small ears and a flattened nose are common. Ophthalmological findings include Brushfield spots and strabismus.

Syringomas are frequently seen in Down syndrome and affect the eyelids and upper cheeks. Elastosis perforans serpiginosa (EPS) is a rare disease caused by the transepidermal elimination of fragmented elastic tissue. EPS is seen with a higher incidence in Down syndrome. The appearance is often that of a thin patch with a peripheral elevated rim and a polycyclic border or serpentine course. Acanthosis nigricans was shown to be present in approximately 50% of individuals with Down syndrome. It can be located in any flexural area, and the etiology is unknown. The external ear canal has been shown to be narrowed in a most patients with Down syndrome; this predisposes them to an increased number of external and middle ear infections. Macroglossia with a scrotal tongue is frequently encountered.

A single transverse palmar crease (simian crease) is unique to patients with Down syndrome. Shortened metacarpal bones lead to smaller-than-normal hands, and an extra-wide gap between the first and second toes

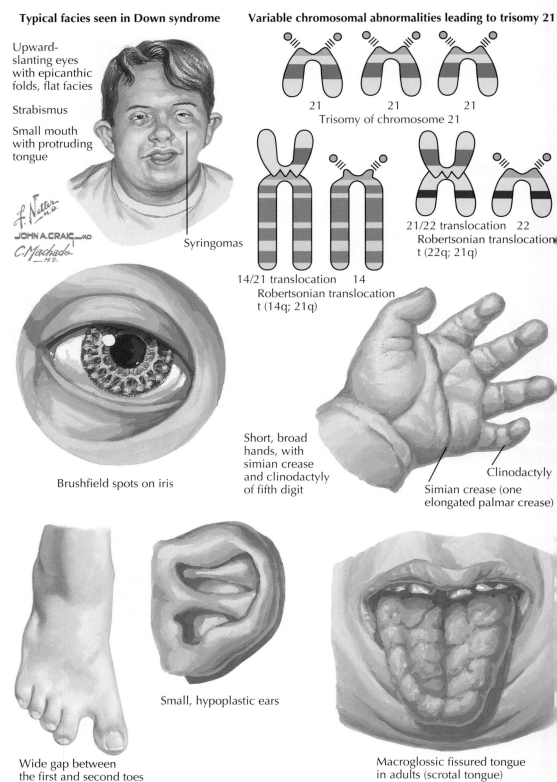

Typical facies seen in Down syndrome

Upward-slanting eyes with epicanthic folds, flat facies

Strabismus

Small mouth with protruding tongue

Syringomas

Variable chromosomal abnormalities leading to trisomy 21

21 21 21

Trisomy of chromosome 21

14/21 translocation   14
Robertsonian translocation
t (14q; 21q)

21/22 translocation   22
Robertsonian translocation
t (22q; 21q)

Brushfield spots on iris

Short, broad hands, with simian crease and clinodactyly of fifth digit

Clinodactyly

Simian crease (one elongated palmar crease)

Small, hypoplastic ears

Wide gap between the first and second toes

Macroglossic fissured tongue in adults (scrotal tongue)

is usually prominent. Alopecia areata is found with increased incidence in Down syndrome.

Treatment: Patients with Down syndrome require a multidisciplinary approach. Cardiac defects tend to cause the most morbidity and mortality, and surgical intervention to correct underlying heart defects is often required. Patients need to be monitored regularly by a pediatrician and then an internist or family physician who is well aware of the complications and care of patients with Down syndrome. The dermatological manifestations are treated as in any other individual, and no special considerations are needed. Xerosis should be managed with excellent daily skin care. It is important for clinicians to recognize the common cutaneous findings in Down syndrome so that they can educate parents and patients alike.

Plate 9-8

Genodermatoses and Syndromes

EHLERS-DANLOS SYNDROME

Ehlers-Danlos syndrome is a heterogeneous disease of defective connective tissue production. There are many subtypes, most caused by defects in collagen formation or in the posttranslational modification of collagen. This grouping of diseases has been confusing because of the variable nature of the subtypes and the lack of a universally adopted classification system. Under the most recent system, there are 7 distinct subtypes; under the historical classification, there were 11 types. The new classification system has not been universally adopted, which contributes to the confusion. As the genetic defects behind each subtype are determined, researchers and clinicians will gain a better understanding of the syndrome.

Clinical Findings: Ehlers-Danlos syndrome is a grouping of connective tissue diseases. Each subtype is distinct and has a unique underlying genetic defect. Taken as a whole, the syndrome is estimated to occur in approximately 1 of every 400,000 persons. Because of the variation in phenotypic expression, the syndrome is likely underreported. Most cases are termed *classic Ehlers-Danlos syndrome* (formerly designated types I and II). The onset of signs and symptoms occurs in early childhood and can even be manifested at birth. Each subtype has a different mode of inheritance. Most are inherited in an autosomal dominant manner, with autosomal recessive inheritance the next most prolific mode of transmission. X-linked inheritance has been described. Ehlers-Danlos syndrome affects males and females equally.

Cutaneous findings are seen in most subtypes of the syndrome. The skin when stretched is hyperextensible, but it recoils to its resting position promptly and entirely after being released. Easy bruisability and excessive scarring are noticed soon after the child begins to crawl. The scarring has a characteristic "fish mouth" appearance, in that the normally thin linear scars stretch abnormally and leave a profoundly wider scar than would have been predicted. The scar tissue is extremely thinned and can appear translucent. The underlying vasculature can be seen prominently through the atrophic skin, further worsening the appearance of the scar tissue. Molluscoid pseudotumors and calcified subcutaneous nodules (spheroids) occur along regions of repetitive trauma. Epicanthic folds and elastosis perforans serpiginosa are two cutaneous findings that can be seen in cases of Ehlers-Danlos syndrome. Rare occurrences of blue sclerae have been reported.

The major morbidity and mortality in Ehlers-Danlos syndrome is seen in the vascular subtype (type IV). Vascular-type Ehlers-Danlos is subdivided into three similar variants and is caused by a defect in the *COL3A1* gene. The skin in this subtype is not hyperextensible but is rather translucent. Joint laxity is minimally present or not at all. Individuals with this subtype are more prone than others with Ehlers-Danlos syndrome to arterial aneurysms and rupture leading to death. Both large and medium-sized vessels are involved. The wall of the colon is easily ruptured, and abdominal pain in these patients can be an impending sign of colonic rupture.

Pathogenesis: Most forms of Ehlers-Danlos syndrome are caused directly by a genetic defect in collagen synthesis or indirectly by a defect in posttranslational modification of collagen. These defects lead to an abnormal amount as well as abnormal functioning of the underlying collagen and the properties it imparts to the connective tissue. The vascular subtype is caused by a defect in the *COL3A1* gene that leads to minimal or

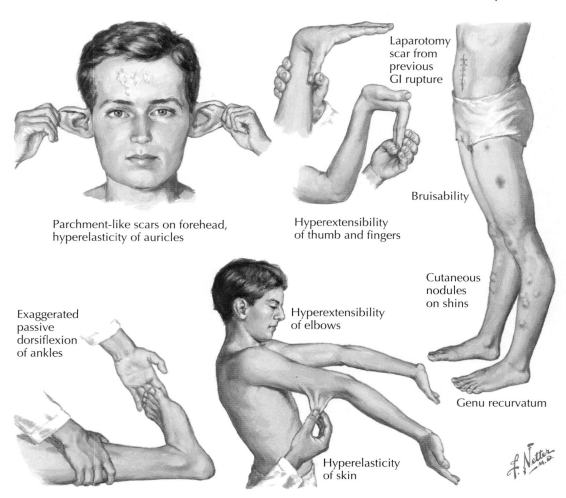

Parchment-like scars on forehead, hyperelasticity of auricles

Laparotomy scar from previous GI rupture

Hyperextensibility of thumb and fingers

Bruisability

Exaggerated passive dorsiflexion of ankles

Hyperextensibility of elbows

Cutaneous nodules on shins

Hyperelasticity of skin

Genu recurvatum

Type	Inheritance	Gene defect (protein)
Classic	AD, AR	*COL5A1, COL5A2* (collagen V)
Hypermobility	AD	Unknown, *TNXB* (tenascin XB) in a small subset
Vascular	AD, AR	*COL3A1* (collagen III)
Kyphoscoliosis	AR	*PLOD1* (lysyl hydroxylase)
Arthrochalasis	AD	*COL1A1, COL1A2* (collagen I)
Dermatosparaxis	AR	*ADAMTS2* (procollagen In-propeptidase)
Other	AR, AD, X	*FN1* (fibronectin), and some unknown

AD, autosomal dominant; AR, autosomal recessive; X, X-linked

no functional type III collagen. Because type III collagen is a critical component of the walls of the vasculature and colon, these structures are weakened and are prone to distention and breakage. Classic Ehlers-Danlos syndrome is caused by defects in the *COL5A1* and *COL5A2* genes that lead to defective type V collagen. Defects in the enzymes lysyl hydroxylase and procollagen peptidase, which are responsible for posttranslational modifications of collagen, are present, respectively, in the kyphoscoliosis and dermatosparaxis subtypes of Ehlers-Danlos syndrome.

Treatment: Patients with Ehlers-Danlos syndrome need to be under the supervision of a pediatrician who understands the disease. Referral to tertiary care centers is an appropriate course of action. Patients need to avoid unnecessary trauma. They should refrain from contact sports. The orthopedic complications can be treated by an experienced orthopedic surgeon. Patients with vascular-type Ehlers-Danlos syndrome need to be monitored routinely by a cardiologist and a cardiothoracic surgeon. This subtype is the most difficult to manage because of its unpredictable nature.

Plate 9-9

Integumentary System

MARFAN SYNDROME

Marfan syndrome is an autosomal dominantly inherited disorder of connective tissue that is caused by a genetic defect in the *FBN1* gene located on chromosome 15. The disorder leads to a defect in the fibrillin-1 protein, which is a component of the extracellular matrix of connective tissue. The defect leads to many clinical findings in the cardiovascular, ocular, skeletal, integumentary, and respiratory systems. The diagnosis is made based on multiple criteria that include major and minor features of the syndrome. Cardiovascular disease is a major cause of morbidity and mortality in this syndrome.

Clinical Findings: Marfan syndrome has an estimated incidence of approximately 1 per 7500 people. It affects all populations and has no gender differential. Many of the manifestations of the syndrome are present at the time of birth. As the child grows, the findings become more evident and the severity may worsen. The diagnosis of Marfan syndrome does not imply any specific prognosis, because the syndrome has a range of clinical manifestations. On one end of the spectrum is the patient with life-threatening disease, and at the other end is the patient who has only the musculoskeletal clinical features of the syndrome.

Many skeletal anomalies can be seen, including arachnodactyly, pectus excavatum, scoliosis, pes planus, high palate, and an increased lower body to upper body ratio. The most striking features are tall stature, thin body habitus, long arms, and disproportionate lower-to-upper body ratio.

Cutaneous findings of Marfan syndrome may be subtle. The presence of striae distensae is almost universal. Adipose tissue is decreased, and patients often appear extremely thin. Elastosis perforans serpiginosa is seen with a high incidence in Marfan syndrome and is caused by the extrusion of abnormal elastic tissue through the epidermis. Ocular involvement often leads to an upward displacement of the lens (ectopia lentis). Myopia is often seen, as well as a decreased ability to constrict the pupil.

The respiratory and cardiovascular systems are commonly affected. Pulmonary blebs can be seen in an apical location. The blebs may spontaneously rupture, causing a pneumothorax. Severity of involvement of the cardiovascular system is the best prognostic indicator in Marfan syndrome. Prolapse of the mitral valve, aortic root dilation, and early-onset calcification of the mitral valve anulus are a few of the cardiovascular findings. The leading cause of mortality is rupture of an aortic aneurysm or aortic dissection.

Pathogenesis: Fibrillin-1 is a glycoprotein found in a wide range of connective tissues. Fibrillin-1 is required for proper elasticity and strength properties of the extracellular matrix. Many hundreds of mutations have been reported in the gene that encodes fibrillin-1. There is a wide phenotypic variability in Marfan syndrome, due in some part to the different mutations of the gene but also to other, as yet undescribed factors. This leads to a large variation in phenotype among individuals with the same genotypic mutation.

Defects in the fibrillin-1 protein lead to a decreased ability to bind to calcium. This ultimately manifests as abnormalities of the microfibrils throughout the connective tissue. These abnormal microfibrils are more susceptible to degradation by matrix metalloproteinases, and when they occur within the connective tissue lining of the vascular walls, the lining's elastic and strength properties are compromised. This may lead to dilation, increased stiffness, aneurysm, and eventual

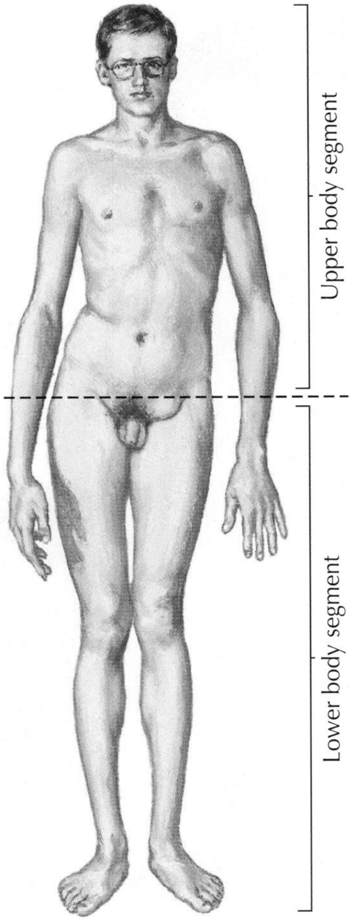

Tall, thin person with skeletal disproportion. Upper body segment (top of head to pubis) shorter than lower body segment (pubis to soles of feet). Fingertips reach almost to knees (arm span-to-height ratio greater than 1.05). Long, thin fingers (arachnodactyly). Scoliosis, chest deformity, inguinal hernia, flatfoot

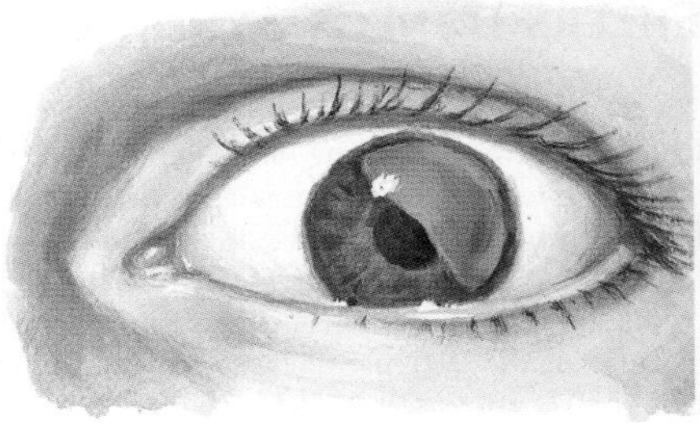

Upper body segment

Lower body segment

Ectopia lentis (upward and temporal displacement of eye lens). Retinal detachment, myopia, and other ocular complications may occur.

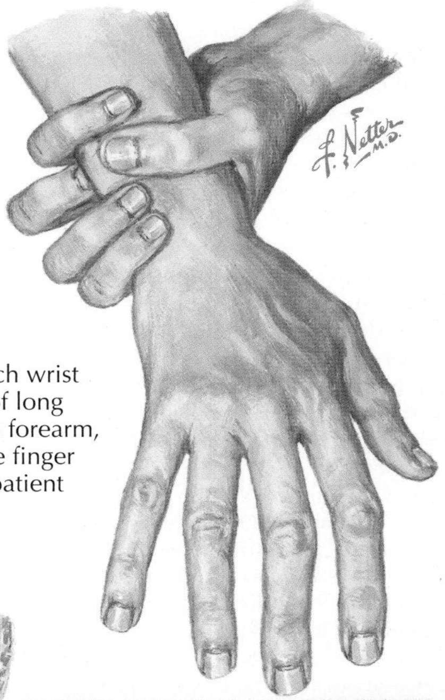

Walker-Murdoch wrist sign. Because of long fingers and thin forearm, thumb and little finger overlap when patient grasps wrist.

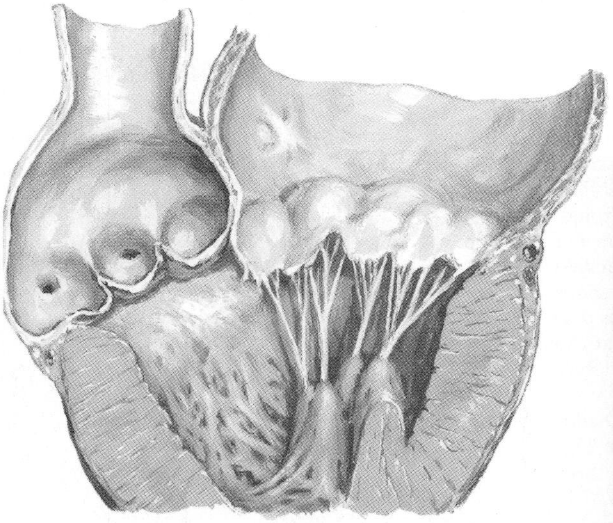

Dilatation of aortic ring and aneurysm of ascending aorta due to cystic medial necrosis cause aortic insufficiency. Mitral valve prolapse causes regurgitation. Heart failure is common.

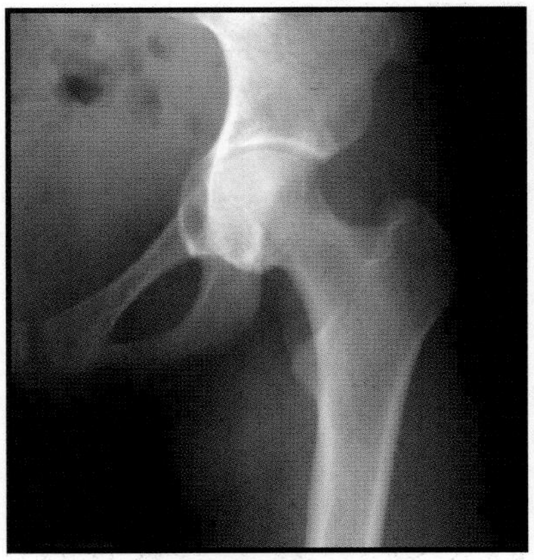

Radiograph shows acetabular protrusion (unilateral or bilateral).

dissection of arterial walls, with the aorta being the most commonly affected vessel.

Treatment: All patients with Marfan syndrome should be monitored directly by a cardiologist and a cardiothoracic surgeon as needed. Routine echocardiograms and evaluations for aortic aneurysms are required. β-Blockade has been shown to be helpful to decrease mean arterial pressure. This reduces the pressure on the weakened vessel walls and subsequently decreases the likelihood of arterial dilation, dissection, and aneurysms.

Calcium channel blockers and angiotensin-converting enzyme (ACE) inhibitors are second-line agents. Patients with Marfan syndrome who are closely followed and treated promptly may live a normal life span. They must be educated to avoid strenuous physical activity and contact sports. Surgery to repair aortic dilation and aneurysm is required once the caliber of the aorta reaches 5.0 cm or if the rate of enlargement is greater than 0.5 cm/year. Ocular disease should be evaluated and treated promptly by an ophthalmologist.

Plate 9-10

Genodermatoses and Syndromes

NEUROFIBROMATOSIS

There are eight distinct clinical forms of neurofibromatosis. The two most studied and clinically important forms are type I and type II. Neurofibromatosis type I (von Recklinghausen disease) and neurofibromatosis type II are autosomal dominant disorders involving the skin, the central nervous system, and various other organ systems. Type II has many overlapping features that are also seen in patients with type I disease. The genetic bases for type I and type II neurofibromatosis have been determined, and the specific gene for each type has been isolated. The skin findings can be instrumental in the diagnosis of neurofibromatosis type I.

Clinical Findings: Type I neurofibromatosis is usually diagnosed in early childhood. It has an estimated incidence of 1 per 3000 births and occurs worldwide. There is no gender or race predilection, and type I accounts for 85% to 90% of all cases of neurofibromatosis. There is wide clinical variability in neurofibromatosis. Diagnostic criteria have been established by the U.S. National Institutes of Health. Two or more of the following seven criteria are needed for diagnosis: (1) six or more café-au-lait macules (≥5 mm in size in prepuberty patients; >1.5 cm in postpuberty patients); (2) one plexiform neurofibroma or two or more neurofibromas; (3) axillary or inguinal freckling; (4) optic glioma; (5) two or more Lisch nodules of the iris; (6) sphenoid dysplasia or other distinctive bone abnormality, such as pseudarthrosis of a long bone; or (7) a first-degree relative with neurofibromatosis.

The cutaneous findings, and in particular the café-au-lait macules, are often the presenting sign of the disease. Solitary café-au-lait macules are seen in a large percentage of the normal population, and the diagnostic criteria for neurofibromatosis require the presence of at least six such lesions. Spinal dysraphism may be present if the skin overlying the spine is involved with a café-au-lait macule. The onset of axillary and inguinal freckling is often during puberty. Axillary freckling is also known as Crowe's sign. Cutaneous neurofibromas are the most common benign tumor found in patients with neurofibromatosis. The tumors tend to be plentiful and to increase in number and size with time. They are soft and often exhibit the "buttonhole" sign when compressed. These tumors may have an overlying pink to light violet coloration. Plexiform neurofibromas are large dermal and subcutaneous tumors specific to type I neurofibromatosis. They can cause compression of underlying structures and wrap themselves around nerves. Compared with the typical neurofibroma, they are firm and larger and have an ill-defined border. Both forms of neurofibromas can produce varying amounts of pruritus. Patients with plexiform neurofibromas have hypertrichosis with and without hyperpigmentation. The presence of multiple neurofibromas can cause psychological disease.

Lisch nodules are hamartomas of the iris. They are observed under slit-lamp examination and can be seen by approximately 6 years of age. Optic gliomas are seen in about 1 of every 8 patients with neurofibromatosis. Optic gliomas may be asymptomatic, or they may cause compression of the pituitary gland, resulting in precocious puberty. Gliomas can also cause visual

CUTANEOUS MANIFESTATIONS OF NEUROFIBROMATOSIS

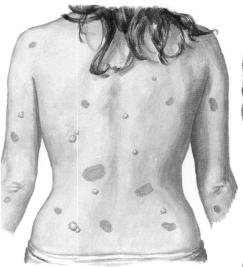

Multiple café-au-lait spots and nodules (fibroma molluscum) are the most common manifestations.

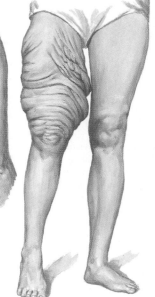

Localized elephantiasis of thigh with redundant skin folds overlying a plexiform neurofibroma.

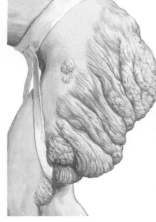

Verrucous hyperplasia. Maceration of velvety-soft skin may cause weeping and infection in crevices overlying a plexiform neurofibroma.

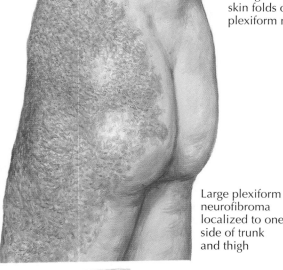

Large plexiform neurofibroma localized to one side of trunk and thigh

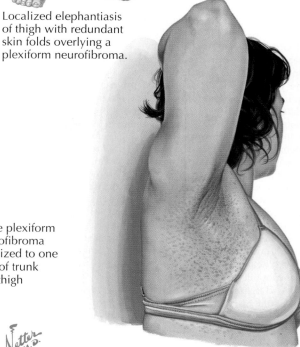

Dense axillary and inguinal freckling is rarely found in the absence of NF1.

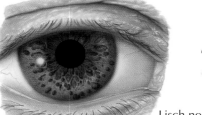

Lisch nodules are hamartomas of the iris. They are raised and frequently pigmented.

disturbance and proptosis. The best method to detect an optic glioma is with brain magnetic resonance imaging (MRI). Other ophthalmological findings that may be present include hypertelorism and congenital glaucoma.

Type II neurofibromatosis has a completely different phenotype than type I disease, with some overlap. Onset of disease is often not until the second or third decade of life. The main aspect of type II neurofibromatosis is the formation of bilateral acoustic neuromas (vestibular schwannomas). These tumors can lead to headaches, vertigo, and various degrees of hearing loss. Schwannomas may occur in any cranial nerve. The criteria used to establish the diagnosis are (1) the presence of bilateral schwannomas; (2) the combination of a first-degree relative with type II neurofibromatosis and a unilateral vestibular schwannoma; or (3) a first-degree relative with type II neurofibromatosis

Plate 9-11   Integumentary System

CUTANEOUS AND SKELETAL MANIFESTATIONS OF NEUROFIBROMATOSIS

NEUROFIBROMATOSIS
(Continued)

and any two of the following tumors: neurofibroma, glioma, schwannoma, meningioma, or juvenile posterior subcapsular lenticular opacity.

Cutaneous findings in type II neurofibromatosis include neurofibromas and café-au-lait macules. Although both findings are less numerous than in type I neurofibromatosis, most patients have only one or two café-au-lait macules. Cutaneous schwannomas are common in type II disease but are not seen in type I disease. A unique form of cataracts can be seen in neurofibromatosis type II; these are termed *juvenile posterior subcapsular lenticular cataracts.*

Histology: Skin biopsies of café-au-lait macules show epidermal hyperpigmentation. There is no increase in the number of melanocytes, and no nevus cells are present. Macromelanosomes can be seen. Neurofibromas can be located within the dermis or subcutaneous tissue. Histological evaluation shows a well-circumscribed tumor composed of uniform-appearing spindle cells of nerve origin. Special immune histochemical stains can be performed to confirm the nerve derivation of the tumors. Many mast cells are seen intermingled within the spindle cell tumor.

Pathogenesis: Type I neurofibromatosis is caused by a mutation in the *NF1* gene. This gene is located on the long arm of chromosome 17 and encodes the protein neurofibromin. Defects in *NF1* are responsible for most cases of neurofibromatosis, making type I neurofibromatosis the most common type of neurofibromatosis. Because of the large size of the *NF1* gene, many spontaneous mutations occur and result in cases of neurofibromatosis. The neurofibromin protein has been determined to be a tumor suppressor protein. It regulates the *ras* family of protooncogene. When neurofibromin is defective, the *ras* protooncogene loses its negative regulatory protein and is able to signal continuously.

Type II neurofibromatosis is caused by a genetic defect in the *SCH (NF2)* gene on the long arm of chromosome 22. The *NF2* gene is approximately one third the size of *NF1*. It encodes the schwannomin (merlin) protein, a tumor suppressor protein that helps act as a go-between in the interactions between the cell cytoskeleton/membrane and the extracellular matrix. Loss of function of the protein results in abnormal cell signaling and unabated cell growth in various tissues.

Treatment: Once the diagnosis has been established, patients need lifelong monitoring for the development of various complications related to their disease. Family members should be screened for the disease, and genetic counseling should be offered to affected patients. Adolescents and young adults may benefit from annual physical examinations, and routine ophthalmological examinations should be recommended. Screening in childhood for the development of scoliosis should be recommended. Patients should be screened for hypertension at each visit because of the increased incidence of pheochromocytoma. Patients with neurofibromatosis are at increased risk for development of malignant transformation of their neurofibromas into neurofibrosarcomas. These rare sarcomas can be located anywhere, and any major change, pain, or

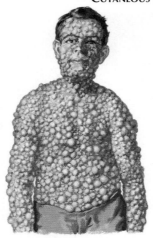

Neurofibromatosis. One of von Recklinghausen's original patients, who had extensive subcutaneous nodules but no neurological symptoms. Such wide-spread skin involvement is uncommon.

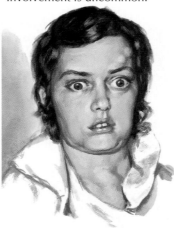

Young woman with bilateral facial palsy. Note drooping of cheeks due to compression of both facial (VII) nerves by acoustic neuromas, which also caused hearing loss. Proptosis resulted from bilateral optic (II) nerve tumors. Subcutaneous nodules developed on her forehead, and masses in her neck compressed the trachea. Disease was fatal in this patient.

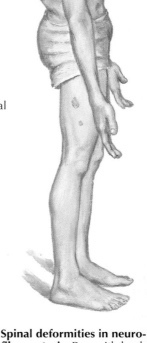

Spinal deformities in neurofibromatosis. Boy with kyphoscoliosis. Foreshortening of trunk secondary to kyphosis gives appearance of longer upper limbs.

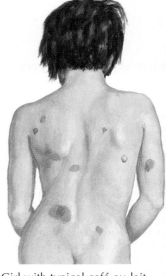

Girl with typical café-au-lait spots but only a few skin nodules. Relatively mild neurofibromatous scoliosis is present.

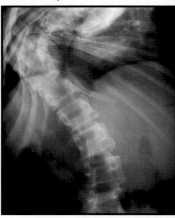

Severe scoliosis. Radiograph shows typical sharp angulation unresponsive to corrective measures, often seen in neurofibromatosis.

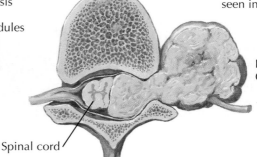

Dumbbell tumor Of spinal nerve root

Spinal cord

growth of a preexisting neurofibroma should make the clinician consider performing a biopsy to rule out malignant degeneration. Optic gliomas are best surgically excised if indicated, even though removal of the optic glioma typically results in blindness.

Patients with type II disease should have screening MRI studies of the brain and the rest of the central nervous system to look for schwannomas. Type II

disease, because of the presence of bilateral schwannomas, is a much more serious and life-altering disease than type I. The follow-up management of type II neurofibromatosis requires a multidisciplinary approach. Ophthalmology, otolaryngology, neurosurgery, and internal medicine physicians need to coordinate care for these patients. Neurosurgery and localized radiotherapy have been used to treat the brain tumors.

Plate 9-12

Genodermatoses and Syndromes

TUBEROUS SCLEROSIS

Tuberous sclerosis (Bourneville's syndrome) is a multisystem disease that often manifests with cutaneous findings. It is inherited in an autosomal dominant manner and is directly caused by a defect in one of two genes, *TSC1* or *TSC2*, usually due to a spontaneous mutation. *TSC1* has been shown to encode the hamartin protein, whereas *TSC2* gene encodes the tuberin protein. The skin, central nervous system (CNS), cardiovascular, respiratory, visual, and musculoskeletal systems are affected. This genodermatosis has an extremely variable phenotype. At one extreme is the severely disabled and mentally delayed individual with severe seizure disorders; at the other end of the spectrum is the individual with mild skin disease and unappreciable CNS disease.

Clinical Findings: The incidence of tuberous sclerosis is approximately 1 in 15,000, and the disease affects all races and genders equally. Infants and young children may present with primary CNS disease with the onset of seizures. All children with new-onset seizures should be evaluated for the cutaneous findings of tuberous sclerosis; if these are located, the child should be further evaluated for the possibility of this diagnosis. Mental delay may be noticeable, because the child may not meet normal developmental milestones. Other brain anomalies have been reported to occur in tuberous sclerosis, including astrocytomas, hydrocephalus, cortical tubers, and subependymal tumors. Cardiac rhabdomyomas may manifest with a murmur and are best evaluated with the use of an echocardiogram. The lungs are rarely involved with lymphangiomyomatosis.

Cutaneous findings are often the earliest findings of the disease, even before the onset of CNS disease. The "ash leaf" macule is the first cutaneous finding; it is represented by a hypopigmented to depigmented macule in the shape of an ash leaf. Other hypopigmented macules are prominent components of tuberous sclerosis and include "confetti" macules and polygonal hypopigmented macules. The isolated finding of a hypopigmented macule in infants should make one consider and evaluate for the diagnosis of tuberous sclerosis. Approximately 0.25% of normal newborns have a hypopigmented macule with no other evidence of tuberous sclerosis.

Connective tissue nevi are frequently seen in this disease and can manifest as small plaques or dermal nodules. These nevi have been termed "shagreen patches." Skin biopsies are required to diagnose a connective tissue nevus. Koenen tumors, a type of periungual fibroma, are a feature of the disease and can be seen on a solitary digit or on multiple digits of the hands and feet. Café-au-lait macules are occasionally seen. At puberty or slightly before, the presence of facial angiofibromas may become noticeable. These facial tumors tend to increase in size and number over time. They cause significant morbidity and psychological harm to the affected individual. These angiofibromas have been given the name *adenoma sebaceum*, and in some cases they are the initial sign of the disease. They are frequently misdiagnosed as early acne, and only after lack of response to therapy or referral to a dermatologist are they accurately identified. These facial growths cause significant disfigurement, and many individuals seek therapy to lessen the appearance of these tumors.

Pathogenesis: When defective, hamartin and tuberin have been shown to cause tuberous sclerosis. They are both tumor suppressor proteins that function by interacting with a G protein. This interaction inhibits the so-called mammalian target of rapamycin (mTOR)

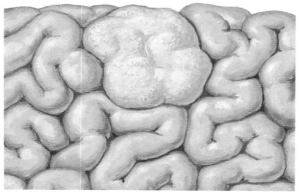

Tuber of cerebral cortex. Consisting of many astrocytes, scanty nerve cells, some abnormal sites

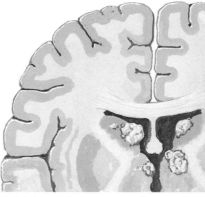

Multiple small tumors. Caudate nucleus and thalamus projecting into ventricles

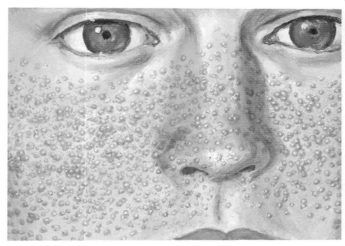

Adenoma sebaceum. Over both cheeks and bridge of nose

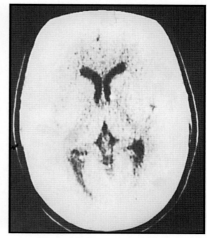

CT scan. Showing one of many calcified lesions in periventricular area

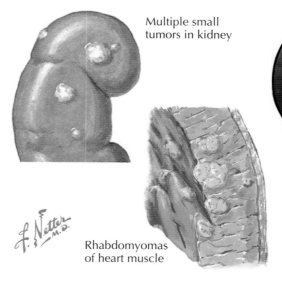

Multiple small tumors in kidney

Rhabdomyomas of heart muscle

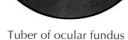

Tuber of ocular fundus

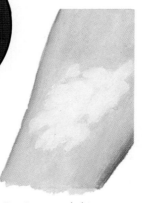

Depigmented skin area

signaling pathway. When these proteins are mutated, the inhibition is removed, and the mTOR pathway is allowed to signal uncontrolled. This leads to unregulated cell division and the production of various tumors.

Treatment: Therapy needs to be individualized for each patient. Those with seizure disorders and CNS tumors require the expertise of a neurologist or neurosurgeon or both. Antiseizure medications are frequently required for prolonged periods. Routine ophthalmological examinations should be recommended to evaluate for the possibility of retinal astrocytic hamartomas (phakomas). Facial angiofibromas can be surgically removed by many means. Laser vaporization and more traditional surgical methods have been used to remove or lessen the appearance of these tumors. No therapy is required for the hypopigmented macules or the connective tissue nevi. All patients should be monitored routinely by their pediatrician for evaluation of developmental milestones and physical examinations.

REFERENCES

Section 1: Anatomy, Physiology, and Embryology

Bolognia J, Jorizzo JL, Rapini RP. *Dermatology*. 2nd ed. St. Louis: Mosby; 2008:664-666.

Elias PM, Hatano Y, Williams ML. Basis for the barrier abnormality in atopic dermatitis: Outside-inside-outside pathogenic mechanisms. *J Allergy Clin Immunol*. 2008;121:1337-1343.

Eming SA, Krieg T, Davidson JM. Inflammation in wound repair: molecular and cellular mechanisms. *J Invest Dermatol*. 2007;127: 514-525.

Ferguson J, Dover J. *Photodermatology*. London: Manson Publishing; 2006 [chapter 4].

Fitzpatrick TB, Freedberg IM, Eisen AZ, et al, eds. *Dermatology in General Medicine*. 5th ed. New York: McGraw-Hill; 1999 [chapter 7].

Harber LC, Brickers DR. *Photosensitivity Diseases: Principles of Diagnoses and Treatment*. 2nd ed. Toronto: BC Decker; 1989 [chapters 1-5].

James WD, Berger TG, Elston DM. *Andrews' Diseases of the Skin: Clinical Dermatology*. 10th ed. Philadelphia: Saunders; 2006 [chapter 1].

Kalinin AE, Kajava AV, Steinert PM. Epithelial barrier function: assembly and structural features of the cornified cell envelope. *BioEssays*. 2002;24:789-800.

Kragballe K. *Vitamin D in Dermatology*. New York: Marcel Dekker; 2000.

Kuritzky LA, Finlay-Jones JJ, Hart PH. The controversial role of vitamin D in the skin: immunosuppression vs. photoprotection. *Clin Exp Dermatol*. 2008;33:167-170.

Moreau M, Leclerc C. The choice between epidermal and neural fate: a matter of calcium. *Int J Dev Biol*. 2004;48:75-84.

Neas JF. *Human Anatomy. Development of the Integumentary System*. San Francisco: Benjamin Cummings; 2003 [chapter 4].

Segeart S, Simonart T. The epidermal vitamin D system and innate immunity: some more light shed on this unique photoendocrine system? *Dermatology*. 2008;217:7-11.

Steed DL. The role of growth factors in wound healing. *Surg Clin North Am*. 1997;77:576-586.

Section 2: Benign Growths

Agero AL, Lahmer JJ, Holzborn RM, et al. Naevus of ota presenting in two generations: a mother and daughter. *J Eur Acad Dermatol Venereol*. 2009;23:102-104.

Arneja JS, Gosain AK. Giant congenital melanocytic nevi. *Plast Reconstr Surg*. 2007;120:26e-40e.

Bakri SJ, Carlson JA, Meyer DR. Recurrent solitary reticulohistiocytoma of the eyelid. *Ophthal Plast Reconstr Surg*. 2003;19: 162-164.

Bansal C, Stewart D, Li A, et al. Histologic variants of fibrous papule. *J Cutan Pathol*. 2005;32:424-428.

Barnhill RL, Crowson AN. *Textbook of Dermatopathology*. 2nd ed. New York: McGraw-Hill; 2004:561-563.

Berk DR, Bayliss SJ. Milia: a review and classification. *J Am Acad Dermatol*. 2008;59:1050-1063.

Bolognia J, Jorizzo JL, Rapini RP. *Dermatology*. 2nd ed. St. Louis: Mosby; 2008.

Boon LM, Mulliken JB, Enjolres O, et al. Glomuvenous malformation (glomangioma) and venous malformation: distinct clinicopathologic and genetic entities. *Arch Dermatol*. 2004;140: 971-976.

Brodsky J. Management of benign skin lesions commonly affecting the face: actinic keratosis, seborrheic keratosis, and rosacea. *Curr Opin Otolaryngol Head Neck Surg*. 2009;17:315-320.

Brown CW, Dy LC. Eccrine porocarcinoma. *Dermatol Ther*. 2008;21:433-438.

Burroni M, Nami N, Rubegni P. Like milia-like cysts. *Skin Res Technol*. 2009;15:250-251.

Cardoso R, Freitas JD, Reis JP, et al. Median raphe cyst of the penis. *Dermatol Online J*. 2005;11:37.

Chang JK, Lee DC, Chang MH. A solitary fibrofolliculoma in the eyelid. *Korean J Ophthalmol*. 2007;21:169-171.

Chen TJ, Chou YC, Chen CH, et al. Genital porokeratosis: a series of 10 patients and review of the literature. *Br J Dermatol*. 2006;155:325-329.

Cota C, Sinagra J, Donati P, et al. Milia en plaque: three new pediatric cases. *Pediatr Dermatol*. 2009;26:717-720.

Dubovy SR, Clark BJ. Palisaded encapsulated neuroma (solitary circumscribed neuroma of the skin) of the eyelid: report of two cases and review of the literature. *Br J Ophthalmol*. 2001;85: 949-951.

Eiberg H, Hansen L, Hansen C, et al. Mapping of hereditary trichilemmal cyst (*TRICY1*) to chromosome 3p24–p21.2 and exclusion of beta-*CATENIN* and *MLH1*. *Am J Med Genet A*. 2005;133A:44-47.

Fink AM, Filz D, Krajnik G, et al. Seborrhoeic keratoses in patients with internal malignancies: a case-control study with prospective accrual of patients. *J Eur Acad Dermatol Venereol*. 2009;23: 1316-1319.

Folpe AL, Reisenauer AK, Mentzel T, et al. Proliferating trichilemmal tumors: clinicopathologic evaluation as a guide to biological behavior. *J Cutan Pathol*. 2003;30:492-498.

Gao J, Li C, Liu L, et al. Nevus lipomatosus cutaneous superficialis with angiokeratoma. *Int J Dermatol*. 2007;46:611-612.

Golod O, Soriano T, Craft N. Palisaded encapsulated neuroma—a classic presentation of a commonly misdiagnosed neural tumor. *J Drugs Dermatol*. 2005;4:92-94.

Grande Sarpa H, Harris R, Hansen CD, et al. Androgen receptor expression patterns in Becker's nevi: an immunohistochemical study. *J Am Acad Dermatol*. 2008;59:834-838.

Haberland-Carrodeguas C, Allen CM, Lovas JGL, et al. Review of linear epidermal nevus with oral mucosal involvement—series of five new cases. *Oral Dis*. 2008;14:131-137.

Hafner C, Stoehr R, van Oers JM, et al. The absence of BRAF, FGFR3, PIK3CA mutations differentiates lentigo simplex from malanocytic nevus and solar lentigo. *J Invest Dermatol*. 2009;129: 2730-2735.

Hafner C, Vogt T. Seborrheic keratosis. *J Dtsch Dermatol Ges*. 2008;8:664-677.

Hamel J, Burgdorf WH, Brauninger W. The man behind the eponym: Hans Biberstein and follicular hyperplasia overlying dermatofibroma. *Am J Dermatopathol*. 2009;31:710-714.

Handa Y, Yamanaka N, Inagaki H, et al. Large ulcerated perianal hidradenoma papilliferum in a young female. *Dermatol Surg*. 2003;29:790-792.

Hann SK, Im S, Chung WS, et al. Pigmentary disorders in the South East. *Dermatol Clin*. 2007;25:431-438.

Hara N, Kawaguchi M, Koike H, et al. Median raphe cyst in the scrotum, mimicking a serous borderline tumor, associated with cryptorchidism after orchiopexy. *Int J Urol*. 2004;11:1150-1152.

Haro R, Revelles JM, Angulo J, et al. Plaque-like osteoma cutis with transepidermal elimination. *J Cutan Pathol*. 2009;36:591-593.

Harvell JD, Kerschmann RL, LeBoit PE. Eccrine or apocrine poroma? Six poromas with divergent adnexal differentiation. *Am J Dermatopathol*. 1996;18:1-9.

Henderson CA, Ruban E, Porter DI. Multiple leiomyomata presenting in a child. *Pediatr Dermatol*. 1997;14:287-289.

Hernandez-Martin A, Perez-Mies B, Torrelo A. Congenital platelike osteoma cutis in an infant. *Pediatr Dermatol*. 2009;26: 479-481.

Herranz P, Pizarro A, De Lucas R, et al. High incidence of porokeratosis in renal transplant recipients. *Br J Dermatol*. 1997; 136:176-179.

Hugel H. Fibrohistiocytic skin tumors. *J Dtsch Dermatol Ges*. 2006;4:544-555.

Ilango NG, Sachi K, Therese M, et al. Nevus lipomatosus cutaneous superficialis: a rare giant variant in an unusual location. *Dermatol Surg*. 2008;34:1695.

James WD, Berger TG, Elston DM. *Andrews' Diseases of the Skin: Clinical Dermatology*. 10th ed. Philadelphia: Saunders; 2006.

Juckett G, Hartman-Adams H. Management of keloids and hypertrophic scars. *Am Fam Physician*. 2009;80:253-260.

Kapoor S, Gogia S, Paul R, et al. Albright's hereditary osteodystrophy. *Indian J Pediatr*. 2006;73:153-156.

Kavak A, Parlak AH, Yesildal N, et al. Preliminary study among truck drivers in Turkey: effects of ultraviolet light in some skin entities. *J Dermatol*. 2008;35:146-150.

Kim HJ, Lee JY, Kim SH, et al. Stromelysin-3 expression in the differential diagnosis of dermatofibroma and dermatofibrosarcoma protuberans: comparison with Factor XIIIa and CD34. *Br J Dermatol*. 2007;157:319-324.

Lee HJ, Chun EY, Kim YC, et al. Nevus comedonicus with hidradenoma papilliferum and syringocystadenoma papilliferum in the female genital area. *Int J Dermatol*. 2002;41:933-936.

Liu K, DeAngelo P, Mahmet K, et al. Cytogenetics of neurofibromas: two case reports and literature review. *Cancer Genet Cytogenet*. 2010;196:93-95.

Losee JE, Serletti JM, Pennino RP. Epidermal nevus syndrome: a review and case report. *Ann Plast Surg*. 1999;43:211-214.

Manonukul J, Omeapinyan P, Vongjirad A. Mucoepidermoid (adenosquamous) carcinoma, trichoblastoma, trichilemmoma, sebaceous adenoma, tumor of the follicular infundibulum and syringocystadenoma papilliferum arising within 2 persistent lesions of nevus sebaceous: report of a case. *Am J Dermatopathol*. 2009;31:658-663.

Matsushita S, Higashi Y, Uchimiya H, et al. Case of giant eccrine hidrocystoma of the scalp. *J Dermatol*. 2007;34:586-587.

Menascu S, Donner EJ. Linear sebaceous syndrome: case reports and review of the literature. *Pediatr Neurol*. 2008;38:207-210.

Miettinen M, Fetsch JF. Reticulohistiocytoma (solitary epitheloid histiocytoma): a clinicopathologic and immunohistochemical study of 44 cases. *Am J Surg Pathol*. 2006;30:521-528.

Misago N, Kimura T, Narisawa Y. Fibrofolliculoma/trichodiscoma and fibrous papule (perifollicular fibroma/angiofibroma): a reevaluation of the histopathological and immunohistochemical features. *J Cutan Pathol*. 2009;36:943-951.

Miteva M, Ziemer M. Lichenoid keratosis—a clinicopathological entity with lupus erythematosus-like features? *J Cutan Pathol*. 2007;34:209-210.

Mones JM, Ackerman AB. "Atypical" Spitz's nevus, "malignant" Spitz's nevus and "metastasizing" Spitz's nevus: a critique in historical perspective of three concepts flawed fatally. *Am J Dermatopathol*. 2004;26:310-333.

Morgan MB, Stevens GL, Switlyk S. Benign lichenoid keratosis, a clinical and pathologic reappraisal of 1040 cases. *Am J Dermatopathol*. 2005;27:387-388.

Murali R, McCarthy SW, Scolyer RA, et al. Blue nevi and related lesions: a review highlighting atypical and newly described variants, distinguishing features and diagnostic pitfalls. *Adv Anat Pathol*. 2009;16:365-382.

Myers RS, Lo AK, Pawel BR. The glomangioma in the differential diagnosis of vascular malformations. *Ann Plast Surg*. 2006;57: 443-446.

Nemeth AJ, Penneys NS, Bernstein HB. Fibrous papule: a tumor of fibrohistiocytic cells that contain factor XIIIa. *J Am Acad Dermatol*. 1988;19:1102-1106.

Newman MD, Milgraum S. Palisaded encapsulated neuroma (PEN): an often misdiagnosed neural tumor. *Dermatol Online J*. 2008;14:12.

Ogawa R, Yoshitatsu S, Yoshida K, et al. Is radiation therapy for keloids acceptable? The risk of radiation-induced carcinogenesis. *Plast Reconstr Surg*. 2009;124:1196-1201.

Pandya KA, Radke F. Benign skin lesions: lipomas, epidermal inclusion cysts, muscle and nerve biopsies. *Surg Clin North Am*. 2009;89:677-687.

Parrinello S, Lloyd AC. Neurofibroma development in NF1—insights into tumour initiation. *Trends Cell Biol*. 2009;19:395-403.

Person JP, Longcope C. Becker's nevus: an androgen-mediated hyperplasia with increased androgen receptors. *J Am Acad Dermatol*. 1984;10:235-238.

Requena C, Requena L, Kutzner H, et al. Spitz nevus: a clinicopathological study of 349 cases. *Am J Dermatopathol*. 2009;31: 107-116.

Saravana GH. Oral pyogenic granuloma: a review of 137 cases. *Br J Oral Maxillofac Surg*. 2009;47:318-319.

Seirafi HH, Akhyani M, Naraghi ZS, et al. Eruptive syringomas. *Dermatol Online J*. 2005;11:13.

Sowa J, Kobayashi H, Ishii M, et al. Histopathologic findings in Unna's nevus suggest it is a tardive congenital nevus. *Am J Dermatopathol*. 2008;30:561-566.

Sperling LC, Sakas EL. Eccrine hidrocystomas. *J Am Acad Dermatol*. 1982;7:763-770.

Spitz JL. *Genodermatosis: A Clinical Guide to Genetic Skin Disorders*. 2nd ed. Philadelphia: Lippincott Williams & Wilkins; 2005: 78-79.

Srinivas UM, Tourani KL. Epidermal nevus syndrome with hypophosphatemic renal rickets with hypercalciuria: a bone marrow diagnosis. *Int J Hematol*. 2008;88:125-126.

Stewart L, Glenn GM, Stratton P, et al. Association of germline mutations in the fumarate hydratase gene and uterine fibroids in women with hereditary leiomyomatosis and renal cell cancer. *Arch Dermatol*. 2008;144:1584-1592.

Sudy E, Urbina F, Maliqueo M, et al. Screening of glucose/insulin metabolic alterations in men with multiple skin tags on the neck. *J Dtsch Dermatol Ges*. 2008;6:852-855.

Suzuki H, Anderson RR. Treatment of melanocytic nevi. *Dermatol Ther*. 2005;18:217-226.

Tang S, Hoshida H, Kamisago M, et al. Phenotype-genotype correlation in a patient with co-occurrence of Marfan and LEOPARD syndromes. *Am J Med Genet A*. 2009;149A:2216-2219.

Ter Poorten MC, Barrett K, Cook J. Familial eccrine spiradenoma: a case report and review of the literature. *Dermatol Surg*. 2003;29:411-414.

Walsh JJ, Eady JL. Vascular tumors. *Hand Clin*. 2004;20:261-268.

Weedon D. *Skin Pathology*. New York: Churchill Livingstone; 1997.

Yamamato T. Dermatofibroma: a possible model of local fibrosis with epithelial/mesenchymal cell interaction. *J Eur Acad Dermatol Venereol*. 2009;23:371-375.

Yung C, Soltani K, Bernstein JE, et al. Unilateral linear nevoidal syringoma. *J Am Acad Dermatol*. 1981;4:412-416.

Zaballos P, Blazquez S, Puig S, et al. Dermoscopic pattern of intermediate stage in seborrhoeic keratosis regressing to lichenoid keratosis: report of 24 cases. *Br J Dermatol*. 2007;157:266-272.

Zalaudek I, Hofmann-Wellenhof R, Kittler H, et al. A dual concept of nevogenesis: theoretical considerations based on dermoscopic features of melanocytic nevi. *J Dtsch Dermatol Ges.* 2007;5:985-992.

Zarineh A, Kozovska ME, Brown WG, et al. Smooth muscle hamartoma associated with a congenital pattern of melanocytic nevus: a case report and review of the literature. *J Cutan Pathol.* 2008;35:83-86.

Section 3: Malignant Growths

Abrams TA, Schuetze SM. Targeted therapy for dermatofibrosarcoma protuberans. *Curr Oncol Rep.* 2006;8:291-296.

Aydin F, Senturk N, Sabanciler MT, et al. A case of Ferguson-Smith type multiple keratoacanthomas associated with keratoacanthoma centrifugum marginatum: response to oral acitretin. *Clin Exp Dermatol.* 2007;32:683-686.

Bhawan J. Squamous cell carcinoma in situ in skin: what does it mean? *J Cutan Pathol.* 2007;34:953-955.

Black APB, Ogg GS. The role of p53 in the immunobiology of cutaneous squamous cell carcinoma. *Clin Exp Immunol.* 2003; 132:379-384.

Bleeker MCG, Heideman DAM, Snijders PJF, et al. Penile cancer: epidemiology, pathogenesis and prevention. *World J Urol.* 2009;27:141-150.

Bongiorno MR, Doukaki S, Ferro G, et al. Matrix metalloproteinases 2 and 9, and extracellular matrix in Kaposi's sarcoma. *Dermatol Ther.* 2010;23:S33-S36.

Budd GT. Management of angiosarcoma. *Curr Oncol Rep.* 2002;4: 515-519.

Buitrago W, Joseph AK. Sebaceous carcinoma: the great masquerader: emerging concepts in diagnosis and treatment. *Dermatol Ther.* 2008;21:459-466.

Catena F, Santini D, Di Saverio S, et al. Skin angiosarcoma arising in an irradiated breast: case-report and literature review. *Dermatol Surg.* 2006;32:447-455.

Cox NH, Eedy DJ, Morton CA. Guidelines for management of Bowen's disease: 2006 update. *Br J Dermatol.* 2007;156:11-21.

Criscione VD, Weinstock MA, Naylor MF, et al. Actinic keratosis: natural history and risk of malignant transformation in the Veterans Affairs Topical Tretinoin Chemoprevention Trial. *Cancer.* 2009;115:2523-2530.

DiLorenzo G. Update on classic Kaposi sarcoma therapy: new look at an old disease. *Crit Rev Oncol/Hematol.* 2008;68:242-249.

Dimitropoulos VA. Dermatofibrosarcoma protuberans. *Dermatol Ther.* 2008;21:447-451.

Donovan J. Review of the hair follicle origin hypothesis for basal cell carcinoma. *Dermatol Surg.* 2009;35:1311-1323.

Dubina M, Goldenberg G. Viral-associated nonmelanoma skin cancers: a review. *Am J Dermatopathol.* 2009;31:561-573.

Duvic M, Donato M, Dabaja B, et al. Total skin electron beam and non-myeloablative allogeneic hematopoietic stem-cell transplantation in advanced mycosis fungoides and Sezary syndrome *J Clin Oncol.* 2010;28:2365-2372.

Egmond SV, Hoedemaker C, Sinclair R. Successful treatment of perianal Bowen's disease: imiquimod. *Int J Dermatol.* 2007;46: 318-319.

Eisen DB, Michael DJ. Sebaceous lesions and their associated syndromes: part I. *J Am Acad Dermatol.* 2009;61:549-560.

Elder DE, Gimotty PA, Guerry D. Cutaneous melanoma: estimating survival and recurrence risk based on histopathologic features. *Dermatol Ther.* 2005;18:369-385.

Epstein EH. Basal cell carcinomas: attack of the hedgehog. *Nat Rev Cancer.* 2008;8:743-754.

Gaertner WB, Hagerman GF, Goldberg SM, et al. Perianal Paget's disease treated with wide excision and gluteal skin flap reconstruction: report of a case and review of the literature. *Dis Colon Rectum.* 2008;51:1842-1845.

Grange JM, Krone B, Stanford JL. Immunotherapy for malignant melanoma—tracing Ariadne's thread through the labyrinth. *Eur J Cancer.* 2009;45:2266-2273.

Gremel G, Rafferty M, Lau TY, et al. Identification and functional validation of therapeutic targets for malignant melanoma. *Crit Rev Oncol/Hematol.* 2009;72:194-214.

Han A, Ratner D. What is the role of adjuvant radiotherapy in the treatment of cutaneous squamous cell carcinoma with perineural invasion? *Cancer.* 2007;109:1053-1059.

Houben R, Schrama D, Becker JC. Molecular pathogenesis of Merkel cell carcinoma. *Exp Dermatol.* 2009;18:193-198.

Ivan D, Diwan AH, Lazar AJF, et al. The usefulness of p63 detection for differentiating primary from metastatic skin adenocarcinomas. *J Cutan Pathol.* 2008;35:880-881.

Jones B, Oh C, Mangold E, et al. Muir-Torre syndrome: diagnostic and screening guidelines. *Aust J Dermatol.* 2006;47:266-269.

Kaehler KC, Sondak VK, Schadendorf D, et al. Pegylated interferons: prospects for the use in the adjuvant and palliative therapy of metastatic melanoma. *Eur J Cancer.* 2010;46:41-46.

Kanitakis J. Mammary and extramammary Paget's disease. *J Eur Acad Dermatol Venereol.* 2007;21:581-590.

Kirkwood JM, Jukic DM, Averbook BJ, et al. Melanoma in pediatric, adolescent and young adults. *Semin Oncol.* 2009;36:419-431.

Kossard S, Tan KB, Choy C. Keratoacanthoma and infundibulocystic squamous cell carcinoma. *Am J Dermatopathol.* 2008;30: 127-134.

Lansigan F, Foss FM. Current and emerging treatment strategies for cutaneous T-cell lymphoma. *Drugs.* 2010;70:273-286.

Liao PB. Merkel cell carcinoma. *Dermatol Ther.* 2008;21:447-451.

Lookingbill DP, Spangler N, Helm KF. Cutaneous metastases in patients with metastatic carcinoma: a retrospective study of 4020 patients. *J Am Acad Dermatol.* 1993;29:228-236.

Mendenhall WM, Mendenhall CM, Werning JW, et al. Cutaneous angiosarcoma. *Am J Clin Oncol.* 2006;29:524-528.

Ming M, He YY. PTEN: new insights into its regulation and function in skin cancer. *J Invest Dermatol.* 2009;129:2109-2112.

Minicozzi A, Borzellino G, Momo R, et al. Perianal Paget's disease: presentation of six cases and literature review. *Int J Colorectal Dis.* 2010;25:1-7.

Murphy GF. *Dermatopathology.* Philadelphia: Saunders; 1995: 192-194.

Ntomouchtsis A, Vahtsesevanos K, Patrikidou A, et al. Adnexal skin carcinomas of the face. *J Craniofac Surg.* 2009;20:134-137.

Odom RB, James WB, Berger TG. *Andrews' Disease of the Skin: Clinical Dermatology.* 9th ed. Philadelphia: Saunders; 2000: 756-760.

Paradisi A, Abeni D, Rusciani A, et al. Dermatofibrosarcoma protuberans: wide local excision vs. mohs micrographic surgery. *Cancer Treat Rev.* 2008;34:728-736.

Richter ON, Petrow W, Wardelmann E, et al. Bowenoid papulosis of the vulva—immunotherapeutical approach with topical imiquimod. *Arch Gynecol Obstet.* 2003;268:333-336.

Rigel DS, Friedman RJ, Dzubow LM, et al. *Cancer of the Skin.* Philadelphia: Saunders; 2005.

Riou-Gotta MO, Fournier E, Danzon A, et al. Rare skin cancer: a population-based cancer registry descriptive study of 151 consecutive cases diagnosed between 1980 and 2004. *Acta Oncol.* 2009;48:605-609.

Schwartz RA, Bridges TM, Butani AK, et al. Actinic keratosis: an occupational and environmental disorder. *J Eur Acad Dermatol Venereol.* 2008;22:606-615.

Shalin SC, Lyle S, Calonje E, et al. Sebaceous neoplasia and the Muir-Torre syndrome: important connections with clinical implications. *Histopathology.* 2010;56:133-147.

Tai P, Yu E, Assouline A, et al. Management of Merkel cell carcinoma with emphasis on small primary tumors: a case series and review of the current literature. *J Drugs Dermatol.* 2010;9: 105-110.

Telfer NR, Clover GB, Morton CA. Guidelines for the management of basal cell carcinoma. *Br J Dermatol.* 2008;159:35-48.

Vergilis-Kalner IJ, Kriseman Y, Goldberg LH. Keratoacanthomas: overview and comparison between Houston and Minneapolis experiences. *J Drugs Dermatol.* 2010;9:117-121.

Weedon D. *Skin Pathology.* New York: Churchill Livingstone; 1997.

Weinberg AS, Ogle CA, Shim EK. Metastatic cutaneous squamous cell carcinoma: an update. *Dermatol Surg.* 2007;33:885-899.

Wood AJ, Lappinga PJ, Ahmed I. Hepatocellular carcinoma metastatic to skin: diagnostic utility of antihuman hepatocyte antibody in combination with albumin in situ hybridization. *J Cutan Pathol.* 2009;36:262-266.

Wu XS, Lonsdorf AS, Hwang ST. Cutaneous T-cell lymphoma: roles for chemokines and chemokine receptors. *J Invest Dermatol.* 2009;129:1115-1119.

Yu F, Finn DT, Rogers GS. Microcystic adnexal carcinoma: a rare locally aggressive cutaneous tumor. *Am J Clin Oncol.* 2010:33: 196-197.

Yu W, Tsoukas MM, Chapman SM, et al. Surgical treatment of dermatofibrosarcoma protuberans: the Dartmouth experience and literature review. *Ann Plastic Surg.* 2008;60:288-293.

Zinzani PL, Ferreri AJM, Cerroni L. Mycosis fungoides. *Crit Rev Oncol/Hematol.* 2008;65:172-182.

Zwenzner EM, Kaatz M, Ziemer M. Skin metastasis of 'nested type' of urothelial carcinoma of the urinary bladder. *J Cutan Pathol.* 2006;33:754-755.

Section 4: Rashes

Abla O, Egeler RM, Weitzman S. Langerhans cell histiocytosis: current concepts and treatments. *Cancer Treat Rev.* 2010;36: 354-359.

Ahdout J, Haley JC, Chiu MW. Erythema multiforme during antitumor necrosis factor treatment for plaque psoriasis. *J Am Acad Dermatol.* 2010;62:874-879.

Ahmadi S, Powell FC. Pruritic urticarial papules and plaques of pregnancy: current status. *Australas J Dermatol.* 2005;46:53-58.

Akin C, Valent P, Escribano L. Urticaria pigmentosa and mastocytosis: the role of immunophenotyping in diagnosis and determining response to treatment. *Curr Allergy Asthma Rep.* 2006;6: 282-288.

Al Hammadi A, Asai Y, Patt ML, et al. Erythema annulare centrifugum secondary to treatment with finasteride. *J Drugs Dermatol.* 2007;6:460-463.

Ale IS, Maibacht HA. Diagnostic approach in allergic and irritant contact dermatitis. *Expert Rev Clin Immunol.* 2010;6:291-310.

Alikhan A, Kurek L, Feldman SR. The role of tetracyclines in rosacea. *Am J Clin Dermatol.* 2010;11:79-87.

Al-Mahfoudh R, Clark S, Buxton N. Alkaptonuria presenting with ochronotic spondyloarthropathy. *Br J Neurosurg.* 2008;22: 805-807.

Antoniu SA. Targeting the TNF-alpha pathway in sarcoidosis. *Expert Opin Ther Targets.* 2010;14:21-29.

Aractingi S, Chosidow O. Cutaneous graft-versus-host disease. *Arch Dermatol.* 1998;134:602-612.

Araki K, Sudo A, Hasegawa M, et al. Devastating ochronotic arthropathy with successful bilateral hip and knee arthroplasties. *J Clin Rheumatol.* 2009;15:138-140.

Arias-Santiago S, Aneiros-Fernandez J, Girón-Prieto MS, et al. Palpable purpura. *Cleve Clin J Med.* 2010;77:205-206.

Auerbach PS, ed. *Wilderness Medicine.* 5th ed. Philadelphia: Mosby; 2007:1262-1286.

Ayangco L, Rogers RS 3rd. Oral manifestations of erythema multiforme. *Dermatol Clin.* 2003;21:195-205.

Badea I, Taylor M, Rosenberg A, et al. Pathogenesis and therapeutic approaches for improved topical treatment in localized scleroderma and systemic sclerosis. *Rheumatology.* 2009;48:213-221.

Bandino JP, Wohltmann WE, Bray DW, et al. Naproxen-induced generalized bullous fixed drug eruption. *Dermatol Online J.* 2009;15:4.

Banikazemi M, Bultas J, Waldek S, et al. Agalsidase-beta therapy for advanced Fabry disease: a randomized trial. *Ann Intern Med.* 2007;146:77-86.

Ben-Amitai D, Metzker A, Cohen HA. Pediatric cutaneous mastocytosis: a review of 180 patients. *Isr Med Assoc J.* 2005;7: 320-322.

Ben Rayana N, Chahed N, Khochtali S, et al. Ocular ochronosis. A case report. *J Fr Ophtalmol.* 2008;31:624.

Bernier J, Booner J, Vermorken JB, et al. Consensus guidelines for the management of radiation dermatitis and co-existing acne-like rash in patients receiving radiotherapy plus EGRF inhibitors for the treatment of squamous cell carcinoma of the head and neck. *Ann Oncol.* 2008;19:142-149.

Bieber T, Novak N. Pathogenesis of atopic dermatitis: new developments. *Curr Allergy Asthma Rep.* 2009;9:291-294.

Blair JE. State-of-the-art treatment of coccidioidomycosis: skin and soft-tissue infections. *Ann N Y Acad Sci.* 2007;1111:411-421.

Boguniewicz M, Leung DY. Recent insights into atopic dermatitis and implications for management of infectious complications. *J Allergy Clin Immunol.* 2010;125:4-13.

Boissan M, Feger F, Guillosson J, et al. c-Kit and c-kit mutations in mastocytosis and other hematological diseases. *J Leukoc Biol.* 2000;67:135-148.

Bolognia JL, Jorizzo JL, Rapini RP. *Dermatology.* 2nd ed. St. Louis: Mosby; 2008.

Brahimi N, Routier E, Raison-Peyron N, et al. A three-year-analysis of fixed drug eruptions in hospital settings in France. *Eur J Dermatol.* 2010;20:461-464.

Bremec T, Demsar J, Luzar B, et al. Longstanding truncal hyperpigmented patches in a young man. Multiple fixed drug eruption caused by acetaminophen. *Clin Exp Dermatol.* 2010;35:e56-e57.

Brickman WJ, Huang J, Silverman BL, et al. Acanthosis nigricans identifies youth at high risk for metabolic abnormalities. *J Pediatr.* 2010;156:87-92.

Briley LD, Phillips CM. Cutaneous mastocytosis: a review focusing on the pediatric population. *Clin Pediatr (Phila).* 2008;47: 757-761.

Brockow K. Urticaria pigmentosa. *Immunol Allergy Clin North Am.* 2004;24:287-316.

Buck T, González LM, Lambert WC, et al. Sweet's syndrome with hematologic disorders: a review and reappraisal. *Int J Dermatol.* 2008;47:775-782.

Burrall B. Sweet's syndrome (acute neutrophilic febrile dermatosis). *Dermatol Online J.* 1999;5:8.

Buyon JP, Clancy RM, Friedman DM. Cardiac manifestations of neonatal lupus erythematosus: guidelines to management, integrating clues from the bench and bedside. *Nat Clin Pract Rheumatol.* 2009;5:139-148.

Camelo-Piragua S, Zambrano E, Pantanowitz L. Langerhans cell histiocytosis. *Ear Nose Throat J.* 2010;89:112-113.

Cario H, McMullin MF, Pahl HL. Clinical and hematological presentation of children and adolescents with polycythemia vera. *Ann Hematol.* 2009;88:713-719.

Carlson JA. The histological assessment of cutaneous vasculitis. *Histopathology.* 2010;56:3-23.

Chang HY, Ridky TW, Kimball AB, et al. Eruptive xanthomas associated with olanzapine use. *Arch Dermatol.* 2003;139: 1045-1048.

Chang KL, Snyder DS. Langerhans cell histiocytosis. *Cancer Treat Res.* 2008;142:383-398.

Chassaing N, Martin L, Calvas P, et al. Pseudoxanthoma elasticum: a clinical, pathophysiological and genetic update including 11 novel ABCC6 mutations. *J Med Genet.* 2005;42:881-892.

Chen YJ, Wu CY, Huang YL, et al. Cancer risks of dermatomyositis and polymyositis: a nationwide cohort study in Taiwan. *Arthritis Res Ther.* 2010;12:R70.

Chkoura A, El Alloussi M, Taleb B, et al. Resolution of eosinophilic granuloma after minimal intervention. Case report and review of literature. *N Y State Dent J*. 2010;76:43-46.

Clark SC, Zirwas MJ. Management of occupational dermatitis. *Dermatol Clin*. 2009;27:365-383.

Cohen PR. Sweet's syndrome—a comprehensive review of an acute febrile neutrophilic dermatosis. *Orphanet J Rare Dis*. 2007;26:34.

Cohen PR. Neutrophilic dermatoses: a review of current treatment options. *Am J Clin Dermatol*. 2009;10:301-312.

Cooper JS, Lee BT. Treatment of facial scarring: lasers, filler and nonoperative techniques. *Facial Plast Surg*. 2009;25:311-315.

Cox V, Lesesky EB, Garcia BD, et al. Treatment of juvenile pityriasis rubra pilaris with etanercept. *J Am Acad Dermatol*. 2008;59(Suppl 5):S113-S114.

Crispín JC, Liossis SN, Kis-Toth K, et al. Pathogenesis of human systemic lupus erythematosus: recent advances. *Trends Mol Med*. 2010;16:47-57.

Crowson AN, Mihm MC Jr, Magro CM. Cutaneous vasculitis: a review. *J Cutan Pathol*. 2003;30:161-173.

Dahl M. Granuloma annulare: long-term follow up. *Arch Dermatol*. 2007;143:946-947.

Dali-Youcef ND, Andrès E. An update on cobalamin deficiency in adults. *Q J Med*. 2009;102:17-28.

Das AM, Naim HY. Biochemical basis of Fabry disease with emphasis on mitochondrial function and protein trafficking. *Adv Clin Chem*. 2009;49:57-71.

da Silva Santos PS, Fontes A, Andrade F, et al. Gingival leukemic infiltration as the first manifestation of acute myeloid leukemia. *Otolaryngol Head Neck Surg*. 2010;143:465-466.

Deeg HJ, Antin JH. The clinical spectrum of acute graft-versus-host disease. *Semin Hematol*. 2006;43:24-31.

Del Rosso JQ. Perspectives on seborrheic dermatitis: looking back to move ahead. *Clin Dermatol*. 2009;27(Suppl 6):S39-S40.

Demirer S, Ozdemir H, Sencan M, et al. Gingival hyperplasia as an early diagnostic oral manifestation of acute monocytic leukemia. *Eur J Dent*. 2007;1:111-114.

Desnick RJ, Brady R, Barranger J, et al. Fabry disease, an under-recognized multisystemic disorder: expert recommendations for diagnosis, management, and enzyme replacement therapy. *Ann Intern Med*. 2003;138:338-346.

Díaz-Pérez JL, De Lagrán ZM, Díaz-Ramón JL, et al. Cutaneous polyarteritis nodosa. *Semin Cutan Med Surg*. 2007;26:77-86.

Drago F, Rebora A. Treatments for pityriasis rosea. *Skin Therapy Lett*. 2009;14:6-7.

Dubrey SW, Falk RH. Diagnosis and management of cardiac sarcoidosis. *Prog Cardiovasc Dis*. 2010;52:336-346.

Eberle FC, Ghoreschi K, Hertl M. Fumaric acid esters in severe ulcerative necrobiosis lipoidica: a case report and evaluation of current therapies. *Acta Derm Venereol (Oslo)*. 2010;90:104-106.

Egeler RM, van Halteren AG, Hogendoorn PC, et al. Langerhans cell histiocytosis: fascinating dynamics of the dendritic cell-macrophage lineage. *Immunol Rev*. 2010;234:213-232.

Eisendle K, Zelger B. The expanding spectrum of cutaneous borreliosis. *G Ital Dermatol Venereol*. 2009;144:157-171.

Elewski BE. Safe and effective treatment of seborrheic dermatitis. *Cutis*. 2009;83:333-338.

Elston DM. What's eating you? Chiggers. *Cutis*. 2006;77:350-352.

Elston DM. Tick bites and skin rashes. *Curr Opin Infect Dis*. 2010;23:132-138.

Esler-Brauer L, Rothman I. Tender nodules on the palms and soles: palmoplantar eccrine hidradenitis. *Arch Dermatol*. 2007;143:1201-1206.

Espírito Santo J, Gomes MF, Gomes MJ, et al. Intravenous immunoglobulin in lupus panniculitis. *Clin Rev Allergy Immunol*. 2010;38:307-318.

Farasat S, Aksentijevich I, Toro J. Autoinflammatory diseases: clinical and genetic advances. *Arch Dermatol*. 2008;144:392-402.

Ferreira M, Sanches M, Lobo I, et al. Alkaptonuric ochronosis. *Eur J Dermatol*. 2007;17:336-337.

Filipovich A, McClain K, Grom A. Histiocytic disorders: recent insights into pathophysiology and practical guidelines. *Biol Blood Marrow Transplant*. 2010;16(Suppl 1):S82-S89.

Finazzi G, Barbui T. How I treat patients with polycythemia vera. *Blood*. 2007;109:5104-5111.

Finger RP, Charbel Issa P, Ladewig MS, et al. Pseudoxanthoma elasticum: genetics, clinical manifestations and therapeutic approaches. *Surv Ophthalmol*. 2009;54:272-285.

Fred HL, Accad M. Images in clinical medicine. Lipemia retinalis. *N Engl J Med*. 1999;340:1969.

Frigerio E, Franchi C, Garutti C, et al. Multiple localized granuloma annulare: ultraviolet A1 phototherapy. *Clin Exp Dermatol*. 2007;32:762-764.

Funabiki M, Tanioka M, Miyachi Y, et al. Sudden onset of calciphylaxis: painful violaceous livedo in a patient with peritoneal dialysis. *Clin Exp Dermatol*. 2009;34:622-624.

Gencoglan G, Inanir I, Gunduz K. Therapeutic hotline: treatment of prurigo nodularis and lichen simplex chronicus with gabapentin. *Dermatol Ther*. 2010;23:194-198.

Gendernalik SB, Galeckas KJ. Fixed drug eruptions: a case report and review of the literature. *Cutis*. 2009;84:215-219.

Geyer AS, MacGregor JL, Fox LP, et al. Eruptive xanthomas associated with protease inhibitor therapy. *Arch Dermatol*. 2004;140:617-618.

Gupta N, Phadke SR. Cutis laxa type II and wrinkly skin syndrome: distinct phenotypes. *Pediatr Dermatol*. 2006;23:225-230.

Hacihamdioglu B, Ozcan A, Kalman S. Subcutaneous granuloma annulare in a child: a case report. *Clin Pediatr*. 2008;47:306-308.

Häusermann P, Walter RB, Halter J, et al. Cutaneous graft-versus-host disease: a guide for the dermatologist. *Dermatology*. 2008;216:287-304.

Hayes J, Koo J. Psoriasis: depression, anxiety, smoking, and drinking habits. *Dermatol Ther*. 2010;23:174-180.

Heffernan MP. Combining traditional systemic and biological therapies for psoriasis. *Semin Cutan Med Surg*. 2010;29:67-69.

Hengstman GJ, van den Hoogen FH, van Engelen BG. Treatment of the inflammatory myopathies: update and practical recommendations. *Expert Opin Pharmacother*. 2009;10:1183-1190.

Henry MF, Maender JL, Shen Y, et al. Fluoroscopy-induced chronic radiation dermatitis: a report of three cases. *Dermatol Online J*. 2009;15:3.

Herbert CR, Russo GG. Polyarteritis nodosa and cutaneous polyarteritis nodosa. *Skinmed*. 2003;2:277-285.

Hida Y, Kubo Y, Nishio Y, et al. Malignancy acanthosis nigricans with enhanced expression of fibroblast growth factor receptor 3. *Acta Derm Venereol*. 2009;89:435-437.

Higgins SP, Freemark M, Prose NS. Acanthosis nigricans: a practical approach to evaluation and management. *Dermatol Online J*. 2008;14:2.

Hoesly FJ, Huerter CJ, Shehan JM. Purpura annularis telangiectodes of Majocchi: case report and review of the literature. *Int J Dermatol*. 2009;48:1129-1133.

Hoffman HM. Therapy of autoinflammatory syndromes. *J Allergy Clin Immunol*. 2009;124:1129-1138.

Hoffmann B. Fabry disease: recent advances in pathology, diagnosis, treatment and monitoring. *Orphanet J Rare Dis*. 2009;4:21.

Hosaka H, Ohtoshi S, Nakada T, et al. Erythema multiforme, Stevens-Johnson syndrome and toxic epidermal necrolysis: frozen-section diagnosis. *J Dermatol*. 2010;37:407-412.

Hossani-Madani AR, Halder RM. Topical treatment and combination approaches for vitiligo: new insights, new developments. *G Ital Dermatol Venereol*. 2010;145:57-78.

Humphrey S, Hemmati I, Randhawa R, et al. Elastosis perforans serpiginosa: treatment with liquid nitrogen cryotherapy and review of the literature. *J Cutan Med Surg*. 2010;14:38-42.

Hymes SR, Strom EA, Fife C. Radiation dermatitis: clinical presentation, pathophysiology, and treatment. *J Am Acad Dermatol*. 2006;54:28-46.

Hymes SR, Turner ML, Champlin RE, et al. Cutaneous manifestations of chronic graft-versus-host disease. *Biol Blood Marrow Transplant*. 2006;12:1101-1113.

Imanishi H, Tsuruta D, Ishii M, et al. Annular leucocytoclastic vasculitis. *Clin Exp Dermatol*. 2009;34:e120-e122.

Ishiguro N, Kawashima M. Cutaneous polyarteritis nodosa: a report of 16 cases with clinical and histopathological analysis and a review of the published work. *J Dermatol*. 2010;37:85-93.

James WD, Berger TG, Elston DM. *Andrews' Diseases of the Skin: Clinical Dermatology*. Philadelphia: Saunders; 2006.

Jessop S, Whitelaw DA, Delamere FM. Drugs for discoid lupus erythematosus. *Cochrane Database Syst Rev*. 2009;7:CD002954.

Jones RO. Lichen simplex chronicus. *Clin Podiatr Med Surg*. 1996;13:47-54.

Kacker A, Huo J, Huang R, et al. Solitary mastocytoma in an infant—case report with review of literature. *Int J Pediatr Otorhinolaryngol*. 2000;52:93-95.

Kanazawa N, Furukawa F. Autoinflammatory syndromes with a dermatological perspective. *J Dermatol*. 2007;34:601-618.

Katoh N. Future perspectives in the treatment of atopic dermatitis. *J Dermatol*. 2009;36:367-376.

Kelly AP. Pseudofolliculitis barbae and acne keloidalis nuchae. *Dermatol Clin*. 2003;21:645-653.

Kennedy Carney C, Cantrell W, Elewski BE. Rosacea: a review of current topical, systemic and light-based therapies. *G Ital Dermatol Venereol*. 2009;144:673-688.

Khan IJ, Azam NA, Sullivan SC, et al. Necrobiotic xanthogranuloma successfully treated with a combination of dexamethasone and oral cyclophosphamide. *Can J Ophthalmol*. 2009;44:335-336.

Khanna S, Reed AM. Immunopathogenesis of juvenile dermatomyositis. *Muscle Nerve*. 2010;41:581-592.

King CS, Kelly W. Treatment of sarcoidosis. *Dis Mon*. 2009;55:704-718.

Kiss JE. Thrombotic thrombocytopenic purpura: recognition and management. *Int J Hematol*. 2010;91:36-45.

Klein A, Landthaler M, Karrer S. Pityriasis rubra pilaris: a review of diagnosis and treatment. *Am J Clin Dermatol*. 2010;11:157-170.

Knowles S, Shear NH. Clinical risk management of Stevens-Johnson syndrome/toxic epidermal necrolysis spectrum. *Dermatol Ther*. 2009;22:441-451.

Kocaturk E, Kavala M, Zindanci I, et al. Narrowband UVB treatment of pigmented purpuric lichenoid dermatitis (Gougerot-Blum). *Photodermatol Photoimmunol Photomed*. 2009;25:55-56.

Krasin MJ, Hoth KA, Hua C, et al. Incidence and correlates of radiation dermatitis in children and adolescents receiving radiation therapy for the treatment of paediatric sarcomas. *Clin Oncol*. 2009;21:781-785.

Krawczyk M, Mykala-Ciesla J, Kolodziej-Jaskula A. Acanthosis nigricans as a paraneoplastic syndrome. Case reports and review of literature. *Pol Arch Med Wewn*. 2009;119:180-183.

Krueger JG, Bowcock A. Psoriasis pathophysiology: current concepts of pathogenesis. *Ann Rheum Dis*. 2005;64(Suppl ii):30-36.

Kung AC, Stephens MB, Darling T. Phytophotodermatitis: bulla formation and hyperpigmentation during spring break. *Mil Med*. 2009;174:657-661.

Kwaku MP, Burman KD. Myxedema coma. *J Intensive Care Med*. 2007;22:224-231.

Landau M, Metzker A, Gat A, et al. Palmoplantar eccrine hidradenitis: three new cases and review. *Pediatr Dermatol*. 1998;15:97-102.

Langley RGB, Krueger GG, Griffiths CEM. Psoriatic arthritis and psoriasis: classifications, clinical features, pathophysiology, immunology, genetics. *Ann Rheum Dis*. 2005;64:18-23.

Larsen S, Bendtzen K, Nielsen OH. Extraintestinal manifestations of inflammatory bowel disease: epidemiology, diagnosis, and management. *Ann Med*. 2010;42:97-114.

Laube S, Moss C. Pseudoxanthoma elasticum. *Arch Dis Child*. 2005;90:754-756.

Laufer F. The treatment of progressive pigmented purpura with ascorbic acid and a bioflavonoid rutoside. *J Drugs Dermatol*. 2006;5:290-293.

Lavogiez C, Delaporte E, Darras-Vercambre S, et al. Clinicopathological study of 13 cases of squamous cell carcinoma complicating hidradenitis suppurativa. *Dermatology*. 2010;220:147-153.

Leask A. Signaling in fibrosis: targeting the TGF beta, endothelin-1 and CCN2 axis in scleroderma. *Front Biosci*. 2009;1:115-122.

Lee DY, Lee JH. Epidermal grafting for vitiligo: a comparison of cultured and noncultured grafts. *Clin Exp Dermatol*. 2010;35:325-326.

Lee LA. The clinical spectrum of neonatal lupus. *Arch Dermatol Res*. 2009;301:107-110.

Lee WJ, Kim CH, Chang SE, et al. Generalized idiopathic neutrophilic eccrine hidradenitis in childhood. *Int J Dermatol*. 2010;49:75-78.

Leung DY, Boguniewicz M, Howell MD, et al. New insights into atopic dermatitis. *J Clin Invest*. 2004;113:651-657.

Leung PC. Diabetic foot ulcers—a comprehensive review. *Surgeon*. 2007;5:219-231.

Levi M. Disseminated intravascular coagulation in cancer patients. *Best Pract Res Clin Haematol*. 2009;22:129-136.

Levy Bencheton A, Pagès F, Berenger JM, et al. Bedbug dermatitis (cimex lectularius). *Ann Dermatol Venereol*. 2010;137:53-55.

Li Q, Jiang Q, Pfendner E, et al. Pseudoxanthoma elasticum: clinical phenotypes, molecular genetics and putative pathomechanisms. *Exp Dermatol*. 2009;18:1-11.

Lim SH, Kim SM, Oh BH, et al. Low-dose ultraviolet A1 phototherapy for treating pityriasis rosea. *Ann Dermatol*. 2009;21:230-236.

Lipozenci J, Wolf R. The diagnostic value of atopy patch testing and prick testing in atopic dermatitis: facts and controversies. *Clin Dermatol*. 2010;28:38-44.

Lo YH, Cheng GS, Huang CC, et al. Efficacy and safety of topical tacrolimus for the treatment of face and neck vitiligo. *J Dermatol*. 2010;37:125-129.

Lolis MS, Bowe WP, Shalita AR. Acne and systemic disease. *Med Clin North Am*. 2009;93:1161-1181.

Lowes MA, Bowcock AM, Krueger JG. Pathogenesis and therapy of psoriasis. *Nature*. 2007;445:866-873.

Luch A. Mechanistic insights on spider neurotoxins. *EXS*. 2010;100:293-315.

Lynch PJ. Lichen simplex chronicus (atopic/neurodermatitis) of the anogenital region. *Dermatol Ther*. 2004;17:8-19.

Madan V, Chinoy H, Griffiths CE, et al. Defining cancer risk in dermatomyositis. Part I. *Clin Exp Dermatol*. 2009;34:451-455.

Madrigal-Martínez-Pereda C, Guerrero-Rodríguez V, Guisado-Moya B, et al. Langerhans cell histiocytosis: literature review and descriptive analysis of oral manifestations. *Med Oral Patol Oral Cir Bucal*. 2009;14:E222-E228.

Magro CM, Schaefer JT, Crowson AN, et al. Pigmented purpuric dermatosis: classification by phenotypic and molecular profiles. *Am J Clin Pathol*. 2007;128:218-229.

Makdsi F, Fall A. Acute pancreatitis with eruptive xanthomas. *J Hosp Med*. 2010;5:115.

Mammen AL. Dermatomyositis and polymyositis: clinical presentation, autoantibodies, and pathogenesis. *Ann N Y Acad Sci*. 2010;1184:134-153.

Mana J, Marcoval J. Erythema nodosum. *Clin Dermatol*. 2007;25:288-294.

Marks JG, Elsner P, DeLeo V. *Contact & Occupational Dermatology*. 3rd ed. St. Louis: Mosby; 2002.

Marqueling AL, Gilliam AE, Prendiville J, et al. Keratosis pilaris rubra. A common but underrecognized condition. *Arch Dermatol.* 2006;142:1611-1616.

Martín-Brufau R, Corbalán-Berná J, Ramirez-Andreo A, et al. Personality differences between patients with lichen simplex chronicus and normal population: a study of pruritus. *Eur J Dermatol.* 2010;20:359-363.

Marzano AV, Vezzoli P, Crosti C. Drug-induced lupus: an update on its dermatologic aspects. *Lupus.* 2009;18:935-940.

Mataix J, Betlloch I. Langerhans cell histiocytosis: an update. *G Ital Dermatol Venereol.* 2009;144:119-134.

Matusiak Ł, Bieniek A, Szepietowski JC. Hidradenitis suppurativa markedly decreases quality of life and professional activity. *J Am Acad Dermatol.* 2010;62:706-708.

Matz H, Orion E, Wolf R. Pruritic urticarial papules and plaques of pregnancy: polymorphic eruption of pregnancy (PUPPP). *Clin Dermatol.* 2006;24:105-108.

Mazereeuw-Hautier J, Bezio S, Mahe E, et al. Segmental and non-segmental childhood vitiligo has distinct clinical characteristics: a prospective observational study. *J Am Acad Dermatol.* 2010; 62:945-949.

McIntosh BC, Lahinjani S, Narayan D. Necrobiosis lipoidica resulting in squamous cell carcinoma. *Conn Med.* 2005;69: 401-403.

Mill J, Wallis B, Cuttle L, et al. Phytophotodermatitis: case reports of children presenting with blistering after preparing lime juice. *Burns.* 2008;34:731-733.

Mizukawa Y, Shiohara T. Fixed drug eruption: a prototypic disorder mediated by effector memory T cells. *Curr Allergy Asthma Rep.* 2009;9:71-77.

Mok CC. Update on emerging drug therapies for systemic lupus erythematosus. *Expert Opin Emerg Drugs.* 2010;15:53-70.

Mold JW, Thompson DM. Management of brown recluse spider bites in primary care. *J Am Board Fam Pract.* 2004;17:347-352.

Morava E, Guillard M, Lefeber DJ, et al. Autosomal recessive cutis laxa syndrome revisited. *Eur J Hum Genet.* 2009;17: 1099-1110.

Mosher DB, Parrish JA, Fitzpatrick TB. Monobenzylether of hydroquinone: a retrospective study of treatment of 18 vitiligo patients and a review of the literature. *Br J Dermatol.* 1977;97: 669-679.

Musso CG, Enz PA, Guelman R, et al. Non-ulcerating calcific uremic arteriolopathy skin lesion treated successfully with intravenous ibandronate. *Perit Dial Int.* 2006;26:717-718.

Neoh CY, Tan AW, Mohamed K, et al. Characterization of the inflammatory cell infiltrate in herald patches and fully developed eruptions of pityriasis rosea. *Clin Exp Dermatol.* 2010;35: 300-304.

Neogi T. Clinical practice. Gout. *N Engl J Med.* 2011;364: 443-452.

Newman JS, Fung MA. Elastosis perforans serpiginosa in a patient with trisomy 21. *Dermatol Online J.* 2006;12:5.

Ng ES, Aw DC, Tan KB, et al. Neutrophilic eccrine hidradenitis associated with decitabine. *Leuk Res.* 2010;34:e130-e132.

Nigliazzo A, Khoo S, Saxe A. Calciphylaxis. *Am Surg.* 2009;75: 516-518.

Nishiyama M, Kanazawa N, Hiroi A, et al. Lupus erythematosus tumidus in Japan: a case report and a review of the literature. *Mod Rheumatol.* 2009;19:567-572.

Nosbaum A, Vocanson M, Rozieres A, et al. Allergic and irritant contact dermatitis. *Eur J Dermatol.* 2009;19:325-332.

Obradovi R, Kesi L, Mihailovi D, et al. Malignant transformation of oral lichen planus. A case report. *West Indian Med J.* 2009;58:490-492.

O'Connell S. Lyme borreliosis: current issues in diagnosis and management. *Curr Opin Infect Dis.* 2010;23:231-235.

Oh BH, Lee YW, Choe YB, et al. Epidemiologic study of malassezia yeasts in seborrheic dermatitis patients by the analysis of 26S rDNA PCR-RFLP. *Ann Dermatol.* 2010;22:149-155.

Ohel I, Levy A, Silberstein T, et al. Pregnancy outcome of patients with pruritic urticarial papules and plaques of pregnancy. *J Matern Fetal Neonatal Med.* 2006;19:305-308.

Ong VH, Denton CP. Innovative therapies for systemic sclerosis. *Curr Opin Rheumatol.* 2010;22:264-272.

Osterne RL, Matos Brito RG, Pacheco IA, et al. Management of erythema multiforme associated with recurrent herpes infection: a case report. *J Can Dent Assoc.* 2009;75:597-601.

Owlia MB, Eley AR. Is the role of Chlamydia trachomatis underestimated in patients with suspected reactive arthritis? *Int J Rheum Dis.* 2010;13:27-38.

Panasiti V, Devirgiliis V, Curzio M, et al. Erythema annulare centrifugum as the presenting sign of breast carcinoma. *J Eur Acad Dermatol Venereol.* 2009;23:318-320.

Pardanani A, Tefferi A. Systemic mastocytosis in adults: a review on prognosis and treatment based on 342 Mayo Clinic patients and current literature. *Curr Opin Hematol.* 2010;17:125-132.

Parrillo SJ. Stevens-Johnson syndrome and toxic epidermal necrolysis. *Curr Allergy Asthma Rep.* 2007;7:243-247.

Paul AY, Creel N, Benson PM. What is your diagnosis? Solitary mastocytoma. *Cutis.* 2004;74:227, 234-236.

Peñas PF, Fernández-Herrera J, García-Diez A. Dermatologic treatment of cutaneous graft versus host disease. *Am J Clin Dermatol.* 2004;5:403-416.

Peyri J, Moreno A, Marcoval J. Necrobiosis lipoidica. *Semin Cutan Med Surg.* 2007;26:87-89.

Phornphutkul C, Introne WJ, Perry MB, et al. Natural history of alkaptonuria. *N Engl J Med.* 2002;347:2111-2112.

Pitt JJ. Newborn screening. *Clin Biochem Rev.* 2010;31:57-68.

Plomp AS, Toonstra J, Bergen AA, et al. Proposal for updating the pseudoxanthoma elasticum classification system and a review of the clinical findings. *Am J Med Genet A.* 2010;152A:1049-1058.

Poindexter GB, Burkhart CN, Morrell DS. Therapies for pediatric seborrheic dermatitis. *Pediatr Ann.* 2009;38:333-338.

Postlethwaite AE, Harris LJ, Raza SH, et al. Pharmacotherapy of systemic sclerosis. *Expert Opin Pharmacother.* 2010;11:789-806.

Powell AM, Sakuma-Oyama Y, Oyama N, et al. Usefulness of BP180 NC16a enzyme-linked immunosorbent assay in the serodiagnosis of pemphigoid gestationis and in differentiating between pemphigoid gestationis and pruritic urticarial papules and plaques of pregnancy. *Arch Dermatol.* 2005;141:705-710.

Raju S, Hollis K, Neglen P. Use of compression stockings in chronic venous disease: patient compliance and efficacy. *Ann Vasc Surg.* 2007;21:790-795.

Ranque B, Mouthon L. Geoepidemiology of systemic sclerosis. *Autoimmun Rev.* 2010;9:A311-A318.

Rath N, Bhardwaj A, Kar HK, et al. Penicillamine induced pseudoxanthoma elasticum with elastosis perforans serpiginosa. *Indian J Dermatol Venereol Leprol.* 2005;71:182-185.

Ratzinger G, Burgdorf W, Zelger BG, et al. Acute febrile neutrophilic dermatosis: a histopathologic study of 31 cases with review of literature. *Am J Dermatopathol.* 2007;29:125-133.

Raymond CB, Wazny LD, Sood AR. Sodium thiosulfate, bisphosphonates, and cinacalcet for calciphylaxis. *CANNT J.* 2009; 19:25-29.

Renner R, Sticherling M. The different faces of cutaneous lupus erythematosus. *G Ital Dermatol Venereol.* 2009;144:135-147.

Requena L, Yus ES. Erythema nodosum. *Dermatol Clin.* 2008; 26:425-438.

Rigopoulos D, Larios G, Katsambas AD. The role of isotretinoin in acne therapy: why not as first-line therapy? Facts and controversies. *Clin Dermatol.* 2010;28:24-30.

Rijal A, Agrawal S. Outcome of Stevens Johnson syndrome and toxic epidermal necrolysis treated with corticosteroids. *Indian J Dermatol Venereol Leprol.* 2009;75:613-614.

Ringpfeil F. Selected disorders of connective tissue: pseudoxanthoma elasticum, cutis laxa, and lipoid proteinosis. *Clin Dermatol.* 2005;23:41-46.

Rodrigue-Gervais IG, Saleh M. Generics of inflammasome-associated disorders: a lesson in the guiding principles of inflammasome function. *Eur J Immunol.* 2010;40:643-648.

Rodriguez-Revenga L, Iranzo P, Badenas C, et al. A novel elastin gene mutation resulting in an autosomal dominant form of cutis laxa. *Arch Dermatol.* 2004;140:1135-1139.

Rosen LB, Muellenhoff M, Tran TT, et al. Elastosis perforans serpiginosa secondary to D-penicillamine therapy with coexisting cutis laxa. *Cutis.* 2005;76:49-53.

Runge MS, Greganti MA. *Netter's Internal Medicine.* 2nd ed. Philadelphia: Saunders; 2009:1045-1051.

Ryan C, Menter A, Warren RB. The latest advances in pharmacogenetics and pharmacogenomics in the treatment of psoriasis. *Mol Diagn Ther.* 2010;14:81-93.

Saeki H, Tomita M, Kai H, et al. Necrobiotic xanthogranuloma with paraproteinemia successfully treated with melphalan, prednisolone and skin graft. *J Dermatol.* 2007;34:795-797.

Sălăvăstru C, Tiplica GS. Therapeutic hotline: ulcerative lichen planus—treatment challenges. *Dermatol Ther.* 2010;23:203-205.

Sarkany RP, Monk BE, Handfield-Jones SE. Telangiectasia macularis eruptiva perstans: a case report and review of the literature. *Clin Exp Dermatol.* 1998;23:38-39.

Sasseville D. Clinical patterns of phytodermatitis. *Dermatol Clin.* 2009;27:299-308.

Satter EK, High WA. Langerhans cell histiocytosis: a review of the current recommendations of the Histiocyte Society. *Pediatr Dermatol.* 2008;25:291-295.

Sawamura A, Hayakawa M, Gando S, et al. Disseminated intravascular coagulation with a fibrinolytic phenotype at an early phase of trauma predicts mortality. *Thromb Res.* 2009;124:608-613.

Saxena M, Tope WD. Response of elastosis perforans serpiginosa to pulsed CO_2, Er: YAG, and dye lasers. *Dermatol Surg.* 2003; 29:677-678.

Schaffer JV. The changing face of graft-versus-host disease. *Semin Cutan Med Surg.* 2006;25:190-200.

Scheinfeld N. Pruritic urticarial papules and plaques of pregnancy wholly abated with one week twice daily application of fluticasone propionate lotion: a case report and review of the literature. *Dermatol Online J.* 2008;15;14:4.

Scheinfeld N, Berk T. A review of the diagnosis and treatment of rosacea. *Postgrad Med.* 2010;122:139-143.

Schiano Lomoriello D, Parravano MC, Chiaravalloti A, et al. Choroidal neovascularization in angioid streaks and pseudoxanthoma elasticum: 1 year follow-up. *Eur J Ophthalmol.* 2009;19: 151-153.

Schlieper G, Brandenburg V, Ketteler M, et al. Sodium thiosulfate in the treatment of calcific uremic arteriolopathy. *Nat Rev Nephrol.* 2009;5:539-543.

Schwartz RA, Nervi SJ. Erythema nodosum: a sign of systemic disease. *Am Fam Physician.* 2007;75:695-700.

Scott AT, Metzig AM, Hames RK, et al. Acanthosis nigricans and oral glucose tolerance in obese children. *Clin Pediatr.* 2010;49:69-71.

Segelmark M, Selga D. The challenge of managing patients with polyarteritis nodosa. *Curr Opin Rheumatol.* 2007;19:33-38.

Selva-O'Callaghan A, Grau JM, Gámez-Cenzano C, et al. Conventional cancer screening versus PET/CT in dermatomyositis/ polymyositis. *Am J Med.* 2010;123:558-562.

Shamban AT, Narurkar VA. Multimodal treatment of acne, acne scars and pigmentation. *Dermatol Clin.* 2009;27:459-471.

Shaw MG, Burkhart CN, Morrell DS. Systemic therapies for pediatric atopic dermatitis: a review for the primary care physician. *Pediatr Ann.* 2009;38:380-387.

Shen Z, Hao F, Wei P. HAIR-AN syndrome in a male adolescent with concomitant vitiligo. *Arch Dermatol.* 2009;145:492-494.

Shenefelt PD. Biofeedback, cognitive-behavioral methods, and hypnosis in dermatology: is it all in your mind? *Dermatol Ther.* 2003;16:114-122.

Shimizu S, Yasui C, Shiroshita K, et al. Calciphylaxis with unusual skin manifestations. *Eur J Dermatol.* 2010;20:241-242.

Shinkai K, McCalmont TH, Leslie KS. Cryopyrin-associated periodic syndromes and autoinflammation. *Clin Exp Dermatol.* 2008;33:1-9.

Shiohara T. Fixed drug eruption: pathogenesis and diagnostic tests. *Curr Opin Allergy Clin Immunol.* 2009;9:316-321.

Silapunt S, Chon SY. Generalized necrobiotic xanthogranuloma successfully treated with lenalidomide. *J Drugs Dermatol.* 2010; 9:273-276.

Silver MJ, Ansel GM. Femoropopliteal occlusive disease: diagnosis, indications for treatment, and results of interventional therapy. *Catheter Cardiovasc Interv.* 2002;56:555-561.

Silver RM, Major H. Maternal coagulation disorders and postpartum hemorrhage. *Clin Obstet Gynecol.* 2010;53:252-264.

Simpson EL. Atopic dermatitis: a review of topical treatment options. *Curr Med Res Opin.* 2010;26:633-640.

Soter NA. Mastocytosis and the skin. *Hematol Oncol Clin North Am.* 2000;14:537-555.

Sotozono C, Ueta M, Kinoshita S. Systemic and local management at the onset of Stevens-Johnson syndrome and toxic epidermal necrolysis with ocular complications. *Am J Ophthalmol.* 2010; 149:354.

Sperling LC, Nguyen JV. Commentary: treatment of lichen planopilaris: some progress, but a long way to go. *J Am Acad Dermatol.* 2010;62:398-401.

Spicknall KE, Mehregan DA. Necrobiotic xanthogranuloma. *Int J Dermatol.* 2009;48:1-10.

Spitz JL. *Genodermatoses: A Clinical Guide to Genetic Skin Disorders.* 2nd ed. Philadelphia: Lippincott Williams & Wilkins; 2005: 334-337.

Stefanaki I, Katsambas A. Therapeutic update on seborrheic dermatitis. *Skin Therapy Lett.* 2010;15:1-4.

Sugandhan S, Khandpur S, Sharma VK. Familial chylomicronemia syndrome. *Pediatr Dermatol.* 2007;24:323-325.

Takai T, Matsunaga A. A case of neutrophilic eccrine hidradenitis associated with streptococcal infectious endocarditis. *Dermatology.* 2006;212:203-205.

Tchernev G, Patterson JW, Nenoff P, et al. Sarcoidosis of the skin—a dermatological puzzle: important differential diagnostic aspects and guidelines for clinical and histopathological recognition. *J Eur Acad Dermatol Venereol.* 2010;24:125-137.

Thiboutot DM, Fleischer AB, Del Rosso JQ Jr, et al. Azelaic acid 15% gel once daily versus twice daily in papulopustular rosacea. *J Drugs Dermatol.* 2008;7:541-546.

Thiboutot DM, Gollnick H, Bettoli V, et al. New insights into the management of acne: an update from the global alliance to improve outcomes in acne group. *J Am Acad Dermatol.* 2009; 60:S1-S50.

Thompson DF, Montarella KE. Drug-induced Sweet's syndrome. *Ann Pharmacother.* 2007;41:802-811.

Thyssen JP, Johansen JD, Linneberg A, et al. The epidemiology of hand eczema in the general population—prevalence and main findings. *Contact Dermatitis.* 2010;62:75-87.

Tlougan BE, Podjasek JO, Dickman PS, et al. Painful plantar papules and nodules in a child. Palmoplantar eccrine hidradenitis (PEH). *Pediatr Ann.* 2008;37:83-84.

Toh CH, Hoots WK. SSC on disseminated intravascular coagulation of the ISTH. The scoring system of the Scientific and Standardisation Committee on Disseminated Intravascular Coagulation of the International Society on Thrombosis and Haemostasis: a 5-year overview. *J Thromb Haemost.* 2007;5: 604-606.

Tsai H. Pathophysiology of thrombotic thrombocytopenic purpura. *Int J Hematol.* 2010;91:1-9.

Uzzan B, Konate L, Diop A, et al. Efficacy of four insect repellents against mosquito bites: a double-blind randomized placebo-controlled field study in Senegal. *Fundam Clin Pharmacol*. 2009; 23:589-594.

Valencia IC, Falabella A, Kirsner RS, et al. Chronic venous insufficiency and venous leg ulceration. *J Am Acad Dermatol*. 2001; 44:401-421.

Valent P, Horny HP, Escribano L, et al. Diagnostic criteria and classification of mastocytosis: a consensus proposal. *Leuk Res*. 2001;25:603-625.

van der Hilst JC, Bodar EJ, Barron KS. Long-term follow up, clinical features, and quality of life in a series of 103 patients with hyperimmunoglobulinemia D syndrome. *Medicine*. 2008; 87:301-310.

Vanderhooft SL, Francis JS, Holbrook KA, et al. Familial pityriasis rubra pilaris. *Arch Dermatol*. 1995;131:448-453.

Ventura F, Vilarinho C, da Luz Duarte M, et al. Two cases of annular elastolytic granuloma: different response to the treatment. *Dermatol Online J*. 2010;16:11.

Vergilis-Kalner IJ, Mann DJ, Wasserman J, et al. Pityriasis rubra pilaris sensitive to narrow band-ultraviolet B light therapy. *J Drugs Dermatol*. 2008;8:270-273.

Villalón G, Martin JM, Monteagudo C, et al. Eruptive xanthomas after onset of diabetes mellitus. *Actas Dermosifiliogr*. 2008; 99:426-427.

Wada H, Asakura H, Okamoto K, et al. Expert consensus for the treatment of disseminated intravascular coagulation in Japan. Japanese Society of Thrombosis Hemostasis/DIC subcommittee. *Thromb Res*. 2010;125:6-11.

Walling HW, Sontheimer RD. Cutaneous lupus erythematosus: issues in diagnosis and treatment. *Am J Clin Dermatol*. 2009;10:365-381.

Walling HW, Swick BL. Pityriasis rubra pilaris responding rapidly to adalimumab. *Arch Dermatol*. 2009;145:99-101.

Walton KE, Bowers EV, Drolet BA, et al. Childhood lichen planus: demographics of a U.S. population. *Pediatr Dermatol*. 2010;27: 34-38.

Warren RB, Griffiths CE. The future of biological therapies. *Semin Cutan Med Surg*. 2010;29:63-66.

Wedderburn LR, Rider LG. Juvenile dermatomyositis: new developments in pathogenesis, assessment and treatment. *Best Pract Res Clin Rheumatol*. 2009;23:665-678.

Weedon D. *Skin Pathology*. Edinburgh: Churchill Livingstone; 1997.

Wetter DA, Camilleri MJ. Clinical, etiologic, and histopathologic features of Stevens-Johnson syndrome during an 8-year period at Mayo Clinic. *Mayo Clin Proc*. 2010;85:131-138.

Whitton ME, Pinart M, Batchelor J, et al. Interventions for vitiligo. Cochrane Database Syst Rev. 2010;CD003263.

Wilmer WA, Magro CM. Calciphylaxis: emerging concepts in prevention, diagnosis, and treatment. *Semin Dial*. 2002;15: 172-186.

Windebank K, Nanduri V. Langerhans cell histiocytosis. *Arch Dis Child*. 2009;94:904-908.

Wolinsky CD, Waldorf H. Chronic venous disease. *Med Clin North Am*. 2009;93:1333-1346.

Wood AJ, Wagner MV, Abbott JJ, et al. Necrobiotic xanthogranuloma: a review of 17 cases with emphasis on clinical and pathologic correlation. *Arch Dermatol*. 2009;145:279-284.

Yang CC, Shih IH, Lin WL, et al. Juvenile pityriasis rubra pilaris: report of 28 cases in Taiwan. *J Am Acad Dermatol*. 2008; 59:943-948.

Yang Y, Xu J, Li F, et al. Combination therapy of intravenous immunoglobulin and corticosteroid in the treatment of toxic epidermal necrolysis and Stevens-Johnson syndrome: a retrospective comparative study in China. *Int J Dermatol*. 2009; 48:1122-1128.

Youn SW. The role of facial sebum secretion in acne pathogenesis: facts and controversies. *Clin Dermatol*. 2010;28:8-11.

Zancanaro PC, Isaac AR, Garcia LT, et al. Localized scleroderma in children: clinical, diagnostic and therapeutic aspects. *An Bras Dermatol*. 2009;84:161-172.

Zetterström R. Kostman disease—infantile genetic agranulocytosis: historical views and new aspects. *Acta Pædiatr*. 2002;91: 1279-1281.

Ziemer M, Eisendle K, Zelger B. New concepts on erythema annulare centrifugum: a clinical reaction pattern that does not represent a specific clinicopathological entity. *Br J Dermatol*. 2009;160:119-126.

Zulian F. New developments in localized scleroderma. *Curr Opin Rheumatol*. 2008;20:601-607.

Section 5: Autoimmune Blistering Diseases

Al-Amoudi A, Frangakis AS. Structural studies on desmosomes. *Biochem Soc Trans*. 2008;36(Pt 2):181-187.

Alonso-Llamazares J, Gibson LE, Rogers RS 3rd. Clinical, pathologic, and immunopathologic features of dermatitis herpetiformis: review of the Mayo Clinic experience. *Int J Dermatol*. 2007;46:910-919.

Amagai M. Non-pathogenic anti-desmoglein 3 IgG autoantibodies in Fogo Selvagem. *J Invest Dermatol*. 2006;126:1931-1932.

Anhalt GJ, Kim SC, Stanley JR, et al. Paraneoplastic pemphigus—an autoimmune mucocutaneous disease associated with neoplasia. *N Engl J Med*. 1990;323:1729-1735.

Barnadas M, Roe E, Brunet S, et al. Therapy of paraneoplastic pemphigus with rituximab: a case report and review of literature. *J Eur Acad Dermatol Venereol*. 2006;20:69-74.

Baroni A, Lanza A, Cirillo N, et al. Vesicular and bullous disorders: pemphigus. *Dermatol Clin*. 2007;25:597-603.

Billet SE, Grando SA, Pittelkow MR. Paraneoplastic autoimmune multiorgan syndrome: review of the literature and support for a cytotoxic role in pathogenesis. *Autoimmunity*. 2006;39:617-630.

Bolognia JL, Jorizzo JL, Rapini RP. *Dermatology*. 2nd ed. Philadelphia: Mosby; 2008:403-446.

Bruch-Gerharz D, Hertl M, Ruzicka T. Mucous membrane pemphigoid: clinical aspects, immunopathological features and therapy. *Eur J Dermatol*. 2007;17:191-200.

Caldarola G, Annese V, Bossa F, et al. Linear IgA bullous dermatosis and ulcerative colitis treated by proctocolectomy. *Eur J Dermatol*. 2009;19:651.

Caproni M, Antiga E, Melani L, et al. Guidelines for the diagnosis and treatment of dermatitis herpetiformis. *J Eur Acad Dermatol Venereol*. 2009;23:633-638.

Chang JH, McCluskey PJ. Ocular cicatricial pemphigoid: manifestations and management. *Curr Allergy Asthma Rep*. 2005;5: 333-338.

Chung HJ, Uitto J. Type VII collagen: the anchoring fibril protein at fault in dystrophic epidermolysis bullosa. *Dermatol Clin*. 2010;28:93-105.

Culton DA, Qian Y, Li N, et al. Advances in pemphigus and its endemic pemphigus foliaceus (Fogo Selvagem) phenotype: a paradigm of human autoimmunity. *J Autoimmun*. 2008;31: 311-324.

Daniel E, Thorne JE. Recent advances in mucous membrane pemphigoid. *Curr Opin Ophthalmol*. 2008;19:292-297.

Dart J. Cicatricial pemphigoid and dry eye. *Semin Ophthalmol*. 2005;20:95-100.

Dasher D, Rubenstein D, Diaz LA. Pemphigus foliaceus. *Curr Dir Autoimmun*. 2008;10:182-194.

de Pereda JM, Lillo MP, Sonnenberg A. Structural basis of the interaction between integrin alpha6beta4 and plectin at the hemidesmosomes. *EMBO J*. 2009;28:1180-1190.

Edgin WA, Pratt TC, Grimwood RE. Pemphigus vulgaris and paraneoplastic pemphigus. *Oral Maxillofac Surg Clin North Am*. 2008;20:577-584.

Egan CA, Zone JJ. Linear IgA bullous dermatosis. *Int J Dermatol*. 1999;38:818-827.

Eschle-Meniconi ME, Ahmad SR, Foster CS. Mucous membrane pemphigoid: an update. *Curr Opin Ophthalmol*. 2005;16: 303-307.

Flores G, Qian Y, Díaz LA. The enigmatic autoimmune response in endemic pemphigus foliaceus. *Actas Dermosifiliogr*. 2009;100 (Suppl 2):40-48.

Hernandez L, Green PH. Extraintestinal manifestations of celiac disease. *Curr Gastroenterol Rep*. 2006;8:383-389.

Hingorani M, Lightman S. Ocular cicatricial pemphigoid. *Curr Opin Allergy Clin Immunol*. 2006;6:373-378.

Humbert P, Pelletier F, Dreno B, et al. Gluten intolerance and skin diseases. *Eur J Dermatol*. 2006;16:4-11.

James WD, Berger TG, Elston DM. *Andrews' Diseases of the Skin: Clinical Dermatology*. Philadelphia: Saunders; 2006:464-465.

Joly P, Roujeau JC, Benichou J, et al. A comparison of oral and topical corticosteroids in patients with bullous pemphigoid. *N Eng J Med*. 2002;346:321-327.

Kasperkiewicz M, Schmidt E. Current treatment of autoimmune blistering diseases. *Curr Drug Discov Technol*. 2009;6:270-280.

Kasperkiewicz M, Zillikens D. The pathophysiology of bullous pemphigoid. *Clin Rev Allergy Immunol*. 2007;33:67-77.

Kharfi M, Khaled A, Karaa A, et al. Linear IgA bullous dermatosis: the more frequent bullous dermatosis of children. *Dermatol Online J*. 2010;16:2.

Kitajima Y. Cross-talk between hemidesmosomes and focal contacts: understanding subepidermal blistering diseases. *J Invest Dermatol*. 2010;130:1493-1496.

Korman NJ. New and emerging therapies in the treatment of blistering diseases. *Dermatol Clin*. 2000;18:127-137.

Lehman JS, Camilleri MJ, Gibson LE. Epidermolysis bullosa acquisita: concise review and practical considerations. *Int J Dermatol*. 2009;48:227-236.

Lessey E, Li N, Dias L, et al. Complement and cutaneous autoimmune blistering diseases. *Immunol Res*. 2008;41:223-232.

McDonald HC, York NR, Pandya AG. Drug-induced linear IgA bullous dermatosis demonstrating the isomorphic phenomenon. *J Am Acad Dermatol*. 2010;62:897-898.

McMillan JR, Akiyama M, Shimizu H. Epidermal basement membrane zone components: ultrastructural distribution and molecular interactions. *J Dermatol Sci*. 2003;31:169-177.

Mellerio JE. Molecular pathology of the cutaneous basement membrane zone. *Clin Exp Dermatol*. 1999;24:25-32.

Onodera H, Mihm MC Jr, Yoshida A, et al. Drug-induced linear IgA bullous dermatosis. *J Dermatol*. 2005;32:759-764.

Ozawa T, Tsuruta D, Jones JC, et al. Dynamic relationship of focal contacts and hemidesmosome protein complexes in live cells. *J Invest Dermatol*. 2010;130:1624-1635.

Remington J, Chen M, Burnett J, et al. Autoimmunity to type VII collagen: epidermolysis bullosa acquisita. *Curr Dir Autoimmun*. 2008;10:195-205.

Sehgal VN, Srivastava G. Paraneoplastic pemphigus/paraneoplastic autoimmune multiorgan syndrome. *Int J Dermatol*. 2009;48: 162-169.

Shimizu H. New insights into the immunoultrastructural organization of cutaneous basement membrane zone molecules. *Exp Dermatol*. 1998;7:303-313.

Shinkuma S, Nishie W, Shibaki A, et al. Cutaneous pemphigus vulgaris with skin features similar to the classic mucocutaneous type: a case report and review of the literature. *Clin Exp Dermatol*. 2008;33:724-728.

Stirling L, Kirsner RS. Evidence-based pemphigus treatment? *J Invest Dermatol*. 2010;130:1963.

Stokes DL. Desmosomes from a structural perspective. *Curr Opin Cell Biol*. 2007;19:565-571.

Templet JT, Welsh JP, Cusack CA. Childhood dermatitis herpetiformis: a case report and review of the literature. *Cutis*. 2007; 80:473-476.

Woodley DT, Remington J, Chen M. Autoimmunity to type VII collagen: epidermolysis bullosa acquisita. *Clin Rev Allergy Immunol*. 2007;33:78-84.

Zhu X, Zhang B. Paraneoplastic pemphigus. *J Dermatol*. 2007;34: 503-511.

Section 6: Infectious Diseases

Adams BB. New strategies for the diagnosis, treatment, and prevention of herpes simplex in contact sports. *Curr Sports Med Rep*. 2004;3:277-283.

Adams EN, Parnapy S, Bautista P. Herpes zoster and vaccination: a clinical review. *Am J Health Syst Pharm*. 2010;67:724-727.

Alfa M. The laboratory diagnosis of *Haemophilus ducreyi*. *Can J Infect Dis Med Microbiol*. 2005;16:31-34.

Anderson AL, Chaney E. Pubic lice (*Pthirus pubis*): history, biology and treatment vs. knowledge and beliefs of US college students. *Int J Environ Res Public Health*. 2009;6:592-600.

Andrews MD, Burns M. Common tinea infections in children. *Am Fam Physician*. 2008;77:1415-1420.

Ayyadurai S, Sebbane F, Raoult D, et al. Body lice, *Yersinia pestis* orientalis, and black death. *Emerg Infect Dis*. 2010;16: 892-893.

Bacelieri R, Johnson SM. Cutaneous warts: an evidence-based approach to therapy. *Am Fam Physician*. 2005;72:647-652.

Bachmeyer C, Buot G, Binet O, et al. Fixed cutaneous sporotrichosis: an unusual diagnosis in West Europe. *Clin Exp Dermatol*. 2006;31:479-481.

Bansal R, Tutrone WD, Weinberg JM. Viral skin infections in the elderly: diagnosis and management. *Drugs Aging*. 2002;19: 503-514.

Baringer JR. Herpes simplex infections of the nervous system. *Neurol Clin*. 2008;26:657-674.

Baughn RE, Musher DM. Secondary syphilitic lesions. *Clin Microbiol Rev*. 2005;18:205-216.

Bechah Y, Capo C, Mege JL, et al. Epidemic typhus. *Lancet Infect Dis*. 2008;8:417-426.

Benard G. An overview of the immunopathology of human paracoccidioidomycosis. *Mycopathologia*. 2008;165:209-221.

Biolcati G, Alabiso A. Creeping eruption of larva migrans—a case report in a beach volley athlete. *Int J Sports Med*. 1997;18: 612-613.

Bolognia JL, Jorizzo JL, Rapini RP. *Dermatology*. 2nd ed. St. Louis: Mosby; 2008.

Bonilla DL, Kabeya H, Henn J, et al. *Bartonella quintana* in body lice and head lice from homeless persons in San Francisco, California, USA. *Emerg Infect Dis*. 2009;15:912-915.

Borelli C, Korting HC, Bödeker RH, et al. Safety and efficacy of sertaconazole nitrate cream 2% in the treatment of tinea pedis interdigitalis: a subgroup analysis. *Cutis*. 2010;85:107-111.

Bouvresse S, Chosidow O. Scabies in healthcare settings. *Curr Opin Infect Dis*. 2010;23:111-118.

Bowman DD, Montgomery SP, Zajac AM, et al. Hookworms of dogs and cats as agents of cutaneous larva migrans. *Trends Parasitol*. 2010;26:162-167.

Bradsher RW, Chapman SW, Pappas PG. Blastomycosis. *Infect Dis Clin North Am*. 2003;17:21-40.

Bratton RL, Whiteside JW, Hovan MJ, et al. Diagnosis and treatment of Lyme disease. *Mayo Clin Proc*. 2008;83:566-571.

Brown M, Paulson C, Henry SL. Treatment for anogenital molluscum contagiosum. *Am Fam Physician*. 2009;80:864.

Burgess IF. Current treatments for pediculosis capitis. *Curr Opin Infect Dis*. 2009;22:131-136.

Carpenter JB, Feldman JS, Leyva WH, et al. Clinical and pathologic characteristics of disseminated cutaneous coccidioidomycosis. *J Am Acad Dermatol*. 2010;62:831-837.

Clarridge JE 3rd, Zhang Q. Genotypic diversity of clinical *Actinomyces* species: phenotype, source, and disease correlation among genospecies. *J Clin Microbiol.* 2002;40:3442-3448.
Coates CM, Boehm AP Jr, Leonheart EE, et al. Malignant transformation of plantar verrucae. *Adv Skin Wound Care.* 2006;19:384-385.
Coloe J, Burkhart CN, Morrell DS. Molluscum contagiosum: what's new and true? *Pediatr Ann.* 2009;38:321-325.
Creed R, Satyaprakash A, Ravanfar P. Varicella zoster vaccines. *Dermatol Ther.* 2009;22:143-149.
Currie BJ, McCarthy JS. Permethrin and ivermectin for scabies. *N Eng J Med.* 2010;362:717-725.
Davies HD, Sakuls P, Keystone JS. Creeping eruption. A review of clinical presentation and management of 60 cases presenting to a tropical disease unit. *Arch Dermatol.* 1993;129:588-591.
Dean D, Bruno WJ, Wan R, et al. Predicting phenotype and emerging strains among *Chlamydia trachomatis* infections. *Emerg Infect Dis.* 2009;15:1385-1394.
Deps P, Lockwood DN. Leprosy presenting as immune reconstitution inflammatory syndrome: proposed definitions and classification. *Lepr Rev.* 2010;81:59-68.
Domantay-Apostol GP, Handog EB, Gabriel MT. Syphilis: the international challenge of the great imitator. *Dermatol Clin.* 2008;26:191-202.
Dourmishev LA, Dourmishev AL. Syphilis: uncommon presentations in adults. *Clin Dermatol.* 2005;23:555-564.
Elston DM. Topical antibiotics in dermatology: emerging patterns of resistance. *Dermatol Clin.* 2009;27:25-31.
Fitzpatrick TB, Eisen AZ, Wolff K, et al., eds. *Dermatology in General Medicine.* 4th ed. New York: McGraw-Hill; 1993: 2753-2756.
Frankowski BL, Bocchini JA Jr. Head lice. *Pediatrics.* 2010;126: 392-403.
Gallo ES, Pehoushek JF, Crowson AN. An exophytic nasal nodule. Coccidioidomycosis. *Arch Dermatol.* 2010;146:789-794.
Garman ME, Orengo I. Unusual infectious complications of dermatologic procedures. *Dermatol Clin.* 2003;21:321-335.
Garvey K, Hinshaw M, Vanness E. Chronic disseminated cutaneous blastomycosis in an 11-year old, with a brief review of the literature. *Pediatr Dermatol.* 2006;23:541-545.
Geria AN, Schwartz RA. Impetigo update: new challenges in the era of methicillin resistance. *Cutis.* 2010;85:65-70.
Ghaninejad H, Hasibi M, Moslehi H, et al. Primary cutaneous actinomycosis of the elbow with an exceptionally long incubation period. *Int J Dermatol.* 2008;47:304-305.
Ghigliotti G, Carrega G, Farris A, et al. Cutaneous cryptococcosis resembling molluscum contagiosum in a homosexual man with AIDS. Report of a case and review of the literature. *Acta Derm Venereol.* 1992;72:182-184.
Goulart LR, Goulart IM. Leprosy pathogenic background: a review and lessons from other mycobacterial diseases. *Arch Dermatol Res.* 2009;301:123-127.
Gould D. An overview of molluscum contagiosum: a viral skin condition. *Nurs Stand.* 2008;22:45-48.
Gräser Y, Scott J, Summerbell R. The new species concept in dermatophytes—a polyphasic approach. *Mycopathologia.* 2008; 166:239-256.
Gupta AK, Cooper EA. Update in antifungal therapy of dermatophytosis. *Mycopathologia.* 2008;166:353-367.
Hardman S, Stephenson I, Jenkins DR, et al. Disseminated *Sporothix schenckii* in a patient with AIDS. *J Infect.* 2005;51:e73-e77.
Harrison LH. Epidemiological profile of meningococcal disease in the United States. *Clin Infect Dis.* 2010;50(Suppl 2):S37-S44.
Haruna K, Shiraki Y, Hiruma M, et al. A case of lymphangitic sporotrichosis occurring on both forearms with a published work review of cases of bilateral sporotrichosis in Japan. *J Dermatol.* 2006;33:364-367.
Hay RJ. Scabies and pyodermas—diagnosis and treatment. *Dermatol Ther.* 2009;22:466-474.
Herman BE, Corneli HM. A practical approach to warts in the emergency department. *Pediatr Emerg Care.* 2008;24:246-254.
Heukelbach J, Wilcke T, Feldmeier H. Cutaneous larva migrans (creeping eruption) in an urban slum in Brazil. *Int J Dermatol.* 2004;43:511-515.
Heukelbach J, Wilcke T, Meier A, et al. A longitudinal study on cutaneous larva migrans in an impoverished Brazilian township. *Travel Med Infect Dis.* 2003;1:213-218.
Hicks MI, Elston DM. Scabies. *Dermatol Ther.* 2009;22:279-292.
Hochedez P, Caumes E. Hookworm-related cutaneous larva migrans. *J Travel Med.* 2007;14:326-333.
Hope-Rapp E, Anyfantakis V, Fouéré S, et al. Etiology of genital ulcer disease. A prospective study of 278 cases seen in an STD clinic in Paris. *Sex Transm Dis.* 2010;37:153-158.
Howell ER, Phillips CM. Cutaneous manifestations of *Staphylococcus aureus* disease. *Skinmed.* 2007;6:274-279.
Janowicz DM, Li W, Bauer ME. Host-pathogen interplay of *Haemophilus ducreyi*. *Curr Opin Infect Dis.* 2010;23:64-69.
Jones S, Kress D. Treatment of molluscum contagiosum and herpes simplex virus cutaneous infections. *Cutis.* 2007;79(Suppl 4): S11-S17.
Kakourou T, Uksal U. Guidelines for the management of tinea capitis in children. *Pediatr Dermatol.* 2010;27:226-228.
Keogh-Brown MR, Fordham RJ, Thomas KS, et al. To freeze or not to freeze: a cost-effectiveness analysis of wart treatment. *Br J Dermatol.* 2007;156:687-692.
Kil EH, Heymann WR, Weinberg JM. Methicillin-resistant *Staphylococcus aureus*: an update for the dermatologist, Part 1: Epidemiology. *Cutis.* 2008;81:227-233.
Kil EH, Heymann WR, Weinberg JM. Methicillin-resistant *Staphylococcus aureus*: an update for the dermatologist. Part 2: Pathogenesis and cutaneous manifestations. *Cutis.* 2008;81: 247-254.
Kim KS. Acute bacterial meningitis in infants and children. *Lancet Infect Dis.* 2010;10:32-42.
Lautenschlager S. Cutaneous manifestations of syphilis: recognition and management. *Am J Clin Dermatol.* 2006;7:291-304.
Leatherman M. What is causing a persistent skin boil? *Adv Skin Wound Care.* 2005;18:30-31.
Lee SY, Kwon HJ, Cho JH, et al. Actinomycosis of the appendix mimicking appendiceal tumor: a case report. *World J Gastroenterol.* 2010;16:395-397.
Li W, Janowicz DM, Fortney KR, et al. Mechanism of human natural killer cell activation by *Haemophilus ducreyi*. *J Infect Dis.* 2009;200:590-598.
Lichon V, Khachemoune A. Plantar warts: a focus on treatment modalities. *Dermatol Nurs.* 2007;19:372-375.
Lübbe J. Secondary infections in patients with atopic dermatitis. *Am J Clin Dermatol.* 2003;4:641-654.
Lundqvist A, Kubler-Kielb J, Teneberg S, et al. Immunogenic and adjuvant properties of *Haemophilus ducreyi* lipooligosaccharides. *Microbes Infect.* 2009;11:352-360.
Malhotra VL, Sharma SK, Laskhmy A, et al. Case of Waterhouse Friderichsen syndrome during outbreak of meningococcal disease in Delhi in May 2005. *J Commun Dis.* 2005;37:159-161.
Martinez-Diaz GJ, Kim J, Bruckner AL. A toddler with facial nodules: a case of idiopathic facial aseptic granuloma. *Dermatol Online J.* 2010;16:9.
McElhaney JE. Herpes zoster: a common disease that can have a devastating impact on patients' quality of life. *Expert Rev Vaccines.* 2010;9(Suppl 3):S27-S30.
McKinnell JA, Pappas PG. Blastomycosis: new insights into diagnosis, prevention, and treatment. *Clin Chest Med.* 2009;30: 227-239.
Mele JA 3rd, Linder S, Capozzi A. Treatment of thromboembolic complications of fulminant meningococcal septic shock. *Ann Plast Surg.* 1997;38:283-290.
Mick G. Vaccination: a new option to reduce the burden of herpes zoster. *Expert Rev Vaccines.* 2010;9(Suppl 3):S31-S35.
Mohammed TT, Olumide YM. Chancroid and human immunodeficiency virus infection—a review. *Int J Dermatol.* 2008;47: 1-8.
Mora DJ, dos Santos CT, Silva-Vergara ML. Disseminated histoplasmosis in acquired immunodeficiency syndrome patients in Uberaba, MG, Brazil. *Mycoses.* 2008;51:136-140.
Morar N, Ramdial PK, Naidoo DK, et al. Lues maligna. *Br J Dermatol.* 1999;140:1175-1177.
Müllegger RR, Glatz M. Skin manifestations of Lyme borreliosis: diagnosis and management. *Am J Clin Dermatol.* 2008;9: 355-368.
Murray TS, Shapiro ED. Lyme disease. *Clin Lab Med.* 2010; 30:311-328.
Mustafa MB, Arduino PG, Porter SR. Varicella zoster virus: review of its management. *J Oral Pathol Med.* 2009;38:673-688.
Naka W, Masuda M, Konohana A, et al. Primary cutaneous cryptococcosis and *Cryptococcus neoformans* serotype D. *Clin Exp Dermatol.* 1995;20:221-225.
Newton HR, Lambiase MC. Disseminated cutaneous coccidioidomycosis masquerading as lupus pernio. *Cutis.* 2010;86:25-28.
Nikkels AF, Pièrard GE. Treatment of mucocutaneous presentations of herpes simplex virus infections. *Am J Clin Dermatol.* 2002;3:475-487.
Nordlund JJ. Cutaneous ectoparasites. *Dermatol Ther.* 2009;22: 503-517.
Odell CA. Community-associated methicillin-resistant *Staphylococcus aureus* (CA-MRSA) skin infections. *Curr Opin Pediatr.* 2010; 22:273-277.
Ohno S, Tanabe H, Kawasaki M, et al. Tinea corporis with acute inflammation caused by *Trichophyton tonsurans*. *J Dermatol.* 2008;35:590-593.
Ooi WW, Srinivasan J. Leprosy and the peripheral nervous system: basic and clinical aspects. *Muscle Nerve.* 2004;30:393-409.
Ozcan A, Senol M, Saglam H, et al. Comparison of the Tzanck test and polymerase chain reaction in the diagnosis of cutaneous herpes simplex and varicella zoster virus infections. *Int J Dermatol.* 2007;46:1177-1179.
Panackal AA, Halpern EF, Watson AJ. Cutaneous fungal infections in the United States: Analysis of the National Ambulatory Medical Care Survey (NAMCS) and National Hospital Ambulatory Medical Care Survey (NHAMCS), 1995-2004. *Int J Dermatol.* 2009;48:704-712.
Patel AR, Romanelli P, Roberts B, et al. Treatment of herpes simplex virus infection: rationale for occlusion. *Adv Skin Wound Care.* 2007;20:408-412.
Patel GA, Wiederkehr M, Schwartz RA. Tinea cruris in children. *Cutis.* 2009;84:133-137.
Patil D, Siddaramappa B, Manjunathswamy BS, et al. Primary cutaneous actinomycosis. *Int J Dermatol.* 2008;47:1271-1273.
Paul AY, Aldrich S, Scott RS, et al. Disseminated histoplasmosis in a patient with AIDS: case report and review of the literature. *Cutis.* 2007;80:309-312.
Peel TN, Bhatti D, De Boer JC, et al. Chronic cutaneous ulcers secondary to *Haemophilus ducreyi* infection. *Med J Aust.* 2010; 192:348-350.
Pietras TA, Baum CL, Swick BL. Coexistent Kaposi sarcoma, cryptococcosis, and *Mycobacterium avium* intracellulare in a solitary cutaneous nodule in a patient with AIDS: report of a case and literature review. *J Am Acad Dermatol.* 2010;62: 676-680.
Pinckney J 2nd, Cole P, Vadapalli SP, et al. *Phthiriasis palpebrarum:* a common culprit with uncommon presentation. *Dermatol Online J.* 2008;14:7.
Ramos-E-Silva M, Saraiva Ldo E. Paracoccidioidomycosis. *Dermatol Clin.* 2008;26:257-269.
Ramos-E-Silva M, Vasconcelos C, Carneiro S, et al. Sporotrichosis. *Clin Dermatol.* 2007;25:181-187.
Reichenbach J, Lopatin U, Mahlaoui N, et al. *Actinomyces* in chronic granulomatous disease: an emerging and unanticipated pathogen. *Clin Infect Dis.* 2009;49:1703-1710.
Restrepo A, Benard G, de Castro CC, et al. Pulmonary paracoccidioidomycosis. *Semin Respir Crit Care Med.* 2008;29: 182-197.
Revenga F, Paricio JF, Merino FJ, et al. Primary cutaneous cryptococcosis in an immunocompetent host: case report and review of the literature. *Dermatology.* 2002;204:145-149.
Romano C, Castelli A, Laurini L, et al. Case report. Primary cutaneous histoplasmosis in an immunosuppressed patient. *Mycoses.* 2000;43:151-154.
Rosen T, Brown TJ. Cutaneous manifestations of sexually transmitted diseases. *Med Clin North Am.* 1998;82:1081-1104.
Rosen T, Hwong H. Pedal interdigital condylomata lata: a rare sign of secondary syphilis. *Sex Transm Dis.* 2001;28:184-186.
Rosen T, Vandergriff T, Harting M. Antibiotic use in sexually transmissible diseases. *Dermatol Clin.* 2009;27:49-61.
Runge MS, Greganti MA, eds. *Netter's Internal Medicine.* 2nd ed. Philadelphia: Saunders; 2009:712-715.
Rutman H. Ivermectin versus malathion for head lice. *N Engl J Med.* 2010;362:2426-2427.
Saberi A, Syed SA. Meningeal signs: Kernig's sign and Brudzinski's sign. *Hosp Physician.* 1999;24:23-24.
Saccente M, Woods GL. Clinical and laboratory update on blastomycosis. *Clin Microbiol Rev.* 2010;23:367-381.
Salazar JC, Hazlett KR, Radolf JD. The immune response to infection with *Treponema pallidum*, the stealth pathogen. *Microbes Infect.* 2002;4:1133-1140.
Scheurich D, Woeltje K. Skin and soft tissue infections due to CA-MRSA. *Mo Med.* 2009;106:274-276.
Schmid DS, Jumaan AO. Impact of varicella vaccine on varicella-zoster virus dynamics. *Clin Microbiol Rev.* 2010;23:202-217.
Schubach A, Barros MB, Wanke B. Epidemic sporotrichosis. *Curr Opin Infect Dis.* 2008;21:129-133.
Sehgal VN, Srivastava G. Chancroid: contemporary appraisal. *Int J Dermatol.* 2003;42:182-190.
Silverberg NB. Human papillomavirus infections in children. *Curr Opin Pediatr.* 2004;16:402-409.
Snoeck R. Papillomavirus and treatment. *Antiviral Res.* 2006;71: 181-191.
Tan HH, Goh CL. Viral infections affecting the skin in organ transplant recipients: epidemiology and current management strategies. *Am J Clin Dermatol.* 2006;7:13-29.
Tan LK, Carlone GM, Borrow R. Advances in the development of vaccines against *Neisseria meningitidis*. *N Engl J Med.* 2010; 362:1511-1520.
Thomas I, Schwartz RA. Cutaneous manifestations of systemic cryptococcosis in immunosupressed patients. *J Med.* 2001;32: 259-266.
Thurnheer MC, Weber R, Toutous-Trellu L, et al. Occurrence, risk factors, diagnosis and treatment of syphilis in the prospective observational Swiss HIV Cohort Study. *AIDS.* 2010;24: 1907-1916.
Tucker JD, Shah S, Jarell AD, et al. Lues maligna in early HIV infection: case report and review of the literature. *Sex Transm Dis.* 2009;36:512-514.
Ulusoy S, Ozkan G, Bekta D, et al. Ramsay Hunt syndrome in renal transplantation recipient: a case report. *Transplant Proc.* 2010;42:1986-1988.
Vázquez M. Varicella infections and varicella vaccine in the 21st century. *Pediatr Infect Dis J.* 2004;23:871-872.
Visbal G, San-Blas G, Murgich J, et al. *Paracoccidioides brasiliensis*, paracoccidioidomycosis, and antifungal antibiotics. *Curr Drug Targets Infect Disord.* 2005;5:211-226.

Walsh DS, Portaels F, Meyers WM. Recent advances in leprosy and Buruli ulcer (*Mycobacterium ulcerans* infection). *Curr Opin Infect Dis*. 2010;23:445-455.

Watkins P. Identifying and treating plantar warts. *Nurs Stand*. 2006;20:50-54.

Welsh RD. Sporotrichosis. *J Am Vet Med Assoc*. 2003;223:1123-1126.

Wolf R, Davidovici B. Treatment of scabies and pediculosis: facts and controversies. *Clin Dermatol*. 2010;28:511-518.

Worobec SM. Treatment of leprosy/Hansen's disease in the early 21st century. *Dermatol Ther*. 2009;22:518-537.

Wu IB, Schwartz RA. Herpetic whitlow. *Cutis*. 2007;79:193-196.

Xue SL, Li L. Oral potassium iodide for the treatment of sporotrichosis. *Mycopathologia*. 2009;167:355-356.

Zargari O, Elpern DJ. Granulomatous diseases of the nose. *Int J Dermatol*. 2009;48:1275-1282.

Zetola N, Francis JS, Nuermberger EL, et al. Community-acquired methicillin-resistant Staphylococcus aureus: an emerging threat. *Lancet Infect Dis*. 2005;5:275-286.

Section 7: Hair and Nail Diseases

Avram M, Rogers N. Contemporary hair transplantation. *Dermatol Surg*. 2009;35:1705-1719.

Burk C, Hu S, Lee C, et al. Netherton syndrome and trichorrhexis invaginata—a novel diagnostic approach. *Pediatr Dermatol*. 2008;25:287-288.

Calderon P, Otberg N, Shapiro J. Uncombable hair syndrome. *J Am Acad Dermatol*. 2009;61:512-515.

Camacho FM, Randall VA, Proce VH, eds. *Hair and Its Disorders: Biology, Pathology, and Management*. London: Martin Dunitz Ltd.; 2000.

Cashman MW, Sloan SB. Nutrition and nail disease. *Clin Dermatol*. 2010;28:420-425.

Chamberlain SR, Odlaug BL, Boulougouris V, et al. Trichotillomania: neurobiology and treatment. *Neurosci Biobehav Rev*. 2009;33:831-842.

Chen W, Yang CC, Todorova A, et al. Hair loss in elderly women. *Eur J Dermatol*. 2010;20:145-151.

Cohen PR, Scher RK. Geriatric nail disorders: diagnosis and treatment. *J Am Acad Dermatol*. 1992;26:521-531.

DeBerker D. Childhood nail diseases. *Dermatol Clin*. 2006;24:355-363.

DeBerker D, Wojnarowska F, Sviland L, et al. Keratin expression in the normal nail unit: markers of regional differentiation. *Br J Dermatol*. 2000;142:89-96.

Duarte AF, Correia O, Barros AM, et al. Nail matrix melanoma in situ: conservative surgical management. *Dermatology*. 2010;220:173-175.

Duke DC, Keeley ML, Geffken GR, et al. Trichotillomania: a current review. *Clin Psychol Rev*. 2010;30:181-193.

Franklin ME, Edson AL, Freeman JB. Behavior therapy for pediatric trichotillomania: exploring the effects of age on treatment outcome. *Child Adolesc Psychiatry Ment Health*. 2010;4:18.

Gupta AK, Cooper EA. Psoriatic nail disease: quality of life and treatment. *J Cutan Med Surg*. 2009;13(Suppl 2):S102-S106.

Hadshiew IM, Foitzik K, Arck PC, et al. Burden of hair loss: stress and the underestimated psychosocial impact of telogen effluvium and androgenetic alopecia. *J Invest Dermatol*. 2004;123:455-457.

Harrison S, Bergfeld WF. Diseases of the hair and nails. *Med Clin North Am*. 2009;93:1195-1209.

Harrison S, Sinclair R. Telogen effluvium. *Clin Exp Dermatol*. 2002;27:389-395.

Heidelbaugh JJ, Lee H. Management of the ingrown toenail. *Am Fam Physician*. 2009;79:303-308.

Jadhav VM, Mahajan PM, Mhaske CB. Nail pitting and onycholysis. *Indian J Dermatol Venereol Leprol*. 2009;75:631-633.

Jaks V, Kasper M, Toftgård R. The hair follicle—a stem cell zoo. *Exp Cell Res*. 2010;316:1422-1428.

Kalish RS. Clues from alopecia areata on the role of neuropeptides in the initiation of autoimmunity. *J Invest Dermatol*. 2007;127:1289-1291.

Kos L, Conlon J. An update on alopecia areata. *Curr Opin Pediatr*. 2009;21:475-480.

Lee JY. Severe 20-nail psoriasis successfully treated with low dose methotrexate. *Dermatol Online J*. 2009;15:8.

Mancini C, Van Ameringen M, Patterson B, et al. Trichotillomania in youth: a retrospective case series. *Depress Anxiety*. 2009;26:661-665.

Mirmirani P, Samimi SS, Mostow E. Pili torti: clinical findings, associated disorders, and new insights into mechanisms of hair twisting. *Cutis*. 2009;84:143-147.

Myung P, Andl T, Ito M. Defining the hair follicle stem cell (Part I). *J Cutan Pathol*. 2009;36:1031-1034.

Myung P, Andl T, Ito M. Defining the hair follicle stem cell (Part II). *J Cutan Pathol*. 2009;36:1134-1137.

Rathnayake D, Sinclair R. Male androgenetic alopecia. *Expert Opin Pharmacother*. 2010;11:1295-1304.

Rigopoulos D, Larios G, Gregoriou S, et al. Acute and chronic paronychia. *Am Fam Physician*. 2008;77:339-346.

Rogers NE, Avram MR. Medical treatments for male and female pattern hair loss. *J Am Acad Dermatol*. 2008;59:547-568.

Schweizer J. More than one gene involved in monilethrix: intracellular but also extracellular players. *J Invest Dermatol*. 2006;126:1216-1219.

Seavolt MB, Sarro RA, Levin K, et al. Mees' lines in a patient following acute arsenic intoxication. *Int J Dermatol*. 2002;41:399-401.

Stefanato CM. Histopathology of alopecia: a clinicopathological approach to diagnosis. *Histopathology*. 2010;56:24-38.

Trüeb RM. Chemotherapy-induced alopecia. *Semin Cutan Med Surg*. 2009;28:11-14.

Wallace MP, de Berker DA. Hair diagnoses and signs: the use of dermatoscopy. *Clin Exp Dermatol*. 2010;35:41-46.

Wasserman D, Guzman-Sanchez DA, Scott K, et al. Alopecia areata. *Int J Dermatol*. 2007;46:121-131.

Wegener EE, Johnson WR. Identification of common nail and skin disorders. *J Hand Ther*. 2010;23:187-198.

Welsh O, Vera-Cabrera L, Welsh E. Onychomycosis. *Clin Dermatol*. 2010;28:151-159.

Wosicka H, Cal K. Targeting to the hair follicles: current status and potential. *J Dermatol Sci*. 2010;57:83-89.

Yun SJ, Kim SJ. Hair loss pattern due to chemotherapy-induced anagen effluvium: a cross-sectional observation. *Dermatology*. 2007;215:36-40.

Section 8: Nutritional and Metabolic Diseases

Adams PC, Barton JC. How I treat hemochromatosis. *Blood*. 2010;116:317-325.

Akikusa JD, Garrick D, Nash MC. Scurvy: forgotten but not gone. *J Paediatr Child Health*. 2003;39:75-77.

Balotti RF Jr, Malone RJ, Schanzer RJ. Warfarin necrosis. *Am J Phys Med Rehabil*. 2009;88:263.

Baron JH. Sailors' scurvy before and after James Lind—a reassessment. *Nutr Rev*. 2009;67:315-332.

Betrosian AP, Thireos E, Toutouzas K, et al. Occidental beriberi and sudden death. *Am J Med Sci*. 2004;327:250-252.

Cederbaum S. Phenylketonuria: an update. *Curr Opin Pediatr*. 2002;14:702-706.

Chacon G, Nguyen T, Khan A, et al. Warfarin-induced skin necrosis mimicking calciphylaxis: a case report and review of the literature. *J Drugs Dermatol*. 2010;9:859-863.

Chalmers EA. Neonatal coagulation problems. *Arch Dis Child Fetal Neonatal Ed*. 2004;89:F475-F478.

Champe PC, Harvey RA. *Biochemistry*. 2nd ed. Philadelphia: Lippincott; 1994:338-340.

Chaudhry SI, Newell EL, Lewis RR, et al. Scurvy: a forgotten disease. *Clin Exp Dermatol*. 2005;30:735-736.

Chu WC, Leung TF, Chan KF, et al. Wilson's disease with chronic active hepatitis: monitoring by in vivo 31-phosphorus MR spectroscopy before and after medical treatment. *Am J Roentgenol*. 2004;183:1339-1342.

Cope-Yokoyama S, Finegold MJ, Sturniolo GC, et al. Wilson disease: histopathological correlations with treatment on follow-up liver biopsies. *World J Gastroenterol*. 2010;16:1487-1494.

Delgado-Sanchez L, Godkar D, Niranjan S. Pellagra: rekindling of an old flame. *Am J Ther*. 2008;15:173-175.

Dolberg OJ, Elis A, Lishner M. Scurvy in the 21st century. *Isr Med Assoc J*. 2010;12:183-184.

Englander L, Friedman A. Iron overload and cutaneous disease: an emphasis on clinicopathological correlations. *J Drugs Dermatol*. 2010;9:719-722.

Feillet F, van Spronsen FJ, MacDonald A, et al. Challenges and pitfalls in the management of phenylketonuria. *Pediatrics*. 2010;126:333-341.

Gabbay KH, Bohren KM, Morello R, et al. Ascorbate synthesis pathway: dual role of ascorbate in bone homeostasis. *J Biol Chem*. 2010;285:19510-19520.

Graham JB, Fagan B, Latessa R. Painful plaques shortly after hospital discharge. Warfarin plaques. *Am Fam Physician*. 2008;77:675-676.

Gupta A, Aikath D, Neogi R, et al. Molecular pathogenesis of Wilson disease: haplotype analysis, detection of prevalent mutations and genotype-phenotype correlation in Indian patients. *Hum Genet*. 2005;118:49-57.

Hanley WB. Adult phenylketonuria. *Am J Med*. 2004;117:590-595.

Hegyi J, Schwartz RA, Hegyi V. Pellagra: dermatitis, dementia, and diarrhea. *Int J Dermatol*. 2004;43:1-5

Inayatullah S, Phadke G, Vilenski L, et al. Warfarin-induced skin necrosis. *South Med J*. 2010;103:74-75.

Ishii N, Nishihara Y. Pellagra among chronic alcoholics: clinical and pathological study of 20 necropsy cases. *J Neurol Neurosurg Psychiatry*. 1981;44:209-215.

Kannourakis G. Glycogen storage disease. *Semin Hematol*. 2002;39:103-106.

Kim HK, Ha SH, Han J. Potential therapeutic applications of tetrahydrobiopterin: from inherited hyperphenylalaninemia to mitochondrial diseases. *Ann N Y Acad Sci*. 2010;1201:177-182.

Koch RK. Issues in newborn screening for phenylketonuria. *Am Fam Physician*. 1999;60:1462-1466.

Kountchev J, Bijuklic K, Bellmann R, et al. A patient with severe lactic acidosis and rapidly evolving multiple organ failure: a case of shoshin beri-beri. *Intensive Care Med*. 2005;31:1004.

Lau H, Massasso D, Joshua F. Skin, muscle and joint disease from the 17th century: scurvy. *Int J Rheum Dis*. 2009;12:361-365.

Levy PA. An overview of newborn screening. *J Dev Behav Pediatr*. 2010;31:622-631.

Lind, J. *A Treatise of the Scurvy. In Three Parts*. Edinburgh: Sands Murray and Cochran; 1753.

López Piñero JM. Gaspar Casal: ecological description of pellagra, the leading deficiency disease. *Rev Esp Salud Publica*. 2006;80:411-415.

Moini M, Mistry P, Schilsky ML. Liver transplantation for inherited metabolic disorders of the liver. *Curr Opin Organ Transplant*. 2010;15:269-276.

Morabia A. Joseph Goldberger's research on the prevention of pellagra. *J R Soc Med*. 2008;101:566-568.

Morin K. Thiamine (vitamin B1) revisited. *MCN Am J Matern Child Nurs*. 2004;29:200.

Nazarian RM, Van Cott EM, Zembowicz A, et al. Warfarin-induced skin necrosis. *J Am Acad Dermatol*. 2009;61:325-332.

Nguyen RT, Cowley DM, Muir JB. Scurvy: a cutaneous clinical diagnosis. *Australas J Dermatol*. 2003;44:48-51.

Okan G, Yaylaci S, Alzafer S. Pellagra: will we see it more frequently? *J Eur Acad Dermatol Venereol*. 2009;23:365-366.

Pitsavas S, Andreou C, Bascialla F, et al. Pellagra encephalopathy following B-complex vitamin treatment without niacin. *Int J Psychiatry Med*. 2004;34:91-95.

Popovich D, McAlhany A, Adewumi AO, et al. Scurvy: forgotten but definitely not gone. *J Pediatr Health Care*. 2009;23:405-415.

Rajakumar K. Pellagra in the United States: a historical perspective. *South Med J*. 2000;93:272-277.

Ridel KR, Leslie ND, Gilbert DL. An updated review of the long-term neurological effects of galactosemia. *Pediatr Neurol*. 2005;33:152-161.

Shah GM, Shah RG, Veillette H, et al. Biochemical assessment of niacin deficiency among carcinoid cancer patients. *Am J Gastroenterol*. 2005;100:2307-2314.

Sommer A. Vitamin A deficiency and clinical disease: an historical overview. *J Nutr*. 2008;138:1835-1839.

Spits Y, De Laey JJ, Leroy BP. Rapid recovery of night blindness due to obesity surgery after vitamin A repletion therapy. *Br J Ophthalmol*. 2004;88:583-585.

Spitz JL. *Genodermatoses: A Clinical Guide to Genetic Skin Disorders*. 2nd ed. Philadelphia: Lippincott Williams & Wilkins; 2005.

Tanumihardjo SA. Assessing vitamin A status: past, present and future. *J Nutr*. 2004;134:290s-293s.

Towbin A, Inge TH, Garcia VF, et al. Beriberi after gastric bypass surgery in adolescence. *J Pediatr*. 2004;145:263-267.

Underwood BA. Vitamin A deficiency disorders: international efforts to control a preventable "pox." *J Nutr*. 2004;134:231s-236s.

van Spronsen FJ. Phenylketonuria: a 21st century perspective. *Nat Rev Endocrinol*. 2010;6:509-514.

Vanier MT. Prenatal diagnosis of Niemann-Pick diseases types A, B, and C. *Prenat Diagn*. 2002;22:630-632.

Vanier MT, Millat G. Niemann-Pick disease type C. *Clin Gent*. 2003;64:269-281.

Walshe JM. Monitoring copper in Wilson's disease. *Adv Clin Chem*. 2010;50:151-163.

Zacharski LR. Hemochromatosis, iron toxicity and disease. *J Intern Med*. 2010;268:246-248.

Section 9: Genodermatoses and Syndromes

Antal Z, Zhou P. Addison disease. *Pediatr Rev*. 2009;30:491-493.

Barbagallo JS, Kolodzieh MS, Silverberg NB, et al. Neurocutaneous disorders. *Dermatol Clin*. 2002;20:547-560.

Bleicken B, Hahner S, Ventz M, et al. Delayed diagnosis of adrenal insufficiency is common: a cross-sectional study in 216 patients. *Am J Med Sci*. 2010;339:525-531.

Bolognia JL, Jorizzo JL, Rapini RP. *Dermatology*. 2nd ed. St. Louis: Mosby; 2008:623-631.

Burrows NP. The molecular genetics of the Ehlers-Danlos syndrome. *Exp Dermatol*. 1999;24:99-106.

Callewaert B, Malfait F, Loeys B, et al. Ehlers-Danlos syndromes and Marfan syndrome. *Best Pract Res Clin Rheumatol*. 2008;22:165-189.

Casaletto JJ. Is salt, vitamin, or endocrinopathy causing this encephalopathy? A review of endocrine and metabolic causes of altered level of consciousness. *Emerg Med Clin North Am*. 2010;28:633-662.

Castori M, Camerota F, Celletti C, et al. Natural history and manifestations of the hypermobility type Ehlers-Danlos syndrome: a pilot study on 21 patients. *Am J Med Genet A*. 2010;152A:556-564.

Chakera AJ, Vaidya B. Addison disease in adults: diagnosis and management. *Am J Med*. 2010;123:409-413.

Ehninger D, de Vries PJ, Silva AJ. From mTOR to cognition: molecular and cellular mechanisms of cognitive impairments in tuberous sclerosis. *J Intellect Disabil Res*. 2009;53:838-851.

Feldman DS, Jordan C, Fonseca L. Orthopaedic manifestations of neurofibromatosis type 1. *J Am Acad Orthop Surg*. 2010;18: 346-357.

Ferner RE. The neurofibromatoses. *Pract Neurol*. 2010;10: 82-93.

Figueroa A, Correnti M, Avila M, et al. Keratocystic odontogenic tumor associated with nevoid basal cell carcinoma syndrome: similar behavior to sporadic type? *Otolaryngol Head Neck Surg*. 2010;142:179-183.

Fujimoto N, Yajima M, Ohnishi Y, et al. Advanced glycation end product-modified? beta2-microglobulin is a component of amyloid fibrils of primary localized cutaneous nodular amyloidosis. *J Invest Dermatol*. 2002;118:479-484.

García de Marcos JA, Dean-Ferrer A, Arroyo Rodríguez S, et al. Basal cell nevus syndrome: clinical and genetic diagnosis. *Oral Maxillofac Surg*. 2009;13:225-230.

Gawthrop F, Mould R, Sperritt A, et al. Ehlers-Danlos syndrome. *BMJ*. 2007;335:448-450.

Giordano R, Picu A, Broglio F, et al. Ghrelin, hypothalamus-pituitary-adrenal (HPA) axis and Cushing's syndrome. *Pituitary*. 2005;7:243-248.

Goldberg LH, Firoz BF, Weiss GJ, et al. Basal cell nevus syndrome: a brave new world. *Arch Dermatol*. 2010;146:17-19.

Gonzales EA. Marfan syndrome. *J Am Acad Nurse Pract*. 2009; 21:663-670.

Greene WB. *Netter's Orthopaedics*. Philadelphia: Saunders; 2006: 131-133.

Hamidi Asl K, Liepnieks JJ, Nakamura M, et al. A novel apolipoprotein A-1 variant, Arg173Pro, associated with cardiac and cutaneous amyloidosis. *Biochem Biophys Res Commun*. 1999;257: 584-588.

Horvath A, Bertherat J, Groussin L, et al. Mutations and polymorphisms in the gene encoding regulatory subunit type 1-alpha of protein kinase A (PRKAR1A): an update. *Hum Mutat*. 2010;31: 369-379.

Isaacs H. Perinatal (fetal and neonatal) tuberous sclerosis: a review. *Am J Perinatol*. 2009;26:755-760.

Jacobson L. Hypothalamic-pituitary-adrenocorticol axis regulation. *Endocrinol Metab Clin North Am*. 2005;34:271-292.

James WD, Berger TG, Elston DM. *Andrews' Diseases of the Skin: Clinical Dermatology*. Philadelphia: Saunders; 2006:650-652.

Jett K, Friedman JM. Clinical and genetic aspects of neurofibromatosis 1. *Genet Med*. 2010;12:1-11.

Keane MG, Pyeritz RE. Medical management of Marfan syndrome. *Circulation*. 2008;117:2802-2813.

Madan V, Williams J, Lear JT. Dermatological manifestations of Down's syndrome. *Clin Exp Dermatol*. 2006;31:623-629.

Mann JA, Siegel DH. Common genodermatoses: what the pediatrician needs to know. *Pediatr Ann*. 2009;38:91-98.

Muñoz-Pérez MA, Camacho F. Acanthosis nigricans: a new cutaneous sign in severe atopic dermatitis and Down syndrome. *J Eur Acad Dermatol Venereol*. 2001;15:325-327.

Newell-Price J, Bertagna X, Grossman AB, et al. Cushing's syndrome. *Lancet*. 2006;367:1605-1617.

Oldfeld EH. Cushing disease. *J Neurosurg*. 2003;98:948-951.

Orlova KA, Crino PB. The tuberous sclerosis complex. *Ann N Y Acad Sci*. 2010;1184:87-105.

Pitak-Arnnop P, Chaine A, Oprean N, et al. Management of odontogenic keratocysts of the jaws: a ten-year experience with 120 consecutive lesions. *J Craniomaxillofac Surg*. 2010;38:358-364.

Pivonello R, De Martino MC, De Leo M, et al. Cushing's syndrome. *Endocrinol Metab Clin Nprth Am*. 2008;37:135-149.

Pursnani AK, Levy NK, Benito M, et al. Carney's complex. *J Am Coll Cardiol*. 2010;55:1395.

Rabin KR, Whitlock JA. Malignancy in children with trisomy 21. *Oncologist*. 2009;14:164-173.

Raff H, Findling JW. A physiological approach to diagnosis of the Cushing syndrome. *Ann Intern Med*. 2003;138:980-991.

Ruggieri M. The different forms of neurofibromatosis. *Childs Nerv Syst*. 1999;15:295-308.

Santos-Briz A, Cañueto J, Antúnez P, et al. Primary cutaneous localized amyloid elastosis. *Am J Dermatopathol*. 2010;32: 86-90.

Shott SR. Down syndrome: common otolaryngologic manifestations. *Am J Med Genet C Semin Med Genet*. 2006;142:131-140.

Siraqusa M, Romano C, Cavallari V, et al. Localized elastosis perforans serpiginosa in a boy with Down syndrome. *Pediatr Dermatol*. 1997;14:244-246.

Spitz JL. *Genodermatoses: A Clinical Guide to Genetic Skin Disorders*. 2nd ed. Philadelphia: Lippincott Williams & Wilkins; 2005.

Staser K, Yang FC, Clapp DW. Mast cells and the neurofibroma microenvironment. *Blood*. 2010;116:157-164.

Storr HL, Chan LF, Grossman AB, et al. Paediatric Cushing's syndrome: epidemiology, investigation and therapeutic advances. *Trends Endocrinol Metab*. 2007;18:167-174.

Valin N, De Castro N, Garrait V, et al. Iatrogenic Cushing's syndrome in HIV-infected patients receiving ritonavir and inhaled fluticasone: description of 4 new cases and review of the literature. *J Int Assoc Physicians AIDS Care*. 2009;8:113-121.

Vandersteen A, Turnbull J, Jan W, et al. Cutaneous signs are important in the diagnosis of the rare neoplasia syndrome Carney complex. *Eur J Pediatr*. 2009;168:1401-1404.

Weyers W, Weyers I, Bonczkowitz M, et al. Lichen amyloidosus: a consequence of scratching. *J Am Acad Dermatol*. 1997;37: 923-928.

Williams A, Davies S, Stuart AG, et al. Medical management of Marfan syndrome: a time for change. *Heart* 2008;94: 414-421.

Wiseman FK, Alford KA, Tybulewicz VL, et al. Down syndrome—recent progress and future prospects. *Hum Mol Genet*. 2009; 18:R75-R83.

Zhang L, Smyrk TC, Young WF, et al. Gastric stromal tumors in Carney triad are different clinically, pathologically, and behaviorally from sporadic gastric gastrointestinal stromal tumors: findings in 104 cases. *Am J Surg Pathol*. 2010;34:53-64.

masassin

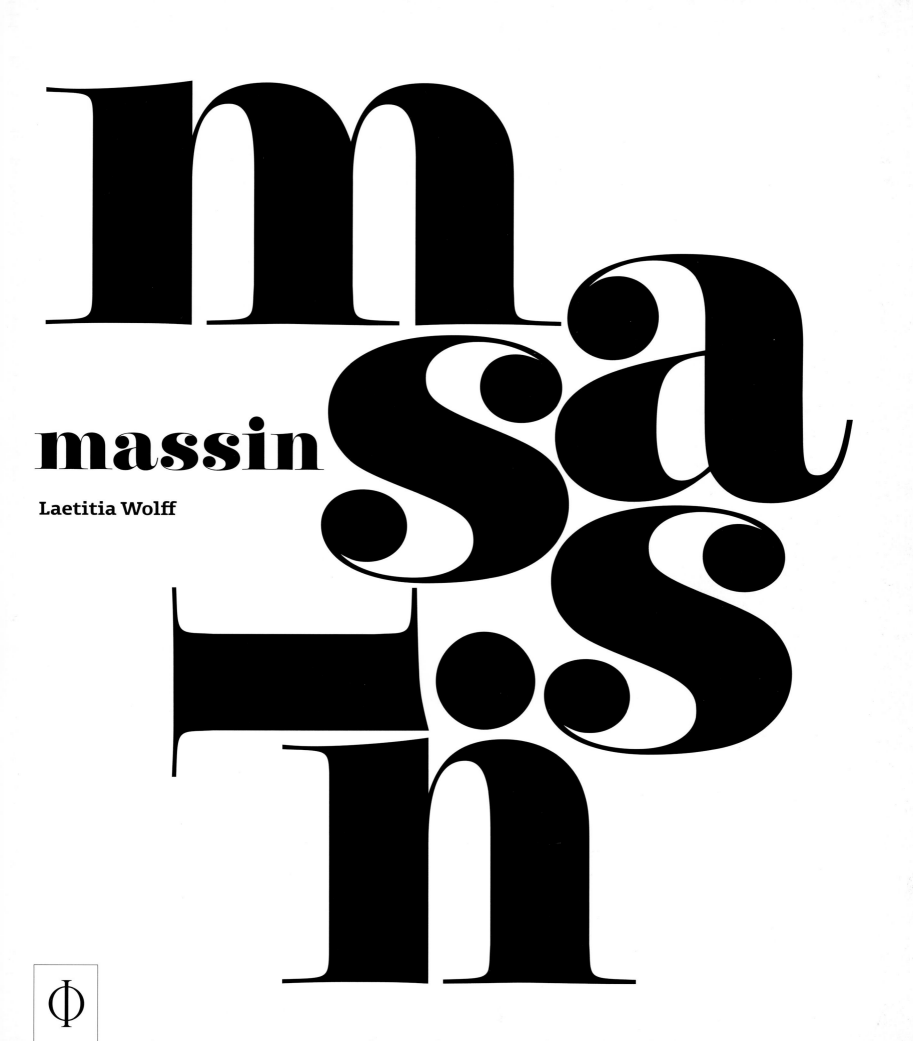

massin

Laetitia Wolff

Phaidon Press Ltd
Regent's Wharf
All Saints Street
London N1 9PA

Phaidon Press Inc.
180 Varick Street
New York, NY 10014

www.phaidon.com

First published 2007
© 2007 Phaidon Press Limited

ISBN 978 0 7148 4811 2
A CIP catalogue record for this book is available from the British Library.

Translated from the French by Trista Selous
Graphic design: Roger Fawcett-Tang, Struktur Design
Printed in China

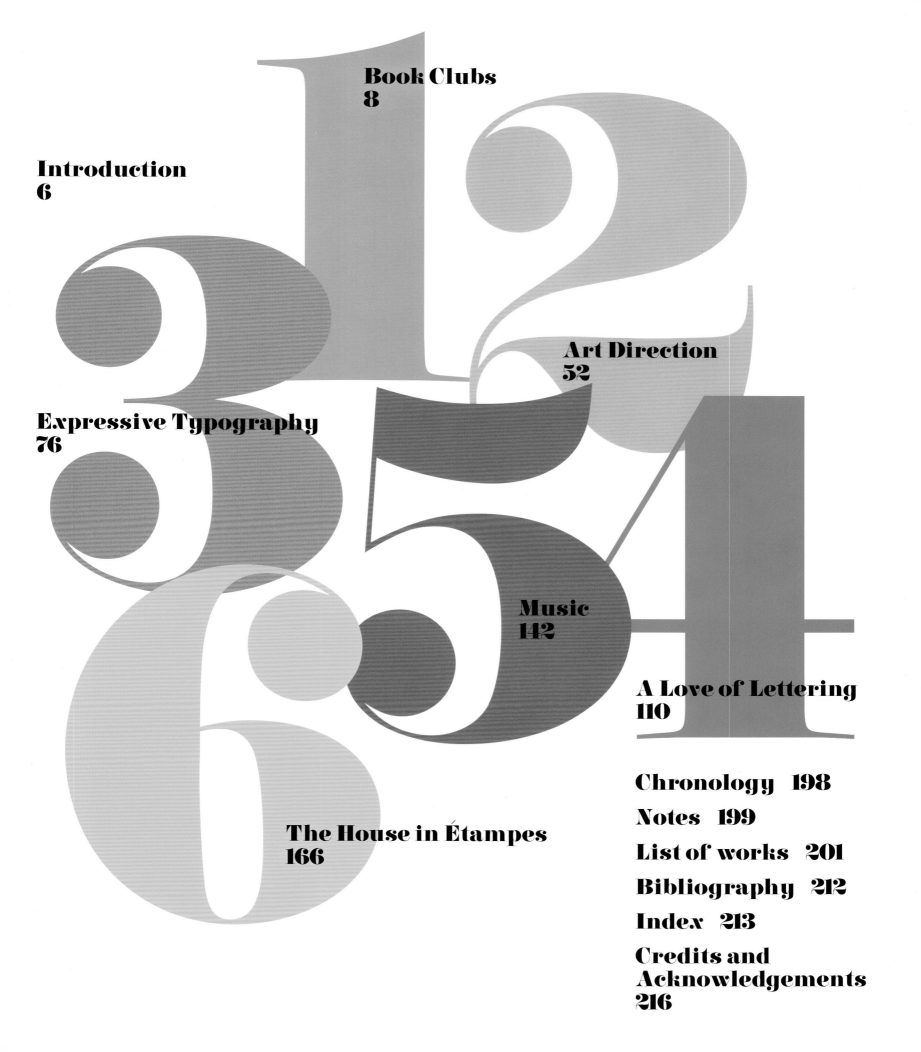

Introduction

Massin: interpretations and variations

Massin is first and foremost a man of culture, fascinated by words, letters, writing and the printed image. Insatiably curious, keen to make things visible and hungry for knowledge, he steers his very own path through the varied territories of graphic art, baroque music, cultural history and the art of writing, with all the ease of the self-taught scholar and the light touch of a man in a hurry. His work is the fruit of interaction between the arts: over the last fifty years he has sought to break down boundaries of specialization and establish similarities between the artistic domains, which he sees with his own, singular, 'absolute typographic eye'. Without actually creating fonts, he plays with lettering to explore its power of gleeful transformation and representation. He collects alphabets, describes their evolution from their beginnings and discusses their visual and illustrative properties in what has become a landmark work on the subject, *La Lettre et l'Image* (Letter and Image). Typography is his means of expression, his second mother tongue; he pulls it to pieces, distorts and distends it, seeking to give it a new identity. It is the tool of his artistic expression and enables him to invent his own vocabulary.

In the fabric of French publishing Massin has lovingly and stubbornly woven extraordinary connections between writing and graphic art, between the letter and the image, always stretching the potentials of the book, that quintessential medium of knowledge, to the limit. Adept in book crafts, by turns graphic artist, layout artist, writer, photographer and art director – to the dismay of the specialists – he has won a unique place in France's cultural heritage, particularly through his long period as art director at Gallimard, where he shaped the graphic design of some twenty literary series in paperback, including 'Poésie/Gallimard', 'Folio' and 'L'Imaginaire', which are still familiar to all French readers today. Books, for which he has designed thousands of covers and layouts, are the primary object of his research, while also the means by which he becomes the spokesman and propagator of this emblematic vehicle of cultural democratization. His own writings have also helped to establish his reputation as a popularizer, particularly his essays on aesthetics and cultural history, including *Les Cris de la ville* (The cries of the city), and his historical novels such as *Les Compagnons de la marjolaine* (The companions of the marjoram). In both the subject of his books and the readability of his designs, in other people's books and his own, he always demonstrates a sincere interest in popular culture, to which he endlessly pays homage for its rich and unexploited capacity for expression.

But it is in his series of typographical interpretations of dramatic and musical works that Massin radically challenges the linear structure of books, breaks with layout conventions and creates a new means of expression. Having launched an experimental approach that spectacularly altered relationships to the writing and reading of a text, Massin took his role as interpreter still further. Around 1964, in an unpublished letter to Gaston Gallimard, he wrote, 'At the risk of appearing an abusive interpreter, I have constantly tried to identify with the writer whose layout I was to create, striving to "express", dreaming of taking his place, like those valets in comedies who try out their masters' armchairs or beds in their absence.' In all his typographical gymnastics, from those he created for Eugène Ionesco's play *La Cantatrice chauve* (The Bald Soprano/The Bald Prima Donna), now famous in the graphic arts community, to the photographic transcriptions of Édith Piaf's voice in *La Foule* (The crowd) or those that arose out of his friendship with Raymond Queneau in *Cent mille milliards de poèmes* (A hundred thousand billion poems), Massin practises what he calls an 'activity of substitution', substituting skills that he has not mastered, but which he intends to explore by means of typographical variation. In his graphic work as in his explorations of musical works, it is this opportunity for a typographic interpretation that fascinates him, since it allows him to enter into the work and gives him the chance to bring to it his own artistic variation. The question of variants in interpretation is therefore many-faceted and endless, representing the guiding thread of his entire work. And, to continue the metaphor of variation, we shall suggest that Massin's work is to expressive typography what Bach's *Art of Fugue* is to music: a long, in-depth study of a theme (for Massin, the graphic transcription of a literary or dramatic work), whose meaning becomes more complex with each improvisation and variant to which it gives rise.

Because he has never taught (he does not have the *baccalauréat*) nor run a major design agency, because he has never either founded or participated in any movement, this compulsive creator remains, like the artists of the Renaissance, a free spirit of French culture and the unknown hero of a vast graphic heritage now ripe for (re)discovery.

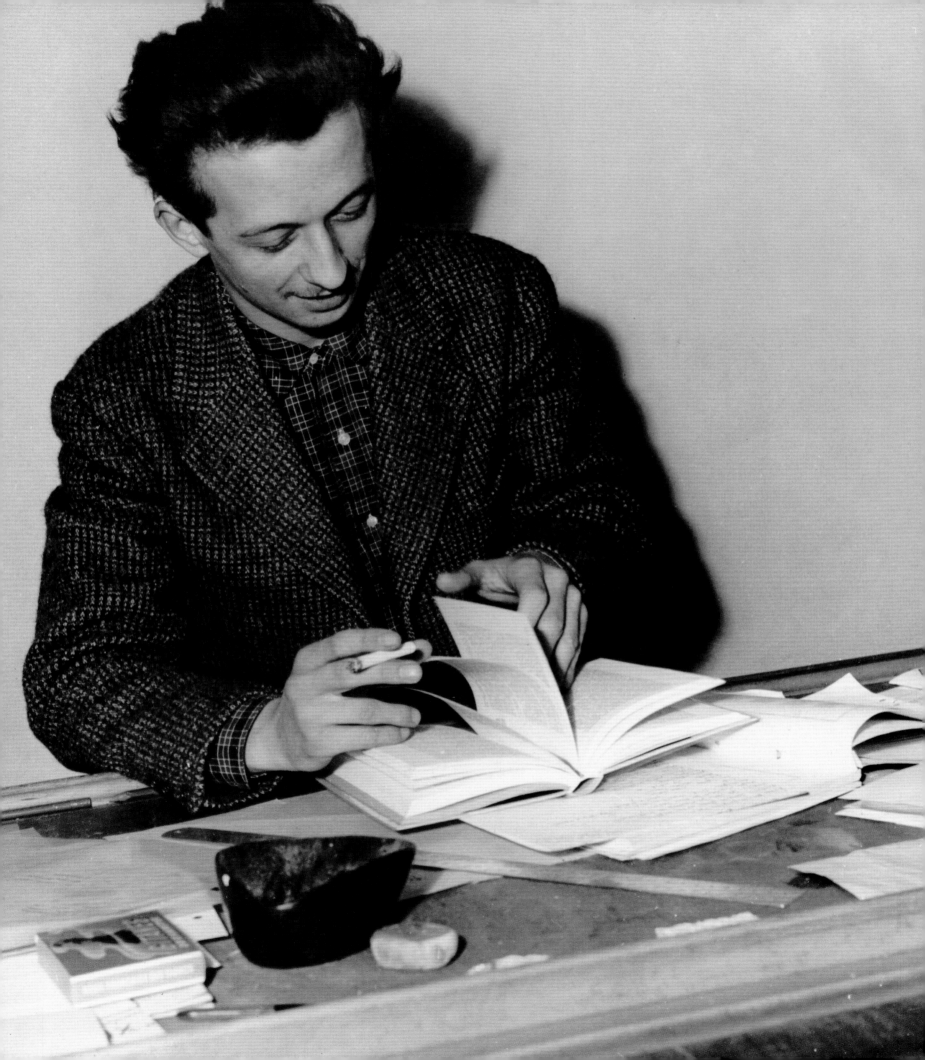

Book Clubs

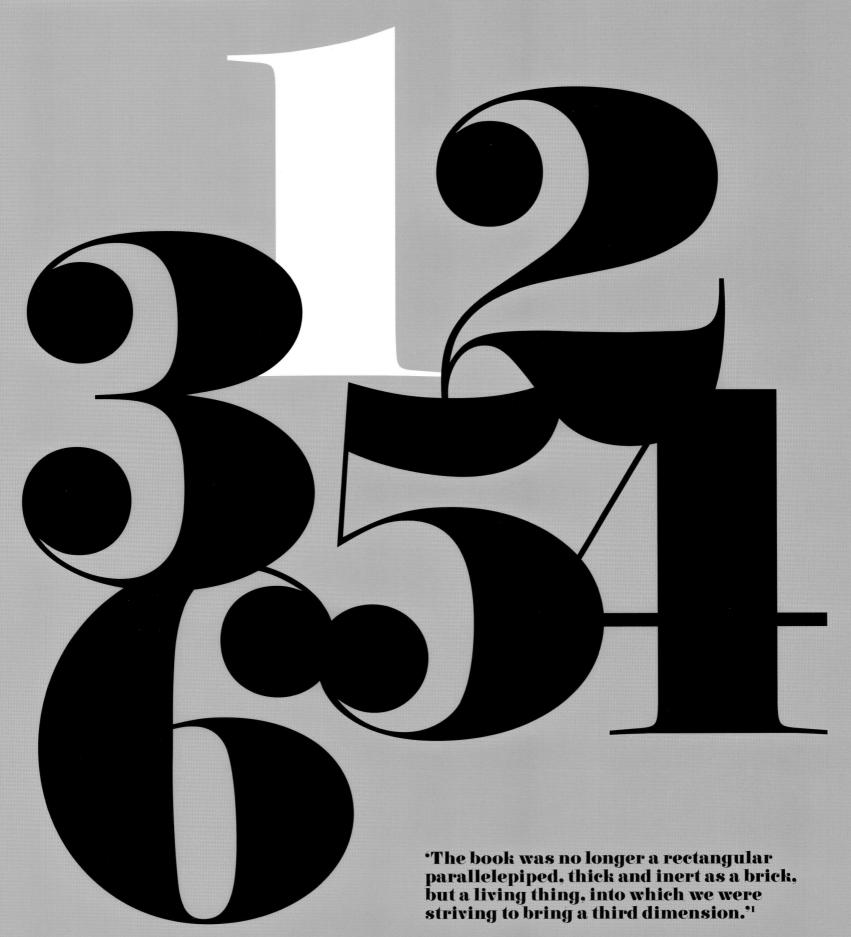

1 2 3 4 5 6

'The book was no longer a rectangular parallelepiped, thick and inert as a brick, but a living thing, into which we were striving to bring a third dimension.'

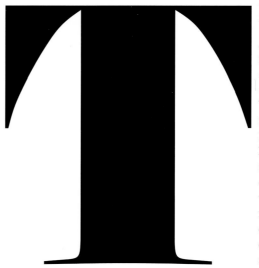

The formation of the book clubs

After World War II, when the library network had collapsed and the reputations of many publishing houses had been damaged by accusations of collaboration, book clubs provided a means of reintroducing books into middle-class French homes. Although publishers were keen to launch new titles (over 12,000 in 1947), bringing out their own new editions of French and foreign literary classics, the clubs were filling a void that was due in part to a lack of paper and the total destruction, caused by the war, of the distribution system. The new concept of selling by mail order, introduced by the American Book of the Month Club (BOMC, 1926) and the Swiss co-operative Guilde du livre, enabled the clubs to offer an average of four books a month (to be chosen from an annual publication total of around forty titles) per subscription. In this way the clubs took over the role of cultural advisors, which the booksellers had fulfilled before the war.

The foremost book club in France was the Club français du livre, founded by Stéphane Aubry and Jean-Paul Lhopital in October 1946. Massin, who began his career at the Club français du livre in 1948 editing its newsletter, *Liens*, describes how it 'started in an attic room in avenue de l'Opéra, then moved to a former bank in rue de Lisbonne, before becoming established in more luxurious surroundings in rue de la Paix in 1951'.[2]

The club's output marked a return to bound books, which had long been abandoned in France, and whose fabric covers with their bright expanses of colour enlivened many domestic bookshelves. Like the BOMC, the Club français du livre prided itself on having an editorial committee made up of literary figures, including Francis Carco, Jean Cocteau, Colette and Henri Calet. But in reality the books to be published were selected by the club's editorial team, headed by the visionary Robert Carlier. Carlier's winning formula consisted of offering a wide variety of literary classics,

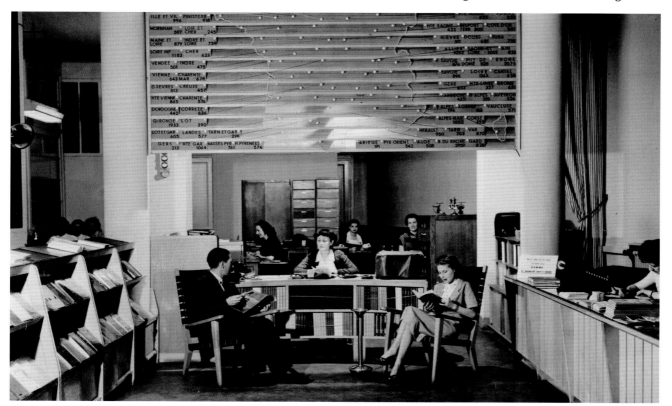

Page 8: photograph of Massin by Roger Roche, in his studio at 20, rue Delambre, Paris, c.1954.

Left: view of the office reception at the Club français du livre, rue de Lisbonne, Paris, in 1951, with Robert Carlier (left) and Huguette Hédouin (centre), Massin's future wife.

foreign works and new editions of books that had gone out of print. Throughout his career in the clubs he maintained a scholarly approach, respectful
of the genesis of the works, and encouraged critical enhancements to texts
by publishing classic works in a format similar to that of critical editions,
notably with the 'Les Portiques' series. Each book was typeset with great
care, printed on bible paper, and included a new preface, notes and additional
matter such as attractive historical illustrations to accompany the text.
Carlier often disagreed with Jean-Paul Lhopital and, by his own admission,
sought to 'encroach on the territory of the Pléiade'.[3] This informative
approach, which also underpinned the graphic innovations of its layout
artist Pierre Faucheux, soon earned the Club français du livre a reputation
as a quality publisher.

   To a greater or lesser extent the many clubs that flourished in the
early 1950s (at one time there were as many as twelve) copied the formula
of Carlier and Faucheux, and competition between them was heightened by
the fact that graphic artists, illustrators and art directors tended to move
from club to club.

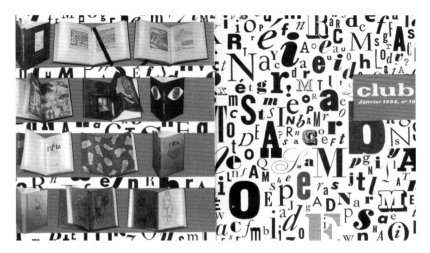

Massin's first steps: from one club to the next

Massin cut his teeth at the Club français du livre, where he also met Huguette
Hédouin, whom he later married and who was then in charge of relations
with the club's members. At its height the Club français du livre had 300,000
members, of whom forty per cent lived in rural areas, where there were
fewer bookshops. 'Seeking out home-based clients is the best way to sell
books'[4] was the mantra of Jean-Paul Lhopital, the director of the Club français
du livre.

   So, in a manner symbolic of the orientation of his entire œuvre, it was
through literature that Massin was able to take his first steps as a graphic
artist. For a short time he was editor of the newsletter *Liens*, for which Pierre
Faucheux designed a new standard layout in 1950. 'For my part, within this
framework I had total freedom to lay out the pages, which I made to look like
a little newspaper,' explains Massin.[5] As he was responsible for laying out
the pieces he was writing, he had to learn the basic techniques of typesetting
and so was sent to the printer's, where, in six weeks, he learned to set text
using cases of metal type. In 1949 he designed his first bound cover for
Arthur Rimbaud's *Œuvres*, in black board with geometric lines intersected
by extracts from Rimbaud's poems. Carlier later regarded this as too
interpretative to be truly successful, given the objectivity he regarded as
indispensable to the graphic design of a book. This was a lesson Massin
quickly learned from Carlier: never over-interpret a cover, never tell the
reader too much.[6]

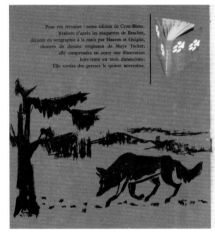
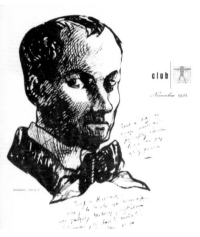

Two-colour covers of *Club*, the monthly
newsletter for members of the Club du
meilleur livre (no. 10, January 1954;
no. 18, November 1954).

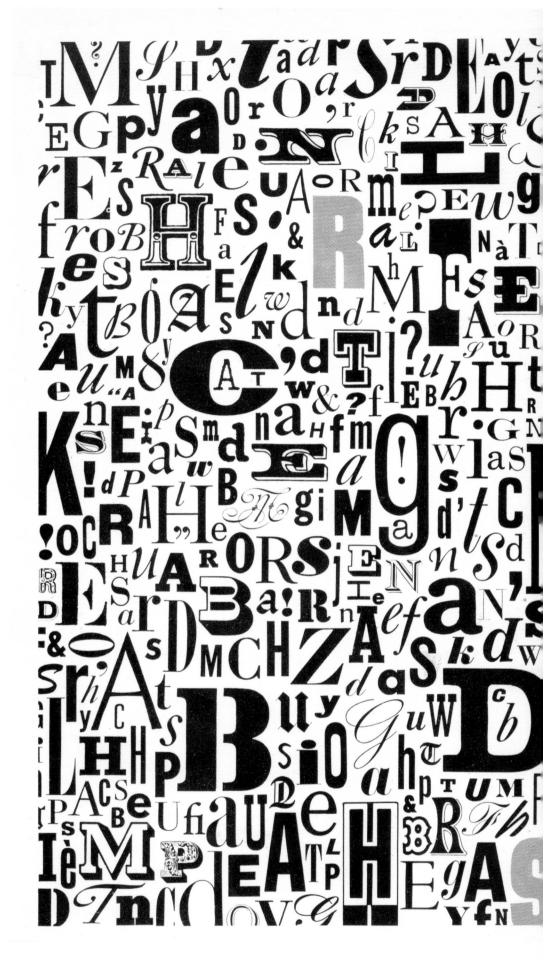

Two-colour wrapping paper for the Club du meilleur livre (1954), made entirely by hand.

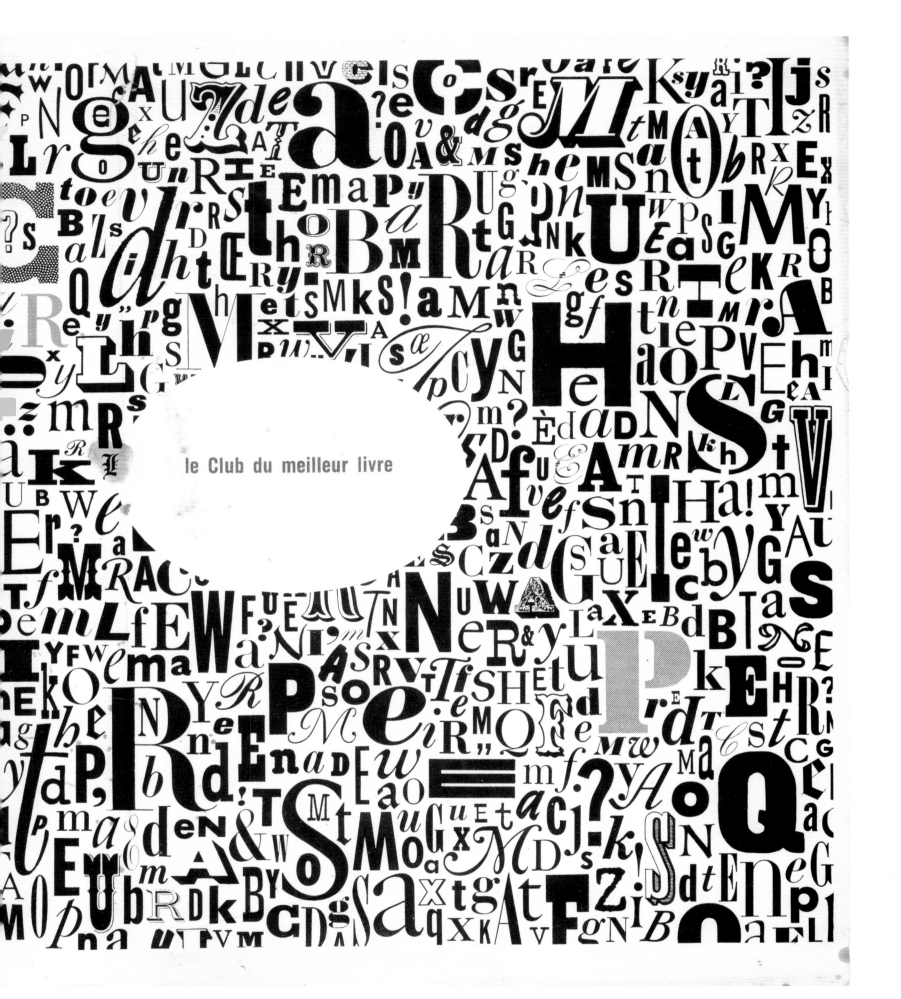

le Club du meilleur livre

LE CLUB DU MEILLEUR LIVRE

3, rue de Grenelle   Paris 6e

Cher lecteur,

Vous aimez les livres et la formule des Clubs ne vous est sans doute pas inconnue; vous savez que les Clubs représentent la forme la plus moderne de l'édition et qu'ils prétendent répondre aux besoins de ce large public qui désire acquérir de beaux livres à un prix accessible.

Nous avons voulu, en créant le CLUB DU MEILLEUR LIVRE, répondre à deux exigences par quoi se marque l'originalité de notre effort : éditer chaque mois pour vous les textes les meilleurs, garantie que seuls, nous pouvons vous offrir; donner à ce club, avec votre concours actif, l'agrément et la richesse d'un club véritable qui sera votre club, et non une simple maison d'édition par correspondance.

Il nous a paru essentiel de prévoir pour vous dans le fonctionnement de notre club, tous les avantages qu'autorise cette formule. En premier lieu, nous vous proposons un choix mensuel de quatre livres reliés. Ces ouvrages sont édités spécialement pour vous. Vous bénéficiez de la gratuité d'inscription et vous recevez sans frais la revue mensuelle "CLUB" où vous pouvez librement choisir ceux des livres que vous désirez commander.

Mais, pour la première fois, un club de livres peut proposer à ses adhérents les oeuvres maîtresses de chacun de ces auteurs : Gide, Mauriac, Graham Greene, André Malraux, Bernanos, Charles Morgan, Saint-Exupéry, Blaise Cendrars, Marcel Proust, etc.

Le Club du Meilleur Livre entend donc éditer pour vous les grands classiques de la littérature contemporaine, sans négliger pour autant les chefs-d'oeuvre rarement édités des siècles passés.

A des textes d'une valeur littéraire incontestable, notre club - votre club, nous l'espérons, bientôt - apporte l'enrichissement d'une typographie et d'une reliure étudiées, respectueuses du caractère propre de chaque oeuvre.

Votre bibliothèque comprendra ainsi un ensemble harmonieux d'ouvrages tous numérotés, dont la variété ne nuira pas à l'unité du bon goût.

Le fonctionnement du Club est simple et vous est exposé en page 7. Il n'exige de vous ni cotisation, ni avance de fonds. Votre adhésion vous assurera pendant un an le service gratuit de "CLUB" qui vous tiendra au courant de l'actualité littéraire.

Nous souhaitons surtout en faire l'intermédiaire vivant au moyen duquel nous entendons animer le Club et lui donner l'essor culturel pour lequel nous réclamons déjà votre amical concours.

Above: open letter to subscribers of the Club du meilleur livre (January 1954).

Opposite: two-colour cover and inside spread from the first issue of *Club* (January 1953) describing the organisation's activities and function.

Below: photograph of Robert Carlier by Massin, Paris, 1956.

Robert Carlier
(1910–2002)

Carlier started out as a maths teacher and worked during World War II at the Ministry of Youth in Vichy. During the war, he shielded Paul Stein, who was of Jewish origin and who subsequently took the name Jean-Paul Lhopital. When Lhopital founded the Club français du livre in 1946, he asked Carlier to be its literary director, knowing that he had been involved with the art world during the 'Libération' while advisor to Odette Arnaud's literary agency. Carlier published the French translation of Malcolm Lowry's Under the Volcano *(Club français du livre, 1950).*

Massin's career ran parallel to that of Carlier, who was like a guardian angel to him. Massin declared, 'I owe him everything', including his work for the Club français du livre and the Club du meilleur livre, and the many recommendations Carlier gave him from 1951 onwards, when he was asked, in addition to his work for the clubs, to create covers for Calmann-Lévy, Julliard and Corrêa. In 1950 Carlier established the Prix du meilleur livre étranger (Prize for the best foreign book). From 1961 to 1971 he was literary director for Gallimard, where he edited the series

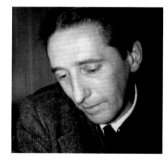

'Bibliothèque idéale' and 'Poésie/Gallimard', and later the classics section of 'Livre de poche'. Carlier remains a key figure in post-war French publishing, efficient but highly erudite, and always abreast of everything. He had a great and subtle knowledge of the Paris publishing world, notably bringing Beckett to Éditions de Minuit after Jean Paulhan had turned him down at Gallimard.

In 1952, Massin joined Carlier when the latter fell out with Lhopital and went off to found the Club du meilleur livre. Massin started by working as a freelance graphic artist in charge of the newsletter, *Club*, and very soon became the club's art director. His wife went with him to the Club du meilleur livre and, from 1953 to 1960, was in charge of customer relations and mail orders from the 90,000 subscribers, who provided ninety-five per cent of the club's turnover.

The quality of its products led the Club du meilleur livre to be regarded as one of the most prestigious of all book clubs. As its manager and publishing director, Carlier pursued the policy of bringing out new editions of classic works that he had initiated while at the Club français du livre. As Massin said at the time, 'In practice, besides the publication of contemporary literary works (enhanced only by the graphic boldness of the covers), [Carlier] had a free hand on a few exceptional volumes, where the new editions were more completely reworked',[7] for example, the 'Le Nombre d'or' series was 'a club publication revealing the master works of world literature in a new light'.[8] Today Massin confirms that Raymond Gallimard had 'Le Nombre d'or' discontinued because it was in direct competition with 'La Bibliothèque de la Pléiade', a prestigious collection of books and an imprint of Gallimard for which he was responsible.

Carlier set up Le Club du meilleur livre with the support of seven shareholders, including three publishers already well established in the book market, whose names were kept secret for reasons of commercial strategy. These were Gallimard, Hachette and Robert Laffont (who was to pull out a year later).

Carlier remembers: 'We had a big challenge ahead of us. We had just left the Club français du livre at a time when it was doing very well and when, in 1947, I had brought in Pierre Faucheux who, with Jacques Darche, reigned supreme over the graphic side. So it was imperative for us to find a way of presenting ourselves, for both our books and our newsletter, that would set us apart unambiguously from the one we had worked on for so long.'[9]

So Massin was charged with a major task: he was to develop the brand image of a new publishing house, in an atmosphere of strong competition between clubs and at a time of rapid reconstruction of the bookshop network and a general revival of interest in books. Paperbacks, in particular, played an important role in the post-war democratization of culture.

blaise cendrars

julien green

françois mauriac

andré maurois

georges bernanos

daphné du maurier

j. de la varende

andré malraux

charles morgan

andré gide

thomas mann

élizabeth goudge

graham greene

marcel proust

Chaque mois, le club du meilleur livre vous présente les grands «classiques» de la littérature contemporaine

club

bulletin du club du meilleur livre janvier 1953 n° 1

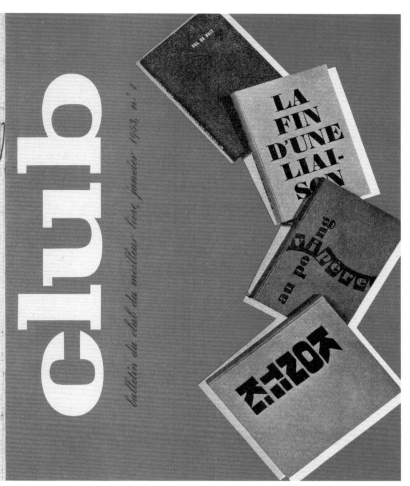

VOL DE NUIT

Guerre à *Citadelle*, il parlera de plus en plus pour lui. Jamais il ne sera aussi simple que dans *Vol de Nuit*, aussi commun à tous.

Le Club est fier de présenter dans son premier choix, ce grand « classique » de l'humanisme héroïque, accompagné d'une préface d'André Gide, et d'avoir réalisé pour ces textes précieux une édition digne d'eux par son élégance et sa sobriété.

LA FIN D'UNE LIAISON

Club : « Ecrivain anglais, écrivain catholique, Graham Greene se situe au-delà des limites nationales ou religieuses. C'est un romancier universel, non seulement par la diffusion de son œuvre dans tous les pays et l'accueil qu'elle reçoit, mais aussi et surtout par la force avec laquelle se pose, dans un « climat » essentiellement moderne, des problèmes qui touchent et qui concernent, qu'ils le veuillent ou non, tous les individus. »

VIPÈRE AU POING

naître qu'Hervé Bazin possédait les qualités sur lesquelles se fondent les réputations littéraires durables : des dons d'écrivain de premier ordre, une puissance et une souplesse d'expression peu communes, une originalité indéniable que ses œuvres ultérieures devaient confirmer.

On comprendra aisément que le Club du Meilleur Livre ait tenu à vous présenter ce livre parmi les tout premiers ouvrages qu'il publie.

L'EXPÉDITION DU "KON-TIKI"

vivre, dans un style tour à tour poignant et plein d'humour, cette navigation périlleuse dont le succès a fait mentir savants et marins. L'auteur a rapporté de son voyage un film qui a connu, comme son livre, traduit en sept langues, un triomphe mondial. Le Club en a extrait plus de soixante-dix photographies qui font de sa belle édition un album-souvenir de prix, et le livre cadeau idéal pour tous les âges et tous les publics.

N° 1
Un volume relié pleine toile. Format 13,5×20. Fers originaux. Impression en 2 couleurs sur Bouffant alfa du Marais. Gardes illustrées. Maquettes de Michel Daniel. 168 pages .... Fr. 730

N° 2
Un volume relié pleine toile. Format 13,5×20. Fers originaux. Impression en 2 couleurs sur Bouffant alfa du Marais. Gardes illustrées. Maquettes de Robert Massin. 344 pages .... Fr. 790

N° 3
Un volume relié pleine toile. Format 13,5×20. Fers originaux. Impression en 2 couleurs sur Bouffant alfa du Marais. Gardes illustrées. Maquettes de Jacques Darche. 320 pages .... Fr. 750

N° 4
Un volume relié, pleine toile. Format 17×20. Fers originaux. Impression en typo et offset 2 couleurs sur papier Offset du Pacifique. Illustré de 72 photographies et d'une carte dépliante. Gardes en 2 couleurs. Maquettes de Robert Massin. 400 pages .. Fr. 1.280

« Club », 3, rue de Grenelle, Paris-6e — Le gérant : R. CARLIER — Tirage : 25.000 ex. — Imprimerie NICEA, Paris.

Activité et fonctionnement du club du meilleur livre

Chaque mois, le Club du Meilleur Livre édite 4 volumes, à tirage limité, tous numérotés, qui sont annoncés et présentés dans « CLUB ». Vous avez toute liberté de choisir ceux des livres que vous désirez commander.

L'adhésion au Club du Meilleur Livre est gratuite. Aucun droit d'entrée, aucune cotisation, aucune avance de fonds ne vous sont demandés. L'adhésion au Club vous donne droit au service gratuit de notre bulletin littéraire mensuel, pendant un an.

Comment faire partie du Club

L'adhésion au Club n'entraîne aucune obligation, *ni engagement* quelconque d'acheter un nombre minimum de volumes.

Pour devenir membre du Club, il vous suffit de commander un volume choisi parmi les titres disponibles.

Comment bénéficier de ses avantages

Si nous désirons vous laisser toute liberté, il va de soi que nous favoriserons ceux d'entre vous qui nous auront manifesté la fidélité la plus active.

Livre-dividende : Tous nos amis ayant adhéré au Club en 1953 et ayant acquis 6 volumes au cours de cette année, auront droit à un 7e volume gratuit. Ce « livre-dividende » qu'ils recevront sans frais, pourra être choisi librement dans nos sélections parmi les volumes d'un prix inférieur à 1.000 francs.

Le dividende sera porté à 2 volumes pour 12 livres commandés dans la même période, et ainsi de suite...

Ainsi, chaque mois, nous nous efforcerons de vous apporter des avantages et de vous ménager des surprises agréables.

Dès à présent, vous trouverez dans les premiers volumes que vous recevrez, l'indication des privilèges réservés à nos propagandistes les plus actifs.

Comment recevoir ses ouvrages

Pour recevoir les ouvrages du Club du Meilleur Livre, utilisez l'enveloppe-réponse ci-jointe, en cochant d'une croix les cases figurant en regard des titres que vous désirez recevoir.

Pour faciliter notre travail et vous assurer une prompte expédition de votre commande, joignez le règlement dans l'enveloppe-réponse, sous la forme d'un mandat-carte, d'un chèque bancaire, ou d'un chèque postal (chèque de virement postal, comprenant les trois feuillets que nous présenterons nous-mêmes à l'encaissement). Ajoutez au montant de chaque commande la somme de 40 francs pour frais d'envoi.

Nous pouvons aussi vous expédier les livres contre remboursement, mais, n'oubliez pas que des frais postaux élevés grèvent ce mode d'envoi (approximativement 100 francs par expédition).

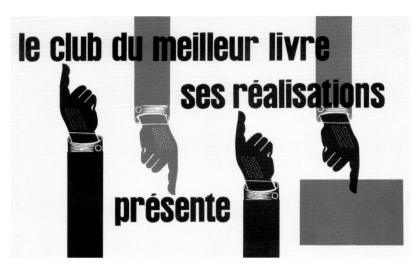

Two-colour poster for the Club du meilleur livre (Paris, 1954).

Like many layout artists (graphic artists, and particularly graphic designers, had yet to be invented) such as Jacques Darche, Jacques Daniel, Jeanine Fricker and William Klein, Massin was working, initially at least, very much in the wake of the pioneer Pierre Faucheux, a father figure and highly influential personality in the world of book design. 'Indeed, curiously, it was watching Faucheux "sell" his layouts, explaining and justifying them with the same fire, that I started to want to make some myself', remembers Massin.[10] And he admits, 'When I was making my first layouts I used to ask myself, "What will Faucheux think?"'.[11] Faucheux had been one of the first graphic artists working to stress the importance of creating a cover with dynamic typography and narrative illustration at a time when photography had not yet replaced illustration.

Over the period 1952–8, Massin's work at the Club du meilleur livre established his reputation as a layout artist and art director, surpassing even the creations of the master Faucheux. Massin drew on the widest possible range of influences, from Dutch graphic artists such as Dick Eiffers to drawings by Saul Steinberg, album covers, newspaper headlines and even, later on, the credits of American films, which he greedily absorbed, cartoons by Tex Avery and title sequences by Saul Bass, which did not become known among the wider French public until the late 1950s.

The materiality of the book

Beyond the flagrant stylistic disparity of the clubs' books, which were characterized by an absence of overall formula or an easily identifiable look – unlike some of the series that Massin would later head at Gallimard – overall homogeneity was assured by a standard size, which ensured that the books all stood on the shelves in perfect alignment.

However, Massin explains, 'The book was no longer a rectangular parallelepiped, thick and inert as a brick, but a living thing, into which we

Four-colour cover of *Club* (no. 12, April 1954), showing a photograph of the Club du meilleur livre's showroom, decorated with modern furniture (Knoll sofa and Mouille lamp).

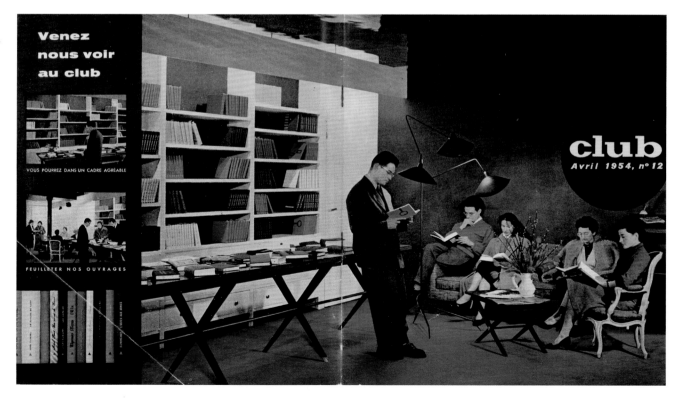

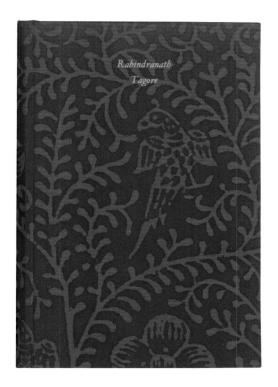

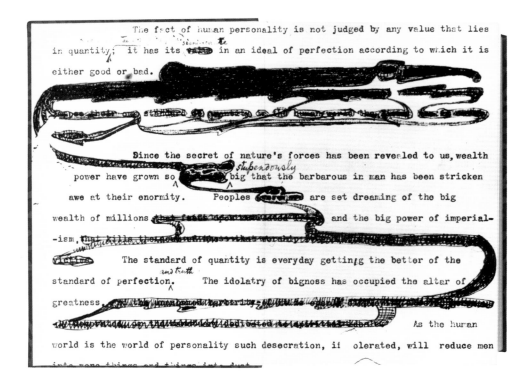

The fact of human personality is not judged by any value that lies in quantity; it has its *standard* in an ideal of perfection according to which it is either good or bad.

Since the secret of nature's forces has been revealed to us, wealth power have grown so *stupendously* big that the barbarous in man has been stricken awe at their enormity. Peoples are set dreaming of the big wealth of millions and the big power of imperial-ism, that kills the

The standard of quantity is everyday getting the better of the standard of perfection *and truth*. The idolatry of bigness has occupied the altar of greatness. As the human world is the world of personality such desecration, if tolerated, will reduce men

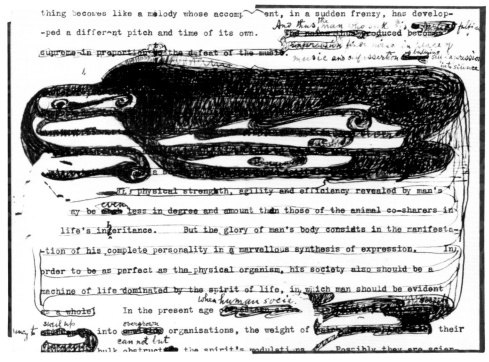

thing becomes like a melody whose accomp ent, in a sudden frenzy, has develop--ped a different pitch and time of its own.

physical strength, agility and efficiency revealed by man's *even* may be less in degree and amount than those of the animal co-sharers in life's inheritance. But the glory of man's body consists in the manifesta--tion of his complete personality in a marvellous synthesis of expression. In order to be as perfect as the physical organism, his society also should be a machine of life dominated by the spirit of life, in which man should be evident *when human socie* as a whole. In the present age *overgrown* into organisations, the weight of their bulk obstruct the spirit's modulation Possibly they are scien-

Pierre Faucheux
(1924–1999)

After working at Flammarion before the war, Pierre Faucheux joined the Club français du livre as art director in 1946, under literary director Robert Carlier. He was a major figure in French publishing for an entire generation of young layout artists, particularly during the period of the book clubs. Massin constantly measured himself against Faucheux and strove to shed his influence throughout his career. In 1972 their friendly rivalry culminated in a meeting on the set of the first show in the television series 'Ouvrez les guillemets' (Open quotation marks), presented by Bernard Pivot.

Trained as a typographer at the École Estienne, Faucheux had studied the first printed books. A year older than Massin, he shared the latter's love of lettering and his passion for music and architecture. Faucheux's originality lies in his art of typographic combination and his inventive, visionary use of letters and printers' vignettes to present characters. His layout for Henri Pichette's Épiphanies, published by K Éditeur in 1948, was a crucial source of inspiration for Massin's work on La Cantatrice chauve. In 1963, at the instigation of Guy Schoeller (collaborator and successor of Henri Filipacchi who founded Hachette's 'Livre de poche' series in 1953), he designed covers for the classics and crime sections of 'Livre de poche'.

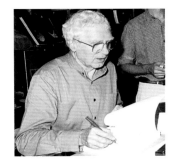

Faucheux established his own studio in 1963, unlike Massin, whose name has almost always been associated with that of a publishing house. Working freelance for many French publishers, he notably designed the 'Libertés' series (1964–8) for Jean-Jacques Pauvert, the 'Pluriel' and 'Livre de poche jeunesse' series for Hachette and 'Points' for Le Seuil. As a press layout artist he created the template and cover for Le Nouvel Observateur (1964) as well as the binding for the Encyclopædia Universalis (1989). Pierre Faucheux, 'bespoke' typographer, was a true magician of the book.

Top left: binding of Rabindranath Tagore's *Œuvres poétiques* (Paris, Club du meilleur livre, 1961) with a decoration of Indian motifs on a two-colour, screen-printed silk binding.

Above: front and back endpapers of *Œuvres poétiques* reproducing Tagore's typescript, with his corrections.

Left: photograph of Pierre Faucheux by Philippe Lavieille at the Imprimerie nationale, Paris, at the time of writing the manifestation 'La Fureur de lire', 1990.

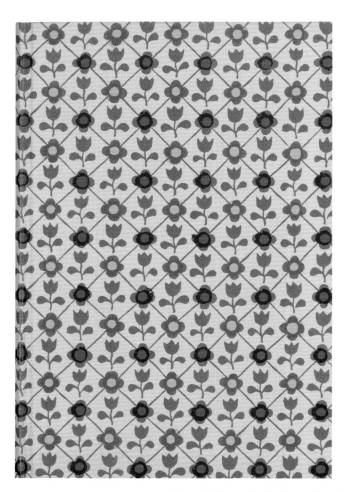

White cloth binding decorated with eighteenth-century patterned paper for Louise de Vilmorin's *Le retour d'Érica* (The return of Érica; Paris, Club du meilleur livre, 1957).

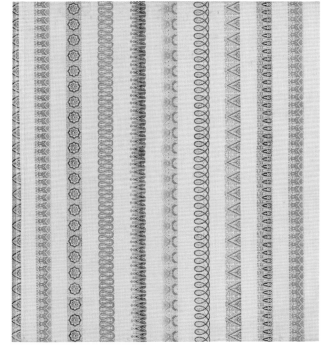

Four-colour cloth binding of André Maurois' *Olympio* (Paris, Club du meilleur livre, 1955).

were striving to bring a third dimension.'[12] The era of the book clubs was the great period of book design. With print runs of 4,000 or 5,000 they were seen as real pieces of art to be touched as well as looked at. The word 'design' is pertinent here, both in relation to the graphic work of the cover, which could be either flat or in relief, and to the design of the inside pages, particularly the endpapers, and their dynamic relationship, which progressed throughout the book. The highly sophisticated production techniques of the time regularly gave rise to unusual innovations, technical tricks and printing methods of a very different order from those on display in bookshops today. These graphic acrobatics, linked as much to the book's rhythm as to its material production, made a considerable contribution to the success of this brief period in the history of books.

Kinetic art

In addition to the bindings, which will be discussed later, the innovations introduced by the clubs to the manufacture of their books included illustrated endpapers (almost the rule at the Club du meilleur livre) and folded pages that opened out to create a kinetic dimension. With Jacques Darche at the Club des éditeurs and now that Pierre Faucheux had moved to the Club des libraires, the graphic artists competed to see who could be the most daring. The first signatures of these bound books provided an opportunity for infinite variations on graphic expertise and playfulness.

At the start of his career Massin had few models of creative, dynamic layout to draw on. The double title page, spread across two pages and replacing the traditional right-hand page, had been invented in the late 1920s and early 1930s by the Americans W. A. Dwiggins and Merle Armitage. But the idea of an unfolding sequence had appeared in Stéphane Mallarmé's legendary final poem *Un coup de dés jamais n'abolira le hasard* (A throw of the dice will never eliminate chance; 1896, posthumously published in 1914). In the context of the late nineteenth-century crisis in poetry, Mallarmé had invented a new form for the alexandrine, based not on poetic structure but the poem's surroundings, in other words the graphic space, the book. So in *Un coup de dés jamais n'abolira le hasard*, the lines of poetry are arranged across double-page spreads and the syntax is reorganized into groups. In what seems more like a musical score than a poem, the typographical arrangement reflects the oral nature of the spoken word so powerfully that it meets the challenge of conveying original speech, which lies at the heart of Mallarmé's poetic quest.

La Prose du Transsibérien et de la petite Jehanne de France (The Prose of the Trans-Siberian and the Little Jeanne of France), the original edition of Blaise Cendrars' 'simultaneous' poem illustrated by Sonia Delaunay (Paris, Éditions des hommes nouveaux, 1913), is another famous example of avant-garde unfolding. *La Prose du Transsibérien et de la petite Jehanne de France* is a conversation poem that leads us in the footsteps of the author who, at the age of sixteen, travelled through Russia and into Siberia. The dialogue is

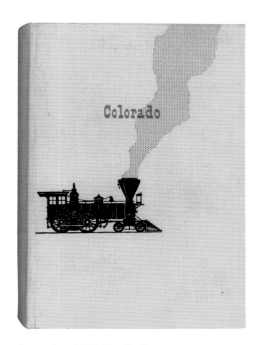

Above: yellow cloth binding of Louis Bromfield's *Colorado* (Paris, Club du meilleur livre, 1953).

Right: multicoloured endpapers and unfolding title page of *Colorado* with die-cut reproductions of saloon doors.

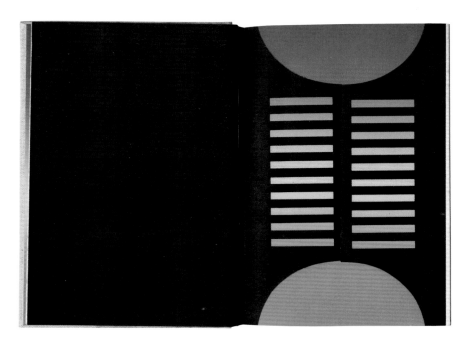

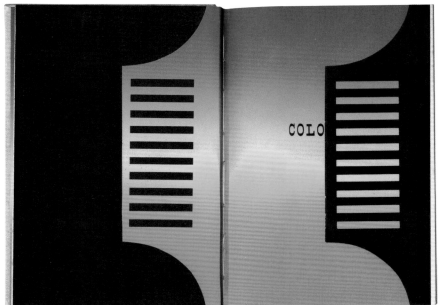

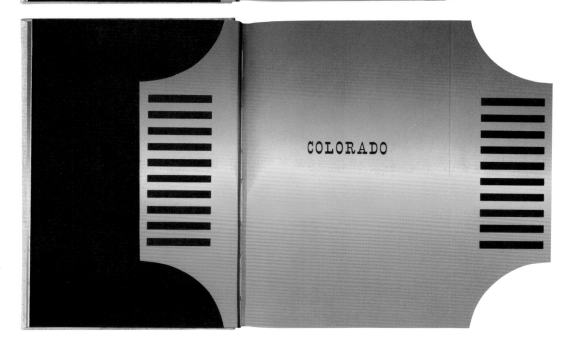

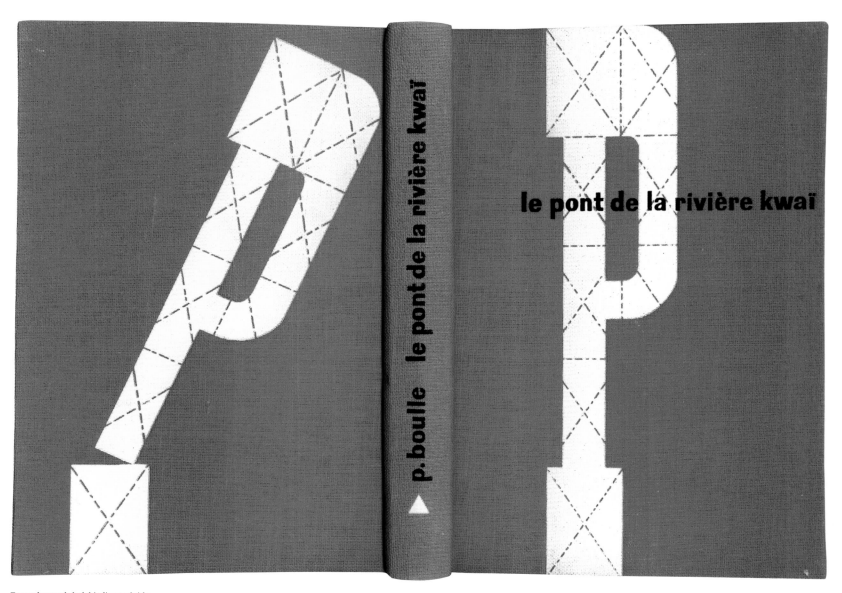

Two-colour red cloth binding and title
pages of Pierre Boulle's *Le Pont de
la rivière Kwaï* (The Bridge over the River
Kwai; Paris, Club du meilleur livre, 1953).

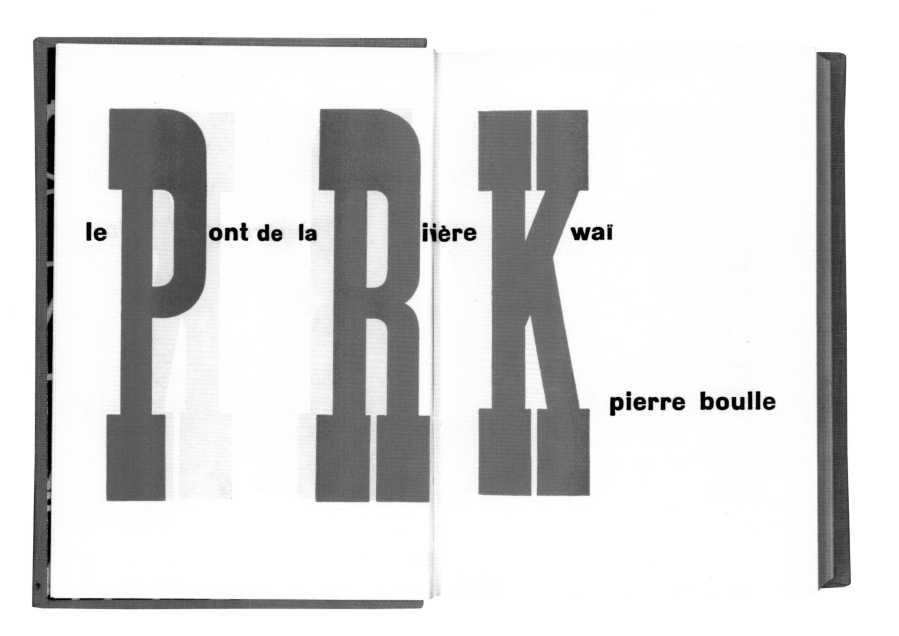

le **P**ont de la **R**ivière **K**waï

pierre boulle

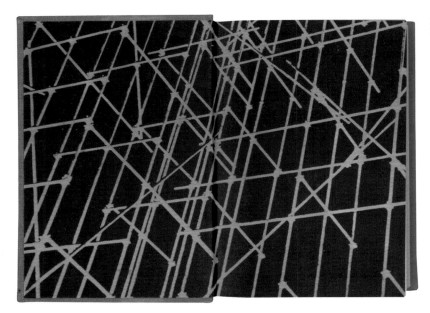

Endpapers, title pages and inside spreads from *Le Pont de la rivière Kwaï*.

le P ont de la R ivière K waï

pierre boulle

PRK

no, it was not funny; it was so representative of the great joke. but the world moves, and so upon the whole. and one would call a good was rather pathetic; he of all the past victims it is by folly alone that it is a respectable thing besides, he was what man. joseph conrad.

1

interrupted by the jerking of the train, suggested by the uneven rhythms of free verse, plunging us into the modernity of familiar language (repeated onomatopoeia) and the vastness to be explored (Siberia), with a background theme of progress (the train). The images twist like hallucinations, opening the way to the fantastical world suggested by Sonia Delaunay's illustrations, which accompany the poem.

Lastly *Jazz* (Paris, Tériade, 1947), by Henri Matisse, is undoubtedly one of the most successful examples of the marriage of word and image. The book comprises twenty plates of colours and words, in which the floating bodies of clowns and dancers appear alongside exotic plant forms and traces of travel memories. *Jazz* reflects the improvisation and vitality that governed its creation and also contains writings by Matisse, copied out using a brush, which resemble aphorisms and which, as the artist put it, 'will be read or not read, but which will be seen […] as a kind of packaging for my colours'. These three major works, in which the art of literature meets that of page layout, remained models for Massin, who continually refers to them in his writings.

When Massin began his work in the late 1940s, the landmarks of publishing were primarily literary in nature. Along the way the influence of cinema and film credits became apparent in the arrangement of his double-page spreads. The space of the page became the screen, with effects

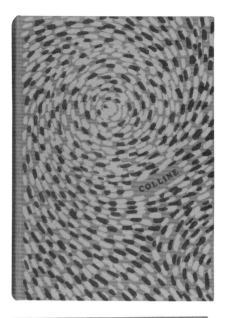

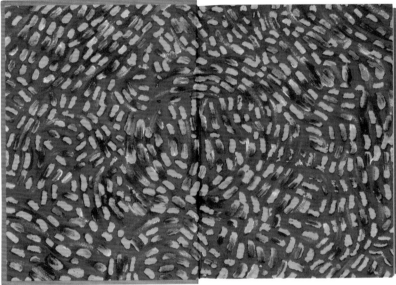

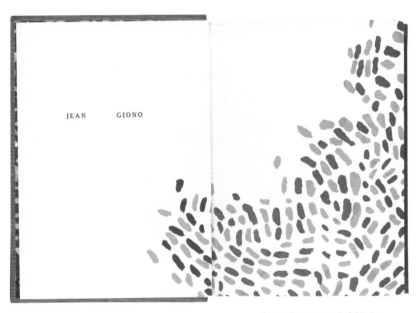

Three-colour orange cloth binding, endpapers and title pages from Jean Giono's *Colline* (Hill of Destiny; Paris, Club du meilleur livre, 1953), illustrated in homage to Van Gogh.

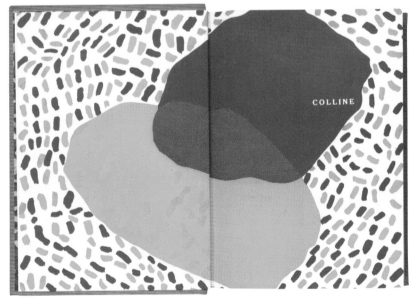

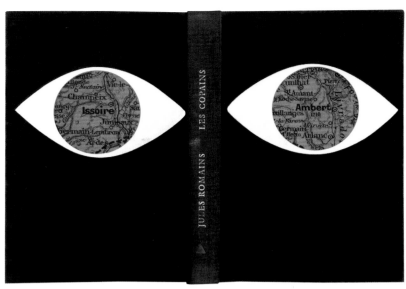

Black cloth binding on to which two-colour labels have been glued, endpapers and title pages of Jules Romains' *Les Copains* (The Buddies; Paris, Club du meilleur livre, 1953).

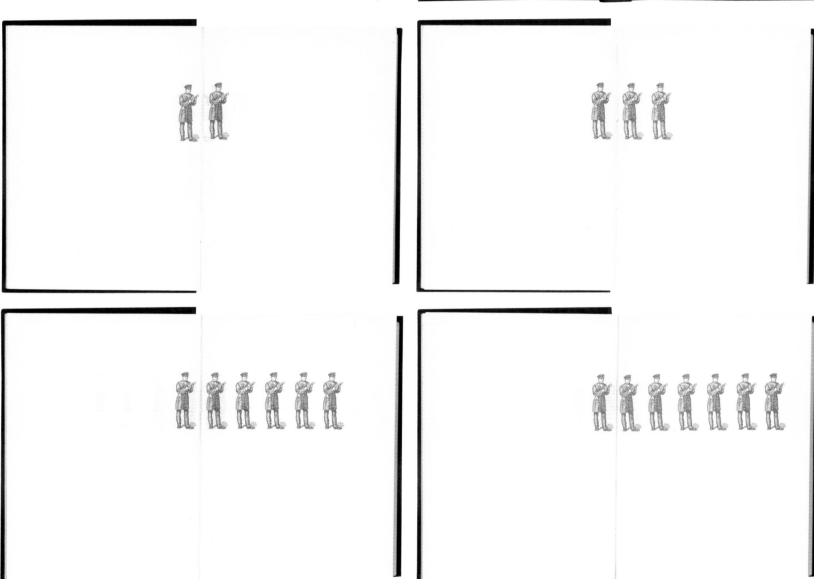

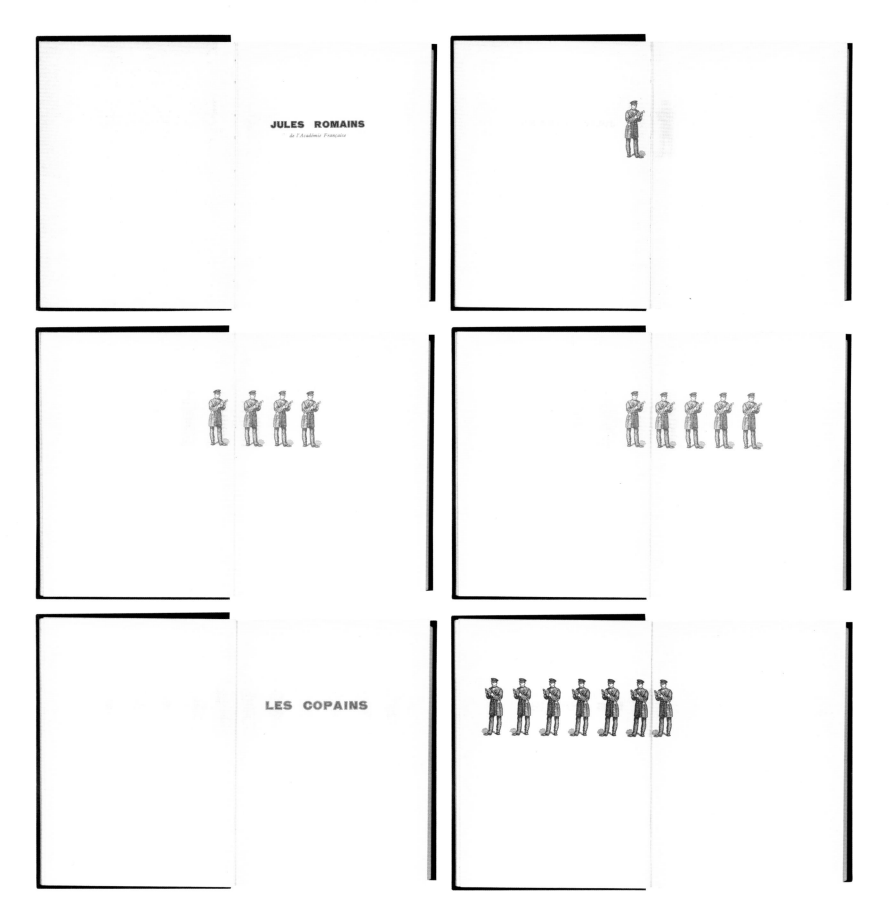

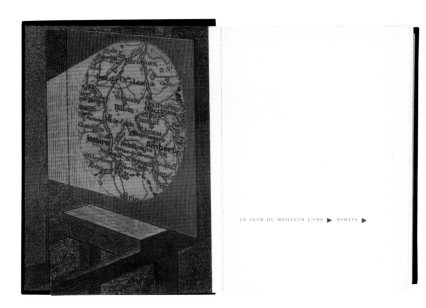

Endpapers of Jules Romains' *Les Copains*
(Paris, Club du meilleur livre, 1953).

analogous to tracking shots highlighting blocks of text or images that would then appear in enlarged or reduced size on the following page. In Jules Romains' *Les Copains* (The Buddies; Paris, Club du meilleur livre, 1953), the title page 'unfolds' over twenty pages, with the seven friends from the l'École normale supérieure appearing one after the other, in a manner reminiscent of one of those small books that you flick through to obtain the impression of movement, creating an animated sequence from a series of illustrations.

Massin has often invoked the cinematic qualities of the book, bringing out the narrative structure through changes of scale and rhythm, alternating zooms, tracking and wide shots. This effect of kinetic progression can be seen in Jean Giono's *Colline* (Hill of Destiny; Paris, Club du meilleur livre, 1953), in which a succession of abstract flecked patterns based on the skies of Provence painted by Van Gogh unfolds in dynamic swirls of colour from one page to the next, as in a film's credit sequence.

Object books: marvellous materials and ingenious production

Fascinated by the possibility of incorporating different elements into the surfaces of his covers, Massin and his colleagues used unusual materials seldom seen in bookbinding, including jute canvas, silk for Marcel Proust's *Un amour de Swann* (Swann in Love; Paris, Club du meilleur livre, 1953), velvet for Francis Jammes' *Jeunes Filles* (Girls; Paris, Club du meilleur livre, 1954), balsa wood and silk ribbon for Thomas Raucat's *L'Honorable Partie de campagne* (The Honourable Picnic; Paris, Club du meilleur livre, 1954), aluminium foil, Cellophane, waxed paper and a long list of other materials, including acetate in the endpapers of Marcel Aymé's *La Vouivre* (Paris, Club du meilleur livre, 1953), whose transparent overlays were individually printed. To create his reliefs and innovatory bindings, Massin set the most unexpected objects into his covers, including a facsimile of a dollar bill for Georges Arnaud's *Le Salaire de la peur* (The Wages of Fear; Paris, Club du meilleur livre, 1953) and the wax seal on the cover of *La Véritable Vie privée du maréchal de Richelieu* (The real private life of the maréchal de Richelieu; Paris, Club du meilleur livre, 1954).

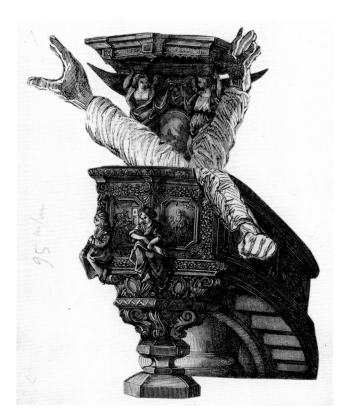

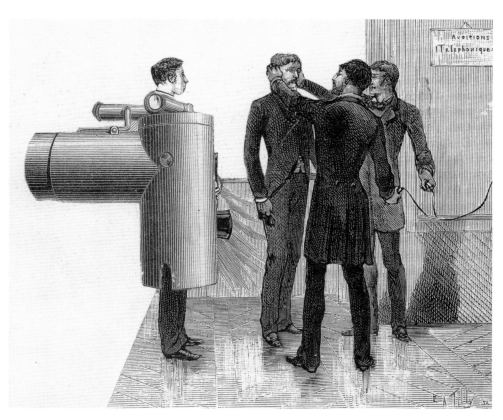

Above and right: original collages by Jacques Sternberg, 1953. Inspired by the work of Max Ernst and made for the inside pages of *Les Copains* by Massin, these collages were inserted into the book.

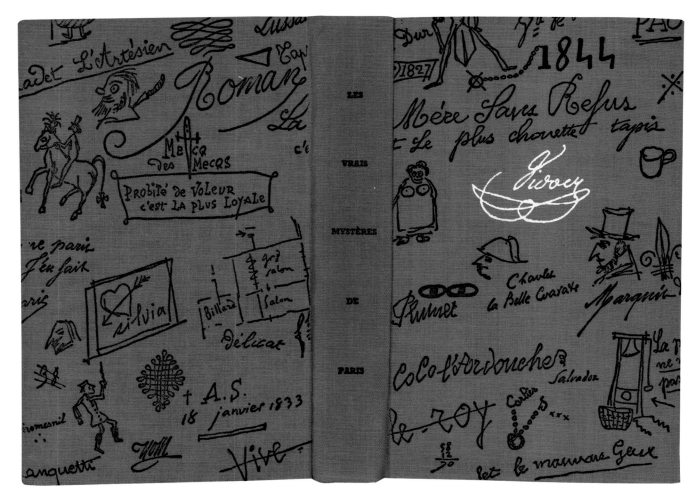

Two-colour red cloth binding and endpapers of Vidocq's *Les Vrais Mystères de Paris* (The True Mysteries of Paris; Paris, Club français du livre, 1950). The hardcover is engraved with imitation graffiti and the endpapers reproduce a detail from a map of Paris dating from 1783.

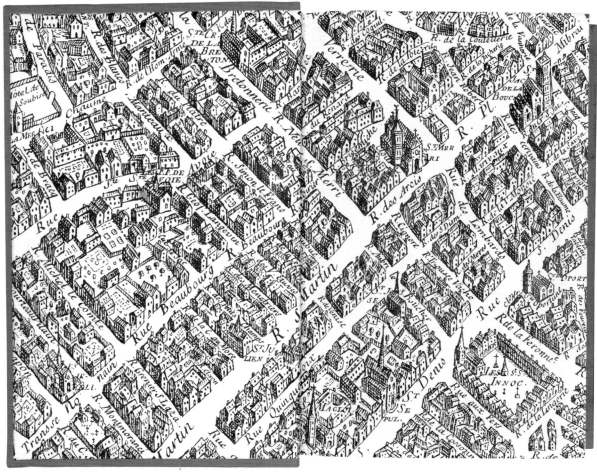

'Massin is a tireless Pygmalion, who keeps on shaping the body of writing to bring it into typographic existence, then, from silk, linen, velvet or leather, tailoring apparel that is most likely to attract us while strictly respecting the reinvigorated spirit of the work', explains Carlier with enthusiasm.[13]

Despite the lack of paper resulting from the war, the layout artists made inspired use of poor materials. Massin confides, 'The truth is that in the early days of the Club français du livre, Lhopital had used sheets of fine pale blue Alfa paper, which had been used by the second armoured division as separators in cases of munitions!'.[14] The layout artists working on standard editions showed much greater ingenuity than those working on the more costly and less imaginative luxury editions, for which engraved leather remained the binding of choice. Their inventive manipulation of unusual materials highlighted the three-dimensional aspect of the 'brick', turning it into something more akin to a craft object, and hence unique, rather than simple printed board.

The traditional hardcover was usually bound with cotton fabric of different colours and weaves. From 1953 onwards most club books, other than those of the Club français du livre, had a protective jacket of transparent acetate (or Rhodoid). The first of these, for Guillaume Apollinaire's *Alcools* (Spirits; Paris, Club du meilleur livre, 1953), was printed with abstract motifs inspired by the paintings of Robert Delaunay and launched a period of new graphic invention for the layout artists, who were interested in its function both as protection (prefiguring the book cover) and as a potential vehicle for other information and graphic elements in addition to those on the decorated binding.

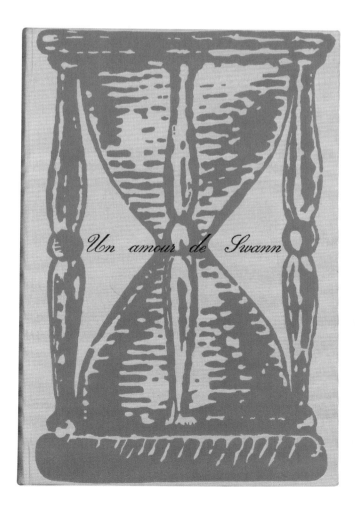

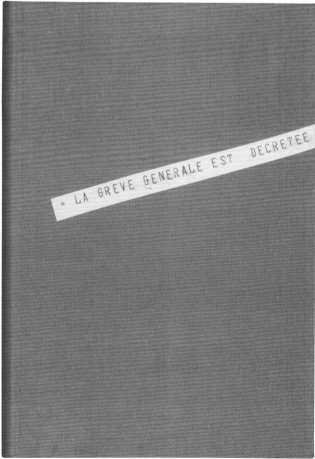

Far Left: two-colour old rose silk binding of Marcel Proust's *Un amour de Swann* (Swann in Love; Paris, Club du meilleur livre, 1953).

Left: orange cloth binding of André Malraux's *Les Conquérants* (The Conquerers; Paris, Club du meilleur livre, 1956) to which is glued a label representing a telexed message.

The fact that the clubs' output consisted primarily of re-editions, notably of literary classics, was almost certainly a factor in the layout artists' predilection for reinterpreting old lettering and the use of original documents. This is true notably of Vidocq's *Les Vrais Mystères de Paris* (The True Mysteries of Paris; Paris, Club français du livre, 1950), in which period illustrations function almost as clues discovered during the hunt for the guilty man, including endpapers showing plans of Paris in 1783, imitation graffiti engraved into the cover, vignettes at the heads of chapters and reproductions of police correspondence.

The role of authentic iconography

In 1952 Faucheux wrote a manifesto on the object book, advocating the making of new from old: 'In trying to create a link between the meaning of the words and the typeface in which they are set, we must find a perfect balance between the text, its meaning and the meaning that the reader will give to the printed words.'[15]

During his typographic explorations in his work for the clubs, Massin showed great respect for fonts, whose history and evolution he knew well. From the classic to the popular, to lettering in the romantic style, he was totally fascinated by their form and evocative power and chose them with great care, often using colour for letters to give greater presence to the text. The quotation from Joseph Conrad across one of the early title pages of Pierre Boulle's *Le Pont de la rivière Kwaï* (The Bridge over the River Kwaï; Paris, Club du meilleur livre, 1953) is printed in bright red alternating with black; the baroque illustrations that punctuate and give rhythm to the text of

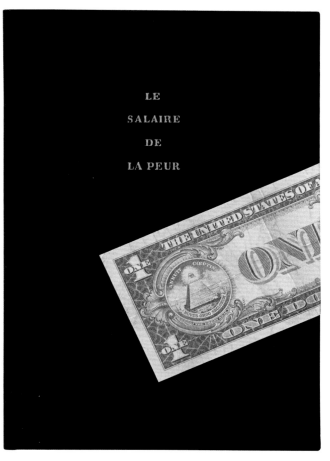

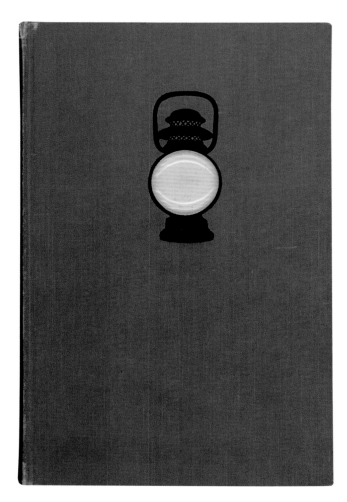

Left to right: green cloth binding of Pierre Mac Orlan's *Sous la lumière froide* (In a cold light; Paris, Club du meilleur livre, 1954); black cloth binding of Georges Arnaud's *Le Salaire de la peur* (The Wages of Fear; Paris, Club du meilleur livre, 1953). Both have three-dimensional effects: a convex watch-glass representing a sailor's lamp on the cover of *Sous la lumière froide* and a facsimile of a dollar bill on *Le Salaire de la peur.*

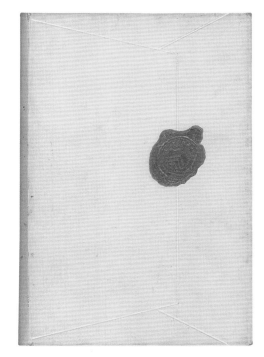

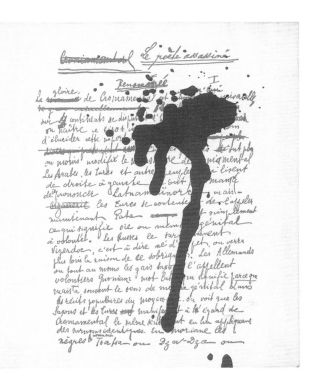

Above: beige cloth binding of *La Véritable Vie privée du maréchal de Richelieu* (The real private life of the maréchal de Richelieu; Paris, Club du meilleur livre, 1954). A wax seal is set into the cover.

Right: three-colour grey-brown cloth binding of Guillaume Apollinaire's *Le Poète assassiné* (The murdered poet; Paris, Club du meilleur livre, 1959), on which a facsimile of an original letter is reproduced.

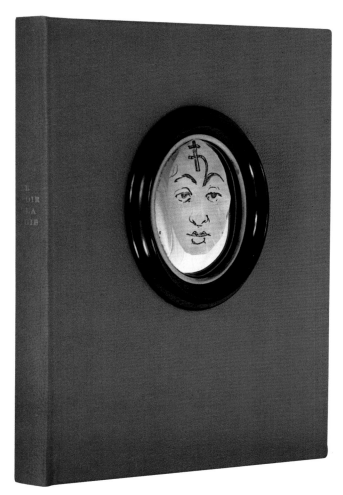

Left: red morocco binding of Kurt Seligmann's *Le Miroir de la magie* (The magic mirror; Paris, Club du meilleur livre, 1956). A 'magic' engraving is set into the front cover: the image does not appear to the naked eye, but by breathing on it the reader can make it appear.

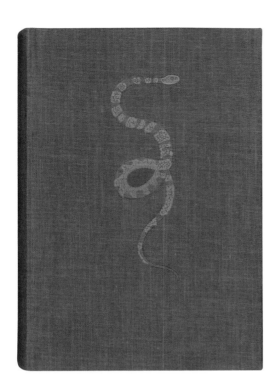

Three-colour cloth binding and preliminary pages of Marcel Aymé's *La Vouivre* (Paris, le Club du meilleur livre, 1953). These pages reproduce the drawing of a woman by Maillol and are printed on Cellophane.

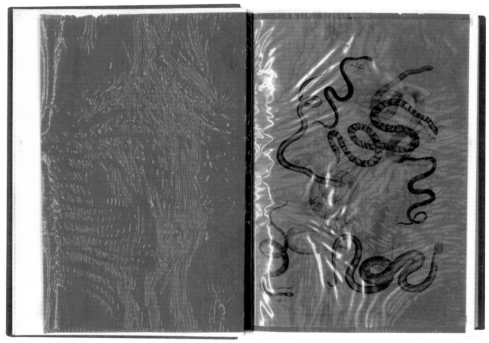

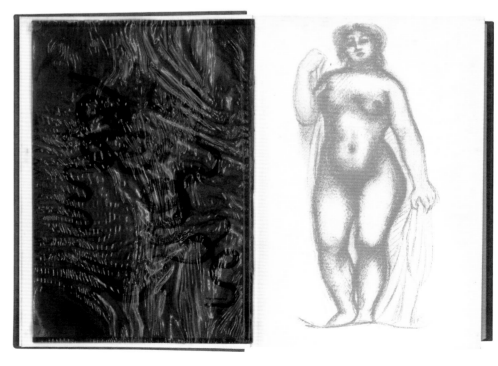

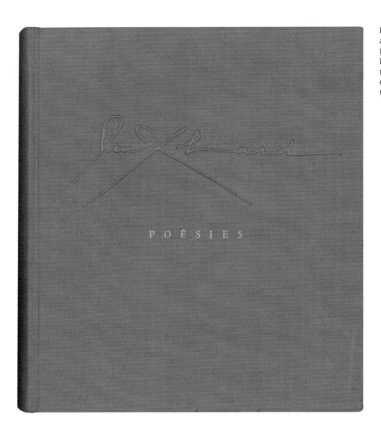

Blue cloth binding, cold-stamped in gold,
and inside pages of Paul Éluard's *Poésies*
(Paris, Club du meilleur livre, 1959).
In addition to the poems, the book
reproduces a series of eighteen portraits
of the poet by Picasso, printed on
tracing paper.

 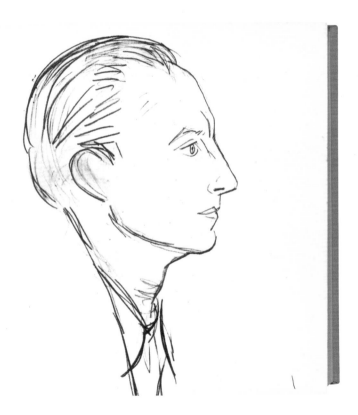

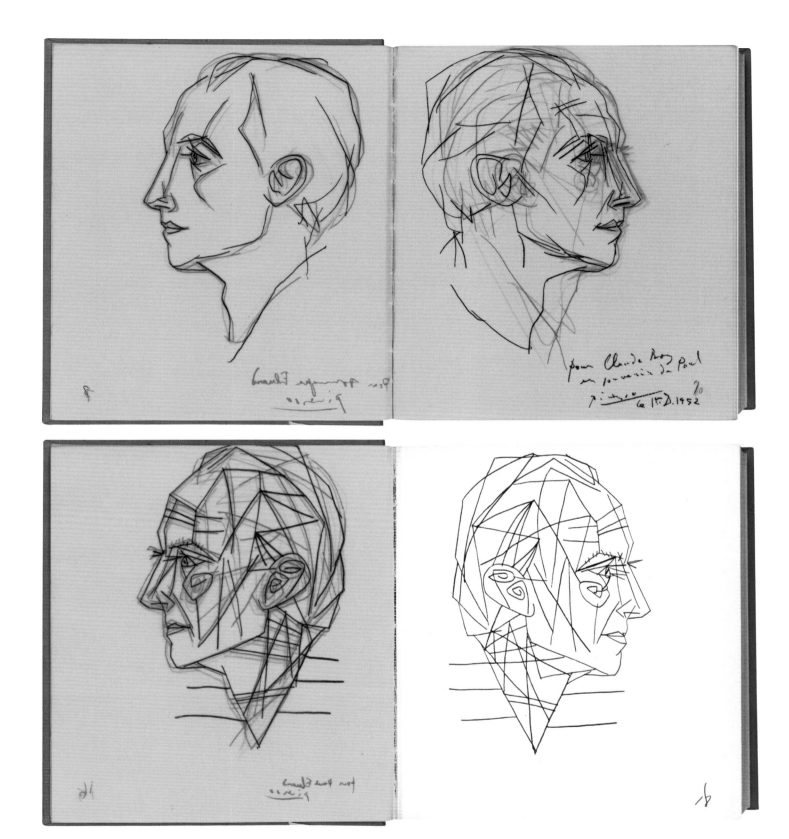

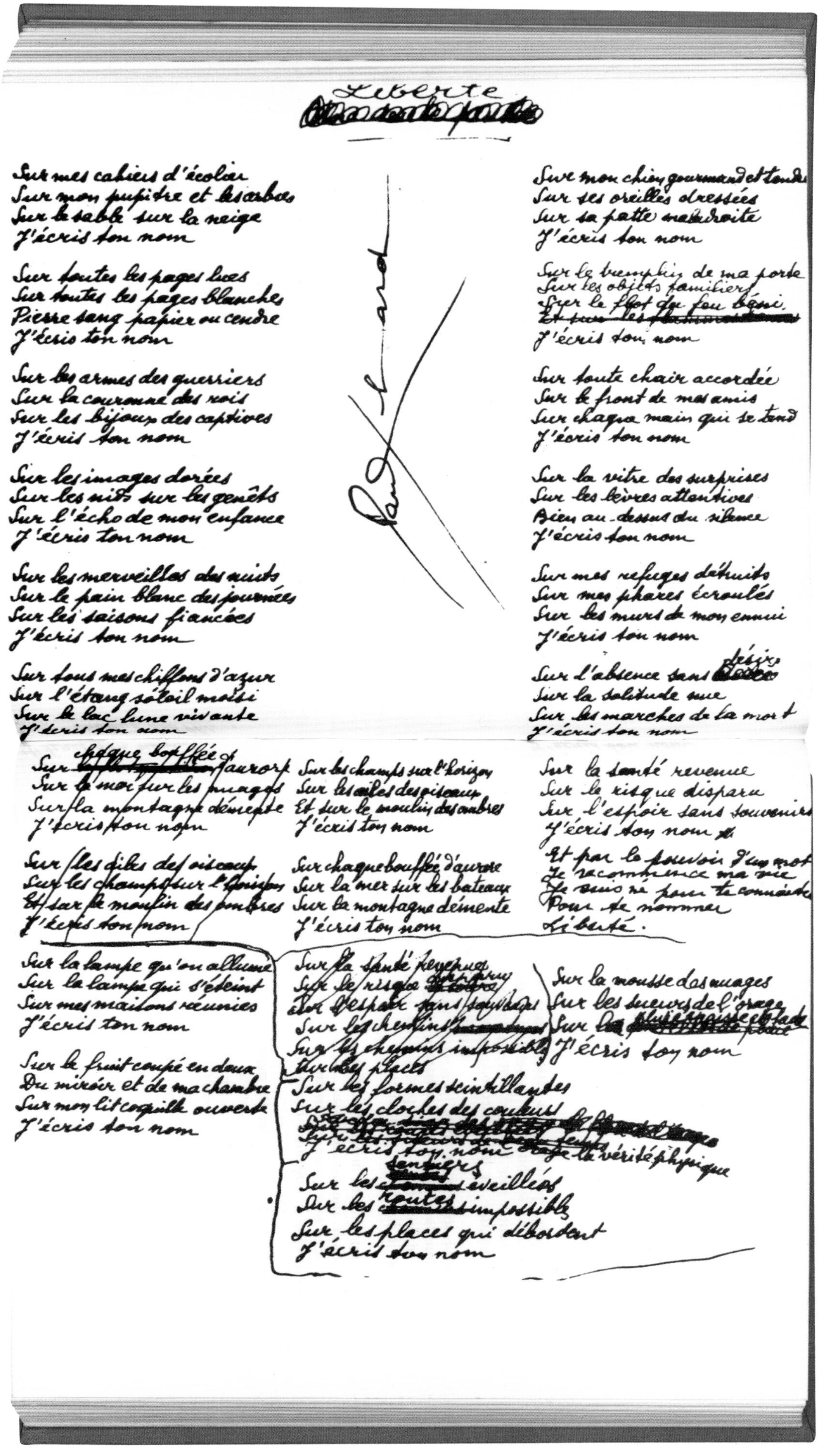

Liberté

Sur mes cahiers d'écolier
Sur mon pupitre et les arbres
Sur le sable sur la neige
J'écris ton nom

Sur toutes les pages lues
Sur toutes les pages blanches
Pierre sang papier ou cendre
J'écris ton nom

Sur les armes des guerriers
Sur la couronne des rois
Sur les bijoux des captives
J'écris ton nom

Sur les images dorées
Sur les nids sur les genêts
Sur l'écho de mon enfance
J'écris ton nom

Sur les merveilles des nuits
Sur le pain blanc des journées
Sur les saisons fiancées
J'écris ton nom

Sur tous mes chiffons d'azur
Sur l'étang soleil moisi
Sur le lac lune vivante
J'écris ton nom

Sur mon chien gourmand et tendre
Sur ses oreilles dressées
Sur sa patte maladroite
J'écris ton nom

Sur le tremplin de ma porte
Sur les objets familiers
Sur le flot du feu béni
Et sur les [rature]
J'écris ton nom

Sur toute chair accordée
Sur le front de mes amis
Sur chaque main qui se tend
J'écris ton nom

Sur la vitre des surprises
Sur les lèvres attentives
Bien au dessus du silence
J'écris ton nom

Sur mes refuges détruits
Sur mes phares écroulés
Sur les murs de mon ennui
J'écris ton nom

Sur l'absence sans désirs
Sur la solitude nue
Sur les marches de la mort
J'écris ton nom

Sur chaque bouffée d'aurore
Sur la mer sur les nuages
Sur la montagne démente
J'écris ton nom

Sur les champs sur l'horizon
Sur les ailes des oiseaux
Et sur le moulin des ombres
J'écris ton nom

Sur la santé revenue
Sur le risque disparu
Sur l'espoir sans souvenirs
J'écris ton nom

Et par le pouvoir d'un mot
Je recommence ma vie
Je suis né pour te connaître
Pour te nommer
Liberté.

Sur la lampe qu'on allume
Sur la lampe qui s'éteint
Sur mes maisons réunies
J'écris ton nom

Sur le fruit coupé en deux
Du miroir et de ma chambre
Sur mon lit coquille ouverte
J'écris ton nom

Sur les chemins impossibles
Sur les formes scintillantes
Sur les cloches des couleurs
J'écris ton nom

Sur les places qui débordent
J'écris ton nom

Paul Claudel's *Le Soulier de satin* (The satin slipper; Paris, Club du meilleur livre, 1953) are multicoloured. 'Faucheux taught me, when I was starting out, that there were no such things as ugly characters, just layout artists who didn't know how to use them', says Massin.[16] A collector of font catalogues, he preferred to use old fonts rather than introduce contemporary type. Today he explains that, 'In doing this I was adopting the same approach as Maximilien Vox who, at Grasset in the 1920s, used to print covers with fonts from the time of Balzac'.[17]

Massin's pastiches are never simple copies but, rather, intelligent and well-informed essences of the fundamental characteristics of a historical period. So, from the romantic period, Massin took the decorative illuminated lettering and a predilection for monochrome wood engravings. For Jean Savant's *Napoléon et Joséphine* (Paris, Club du meilleur livre, 1955), historical associations inspired him to choose a silk binding patterned in the style of the furnishing fabrics of the Empress Joséphine's residence, the château de Malmaison. 'It's hard, even unpleasant, for me to read Rabelais set in Didot and, conversely, Victor Hugo in Garamond, just as I won't use the same font for Proust and Céline, Claudel and Prévert, Balzac and Rimbaud', he explains.[18]

The type, often enlarged and distorted, is treated as a graphic element of the page. It plays the main role, to the detriment of pure illustration, which remains primarily iconographic. The frequent reproduction of handwritten elements, symbolically linked to the work and its author – such as the crossings-out in the poem signed '*Liberté*' (Freedom) in Paul Éluard's *Poésies* (Paris, Club du meilleur livre, 1959) – accentuates the sense of objectivity suggested by this graphic treatment. Massin often used such reproductions of handwritten text and the author's signature on his covers. The examples are many and varied, retaining a subtle balance between the subjectivity of the writing and documentary objectivity. In this way the cover of Jules Roy's *La Vallée heureuse* (The Happy Valley; Paris, Club du meilleur livre, 1956) shows reproductions of war mission plans, while the endpaper shows

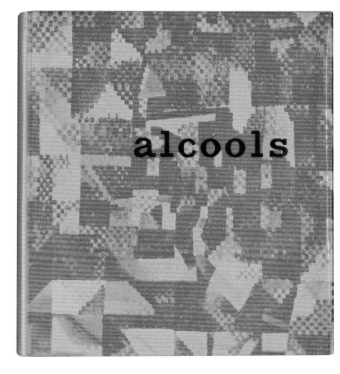

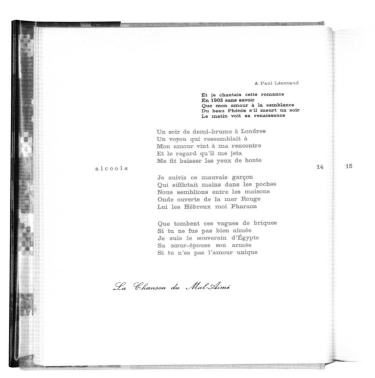

Opposite: 'Liberté', a poem from Paul Éluard's collection *Poésies*, reproduced in its original manuscript version.

Above: acetate (or Rhodoïd) jacket for Guillaume Apollinaire's *Alcools* (Spirits; Paris, Club du meilleur livre, 1953), illustrated with a reproduction of Robert Delaunay's painting *Fenêtres sur la ville no. 3* (Windows on the city). The two colours of the cover also appear on the inside pages (left).

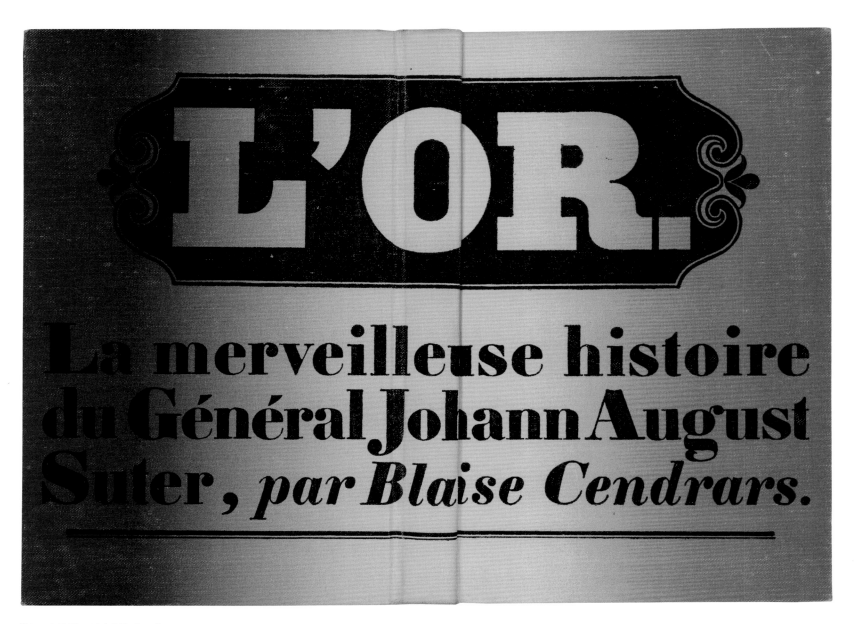

Above: multicoloured cloth binding of Blaise Cendrars' *L'Or* (Gold; Paris, Club du meilleur livre, 1956). This typographical cover is influenced by public notices.

Opposite: five-colour offset white cloth cover of Guillaume Apollinaire's *Calligrammes* (Paris, Club du meilleur livre, 1955). The cover is decorated with one of the poet's calligrams.

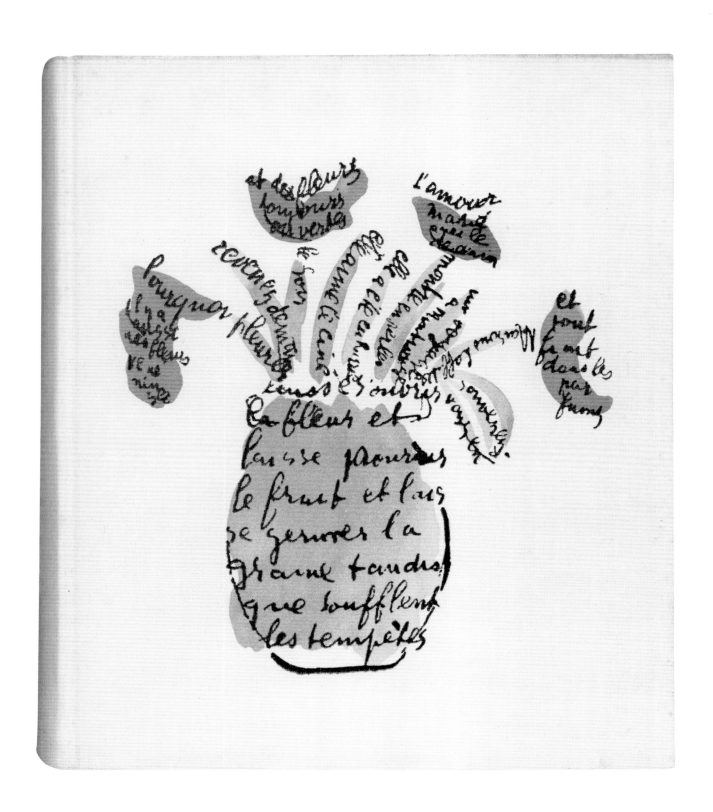

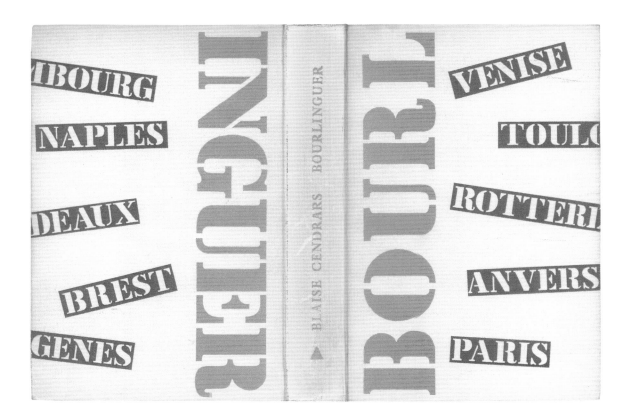

Blaise Cendrars
(1887–1961)

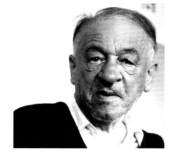

Born Frédéric-Louis Sauser in La Chaux-de-Fonds, Switzerland, Cendrars was a poet of modernity who, with his Les Pâques à New York (Easter in New York; Paris, Éditions des hommes nouveaux, 1912), discovered that writing was his true vocation. Recklessly hurling himself into every adventure of his hectic life, this man 'of the whole world' (the title of his first collection of poems, Du Monde entier, published in 1919) travelled in the most exotic lands and mixed with groups on the margins of society. Cendrars worked as a filmmaker, journalist, art critic, horticulturalist and businessman before devoting himself to writing and becoming one of the key figures of the pre-war French literary avant-garde.

'A contemplative man, quite the opposite of an "intellectual", who is curious about everything, speaks a dozen languages, has deciphered Aztec manuscripts, is abreast of every new development and, like his friend t'Serstevens – another great traveller – knows the whole world's libraries and has read the complete works of unknown authors in their original languages', says Massin.[19] Through such praise we gain the impression of an older brother figure, against whom Massin measured himself and whom he admired for his experimentation (particularly in typography), his interdisciplinary, eclectic approaches and his thirst for a knowledge that was universal rather than academic. 'I met Blaise Cendrars in 1949, after his time in Aix, when he was living in Beaulieu near Villefranche-sur-Mer, in what was, according to him, one of the finest landscapes in the world, and he had travelled

enough for me to take him at his word.'[20]

Massin's collaboration with Cendrars came to fruition in 1956 with his cover for L'Or (Gold), brought out by the Club du meilleur livre. First published in 1925, this book was Cendrars' major international success. It had originally been entitled La Merveilleuse Histoire du général Johann August Suter (The Wonderful Story of General Johann August Suter) but the great typographer Maximilien Vox is said to have thought this too long (this later became its subtitle). The cover of the Club du meilleur livre edition drew on a popular poster from 1848, which Massin had bought from an antiques dealer and which still hangs in the attic of his country house. Meanwhile the Club du meilleur livre's 1953 edition of one of Cendrars' last books, Bourlinguer (Travelling; first published 1948), contains facsimile reproductions of the author's handwritten dedications to each chapter. Cendrars was so pleased with the cover design that he would write it as a post-script in his postcards to Massin.

Top to bottom: two-colour white cloth binding of Blaise Cendrars' Bourlinguer (Travelling; Paris, Club du meilleur livre, 1953); postcard from Cendrars to Massin, 1956; letter from Cendrars to Robert Carlier, May 1956.

Far left: photograph of Cendrars by Massin, at his home in rue Jean-Dolent, Paris, 1956.

flight plan calculations. *Le Soulier de satin* is accompanied by previously unpublished writings by its author, Paul Claudel, and staging sketches by Jean-Louis Barrault, maps of the sky and facsimiles of Nicola Sabbattini's *Pratique pour fabriquer des scènes et machines de théâtre* (Manual for Constructing Theatrical Scenes and Machines; 1638).

The frequent and almost certainly costly reproduction of these facsimiles adds a unique exploratory dimension to the reader's experience of the text. For example, in *La Véritable Vie privée du maréchal de Richelieu* the reader holds a book made thicker by endpapers of imitation suede, which contain an autobiographical letter reproduced by photocollography. Later, in Billie Holiday's autobiography *Lady Sings the Blues* (Paris, Club du meilleur livre, 1960), the reader is invited to leaf through documentary photographs and black and white portraits of the singer in concert before starting to read the text.

Other designers of the period were inspired by a similar desire for historical realism and objective rigour and, rather than hiring contemporary illustrators, preferred to use graphic elements dating from the period of a book's first publication as illustrations, thereby adding to the air of authenticity of the whole. Today Massin says, 'Eventually Faucheux turned this into a kind of dogma or religion to which – he dominated us so much – we all felt obliged to adhere, even though some of us, such as Darche, Bonin and Daniel, would have liked the clubs to take advantage of their talents as illustrators.'[21] Later, in his role as art director, Massin himself used the talents of draughtsmen such as André François, Siné and Jean-Michel Folon.

Four-colour offset white cloth binding of Jules Roy's *La Vallée heureuse* (The Happy Valley; Paris, Club du meilleur livre, 1956), illustrated with plans for war missions.

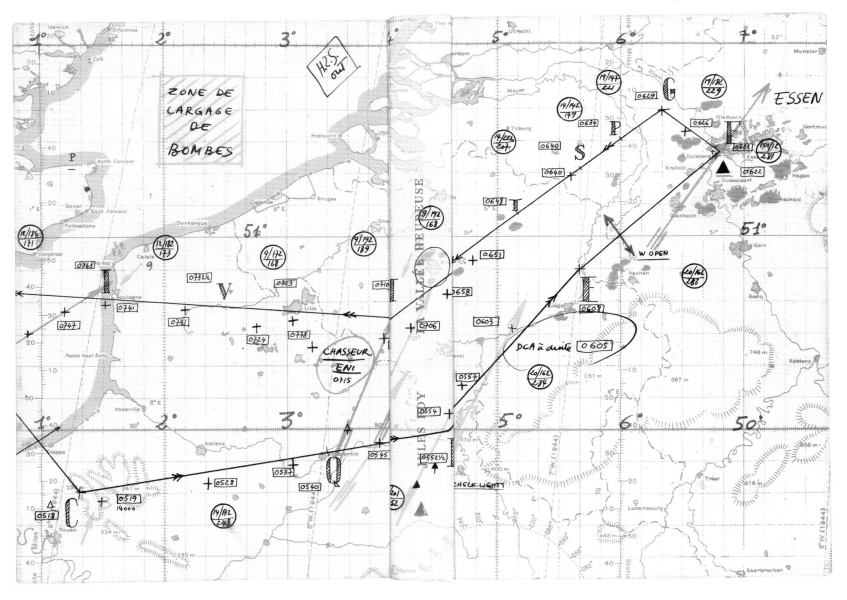

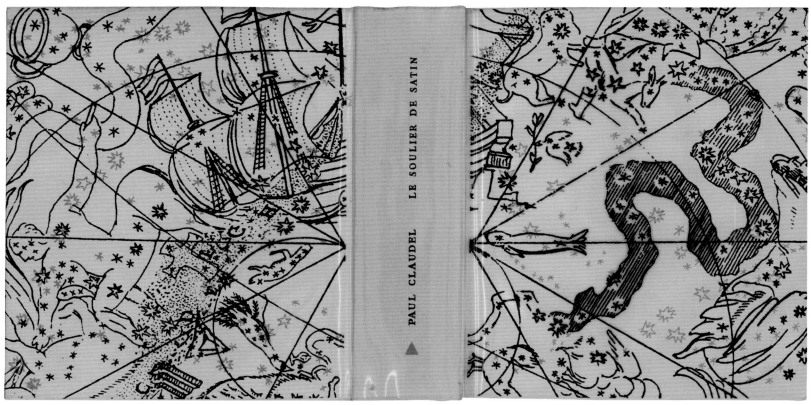

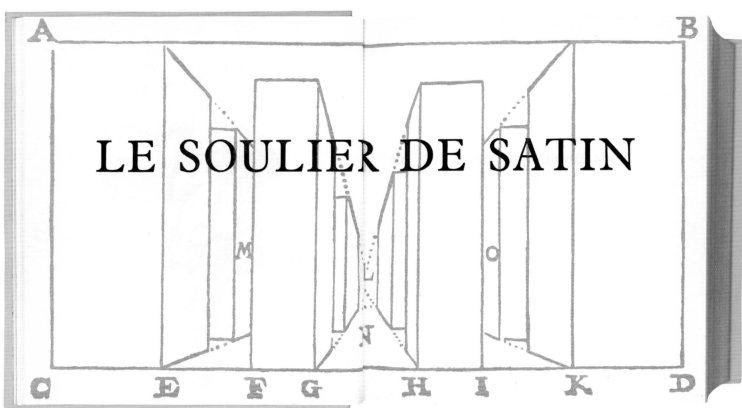

Above and opposite: two-colour yellow
cloth binding of Paul Claudel's *Le Soulier
de satin* (The satin slipper; Paris, Club du
meilleur livre, 1953). The acetate jacket
is illustrated with a star map; inside
spreads from *Le Soulier de satin.*

Je suppose que ma pièce soit jouée par exemple un jour de

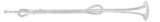

Mardi-Gras à quatre heures de l'après-midi. Je rêve une grande

salle chauffée par un spectacle précédent, que le public envahit et

que remplissent les conversations. Par les portes battantes on entend

le tapage sourd d'un orchestre bien nourri qui fonctionne dans le

foyer. Un autre petit orchestre nasillard dans la salle s'amuse à

imiter les bruits du public en les conduisant et en leur donnant peu

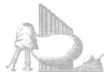

à peu une espèce de rythme et de figure.

Apparaît sur le proscenium devant le rideau baissé l'ANNON-

CIER. C'est un solide gaillard barbu et qui a emprunté aux plus

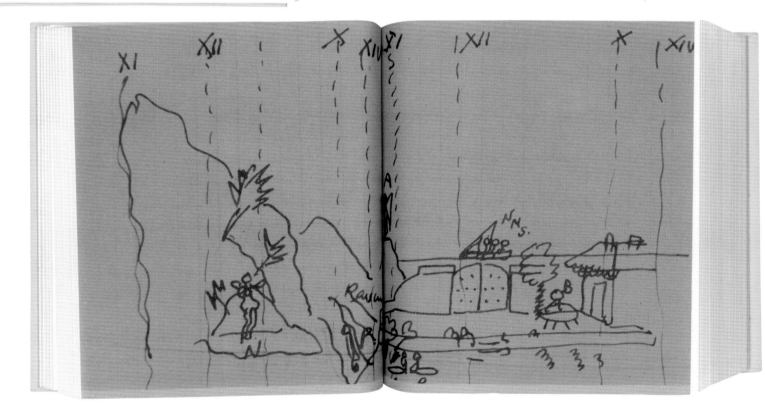

The rise and fall: the collapse of the clubs and the rise of bookshops and distributors

At the height of their success in the early 1950s, the book clubs had around 700,000 members; but their triumph was short-lived, although many survived into the 1960s. The decline began in 1958, when the bookshops had at last been re-established (with support from the publishers) and were able to short-circuit the market. Once club books were available in bookshops, including shops in rural areas, there was no longer a need for the clubs themselves. Books published by the clubs represented serious competition for the publishing houses, being cheaper, generally better produced, printed on paper of a higher quality, laid out, set and printed with great care and protected by board or fabric-covered binding.

Having witnessed the democratic change generated by the clubs and been irritated by their commercial success, the publishers now understood the full importance of the appearance of books to be sold in bookshops. The fate of the 'Nombre d'or' series provides a perfect illustration of the complexity of the post-war landscape of French publishing:

'This was soon understood in the corridors of NRF [Nouvelle Revue française] and the Hachette shipping service […]. Because there was not a single detail that haste had caused us to neglect: the backers of the Club du meilleur livre – and hence the owners of the fine, bound books from 'Nombre d'or' – were none other than… Gallimard and Hachette, the well-known publisher and distributor of the Pléiade! It was too much! And they – if we are to believe Robert Carlier – were partly responsible for the fate of that series.'[22]

Under increasing pressure from the bookshops and weakened by competition from the clubs, the publishers adopted the latter's formulas and methods. By organizing their own distribution networks and increasingly having their layouts designed in-house, they learned how to create harmonious relationships between choice of format, typeface and justified

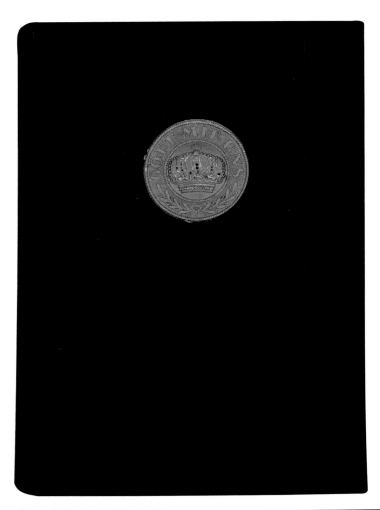

Above and right: black cloth binding of Maxence Van der Meersch's *Invasion 14* (Paris, Club du meilleur livre, 1954). The front cover is decorated with a German belt buckle bearing the words 'Gott Mit Uns'; endpapers of *Invasion 14*.

Opposite, above and below: title pages of *Invasion 14*; inside spread from *Invasion 14*, presenting the characters.

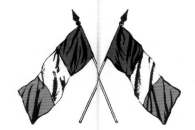

ARMÉE DE TERRE ET ARMÉE DE MER

ORDRE
DE MOBILISATION GÉNÉRALE

Par décret du Président de la République, la mobilisation des armées de terre et de mer est ordonnée, ainsi que la réquisition des animaux, voitures et harnais nécessaires au complément de ces armées.

Le premier jour de la mobilisation est le   Dimanche 2 Août 1914

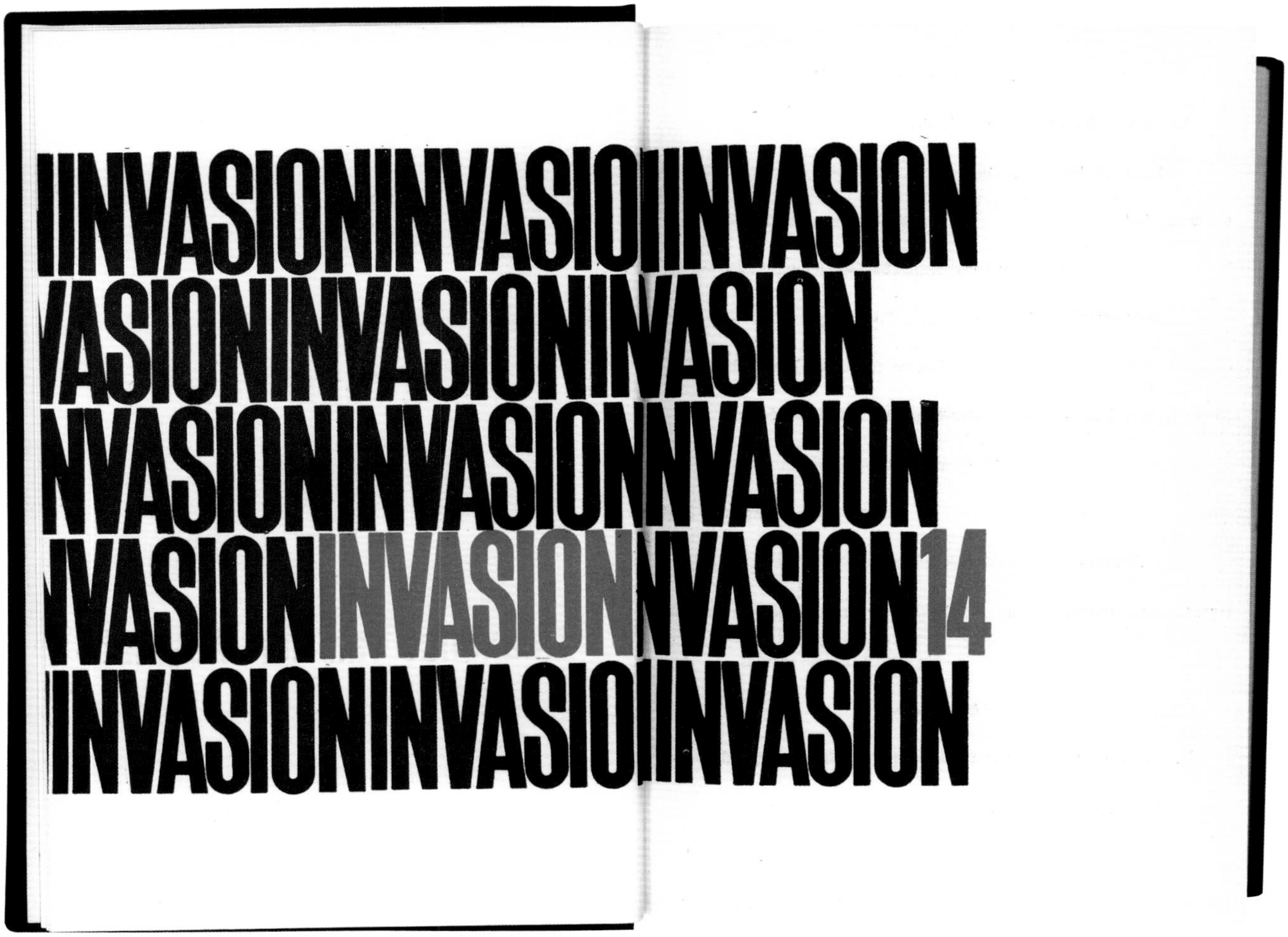

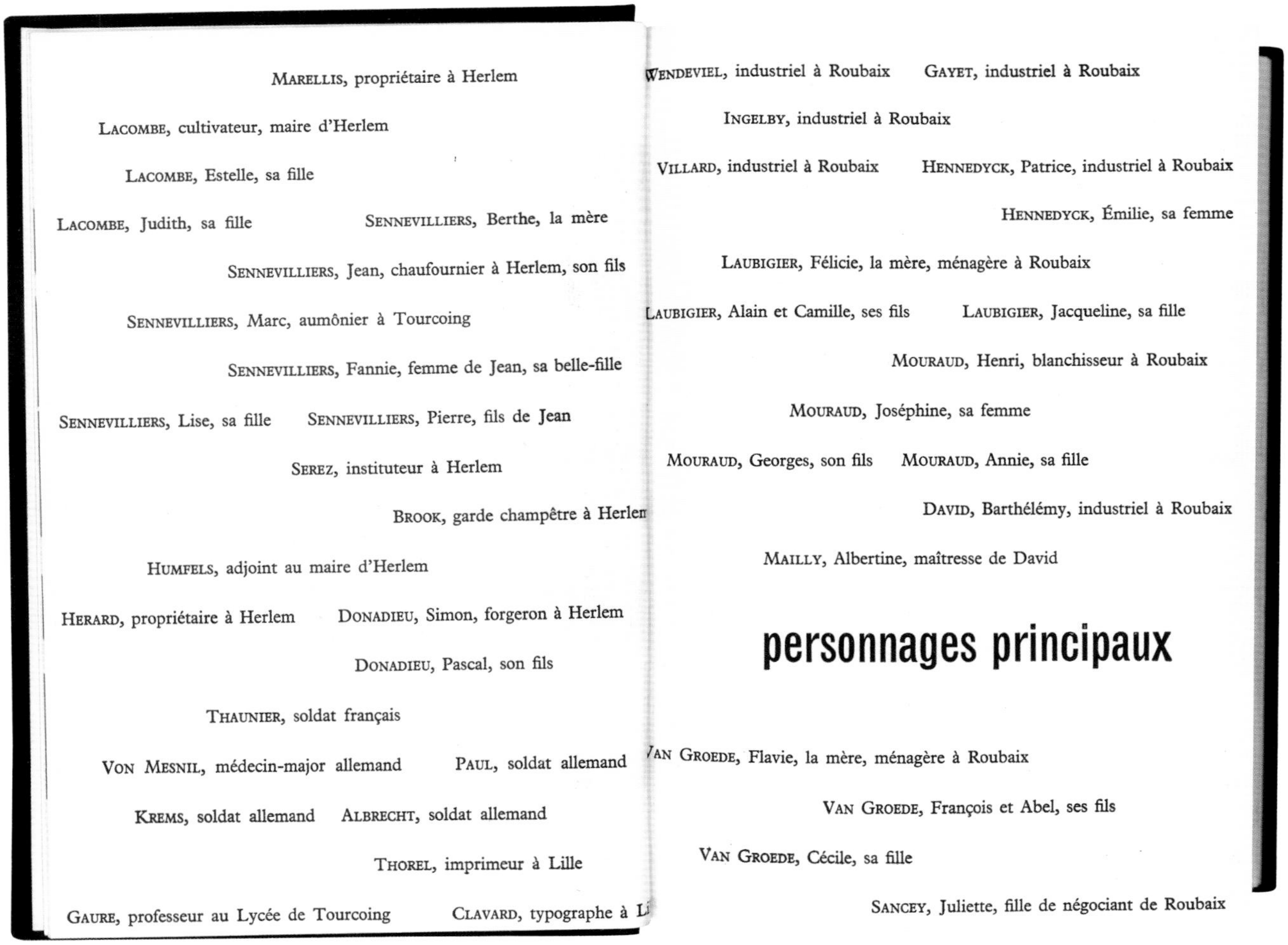

INVASIONINVASIOINVASION
VASIONINVASIONINVASION
NVASIONINVASIONNVASION
NVASIONINVASIONNVASION14
INVASIONINVASIOINVASION

MARELLIS, propriétaire à Herlem

LACOMBE, cultivateur, maire d'Herlem

LACOMBE, Estelle, sa fille

LACOMBE, Judith, sa fille   SENNEVILLIERS, Berthe, la mère

SENNEVILLIERS, Jean, chaufournier à Herlem, son fils

SENNEVILLIERS, Marc, aumônier à Tourcoing

SENNEVILLIERS, Fannie, femme de Jean, sa belle-fille

SENNEVILLIERS, Lise, sa fille   SENNEVILLIERS, Pierre, fils de Jean

SEREZ, instituteur à Herlem

BROOK, garde champêtre à Herlem

HUMFELS, adjoint au maire d'Herlem

HERARD, propriétaire à Herlem   DONADIEU, Simon, forgeron à Herlem

DONADIEU, Pascal, son fils

THAUNIER, soldat français

VON MESNIL, médecin-major allemand   PAUL, soldat allemand

KREMS, soldat allemand   ALBRECHT, soldat allemand

THOREL, imprimeur à Lille

GAURE, professeur au Lycée de Tourcoing   CLAVARD, typographe à L...

WENDEVIEL, industriel à Roubaix   GAYET, industriel à Roubaix

INGELBY, industriel à Roubaix

VILLARD, industriel à Roubaix   HENNEDYCK, Patrice, industriel à Roubaix

HENNEDYCK, Émilie, sa femme

LAUBIGIER, Félicie, la mère, ménagère à Roubaix

LAUBIGIER, Alain et Camille, ses fils   LAUBIGIER, Jacqueline, sa fille

MOURAUD, Henri, blanchisseur à Roubaix

MOURAUD, Joséphine, sa femme

MOURAUD, Georges, son fils   MOURAUD, Annie, sa fille

DAVID, Barthélémy, industriel à Roubaix

MAILLY, Albertine, maîtresse de David

personnages principaux

VAN GROEDE, Flavie, la mère, ménagère à Roubaix

VAN GROEDE, François et Abel, ses fils

VAN GROEDE, Cécile, sa fille

SANCEY, Juliette, fille de négociant de Roubaix

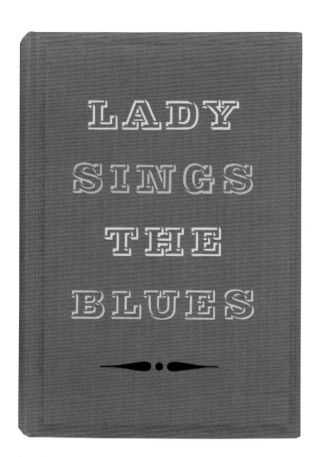

columns of text. Similarly, when it came to the book's external appearance, they brought in commercial artists such as Villemot and well-known illustrators such as André François to design jackets and covers, having understood the power of attraction and commercial importance these elements could have on shelves which were, by that time, laden with books.

In the mid-1950s the clubs' graphic artists also started working with publishers such as Corrêa, Pierre Horay, La Table Ronde, Le Seuil and Calmann-Lévy. Once this happened, graphic virtuosity ceased to be the preserve of the clubs. Massin sincerely believes that the clubs' members grew weary of the graphic excesses of their object books ('experiments that were sometimes rather precious', the journal *Graphis* reported during the 1950s). The time of the book clubs was drawing to a close and, although their members still liked the formula, publishers were seeking out less expensive and equally profitable alternatives. Annoyed by public enthusiasm for the clubs' output, which consisted largely of re-editions that ultimately hindered the launch of new titles, in 1957 Gallimard decided to launch a bound library edition and the 'Soleil' series was born. Its aesthetics deliberately ran counter to the exuberance of the clubs, in which Massin continued to operate officially until 1963. In becoming head of 'Soleil', it was Massin who managed the transition between the end of the clubs and the establishment of art direction at Gallimard.

Above: five-colour brown cloth binding of Billie Holiday's autobiography *Lady Sings the Blues* (Paris, Club du meilleur livre, 1960).

Right, opposite and following two pages: inside pages from *Lady Sings the Blues.*

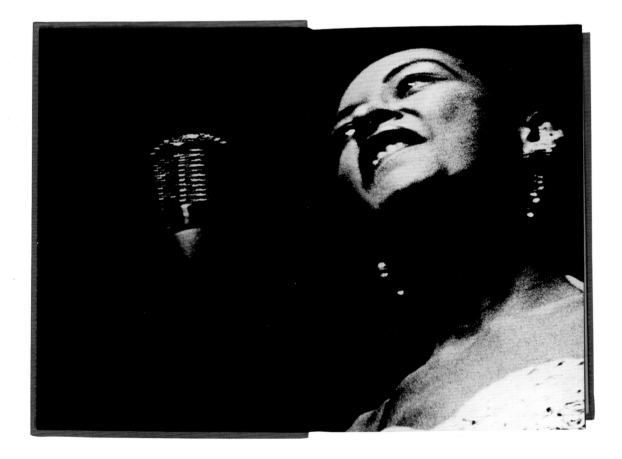

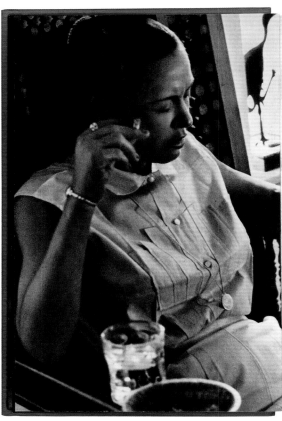

HOMMAGE A « LADY DAY »

A la nouvelle de l'édition française de Lady sings the blues, *plusieurs musiciens américains, qui résident en France ou l'ont récemment traversée, ont tenu à apporter leur témoignage, tant sur la personnalité de la grande chanteuse que sur le livre qu'elle avait écrit trois ans avant sa mort.*

RUBLE BLAKEY

A mon avis, Billie était une des chanteuses les plus extraordinaires de notre époque. Ce fut une grande chance pour moi de l'avoir connue et d'avoir travaillé à ses côtés, en maintes occasions, alors qu'elle était au sommet de sa carrière.

Son art d'imprimer une touche de mélancolie à n'importe quelle

LADY

chanson populaire ou moderne a probablement donné naissance à l'expression « song stylist », expression si fréquemment employée aux États-Unis depuis une dizaine d'années, lorsque nous parlions d'un chanteur ou d'une chanteuse qui improvise d'une manière personnelle sur une mélodie, ou qui donne à une chanson un accent neuf et original.

Dans la vie privée, elle était chaleureuse, compréhensive et toujours prête à apporter son aide à ceux qui avaient besoin d'elle. Mais le meilleur d'un être ne passe-t-il pas souvent inaperçu en regard des incidents malencontreux de sa vie ? Aussi bien que lors de ses apparitions sur scène ou au cabaret, aussi bien que dans ses disques, je la retrouve dans ce livre, et cela me va droit au cœur.

Ci-contre : Billie Holiday, à l'hôpital, peu avant sa mort.

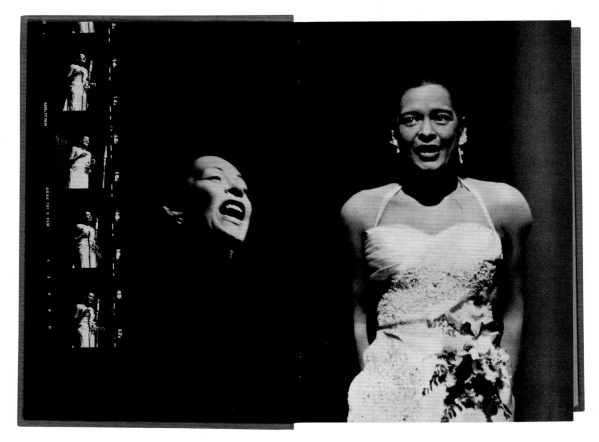

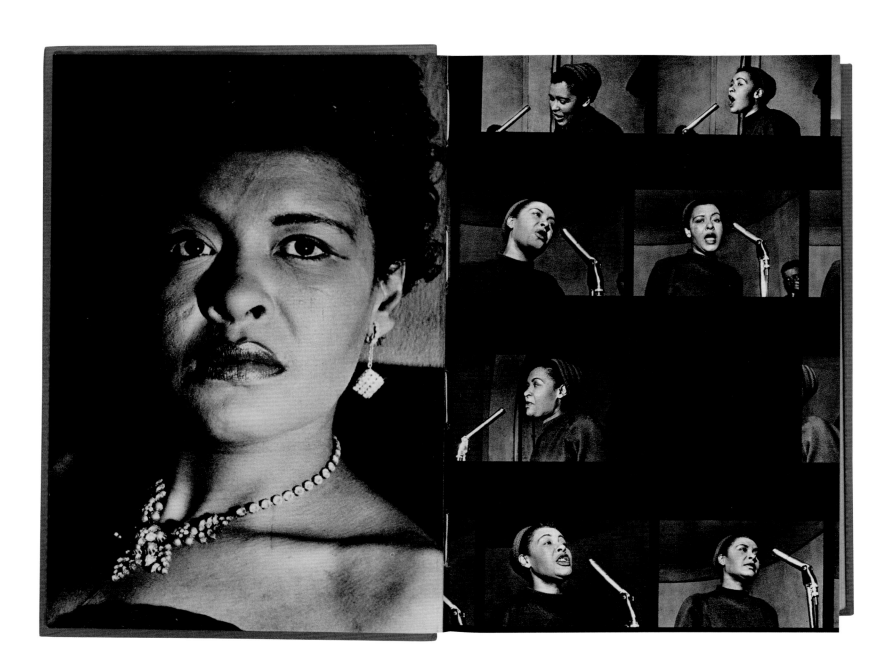

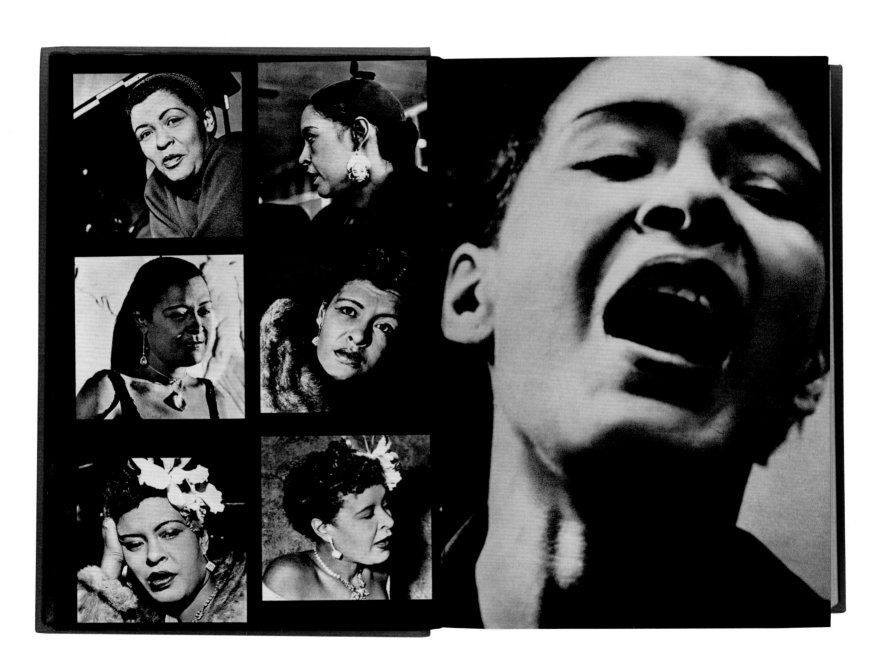

Top right: poster for Alfred Jarry's *Ubu roi ou les Polonais* (King Ubu or the Polish), printed in black on butcher's paper with illustrations by André François.

Left: three-colour black cloth binding for *Ubu roi* (Paris, Club du meilleur livre, 1958), with an illustration by André François printed in relief.

Bottom right: three-colour paper cover for the catalogue of the exhibition 'Ubu roi, cent ans de règne' at the musée-galerie de la Seita (1989), reproducing Alfred Jarry's famous sketch of Père Ubu.

Opposite and following two pages: endpapers from *Ubu roi ou les Polonais*, with illustrations by André François.

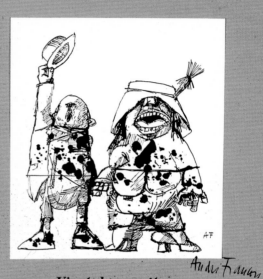

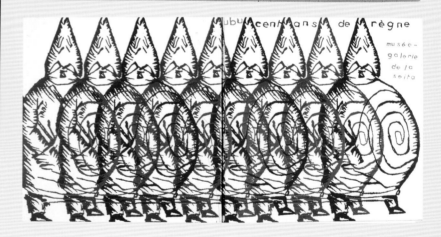

Focus
Ubu roi ou les Polonais
Paris, le Club du meilleur livre, 1958

After its first, turbulent performance in Paris in 1896, Alfred Jarry's *Ubu roi* (Ubu the king), a masterly forerunner of the theatre of the absurd, travelled the world and won over audiences of all kinds by making them laugh. Coming out of burlesque theatre, the play tells the story of the tyrant Ubu, a base, unscrupulous buffoon who, with the support of Mother Ubu, betrays and kills his sovereign to take his place. Once established as an authoritarian king, Ubu spreads discord with cries of 'Merdre!' and 'Open the trapdoor!' and is always on the look out for means to satisfy his greed. Like some vast, joyful, schoolboy farce, *Ubu roi* uses derision as a weapon against dictatorship and foreshadows the coming of totalitarianism in all its forms.

In deciding to revise the layout of *Ubu roi*, which had already been reworked by the master Pierre Faucheux in 1950 for the Club français du livre, Massin added his personal touch to the work, notably in his surprising choice of materials and desire to highlight the illustrations accompanying the text. The use of butcher's paper, with its uneven, dappled surface,

enabled him to evoke all the crudeness of Ubu's bloody character. Massin tells a colourful anecdote from his childhood to explain his fascination with this tripe-shop paper, reddened with ox blood: there was no butcher in his native village (La Bourdinière), but Touchard, a butcher from a village nearby, would come by in his van once a week to sell meat. His daughter had died after swallowing a one-franc piece - the hospital in Chartres was too far away. Massin remembers his parents' quipping, in rather poor taste, 'Poor little thing, she got carved up.'

Massin hired André François, an artist still unknown to the wider public at that time, who made twenty satirical drawings. The character of Captain Bordure seems to have been secretly modelled on General Massu (when the design created by Massin was published in 1958 by the Club du meilleur livre, it was at the height of the Algerian war, in which Massu became famous for his brutal methods, particularly during the Battle of Algiers in 1957). Sketched in the tragi-comic style of the cartoon strip, François' figures

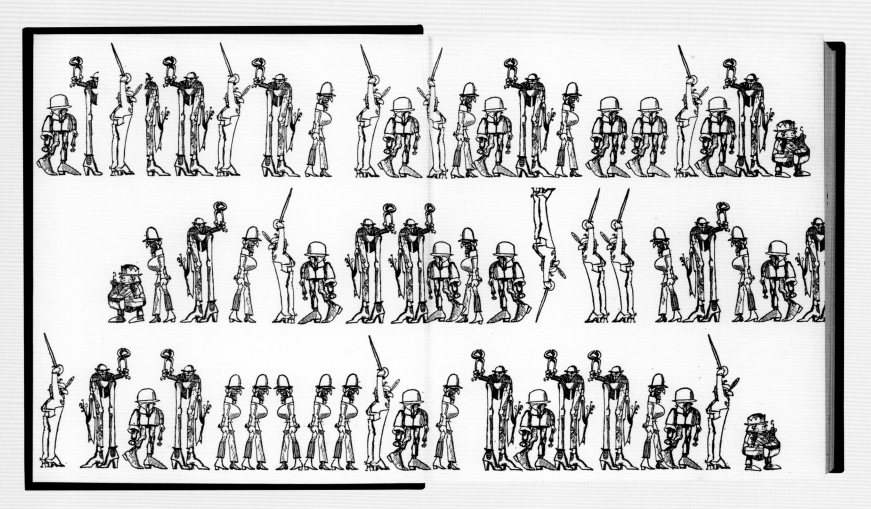

COMPOSITION DE L'ORCHESTRE

Hautbois

Chalumeaux

Cervelas

Grande Basse

Flageolets   Flûtes traversières

Grande Flûte

Petit Basson   Grand Basson

Triple Basson   Petits Cornets noirs

Cornets blancs aigus

Cors   Sacquebutes   Trombones

Oliphans verts   Galoubets

Cornemuses

Bombardes   Timbales

Tambour   Grosse Caisse

Grandes Orgues

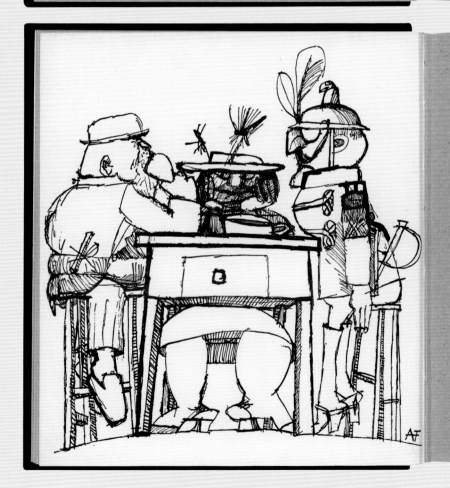

SCÈNE PREMIÈRE

Père Ubu, Mère Ubu

Père Ubu

Merdre!

Mère Ubu

Oh! voilà du joli, Père Ubu, vous estes un fort grand voyou.

Père Ubu

Que ne vous assom-je, Mère Ubu!

Mère Ubu

Ce n'est pas moi, Père Ubu, c'est un autre qu'il faudrait assassiner.

Père Ubu

De par ma chandelle verte, je ne comprends pas.

3

retain the pot-bellied grotesquery of *Le Véritable Portrait de monsieur Ubu* (The real portrait of Mr Ubu) in his pointed hat, the famous woodcut made by Jarry himself for the playbill of the performance of 1896 at the Théâtre de l'Œuvre. Faucheux had used this woodcut for his cover, as did Massin for the cover he later designed in 1989 for *Ubu roi, cent ans de règne* (Ubu the king, a hundred years in power), the catalogue of the exhibition at the musée-galerie de la Seita.

The typeface, a classic 18-point Bodoni, remains deliberately traditional, in total contrast to the roughness of the paper which, itself, contrasts with the white paper on which the drawings are printed. 'This paper, made, they say, from recycled banknotes, had bumps, hollows and even fragments of straw, which moreover made the Bodoni unsuitable. The printer had to send it back for recasting.'[23] Entirely set by hand, composed of lead characters placed one by one on a composing stick, this was a costly project. François' 'score drawing', whose blots of red ink imitate blood and herald the splashes of Eugène Ionesco's *Délire à deux* (Delirium for two; Paris, Gallimard, 1966), were to be stuck on to the board, but Massin gave up the idea of making it into an endpaper, as the glue would have made it too lumpy.

This illustration of Jarry's work became a true interpretation thanks to the invaluable collaboration of François and, despite political references dating from the period of its publication, retains extraordinary artistic importance today.

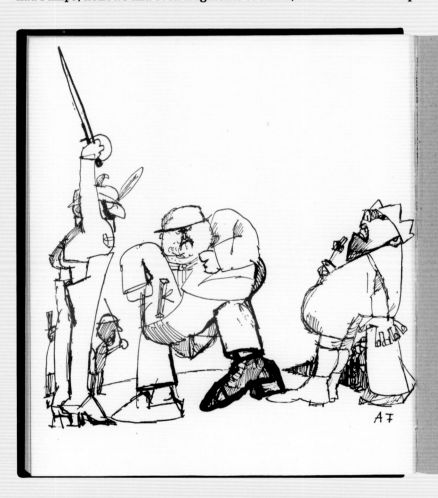

SCÈNE IV

Père Ubu, Mère Ubu, Capitaine Bordure

Père Ubu
Eh bien ! capitaine, avez-vous bien dîné ?

Capitaine Bordure
Fort bien, monsieur, sauf la merdre.

Père Ubu
Eh ! la merdre n'était pas mauvaise.

Mère Ubu
Chacun son goût.

Père Ubu
Capitaine Bordure, je suis décidé à vous faire duc de Lithuanie.

19

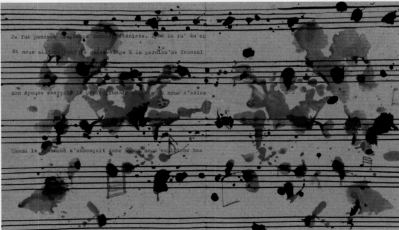

Left: original 'score drawing' by André François for the endpapers (not used) on butcher's paper with blood-red blotches.

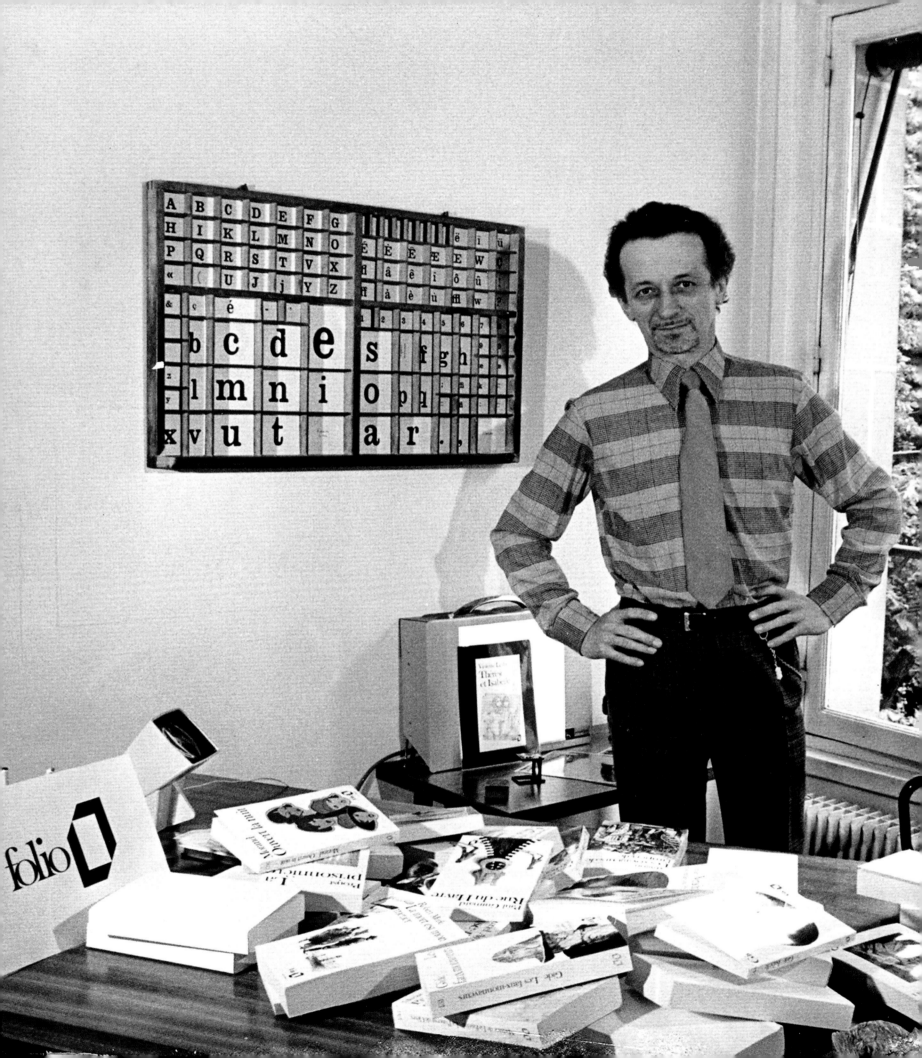

Art Direction

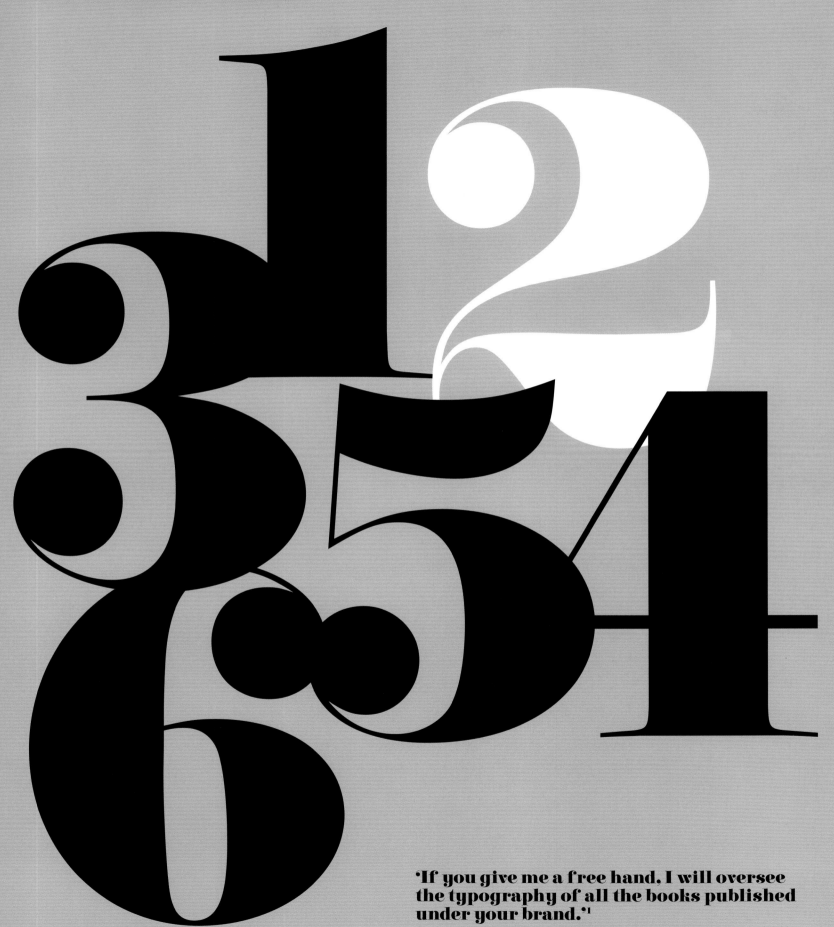

'If you give me a free hand, I will oversee the typography of all the books published under your brand.'[1]

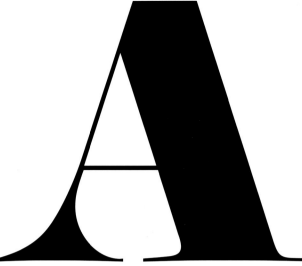

At the heart of the French publishing empire

'I started at the Club français du livre on 1 February 1948. Ten years later, to the day, I stepped through the door of no. 5, rue Sébastien-Bottin', remembers Massin.[2] Gallimard's famous Paris address, close to the boulevard Saint-Germain, still makes an impression today and evokes an entire period of post-war French literary history.

In 1958, while continuing to work at the Club du meilleur livre, where he retained his title of art director, Massin officially joined Gallimard on the recommendation of literary director Robert Carlier. At the time Gallimard had neither a graphic art department, nor an art director, nor any 'house layout' in any real sense. Everything was still being done at the printer's. It was not until the departure of their head of production in 1961 that the foundations were laid for an art department which, for twenty years, was personified by Massin himself. By the time the 'Folio' series was launched in 1972, there were a dozen people working in the department. In his role as art director, Massin proposed to revise the company's image down to its most humble manifestations and minute details, creating a brand identity ahead of its time. He was already aware of the visual impact of books, their logo and presentation in the bookshops. He quickly expressed his panoramic, interdisciplinary vision, seeking to design series that would be sustained over the long term rather than just individual covers of new books about to be launched.

Anecdote has it that Massin challenged Gaston Gallimard in person, by offering to take over all the books the company published: 'If you give me a free hand, I will oversee the typography of all the books published under your brand.' Although initially surprised by the scale of the request, as time went by Gallimard asked Massin to rethink certain aspects and gave him

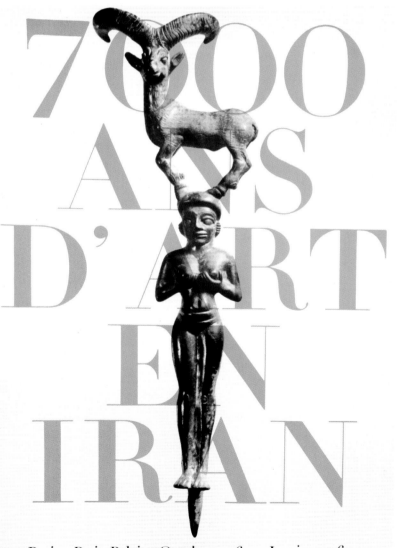

Paris, Petit Palais. Octobre 1961 – Janvier 1962.
Tous les jours, sauf le mardi, de 10 h. à 18 h.

Page 52: photograph of Massin by Jacques Robert, in his studio at Éditions Gallimard, 5, rue Sébastien-Bottin, Paris, c.1972.

Left: Poster for the exhibition '7000 ans d'art en Iran' (Petit Palais, Paris, 1961).

the freedom to 'maintain, restore and renew' (in Massin's words) the some 10,000 titles in the catalogue. Throughout his twenty years at Gallimard Massin, the eternal workaholic, used the stability of his position to explore every possible or imaginable avenue Gallimard offered: from series design to the creation of unique covers, the independent production of experimental typographical projects – which would establish his reputation – and the typographical reworking of the NRF (Nouvelle Revue française) logo. By taking a long view, which often concentrated on details and necessarily took time to bear fruit, his challenge was met and rewarded, notably by giving art direction a real place in the publishing world, which many other French publishing houses strove to imitate as the years went by.

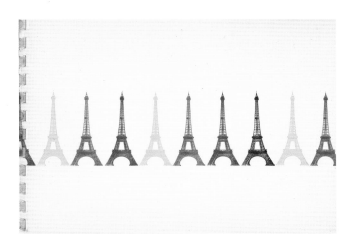

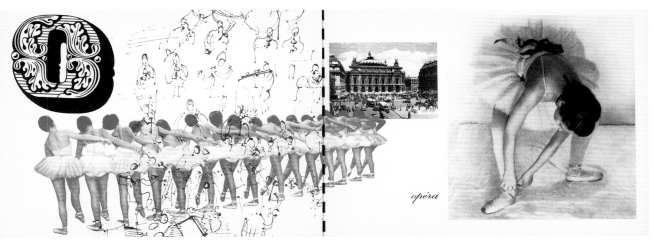

Top to bottom, left to right: four-colour cover and inside pages of *Paris*, brochure for the ministère des Travaux publics, des Transports et du Tourisme (1955), illustrated with photographs and drawings by artists, including Edgar Degas; four-colour offset cover of *Carnet de voyage en France, calendrier des manifestations* (French travel notebook, events calendar) for the ministère des Travaux publics, des Transports et du Tourisme (1958), after a drawing by Georges Braque; four-colour offset cover of *Almanach du touriste, France* (Tourist's almanach, France) for the ministère des Travaux publics, des Transports et du

Tourisme (1957), cover illustration by Jacques Noël; four-colour cover of *France*, year planner for 1959 illustrated by Pierre-Joseph Redouté; four-colour offset cover for *De Bruxelles à Lourdes, routes et pèlerinages de France* (From Brussels to Lourdes, routes and pilgrimages in France), year calendar illustrated by Benedictine monk Frère Yves of La Pierre-qui-Vire, for the ministère des Travaux publics, des Transports et du Tourisme (1956).

Below: photograph of André Malraux by Massin at the ministère des Affaires culturelles, Paris, 1968.

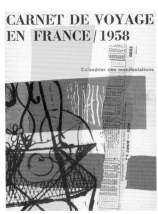

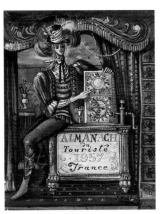

Public or private: a career choice

Hired by Gallimard in 1958, but officially on the payroll only from 1961, Massin initially continued to work freelance for other publishing houses, both private (such as Pierre Horay, Mercure de France and Calmann-Lévy) and public.

It was André Malraux who asked him to revise the typography of all state publications. A former publisher at NRF, in the late 1920s Malraux had preceded Massin in a role foreshadowing that of art director at Gallimard. In 1958 he was appointed Minister of Information by General de Gaulle. An erudite aesthete and author published by Gallimard (La Condition humaine [The Human Condition] is still one of the company's best selling titles) he later headed the ministère des Affaires culturelles from 1959 to 1969. In 1960 Massin was invited to participate in the great project for the art direction and enhancement of the

national heritage, by establishing basic guidelines for the design of exhibition catalogues and museum guides.[3] He redesigned the entrance tickets for the musée du Louvre, the ministry letterheads, posters for major exhibitions at the national museums, invitations and menus for official receptions and information brochures on the restoration of national monuments. A little earlier in his career, he had been asked by Bernard Anthonioz, who was then art director at the French tourist board, to design what were known as prestige leaflets. These were publications aimed at increasing awareness of France throughout the world.

But in 1962, faced with the scale of the task, Massin had to make a choice. Unable to go in both directions at once, he opted for a career at Gallimard.

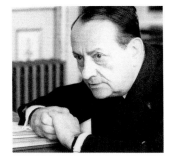

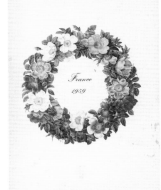

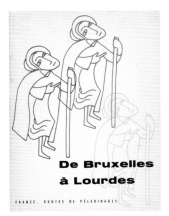

The 'Soleil' series

One of the first manifestations of the 'global vision' that Massin brought in before he even joined Gallimard was the 'Soleil' series, launched in 1957. As a counterweight to the eclecticism of the book clubs (which Gallimard and Hachette were unofficially funding), Massin was invited to design a simple, elegant and homogeneous series consisting entirely of titles from Gallimard's back catalogue, including best sellers such as the French translation of William Faulkner's *Light in August* and André Gide's *La Symphonie pastorale* (The Pastoral Symphony).

While the 'Soleil' series took its overall style, board binding and acetate dust jackets from the tradition of the clubs, its original minimalist concept was based on the colours of the rainbow. 'So everything in the design of this series was the opposite of what I had previously proposed to revolutionize book presentation; but it was in fact another revolution to choose "masses" of colour for sets of books', explains Massin.[4] The books in the series, in a 140 x 205 mm format, were bound in coloured cloth with decoration in bronze and a blind-tooled border (an engraving technique in which a pre-heated tool is pushed across the cover of a book, leaving an impression). In order to make up for the limited choice of colours for the covers (different authors could be published with covers of the same colour), the printed colours of the endpapers varied from author to author. With its small Didot type and well-spaced titles (allowing a larger space between each letter), the 'Soleil' series reflects an updated classicism. In the period 1957–77, 344 titles were published. Massin explains, 'Instead of being designed individually, each book was part of a whole; in short it was a way of reinventing edition binding'.[5] To us today this holistic approach seems particularly bold in its minimalism, given that, at that time, these books with their 'masses' of colour were still being displayed in showrooms where the books of the Club du meilleur livre were on sale and in a few handpicked bookshops that had the facilities to show them properly as a series.

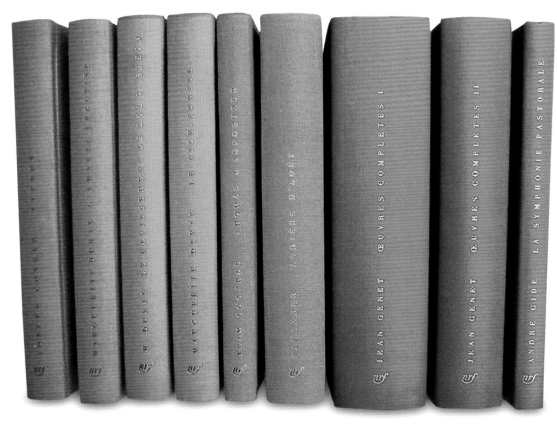

Rainbow-coloured cloth bindings for
the 'Soleil' series (Paris, Gallimard,
from 1957).

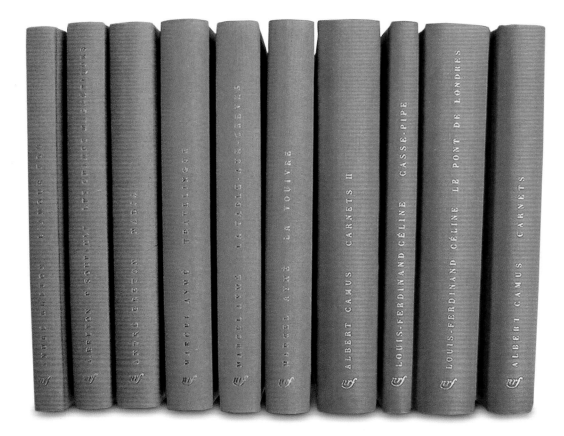

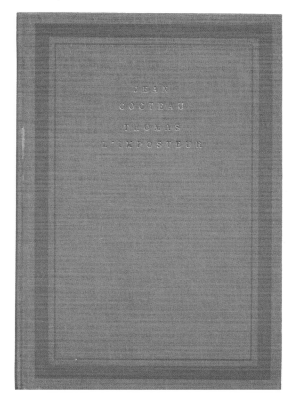

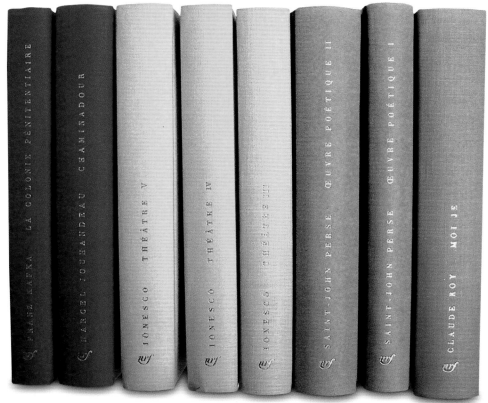

Jacques Prévert
La pluie et le beau temps

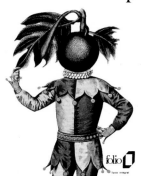

Forsyth ## Chacal

Malaparte ## La peau

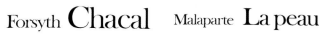

Roald Dahl
Kiss Kiss

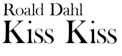
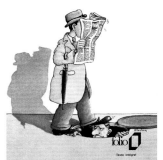
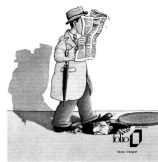

Jorge Semprun
Le grand voyage

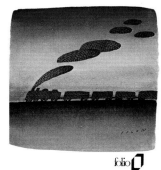

Romain Gary
Lady L.

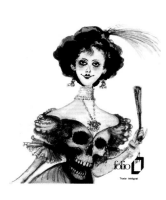

Gide ## Paludes

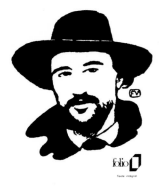

Colette ## La retraite sentimentale

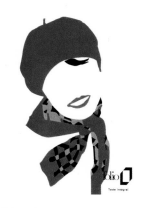

Marcel Aymé ## Le passe-muraille

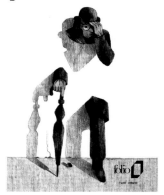

Dostoïevski
Les possédés II

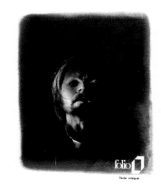

Mérimée ## Carmen
et treize autres nouvelles

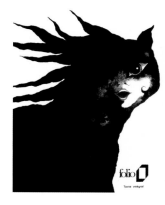

Alejo Carpentier ## Le partage des eaux

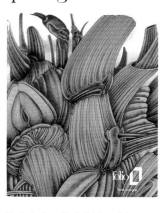

Faulkner
Sartoris

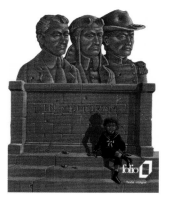

Borges ## Fictions

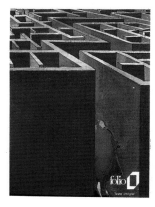

Maurice Genevoix
Bestiaire sans oubli

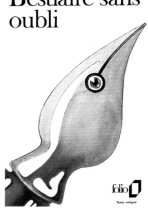

Four-colour paper covers for the 'Folio' series (Paris, Gallimard), with the exception of *Paludes* (cover in black and white).

Top to bottom: Jacques Prévert's *La Pluie et le beau temps* (Rain and fine weather), with collage by Jacques Prévert (1972); Romain Gary's *Lady L.*, with an illustration by Ronald Searle (1973); Prosper Mérimée's *Carmen*, with an illustration by Carlo and Mireille Wieland (1974).

Top to bottom: Frederick Forsyth's *Chacal* (The Day of the Jackal) with an illustration by Dimitri Selesneff (1974); André Gide's *Paludes* with a woodcut by Félix Vallotton (1973); Alejo Carpentier's *Le Partage des eaux* (The watershed) with an illustration by Alain Le Foll (1976).

Top to bottom: Curzio Malaparte's *La Peau* (Skin) with an illustration by Roland Topor (1973); Colette's *La Retraite sentimentale* (Emotional retreat) with an illustration by Walter Zimbrich (1977); William Faulkner's *Sartoris* with an illustration by Jean-Michel Nicollet (1977).

Top to bottom: Roald Dahl's *Kiss Kiss* with an illustration by Roger Blachon (1978); Marcel Aymé's *Le Passe-muraille* (Over the wall) with an illustration by Mireille Wieland (1972); Jorge Luis Borges's *Fictions* with an illustration by José David (1974).

Top to bottom: Jorge Semprun's *Le Grand Voyage* (The great journey) with an illustration by Jean-Michel Folon (1972); Fyodor Dostoyevsky's *Les Possédés* (The Devils) with an illustration by Tibor Csernus (1974); Maurice Genevoix's *Bestiaire sans oubli* (Unforgetting bestiary) with an illustration by Frédérique Courtadon (1974).

The 'Folio' series

Until the early 1970s the NRF catalogue[6] accounted for one third of the books published in the 'Livre de poche' series founded in 1953 by Guy Schoeller and Henri Filipacchi. Gallimard had ceded to Hachette the rights to sell titles by major literary authors such as André Gide, Jean-Paul Sartre and Louis-Ferdinand Céline – in fact, Distribution Hachette-Librairie générale française was Gallimard's distributor. In 1970 the partnership between Gallimard and Hachette came to an abrupt end and they separated. Gallimard set up a new distribution subsidiary, Sodis, which later also distributed other French publishers. At the same time there was a perceived need to create an independent, modern paperback series.

The experiment begun by 'Livre de poche' was bearing fruit: the publishers were realizing that there was a secondary market through which they could make intelligent use of their catalogue and turn books hitherto known only to a select few into commercial successes. And while the small paperback format was not entirely new for Gallimard (the 'Série noire' series dates from 1945, 'Idées' from 1961 and 'Poésie/Gallimard' from 1966), the launch of 'Folio' in 1972 was a risky operation, a commercial riposte to its Hachette-owned competitor 'Livre de poche'.

So 'Folio' was primarily a marketing operation, standing apart from the Gallimard tradition in many ways. The name 'Folio' was the idea of Claude Bonnange, the 'B' of the acronym TBWA, a Paris advertising agency in vogue at the time. The agency launched one of the first advertising campaigns in publishing, with the blessing of its client, Christian Gallimard, grandson of the founder Gaston, who had asked Christian to manage the series. Throughout Massin's time at Gallimard it was Christian who presented the art director's work to his father Claude Gallimard, who was then running the company. Christian had also had to convince his father of the worth of the name 'Folio', which Claude thought too technical.[7]

Around 500 titles were published in 1972–3 and 15 million copies sold in the period 1972–8. Overseen by Massin, the series soon became a benchmark in terms of graphic design and art direction, with white backgrounds, easily recognizable titles, and cover illustrations that were constantly updated. The books were rarely printed in runs of less than 10,000–12,000 and today every French bookshop has shelves full of books from the 'Folio' series. They have become part of the French cultural landscape. The series' typographical formula is like a perfect musical cocktail of basso continuo: Baskerville, a font dating from the late eighteenth century, which never goes out of fashion and was redesigned in the 1920s, is still used on the upper part of the cover. The font size varies according to title length and is printed in a strong yet elegant black. A technological advance in the field of paper (the invention of Kromekote, a matte, semi-rigid paper made by Champion) made it possible to create a glossy cover with a white background. 'The more difficult thing is to take it to the extreme and to title in black on the white ground. In other words to make black act as a colour,' explains Massin.[8]

Analysing the design of the 'Livre de poche' series whose lowbrow cover illustrations were often incongruous, bland or dated and seldom changed from one edition to the next, Massin concludes, 'Our concern was to make it so that these little books could be both read and kept.'[9] Massin likes to give a pleasing shape to everyday objects and, like other supporters of the democratization of culture, was able to put this philosophy into practice throughout his career. While the covers of the 'Folio' series had unity conferred on them by their typography, they also had the diversity of a rich, surprising and often risky choice of illustration, usually placed in the centre of the cover, either silhouetted or extended beyond the edges, creating a block of contrasting colour below the title.

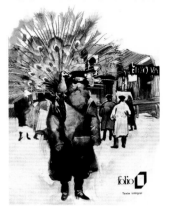

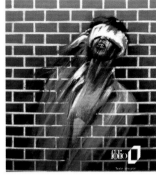

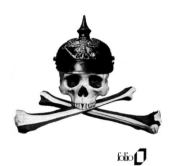

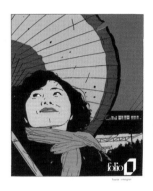

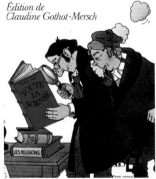

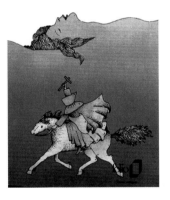

Top to bottom: Isaac Babel's *Contes d'Odessa* (Odessa tales) with an illustration by Tibor Csernus (1979); Léon Bloy's *Sueur de sang* (Sweat of blood) with an illustration by Jean Castel (1972); Gustave Flaubert's *Bouvard et Pécuchet* with an illustration by Philippe Poncet de la Grave (1979).

Top to bottom: Jean-Paul Sartre's *Le Mur* (The wall) with an illustration by Jean Lagarrigue (1976); Yukio Mishima's *Après le banquet* (After the Banquet) with an illustration by Romain Slocombe (1979); Jules Barbey d'Aurevilly's *L'Ensorcelée* (Bewitched) with an illustration by Christine Bassery (1977).

From the outset Massin adopted the more or less systematic approach of using illustrators at a time when the fashion was for typography and photography. This also enabled him to set 'Folio' apart from other small paperback series. But the 1970s marked the start of a revolution in illustration, which became more conceptual, notably through the work of children's book illustrators, such as the American Maurice Sendak in his *Where The Wild Things Are*, Tomi Ungerer and his *Monsieur Racine* and Étienne Delessert in his illustrated *Contes* (Tales) by Ionesco (*Contes no. 1*, Paris, Harlin Quist, 1969; *Contes no. 2*, Paris, J-P Delarge, 1976). 'At that time there was a complete transformation in the way of talking to children, showing that children and adults could share the same point of view and that illustration knew how to play with concepts', says Delessert.[10] Figures such as Alain Le Foll, André François and Jean-Michel Folon introduced a certain imaginative 'cruelty', which was considered subversive at the time, while cartoons aimed at adults were also emerging and the aesthetics of social protest and challenge was at its height. 'The post-68 period was marked by a strong comeback for illustration, from books to magazines to record covers with the arrival of pop music and alternative rock,' explains Michel Wlassikoff.[11]

Massin was always fascinated by the figurative work of illustrators such as Benjamin Rabier, the early twentieth-century illustrator of children's books and creator of well-known images such as the unforgettable 'Laughing cow' and Gédéon the duck. He often used images of this kind for his covers and recruited his illustrators from magazines, with *Playboy*, *Lui* and particularly *Okapi* providing rich seams of emerging talent. There he found artists such as Jean Lagarrigue, Jean-Michel Nicollet, Roger Blachon and Jean Alessandrini, who made names for themselves in children's books. 'I decided to pay them all the same, because how can you put merit on a scale? Searle, François and Folon were no more expensive than a beginner – 900 francs a cover in those days', remembers Massin.[12] He admits not knowing how to draw, but hired a total of over 250 illustrators, including Jean-Michel Folon, André François, Étienne Delessert, Ronald Searle and Roland Topor, not to mention some of his assistants, who sometimes worked under pseudonyms to create a cover at the last minute. Tibor Csernus, an illustrator of Hungarian origin hired by Gallimard to create illustrated books and designer of over a hundred covers for 'Folio', remembers: 'With Massin everything fell into place for me. There was so much freedom with him, I didn't have to

Four-colour paper covers for the 'Folio' series (Paris, Gallimard), with the exception of *La Cantatrice chauve* (cover in black and white).

Below, left to right: André Malraux's *La Condition humaine* (The human condition) with a photograph by Roger Parry (1972); André Malraux's *La Condition humaine* with an illustration by Jean Lagarrigue (2nd edition, 1977); Louis Aragon's *Le Paysan de Paris* (Nightwalker) with an illustration by Massin (c.1972).

Opposite, left to right: Alberto Moravia's *La Désobéissance* (Disobedience) with an illustration by Sylvie Saulnier (1973); Eugène Ionesco's *La Cantatrice chauve* (The Bald Soprano/The Bald Prima Donna), followed by *La Leçon* (The lesson), with an illustration by Saul Steinberg (1972).

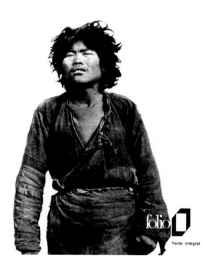

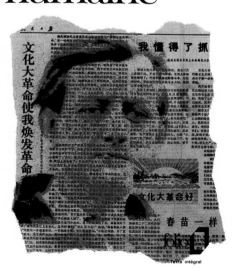

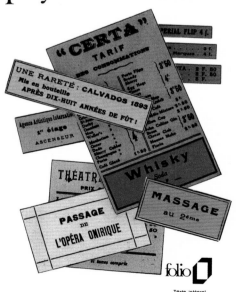

Ionesco **La cantatrice chauve** *suivi de* La leçon

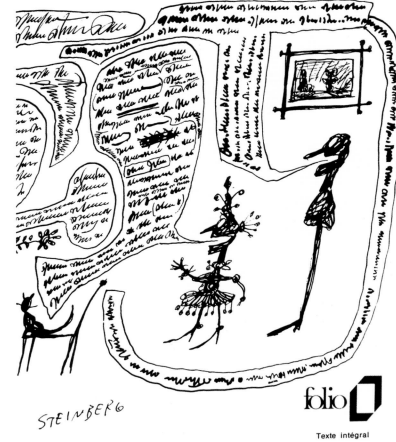

STEINBERG

folio

Texte intégral

Moravia
La désobéissance

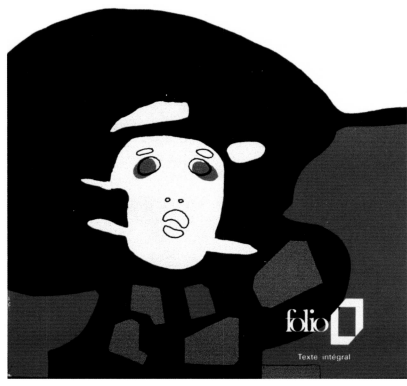

folio

Texte intégral

argue for my choices of figurative illustration.'[13] From Csernus's dark monotypes, heightened in oil, to the poetic watercolours of Georges Lemoine, caricatures by Sempé and Siné and the surrealist figures of Delessert, the artistic direction of illustrators remained a signature for the series, along with the 'Folio' square logo in the bottom right corner. '"Folio" completely changed the field of illustration in France by promoting conceptual illustration in the way Push Pin had done in the United States,' says Delessert.[14]

Sadly, since 1985 image-bank photographs have replaced specially commissioned illustrations, along the lines of the 1,100 or so covers designed by Massin from 1972 until his departure from Gallimard in 1979. The 'Folio' concept was so successful that, in addition to influencing Le Seuil's 'Points' series (launched in 1974 and designed by Pierre Faucheux), it was an important model for 'Livre de poche's 'Biblio' look, launched in 1981.

The white ground

If there is one constant in Massin's work as an art director, and particularly in his work at Gallimard, it is the white ground – an echo of 'the famous and still current cover of the "white" series, the most characteristic example of French publishing today', notes graphic art critic Catherine de Smet.[15]

Integral to the spirit and identity of NRF and with a few famous antecedents – *La Revue blanche* (The white review) in the nineteenth century and Charles Peguy's *Les Cahiers de la quinzaine* (Notebooks of the week) – the white cover, Massin observes, is never completely white, being either ivory or bearing a red strip with the author's name and the title of the book. Christian Gallimard and Massin were familiar with the German paperback series 'DTV', with its white covers, drawings in the style of Rouault and graphic design by Celestino Piatti. Like the first version of the '10/18' series, 'Folio' continued the tradition of the white cover, which, compared to the multicoloured covers of 'Livre de poche', seemed really new in the late 1960s and early 1970s.[16]

Massin knew how to make the most of this white 'canvas' without ever repeating himself from one series to the next, playing with a palette of typefaces and a variety of images, using black reproductions of works of art, collages and more fantastical illustrations than anything Gallimard – a major publisher representing the French intelligentsia – could ever have imagined in the first decades of its existence. Among the great successes of art direction that still stand out, both in the history of Gallimard in particular and the landscape of French publishing in general, we can cite 'Tel', a memorable series of philosophical writings, whose covers, overseen by Massin were decorated with four-colour varnished reproductions of works by Vasarely, at a time when Op Art was in the ascendancy among the shifting sands of abstract art. The 'Poésie/Gallimard' series was also an exercise in variations on a white ground, with a strip of small portrait photographs of the author heightened with areas of monochrome colour. In their different ways each work with the possibilities offered by the white ground.

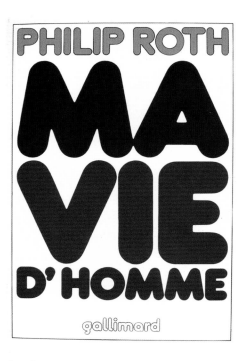

Above: four-colour dust jacket for Philip Roth's *Ma vie d'homme* (My life as a man; Paris, Gallimard, 1976).

Right: two-colour paper cover for Pierre Guyotat's *Bond en avant* (Leap forward; Paris, Gallimard, 1973), design by Jean Castel.

Opposite: three-colour paper cover for Paul Malar's *Tropique du Caducée* (Tropic of caduceus), vol. III (Paris, Éditions du Scorpion, 1954).

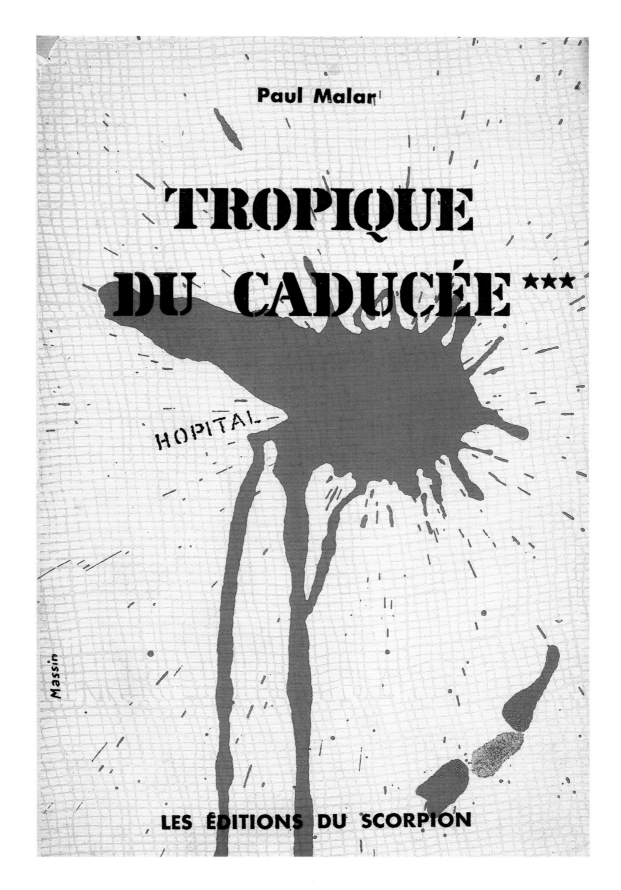

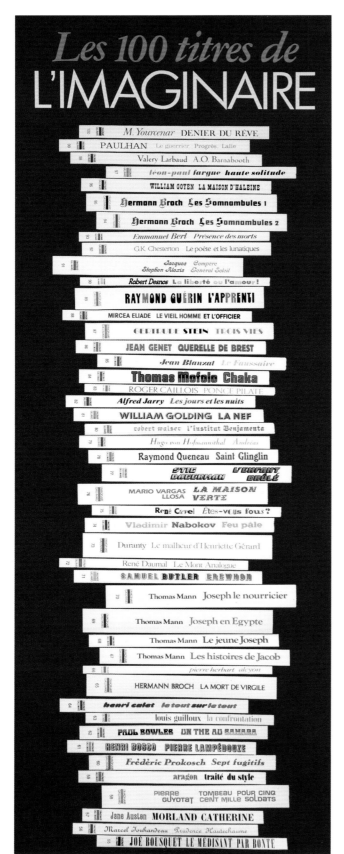

The 'L'Imaginaire' series

The 'L'Imaginaire' series did not buck the trend but also joined the category of covers with a white ground. It remains one of Massin's favourites and the one in which he almost certainly carried typographic experimentation to its furthest point. 'It's probably the cover of covers, and the cover of my entire career as a graphic artist.'[17]

But where did he find the inspiration for a formula even bolder than that of 'Folio'? Massin remembers how, during the summer of 1977, he had amused himself cutting out sample typefaces, creating typographic pictures from rarely-used fonts and digging around in his own collection. In a way he had already put this pure research and compilation of different forms to practical use around ten years earlier, experimenting with typographic illustrations for the different stories of the bus incident in Raymond Queneau's *Exercices de style* (Exercises in style; Paris, Gallimard, 1963).

After 'Folio's success, Gallimard decided to create an entire series of titles that would be less commercial than the new editions of major classics published in 'Folio' and which had not yet been marketed a second time in the small paperback format. Massin himself suggested the name for the series, inspired by the title of a book by Jean-Paul Sartre. The covers of 'L'Imaginaire' used a well-balanced combination of lettering and white background. To explain the subtle balance of a visual rhythm based on differences and similarities, Massin sometimes uses the metaphor of musical variations. The white ground and the logo (a bar above the name Gallimard helping to mark out the territory of white) represent the basso continuo, with the variations provided by the choice of colour for the typeface, which changed with every title and every author's name. When asked today about the names of the fonts he used, Massin stresses his 'absolute typographic eye' (as he likes to call it) but explains, 'I can't give you the names of the typefaces used, because I used precisely those that weren't in common use, and were very distinctive, so that the uninitiated eye could tell the covers apart.'[18] Paradoxically it was this difference between covers that gives the series its homogeneity. 'What I really like, in this case, is that while it always remains mine, this is a creation that escapes its creator', says Massin.[19]

The typographers' 'bible', the font catalogue of pre-war Europe's largest foundry Deberny and Peignot, was still widely used up until the 1960s and influenced the general aesthetics and typography of Gallimard, ninety per cent of whose covers were set in Didot. In 1958, when Gaston Gallimard asked Massin to 'put right' the company's logo, it was only natural to convert the monogram 'nrf' to Didot. The very wide choice of little-used fonts and the imaginative combinations of bright colours on the covers of 'L'Imaginaire' seemed all the more adventurous for their minimalism, while also being very cost-effective, as they were confined to two colours plus black.

max jacob
le cabinet
noir

L'IMAGINAIRE
GALLIMARD

aragon le
libertinage

L'IMAGINAIRE
GALLIMARD

duras le
vice-
consul

L'IMAGINAIRE
GALLIMARD

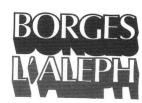

L'IMAGINAIRE
GALLIMARD

jean
giono
fragments
d'un
paradis

L'IMAGINAIRE
GALLIMARD

Drieu La Rochelle
État civil

L'IMAGINAIRE
GALLIMARD

George
du Maurier
Peter
Ibbetson

L'IMAGINAIRE
GALLIMARD

MAURICE
BLANCHOT
L'ARRÊT
DE MORT

L'IMAGINAIRE
GALLIMARD

conrad
jeunesse
SUIVI DE
cœur des ténèbres

L'IMAGINAIRE
GALLIMARD

georges
limbour
les
vanilliers

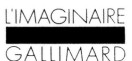
L'IMAGINAIRE
GALLIMARD

Opposite: poster advertising the
'L'Imaginaire' series (Paris,
Gallimard, c.1977–8).

Above: examples of three-colour
covers from the 'L'Imaginaire' series,
characterized by varied coloured
typography and a plain layout. All these
books were published in 1977 except for
Joseph Conrad's *Jeunesse* (Youth; 1978).

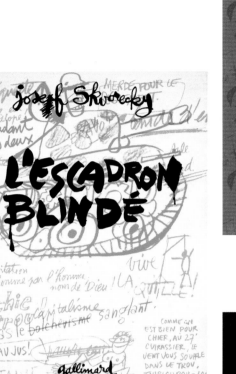

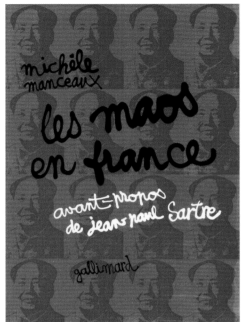

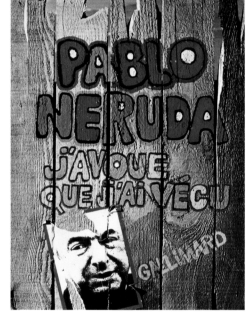

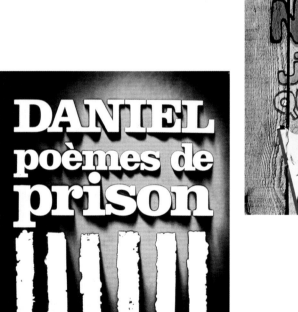

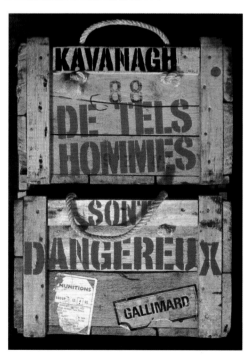

Top row, left to right: three-colour dust jacket for Josef Skvorecky's *L'Escadron blindé* (The armoured squadron; Paris, Gallimard, 1969) with an illustration by Siné; two-colour cover for Michèle Manceaux's *Les Maos en France* (Maos in France; Paris, Gallimard, 1972), design by Philippe Mercier; four-colour dust jacket for Pablo Neruda's *J'avoue que j'ai vécu* (I admit that I've lived; Paris, Gallimard, 1975), design by Jean Castel.

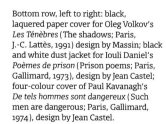

Bottom row, left to right: black, laquered paper cover for Oleg Volkov's *Les Ténèbres* (The shadows; Paris, J.-C. Lattès, 1991) design by Massin; black and white dust jacket for Iouli Daniel's *Poèmes de prison* (Prison poems; Paris, Gallimard, 1973), design by Jean Castel; four-colour cover of Paul Kavanagh's *De tels hommes sont dangereux* (Such men are dangerous; Paris, Gallimard, 1974), design by Jean Castel.

Beyond Massin's Herculean work as art director for original covers (for both novels and essays), for which he always sought high-quality and usually expressive typography, his boundless vision and talent for creating homogeneous, lasting series are particularly striking. A series cover must combine the opposing notions of identity and difference, and establish a dialogue between them. Offering his metaphor of baroque music to anyone willing to grasp it, Massin has often used the term 'counterpoint' to describe an indispensable element in complete success. At a lecture he gave in Seoul in March 2005, he returned to one of his favourite topics of conversation: 'In all these aspects of variation, it is important to stress that variation is not repetition, since every transformation or metamorphosis of the subject entails its renewal, augmenting and enhancing it. So then we might think, perhaps it is the variations that give existence to the theme.'[20] And Massin practices this art of counterpoint with unchanging integrity and elegance in everything he designs, from series covers to the layout of illustrated books to the series of posters designed for the store chain FNAC.

During the course of his twenty years at Gallimard, with the benefit of his experience of working with the company's different managers and generations, Massin left a profound mark on the landscape of French publishing and, in many respects, established the foundations and signposts of art direction, the 'ABC' of a profession that was still unusual in the post-war period. Gallimard offered him his most fertile ground, in terms of both long-term work and his boldest and most experimental projects.

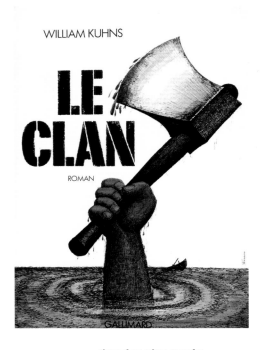

Above: four-colour cover for William Kuhns' *Le Clan* (The clan; Paris, Gallimard, 1975), design by Ferracci.

Left: two-colour dust jacket for Romain Gary's *Chien blanc* (White dog; Paris, Gallimard, 1970), design by Henri Carcaud.

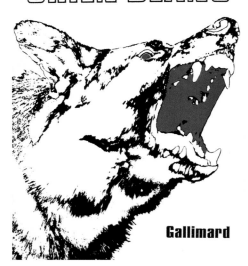

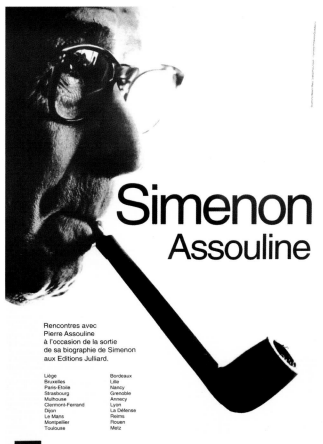

Simenon
Assouline

Rencontres avec
Pierre Assouline
à l'occasion de la sortie
de sa biographie de Simenon
aux Editions Julliard.

Liège	Bordeaux
Bruxelles	Lille
Paris-Etoile	Nancy
Strasbourg	Grenoble
Mulhouse	Annecy
Clermont-Ferrand	Lyon
Dijon	La Défense
Le Mans	Reims
Montpellier	Rouen
Toulouse	Metz

 le choix des libraires

Left to right: posters for the cultural
department of FNAC (1992 and 1993);
poster for the TNS, Théâtre national
de Strasburg, set in a version of Bifur,
a font designed by Cassandre in
1927 (1994).

Opposite: poster for the cultural
department of FNAC (1992).

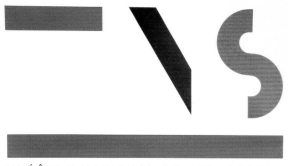

THÉÂTRE NATIONAL DE STRASBOURG

Direction   Jean-Louis Martinelli

Graphisme : Massin

LIVRE
NOIR

crimes de guerre   crimes contre
l'humanité et «purification ethnique»
dans l'ex-yougoslavie   documents
rassemblés par le nouvel observa
-teur et reporters sans frontières

Rencontres à l'occasion de la sortie du livre aux Editions Arléa

Angers	Mulhouse	Angers
Bordeaux	Reims	Bordeaux
Grenoble	Rennes	Grenoble
Marseille	Toulouse	Marseille

Graphisme Massin

Logo Nouvel Obs	Logo Reporters	

Afriue

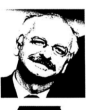

Rencontre avec
Erik Orsenna,
Eric Fottorino
et Christophe Guillemin
à l'occasion de la parution
de leur livre *Besoin d'Afrique*
aux Editions Fayard.

Fnac Bordeaux
Fnac Grenoble
Fnac Librairie internationale
Fnac Metz
Fnac Montpellier
Fnac Orléans
Fnac Reims
Fnac Rennes
Fnac Strasbourg
Fnac Toulouse

fnac

Graphisme Massin : Photo Louis Monier. Imprimerie Primavera-Quotidienne

A shared spirit

In conversations about their experience of the 'Folio' series, illustrators Jean Alessandrini, Étienne Delessert, Jean-Olivier Héron, Jean Lagarrigue, Georges Lemoine and Jean-Michel Nicollet have all described, with deep and sincere respect, the creative freedom that Massin gave them at the start of their careers in the early 1970s.[21] Massin was an enlightened art director, full of curiosity, who well understood the workings of a profession that required him to surround himself with exceptional talents whose imagination must be stimulated.

These illustrators, whose works are now part of the heritage of books in the French language, share with Massin an innate sense of art direction, a precise knowledge of typography and a passion for literature – indeed most are also writers. Their approach to books is primarily cultural rather than commercial, in the tradition of the cultivated graphic artist.

Events such as the exhibition openings at Galerie Delpire in rue de l'Abbaye, Paris, the exhibition 'L'enfant et les images' (1973–4) at the musée des Arts décoratifs and the launch of special issues of the Swiss magazine *Graphis* on children's book illustration enabled Massin to seek out his illustrators and, through the 'Folio' series, to transform the panorama of French illustration.

Jean Alessandrini

Jean Alessandrini was born in Marseilles in 1942 and lives in Strasburg. As a press illustrator, he began working for Gallimard creating covers for the magazine *Pilote* as well as for the publisher Marabout. A writer, layout artist and typographer, he created an original series of typefaces for Hollenstein-Phottype and is the author of technical guides for graphic arts students.

He uses his typographical knowledge to create imaginative word-images for illustrated books and novels for children, which he writes and illustrates, notably for Bayard Presse, Hatier, Hachette, Nathan and L'École des loisirs and is now specializing in writing crime novels for Phébus.

'The cover of a book is a poster, I entirely agree with Massin about that, but the poster has to be good! I remember spending hours in his office discussing typography, because I had designed fonts myself. I liked the title in Baskerville but I hated the "Folio" logo, that monstrosity of a black rectangle bottom right, which in my view sometimes spoilt the illustration. I must have done five or six covers for "Folio", notably Barbey d'Aurevilly's *Le Chevalier des Touches* (The knight of the keys), Dumas's *Les Trois Mousquetaires* (The Three Musketeers) and Romain Gary's *Les Têtes de Stéphanie* (The heads of Stephanie), and I even tried to illustrate Céline's *Voyage au bout de la nuit* (Journey to the End of the Night) – not an easy nut to crack.'

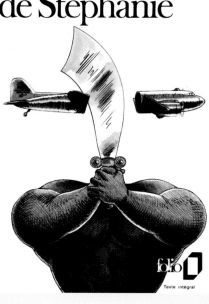

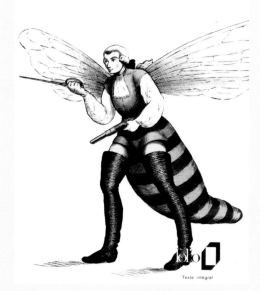

Focus
The 'Folio' Illustrators

Étienne Delessert

Illustrator Étienne Delessert was born in Switzerland in 1941 and lives in the United States. He is the author of over eighty children's books, some translated into fourteen languages with print runs totalling millions. He draws regularly for *The New York Times*, *Atlantic Monthly* and *Le Monde*. In the early 1960s he worked in graphic art and illustration in Paris. In 1970 he met the Swiss psychologist Jean Piaget, a specialist in cognitive development, who was then interested in the question of how young children decode adult imagery. Delessert showed Piaget his famous illustrations for Ionesco's *Contes*, which were very controversial at the time. This fruitful collaboration resulted in *Comment la souris reçoit une pierre sur la tête et découvre le monde* (How the mouse gets a stone on its head and discovers the world; Paris, L'École des loisirs, 1971), an experimental book that demonstrated to art directors and the wider press how illustration could be based on concepts. 'The limitations of children's perception, their faculty of assimilation and their artistic sensitivity exist only in the minds of adults,' he observes.

'After my illustrations for Eugène Ionesco's *Conte no. 1* and *Conte no. 2*, published in America by Harlin Quist – that Don Quixote of children's publishing – I had become a kind of Ionesco specialist. As I knew him personally, Massin had asked me to do the "Folio" cover for his *Rhinocéros*. So I said to Massin, 'I'm going to do a guy with horns.' I really filled the cover – usually there was more white left round the drawing, my illustration was set very high on the page. I think Massin still has the original in his Paris apartment.'

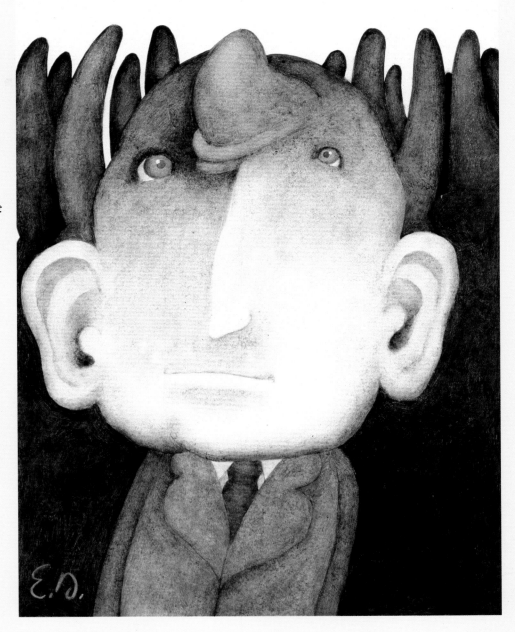

Opposite, left to right: four-colour paper covers for Romain Gary's *Les Têtes de Stéphanie* (The heads of Stéphanie; 1977); Jules Barbey d'Aurevilly's *Le Chevalier des Touches* (The knight of the keys; 1976) with illustrations by Jean Alessandrini.

Above: original watercolour illustration by Étienne Delessert for Eugène Ionesco's *Rhinocéros* (1977).

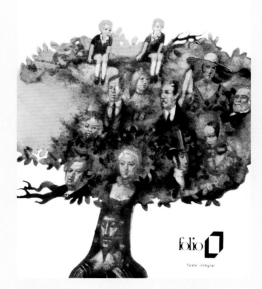

Michel de Saint Pierre
Les aristocrates

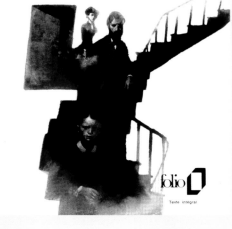

Duhamel Le notaire du Havre

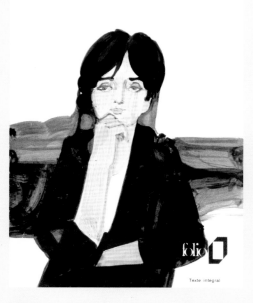

Montherlant
Les jeunes filles

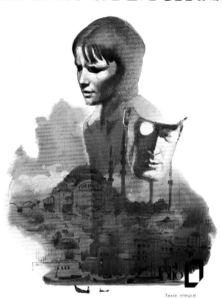

Simenon Les clients d'Avrenos

Top to bottom, left to right: four-colour paper covers for Michel de Saint-Pierre's *Les Aristocrates* (The Aristocrats; 1972); Georges Duhamel's *Le Notaire du Havre* (The notary of Le Havre; 1972); Henry de Montherlant's *Les Jeunes Filles* (Girls; 1972); Georges Simenon's *Les Clients d'Avrenos* (The clients of Avrenos; 1975) with illustrations by Jean-Olivier Héron.

Jean-Olivier Héron

Jean-Olivier Héron was born in 1938 and trained as a journalist. He created the magazine *Voiles et Voiliers* (Sails and sailing boats; 1971), before founding the 'Gallimard Jeunesse' series in 1972 with his friend Pierre Marchand. 'Massin was our guardian angel and Gallimard's ambassador. It was because I worked with him that Pierre and I were able to make the "Gallimard Jeunesse" series into a child's bedroom that was almost as big as the mother house,' explains the painter and illustrator, now living on the île d'Yeu, where he writes, illustrates and publishes children's books with his small publishing house, Gulf Stream.

'The thing I'm most grateful for is that he allowed us to try out several styles. He was open to reading all kinds of things and encouraged us to explore the widest possible range of directions and techniques. My first illustration for "Folio" was Michel de Saint-Pierre's *Les Aristocrates*, my visiting card before Massin gave me the entire run of Duhamel titles. I had the idea of doing something really amusing, a series of fake games of chance. The splashes of Indian ink were thrown on pieces of blotting paper and some areas of the paper were then lightened with white acrylic, which allows the ink pigments to rise in proportion to the thickness of the white. Then I reused these shapes, which seemed to have been made with a single brushstroke, for "Folio"s Simenon titles, then the Montherlants, which gave me an identical graphic impact and technical rigour, while varying the dominant elements for each title.'

Jean Lagarrigue

'Folio' was not the first area of work at Gallimard for the illustrator Jean Lagarrigue (born 1939); Massin asked him to illustrate the cover of *Dear Henry* (a portrait of Henry Kissinger by Danielle Hunebelle, Paris, Gallimard, 1972) on his return from the United States, where he was joint art director (1968–72) with Jean-Paul Goude at the monthly magazine *Esquire*. He continued to work for the American and French press as an illustrator and art director, while also teaching at the École nationale supérieure des arts décoratifs in Paris. In 1982 he created the poster for *Brazil*, the cult film by Terry Gilliam. He is the author of children's books and comic books published by Casterman, while his sketches around the suburban RER rail network of Paris have been shown in exhibitions and published in several books.

'"Folio" – in the tradition of the American Push Pin and in parallel to Christian Bourgois' "10/18" - lifted the graphic art of French publishing out of the rut into which it had fallen after the golden age of Cassandre. It raised it to the level of the successes of English-language publishing at that time,' says Lagarrigue.

'Massin asked me to illustrate some of "Folio"'s best-selling titles, including Malraux's *La Condition humaine* (The human condition; 1977), Sartre's *Le Mur* (The wall; 1976) and Pavese's *Le Métier de vivre* (The business of living; vols 1 and 2, 1977). It goes without saying that I was as happy as a child in a sweet shop. I've never worked with anyone who placed such trust in me, I never had to redo anything. The only graphic constraint he gave us was the white background, against which we had to draw a strong image, or a close-up of a face, and the image was then cut out to leave the top of the cover free for the placement of the title. It was the marriage of a highly present illustration and a recognizable typeface that helped establish the graphic identity of "Folio" – which I really came to appreciate later when I started doing graphics myself and was faced with the same challenge.'

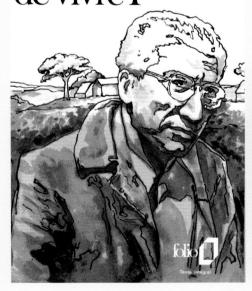
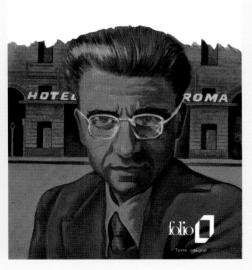

Left to right: four-colour paper covers for Cesare Pavese's *Le Métier de vivre* (The business of living; vols 1 and 2, 1977) with illustrations by Jean Lagarrigue.

Georges Lemoine

Born in 1935, in Rouen, where he now lives, Georges Lemoine began his career as an illustrator of children's comics and advertising through a series of crucial meetings, notably with typographer Marcel Jacno, followed by the publisher Robert Delpire, with whom he worked in his advertising agency, and lastly Étienne Delessert, who commissioned his first illustrated book for children, *Little Lord Blink and His Ice Cream Castle* (New York, 1971), for the American publisher Good Book.

Lemoine met Massin when the 'Folio' series was being set up, and then at the foundation of the 'Jeunesse' department and the 'Folio Junior' section, whose first title he illustrated in 1977. There followed a whole series of illustrations for children's books by renowned authors such as J. M. G. Le Clézio, Marguerite Yourcenar and Michel Tournier. Such illustrations, for which Lemoine has received a series of prizes, occupies a very large place in his life as a painter and draughtsman, but his work as author, illustrator and photographer has recently been focused on special books resembling notebooks of journeys through different neighbourhoods and cities.

'My work with Massin corresponded to a change in my work as an illustrator, when I moved from comics to books. I learned a great deal through my contact with him. We were really of one mind through our shared love of music, lettering and typography: it was a kind of companionship that was beneficial both personally and professionally. But what Massin appreciated was my past as a graphic artist. A cover is a clever assemblage of graphics and illustration, and few of us were really able to design an illustration like a poster.

On Delessert's advice I gave up colouring with inks for watercolours, because of the limitations and unreliability of coloured inks, which are unstable in the light. The cover of Émile Ajar's *Gros-Câlin* is almost certainly one of my happiest memories of that "Folio" period.'

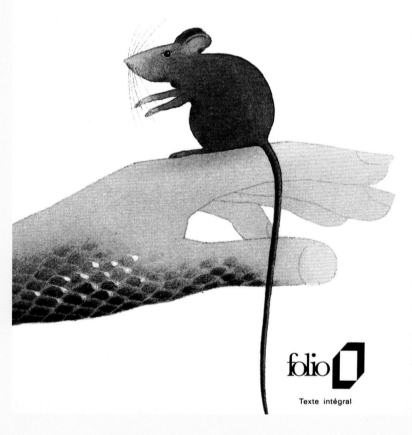

Emile Ajar
Gros-Câlin

folio

Texte intégral

Jean-Michel Nicollet

Jean-Michel Nicollet was born in 1944 in Lyons, where he has taught for the last twenty-three years at the École Émile-Cohl, known for its excellent courses in illustration, animation and graphic art. Today Nicollet divides his time between illustration and painting. Over the years he has forged a solid reputation in the graphics world, notably working for major magazines such as *Playboy*, *Lui* and above all *Métal hurlant*, whose layout he helped to design with Étienne Robial. He also has his own publishing company, Crapule, which publishes popular fiction (fantasy, crime and science fiction). 'Coming from the world of painting and theatre set design, it was Massin who gave me my first opportunity, with a commission for the "Folio" cover of Marcel Aymé's *La Belle Image* (The lovely image). He helped me to position myself in the illustration market.

'I regard Massin as one of the last great art directors of our time, from a bygone period and a rare breed: excellent graphic artists, curious about the work of others and cultivated (preferably outside their chosen fields). I remember meeting all kinds of colourful types in his office, including the author Albert Simonin, for whom I drew the "Folio" cover of *L'Élégant* and a poster.

'When Massin left "Folio" illustration changed a great deal, and not necessarily for the better, particularly with the shift towards photography and doing stuff on computers. In all this superabundance of illustrators and layout artists, which we helped to create, apparently dominated by technical one-upmanship, what has sadly disappeared is the intelligent design of images; the illustrator's imaginary world has been destroyed. Massin always left us a great deal of freedom to explore, particularly in my cover for *Stephen le héros* (Stephen Hero), for which I imagined what a self-portrait by Joyce would look like; or in the cover of Céline's *Casse-pipe* (Killing fields), where, with my fire-breathing cuirassier, I took the risk of experimenting with a caricatured, amusing and provocative interpretation of the subject.'

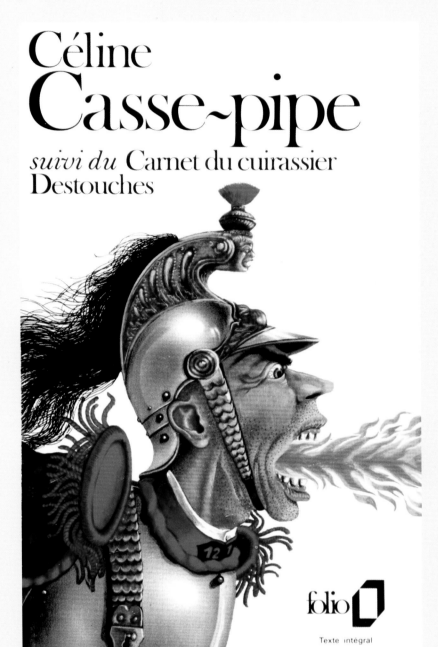

Opposite: four-colour paper cover for Émile Ajar's *Gros-Câlin* (Big hug) with illustration by Georges Lemoine (1976).

Above: four-colour paper cover for Louis-Ferdinand Céline's *Casse-pipe* (Killing fields) with illustration by Jean-Michel Nicollet (1975).

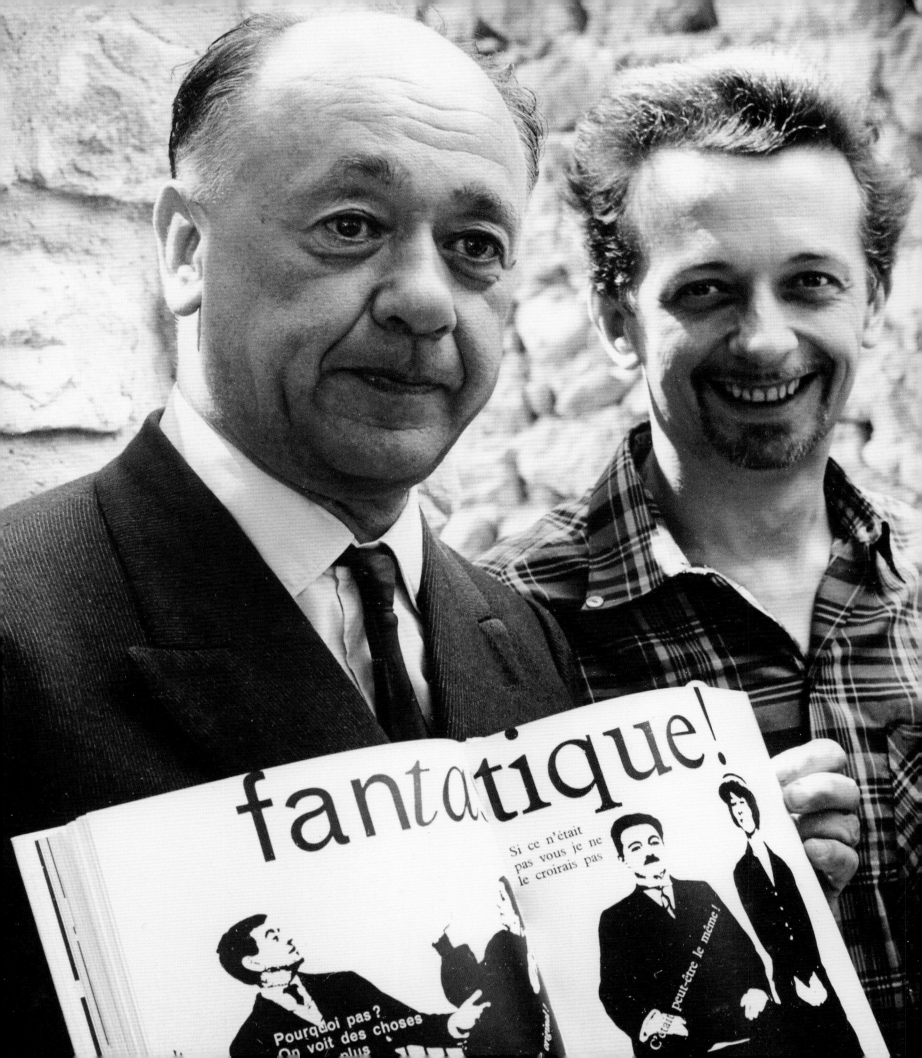

Expressive Typography

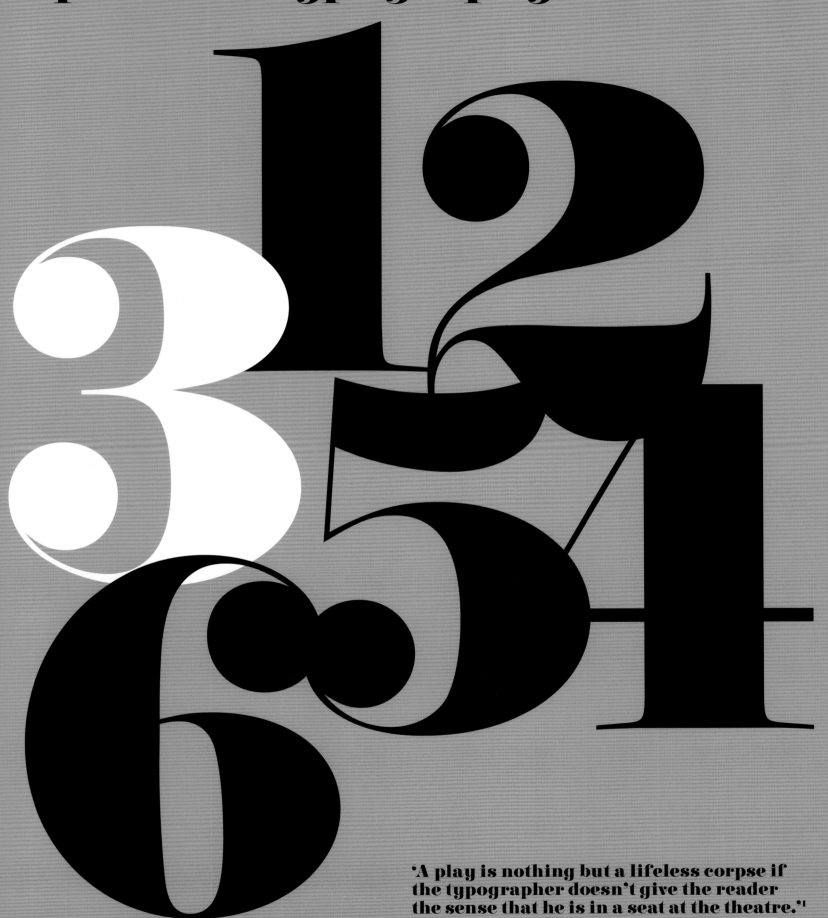

'A play is nothing but a lifeless corpse if the typographer doesn't give the reader the sense that he is in a seat at the theatre.'[1]

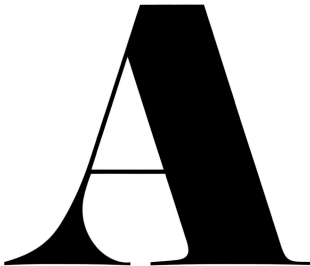

Artistic antecedents

Massin's artistic approach is anchored at one and the same time in the written word and the world of printing and books, and in the specific problems of transcribing a literary or dramatic work on to paper.

Eugène Ionesco's *La Cantatrice chauve* (Paris, Gallimard, 1964) was Massin's first experiment in expressive typography intended to introduce notions of the space and time of theatre into the printed page, and thus upsetting the dialectics of semiological analysis. In this sense Massin's work would seem to contradict the view of Anne Ubersfeld, the great specialist in semiological analysis of contemporary theatre, for whom, 'Whatever the process of spatialization produced by all literary texts, however much a novel's reader reads in a 'spatializing' way, the fact remains that the space of a book is, even materially, a flat space.'[2] It is precisely this view that Massin counters, proving that the space of the book is an architectural space, an allegory of the three-dimensional theatre stage.

Although 'expressive typography' has become a genre now largely associated with the name of Massin, the typographer and calligrapher Paul Shaw recalls that the term was first used by Ed Gottschall in 1961 during a lecture given to the Type Directors Club in New York. In the United States the term was later popularized by the famous art director Herb Lubalin, who, according to Paul Shaw, saw 'the use of typography not just as a mechanical means for laying words out on a page, but more importantly as a creative tool, making it possible to express an idea in order to improve the impact of a graphic utterance.'[3] So Massin's stroke of genius was to appropriate these techniques – hitherto the preserve of advertising messages – in response to the specific challenges posed by the graphic transcription of plays and, at the same time, to question the role of the graphic artist in this creative exercise of interpretative transcription.

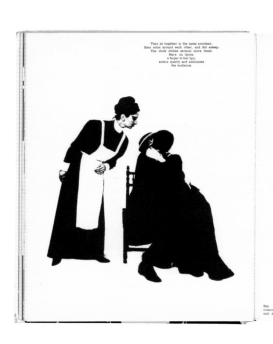

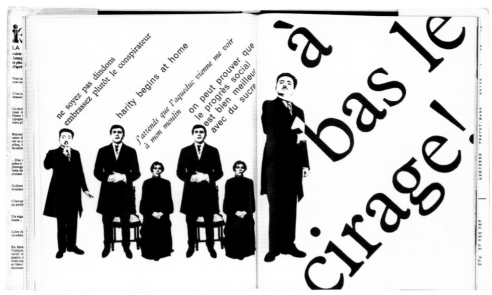

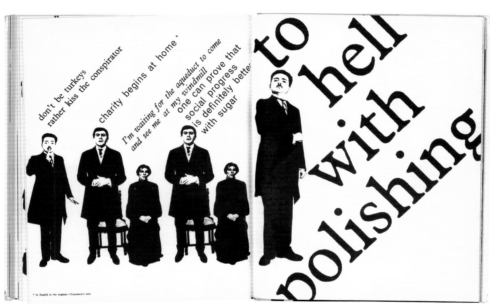

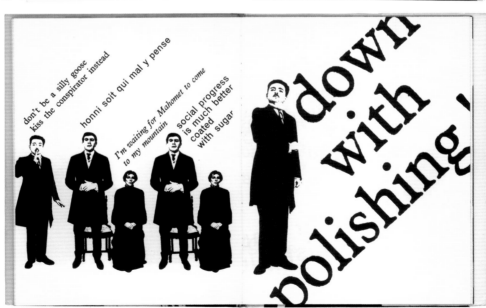

Page 76: photograph by Yan (Jean Dieuziade) of Massin with Eugène Ionesco holding *La Cantatrice chauve* in Lure, August 1965.

Inside pages from Eugène Ionesco's *La Cantatrice chauve* (Paris, Gallimard, 1964).

Opposite: soliloquy by Mary, the maid, presented as a calligram, with a nod to Apollinaire.

Left, top to bottom: one of the play's most famous phrases as published in France, the United States (*The Bald Soprano*, New York, Grove Press, 1965) and Britain (*The Bald Prima Donna*, London, Calder and Boyars, 1966).

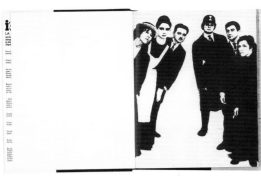
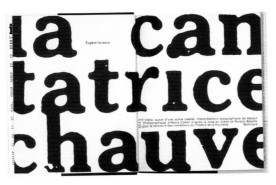
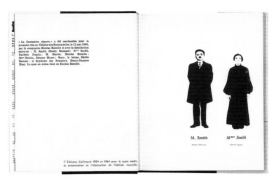

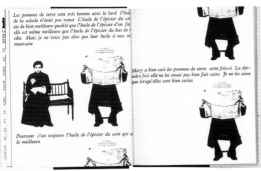
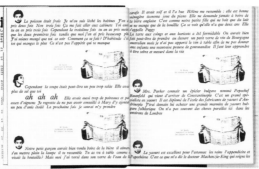
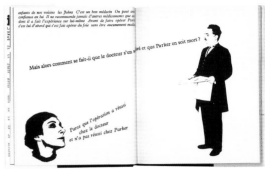

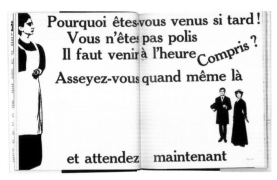
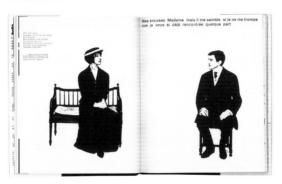
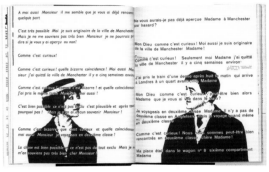

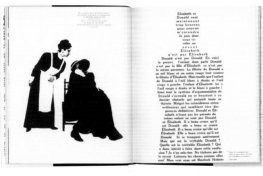
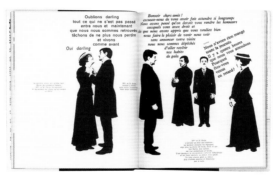
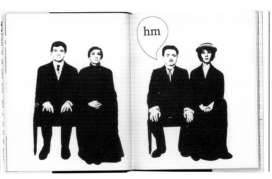

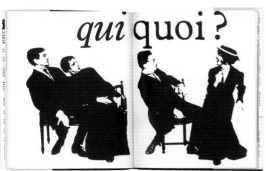
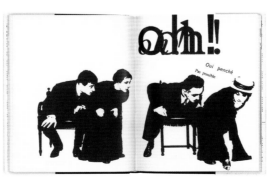
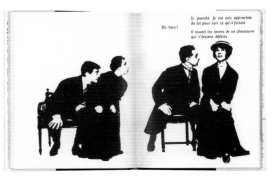

Spreads from *La Cantatrice chauve*
(Paris, Gallimard, 1964): pages 1–17,
24–37, 42–51, 90–7, 100–15, 128–43
and 150–87. The red vertical lines
mark the interruptions in the sequence
of pages.

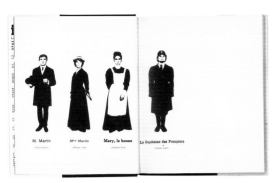

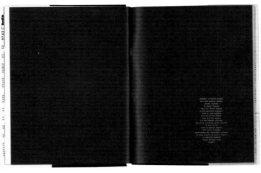

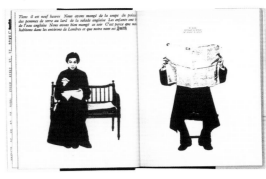

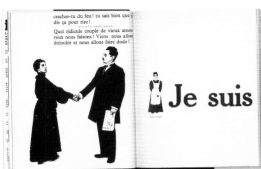

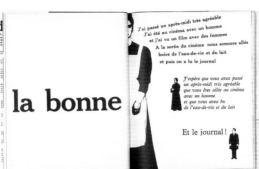

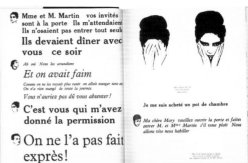

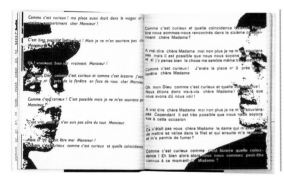

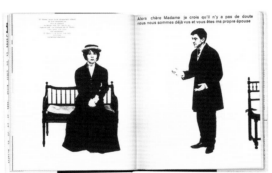

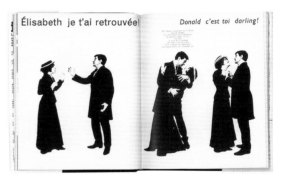

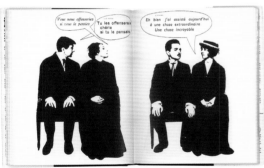

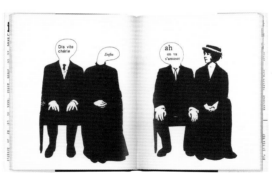

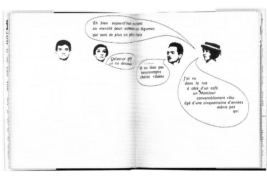

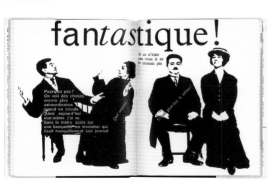

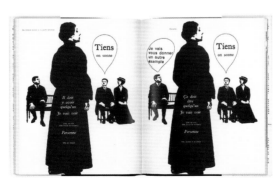

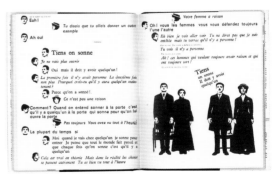

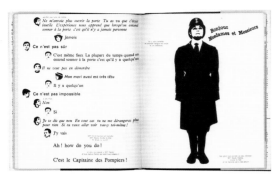 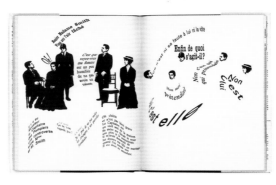 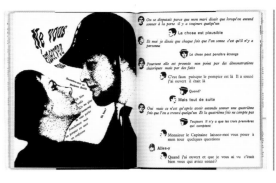

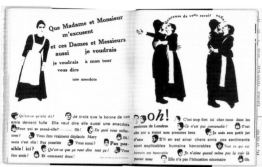 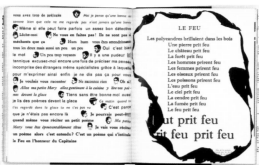 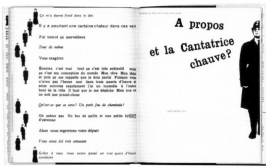

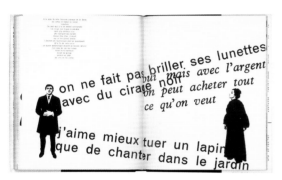 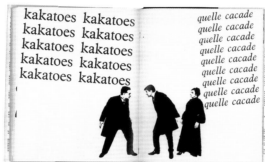 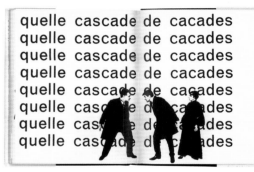

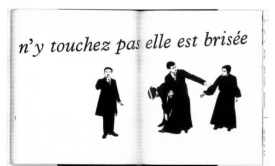 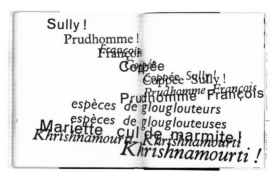 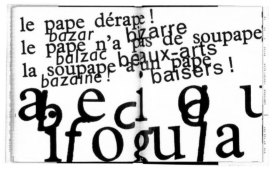

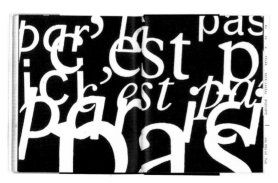 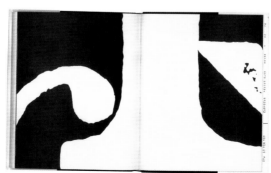 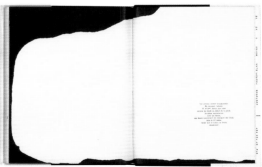

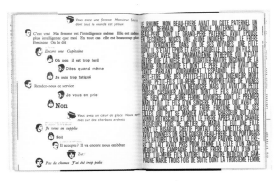

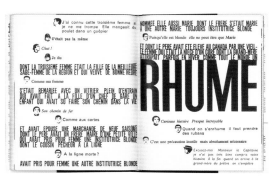

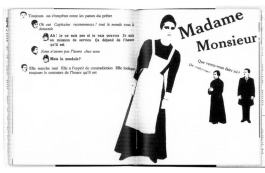

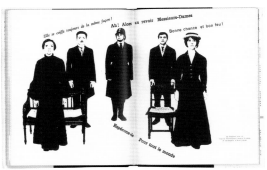

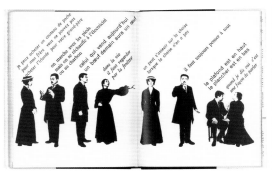

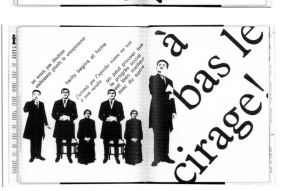

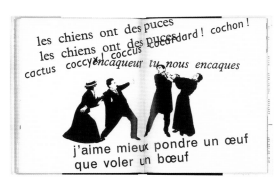

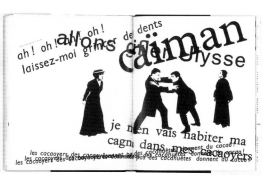

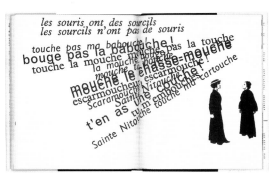

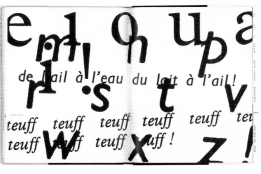

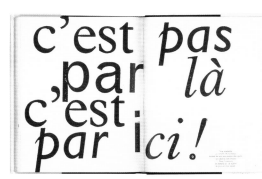

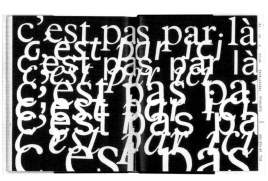

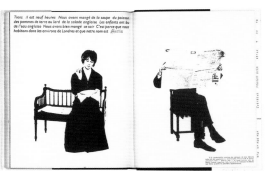

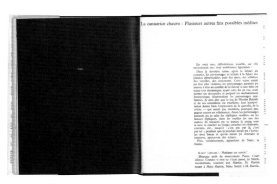

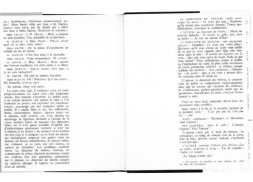

But in other literary and artistic fields concerns had long been raised at the apparent impossibility of giving visual expression to oral language by means of a dynamic relationship between a variety of typographic elements. Massin readily acknowledges this and, being well aware of experiments in poetry and the visual arts, sees Stéphane Mallarmé as the first to have suggested a 'spatialist'-inspired model, with *Un coup de dés jamais n'abolira le hasard* (1896). Michel Melot, curator of the bibliothèque du patrimoine, explains: 'Mallarmé's publishing strategy orientates the book as a total work of art, firstly in the eighteenth-century tradition of the fine book, with contributions from a few illustrators chosen among painters who were his friends, and then simply by the power of the typography, which is used to present the text, into which the reader breathes a dimension of sound.'[4]

Retracing the tradition of expressive typography in art, Massin often mentions the original edition of Blaise Cendrars' 'simultaneous' poem illustrated by Sonia Delaunay, *La Prose du Transsibérien et de la Petite Jehanne de France* (Paris, Éditions des hommes nouveaux, 1913) – he even made a colour photocopy of it to put on the wall of his Paris apartment, an ironic comment on the recent sale at auction of the limited edition, at which bidding started at an exorbitant price. There was also, of course, the work of the Futurists (particularly Filippo Tommaso Marinetti with *Les Mots en liberté futuristes* [Futurist words at liberty], Milan, Edizioni futuriste di poesia, 1919) and the Dadaists (such as Tristan Tzara and his magazine *391*), who had already challenged the rules of layout, with approaches that were perhaps more political and formalist than that of Massin.

Some of the techniques then prescribed by the dissident avant-garde included non-orthogonal orientation (characters set on a diagonal, a curve or simply set freely), reduced spaces between lines or letters, the mixing of fonts, distortion of characters and typography treated as an image (and vice versa). Massin experimented with all these techniques, in several books, in order to express the complexity of human communication.

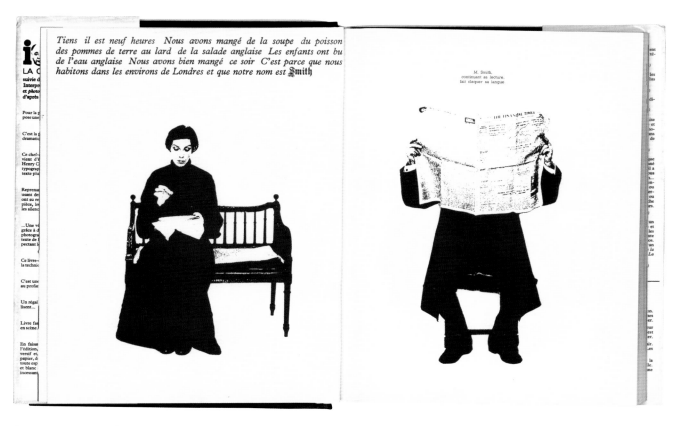

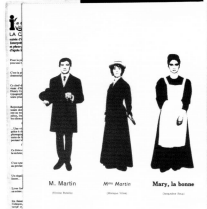
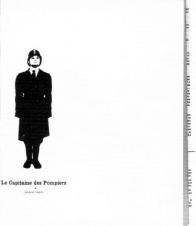
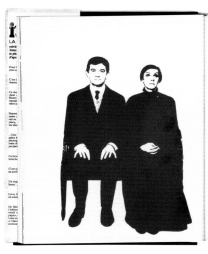
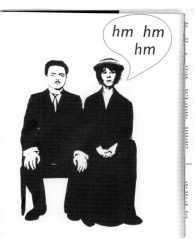

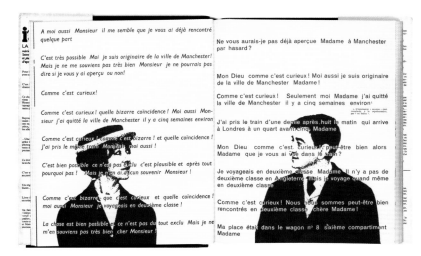

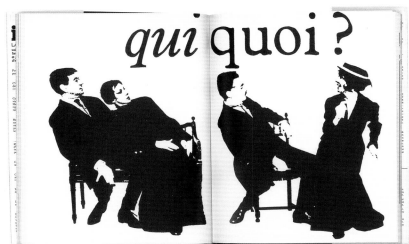

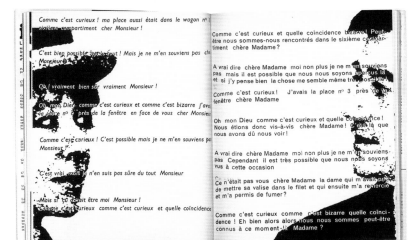

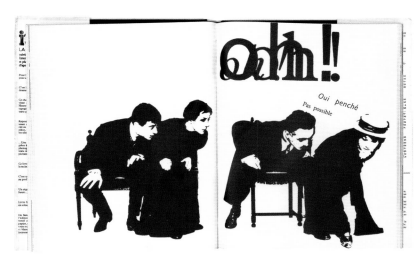

Opposite and above: inside pages from
La Cantatrice chauve (Paris, Gallimard,
1964). The first pages of dialogue reflect
the typical lack of communication
between the characters, who are
absorbed in their own monologues
or reading.

THE HEADCOLD MY BROTHER-IN-LAW HAD ON THE PATER-
NAL SIDE A FIRST COUSIN WHOSE MATERNAL UNCLE HAD A
FATHER-IN-LAW WHOSE PATERNAL GRANDFATHER HAD MARRIED
AS HIS SECOND WIFE A YOUNG NATIVE WHOSE BROTHER HE
HAD MET ON ONE OF HIS TRAVELS A GIRL OF WHOM HE WAS
ENAMORED AND BY WHOM HE HAD A SON WHO MARRIED AN
INTREPID LADY PHARMACIST WHO WAS NONE OTHER THAN
THE NIECE OF AN UNKNOWN FOURTH-CLASS PETTY OFFICER OF
THE ROYAL NAVY AND WHOSE ADOPTED FATHER HAD AN AUNT
WHO SPOKE SPANISH FLUENTLY AND WHO WAS PERHAPS ONE
OF THE GRANDDAUGHTERS OF AN ENGINEER WHO DIED YOUNG
HIMSELF THE GRANDSON OF THE OWNER OF A VINEYARD
WHICH PRODUCED MEDIOCRE WINE BUT WHO HAD A SECOND
COUSIN A STAY-AT-HOME A SERGEANT-MAJOR WHOSE SON
HAD MARRIED A VERY PRETTY YOUNG WOMAN A DIVORCEE
WHOSE FIRST HUSBAND WAS THE SON OF A LOYAL PATRIOT
WHO IN THE HOPE OF MAKING HIS FORTUNE HAD MANAGED
TO BRING UP ONE OF HIS DAUGHTERS SO THAT SHE COULD
MARRY A FOOTMAN WHO HAD KNOWN ROTHSCHILD AND
WHOSE BROTHER AFTER HAVING CHANGED HIS TRADE
SEVERAL TIMES MARRIED AND HAD A DAUGHTER WHOSE
STUNTED GREAT-GRANDFATHER WORE SPECTACLES WHICH
HAD BEEN GIVEN HIM BY A COUSIN OF HIS THE BROTHER-IN-
LAW OF A MAN FROM PORTUGAL NATURAL SON OF A MILLER
NOT TOO BADLY OFF WHOSE FOSTER-BROTHER HAD MARRIED
THE DAUGHTER OF A FORMER COUNTRY DOCTOR WHO WAS
HIMSELF A FOSTER-BROTHER OF THE SON OF A FORESTER

The ars poetica of the theatre of the absurd

The raw material with which Massin was working in fact marked a literary break, questioning the validity of communication and, in the tradition of ars poetica, questioning oneself and language. Perhaps Massin's expressive typography would not have succeeded had it not provided a kind of graphic echo to the questioning of the playwrights of the period. Massin knew the 'absurdists' well: in the corridors of Gallimard he met the literary intelligentsia of Paris (Queneau was a reader there, for example). Étienne Delessert remembers that, when it came to negotiating with certain authors – notably Ionesco – Claude Gallimard, a timid, hesitant person, would often send Massin as company emissary, a kind of ambassador who would represent Gallimard at the highest level.[5] Moreover, as Gallimard's art director it was Massin's privilege to be able to make friends with the company's authors and gain almost direct access to all that was best in the avant-garde theatre of the 1960s.

While, in those years, the literature of the absurd was dealing with the problem of communication – or, more precisely, non-communication and the self-destruction of language – expressive typography found the perfect ground to test the role of graphic art itself, whose main objective is precisely to transmit a message. Whether in Ionesco's *La Cantatrice chauve* and *Délire à deux* (Delirium for two), or Jean Tardieu's *Conversation-sinfonietta*, in his typographical transpositions of theatrical works Massin provides a graphic translation of the conversational void, the explosion and obsessive repetition of words and the omnipresence of silence in the most comical situations. These experiments in expressive typography, begun in the mid-1960s, left a unique stamp on the world of book publishing and graphic art, not only through the scale of explorations sustained throughout entire books, but also through the cultural resonance brought by the translation into English of *La Cantatrice chauve*.

In *Délire à deux* (first performed in 1962), two characters express the breakdown of a relationship between a couple who have been together for seventeen years. There is nothing ordinary or boring here, since it is Ionesco who beats time in this duet, pacing it like a boxing match in which the lines of the adversaries shatter into fragments and situations are taken to an extreme verging on the outrageous. It is only when confronted with complaints and threats from the outside world that the couple come together again. The text of *Délire à deux*, subtitled by Massin 'an essay in the calligraphy of sound', was composed by means of 'transfer lettering'

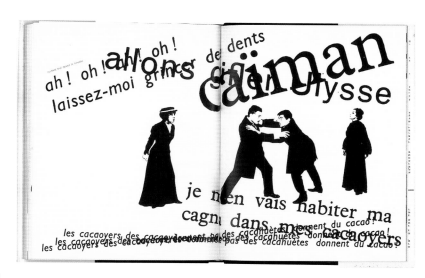

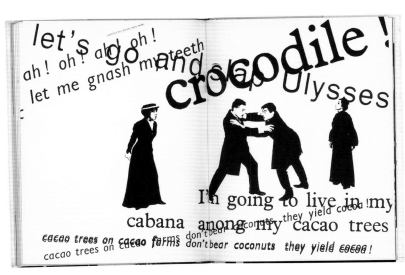

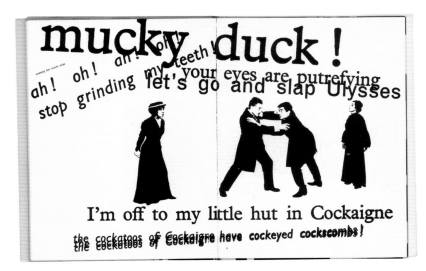

Opposite: page from 'The headcold', an extract from *The Bald Soprano* (New York, Grove Press, 1965) in ironic homage to the typographic rigour of the Swiss school.

Above, top to bottom: the same scene from *La Cantatrice chauve* as it appeared in the French, American and British editions.

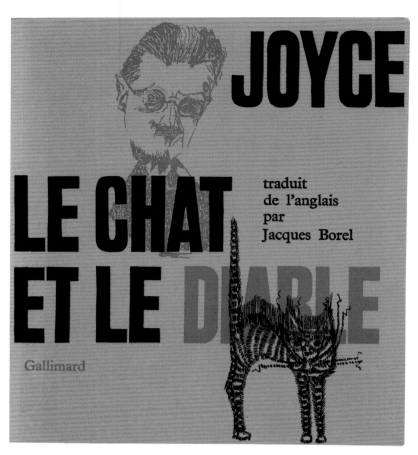

(or decalcomania) using two alphabets designed by Massin. The man's lines are set in a mix of modified Cheltenham and Robur; the woman's in Garamond italic, inclined at five different angles, one of which is the exact opposite of usual italics. In this oral calligraphy Massin translates the human voice with different degrees of typographic bolds, combined with ink blots and graphic accidents, as Richard Hollis explains.[6] Massin adds, '*Délire à deux* extends the approach of *La Cantatrice chauve*. Moreover, I've never been able to go any further, despite all my efforts and research (and even using a computer!) over more than thirty years'.[7]

The vocal sextet of *Conversation-sinfonietta*, subtitled by Massin 'an essay in typographical orchestration', still retains a semblance of visual rationality. In 1955 Jean Tardieu published a new cycle of poems and writings with the title *Théâtre de chambre*, which included *Conversation-sinfonietta*. This was a dramatization of the lyrical, or vocal art, an experiment that enabled Tardieu to render visible and audible the fact that it is but a short step from one genre to the other. In this way he revealed the great musical potential of language, while continuing to explore his favourite themes,

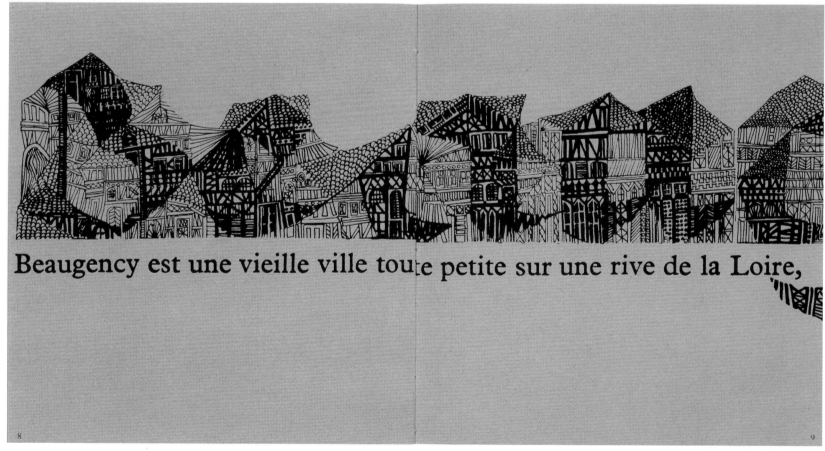

Two-colour cover and inside spread from James Joyce's *Le Chat et le Diable* (The cat and the devil; Paris, Gallimard, 1966) with illustrations by Jean-Jacques Corre; another example, contemporary with *La cantatrice chauve*, of expressive typography.

including fear of the unknown, death and the absurd. In Massin's layout, created in 1966 and imitating a musical score, the harmonious diversity of fonts retains a certain typographical rigour. Voices are set out on the score and defined both by typeface and by the identity of the characters, so that the lettering itself has an extraordinary presence as a living character; in *Délire à deux*, on the other hand, the ink blots interrupt the text to the point of rendering it impossible to read. Effects of dripping ink (created by using the brush or paint-pot itself to throw paint across a flat canvas, a method invented by Jackson Pollock) become symbolic of a violent unconscious, which mumbles, interrupts and erases itself to the point of being incapable of self-expression.

In questioning the very essence of the role of the typographer and graphic artist, in all these experimental projects Massin pushed back the boundaries of the use of typography and its contextualization. We should remember that the intrepid Massin made almost all his works of expressive typography alone, in his own time, returning to the Gallimard studio at the weekend. They are all projects that he conceived himself, with the exception

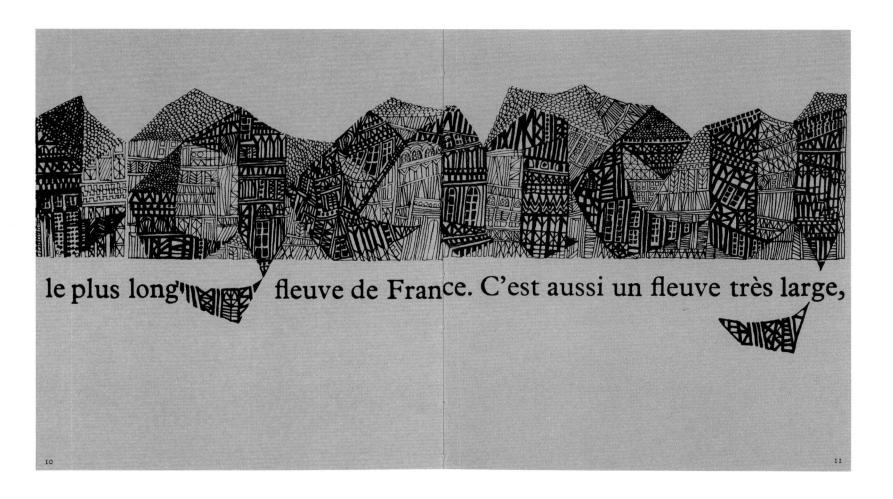

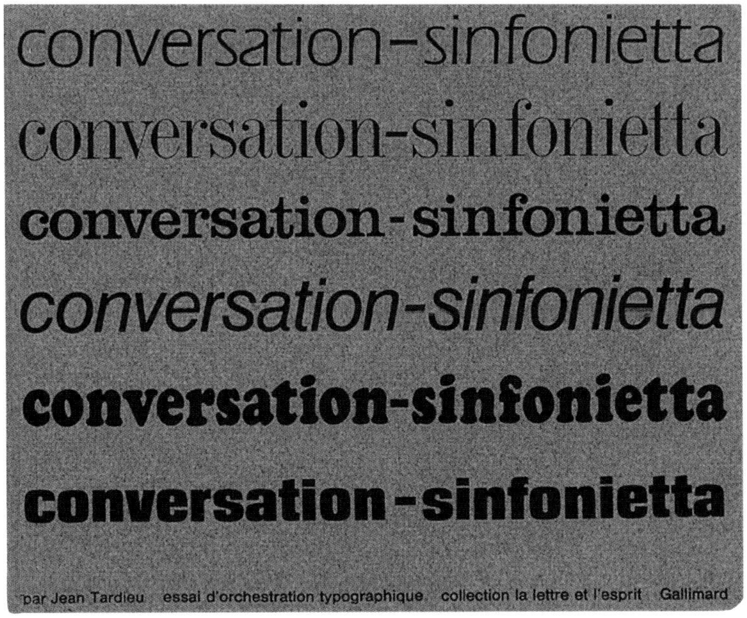

conversation-sinfonietta
conversation-sinfonietta
conversation-sinfonietta
conversation-sinfonietta
conversation-sinfonietta
conversation-sinfonietta

par Jean Tardieu | essai d'orchestration typographique. | collection la lettre et l'esprit | Gallimard

This page and opposite: cover in black and white on brown Ingres paper and inside pages from Jean Tardieu's *Conversation-sinfonietta*, subtitled 'essai d'orchestration typographique' (an essay in typographic orchestration; Paris, Gallimard, 1966).

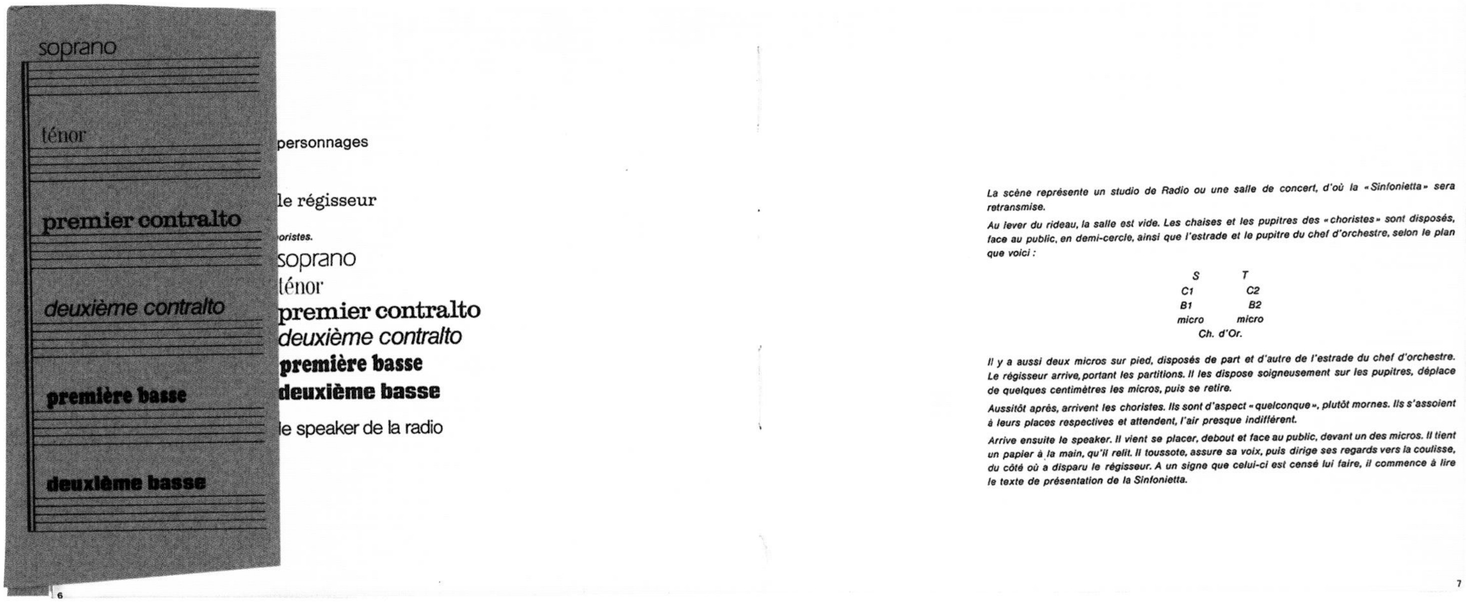

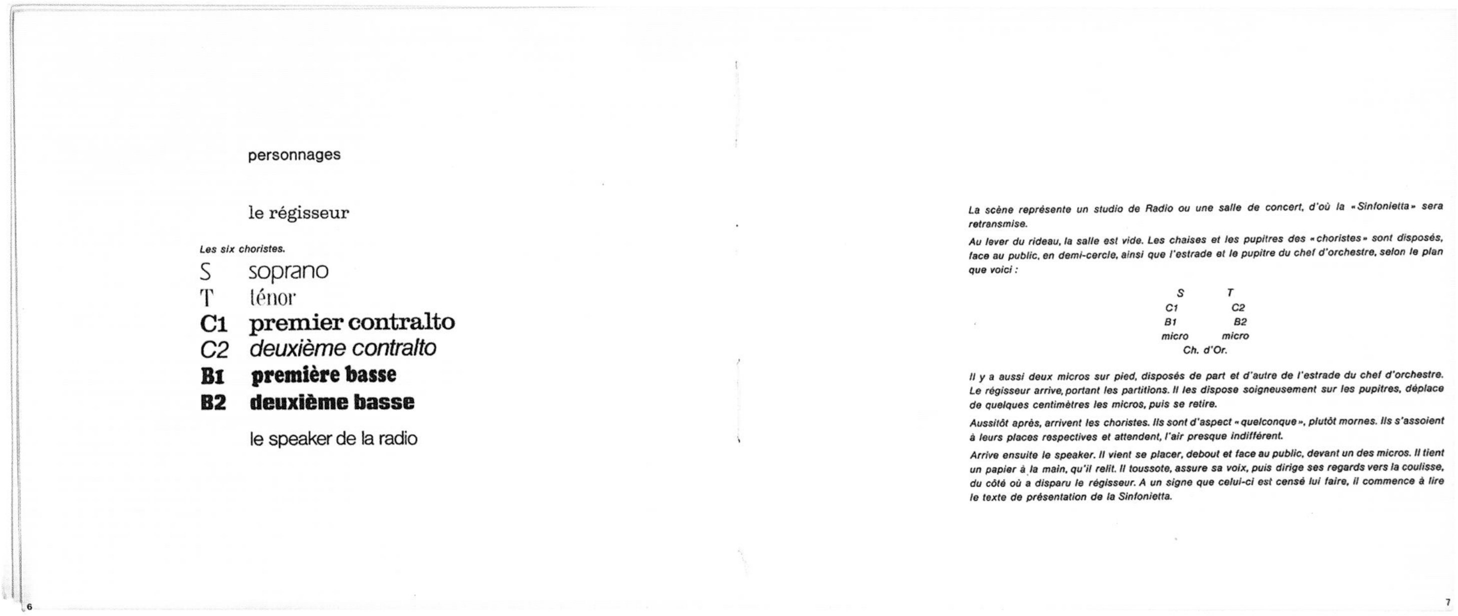

soprano

ténor

premier contralto

deuxième contralto

première basse

deuxième basse

personnages

le régisseur

choristes.

soprano
ténor
premier contralto
deuxième contralto
première basse
deuxième basse

le speaker de la radio

La scène représente un studio de Radio ou une salle de concert, d'où la «Sinfonietta» sera retransmise.

Au lever du rideau, la salle est vide. Les chaises et les pupitres des «choristes» sont disposés, face au public, en demi-cercle, ainsi que l'estrade et le pupitre du chef d'orchestre, selon le plan que voici :

	S	T
	C1	C2
	B1	B2
	micro	micro
	Ch. d'Or.	

Il y a aussi deux micros sur pied, disposés de part et d'autre de l'estrade du chef d'orchestre. Le régisseur arrive, portant les partitions. Il les dispose soigneusement sur les pupitres, déplace de quelques centimètres les micros, puis se retire.

Aussitôt après, arrivent les choristes. Ils sont d'aspect «quelconque», plutôt mornes. Ils s'assoient à leurs places respectives et attendent, l'air presque indifférent.

Arrive ensuite le speaker. Il vient se placer, debout et face au public, devant un des micros. Il tient un papier à la main, qu'il relit. Il toussote, assure sa voix, puis dirige ses regards vers la coulisse, du côté où a disparu le régisseur. A un signe que celui-ci est censé lui faire, il commence à lire le texte de présentation de la Sinfonietta.

6

7

personnages

le régisseur

Les six choristes.

S soprano
T ténor
C1 premier contralto
C2 *deuxième contralto*
B1 **première basse**
B2 **deuxième basse**

le speaker de la radio

La scène représente un studio de Radio ou une salle de concert, d'où la «Sinfonietta» sera retransmise.

Au lever du rideau, la salle est vide. Les chaises et les pupitres des «choristes» sont disposés, face au public, en demi-cercle, ainsi que l'estrade et le pupitre du chef d'orchestre, selon le plan que voici :

	S	T
	C1	C2
	B1	B2
	micro	micro
	Ch. d'Or.	

Il y a aussi deux micros sur pied, disposés de part et d'autre de l'estrade du chef d'orchestre. Le régisseur arrive, portant les partitions. Il les dispose soigneusement sur les pupitres, déplace de quelques centimètres les micros, puis se retire.

Aussitôt après, arrivent les choristes. Ils sont d'aspect «quelconque», plutôt mornes. Ils s'assoient à leurs places respectives et attendent, l'air presque indifférent.

Arrive ensuite le speaker. Il vient se placer, debout et face au public, devant un des micros. Il tient un papier à la main, qu'il relit. Il toussote, assure sa voix, puis dirige ses regards vers la coulisse, du côté où a disparu le régisseur. A un signe que celui-ci est censé lui faire, il commence à lire le texte de présentation de la Sinfonietta.

6

7

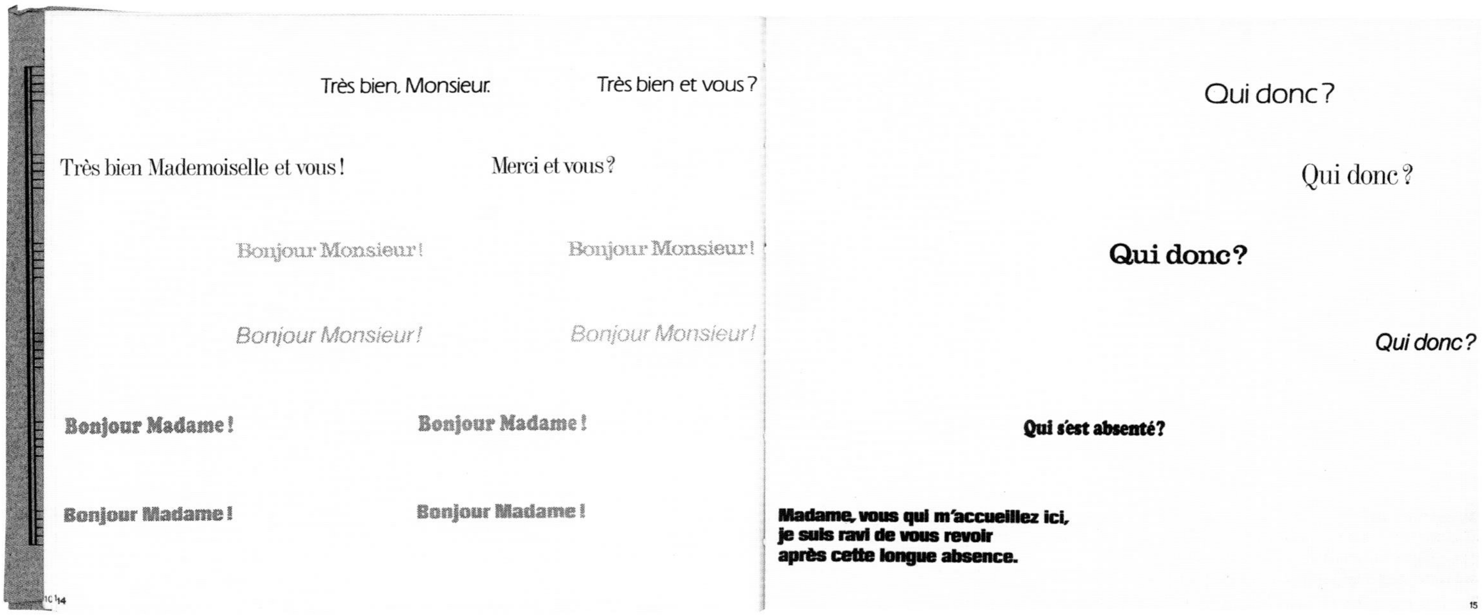

Très bien, Monsieur.   Très bien et vous ?

Très bien Mademoiselle et vous !   Merci et vous ?

Bonjour Monsieur !   Bonjour Monsieur !

Bonjour Monsieur !   Bonjour Monsieur !

Bonjour Madame !   Bonjour Madame !

Bonjour Madame !   Bonjour Madame !

Qui donc ?

Qui donc ?

Qui donc ?

Qui donc ?

Qui s'est absenté ?

**Madame, vous qui m'accueillez ici,
je suis ravi de vous revoir
après cette longue absence.**

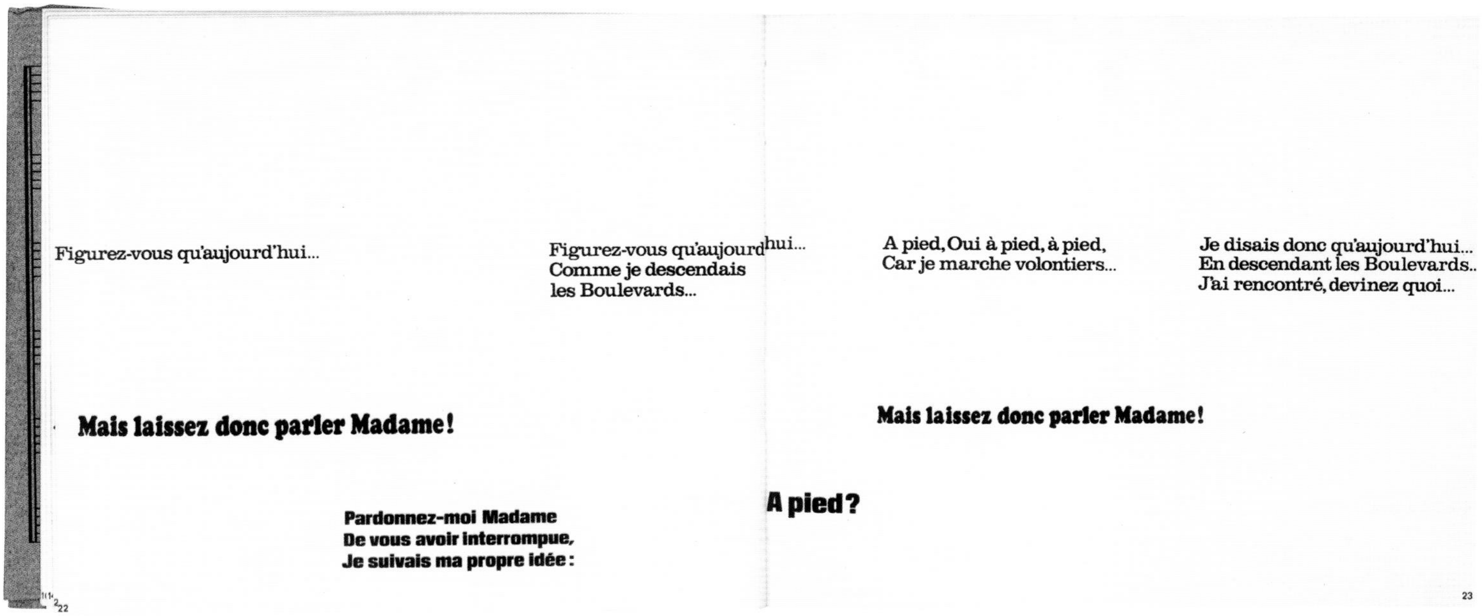

Figurez-vous qu'aujourd'hui...

Figurez-vous qu'aujourd'hui...
Comme je descendais
les Boulevards...

A pied, Oui à pied, à pied,
Car je marche volontiers...

Je disais donc qu'aujourd'hui...
En descendant les Boulevards...
J'ai rencontré, devinez quoi...

Mais laissez donc parler Madame !

Mais laissez donc parler Madame !

A pied ?

**Pardonnez-moi Madame
De vous avoir interrompue,
Je suivais ma propre idée :**

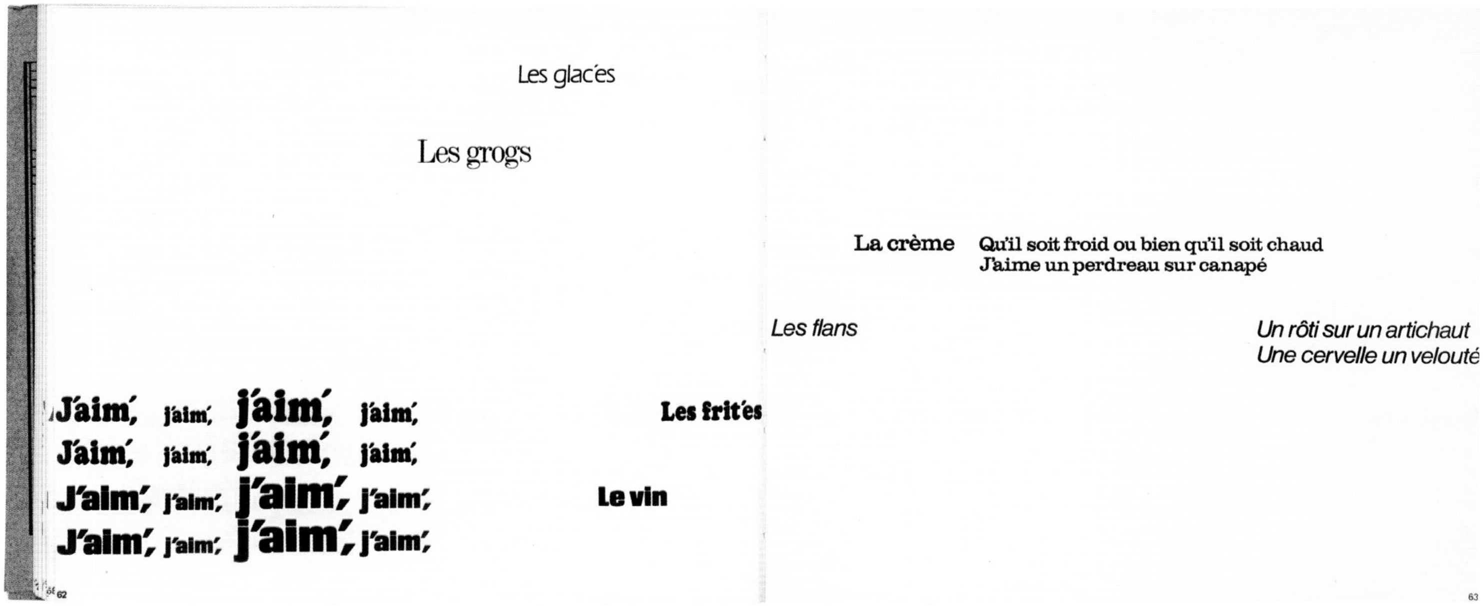

Les glacés

Les grogs

La crème   Qu'il soit froid ou bien qu'il soit chaud
            J'aime un perdreau sur canapé

Les flans   *Un rôti sur un artichaut*
                 Une cervelle un velouté

**J'aim', j'aim', j'aim', j'aim',
J'aim', j'aim', j'aim', j'aim',
J'aim', j'aim', j'aim', j'aim',
J'aim', j'aim', j'aim', j'aim',**

Les frites

Le vin

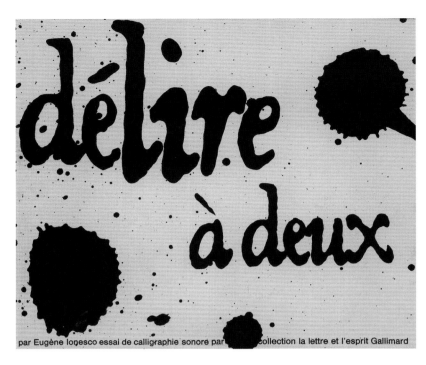

par Eugène Ionesco essai de calligraphie sonoré par ⬛ collection la lettre et l'esprit Gallimard

Above: black and white cover for Eugène Ionesco's *Délire à deux*, subtitled 'essai de calligraphie sonore' (an essay in sound calligraphy; Paris, Gallimard, 1966).

Opposite and following two pages: inside pages from *Délire à deux*. The ink blots are graphic elements that symbolize the violence of the couple, while also representing sound effects: machine guns, breaking glasses, gun shots and exploding bombs.

of *La Foule*, based on the song by Édith Piaf, which was commissioned by the American avant-garde magazine *Evergreen Review* in 1965.

As an artist of graphics and layout, Massin turned typography into a subject in itself rather than simply a means to an end. He made it a theme, a game, a celebration – although he never went so far as to design fonts or illustrations, on the grounds that he was no good with a pencil. A wise successor to Faucheux, who designed the layout of Henri Pichette's *Épiphanies* (Paris, K Éditeur, 1948), it was lettering itself that Massin was laying out, taking first the theatre and then the musical theatre as the arena for his explorations. He rejects the neutrality of traditional layout to give the reader a subjective vision of the plays of Ionesco and Tardieu. Making a break with the traditional linear, diachronic reading of dramatic texts, Massin breaks the message down into meaningful graphic entities. In so doing he alters the neutral function of typography, turning it into the critical material of the layout artist – along the lines of the director who 'interprets' the text – thereby bringing a new definition to the expression 'committed artist'.[8]

The rules of the game

Massin's expressive typography channels space, time, sound and rhythm and seeks to lay them out on an empty page – these are the rules that are broken, messed around and reinvented by the graphic artist. In the club books the notion of duration was intrinsically linked to the reader's experience of the book as an object that 'unfolds', with the graphic artist playing with the notion of sequence as inspired by cinema. In relation to theatre the reader's experience is at once linked to the physical architecture of the book, while also seeking to connect with the narrative unfolding of the play. This time-based lettering that moves is no longer confined to an animated title, illustrated endpaper or credits spread across several endpapers, but let loose throughout the whole book.

The challenge of bringing a page to life by purely typographic means – though these may be enhanced with photographs, bubbles and other graphic accidents such as the ink blots of *Délire à deux* – lies particularly in the evocation of the movement of the actors on stage. The stage directions are no longer enough in a layout that still has to respect the order of lines, which renders the dialogue comprehensible, and the western system of reading from left to right. Massin gives visual expression to oral language through the dynamic relationships between typographic variations (of font family and size), intertwined letters, overlapping lines and bubbles, using different fonts to translate each character's intonation, speed, volume and diction.

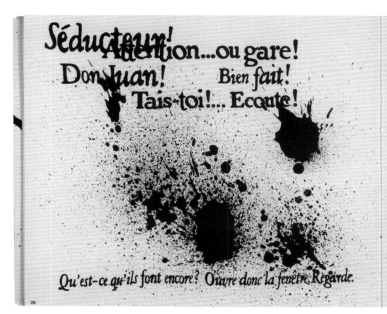

Séducteur! Attention...ou gare!

Don Juan! Bien fait!

Tais-toi!... Ecoute!

Qu'est-ce qu'ils font encore? Ouvre donc la fenêtre. Regarde.

26

Tout à l'heure, tu disais que tu ne voulais pas l'ouvrir. *Je cède.* Tu vois. Je suis **bonne.** C'est vrai, pour une fois c'est vrai, menteuse. D'ailleurs, tu n'auras plus froid. Ça a l'air de chauffer.

Que se passe-t-il? Pas grand chose. Il y a trois morts. Lesquels? Un de chaque côté. Et un neutre, un passant. *Ne reste pas à la fenêtre. Ils vont tirer sur toi.* Je ferme. D'ailleurs, ça s'éloigne. Alors, c'est *qu'ils sont partis.* On va étouffer. On les voit quand même qui s'épient. Il y a leurs têtes là, au coin, aux deux bouts. On va pas encore se promener. On peut pas encore sortir. Nous prendrons les décisions plus tard. **Demain.** Encore une **belle** *occasion de ne pas prendre de décision.* C'est comme ça. *Et ça va continuer, ça va continuer.*

27

choisi la maison. **Comment j'aurais fait si j'en avais pas eu l'idée.** C'est ou bien ou bien. On a fait ça comme ça. *Ils montent. Ferme bien la porte.* Elle est fermée. Elle ferme mal. *Ferme-la bien quand même.* Ils sont sur le palier. *Sur le nôtre?*

Calme-toi, c'est pas à nous qu'ils en veulent. Ils frappent à la porte d'en face.

On les emmène. Ils montent à l'étage au-dessus. *Ils descendent.* Non, ils montent. *Ils descendent.* **Non, ils montent.** Je te

34

dis qu'ils descendent. **Tu veux toujours avoir raison.** Je te dis qu'ils montent.

Ils descendent. Tu ne sais même plus interpréter les bruits. C'est un effet de la peur.

Qu'ils montent ou qu'ils descendent, c'est à peu près pareil. La prochaine fois, c'est chez nous qu'ils viendront. Barricadons-nous. **L'armoire.** Pousse l'armoire devant la porte. Et tu dis que tu as des idées.

J'ai pas dit que j'avais des idées.

Pourtant, de deux choses l'une. L'armoire,

35

exceptions. *L'exception, c'est moi.* C'est ce que tu veux dire? Je ne sais pas. Tu vois bien tu veux dire. Tu m'insultes. Je vais te prouver. J'ai pas envie que tu me prouves quoi que ce soit, laisse-moi tranquille. Laisse-moi tranquille. Moi aussi, je veux être tranquille. Mais avec toi!

Tu vois bien que ce n'est pas possible

52

avec toi. Ce n'est pas possible d'être tranquille, **oui;** mais c'est en dehors de notre volonté. Ce n'est pas possible objectivement. *J'en ai assez de ta* **manie** *de l'objectivité.* **Attention** plutôt au projectile, il va exploser...comme l'autre.

Mais non, mais non, ce n'est plus une grenade. **Attention, tu vas nous tuer, ça va démolir la chambre.** C'est un éclat d'obus. *Justement,*

53

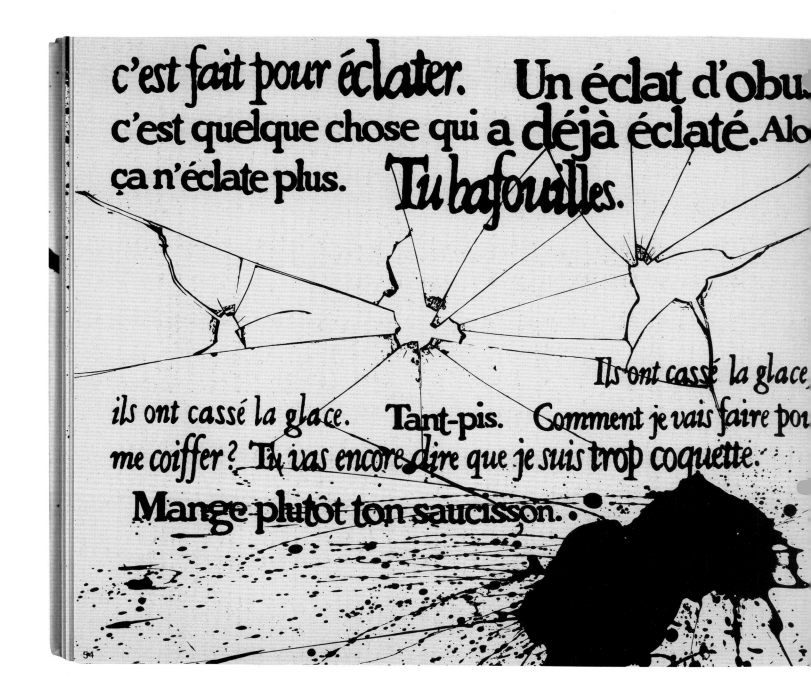

c'est fait pour éclater. Un éclat d'obu...
c'est quelque chose qui a déjà éclaté. Alo...
ça n'éclate plus. Tu bafouilles.

Ils ont cassé la glace,

ils ont cassé la glace. Tant-pis. Comment je vais faire pou...
me coiffer ? Tu vas encore dire que je suis trop coquette.

Mange plutôt ton saucisson.

Quand j'étais petite, j'étais une enfant. Les enfants de mon âge aussi étaient petits. Des petits garçons, des petites filles. On n'était pas tous de la même taille. Il y a toujours des plus petits, des plus grands, des enfants blonds, des enfants bruns, des enfants ni bruns, ni blonds. On apprenait à lire, à écrire, à compter. Des soustractions, des divisions, des multiplications, des additions. Parce qu'on allait à l'école. Il y en a qui apprenaient à la maison. Il y avait un lac, pas loin. Avec des poissons, les poissons vivent dans l'eau. C'est pas comme nous. Nous on ne peut pas, même quand on est petit; pourtant, on devrait. Pourquoi pas ? Si j'avais appris la technique, je serais technicien. Je fabriquerais des objets. Des objets compliqués. Des objets très compliqués,

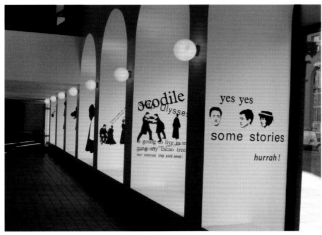

Already revealing his fascination with the spirit of lettering, with the alphabet as a living organism made of pictograms, which he would dissect later in *La Lettre et l'Image*,[9] in a letter to Gaston Gallimard about *La Cantatrice chauve*, Massin concludes:

'So from now on typography will play a role that goes beyond that of simple communication. With the help of images it will strive to fix these privileged moments that seem swollen with a thousand instants. The image, for its part, has already travelled much of the path: it strives to meet up with lettering through the ideogram. So ultimately we no longer really know whether a character's appearance follows the outlines of the letter or whether, conversely, lettering itself has become a character. This ambiguity is most tangible in the last part of the play: helped by the disintegration of language, the reader reinvents the alphabet by moving from sentences to words, from words to syllables and from syllables to letters, while the letters, undressed in this way, magnified and revealed by the spotlight, become once more the characters they have never ceased to be.'[10]

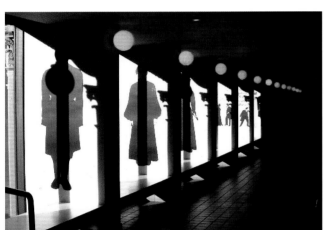

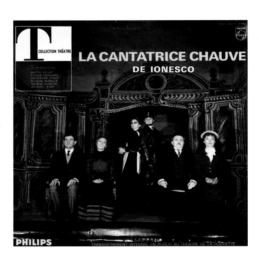

Left, top to bottom: photographs of the exhibition 'Massin in Continuo: A Dictionary', curated by Laetitia Wolff with art direction by Philippe Apeloig at the Herb Lubalin Study Center of Design and Typography at the Cooper Union School of Art, New York, Winter 2001–2; cover for the album *La Cantatrice chauve de Ionesco* (Philips, c.1956), featuring a photograph of the company of the Théâtre de la Huchette, Paris.

Below: photograph of Henry Cohen by Jean-Marie Perret, Auxerre, 1992.

Henry Cohen and graphic techniques using photography

The photographer Henry Cohen was born in 1919 and now lives in retirement in the Yonne. He created over 300 cover illustrations for Gallimard's 'Idées' series. Massin met him at the Club du meilleur livre, for whom he invited Cohen to create his first cover illustrations for a collection of poems by Federico García Lorca (Romancero gitan, The Gypsy Ballads; 1959). Cohen also worked as a photographer and reporter for the magazine Sciences et Avenir and as a catalogue photographer, notably for Daum crystal, and was involved in various advertising and public relations campaigns. During the 1970s he set up a small offset printworks publishing posters and artists' catalogues.

The 'Idées' paperback series, launched in 1961 when Massin was art director, gave Cohen an opportunity to experiment – for almost thirteen years – with his 'photo-graphics'. '"Photo-graphics"? I think it was me who invented the term; it's the creation of graphics using photographic means, the manipulation of images before

Photoshop', explains Cohen.[11] For 'Idées', a series covering the humanities and philosophical writings, his black and white illustrations, whose abstract nature makes them instantly recognizable, were printed under an area of colour and created on transparent monochrome film. These manipulations mark the start of what can be called synthesized images. Sometimes Cohen also practises solarization; a technique of quickly exposing the film under a light during development made famous by the photographer Man Ray in the 1920s. The image obtained is thus partly negative and partly positive. Massin notes, 'When you take a look at these many hundreds of covers, you're astounded by the graphic quality of the whole and the coherent intention in their very diversity, and you're amazed by the photographer's constant inventiveness (even more so when the text is of a philosophical nature that doesn't lend itself to the picturesque), his skilful work with light and shadow and the delicious mix of poetry and a sometimes surrealist humour.'[12]

Cohen also worked with Massin on the design of La Cantatrice chauve *in 1964, for which he designed the photo-graphics, thereby becoming just as much its interpreter as Massin. After seeing the play several times at the théâtre de la Huchette to identify its most graphic scenes and make the most of the characters' poses, Cohen took pictures of the actors in the Gallimard building. These were 'as flat as possible, without any shadows cast and with totally diffuse light'.[13] The high-contrast photographic print was obtained using special lith film and developed in lith developer (diluted or not) which requires a precise amount of time in the enlarger. One of the processes of photo-graphics consists in gradually eliminating all the half-tones – in other words the greys that usually give a photograph its realist aspect – to produce an effect of very high contrast. The interpretative aspect lies in identifying the level (or density) of separation between blacks and whites that will give the most meaningful image. 'Creating high contrast is not an automatic operation', Cohen explains.[14]*

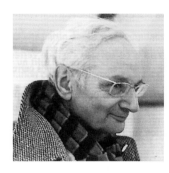

The photographer uses a system of retouching to make high-contrast prints that transform the actors into graphic signs. 'So it is a Manichean approach, as arbitrary as binary language in computer technology: some of the greys become white, the others black.'[15]

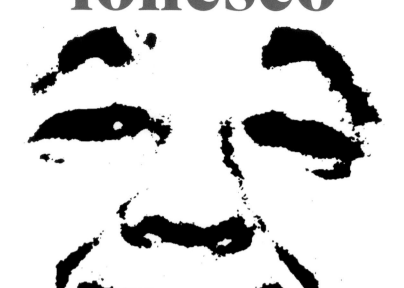

THEATRE DE LA HUCHETTE
23 rue de la huchette 75 005 paris tél. 01 43 26 38 99 métro st michel

ionesco

19 h la cantatrice chauve mise en scène de nicolas bataille
20h la leçon mise en scène de marcel cuvelier
décors de jacques noël

44e année ! 14000e !
location au théâtre et par téléphone de 17h à 21h. relâche le dimanche

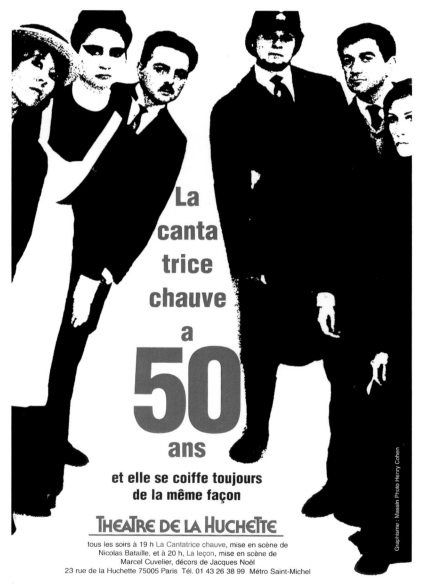

La
canta
trice
chauve
a
50
ans

et elle se coiffe toujours
de la même façon

THEATRE DE LA HUCHETTE
tous les soirs à 19 h La Cantatrice chauve, mise en scène de
Nicolas Bataille, et à 20 h, La leçon, mise en scène de
Marcel Cuvelier, décors de Jacques Noël
23 rue de la huchette 75005 Paris Tél. 01 43 26 38 99 Métro Saint-Michel

Top to bottom: black and white paper covers for the editions published in France (*La Cantatrice chauve*, Paris, Gallimard, 1964), the United States (*The Bald Soprano*, New York, Grove Press, 1965) and Britain (*The Bald Prima Donna*, London, Calder and Boyars, 1966).

Opposite: original edition of *La Cantatrice chauve* (Paris, Gallimard, 1950), with handwritten layout notes by Massin, c.1964.

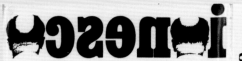
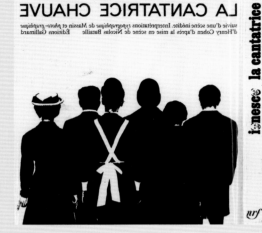
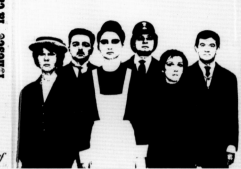
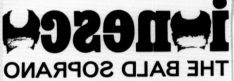
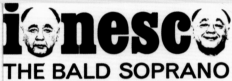
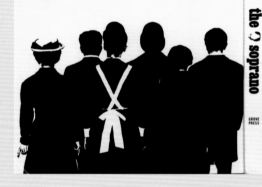
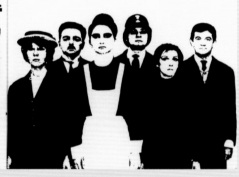
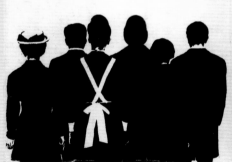
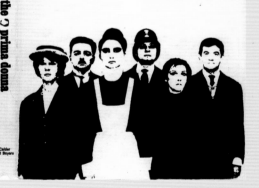

Focus
La Cantatrice chauve
Paris, Gallimard, 1964

Interpreting the word

To this day *La Cantatrice chauve, interprétations typographique de Massin et photographique d'Henry Cohen d'après la mise en scène de Nicolas Bataille* (Paris, Gallimard, 1964) remains Massin's masterpiece. The book was translated and adapted in the United States (*The Bald Soprano*, New York, Grove Press, 1965) and the UK (*The Bald Prima Donna*, London, Calder and Boyars, 1966). Massin's work is an interpretation of Eugène Ionesco's 'anti-play', published by Gallimard in 1950, and has become a classic of the theatre of the absurd, which has powerfully marked the history of modern theatre. *La Cantatrice chauve* formed in its author's mind after his comical experience of learning English. Amused at conversing by means of a simple succession of idiomatic expressions, proverbs, maxims and other

phrases which, placed end to end, became meaningless, he set the play in a bourgeois home in which six characters would play around with linguistic variations. So anachronisms and clichés pass from mouth to mouth, ultimately finding their own logic. Here there is neither a hero, nor a defined dramatic structure of the kind found in the classic theatre with its acts and scenes, but a series of fragmented sketches. As for the prima donna – or soprano – she does not appear, she does not exist, but has received ovation after ovation for more than fifty years at the théâtre de la Huchette in Paris, where the play has been performed continuously since it was first produced.

Explaining the reasons behind his 're-creation' of this classic of the absurd, Massin wrote, 'Ionesco

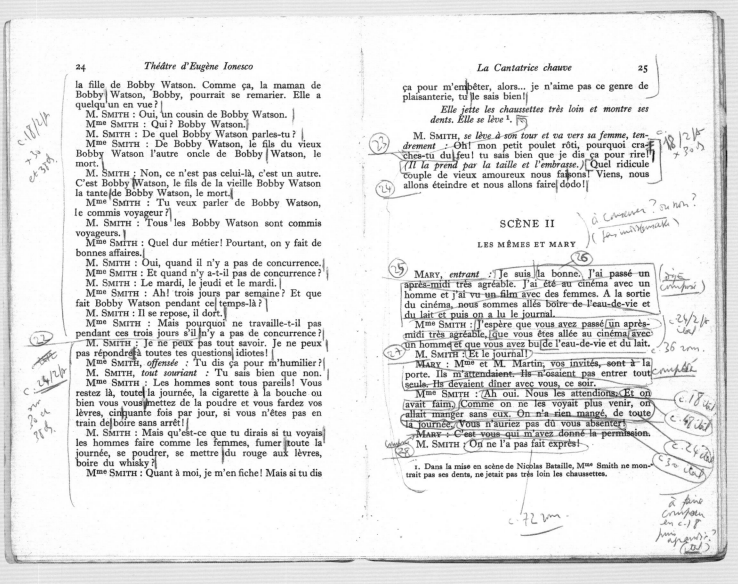

Top to bottom: collage of scenes extracted from *The Bald Soprano* with enlargement percentages and indications for different fonts; handwritten note by Massin to the editor on the punctuation of Mrs Smith.

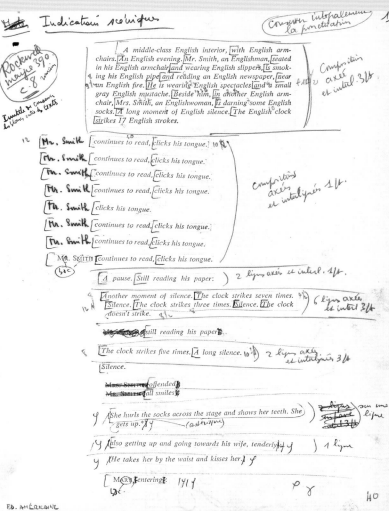

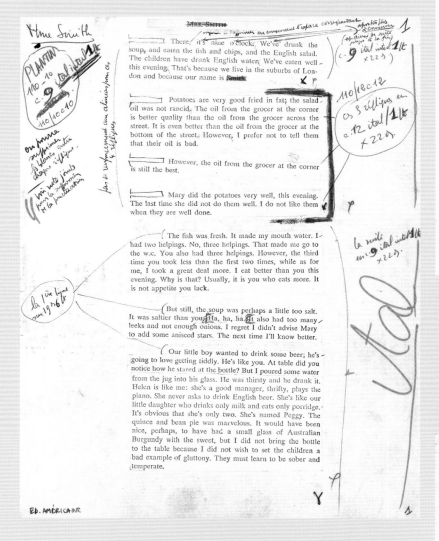

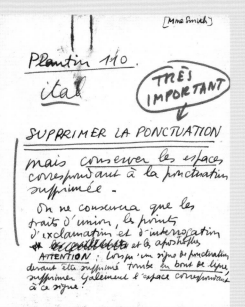

admits he now sees his play only as it exists on paper. This re-creation, seen as an extension of the author's intention, gives his work new life, exorcises familiar demons, amplifies the themes and precipitates the final catastrophe of language'.[16] Massin's version of *La Cantatrice chauve*, designed with Ionesco's blessing, seeks to render the dynamism proper to the representation of time in the theatre, while playing with the static constraints of the book. The only condition that Ionesco politely requested the graphic artist to respect was that the text should remain legible, as the play was on the syllabus for pupils in high school.

This 'typographic interpretation' drew on Nicolas Bataille's pantomime-style version, as performed at the théâtre de la Huchette in Paris since the play's revival in 1957 to the present day (it was first performed in 1950 at the Théâtre des Noctambules). Bataille remains present, in the theatre and on stage, and most of the actors in the play today are from the family of actors of the period by which Massin was inspired. Massin himself has seen the play twenty times and wanted to convey to the reader the actual experience of the theatrical performance. He made a tape recording of the play in order to translate not just the text, but also all the inflexions, intonations and silences of the actors.

GROVE PRESS, INC.
64 UNIVERSITY PLACE
NEW YORK 3, NEW YORK
OREGON 4-7200

CABLE ADDRESS: GROVEPRESS

le 15 janvier 1964

Monsieur Massin:
Editions Gallimard
5, rue Sebastien-Bottin
Paris VII, France

Cher Monsieur:

Barney Rosset m'a demandé de vous écrire concernant notre édition de LA CANTATRICE CHAUVE -- édition d'ailleurs que nous trouvons admirable de tous les points de vue.

Il nous a fallu plusieurs semaines de recherches pour resoudre toutes les questions de fabrication, mais je crois que nous avons maintenant tous les reseignements necéssaires et pourrions procéder selon les conditions que vous avez indiquées dans votre lettre du 15 octobre.

Comme vous l'avez supposé, nous préferons ce que nous appelons "finished mechanicals" plutôt que les "offset flats", c'est à dire les pages terminées "ready for printing" desquelles nous ferons les "offset flats" ici. Quant au format exact, nous vous prions de faire un format pour notre édition de 8 x 10" (au lieu de 8 1/4" x 10 1/2" de l'édition française). Si cela présente un problème, vous pourriez faire le format plus grand, pourvu que la proportion 8:10 soit respectée, car nous pourrions reduire à ce format (qui est important pour la brochage surtout) au moment de faire les "offset flats", c'est à dire on pourrait reduire les pages photographiquement.

Par cette lettre donc nous confirmons que nous voulons procéder a éditer cette édition et que nous vous payerons la somme de deux mille dollars ($2,000) pour votre travail, tout compris jusqu'aux pages prêtes à imprimer.

Pourriez-vous me donner une idée de la date à laquelle vous croyez pouvoir terminer ce travail? Nous aimerions que ce livre sorte ici au plus tard le mois de septembre prochain, c'est à dire bien avant Noel.

Bien amicalement,

Dick Seaver

Top to bottom: airmail letter to Massin from Dick Seaver, of Grove Press, dated 15 January 1964, officially commissioning the American adaptation of *La Cantatrice chauve*; typed letter from Ionesco giving Massin his agreement for the American edition, dated 20 January 1965.

Bottom left: photograph of Eugène Ionesco by Massin, at the latter's home, in front of his daughters' puppet theatre, Paris, 1968.

Paris le 20 Janvier 1965.

E. IONESCO
96 bd du Montparnasse
PARIS XIV.

Monsieur M A S S I N
Editions GALLIMARD
5 rue Sébastien-Bottin
P A R I S   VII

Cher Ami,

D'accord pour la publication de "LA CANTATRICE CHAUVE" chez Barney ROSSET -GROVE PRESS-. (en tenant compte du P.S.)

En ce qui concerne la traduction de Donald Allen, peut-être faudra-il la comparer à celle de Donald WATSON. Je ne vois pas de correction de détail en ce qui concerne la mise en scène typographique et je pense que la post-face doit être publiée car elle fait maintenant partie intégrante du volume publié chez GALLIMARD.

Tenez moi au courant des conditions du contrat. Je vous remercie et espère vous revoir bientôt. Vous viendrez à la maison pour voir les coupures de presse qui m'ont été envoyées par l'Argus.

Bien amicalement, et à bientôt. Hommage chez vous,
E. IONESCO

P.S. Une seule petite mais impérieux exigeance: je désirerais que le texte soit nettement plus lisible. Dans les écoles où on le travaille on trouve qu'il n'est pas sans importance. Priè donc de vouloir bien faire voir toutes épreuves. Merci.

Eugène Ionesco (1909–1994)

Eugène Ionesco, father of the theatre of the absurd, was born in Romania in 1909 to a Romanian father and a French mother. In 1938 he settled permanently in Paris, where he received a state grant to study French poetry. It was comparatively late in his career that Ionesco wrote La Cantatrice chauve (1949), which shatters clichés and commonplaces, turning them into an unbridled, absurd (Ionesco preferred the term 'derision') caricature and reducing language to disconnected words. Ionesco rejected the logic of plot and character development, replacing this with a farce that highlights the senseless existence of modern humanity in a society governed by chance and convention.

A fervent anti-Communist, Ionesco long campaigned against the authoritarian regime of Ceaucescu in Romania, which banned his plays. The revolutionary form of La Cantatrice chauve met with a luke-warm reception in Paris in the first years in which it was performed at the théâtre des Noctambules (1950) and then at la Huchette.
It was only once the theatre of the absurd garnered support from other radical writers, such as Samuel Beckett, and members of the surrealist movement such as André Breton and Luis Buñuel, that the play became a classic. Ionesco's love of adventure, incongruous humour and nihilism, also manifested in his plays La Leçon and Rhinocéros, led him to join the College of 'pataphysics (with Boris Vian, Raymond Queneau, Jacques Prévert, Marcel Duchamp and Michel Leiris). Ionesco was a keen contributor to the Cahiers du Collège de 'Pataphysique, in which most of his plays appeared. He later became a member of the Académie française. Ionesco, Tardieu and Queneau were all playwrights who explored the limits of language, played with words and took lack of communication as a theme. Massin shared their interest in the

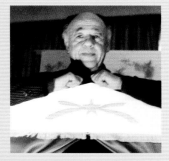

relationship between language and images and between popular, written and spoken words, with all the richness of their incredible visual resonance. Ionesco said that Massin was 'a great artist. Neither painter, nor musician, nor poet, but an artist of typography. The genius of typography.'[17]

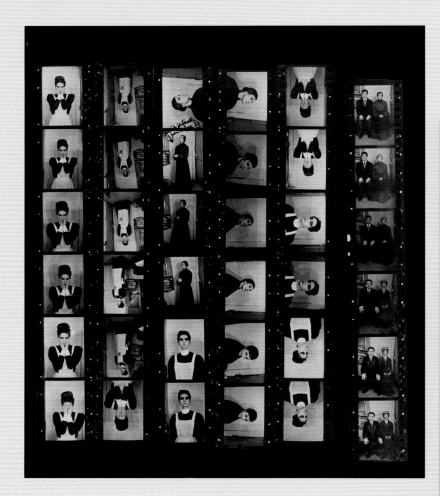

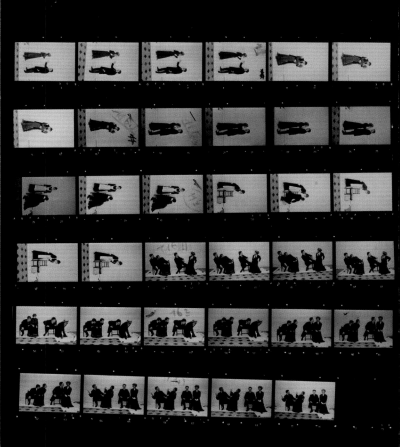

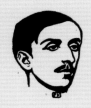

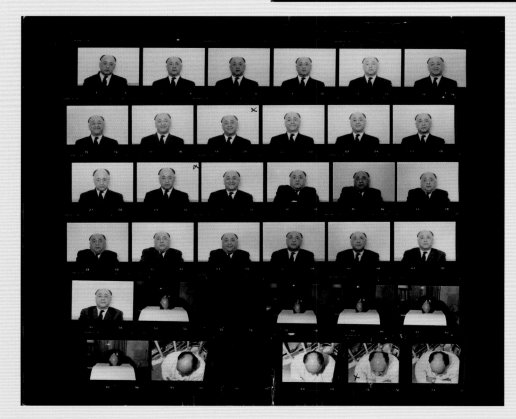

Top to bottom: contact sheets of photographs of the actors of the théâtre de la Huchette and Ionesco, taken on the Gallimard premises by Henry Cohen, Paris, 1964.

Far left: reproduction of a woodcut of Maurice Barrès by Félix Vallotton (early twentieth century), one of the first sources of inspiration for the photographic treatment of *La Cantatrice chauve*.

Photographic collaboration

For graphic artists *La Cantatrice chauve* remains a landmark in Massin's work, but it also grew out of Massin's collaboration with photographer Henry Cohen, who photographed the actors in their original costumes at Gallimard's headquarters at rue Sébastien-Bottin, Paris. On the dramatization of characters and their relationship to the actor who interprets them, Anne Ubersfeld writes: 'We need to look again at the commonplace that the character has concrete existence only through a concrete performance, the textual character being only *virtual*.'[18] Massin proves the opposite.

In the printed dialogue the usual names are replaced by faces and busts (photographs of the actors). Silhouettes of the characters – like the drawings of Saul Steinberg in which features and faces are traced by shadows alone – provide the graphic background in areas of monochrome colour over which Massin's 'typographs' unfold. They also reflect the art of contrast between black and white that Massin has explored throughout his typographical experiments, whether in his various covers or in the poetic compilations of *Typoésie* (Paris, Imprimerie nationale, 1993). Easily

handling black in its infinite nuances, he uses white spaces to represent the breaths in the text, giving them the role of silence as in music.

Gallimard had little faith in the project (from the start the book was very successful in the shops, but it was hard to persuade the publisher that this was an appropriate experiment) and Massin was obliged to use inexpensive techniques. So he replaced the more expensive 'simili' technique, which reproduces half-tones, with un-nuanced black areas and lines. But these budgetary constraints went hand in hand with an aesthetic approach: imperfections and smears from the inking and worn metal could be used to evoke roughness in the voices. So, as Marie-Laure Jaubert de Beaujeu explains, 'the "typo-photo-graphic" richness of the experiment was inversely proportional to the economy of the project'.[19] As François Caradec notes, the high-contrast black and white accentuates the graphic abstraction of the two-dimensional space 'while giving each character a new iconic and physical identity'.[20]

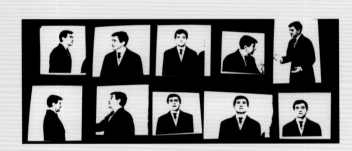

Left to right: cut-out Photostat copies of the character of M. Martin, showing his different bodily attitudes; collage of the faces of the four main characters, representing the range of their feelings.

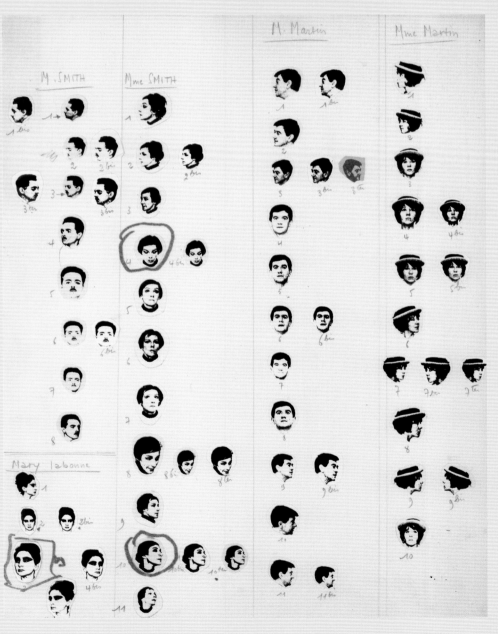

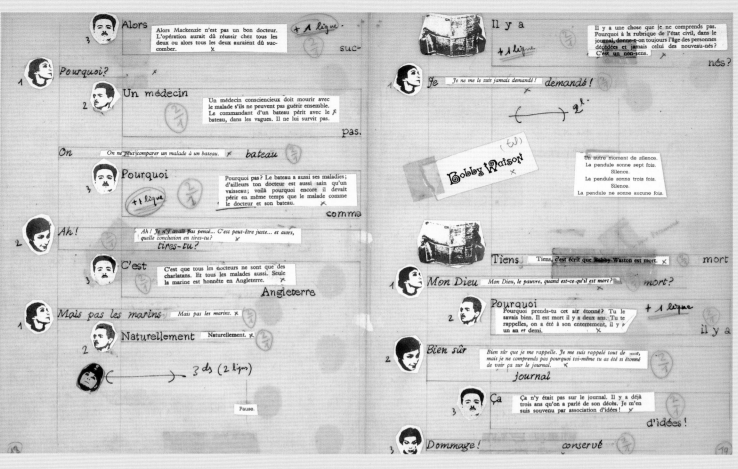

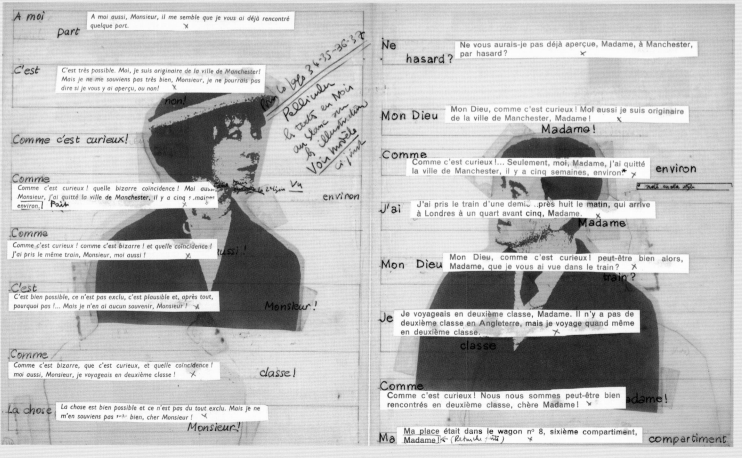

Typographical experimentation

In Massin's 'typo-graphs' each character is given a different font: Plantin for M. Smith, Plantin italic for Mme Smith, Monotype Grotesque 215 for M. Martin, Gill Sans italic for Mme Martin (because there is no Monotype Grotesque 215 italic), Cheltenham for the maid and Monotype Clarendon for the fireman. Marie, the maid, whom Massin sees as a rather masculine character, is represented with Cheltenham bold roman, unlike the other women, who are represented with italics.

In today's digital world, effects of this kind have become commonplace. Massin obtained them without the use of a computer and, moreover, without recourse to the flexibility of Letraset which, being expensive, was rarely used in the early 1960s. He had an epidiascope, which enabled him to project and enlarge the various elements of the text however he wanted (and thus to avoid the intermediate stage between the

finished design and the ozalid – the last printer's proof before the final printing). The lettering was done in pencil and projected on to the wall, providing a model for the size and scale of the letters to be enlarged from a composition in small type (monotype, because it was cheaper). Then the various typographical elements, illustrations and photographs were superimposed, if necessary, with tracing paper.

The whole was then photographed by the printer to create the negatives for the offset plates. As *La Cantatrice chauve* was to be offset printed, Massin had to cut and paste each page by hand. The use of typographical composition – transformed into images – made it possible to adjust the spaces between the words, reflecting the subtle pauses and breaks in the dialogue and so, with Ionesco's approval, to avoid all forms of punctuation other than exclamation and question marks.

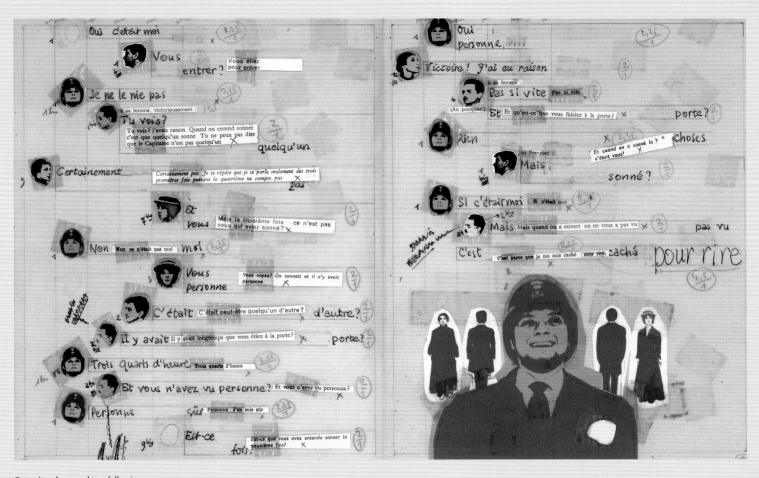

Opposite, above and two following spreads: draft double-page spreads on tracing paper for *La Cantatrice chauve* (pages 18–19, pages 34–5, pages 116–17, pages 160–1, pages 162–3 and pages 188–9). These collages, consisting of cut-up Photostat copies and fragments of text, were made by hand and annotated with layout indications and percentages for enlarging the fonts.

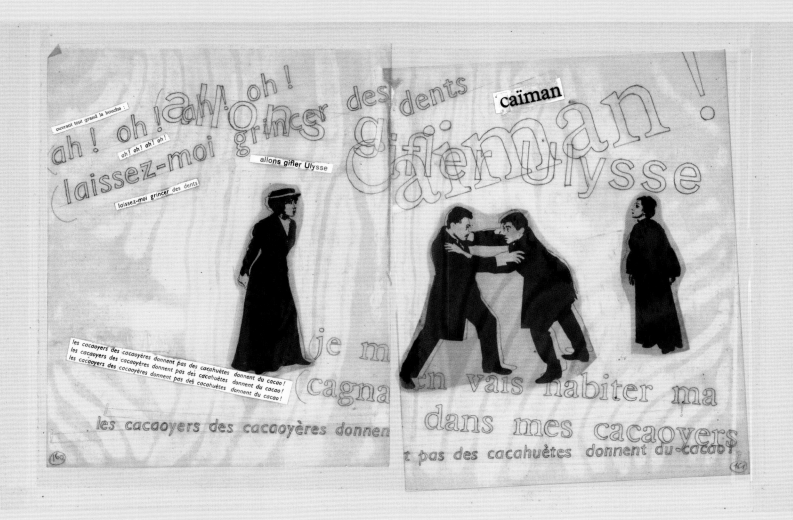

Animation in tempo

Massin was able to combine the aesthetics of comic-strip illustrations with the figurative aesthetics of photo novels and forms of expressive lettering used in the poetry of the Futurists into a masterpiece of 'visual literature'.

He returned to the rhythm of kinetics created by the use of folding pages he had perfected during his years at the book clubs. The illusion begins with the jacket, which bears the author's name on the front, with the two 'o's in 'Ionesco' replaced by his round, clownish face (by turns smiling and crying), and the play's title, with the cast members lined up along the bottom of the cover. On the back the actors are seen from behind, as though bowing, and the type is reversed as in a mirror (with Ionesco's bald head replacing the two 'o's in his name). Massin's *La Cantatrice chauve* begins with the members of the cast looking at the audience, from a frontal viewpoint, that of the audience in the theatre, as though they were poking their noses out from behind the curtain. The double title page, with its Cheltenham lower case enlarged to 150 or 200 points and overflowing the page, breaks with conventions of scale and clearly signals a play that itself is revolutionary. Later on, a black page evokes the darkness of the theatre before the curtain rises and follows a series of double pages in which the lettering has become totally abstract, aside from a few discreet stage directions. The use of cinematic techniques allows for a combination of close-ups, medium close-ups, tracking shots, etc., as in a film, imposed by the pace and action of the staging. The very last page contains Ionesco's head bowing to the audience, representing the triumphant playwright.

It is no surprise that Ionesco thought seriously of transposing this dynamic play into the medium of film, which, by definition, suits the dialectics of time and movement. He developed a film project (thinking of the director Hervé Bromberger) and joked, 'We can add applause to make it 52 minutes.' Massin remembers that Ionesco got himself into a mess by signing three different contracts in the United States for the production of an opera based on *La Cantatrice chauve*, 'to make a little pocket money' (as Ionesco put it).[21] The three production companies each discovered the existence of the other contracts, so nothing came of them. One hardly dare imagine the infinite possibilities that such a 're-re-creation' might have offered readers and viewers. But while Massin worked to translate three dimensions into two using cinematic techniques, he never tried directing for the cinema.

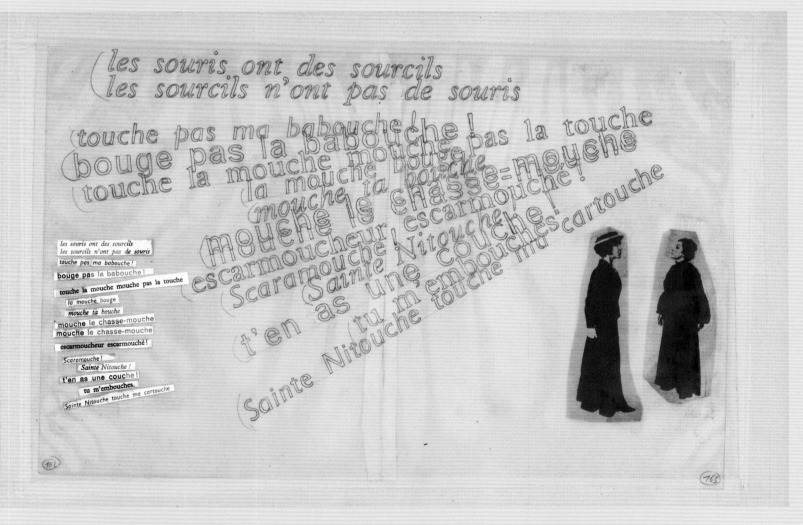

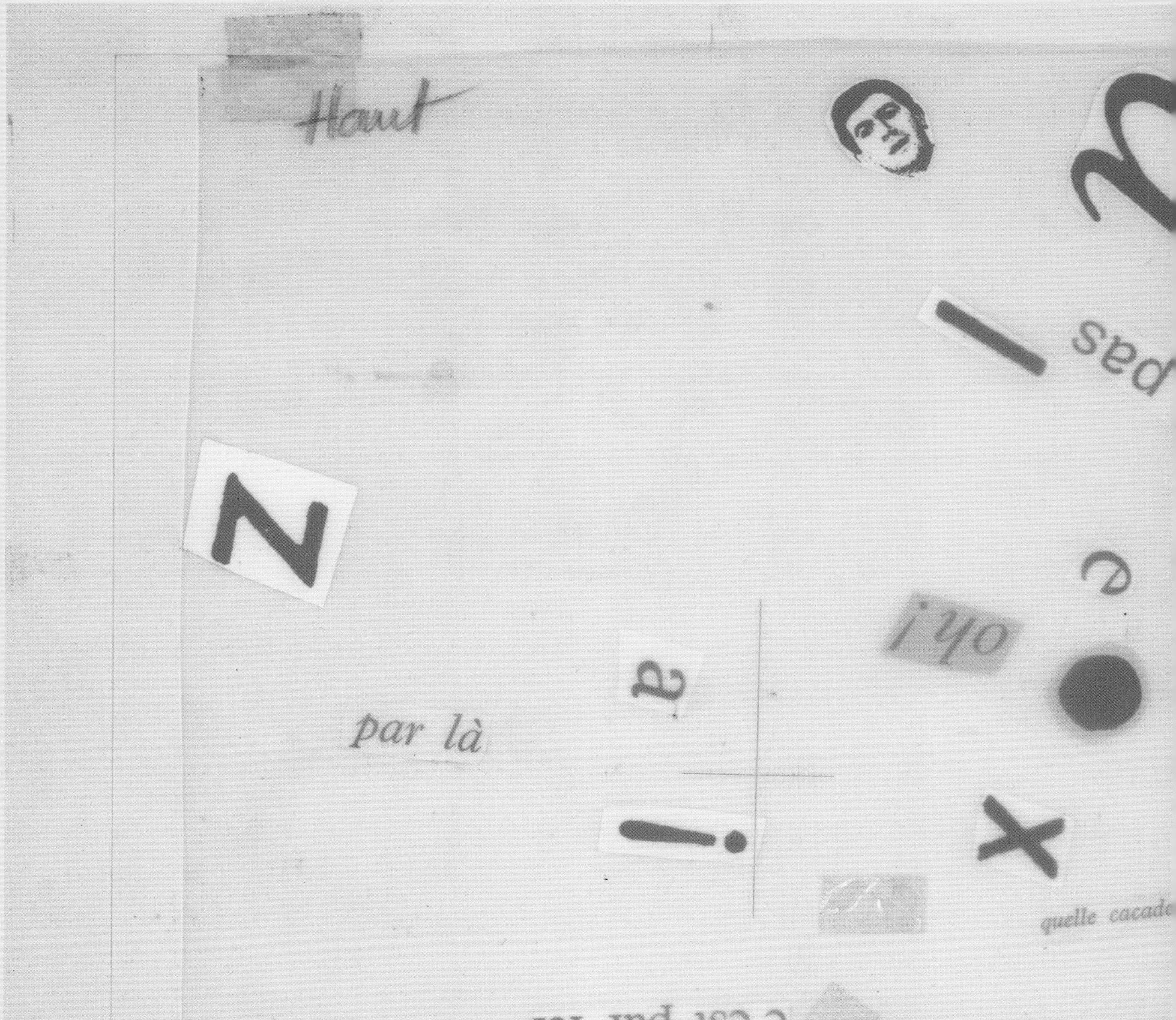

Haut

sed

N

e

¡yo

par là

a

x

i

quelle cacade

c'est par ici

est pas par là

c'est

c'est par

Bas   là c'est par ici

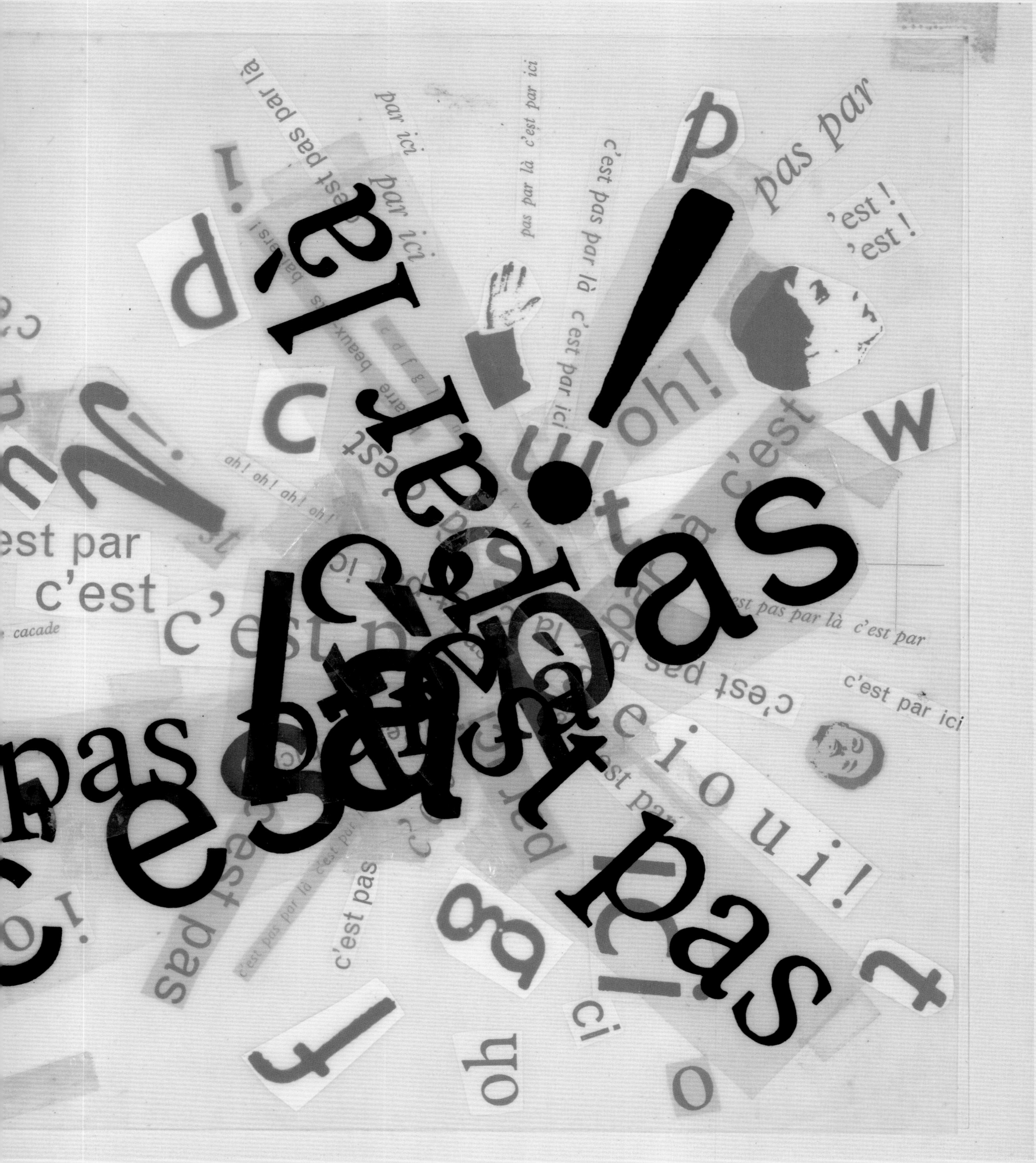
c'est pas par là
par ici
pas par là c'est par ici
c'est pas par là c'est par ici
pas par
'est !
'est !
oh!
c'est
w
est par
c'est
cacade
ah ! oh ! ah ! oh !
c'est pas par là c'est par
c'est par ici
e i o u i!
c'est pas
ci
oh
o

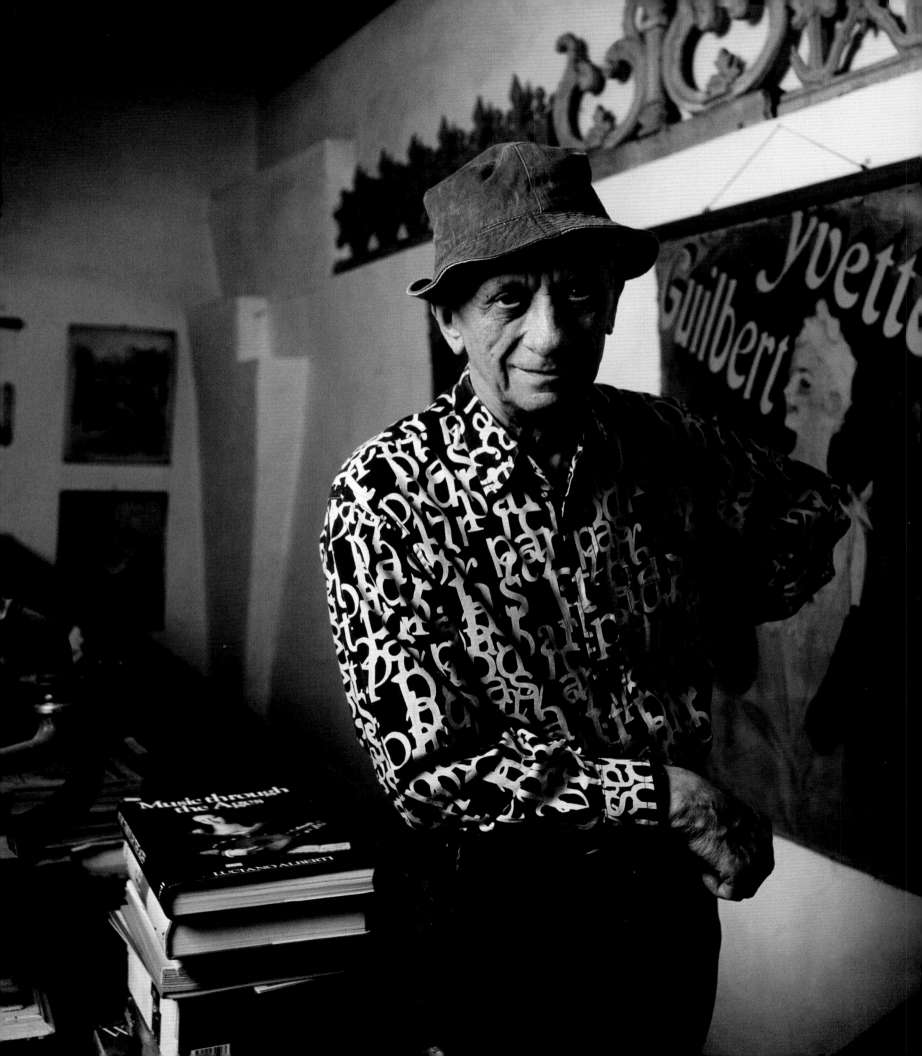

A Love of Lettering

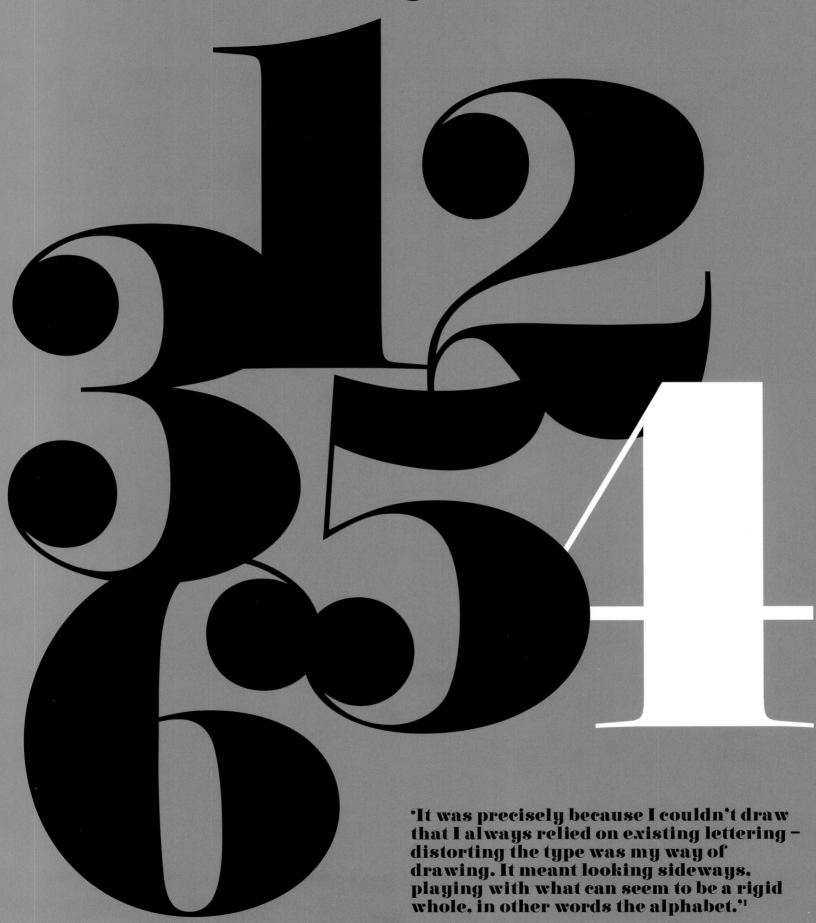

'It was precisely because I couldn't draw that I always relied on existing lettering – distorting the type was my way of drawing. It meant looking sideways, playing with what can seem to be a rigid whole, in other words the alphabet.'

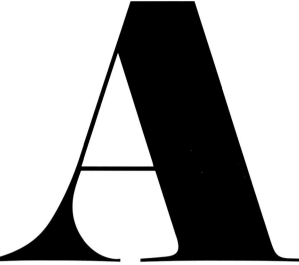

collector of letters and images

Since he was a very small boy Massin has made connections between the act of writing with a pen and typography, between the formation of letters and their graphic manipulation, between 'letters and images'. He likes to tell how his father, an engraver, sculptor and stone carver, taught him to write his name in soft stone when he was only four and a half years old and could not yet recite the alphabet. Indeed he has made this anecdote the founding moment of his typographical vocation. Describing himself as having an 'absolute typographical eye', in the same vein he also tells how, around twenty years ago, he bought a copy of his primary-school reading primer, found by chance in an antiques shop in Montlhéry. 'The details of these designs were so imprinted on my mind that later, when I began to learn the secrets of typography, I was able to state that my reading primer was set in Bodoni.'[2] This reading primer was a crystallization of his 'childhood mythology'[3] in which he discovered that 'a' and 'A' were the same letter, whether in bold or cursive copperplate script.[4] This variation between upper and lower case metaphorically sums up Massin's fascination with letters as forms, with their own lives.

In writing his own story and that of his profession, Massin has often described in detail the visual and typographical influences he received in childhood. The logos of Peugeot and Monsavon could be seen on the wall of his grandmother's shop in a small village in the Beauce region, alongside packets of Bouillon Kub and boxes of Éclipse cream, the smile of the Laughing Cow and the inflated body of the Michelin man, the coloured illustrations of the postal calendars, advertisements for Bitter liqueur and the liner *Normandie* and posters for Nicolas wines. The walls of his Montparnasse apartment are still decorated with these today.[5]

From such everyday images, the printed ephemera and advertising messages that keep paper merchants in business, Massin has created a personal scrapbook, a school of life for the self-taught graphic artist. His collection even includes tickets for the Chartres theatre, where he used to

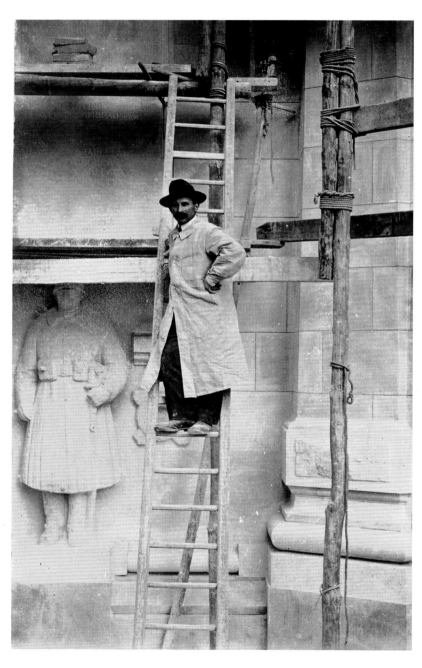

Page 110: photograph of Massin in his house in Étampes by Louis Monier, April 2005.

Left: photograph of Massin's father, Henri Massin, an engraver, sculptor and stone carver, in front of the war memorial in Chartres in the early 1920s.

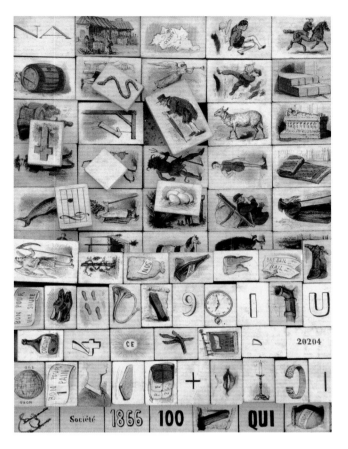

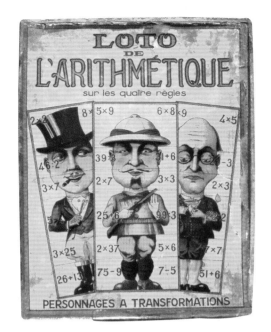

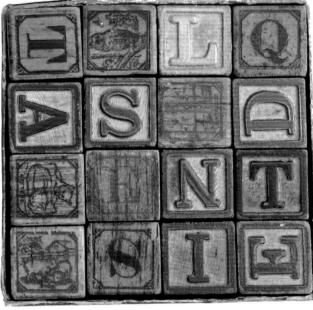

Top to bottom, left to right: educational game with lithographed pieces similar to dominoes (1866); lid of the game 'Loto arithmétique' (late nineteenth century); sixteen carved and illustrated wooden cubes (The Embossing Company, United States, early 1920s); illustrated reading primer (1930s).

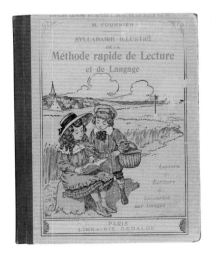

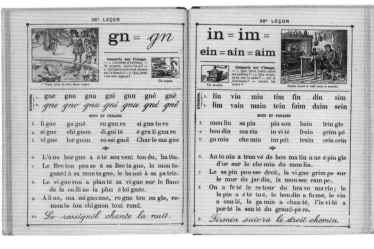

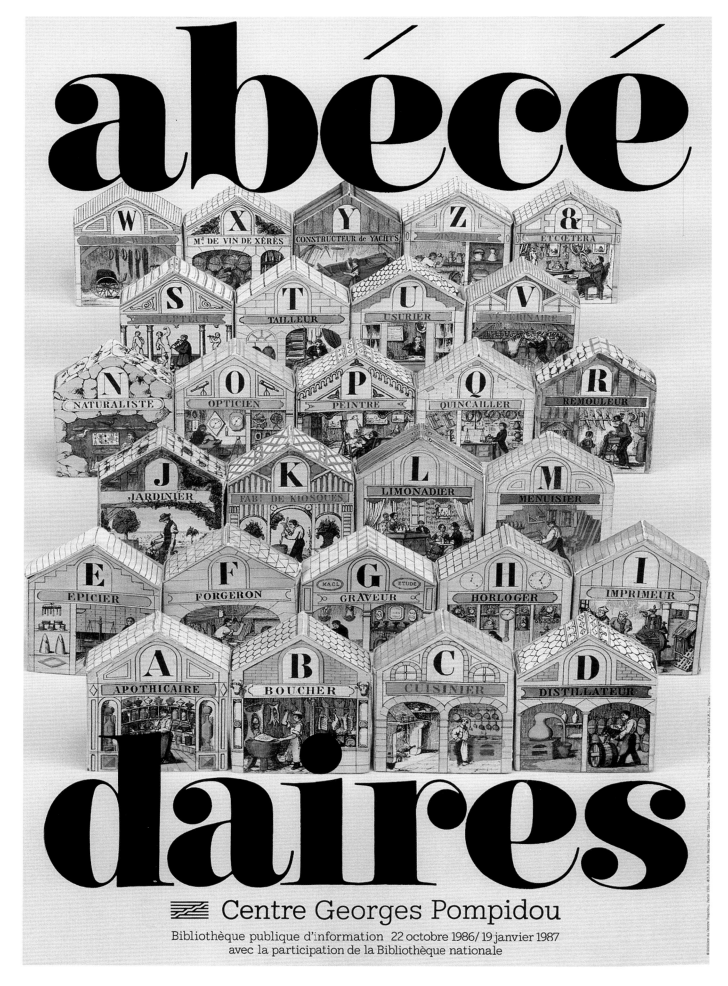

abécé daires

Centre Georges Pompidou

Bibliothèque publique d'information 22 octobre 1986 / 19 janvier 1987
avec la participation de la Bibliothèque nationale

attend performances during the war. His notebooks and bus and cinema tickets are carefully preserved in numbered envelopes. But what stands out, beyond his incredible ability to identify, collect and preserve the tiniest details (see chapter 6) is Massin's talent for putting a personal slant on this graphic collection. His is an intuitive, free and intelligent interpretation, which eventually transformed him from an inveterate collector into an amateur historian, to the dismay of the academics.

He exploits his encyclopaedic inventory in many ways: descriptions of writing in his autobiographical pieces; the secrets of 'communicative' letters, expressive letters, to design poster-like book covers (at the Club du meilleur livre, for the cover of Blaise Cendrars' *L'Or* published in 1956, he was inspired by a poster from 1848 that he had found in a junk shop); cut-out images and words to make collages (*Cortège* and *Dîner de têtes* by Jacques Prévert, a series of illustrated tales; Paris, Gallimard, 1998 and 1997); he makes cut-up poems (Raymond Queneau's *Cent mille milliards de poèmes*; Paris, Gallimard, 1961); he takes part in themed exhibitions ('Abécédaires' and 'Alphabets'); he creates typographical interpretations (Queneau's *Exercices de style;* Paris, Gallimard, 1963, and Jean Cocteau's *Les Mariés de la tour Eiffel*; Paris, Hoëbeke, 1994); lastly, and most importantly, he gives concrete expression to his fascination with expressive lettering in *La Lettre et l'Image* (Paris, Gallimard, 1970), a key work for any understanding of the graphic arts, which explores the delicate balance between image and text in a western culture that increasingly tends to separate the two.

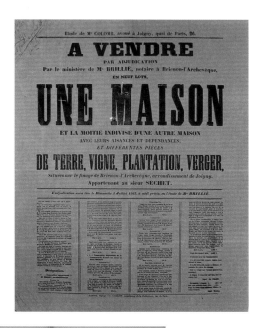

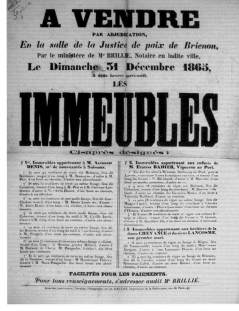

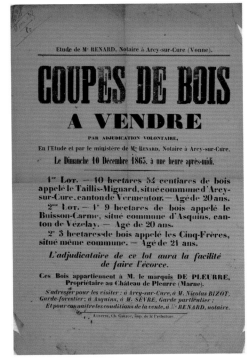

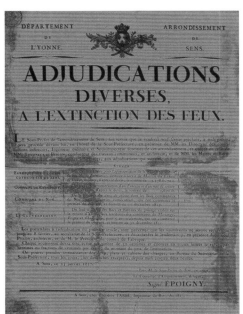

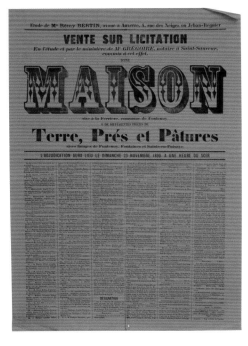

Opposite: four-colour poster for the exhibition 'Abécédaires' (ABCs) at the Bibliothèque publique d'information du Centre Georges-Pompidou, Paris, 1986–7, organised in conjunction with the exhibition 'Alphabets' at the musée-galerie de la Seita, Paris.

Above: posters and public notices (late nineteenth and early twentieth century), sources of inspiration for the coloured pages of Massin's version of Jean Cocteau's *Les Mariés de la tour Eiffel* (Paris, Hoëbeke, 1994).

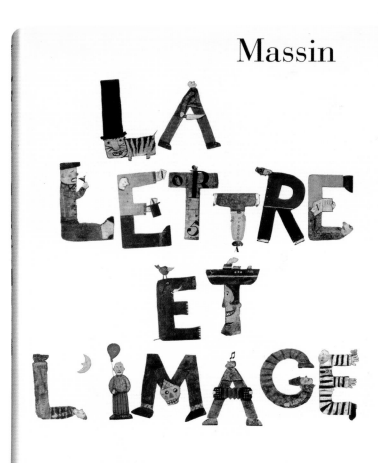

Massin

LA LETTRE ET L'IMAGE

Gallimard

Encyclopaedic knowledge

La Lettre et l'Image (published in 1970 and since reprinted five times, including new images collected by Massin on his travels across the globe) is an in-depth study of the relationship between culture and printed letters in the West through the centuries. Translated into several languages, it has become a major reference book for graphic artists throughout the world.

Rather than thinking of lettering as an accessory to the image, useful only when the latter cannot fully illustrate a concept, Massin celebrates its rhythmical and visual qualities and capacity for transformation. *La Lettre et l'Image* (subtitled *La figuration dans l'alphabet latin du VIIIe siècle à nos jours* [Figuration in the Roman alphabet from the eighth century to the present day]) is as much about literature as about art. As Philippe Schuwer writes, having made 'a book in which it is easy to get lost [...] Massin is the erudite and amusing interpreter of what is almost certainly the richest illustrated anthology in the no man's land where art and lettering meet'.[6]

Serious but never pedantic, this book considers four ways of animating text: lettering in its own context, lettering as symbol, calligrams and lettering in the visual arts. It is an anthology of over a thousand symbols, from Apollinaire's calligrams to medieval illuminations, the billboards of New York's Times Square and street graffiti – not to mention the many different alphabets (grotesque, erotic, architectonic, vegetal, instrumental, formed of figures, silhouettes, and so on). Discussing the Lascaux caves, Massin notes that everything began with images. 'The most ancient form of writing is the pictograph, characterized by talking drawings or 'thing-signs'.[7] Through a process of stylization and schematization, the image became the symbol of the original idea – as with hieroglyphs – constantly becoming more abstract.

Above and right: three-colour dust jacket for the fifth French edition of *La Lettre et l'Image, la figuration dans l'alphabet latin du VIIIe siècle à nos jours* (Paris, Gallimard, 1993), designed by Massin based on three-dimensional letters created by Les Chats Pelés; four-colour dust jacket for the second edition, illustrated by André François (Paris, Gallimard, 1973).

Opposite: four-colour dust jacket for the American edition of *La Lettre et l'Image* (Letter and Image, New York, Van Nostrand Reinhold, 1970).

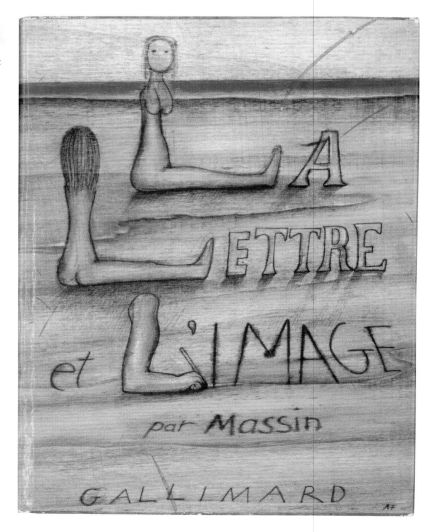

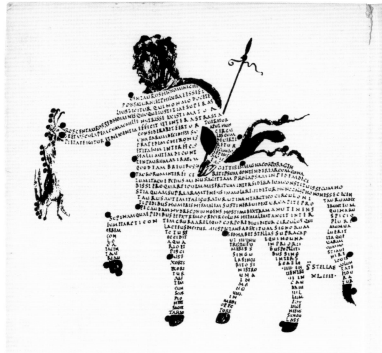

MASSIN / LETTER AND IMAGE

VAN NOSTRAND REINHOLD

LETTER AND IMAGE

by Massin

VAN NOSTRAND REINHOLD

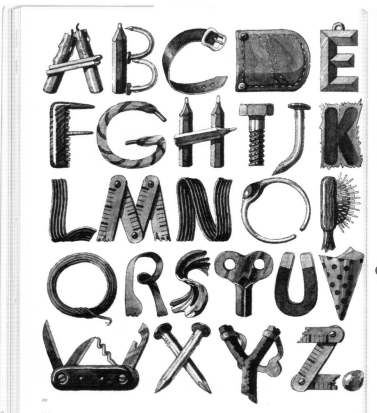

Opposite, top to bottom: animated figures taken from an etching, Italy, early nineteenth century; copperplate engraving in colour, France, 1834; alphabet designed by Bourdet, lithograph, Paris, 1836.

Inside double-page spreads from *La Lettre et l'Image* (Paris, Gallimard, 1970).

Above and right: alphabet of tools drawn by Klaus Bliesener (June 1978) and alphabet of water hydrants, set in Fireplug Gothic, designed by Craig Vosler (December 1979), both published by the International Typeface Corporation; illuminations on parchment showing seraphim and cherubim, Rabanus Maurus's *De Laudibus sanctæ Crucis*, manuscript of the Fulda school, 836–840 AD.

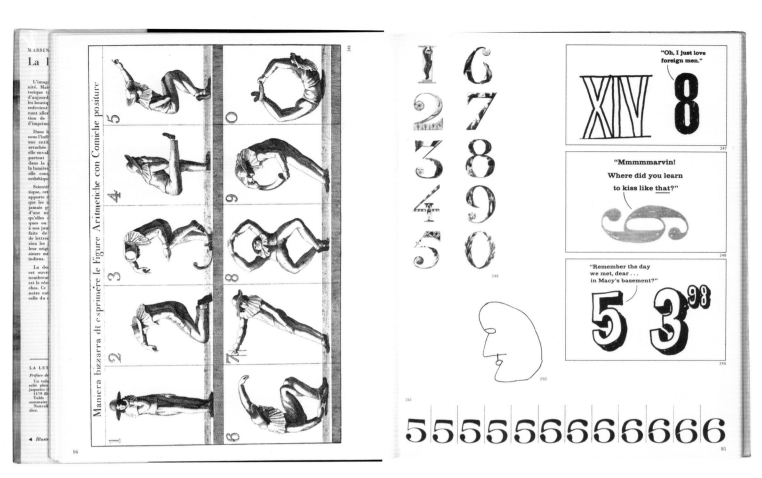

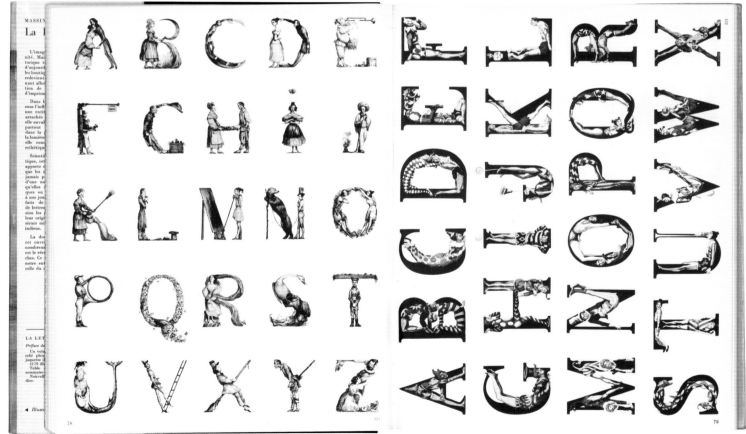

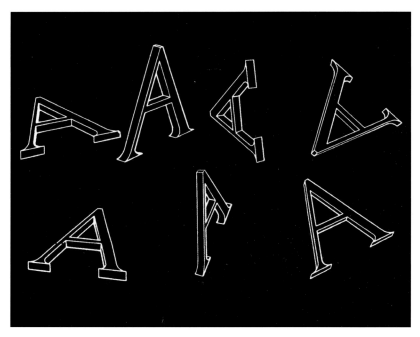

'Massin is a ringmaster of animated lettering. […] There is something almost Rabelaisian in this delight in lettering and signs', adds the literary critic Hubert Juin.[8] With its plethora of images, signs and letters, drawing on both high and popular culture, the book offers an alternative to the rationalist history of typography, influenced by 'modernists' such as Adrian Frutiger and later spread by the Swiss school. With *La Lettre et l'Image*, Massin succeeds in giving lettering back its spirit.

Rationalism versus expressiveness

By the end of the 1960s, when Massin was researching *La Lettre et l'Image*, graphic art had been widely accepted as a profession and was quite distinct from so-called commercial art (advertising). This evolution came about in conjunction with the widespread influence of the 'international typographical style' or 'Swiss school' (the schools of Basle and Zurich), which was very influential in France, notably with figures such as Albert Hollenstein, Peter Knapp and Jean Widmer. This school, which had considerable impact on the training of American graphic artists – the style Katharine McCoy calls 'American Swiss', with Paul Rand and Rudolf DeHarak, for example[9] – generally treated lettering with equal measures of objectivity and neutrality, starting from the principle that the graphic artist is merely the bearer of a message, stripped of all forms of subjectivity. The opposite of this movement is embodied by the Push Pin group, which promotes a more

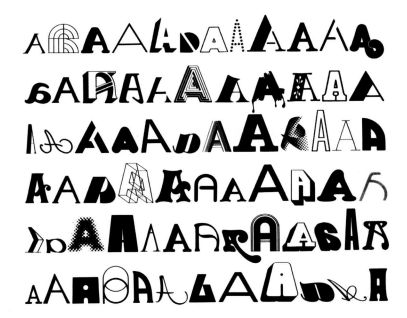

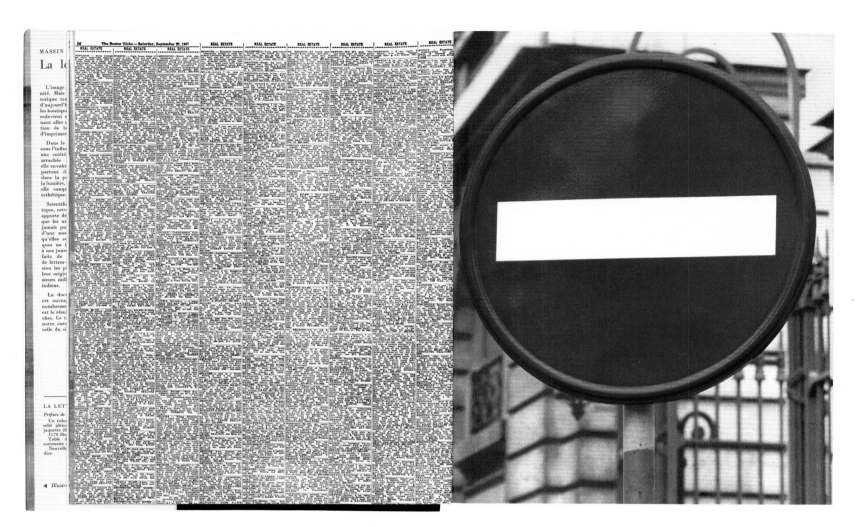

Opposite: extracts and cover of
Variations sur la lettre A (1976),
typographical experiment by Massin,
unpublished. He later returned to this
project in *Azerty, l'alphabet du monde*
(Paris, Gallimard, 2004).

Above: inside double-page spread from
La Lettre et l'Image (Paris, Gallimard,
1970), contrasting a page of classified
advertisements from *The Boston Globe*
(1967) with a no entry sign.

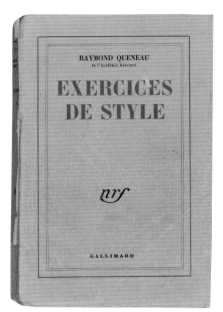

Left and below: cover of the trade edition of Raymond Queneau's *Exercices de style* (Paris, Gallimard, 1947); inside pages from *Exercices de style* annotated by Massin with typographical variations, 1963.

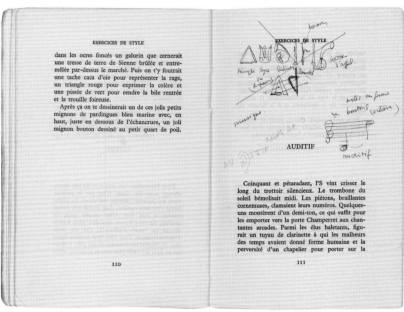

fanciful, though rigorous, expression, summed up in the word 'baroque'. Swiss neutrality is best represented by fonts of the 'sans serif' type promoted a few decades earlier by the Bauhaus. Curiously, what was originally an expression of the graphic avant-garde became, in the 1960s, the norm in the emerging field of corporate graphics for conglomerates and multinationals such as ITT, IBM, Knoll, Olivetti, Bayer and Braun, which were heavily influenced by the Swiss school.

In contrast and in parallel to this evolution, Massin, who was immersed in the Parisian literary world and had a visible penchant for the theatre of the absurd, post-surrealist poetry and the experiments of the OuLiPo group, regarded such formal, intellectualizing approaches as an aberration. Opposed to the despotic reign of the countless lineal sans serif fonts (such as Univers, Arial and Helvetica), he attacked this rationalist tendency in certain pages of *La Cantatrice chauve*. The 'headcold' page, for example (see page 86), with its compact typography and absence of line spacing, becomes the ultimate expression of typographical boredom. In the same period, he summed up the intention manifest in his interpretation of *Les Mariés de la tour Eiffel* with the words, 'It's a pamphlet, a protest against the Alemmanic levelling of typography.'[10]

In their own way Massin's contemporaries, the Americans Herb Lubalin and Edward Gottschall, were also promoting the idea of expressive typography, but in art direction for advertising rather than in business communications. They saw it as a real challenge to the notion of invisible typography integral to the British typographer Beatrice Warde's theory of the 'crystal goblet', which was dominant at the time.[11] In one of the most highly regarded essays on contemporary typography, Warde uses the metaphor of a glass of wine to criticize the fanciful expressionism of avant-garde typography, in opposition to which she advocates a classical typography whose function is to convey the author's ideas as transparently as possible, just as the function of a glass is to show the wine to best effect.

In a total break with the formalist rules of layout, Massin used certain techniques previously advocated by the Futurists (but, in his work, stripped of any political message), including abandoning standardized page orientation, scattering letters diagonally, altering spaces between letters and words, mixing fonts, distorting letter shapes and generally treating typography as image. The Futurist Marinetti declared, 'My revolution is aimed at the so-called typographical harmony of the page, which runs counter to the ebb and flow, the leaps and explosions of style that run across the page. So on the same page we use three or four different coloured inks, and even twenty different fonts if necessary.'[12]

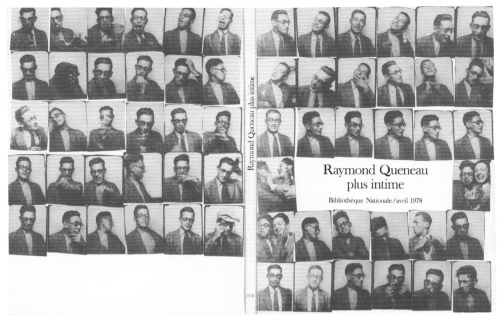

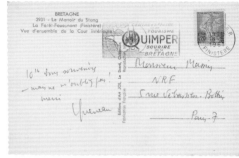

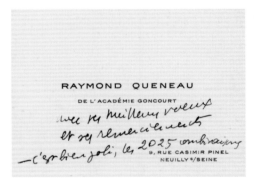

Top to bottom, left to right: two-colour paper cover of the catalogue for the exhibition catalogue *Raymond Queneau plus intime* (The private Raymond Queneau; Paris, Bibliothèque nationale/Gallimard, 1978); postcard and note to Massin from Raymond Queneau on a visiting card congratulating him on his work on *Cent mille milliards de poèmes* (Paris, Gallimard, 1961).

Below: photograph of Raymond Queneau by Massin in his office at Gallimard, Paris, 1961.

Raymond Queneau (1903–1976)

Raymond Queneau was one of the few French writers involved in the development of the pre-war intellectual groups who also became a unique voice in post-war French literature, without ever being part of a specific school of thought. After flirting with Breton's surrealism, Queneau divided his time between his work at Gallimard (in whose corridors he met Massin) as a reader of manuscripts and editor of the 'Encyclopédie de la Pléiade', and his own writing. Queneau was a versatile figure who excelled equally in poetry, essays, fiction, journalism and cinema. His book *Zazie dans le métro* (*Zazie in the Metro*; 1959) was adapted for the cinema by Louis Malle in 1960, bringing Queneau to the attention of the wider public. He was involved in the curious Collège de 'pataphysique and, in 1960, co-founded the OuLiPo (*Ouvroir de Littérature Potentielle*; Workroom for Potential Literature) with François Le Lionnais – who wrote the postface to Cent mille

milliards de poèmes – and around ten friends who were painters and mathematicians; Georges Perec did not join the group until later. The Oulipians were seeking to invent new forms of poetry and the novel by sharing knowledge between writers and mathematicians.

Queneau and Massin began working together in 1961 with *Cent mille milliards de poèmes*, a book designed in the spirit of an 'exquisite corpse' and first concrete manifestation of the OuLiPo research group, combining mathematics (probabilities) and linguistics. Massin made it into an interactive piece before the arrival of computer science, with ten short poems of fourteen lines each, cut into interchangeable strips.

In 1963 their mutual understanding led to the illustrated version of *Exercices de style* (the first edition of the text alone was published in 1947), a Dada-inspired combination of typography and message. A series of

ninety-nine short pieces recount the same banal incident. In a bus the narrator sees a young man with a particularly long neck, then later catches sight of him at a station with a friend who adjusts a button on his coat. This button provided Massin with the inspiration for the box cover of the limited edition. The painter and sculptor Jacques Carelman, a founder member of OuPeinPo (*Ouvroir de Peinture Potentielle*; Workroom for Potential Painting), suggested adding a series of visual 'exercises in style', drawn, painted or sculpted and presented in parallel to the text, adding a new dimension to the book that would go beyond pure visual translation.

Queneau's interest in linguistics and his fascination with phonetic spelling and popular language are apparent throughout his entire œuvre, in which he explores the relationship between the oneirism of surrealism and the notion of the absurd present in existentialism, both of which greatly interested Massin.

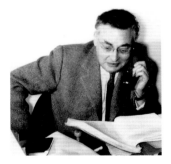

Queneau wrote the preface to La Lettre et l'Image, revealing to the reader that Massin is a member of the S.P.A.: not, as French readers would at first assume, the *Société protectrice des animaux*, but rather the '*Société protectrice de l'alphabet*' (Society for the Protection of the Alphabet).

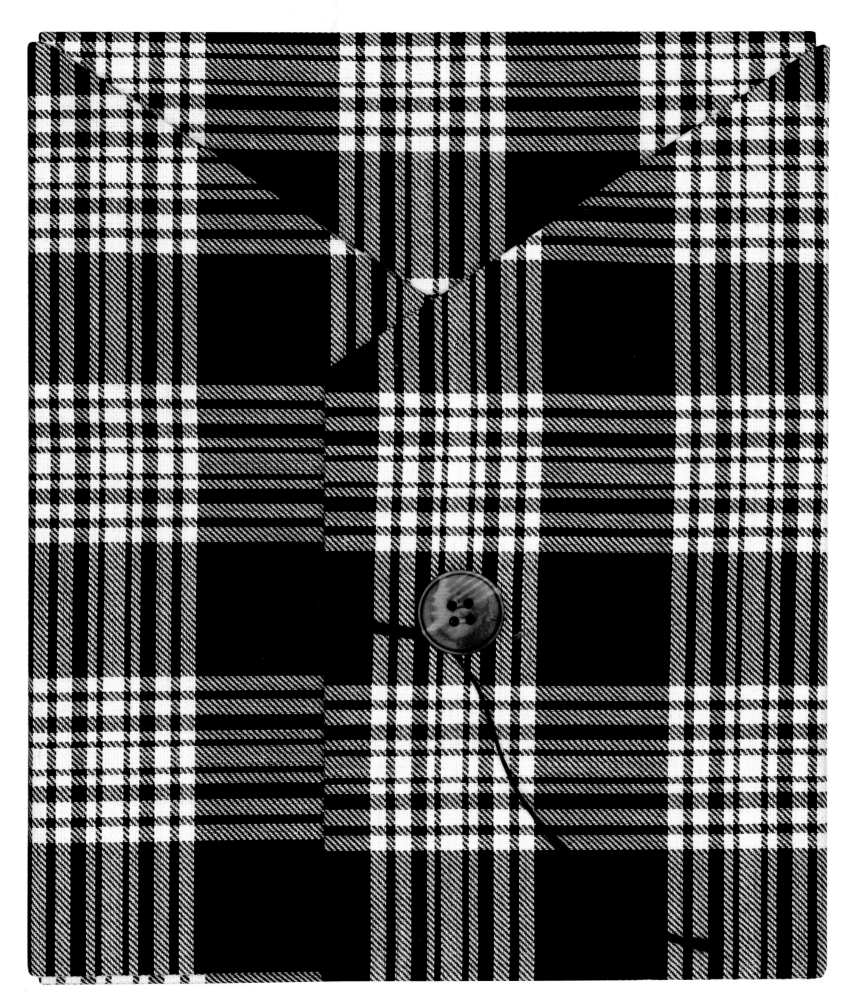

Massin

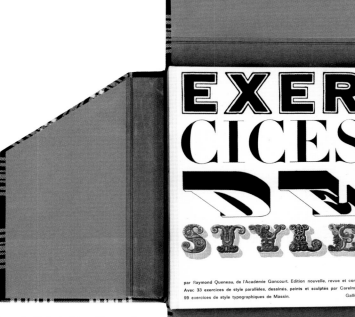

Opposite: limited edition of Raymond Queneau's *Exercices de style* 'avec 33 exercices de style parallèles, dessinés, peints et sculptés par Carelman et 99 exercices typographiques de Massin' (with 33 parallel exercises in style, drawn, painted and sculpted by Carelman and 99 typographic exercises by Massin; Paris, Gallimard, 1963). The box is covered in shirt fabric and fastens with a button (shown open, above).

Right, top to bottom: four-colour cover and inside pages of *Exercices de style*.

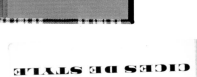

Un jour vers midi du côté du parc Monceau, sur la plate-forme arrière d'un autobus à peu près complet de la ligne S (aujourd'hui 84), j'aperçus un personnage au cou fort long qui portait un feutre mou entouré d'un galon tressé au lieu de ruban. Cet individu interpella tout à coup son voisin en prétendant que celui-ci faisait exprès de lui marcher sur les pieds chaque fois qu'il montait ou descendait des voyageurs. Il abandonna d'ailleurs rapidement la discussion pour se jeter sur une place devenue libre.

Deux heures plus tard, je le revis devant la gare Saint-Lazare en grande conversation avec un ami qui lui conseillait de diminuer l'échancrure de son pardessus en faisant remonter le bouton supérieur par quelque tailleur compétent.

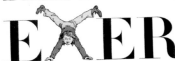

par Raymond Queneau, de l'Académie Goncourt. Edition nouvelle, revue et corrigée. Avec 33 exercices de style parallèles, dessinés, peints et sculptés par Carelman et 99 exercices de style typographiques de Massin. Gallimard.

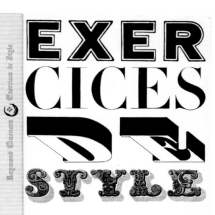

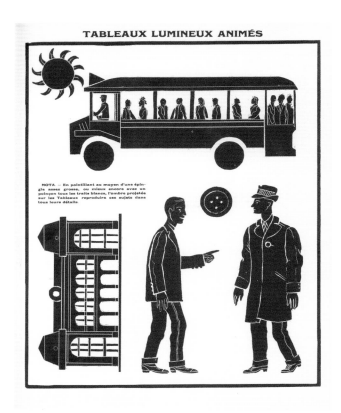

TABLEAUX LUMINEUX ANIMÉS

NOTA. — En pointillant au moyen d'une épingle assez grosse, ou mieux encore avec un poinçon tous les traits blancs, l'ombre projetée sur le Tableau reproduira ces sujets dans tous leurs détails.

Taking Marinetti's words almost to the letter, as it were, in Queneau's *Exercices de style* (Paris, Gallimard, 1963), Massin's expressionist typographical revolution found its ultimate illustration. The book consists of ninety-nine playful feats of literature based on the same banal story told in a multitude of different styles. Queneau's aim was not to demonstrate how to exhaust a subject, but to render the infinite possibilities of imaginable points of view. The banality of the situation is eclipsed by its humour, in a playful use of language akin to that of the OuLiPo movement, which this book heralds. 'In fact I wrote *Exercices de style* quite consciously remembering Bach [*The Art of Fugue*],' observes Queneau in the preface to Massin's series of ninety-nine typographical exercises, which enrich the text[13] with an illustrative dimension and provide an echo (or possibly competition) for the forty-five exercises in style painted, drawn and sculpted by Jacques Carelman that gave rise to the project.[14]

Where the version that Faucheux had published at the Club des libraires de France in 1956 contained only thirteen typographical experiments, consisting more of plates in the form of unfolding pages and illustrated endpapers, Massin's version is a typographical interpretation of the ninety-nine titles. Queneau's main text, a rhetorical sampler written in the spirit of the surrealists' experiments, remains classically set in Didot. Massin has been criticized for not having extended his experimentation to the entire text, but as he says himself, 'the book was already under way when I had the idea of getting involved. So I only had two weeks before me and I had to go to Lurs for the annual typographers' meeting. And I can still see myself in the single sleeper I had taken for the occasion, spending most of the night thinking up typographical gags for those exercises in style.'[15]

Once again we can observe the extraordinary liberty Massin takes in his choice of typefaces and the fact that in so doing he restores an iconographic role to the fonts heading the chapters. Taking variation

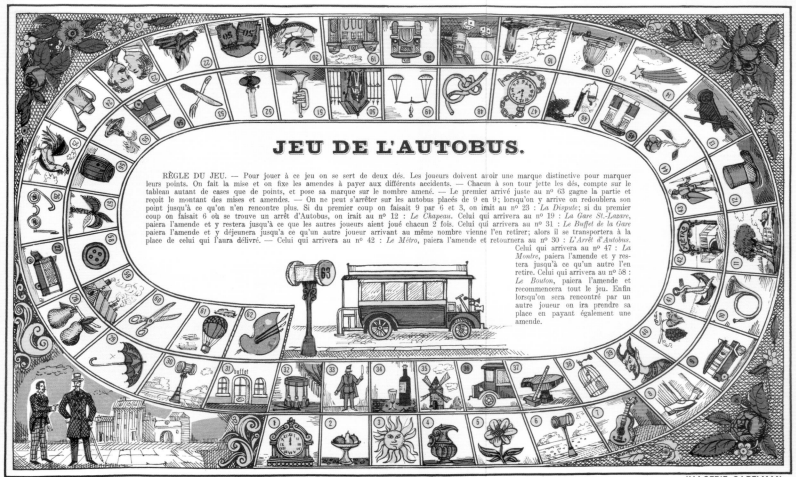

IMAGERIE CARELMAN.

on a theme as his pretext, Massin enjoyed carrying out this typographical exercise, whose systematic nature echoes the principle of series that was then emerging in contemporary art, notably with Andy Warhol, who shows every conceivable way of representing the same subject. 'An atypical work in the array of contemporary literature. Neither poetry, nor theatre, nor essay, nor novel [...] [*Exercices de style*] has something of all the genres at once', notes Emmanuël Souchier.[16]

An aptitude for metamorphosis

Typographical variation, emphasizing lettering's capacity for figurative metamorphosis, creates synaesthetic correspondences and instigates new interactions between lettering and the other arts. As we know, interaction between the arts is a crucial principle for Massin: 'Variation is the same and the other, identity and otherness, woman and all women, a story and the thousand ways to tell it, a particular landscape and all possible landscapes, a tune and all the tunes that flow from it. So variation is inseparable from music, typography and almost certainly all the arts of expression.'[17]

In the same context of this philosophy of synthesis, Massin's typographical works – whether analytical, like *La Lettre et l'Image*, or applied, like *Exercices de style* – seek to grasp the distinction between information and communication. Through his graphic experimentation Massin gives new meanings to everyday language and tests its power of poetic evocation – for example, in *La Lettre et l'Image*, his photographs of advertising hoardings teach us how to see typography in the street and the way in which seemingly unrelated words are in fact linked to our perception of our urban environment and our culture. 'Artifice taken boldly to an extreme has the advantage of generating a visual lyricism that was almost unknown before our own time. This artifice still has a long way to go and can achieve a synthesis

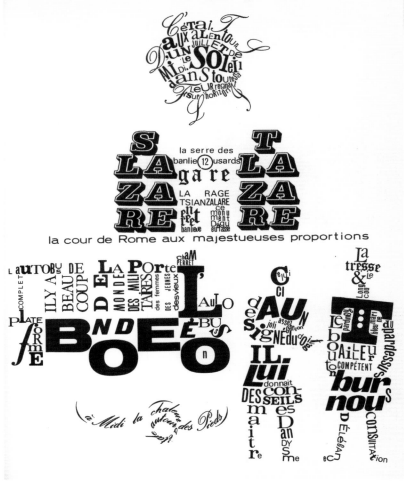

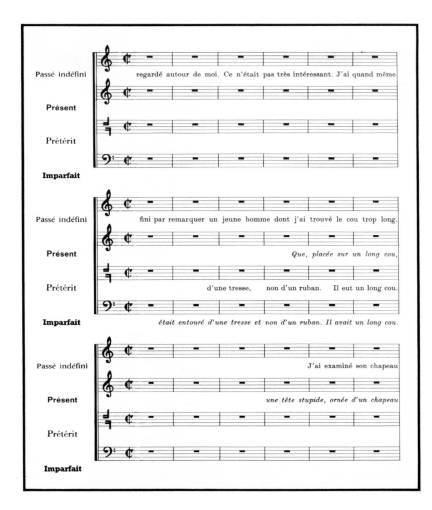

Opposite, top to bottom: Jacques Carelman's visual variations 'ombre chinoise' (shadow play) and 'jeu de l'oie' (board game), extracts from *Exercices de style* (Paris, Gallimard, 1963).

This page, left to right: Massin's typographical variation 'portée musicale' (stave) and Jacques Carelman's visual variation 'calligramme', extracts from *Exercices de style*.

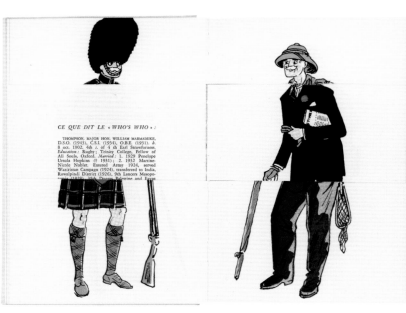

Top to bottom: Pierre Daninos' *Carnets du major Thompson* (Major Thompson's notebooks), design with three strips by Mitschké, illustrations by Walter Goetz (Paris, Club du meilleur livre, 1956); two-colour white cloth binding of the limited edition of Raymond Queneau's *Cent mille milliards de poèmes* (Paris, Gallimard, 1961).

Raymond Queneau

Cent mille milliards de poèmes

of the arts, music, painting and literature,' wrote Guillaume Apollinaire.[18] As the literary critic Marcel Brion concludes, such an 'achievement of synthesis' comes to full fruition in *La Lettre et l'Image*.[19] This fascinating book reproduces a great many calligrams, which were, after all, and as Apollinaire notes in his preface to *Calligrams*, described as 'lyrical ideograms'.

The concrete expression of graphic variation's potential for poetic evocation reaches its height in the collaboration between graphic artist Massin and poet Raymond Queneau. *Cent mille milliards de poèmes* (1961) is a work of 'combinatorial poetry', a vast poetic undertaking consisting of ten sonnets cut horizontally, line by line, enabling the reader to recompose them at will into a hundred thousand billion poems, which is 10 (the original number of poems) to the power of 14 (the number of lines in a sonnet) – an exercise in style in the manner of OuLiPo which has also been tried by others, such as Georges Perec. The idea underlying the OuLiPo movement (Ouvroir de Littérature Potentielle), founded in 1960 by Raymond Queneau and the mathematician François Le Lionnais, was to invent stylistic and rhetorical exercises and to experiment with literary constraints (such as working with a limited number of letters or applying mathematical formulae to the writing of poems). In *Cent mille milliards de poèmes*, Raymond Queneau's fondness for permutation is highlighted by Massin in a remarkable way.[20] 'Here [the sonnets] are serving a project that goes beyond the habitual use of this fixed form in a unique way. The combination set in motion leads to a number that the human imagination cannot really encompass', notes the critic Claude Lebon.[21]

Given the total symbiosis of form and content in this object-cum-book, one might wonder how the system for composing the poems could have worked without the interchangeable paper strips. Using 'comb' binding, for which Massin owes much to the binder, *Cent mille milliards de poèmes* spectacularly altered the relationships involved in both writing and reading a poem. 'Basically it is a machine for making poems, but in a limited number. True this number, though limited, provides reading matter for around two hundred million years (reading round the clock)', jokes Queneau.[22]

Queneau had at once thought of layout in the manner of an exquisite corpse, similar to the 'interactive' children's books containing three separate strips representing the head, body and legs to make different characters. Massin's version, with its fourteen strips of lines of poetry, draws directly on this model but takes it still further. Rarely mentioned in the complete works of Massin and little known to the wider public, *Cent mille milliards de poèmes* is contemporary with the earliest days of the OuLiPo. 'This collection is, in a way, the first concrete manifestation of the research group', explains Queneau.[23] Created at the height of the literature of the absurd, it is an exercise that foreshadows the computer age in its interactive form and a link structure generally associated with the internet.

Typographical variations take on a new dimension when the exercise goes beyond simple formal repetition to invest lettering with entirely new correspondences with other artistic domains and give it the power of transformation. Whether in the scholarly compilation of *La Lettre et l'Image* or his experiments based on the work of Queneau, Massin likes to test the limits of 'communicative' lettering and to prove that it really does exist.

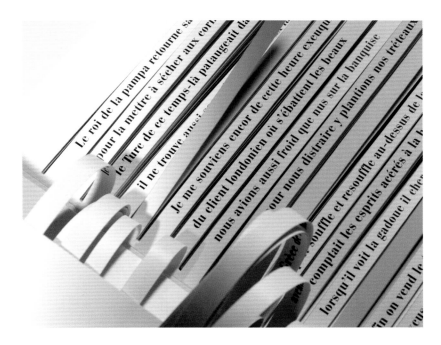

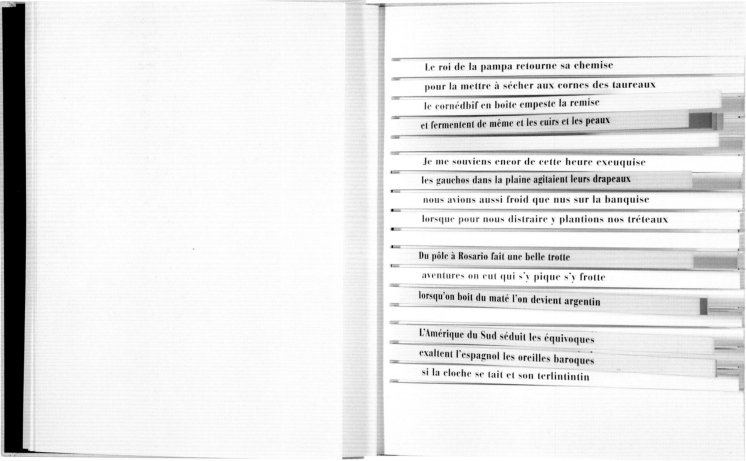

Le roi de la pampa retourne sa chemise

pour la mettre à sécher aux cornes des taureaux

le cornédbif en boîte empeste la remise

et fermentent de même et les cuirs et les peaux

Je me souviens encor de cette heure exeuquise

les gauchos dans la plaine agitaient leurs drapeaux

nous avions aussi froid que nus sur la banquise

lorsque pour nous distraire y plantions nos tréteaux

Du pôle à Rosario fait une belle trotte

aventures on eut qui s'y pique s'y frotte

lorsqu'on boit du maté l'on devient argentin

L'Amérique du Sud séduit les équivoques

exaltent l'espagnol les oreilles baroques

si la cloche se tait et son terlintintin

Above: the fourteen lines are cut into seventeen strips for the limited edition of Raymond Queneau's *Cent mille milliards de poèmes* (Paris, Gallimard, 1961).

Anti-bourgeois literature

Jean Cocteau's play *Les Mariés de la tour Eiffel* (1921)[24] has a thin plot that tells the story of a wedding that takes place on the first platform of the Eiffel tower. The guests are constantly interrupted by a series of comical events and surrealist encounters, notably with an ostrich. A play emblematic of the 1920s, its apparent lightness is misleading, since it expresses a social critique of the bourgeoisie of the roaring twenties and ridicules French colonial expansion in Africa. None of the play's protagonists speak, since the lines are spoken by two gramophones. Speech and movement are disassociated, the better to stress the importance of actions. It is almost certainly one of Cocteau's most controversial plays. Anti-bourgeois in its irreverent tone, revolutionary in its overturning of dramatic structure and experimental in its approach to staging, it is a complete work of art that mounts an all-out attack on cliché and the commonplace.

Massin deliberately chose to 'stage' it typographically by closely following the avant-garde trends of the roaring twenties. As he explains, the play is part of 'the tradition of performances that caused a scandal at the time, from *Les Mamelles de Tirésias* to *Parade*'.[25] Poets, painters and musicians come together in the same desire to break the rules and to experiment in all directions and with all meanings: extraordinary visuals, a cacophony of sound and riotous dialogue combining satire, poetry, dance, mime and orchestral accompaniment.

Pre-dating the theatre of the absurd by some time, Cocteau's ballet-play is characterized by its fragmented rhythm and the dislocation of its characters, who are transformed into mute puppets, animated by phrases emptied of meaning, with a squeaky musical accompaniment in the background. The music was composed by the five members of the famous Groupe des six: Georges Auric, Arthur Honegger, Francis Poulenc, Darius Milhaud and Germaine Tailleferre. Cocteau's sometimes disconcerting aesthetics, a kind of anti-Wagnerianism, is often grounded in a rejection of formalism and mixes the banal and vulgar with spiritual imagery.

The controversy generated by the play, performed at the Théâtre des Champs-Élysées in 1921, arose partly from the fact that Cocteau had created a work in the spirit of Dada without even belonging to the movement, thereby frustrating the Dadaists in their own creativity. We imagine the actors' lines – which cut across each

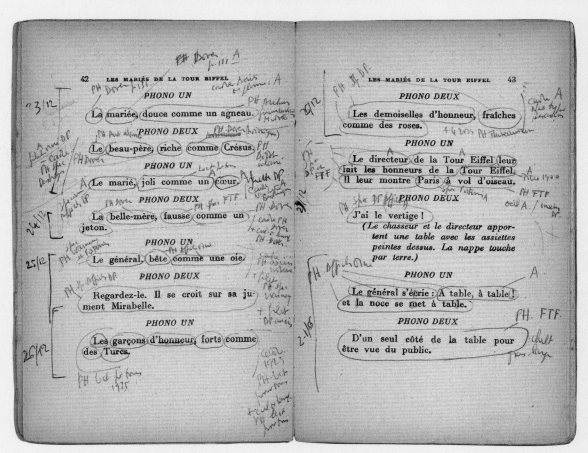

Left: inside pages of the trade edition of Jean Cocteau's *Les Mariés de la tour Eiffel* (Paris, Gallimard, 1921) with layout notes by Massin, c.1966.

Opposite: four-colour dust jacket for *Les Mariés de la tour Eiffel* (Paris, Hoëbeke, 1994).

Focus
Les Mariés de la tour Eiffel
Paris, Hoëbeke, 1994

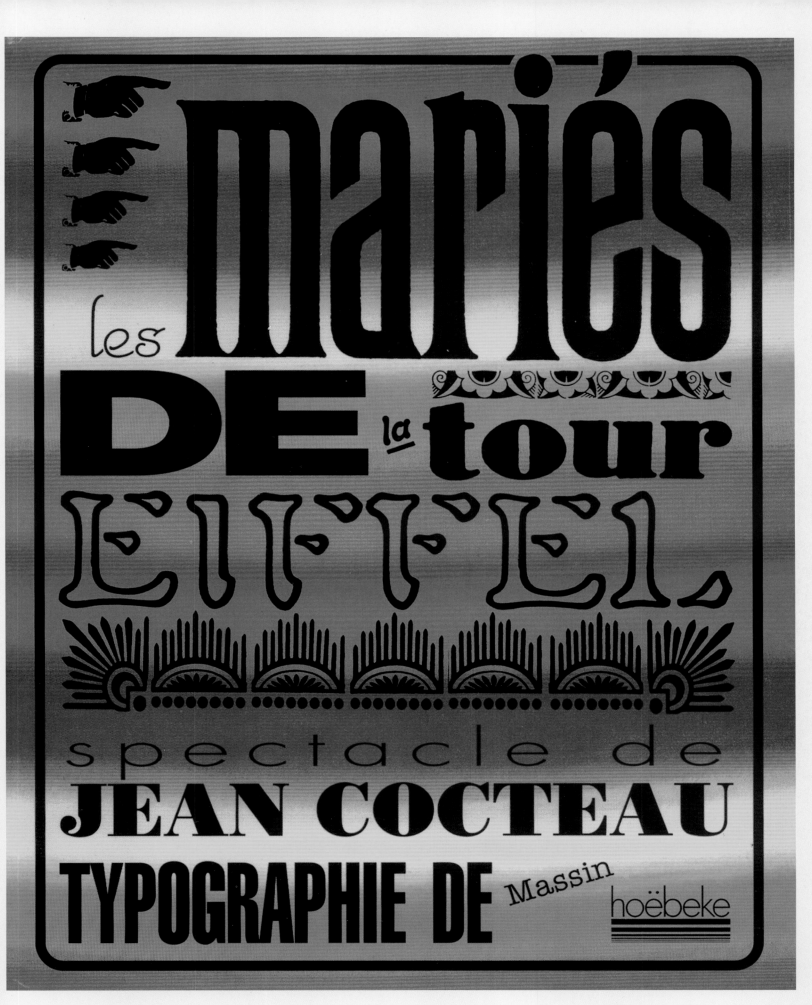

les **mariés DE la tour EIFFEL** spectacle de **JEAN COCTEAU** TYPOGRAPHIE DE *Massin* hoëbeke

Left to right: estimate of production costs for *Les Mariés de la tour Eiffel* with inserted album, dated 13 January 1966; technical note from Massin to John O'Neill, broadcast rights manager at Gallimard, 23 December 1965.

Opposite: extracts from posters and newspaper headlines, 1960s.

LES MARIES DE LA TOUR EIFFEL

Détail du prix proposé par la firme Adès.

(prix calculé sur 3 000 exemplaires).

Galvano-gravure	1 200
Pressage (2 fois 3 000 ex. à 1,35 F pièce)	8 100
Droits d'Auteur du BIEM : 0,65 F par face	7 800
Royalties Darius Milhaud : 5 % sur le prix de vente légal d'un disque de 20 cm, soit sur 19 F	5 700
	22.800

Adès nous ayant demandé 36 000 F au total (soit 6 F par disque), nous estimons que la différence (13.200 F) qui correspond en somme à un bénéfice, est exagérée et devrait être réduite.

Il est peut-être possible également de ramener, d'une part, à 2 000 F les royalties de Milhaud en les *calculant* sur le prix coûtant du disque et, d'autre part, d'obtenir que la redevance du BIEM comptée à partir de la catégorie "artistique" du disque soit faite sur la catégorie "standard" soit, 0,40 F par face. En outre, il faut rappeler que sur les droits prélevés par le BIEM nous reviendront environ 25 % (à partager avec les héritiers Cocteau). → *soit 3250 F.*

MASSIN
Le 13.1.66

O'Neill m'informe que le prix de F.6 par disque a été ramené à F.4.

M/AA

Note pour M. O'NEILL

LES MARIES DE LA TOUR EIFFEL

Etant donné que ce façonnage ressortit probablement à des fournisseurs spécialisés, S. Ducongé aimerait que tu demandes à Adès de bien vouloir se charger lui-même des deux pochettes de disques qui seront encartées dans les deux pages de garde du livre. Le papier sera toutefois fourni par nous, ainsi que la bande gommée. Quant aux dimensions, il faut se baser sur le format 20,8 cm pour le diamètre du disque et prévoir une découpe centrale laissant voir l'étiquette, comme le modèle italien ci-joint que je vous retourne.

Je présume que seront compris dans le devis d'Adès, en outre des gravure et passage spéciaux, les étiquettes, la mise sous enveloppe cristal ou plastique ainsi que la mise sous pochette.

Pierre Gallimard prépare une maquette en blanc du livre, comprenant également les deux pochettes me demande de bien vouloir lui fournir un autre disque 20 cm comme celui qu'Adès nous avait remis il y a quelque temps.

Veux-tu en demander un à Adès rapidement ?

MASSIN
Le 23.12.65

M/AA

other on stage – intersecting like the disordered words of a page by Tristan Tzara. It is a similar expressiveness to that of Ionesco's 'anti-plays', Tardieu's monologue confabulations and Édith Piaf's rasping voice that draws Massin to Cocteau's play. Cocteau himself said about it, 'Here I abandon mystery. I light everything, underline everything. Sunday emptiness, human cattle, ready-made expressions, dissociated ideas in flesh and blood, ferocity of childhood, the poetry and miraculousness of everyday life: that's my play, very well understood by the young musicians who accompany it.'[26] Inspired by Cocteau's vivid words, Massin sought a graphic reflection of this modern aesthetics of fragmentation.

The original staging drew on the most eclectic range of theatrical traditions and artistic forms. Cocteau returned to the tradition of the chorus in ancient Greek tragedy – the newly-weds' lines are here declaimed by two gramophones – making the characters appear as mute puppets. The disembodied lines are a torrent of ready-made phrases, truisms and commonplaces, on which the poet turns a spotlight, just as, Massin notes, Ionesco was later to do in *La Cantatrice chauve*.[27] To these modes from ancient drama the playwright adds the ingredients of tragi-comic realism to depict a truer than true ridiculousness. As the anarchic, colourful action unfolds, an implicit parody of farce takes shape. Charlie Chaplin and Buster Keaton also spring to mind in the play's aesthetics of clowning and, with them, the intertitles of silent films: some of the spreads announcing a new chapter in *Les Mariés de la tour Eiffel* echo the narrative black-outs of silent film in which typographical cartouches appear with decorated frames.

In 1966 Massin, who loves to work with the gap between the speech and performance of words, took this absurd literary material from a time before the literature of the absurd – a direct descendant of Jarry's *Ubu roi* and Apollinaire's *Les Mamelles de Tirésias* – as his starting point for a 192-page exercise in style. His aim was to transform a puppet performance into the visible

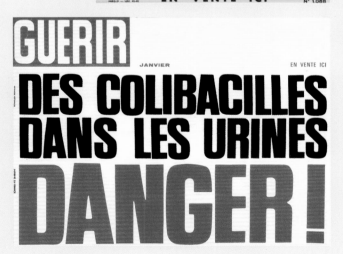

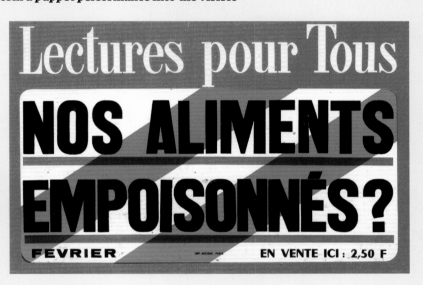

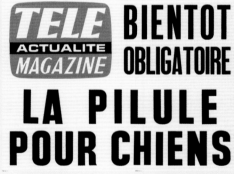

typography of posters; in other words to turn typography into a character, which would come to life over a background of coloured posters.[28]

Once again Massin's literary affinities, his sense of the comic and love of speech and the setting of words influenced his choice of typographical experiment. 'It was a graphic work, a personal work', he explains.[29]

Dadaist inspiration

When Massin began work on this exercise in typographical variations a few months after *La Cantatrice chauve*, the cultural context was rich in coincidences and historical events to fuel his inspiration: Cocteau died in 1963 (born in 1889, he liked to joke that he was the same age as the Eiffel tower) and the score for the ballet of the *Mariés de la tour Eiffel* had just been rediscovered, by chance, in the archives of the Stockholm Dansmuseet. The piece had last been performed by the Swedish ballet, who had kept the score since 1921. Having been found – forty years later in the mid-1960s – it breathed new life into Cocteau's play, its aesthetic pertinence and critical force. Paradoxically Massin designed his best work in one of the most dissent-filled decades in the (graphic) history of France, but has rarely politicized anything in either his work or his life. His personal preference is for a more lateral, subtle approach to artistic and literary subversion.

These major cultural events went hand in hand with a renewed interest in Dada: the year 1966 marked fifty years since the movement began and a retrospective exhibition was mounted by the Kunsthaus in Zurich and presented at the musée national d'Art moderne in Paris. For the first time since the 1920s this exhibition brought the graphic collages of the Dadaists to the wider public. It had a direct influence on women's magazines – the typographic 'calligrams' designed by Peter Knapp for *Elle*, for instance. In 1965 Michel Sanouillet published *Dada à Paris* (Paris, Jean-Jacques Pauvert), a remarkable illustrated study which has now become a crucial work of reference on the subject, presenting the movement's antecedents, influences and protagonists and restoring it to its full importance. To this were added a series of initiatives in Europe, instigated by the New Realists, including artists such as Daniel Spoerri and Arman in France, Piero Manzoni in Italy and the artists of the New Dada in the United States, notably Robert Rauschenberg – all of whom were involved in spreading an international awareness of the Dadaist heritage.[30]

Although Massin remained somewhat apart from the political events of his time, he plunged happily into the gratuitous game of Dadaist graphics – of both the historical movement and its heirs. So, for the wedding procession of *Les Mariés de la tour Eiffel*, he sought to create typographical portraits of the characters that caricatured the fashions of the period, scribbling in a notebook, 'Every font family, every kind, trend, style, variation, even modification and malfiguration are represented – a sort of typographical microcosm'.[31]

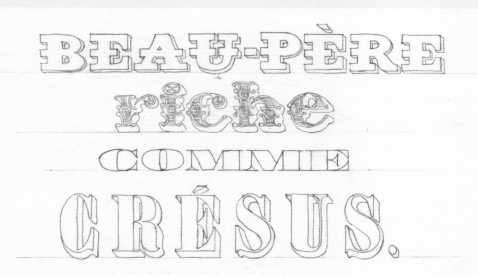

Left: draft layout for *Les Mariés de la tour Eiffel*, pencil on tracing paper, c.1966.

Opposite and following two pages: draft layouts for *Les Mariés de la tour Eiffel*, pencil on tracing paper, with cut-out Photostat copies of letters pasted on to the layout on Canson paper, c.1966.

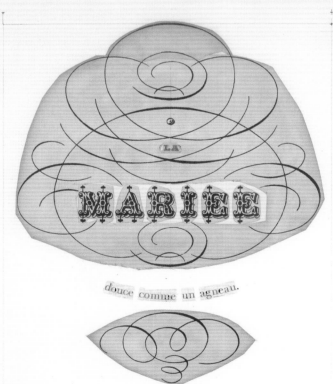

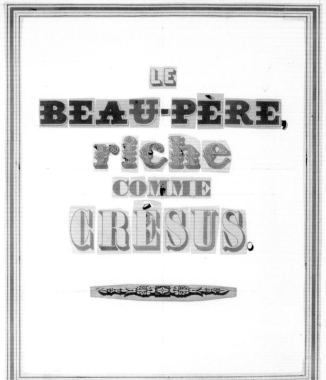

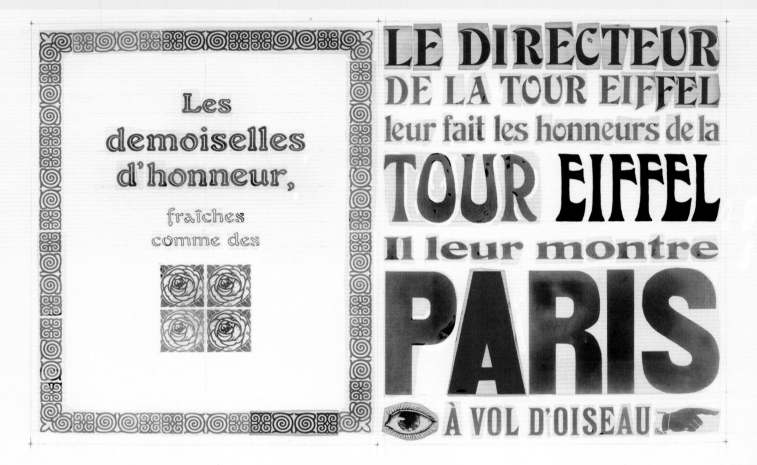

On each page, functioning as a little poster, Massin gleefully sets out the widest possible variety of typographical styles: the page of the '*beau-père riche comme Crésus*' (father-in-law rich as Croesus) recalls the 'Wanted' posters of the American West, with their nineteenth-century fonts 'in relief'; the '*belle-mère fausse comme un jeton*' (mother-in-law fake as a token) is surrounded by decorative garlands in a romantic style; and the page of the '*garçons d'honneur forts comme des Turcs*' (ushers as strong as Turks) is decorated with details in the Art Deco style, with an engraved monotype font, Broadway, whose serifed letters seem very well suited to these forceful, not to say booming messages. Massin notes, 'The enlargement of the lines (in the literal sense) becomes the caricature of a style'.[32]

So the art of variation is expressed in a very heterogeneous typographical palette, giving typography a role that goes beyond reading to become primarily visual, equal to that of the image. The names of some of the fonts used are hard to find, since Massin collects samples in a rather empirical way. Facsimiles of letters were made and photographed in his studio in the country, then pasted in one by one, along with borrowings from the catalogue of Deberny and Peignot, copies of small posters, press announcements, headlines, notices, prospectuses, vignettes from notebooks, restaurant menus and so on.[33]

Massin combined this extraordinary variety of fonts, many of them very well known, to make the most of every line, setting each on a full page so that it looks like a poster. Posters for electoral campaigns and advertising have dense, black, bold fonts which – because the poster was screen-printed – stand out from the thirteen bright hues of the paper in bright, saturated matt colours reminiscent of cheap posters for Bastille Day dances. Cocteau warns, 'Diction black as ink, as bold and clear as the capitals on an advert. Here, surprise surprise, the actors seek to serve the text, instead of making it serve them. Another lyrical novelty that a theatre is not used to'.[34]

Although he did not have the chance to experience it during his own lifetime, the playwright (Cocteau) had found his typographic soulmate (Massin): the words set across the page take their resonance from the size of the lettering, while their absurd agitation evokes that of the characters on stage.

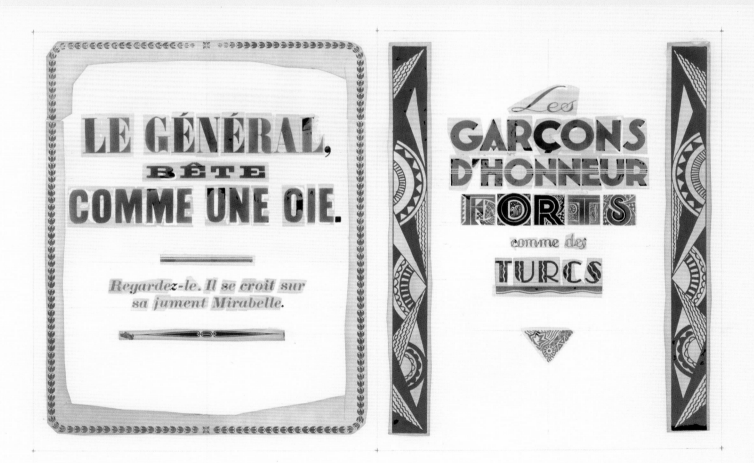

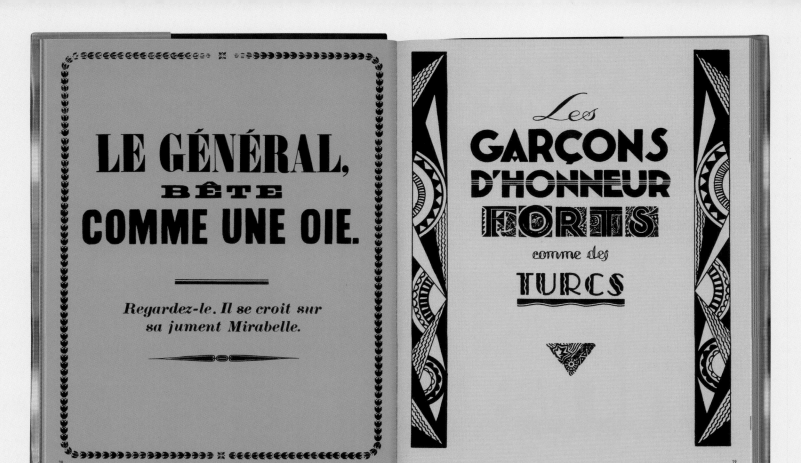

The story of a print run

Les Mariés de la tour Eiffel reflects the developments in book manufacture in the twentieth century, from cut and paste through to digital publishing. A further essay in expressive typography, the book is the result of thirty years' work. It was not until late in Massin's career, in 1994, when *La Cantatrice chauve* had already become a landmark in the history of graphic art, that *Les Mariés de la tour Eiffel* was published, with the blessing of the publisher Lionel Hoëbeke, founder of Éditions Hoëbeke, with whom Massin often worked.[35]

The first thirty pages of the book, made around 1965–6, were put together entirely by hand. Each letter was individually cut out and pasted in from old advertisements found in flea markets and in Massin's collections of everyday printed materials. When he returned to the work in the 1970s, Massin used 'transfer lettering' and then, during the 1980s, photocomposition and photolettering. Lastly, in the 1990s, the last 200 or so pages of the 240-page book were composed on a computer. These changes can be seen and felt: the richness of the decorations,

originality of the everyday fonts and 'handmade' feel contrast visually with the cold, electronic stiffness of the graphic software fonts.

In comparison with Massin's other works of experimental typography, the challenge of *Les Mariés de la tour Eiffel* lay in its extension of the exercise to tackle the entire work (rather than just the titles, as in *Exercices de style*), without even the support of images (aside from two or three small illustrations in a nineteenth-century style showing a fly and a camera), as in *La Cantatrice chauve*.

Musical overture

Whether by pure coincidence or visionary intuition, when Massin was working on the typographical interpretation of *Les Mariés de la tour Eiffel*, the record company Adès bought the rights to make a record of its unique music. The composer Darius Milhaud, a surviving member of the Groupe des six, was to conduct for the recording.

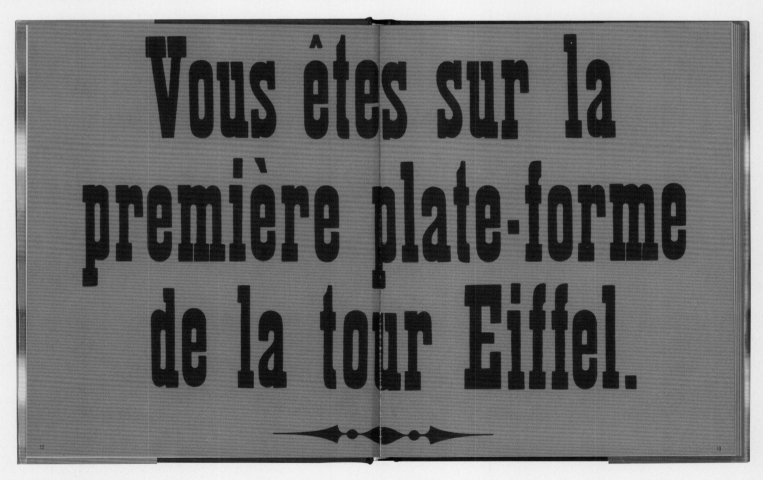

Opposite, above and following two pages: inside pages of *Les Mariés de la tour Eiffel*, screen-printed on thirteen different colours of Pop'set paper, 1994.

LE GÉNÉRAL S'ÉCRIE:

à table, à table!

ET LA NOCE SE MET A TABLE.

D'un seul côté de la table pour être vue du public.

LE GÉNÉRAL SE LÈVE »»—→

A handwritten note shows that Massin was already imagining different possible incarnations for the play – as 'TV programme, Bataille show, Adès record'.[36] As with Édith Piaf's song *La Foule*, he explores its possible theatrical and musical correspondences and envisages a 'total' book, while Nicolas Bataille, who directed *La Cantatrice chauve* at the théâtre de la Huchette, talked of a new staging of *Les Mariés de la tour Eiffel* in Paris. Massin was thinking of a commercial equivalent of the total show: the book could include a recording of the ballet-play and a record in a sleeve inserted into the binding. The inclusion of an LP would have enabled a co-edition by Gallimard and Adès with,

potentially, a special boxed limited edition.[37] But the project never came to anything, not even, strangely, when the book was published in 1994, by which time the insertion of CD-ROMs in books was commonplace in French publishing.

Reflecting an experiment in artistic synthesis, the interdisciplinary vision of *Les Mariés de la tour Eiffel* echoes Massin's typographical experiments inspired strictly by music, which he began to undertake at around the same time.

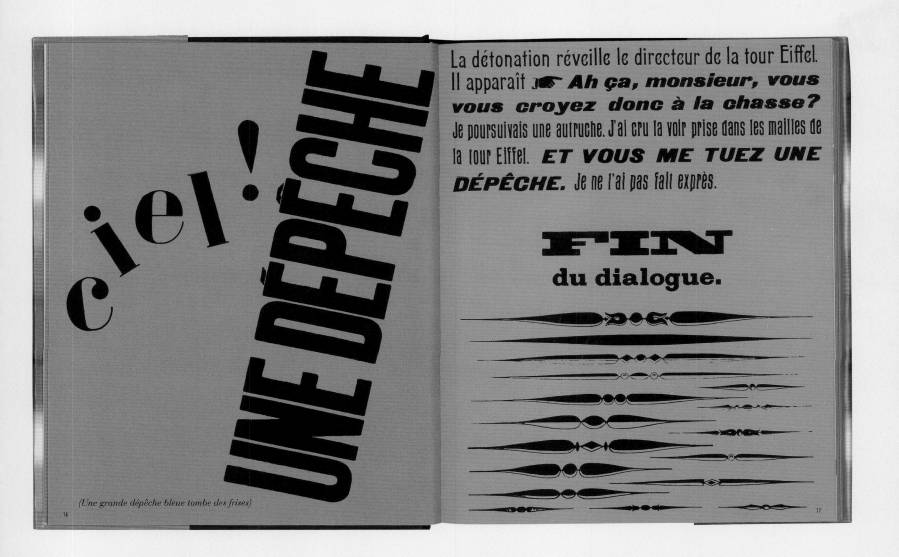

(Une grande dépêche bleue tombe des frises)

16

17

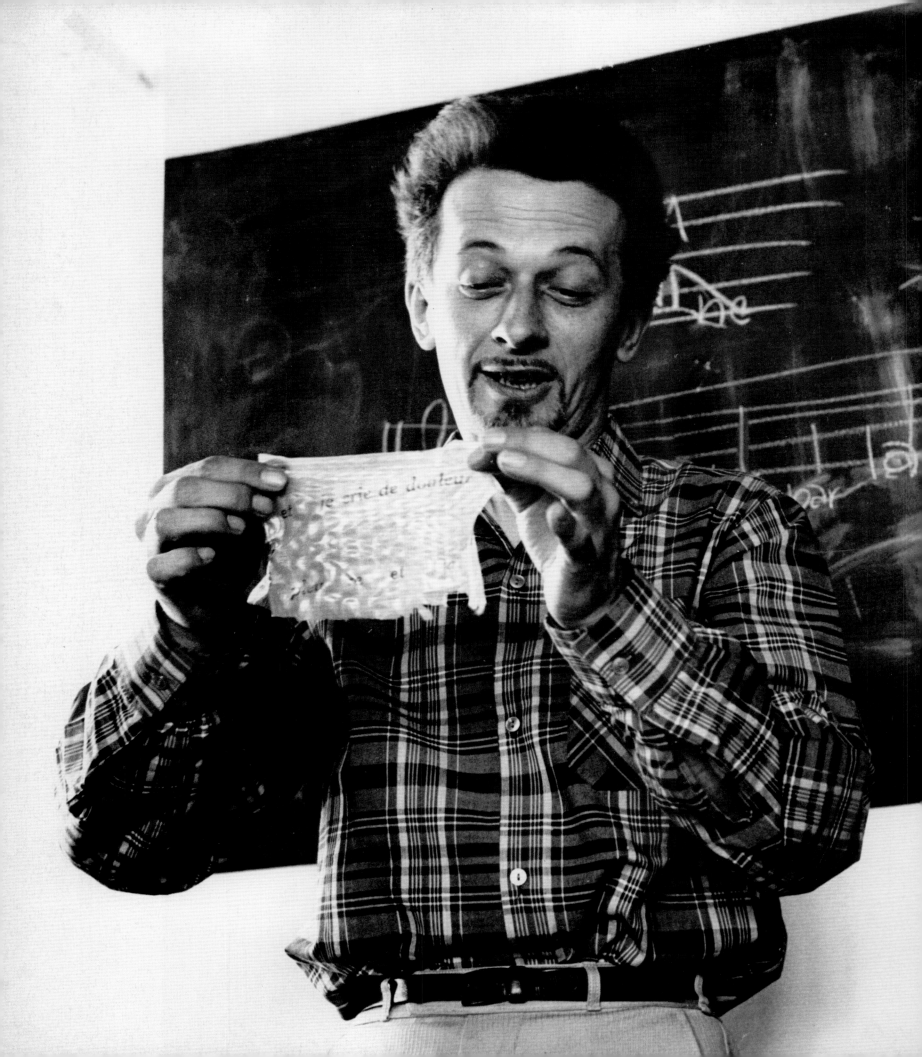

Music

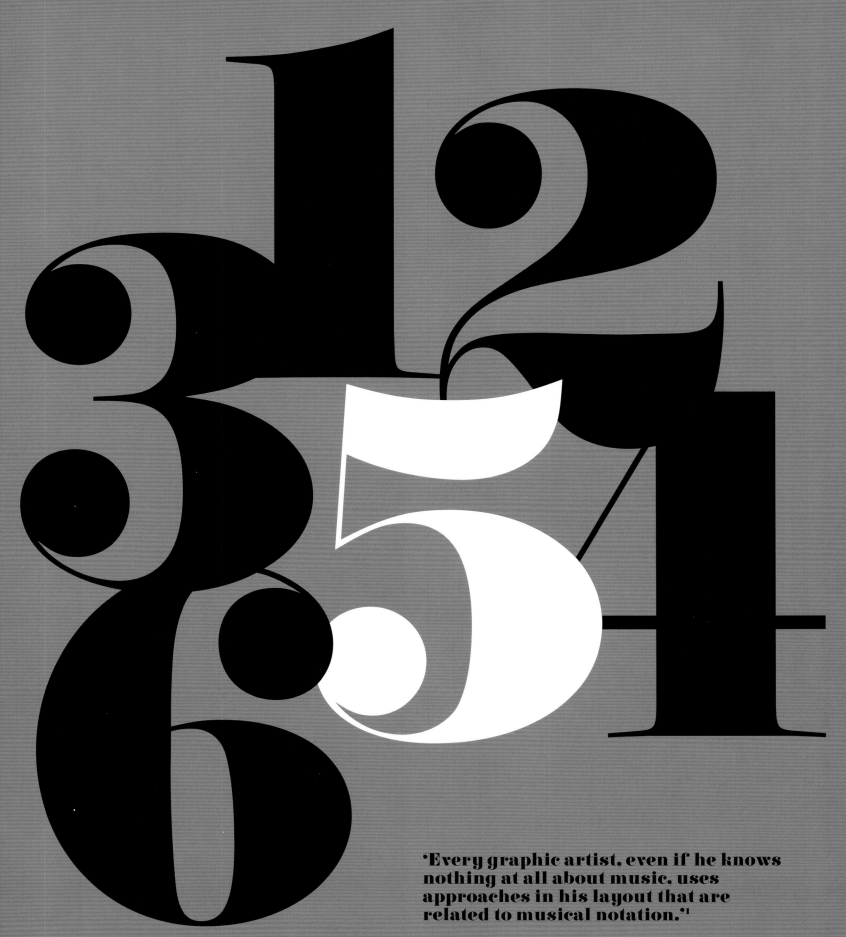

'Every graphic artist, even if he knows nothing at all about music, uses approaches in his layout that are related to musical notation.'

lifelong love

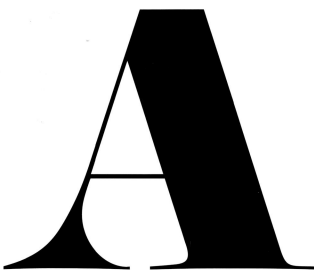

For Massin, music is more than a pastime – it is a passion and, above all, the manifestation of a different kind of graphic writing. Since his earliest days his life has been filled with music, as a listener rather than a player, appreciating it in almost all its forms, particularly those that involve the voice. Above and beyond his personal passion, he also constantly talks and writes about music. He is a knowledgeable music-lover who prefers to make his analyses by listening to recordings rather than going to concerts. Massin also sees music as a method parallel to that of graphics and one which, through the notion of variation proper to the musical domain, has broadly inspired his work.

Brought up on popular songs and dances by his father, Massin began listening to recorded music very early in his life – on the radio, record player and, later, CD player. When he reached the age of reason his older sister gave him a small child's gramophone and a pile of Pathé and Columbia records, recordings of comic dialogues and songs from the years 1900 to 1930. He carefully listed them by hand, in a layout worthy of a record-seller's catalogue. The future junk-shop explorer, compiler of *catalogues raisonnés* and chief archivist of his own history was already emerging.

For a while Massin was a member of the Chartres' Swingtette du Hot Club de l'Île-de-France (a jazz group founded by his schoolmates and directly influenced by the band of Stéphane Grappelli and Django Reinhardt), in which he played the double bass. At the same time, and unconcerned by the opposition of jazz and classical music, he played classical double bass in the ensemble Harmonie Saint-Ferdinand. But the young Massin spent most of his time with his ear glued to his radio, notably throughout the war, during which he discovered the symphonic music of Berlioz and Debussy, of which the Germans were particularly fond.

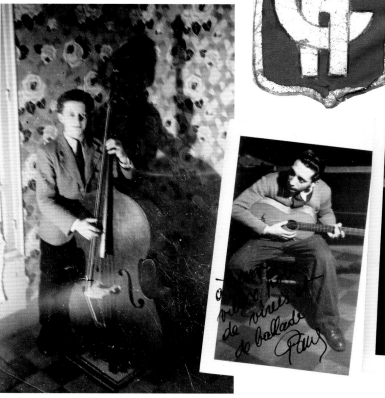

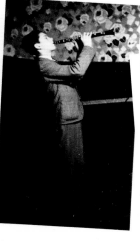

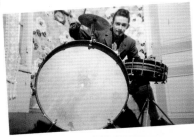

Throughout Massin's life, radio has remained a particular source of information and inspiration. In the 1960s he began listening, with all the fervour of a religious ritual, to 'Le matin des musiciens' (the musicians' morning), a programme presented by Jacques Merlet on France-Musique (1970–1990). His recordings of this programme (almost 2,000 kilometres of tape) are, moreover, kept preserved in his house in Étampes and he listens to them regularly. Inspired by these scholarly themed programmes, in which

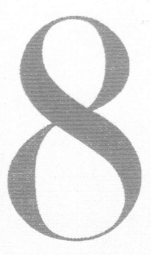

BEETHOVEN : HUITIÈME ET NEUVIÈME SYMPHONIES

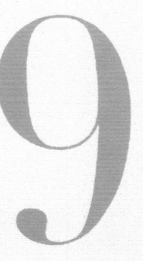

Page 142: photograph of Massin by Yan (Jean Dieuzaide), explaining the process of printing on condoms at the Rencontres internationales de Lure, summer 1965.

Opposite, top to bottom, left to right: badge of the Swingtette du Hot Club de l'Île-de-France de Chartres, designed by Massin, 1943–4; Massin playing double bass in the Swingtette, c.1944; photographs of members of the Swingtette, 1943–4.

Above: three-colour, grey/brown cloth cover for album of the eighth and ninth symphonies of Ludwig van Beethoven (Paris, Club des disquaires de France, 1958).

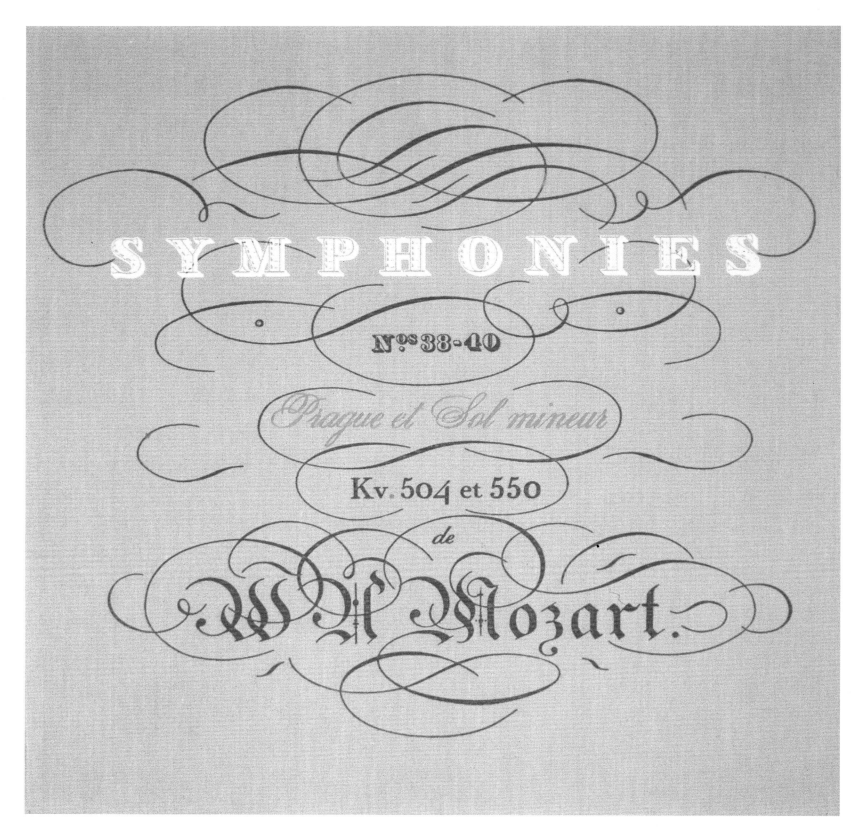

Above: two-colour, violet cloth cover with gold for album of *symphonies nos 38–40* by Wolfgang Amadeus Mozart (Paris, Club des disquaires de France, 1958).

Opposite: sheet music for popular songs, 1930s.

musicological essays alternate with interviews with makers of early instruments, musical extracts, commentary, interviews with musicians and entire operas, Massin developed a true passion for music. At the same time he delighted in the socio-cultural approach that was taking shape in intellectual and academic circles, and which he adopted himself in *La Lettre et l'Image*, in the series of thematic works for the 'Atelier Massin' published by Hachette[2] and in his various historical novels.

Massin was an enthusiastic witness to the renewal of interest in baroque music, which regained its importance in the 1970s. 'Today, after twenty or thirty years of concerted effort by musicologists, instrument makers, musicians and those who are rather disparagingly termed the "*baroqueux*", we have seen the rediscovery of entire continents of Elizabethan, Tudor and Italian music', he wrote.[3] This revival manifested itself notably in the return to favour of composers who had remained in the shadows for centuries, such as Monteverdi, Purcell, Vivaldi and Couperin, and also in a new appreciation of period instruments and a new way of looking at the architecture linked to the performance of this music (in Italy in the 1970s Massin discovered the rococo palaces and, in Bavaria, the church in Wies and the abbey in Ottobeuren). Unlike 'traditionalist' France-Musique broadcasts such as 'La tribune des critiques de disques' (Jury of record critics) or 'Le pavé dans la mare' (Stepping-stone), 'Le matin des musiciens' rehabilitated composers forgotten by the classical musicologists, who concentrated on the romantic period. Massin followed this renaissance and drew personal and professional inspiration from it, since it closely resembled his own approach in his typographical experiments and also, of course, his idea of interaction between the arts.

Later, Massin also ventured into radio himself as a commentator. Claude Maupomé invited him to participate in the programme 'Le concert égoïste' (The selfish concert') on France-Musique (later renamed 'Comment l'entendez-vous?' [How does it sound to you?]), in which people of the written word talk about music. Between 1979 and 1983 Massin took part in seven two-hour programmes, in which the discussion was about a mixture of music, graphic art and art, with the launch of Massin's books providing the pretext for a pleasant, informal conversation about culture in general.

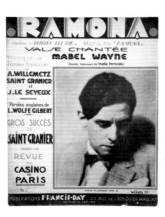
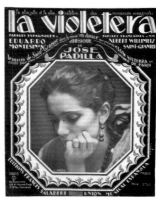
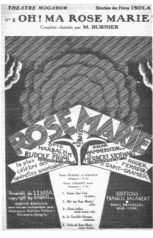
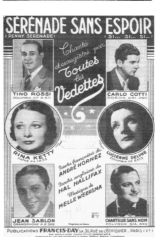
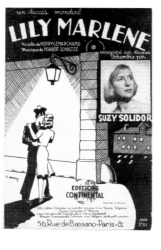
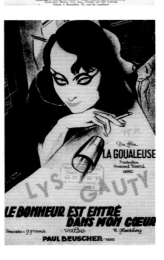

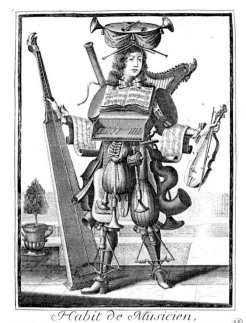

ELEGIACA:

Elegiaca harmonia é qua in elegiacis miseriscg; carminib.decantandis utimur:cuius numeri sunt tales.

Tempora labuntur tacitisq; senescimus annis

Et fugiunt freno non remorante dies

Prospera lux oritur:linguis animisq; fauete.

Nunc dicenda bona Sunt bona uerba die

Habit de Musicien.

A Paris Chez N. de Larmessin. Rue S.t Iacques, à la Pome d'Or. Avec. Priuil. du Roy.

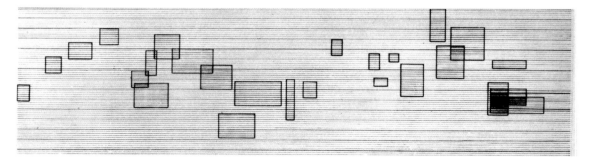

Extracts from *Azerty, l'alphabet du monde* (Paris, Gallimard, 2004).

Top to bottom: page from *Elegiaca*, neumes for Gregorian plain chant, one of the earliest attempts at the transcription of medieval vocal music; engraving by Nicolas de Larmessin, musician's dress, eighteenth century; extract from *Franchinus Gafurius* (Milan, Theorica Musicae, 1492), one of the first musical treatises of the Renaissance; extract from the first edition of Karlheinz Stockhausen's *Studie II*, a score for electronic music (1956).

Writing about music

Asked about his transition from knowledgeable music-lover to musicologist, Massin answered with the aplomb of the self-taught: 'Through listening to music I eventually learned to talk about it.'[4] True, he was a non-specialist who had forgotten how to read music, but he knew how to choose the right words (and images) to discuss it, exploring both his own sensibility and great swathes of cultural history from a perspective that remains central to an understanding of his own work: 'Talking about music means talking about the question of variation, which is fundamental in my work and the basis of everything'.[5] It is no surprise that he chose Johann Sebastian Bach as the model and undisputed master of variation: *The Goldberg Variations* are often regarded as the most ambitious work ever composed for the harpsichord, representing an encyclopaedic overview of the entire development of baroque variation. So, from work that was of a highly personal nature – a third of his autobiographical writings are about music – Massin came to write essays that are more substantial.

In his journal *Continuo* (Paris, Balbec, 1988), which contains his first piece on the subject, Massin expresses his amazement, for example, that the baroque musicians managed to harmonize controlled dissonances. In *Journal en désordre* (Disorderly journal; Paris, Robert Laffont, 1996) he combines his memories with a series of music-lover's musings on the aesthetics common to images and sounds. In his free essays *De la variation* (On variation; Paris, Le Promeneur, 2000) and *Style et écriture. Du rococo aux arts deco* (Style and writing. From the rococo to art deco; Paris, Albin Michel, 2001), he focuses on the history of music. In his own light, accessible style, he reveals the points where different forms of art converge, discusses the unity of styles and shows how music often echoes ideological standpoints. In *De la variation* he suggests that improvisation precedes the establishment of artistic canons, in all fields of creativity.

Lastly, in some chapters of *Azerty, l'alphabet du monde* (Qwerty, the world's alphabet; Paris, Gallimard, 2004) Massin puts forward an interpretation that seeks to measure the importance of music in relation to its graphic representation. The chapter 'M' is dedicated to the development of the writing of music and its graphic notation. Massin traces the development of transcription of a score of notes that were initially square, and then rhomboid, before acquiring their contemporary oval shape. In addition to the quality of the graphic composition of the score – which is, moreover, handwritten and therefore naturally expressive – at a fundamental level it is the margin for interpretation left to the musicians (to whom the composer rarely gives precise instructions) that intrigues Massin. And if the indications of tempo in music correspond to stage directions in the theatre, it is once more this narrow opportunity for interpretation that fascinates Massin, for it gives to him too the right to enter into the work and the chance to provide a variation.

Above: two-colour, brown cloth cover for
the album *Negro Spirituals* (Paris, Club
des disquaires de France, 1958).

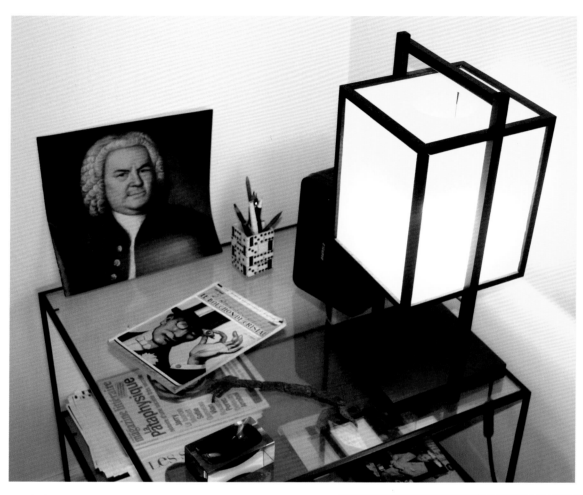

Portrait of Johann Sebastian Bach,
Massin's soulmate, in the living room
of his Paris apartment.

Johann Sebastian Bach

*If there is one composer who embodies
both Massin's enthusiasm for music in
general and baroque music in particular,
together with his fascination with
variation, it is Johann Sebastian Bach
(1685–1750). Bach's work is music of
infinite variation – the art of fugue, the
art of counterpoint – which Massin has
discussed at length in relation to his role
as a layout artist.[6] Counterpoint is often
mentioned in his writings as a musical
metaphor for a layout that, in spatial
terms, works, displaying a subtle balance
of interrelated images and graphic signs
that are mutually enriching and that
create a dialogue expressed through
interdependence and correspondence.
What Massin says about the principles
of designing the space on album covers
seems relevant to his work as a whole:
'Because the layout of an illustrated
book is made of images moving to the
right (the direction in which we read,
as users of the Latin alphabet) and
others arranged from top to bottom, it
precisely illustrates the principle of
musical composition, which is based
on both vertical structures (determining*

*harmony) and other horizontal,
superimposed structures that form
the counterpoint.'[7]
In De la variation[8] Massin suggests
that variation is perhaps the precondition
of style. In this subtle, informed and
eclectic book, he reviews variation in
its different incarnations, from the
development of music, to architecture
and the so-called minor arts. Massin
has often proclaimed his desire not to
follow any particular style; it might
be suggested that his various graphic
transcriptions of dramatic or musical
works are a response to Bach's Art
of Fugue.
Bach, the musical alchemist, has
become something of a travelling
companion to Massin throughout his life,
inspiring him every day. The portrait of
Proust on his bedside table has its echo
in the portrait of Bach enthroned in his
sitting room. Massin himself devoted an
entire chapter of his most recent book,
Azerty, l'alphabet du monde, to the
letter 'B': 'I love his joyful, dancing
cantatas, such as the BWV 134 for the
third day of Easter. […] I prefer to listen*

*to these cantatas in the morning, because
they have the same effect on me as a
bath. I listen to them in my car, all along
the way, because what else can you do
at the wheel? Driving is so boring.'[9]
Bach also provides a perfect case
study in the difficulty of interpreting
a written work, which is our subject in
this chapter. Glenn Gould played* The
Goldberg Variations *on the piano,
although they were written for the
harpsichord, the instrument on which
Massin now exclusively listens to
interpretations of baroque music (he
makes an exception for Gould, whom
he finds extraordinary). 'Played by Pablo
Casals, Wanda Landowska or Ton
Koopman, Bach is always Bach, even if
Glenn Gould appropriates him sometimes
to the point of re-creating him almost
completely,' he observes.[10] So Bach is a
kind of musical alter ego, an inspirational
model for his own graphic compositions
and interpretations.*

A question of interpretation

For Massin, exploring early music means entering a different world, a forgotten period, an art of living, and accepting a new way of understanding (musical) art and its practice. The re-emergence of baroque music in the 1970s marks the return of the performer, the intermediary and, so, of unpredictability. Massin often mentions the performers and promoters of baroque music with almost more admiration than he shows in relation to the composers themselves: the American conductor William Christie, founder of the Arts Florissants and figurehead of the movement; the Canadian harpsichordist Scott Ross, brilliant interpreter of Couperin and Rameau; Nikolaus Harnoncourt, player of the viola da gamba; and the organist Rinaldo Alessandrini – all have helped popularize the music of the period. They pay daily visits to Massin, as his television is always on. 'I discovered them thanks to cable. With these high-quality images you get an irreplaceable view of the playing, with close-ups of the pianist's hands for example, or the movements of the violinists' fingers.'[11]

Above and beyond the margin of variation left by the performers' playing, Massin, always on the lookout for the cultural context that might illuminate a work, is also interested in the historical conditions of this musical practice, which are themselves unpredictable. Not only have hitherto neglected scores been rediscovered (including Vivaldi's concertos, the sonatas of the virtuoso Heinrich von Biber and Neapolitan operettas that were often performed only once), but modern musicologists now stress the importance of the craft of making the instruments themselves, in order to respect their original tone and sound colour. The instrument makers are reconstructing violas da gamba and lutes using authentic techniques. 'I can't listen to Bach as he was played in the 1950s, with no regard for instruments of the period', says Massin.[12]

Contemporary with the advocates of synchronic as opposed to event-led cultural history, the artisans of this renaissance of baroque music, like Massin himself, appreciated the writings of the historians of the Annales School – whose best-known initiators were Fernand Braudel, Lucien Febvre and Emmanuel Le Roy Ladurie – which offered them a way of thinking that emphasizes the historical context in which music was written and the material conditions in which it was performed. In his own field of typography Massin shows the same respect for authentic techniques in the subject he is treating. For example, in decorating his luxury, leather-bound edition of the *Œuvres complètes de Molière* (Paris, Club du meilleur livre, 1954) he paid particular attention to seventeenth-century decorative motifs, which he reproduced in pastiche for the borders of the cover and endpapers.

The question of variation in interpretation is many-faceted and endless – and the guiding thread of Massin's work – whether as the subject of a conversation about music, or practised in his art of pastiche, or in his various typographical translations. All his graphic work is imbued with the baroque spirit: it honours lettering, celebrating it for its power of transformation. In baroque music, which is the art of movement, nothing is fixed, explains Massin.[13] From the scribes with their letters of lead to today's computers, the transcription of music has also always been in process, dependent on its graphic translation.

The written score acquires a new life with each new musician, like a play performed by an actor or like a text in a foreign language that speaks through a translator. One problem peculiar to early music is that it was not notated (the length of notes was not indicated on the scores). Contemporary musicians can interpret scores from the past and, without any 'scientific'

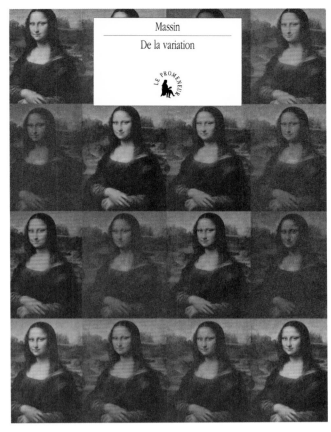

Top to bottom: four-colour cover of *De la variation* (Paris, Le Promeneur, 2000), inspired by the screen-printed portraits of Andy Warhol; hand written list of records Massin collected as a child, 1930s.

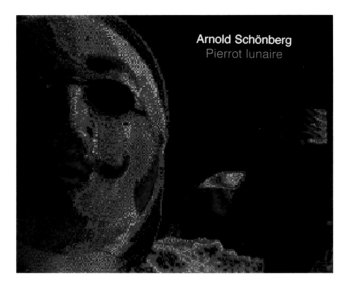

references, appropriate them. So the door is open to personal expression. 'But where did the habit come from, in music, of not playing what is written?', wonders Massin, speaking of the medieval and ecclesiastical origins of the trend for improvisation, a theme which has always captivated his eye and his thinking.[14] He goes on: 'Improvisation, in every creative field, is as old as the world, since it precedes the establishment of artistic canons'.[15]

Throughout his career Massin has chosen the role of the interpreter who honours the work of others; like the jazz artist who plays the theme or the basso continuo that accompanies a baroque melody, his position is that of the creative intermediary and he often rejects the title of creative artist. As their subtitles suggest, his typographical works are interpretations, translations or transcriptions – in other words, variations improvised on an existing idea. In the case of *La Cantatrice chauve* (Paris, Gallimard, 1964) there is a dual interpretation, since it consists of a typographical and photographic variation on the characters in Ionesco's play; in *Délire à deux* (Paris, Gallimard, 1966) the interpretation is expressed through the fortuitous presence of expressionist blotches that are also signs; in *Exercices de style* (Paris, Gallimard, 1963) it is expressed through the search for fonts equivalent to the ninety-nine tones and styles of Queneau's text. In improvisation, which always goes hand in hand with variation – for the graphic artist as for the performing musician – Massin finds the keys to an artistic expressiveness that enables him to invent his own canons.

An experiment in expressive typography, *Pierrot lunaire*, the graphic transposition of the first atonal work by Arnold Schoenberg, unpublished project.

Above: cover of *Pierrot lunaire*.

Below and opposite, bottom: inside spreads (*Der kranke Mond, Der Mondfleck* and *Heimfahrt*).

Opposite, top: musical scale illustrating correspondences between musical notes and colours across the range of the voice of the mezzo-soprano who performs *Pierrot lunaire*. The choice of colours is subjective: the high notes are represented by yellow, the low notes by a violet-red.

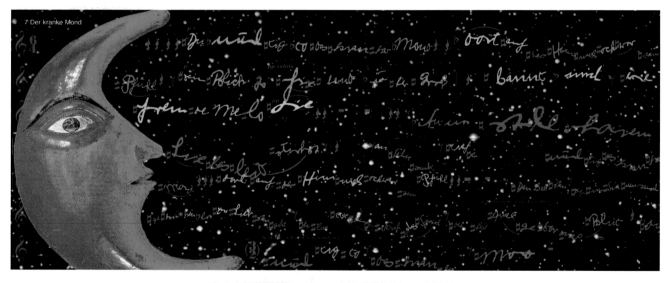

Music is visual

So the love of music is not confined to a purely cerebral, scholarly experience but is also physical, visual and tangible. In addition to the radio, Massin's great discovery of the early 1950s was the gramophone and the long-playing record which, in France, were late in replacing the phonograph. This invention led to a shift from the use of universal sleeves to protective cardboard covers for discs, a phenomenon concomitant with the creation of the dust jacket for books, which required the collaboration of graphic artists. Influenced by the covers of the 10- and 12-inch jazz records that arrived from the United States in the early 1950s, Massin saw them as 'wonders of invention in the field of graphic art'.[16]

With good advice from a sales assistant in Durand (a record shop on place de la Madeleine, Paris), Massin's musical world was expanded to embrace new styles and periods, while his taste led him, initially at least, to chamber music (particularly Beethoven's piano sonatas and Schubert's string quartets). 'Each time I would stop short in front of the releases from Erato; the intelligence and taste shown in their selection of music had their equivalent in the presentation, whose quality was instantly apparent. It was Haydn's *Creation* decorated by a detail from Michelangelo's Sistine Chapel.'[17] The first synaesthetic correspondences very soon began to emerge: Massin also explored music through its visual presentation on the record cover, before plunging seriously into the study of its graphic translation, which he

addressed, as we have seen, in his writings on aesthetics. Commenting on the reproduction of musical scores in *Azerty, l'alphabet du monde*, Massin cites the performer of early music Rinaldo Alessandrini, for whom Bach's music does not need to be played: it is enough to read it,[18] since the quality of the score is reminiscent of a graphic composition equivalent to a successful book cover.

When the Club du meilleur livre was supplemented by the Club des disquaires de France (established in 1958 and headed, of course, by Carlier), Massin designed coloured covers for long-playing records, whose elegant simplicity recalls that of the 'Soleil' series. 'To break the monotony [...] I used unusual colours, I sought out combinations that were sometimes grating – red and violet, blue and green, and so on. To tell the truth, it wasn't hard for me to stand out, given the conformism that was the rule in the presentation of covers in the late 1940's', he remembers.[19] The chromatic range of these covers remains, nevertheless, fairly sober and the graphic line is rarely figurative or referential, aside from a few illustrations in the baroque spirit here and there. But whatever his efforts to find correspondences between image and sound, touch and tone, Massin always addresses all the senses, thereby extending his field of graphic investigation.

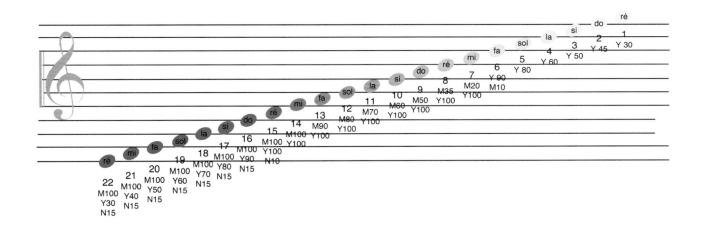

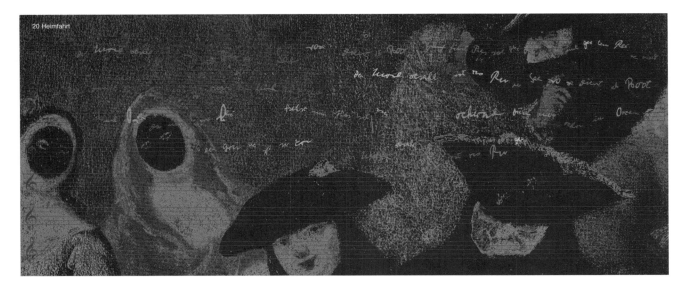

A work of substitution

The interpreter's role, like that of some chameleon–like actor, almost certainly remains a mask that Massin needs in order to try on other roles, a way for him to test out every possible means of expression: 'Interpretation is an activity that substitutes for things I don't know how to do.'[20]

Substituting interpretation for music that he can neither play nor sing, Massin set about creating a graphic transposition of *Pierrot lunaire*, the first atonal work by Arnold Schoenberg. He was inspired by the twelve-tone construction of the work (it was written using the twelve semi-tones of the western scale; unlike classical writing, which primarily uses its 'traditional', unmodified tones – do, re, mi, fa, sol, la, ti) and the recitation used in its performance; his challenge was to find a graphic and typographical equivalent of the vocal register, tone and intensity of the piece.

Massin chose *Pierrot lunaire* for its expressive, dramatic qualities, notably the evocative power of the voice, and went right to the source of the term 'expressionist' by choosing the period of German expressionism to illustrate his graphic interpretation. Having already and successfully taken on avant-garde theatre, here Massin was directly addressing musical material. He started this project in the year of his lucky star (1966 was the year in which he created his greatest works), abandoned and then reworked it over and over again, by hand and on computer. It is still in progress today, as he fine-tunes its typography. 'This work permits all kinds of distortions. But it seems that even computers are powerless to solve the problem', he admits in a moment of doubt.[21]

Pierrot lunaire was composed in 1911–12 and performed in a Berlin cabaret in 1912 with a libretto (translated into German) based on a symbolist poem by the Belgian poet Albert Giraud. The melodrama is set against a decadent version of Watteau-style *fêtes galantes* (with streams of blood, absinthe, ghosts and vampires). The piece is spoken with a musical accompaniment and the single vocalist may not necessarily be a singer, but is rather a recitator (more precisely, the performer speaks the text over a vocal range of two octaves), of a kind often seen in the literary cabarets of the inter-war period.[22]

The critic Antoine Goléa regards *Pierrot lunaire* as the first-ever piece of aleatory music, since each vocalist sings or reads it in their own individual voice, which is thus necessarily different from all others.[23] It is by definition a work that exists through its 'room to manœuvre', in which performance and its variants are more important than the written work. In this sort of modern baroque music, Massin is fascinated by the element that is left to improvisation, which is dizzyingly seductive and full of meaning. In his view, 'Each transformation or metamorphosis of the subject renews and expands it, enriches it, because, as Schoenberg said, what matters is not the subject, but the commentary on it, which takes the form of a counter-subject; because it is the commentary itself that is the subject and not the other way round'.[24]

In this ambitious project Massin has set himself the goal of respecting the position of the notes on the staves as closely as possible (with yellows for the high notes and violet reds for the low notes), so that a performer can reconstruct the music from the typography and the undulating movement traced by the text. But he had already come up against the difficulty of transcription in his typographical experiment with playwright Jean Tardieu's *La Sonate et les trois messieurs* (The sonata and the three gentlemen; also begun in 1966, then continued on computer in 1993 but not finished). Moreover, all of Tardieu's work consists of placing words in the service of music. For Tardieu, words are sounds first and foremost, which must find their place through the harmony they produce when they are juxtaposed with other words. *La Sonate et les trois messieurs* is a stunning and amusing demonstration of this: each of the three characters takes the part of an instrument and shares words among themselves according to the mood of the movement – *largo* or *andante*, for example – to be created. Massin chose to represent each instrument in the trio with a particular typeface or colour, whereas in *Pierrot lunaire* he emphasizes the visual treatment of each page.

The size of the lettering changes depending on the volume of the voice and the vocalized words that cross the spreads, moved by the sudden vocal shifts and leaps of a singer who can cover two octaves, are set in Mistral, a font inspired by the handwriting of its creator, typographer Roger Excoffon. But Mistral's slightly 1950s mood did not entirely satisfy Massin, who is always on the lookout for an appropriate, expressive typographical equivalent. In 2006 he began work on a fifth version based on a feminine, German handwriting style, whose serifed letters are typical of the Germanic, gothic influence – which should, he hopes, be more expressive and personal to each character.

This exploration, which has obsessed Massin for forty years, is akin to the typographical interpretation of *La Cantatrice chauve*: in reality in both cases he is trying to fix on paper the written trace of an intrinsically ephemeral artistic performance. To this day Massin is still working on the relationship between the human voice and typography, always drawing on new materials, as shown by his limited edition of *Viens Poupoule!* (Come on, Poupoule!), a popular song of the early twentieth century. In the preface to this little book Massin explains, 'Here the staves of the musical score do not appear, the words are in the air, as though thrown out by the singer's mouth. The proportion of the letters and their colour still follow the same system used for *Pierrot lunaire* and *Les Cris de Paris* (The cries of Paris).'[25] In *Pierrot lunaire* the soprano's voice is underpinned by a background richly illustrated with the works of expressionist artists, whom Schoenberg may have known or even associated with, including the Germans Emil Nolde and Oskar Kokoschka and the Norwegian Edvard Munch. These pictures are often cropped by Massin so that they are not directly recognizable, and their colours are heightened, even corrected, for greater expressiveness, while enlargement renders the now pixelized images more abstract. Here illustration has the poetic power to evoke the historical and cultural context of Germany before the Weimar republic. The iconography, used as a background to the typographical manipulations, brings a second level of interpretation to this musical work, an interpretation whose three-dimensional aspect sets it apart among Massin's experiments as a whole. Depending on whether he is typographically transposing dramatic or musical works, Massin uses a vast array of iconographic registers: from the purely graphic treatment of the ink blots in *Délire à deux* to the lyrical effects of *Pierrot lunaire* and the 'photo-graphic' manipulation of *La Cantatrice Chauve*.

Opposite: experiment in expressive typography, 'Là ci darem la mano', aria from Mozart's *Don Giovanni* (2006, unpublished). The cut-out faces of the figures represent musical notes.

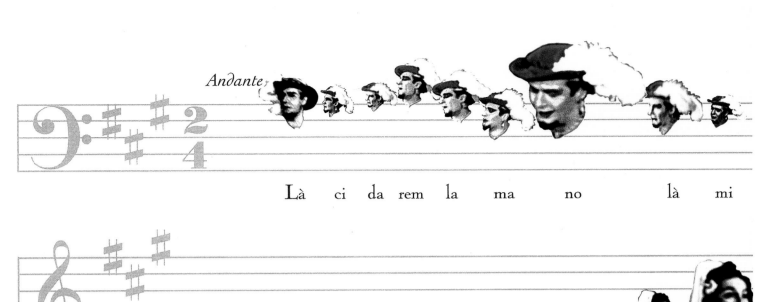

Andante

Là   ci   da rem   la   ma   no   là   mi

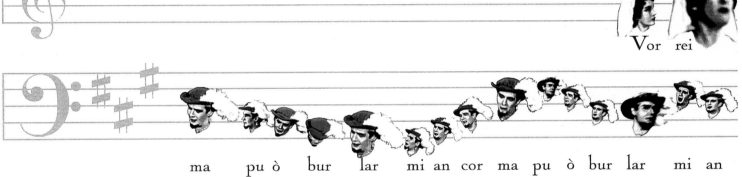

Vor rei

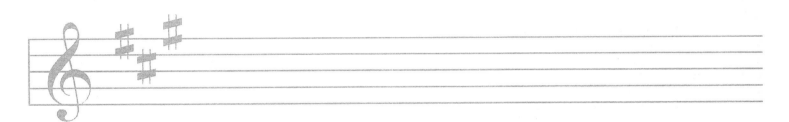

ma   pu ò   bur   lar   mi an cor   ma   pu   ò   bur   lar   mi   an

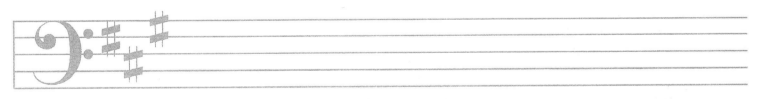

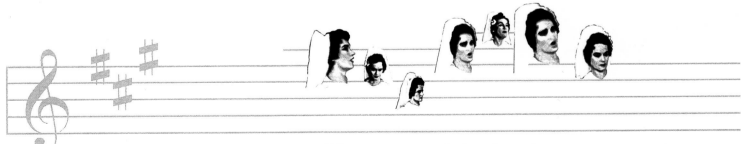

Vie   ne   mio   bel   di   let   to

69

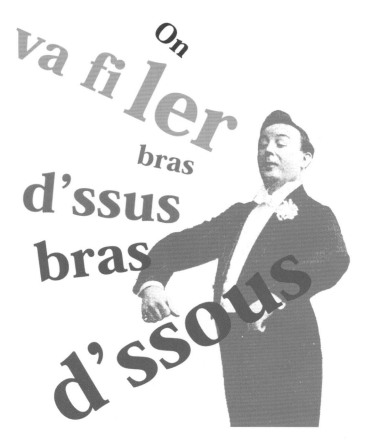

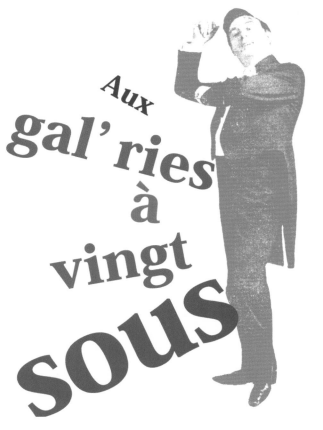

On va fi ler bras d'ssus bras d'ssous

Aux gal'ries à vingt sous

Quand j'en tends des chan sons

Ça m'rend tout po lis son

22 23

156   Massin

Experiment in expressive typography, *Viens Poupoule!*, song written by Mayol in 1902 (Paris, Typographies expressives, 2006).

Sou viens toi qu'c'est comm' ça

Que j'suis dev' nu pa pa

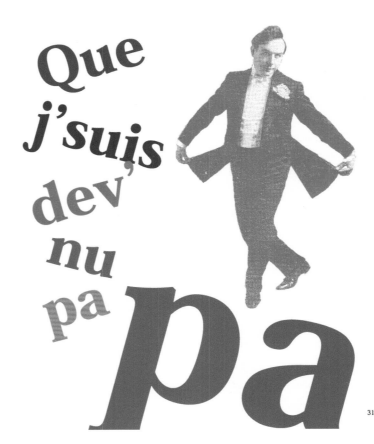

30

31

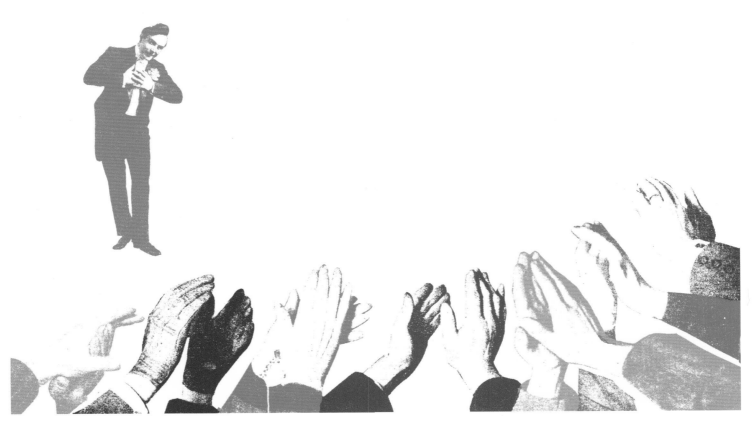

EVERGREEN

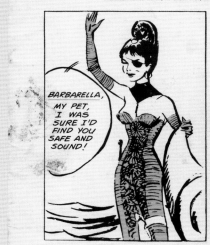

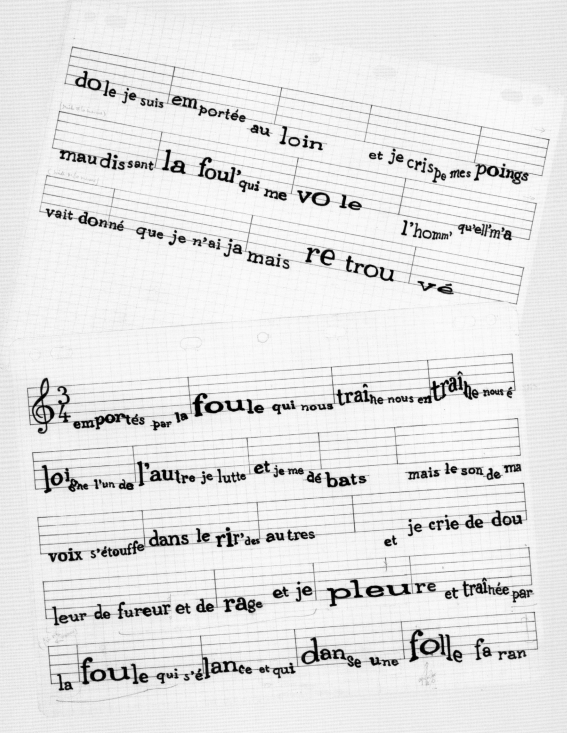

Above: cover of *Evergreen Review* (New York, Grove Press, no. 38, November 1965), featuring an illustration from Jean-Claude Forest's well-known cartoon strip *Barbarella*.

Right: typographical transcription on a score of the lyrics to Édith Piaf's song *La Foule*, 1965.

Opposite, left to right: letters from Massin to Barney Rosset, head of Grove Press (8 July and 17 August 1965) explaining the details of the project for *La Foule*.

Focus
'La Foule'
Evergreen Review, New York, Grove Press, 1965

A unique commission

Unlike many of the typographical projects Massin undertook in the 1960s – a great period of inspiration – *La Foule* (The crowd) was the result of a commission and was not based on a purely literary work. But this did not stop Massin from experimenting with the most surprising printing techniques.

La Foule is a typographical interpretation, across three double-page spreads, of the song by Édith Piaf, accompanied by photographic interpretations by Emil Cadoo, an American photographer living in Paris. The project was started in October 1964, finished in August 1965 and published in *Evergreen Review*, a progressive American literary magazine from Grove Press. In the decade 1960–70, Barney Rosset, owner of *Evergreen Review* and Grove Press, combined radical activism with experimental art in both his life and his publications. With great verve and a nose for the controversial, he published the beatnik poets, plays by the British playwright Harold Pinter, conversations with filmmaker John Cassavetes and the writings of Che Guevara.

Rosset was also the publisher in the United States of Michel Butor, Marguerite Duras, Eugène Ionesco and other authors who were much talked about at the time. He paid great attention to new developments in publishing in Paris and, although Gallimard's foreign rights department was more than embryonic at the time, published the American edition of *La Cantatrice chauve*, having bought the rights a year after the French edition came out. The American edition appeared in 1965 with the title *The Bald Soprano*, followed the next year by the English edition from British publisher Calder and Boyars with the title *The Bald Prima Donna*. Massin had to compose entirely separate layouts for these two versions. 'It was when the American edition was announced in 1965 that Barney – or rather Richard Seaver, who was his assistant and spoke perfect French – suggested I should do a similar piece for *Evergreen*', remembers Massin.[26]

Thus the work on *La Foule* was primarily intended to promote Grove Press, who wanted to announce their publication of *The Bald Soprano* and get the best possible publicity in the United States. It was for this reason that Rosset ensured that *The Bald Soprano* became a landmark work in American graphic art circles.

Photoreportage

With *La Foule*, Massin experimented still further with the typographical manipulation he had explored in his earlier works, while combining it with a new, documentary-related photographic aesthetic. The iconography is no longer confined to graphic treatment, as in *La Cantatrice chauve*. He had done an initial experiment along similar lines, with collages of black and white photographs, in his layout for Billie Holiday's

Paris, le 8 juillet 1965

Monsieur Barney Rosset
c/o Grove Press
80 University Place
New York 1003

Cher Monsieur,

Tout arrive : je suis en train de réaliser les 6 pages de la chanson d'Edith Piaf illustrées par les photos d'Emil Cadoo.

C'est un travail très difficile, qui relève du laboratoire et sur la réussite duquel (si réussite il y a), je compte beaucoup, comme démonstration de haute voltige.

Ces difficultés n'expliquent pas à elles seules le retard mis à entreprendre ce travail et je vous prie de m'en excuser.

Je serai à New York vers la mi-septembre. J'espère que j'aurai le plaisir de vous y rencontrer si vous y êtes à cette époque.

Croyez, Cher Monsieur, à tous mes meilleurs sentiments.

MASSIN

P. S. : J'ai envoyé aujourd'hui à Dick Seaver les dernières pages de The Bald Soppano.

M/AA

Paris, le 17 août 1965

Monsieur Barney Rosset
c/o Grove Press
80 University Place
New York 10-003

Cher Monsieur,

Je vous envoie, par pli séparé et par avion, les "offset mechanicals" des 6 pages sur Edith Piaf.

J'ai réservé une demi-page pour un texte de commentaire et, si vous jugez bon de le faire, pour la reproduction inté-grale de la chanson dont je vous envoie la partition. (C'est l'interprète qui a introduit quelques légères différences dans le texte).

Je suis assez content de cet essai qui m'a demandé beaucoup d'efforts car j'ai eu à résoudre de nombreuses difficultés lors de la réalisation. Le procédé que j'ai utilisé et qui est de mon invention ne comporte pas, comme on pourrait le croire, de déformations optiques comme dans "The bald soprano". Il s'agit tout simplement de... Mais je vous expliquerai cela de vive voix à New York : cela vous amusera, je pense. Je suis prêt à en vendre le brevet aux graphistes et publicitaires américains.

Comme vous verrez, j'ai essayé dans cette "musique typographiée", de tenir compte à la fois de la durée, et de la hauteur des notes, ainsi que du volume de la voix, du timbre, de la diction et de l'accent tonique de l'interprète. J'espère que Emil Cadoo, pour sa part, sera satisfait de la mise en page des photos.

Je serai le 15 septembre à New York. Je me réjouis de vous rencontrer et de faire la connaissance de votre art director.

Bien cordialement,

MASSIN

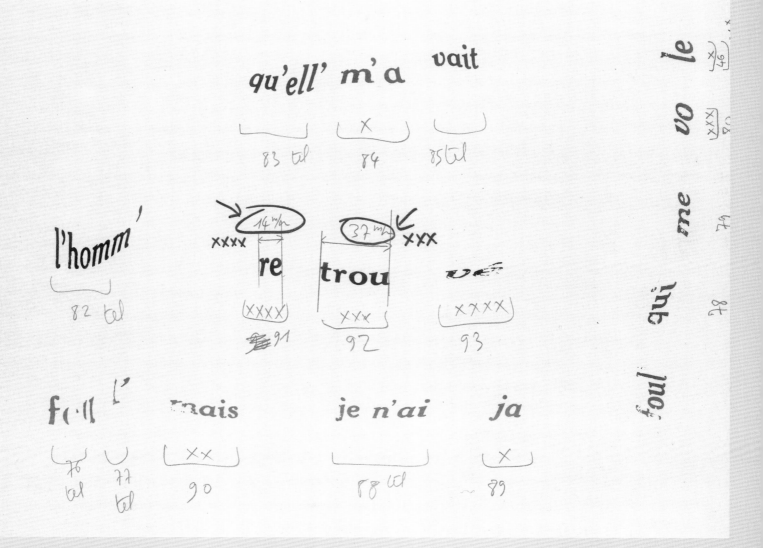

Above and right: layout instructions for *La Foule*, with percentages for the stretching of the letters; initial layout with distorted letters pasted on paper.

Lady Sings the Blues (Club du meilleur livre, 1960; see chapter 1). Using the sequence effect of a strip of negatives, he heightened the dramatic expressiveness of the images of the singer while giving them a cinematic narrative thread. For *La Foule* he quickly persuaded Cadoo to remove all half-tones from his photographs – as Henry Cohen had done for the photos of the actors in *La Cantatrice chauve* – to give a more dramatic feel to Édith Piaf's face.[27]

So it all started with the photographs. Rosset was in possession of a series of shots of Piaf taken by Cadoo. In honour of the French star who had died a few years earlier (1963), Rosset had made two vain attempts to present a combination of photographs and words from her songs using American graphic artists.[28] As Cadoo had taken photographs throughout an entire concert, Massin now had to choose which song to work on: 'I had a choice between *La Vie en rose* and *La Foule*. I chose the latter, mainly because of its Peruvian waltz tempo, which was easier to represent.'[29] He also had to select

the images and, crucially, classify them according to the order of the song. Massin often alludes to this in his correspondence and his work notes, as though respect for chronological order could guarantee a degree of credibility.

For the American public, who discovered Piaf after the war and then during a memorable series of concerts in New York in the mid-1950s, 'la môme Piaf' (The Piaf kid) was the embodiment of the feisty, knowing girl from the Paris streets and Cadoo's photographs provided the melodramatic expression that made her famous. These representations of a face distorted by singing, appearing like death masks, seem to come closer as we turn the pages of the magazine, with a calculated zoom effect, while her hands, like those of a mime artist, reproduced in high contrast, accentuate the theatricality. By cutting up and reprinting negatives to disguise any faults, Massin heightened the effect of a spotlight trained on Piaf's white figure against the blackness of the concert hall.

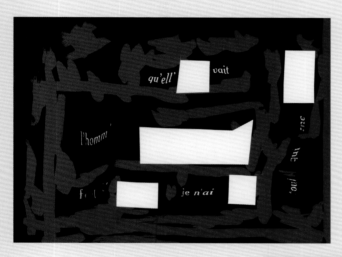

Above and right: negatives of the lyrics to *La Foule* cut out and repainted to remove any faults; typographic experiment to stretch letters on rubber sheet, inconclusive.

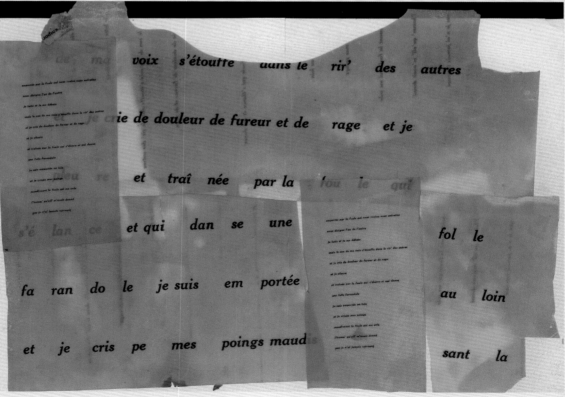

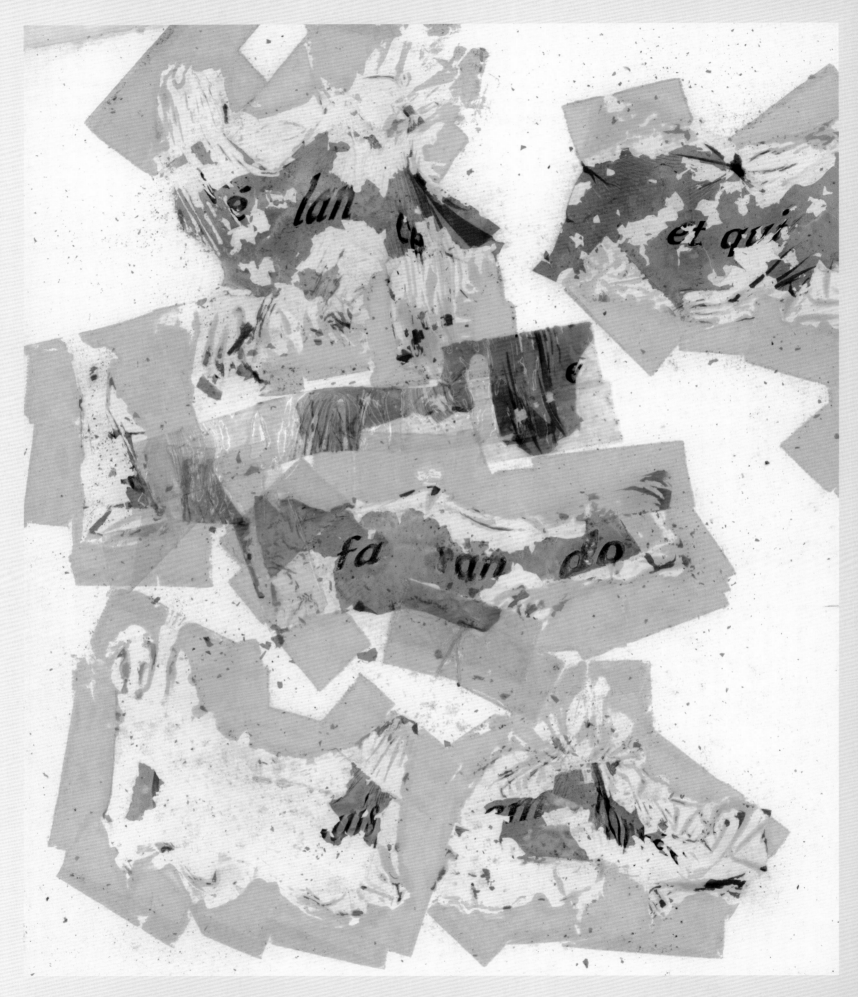

A laboratory of typographic distortions

Returning to his technique of distorting letters, Massin emphasizes the rasping tone and volume of Piaf's voice, and the length and height of the notes in her highly emotional phrasing. Indeed he made this into a kind of manifesto, methodology or instruction manual, as though to clarify his intentions, identifying nine problems for which he had to find solutions. He takes his technique of distorted typography even further than in *La Cantatrice chauve*, manipulating surprising materials, as he had in the good old days of the book clubs. He confided, 'I'm in the process of creating the six pages of Édith Piaf's song illustrated with photos by Emil Cadoo. It's a very difficult task, laboratory work, on whose success (if success there be) I am counting a great deal, as a very daring demonstration'.[30]

After a few fruitless experiments with photographic distortion, Massin decided to use a flexible, rubber material in order to distort the printed letters. Initially he bought rubber sheeting of the kind used on children's beds, but the latex proved too thick to be easy to stretch. 'When I tried it out it emerged that the latex tore as soon as I put in a nail or a pin before I could take the picture, which required a fairly long exposure to take out all the half-tones.'[31] He then tried commercial rubber balloons, but it proved impossible to print the song's lyrics over the pre-existing advertising slogans on all the available types.

Eventually Massin had the idea of trying condoms (known then as 'French letters' in English and '*capotes anglaises*' ['English hoods'] in French), which could not legally be put on open sale in chemists' shops at that time. The first samples proved too lubricated to hold the ink, but the second, with talcum powder, a little thicker but still flexible, worked better: 'Although this time it worked (because Sellotape was strong enough to hold the latex in place to take the photograph), there were never enough of them, because to get the right distortions I had to print one syllable at a time, with big spaces on either side.'[32] Massin often likes to tell the unique, if slightly mad story of his repeated purchasing of condoms to the bemusement of his chemist.

What would today's graphic artist, expert in the use of Photoshop, do to counter the stiffness of lettering? This is a question that Massin – who started using computerized tools twenty years ago and knows their limitations – asks himself. His approach in *La Foule*, as in his other typographical experiments, reminds us just how deeply his work is rooted in a manual tradition of graphic art, requiring the physical manipulation of simple means, in this case an everyday product that he put to use in a way that has little to

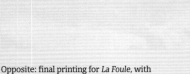

Opposite: final printing for *La Foule*, with type stretched on condoms that are glued, stretched, then laid flat on card.

Left to right: Massin at the Rencontres internationales de Lure, summer 1965, with Germano Facetti, art director at Penguin Books, explaining the different stages in his printing experiments for *La Foule*; detail of printing on condom.

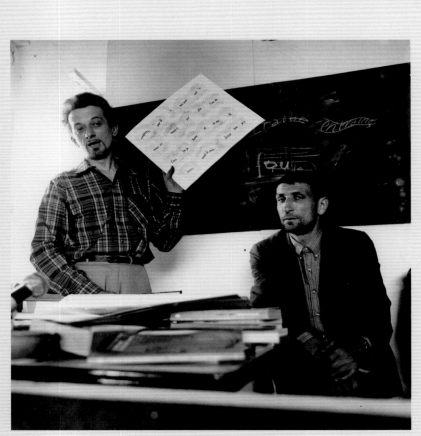

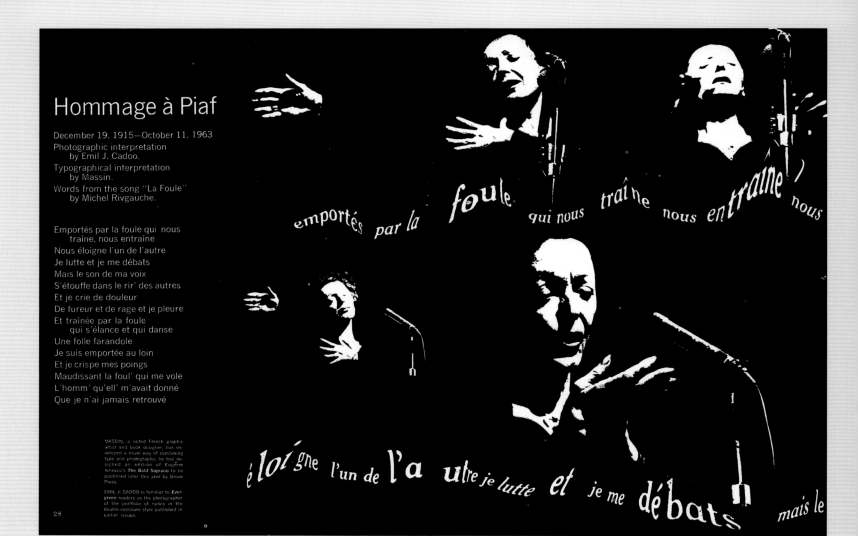

Above and opposite: final layout of
La Foule (Evergreen Review, New York,
Grove Press, 1965), a typographic
interpretation of the song by Édith Piaf,
with photographic interpretations
by Emil Cadoo.

do with its original function. Throughout his many experiments he never used a laboratory specializing in innovatory materials or special printing processes, as would almost certainly be the case today. The cutting and pasting of *La Foule* displays a low-tech ingenuity, almost akin to found art, that is full of humour and a long way from the formal, de-personalized experiments carried out on a computer.

'I'm quite pleased with this experiment, which demanded a lot of effort on my part, because I managed to resolve a great many problems while I was making it. The approach I used and which is my own invention doesn't, as you might think, involve any optical distortions as in *The Bald Soprano*', says Massin.[33] Once photographed, the letters were stuck on to paper, to recompose words and phrases. In his preparatory drawings, annotated with coefficients for the enlargement of the characters, Massin indicates the specific distortion of certain syllables, which the singer draws out. 'The typography must certainly follow an undulating movement

dominated by a strong beat (the tempo of the waltz) that is clearly marked. However that doesn't mean eliminating the breaks in diction, which may be deliberate or required for breathing (taking a breath)', he explains.[34]

Through their obvious faults, the handmade collages make it possible to evoke the rasping grain of Piaf's voice while respecting the melodic line of the song. This typographical exercise also honours the spirit of the musical genre through a more direct equivalence between the aesthetics of the photographic visuals and the words of *La Foule*. This Baudelairean approach to synaesthetic correspondence (photographs of the singer in concert allied with lyrics of the song) seems easier for the reader to grasp than that adopted in *Pierrot lunaire*, with its essentially referential background of images from paintings.

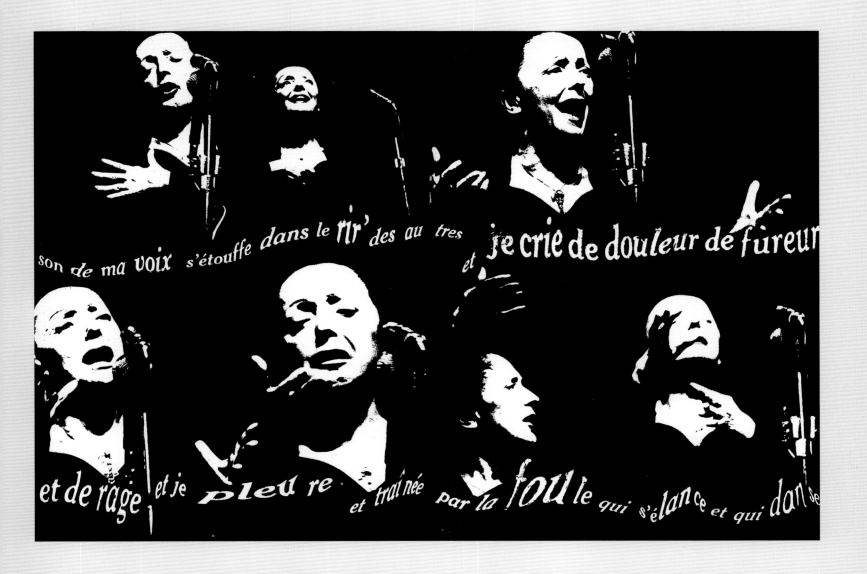

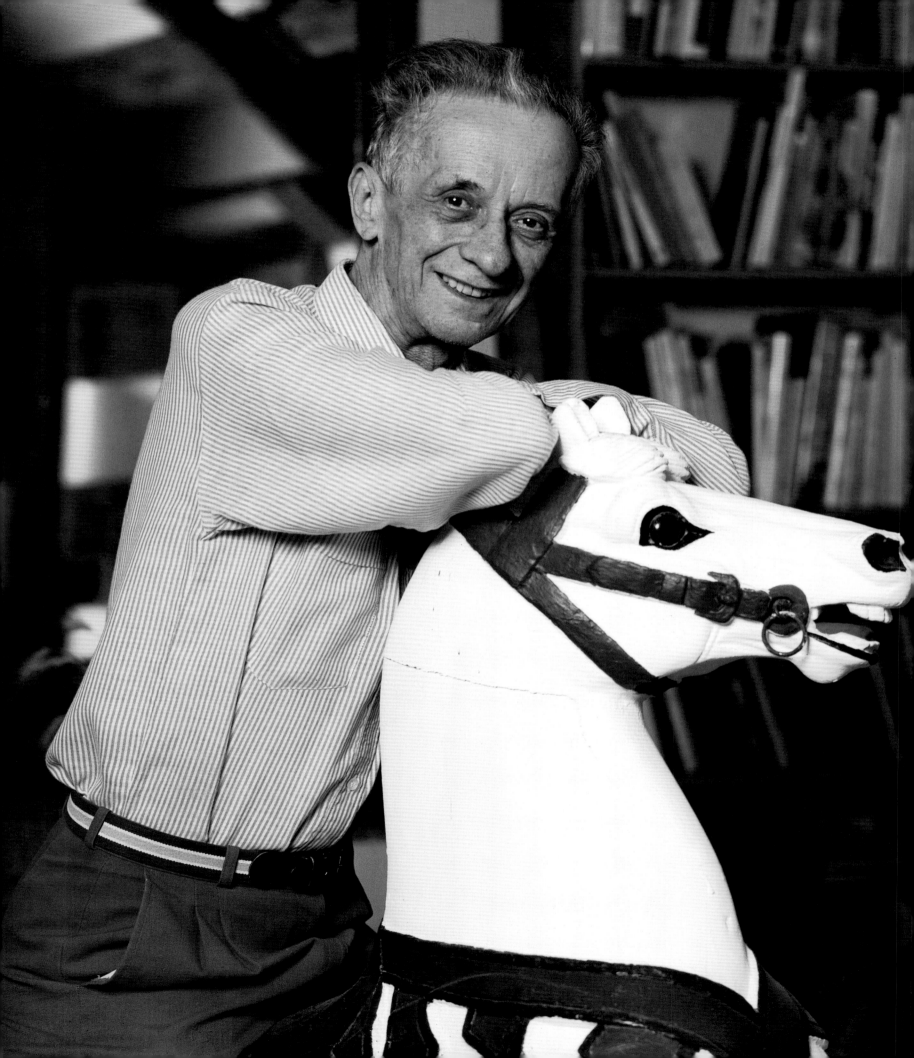

The House in Étampes

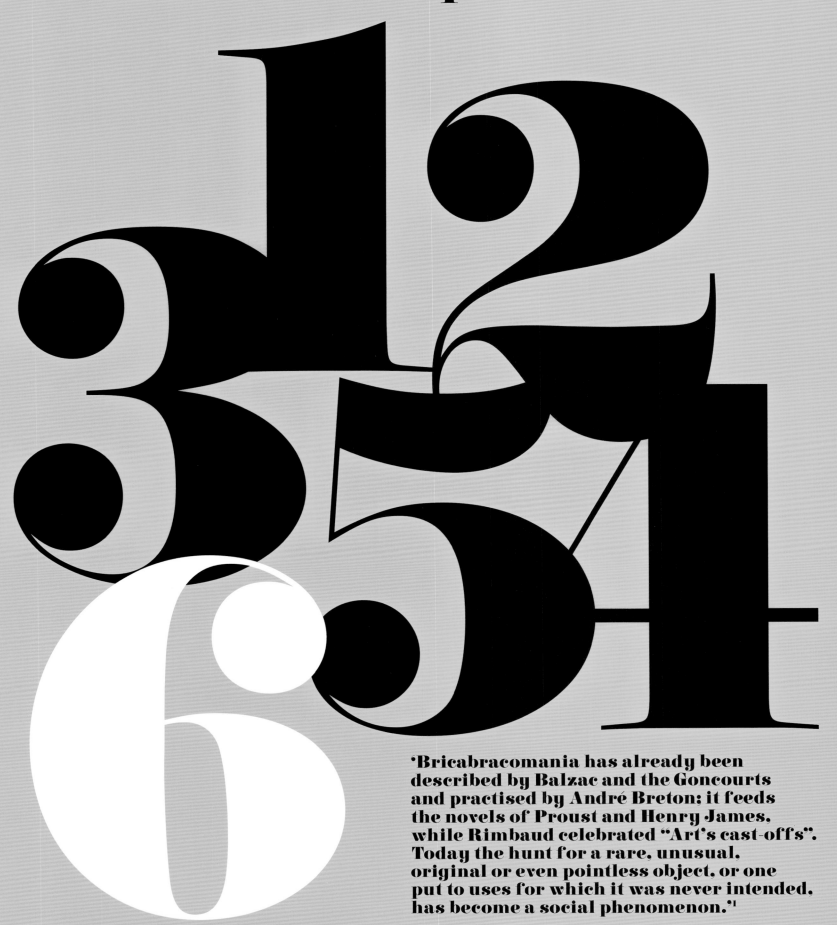

1 2 3 4 5 6

'Bricabracomania has already been described by Balzac and the Goncourts and practised by André Breton: it feeds the novels of Proust and Henry James, while Rimbaud celebrated "Art's cast-offs". Today the hunt for a rare, unusual, original or even pointless object, or one put to uses for which it was never intended, has become a social phenomenon.'[1]

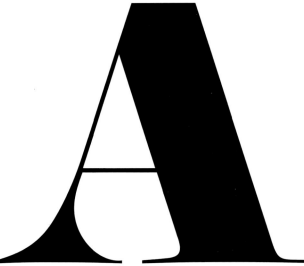

museum of personal history

'Pierrefitte', Massin's house in Étampes, located fifty kilometres south of Paris in the Essonne region, is a kind of magic mirror, an invented museum of his childhood, the secret store of a graphic imagination inspired by popular culture.

Bought as a second home in 1960, the house, which acts as a weekend studio, now contains all the books Massin has created or whose covers he has designed. His own collection is separate from the fonds Massin, the official archive housed since 1997 in the médiathèque l'Apostrophe in Chartres under the auspices of the city authorities. Massin was heavily involved in the establishment of the fonds Massin, for which he compiled his own *catalogue raisonné*. It is a cultural tie for this child of what he fondly calls the '*Beau-ce*' ('beautiful-this' – a play on the name of the Beauce region, south of Paris).[2]

The walls of the Étampes house, its every shelf and the stacks of paper it contains, all tell of Massin's lifelong passion for the alphabet – and more precisely for animated letters – and of his interest in popular forms of expression of all kinds. He shared this passion with his wife Huguette (now deceased), who loved secondhand shops and was fascinated by 1925, the year of Massin's birth. The 'year 1925' collection, housed primarily in the main room of their Montparnasse apartment and comprising a mix of curiosities, cellulose dolls, Tiffany-style flasks, extravagant hats and lamé dresses, is supplemented by a variety of objects scattered here and there in the house in Étampes. This magical place is filled with history – Massin's own, that of his family, of his past and the one he has reconstructed in a real museum of personal history.

In this Ali Baba's cave of a house, containing around 2,000 unusual and lovingly collected objects, reading and writing provide two paradigms for an understanding of both the place itself and Massin's relationship to the past. Reading is a crucial activity for this artist of graphic design skilled in depiction and revelation; reading and writing are the tools of the journal writer; children's books revisited by the adult reader are read and reread. Massin writes for the pleasure of commenting on what he has read and, through this activity, to remember and relive the sensations of yesteryear that this house evokes and arouses.

The eventful history of this former farmhouse has generated a wealth of vivid memories and has passed into local legend. When Massin bought it the place was in a pitiful state. The former owner had transformed it – literally – into a hen house, using it to raise 5,000 chickens until his neighbours finally had him evicted, after which it became a haunt for drug

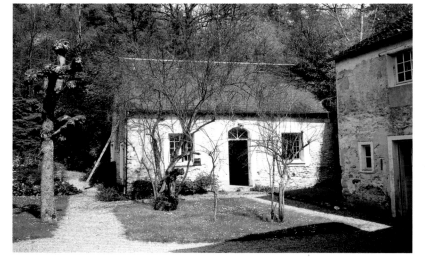

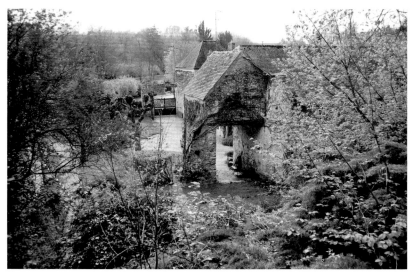

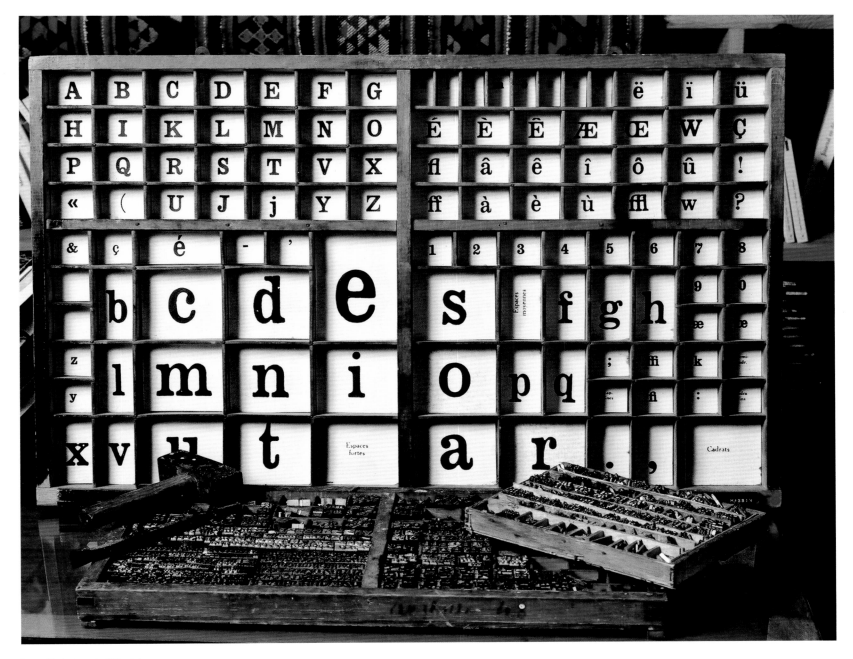

Page 166: photograph of Massin by
Louis Monier at his house in Étampes,
April 2005. All photographs in this
chapter were taken by Louis Monier.

Opposite: 'Pierrefitte', Massin's house
in Étampes.

Above: a case of printer's type in
Massin's studio, twentieth century.

Below, top to bottom: side table with a collection of ashtrays; collection of boxes, both early twentieth century.

Opposite: side tables with various collections: ashtrays and bookmarks; a shoemaker's sign turned into a lamp; skeins of yarn; a marble lion sculpted by Massin's father, surrounded by baskets and everyday images, late nineteenth and early twentieth century.

addicts. But its more distant past was far more glorious: the farm was a post house for stage coaches in the late eighteenth century and, in 1921, became an inn whose restaurant ranked as one of the finest in the Île-de-France. In the 1930s it became the favourite restaurant of Parisian celebrities, where the Folies-Bergère entertainer Mistinguett, singer Maurice Chevalier and painter Léonard Foujita would come to have their Sunday lunch.

Over the years the four buildings surrounding the central courtyard have been renovated. One houses Massin's studio on the first floor, as well as a library; another has two further libraries and a room formerly used as a darkroom; the third contains his daughters' bedrooms; while the main building comprises the kitchen, living room and Massin's own bedroom, 'the number one master bedroom'.[3] Objects have invaded every available surface in the place and a charming, calculated disorder has arisen in which items are combined in unusual ways and treated as antiques rather than museum pieces. There is not a wall that does not have a picture on it, not a mantelpiece without its row of statuettes and other ornaments, not a side table that is not covered in an orderly display of snuff boxes or animal-shaped ashtrays, not the slightest nook which does not have its store of broken puppets, skittles with their original packaging or rusty weather-vanes. Massin explains, 'In principle I never move them, they are part of an immutable set design. A cleaning lady would never understand that one object must be out of line in terms of symmetry and another deliberately placed awry'.[4] In this impromptu yet carefully planned set design, the nostalgic world of childhood coexists with the three-dimensional *mondo materialis* of the collector and graphic artist.

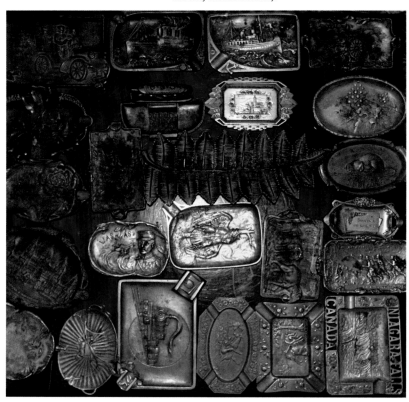

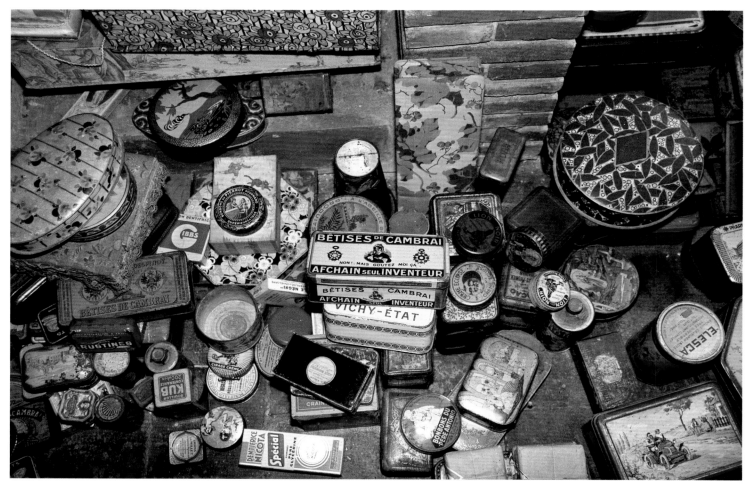

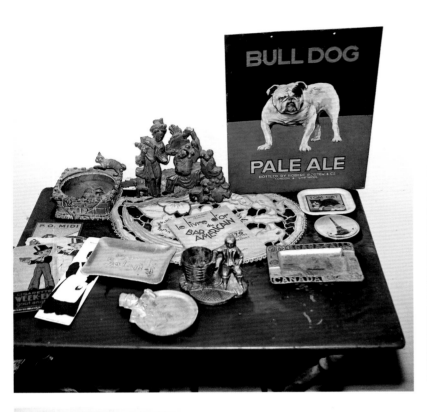

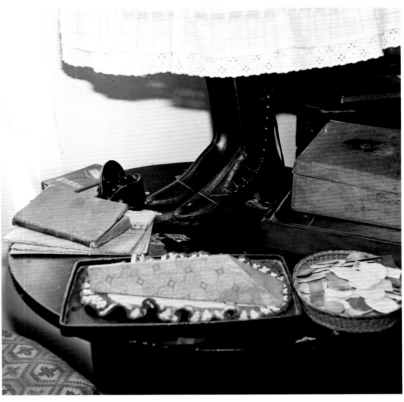

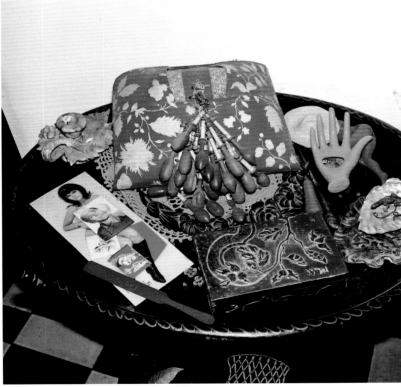

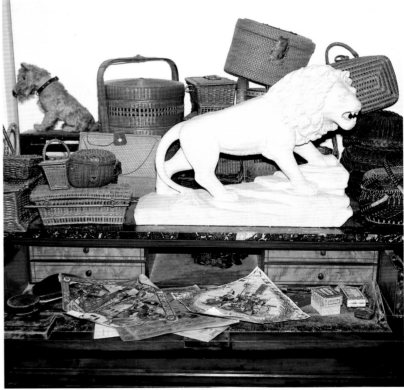

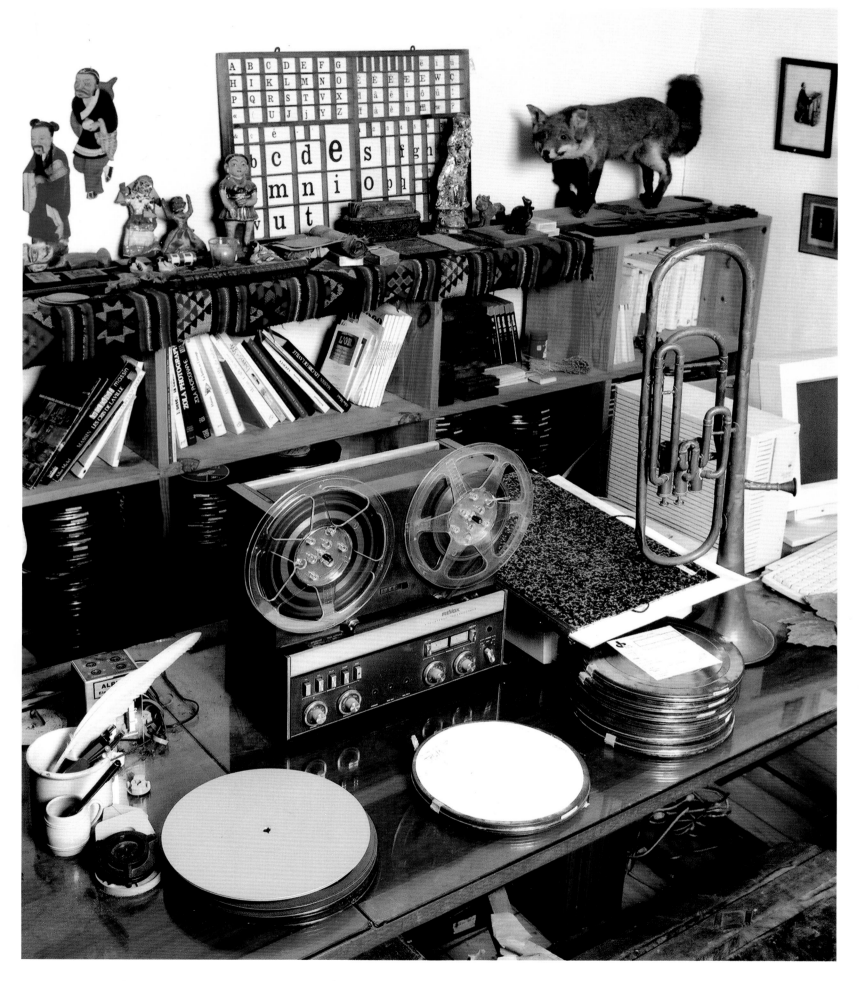

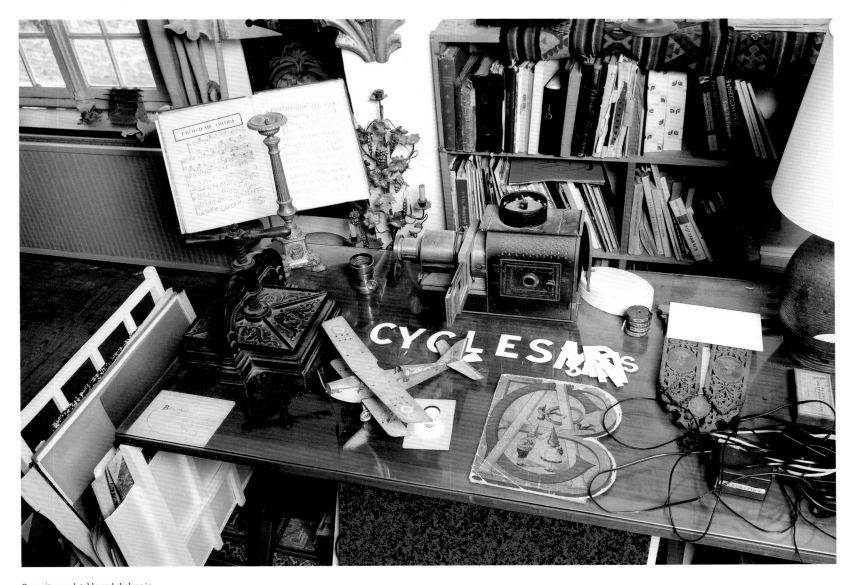

Opposite: work table and shelves in the studio, on which are stored some 2,000 kilometres of music tapes recorded since 1970.

Above: the work table in the studio notably features an English reading primer in the shape of a letter 'B', dating from 1880, an eighteenth-century hand-written score by Couperin and the magic lantern that belonged to Massin's father, Henri Massin.

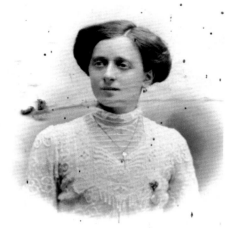

Left: photograph of Massin's mother Palmyre Massin (née Foiret), c.1910.

Below, top to bottom: Robert Massin's exercise books, 1930s; various drawings and layouts by Massin as a child, 1930s; handwritten draft of a play, 1942–3.

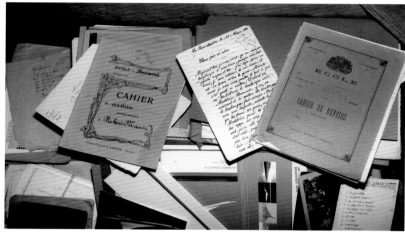

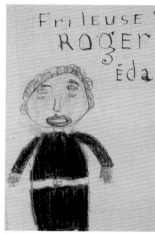

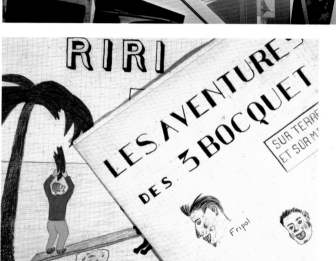

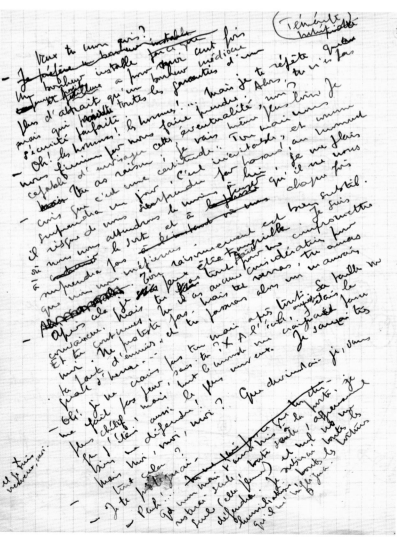

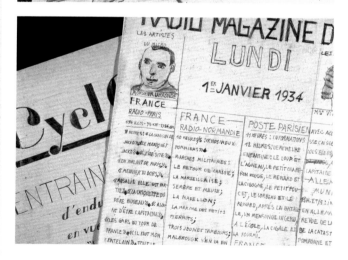

Preserving and reinventing a child-like vision

Although Massin grew up in the Beauce – in Chartres itself and the surrounding area – he has not inherited a family home in any real sense. So 'Pierrefitte' has become a reconstruction of the world he saw as a child. It contains not only writings and drawings from his own childhood, but also all the old books and objects that he has acquired down the years and which were or could have been part of his graphic world in the 1920s and 30s. Just as people remember events that happened in their childhood from photographs they have seen in the family album, so Massin remembers his past through objects – rewriting, analysing and reliving it by immersing himself in the things he read as a child.

In an antique shop in Montlhéry, on the road from Paris to Étampes, he found his primary-school reading primer – a book he often credits for sparking his interest in typography and layout.[5] It is hard to believe that the reading matter of this day-dreamer, the son of a primary-school teacher, consisted mainly of school text books; but he admits, 'I spent most of my time looking at my alphabet book, and later primary-school reading books such as *Line et Pierrot* and *Jeannot et Jeannette*. I was fascinated by their layout, illustrations, engravings and lithographs and the calligraphic writing with bold and thin type. I became passionate for written letters very early and I understood the direct link between the writing and the content.'[6]

The young Robert Massin's illustrated books and handwriting books, with their covers of pink, absorbent paper and flowery art nouveau borders, have been carefully preserved in trunks, partly thanks to his father's curatorial instinct. Massin explains, 'Any old drawing done on the back of an electoral notice or a cake box, the slightest bit of paper I'd scribbled something on, he'd date it on the back and classify it all. He was so fond of me that he kept everything and organized it'.[7] So the treasures in the collection of his personal museum range from books of poems in alexandrines, which he never showed to anyone, to lists of the records he played on his phonograph, calligraphic exercises (sometimes in German blackletter), collages and paper folding with borrowings from commercial layouts, geographical maps of the region with captions commemorating the German attack on his native village, La Bourdinière, in 1940, and even little illustrated books, handmade and bound. When asked about the first books he made he replies, 'I was around seven when I made my first books. Because

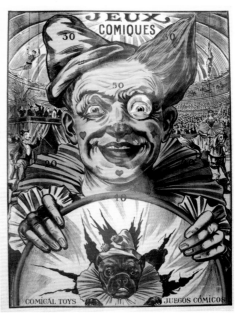

Left to right: board for the game 'Les mystères de Paris', nineteenth century; lid for 'Jeux comiques' games box, second half of the nineteenth century.

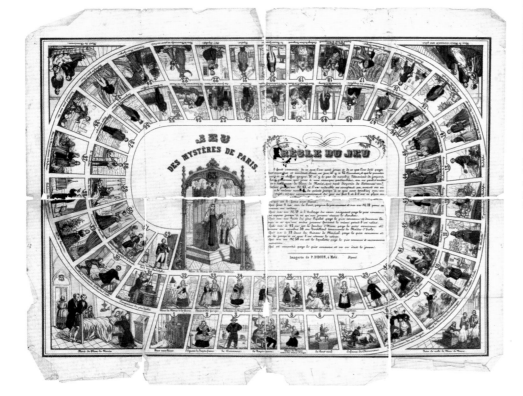

I'd seen it in books I used to sign my own works "Robert Massin, author, photographer, bookseller". I acquired a liking for making books – a kind of premonition – at a very young age. I was inspired by newspaper headlines, radio schedules, commercial catalogues, notices and the postal calendars that I saw in my grandmother's café and grocery shop in La Frileuse. I used to draw the illustrations and tell stories.'[8] His early illustrated writings also reflect his enthusiasm for the Tour de France and the radio. He remembers, 'I used to listen to the wireless every day, at 4 p.m., the arrival time. I used to go to the other end of the village to buy *Le Miroir des sports* (The sporting mirror), a publication produced by photogravure, a remarkable monochrome printing process, then I would write radio reports, with illustrations of racing cyclists'.[9]

In *L'ABC du metier* (The ABC of the profession) and his many memoirs and journals, Massin tells his own story and, in so doing, reveals a sensitive person who relives his life through the memory of the objects around him, the smells and colours associated with them, even the creaking of the house and the music of the period. Sometimes the graphic translation of music becomes more important than the music itself: old polka scores and songs from the 1930s are preserved for their typography, just as he chose his books in the school library according to the eminently mysterious words '*de l'Académie Française*' (of the Académie Française) after the author's name, because these words fired his imagination. So he blurs the boundaries between reality and imagination, between the memory of his past and the endless reconstruction of a distant memory. 'I love to remember; I live in the past, not in the present.'[10]

The visual culture of the boy Massin in La Bourdinière, a village in the rural Beauce, consisted primarily of banal commercial printed matter. It was almost certainly less book-based than that of an urban child, since he did not have everyday access to bookshops. And although he read all the classics in the library of the school where his mother taught, his early interest in layout was nurtured mainly through the almanacs that his father received, such as the popular *Almanach Vermot*, a well-known compilation of puns and recipes full of rural humour, and the *Almanach du combattant*, a conservative annual launched in 1922 to uphold veterans' rights, full of heroic war stories and satirical strip cartoons. He also read the illustrated children's magazine *Benjamin*, to which he subscribed; reviews and magazines such as *Miroir du monde*, a general interest, news-based illustrated weekly of the 1930s; and the patriotic weekly *L'Illustration*, the most prestigious and widely read periodical during World War I, known for its large format, high-quality printing and striking black and white photographs of war scenes. All these publications, richly illustrated with drawings and photographs, were an early source of visual influence on the young Massin. He was particularly inspired by the imaginary world of *Lectures pour tous* (Reading for all), a weekly of the 1920s which he 'read through in all directions, reading and re-reading little tales, comic sketches, personal stories, news features, all accompanied by images, chopped initials and vignettes in the art deco style.'[11]

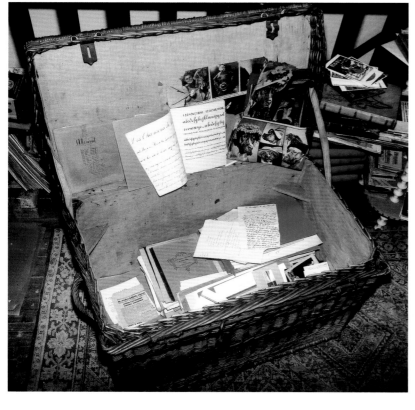

Left: wicker basket in the room adjoining the studio containing childhood souvenirs, exercise books, press cuttings and a variety of documents.

Opposite: cellulose mannequins, 1930s and 50s, posters by Massin and his colleagues and a late-nineteenth century pram, in the room adjoining the studio.

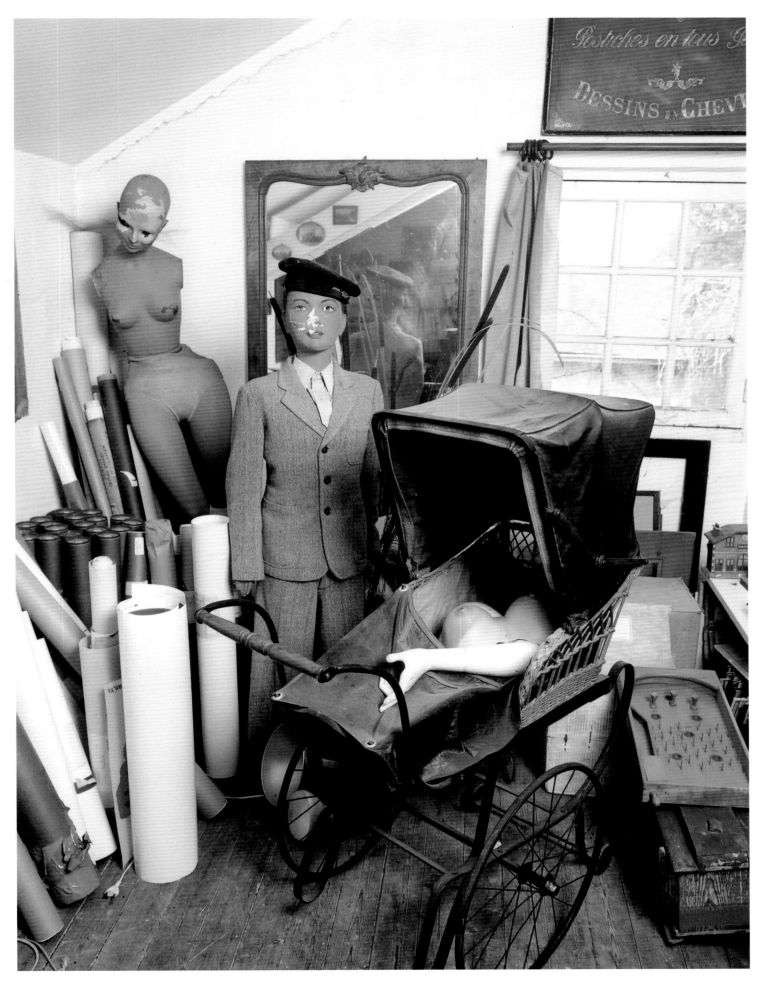

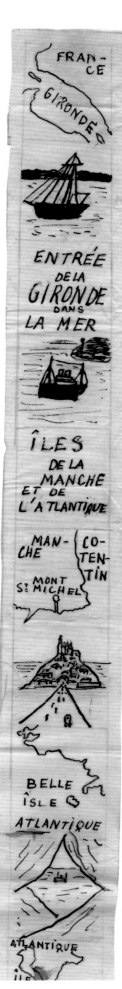

Top to bottom, left to right: drawing of the Gironde by Massin, c.1930; book of poems, 1937; notebook containing a list of his getting-up times, a truly Proustian exercise, 1941.

It is almost surprising that Massin should have orientated his career towards books rather than art direction in the generalist press. He turned seventy before contributing to the Strasburg review *Les Saisons d'Alsace* (Alsace seasons), for which he created the standard layout when it changed format in 1998. All the same it was the popular press that acted as the catalyst for the young Massin's professional ambitions. He recalls, 'I had read over three hundred pieces in *La Petite Illustration* and closely followed its theatrical supplement, which offered subscribers a twenty-four-page booklet with photos and reviews of plays'.[12] He began working as a journalist, writing columns about music hall and the circus for the newspaper *Gavroche* and notes on plays and other cultural news in Paris for *Le Populaire*.

His sensibility frequently expressed itself through associations of ideas. He has often described the graphic world of his grandmother's general grocery store in the village of La Frileuse (with its enamelled advertising panels, packaging and promotional leaflets) but, as his career took off, he brought his own graphic touch to the process of remembering, his 'absolute typographic eye', his fascination with expressive lettering and the dynamic layout of words and images: 'Years later I started to collect postal calendars, and in that way, year on year, images marking out the time when I was little resurfaced in my memory. Of course I didn't think I would go back so far in

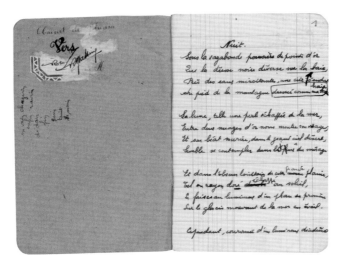

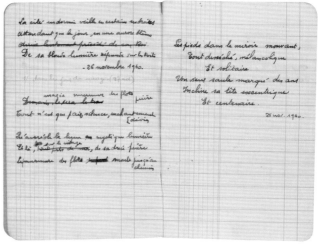

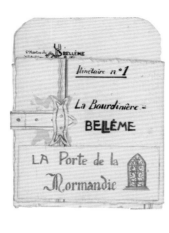

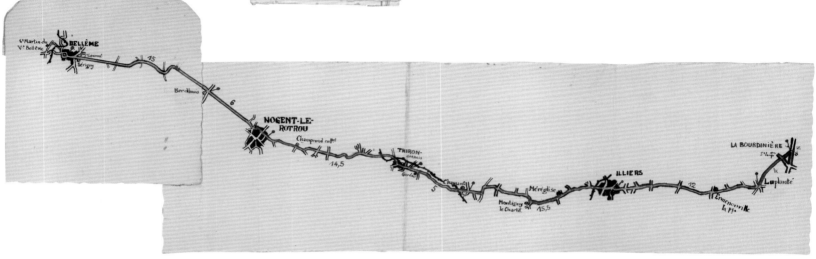

Top to bottom, left to right: drawing-cum-sleeve with a folding map illustrating the bicycle journey undertaken by Massin and his sister from La Bourdinière to Bellême (Eure-et-Loir) two months after the German bombardment of 14 June 1940, made by hand by Massin, early September 1940; letter from Massin to his sister with a plan of the German bombardment of 14 June 1940 drawn on the back, 12 July 1940.

time (the earliest pieces date from 1830).'[13] What could be more meaningful than to collect calendars, the printed object which, by definition, preserves a two-dimensional trace of the passing of time?

Massin has spoken at length about the advertisements and logos that surrounded him when he was a little boy,[14] and the house in Étampes holds archives of these printed images, whose quality is almost worthy of a museum: the kitchen shelves are filled with camembert box lids and painted metal boxes (including the famous Bouillon Kub): 'We are living in a world saturated with mass-produced objects, reproduced a thousand times by advertising and the media. Objects are the companions of our lives, whether they are designed for utilitarian purposes or simply for fun or decoration. Above and beyond relationships of possession and use, an object is a mirror, a cultural sign, a witness, a silent presence that makes up our everyday world.'[15]

In search of Ali Baba's cave

The house in Étampes is primarily a treasure store of books, a place where Massin's works are exhaustively archived, in rooms entirely lined from floor to ceiling with shelves, some double, all filled with books. 'There are around twenty themed libraries of very different sizes: club books and the 'Folio' series in my bedroom, books of literature and the humanities, history, illustrated books on art, photography, techniques in graphic art, typeface catalogues, kitsch books and so on,' he explains.[16]

Above the door to one of the rooms, cast-iron letters make the word 'LIRE' (to read). In the same part of the building the studio – where he works all weekend – also contains illustrated books (on the history of art from antiquity to the present day and books of photographs by Robert Doisneau, Jeanloup Sieff and others), collections of illustrated newspapers from the romantic period to around 1900, technical documentation (on the history of printing and graphic art and font catalogues from 1830 to 1995), not to mention around 2,000 kilometres of music tapes recorded since 1970. But Massin's world of books is far from mere decorative wallpaper: all the volumes are classified, noted in an inventory and located purely by means of visual memory. This archivist syndrome undoubtedly facilitated the preparation of the three-volume *catalogue raisonné* of his work, annotated with personal comments in the margins and written with the distance conferred by time and wisdom.

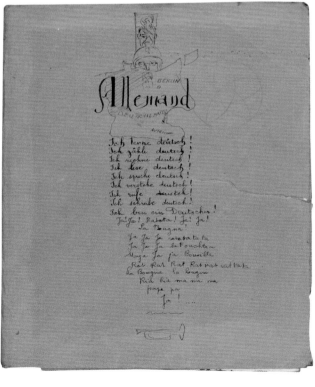

Left: cover of a German book, c.1936–7.

Opposite: map detailing the route of the exodus from La Bourdinière to the south of the Loire, just after the bombardment of June 1940, made in 1940.

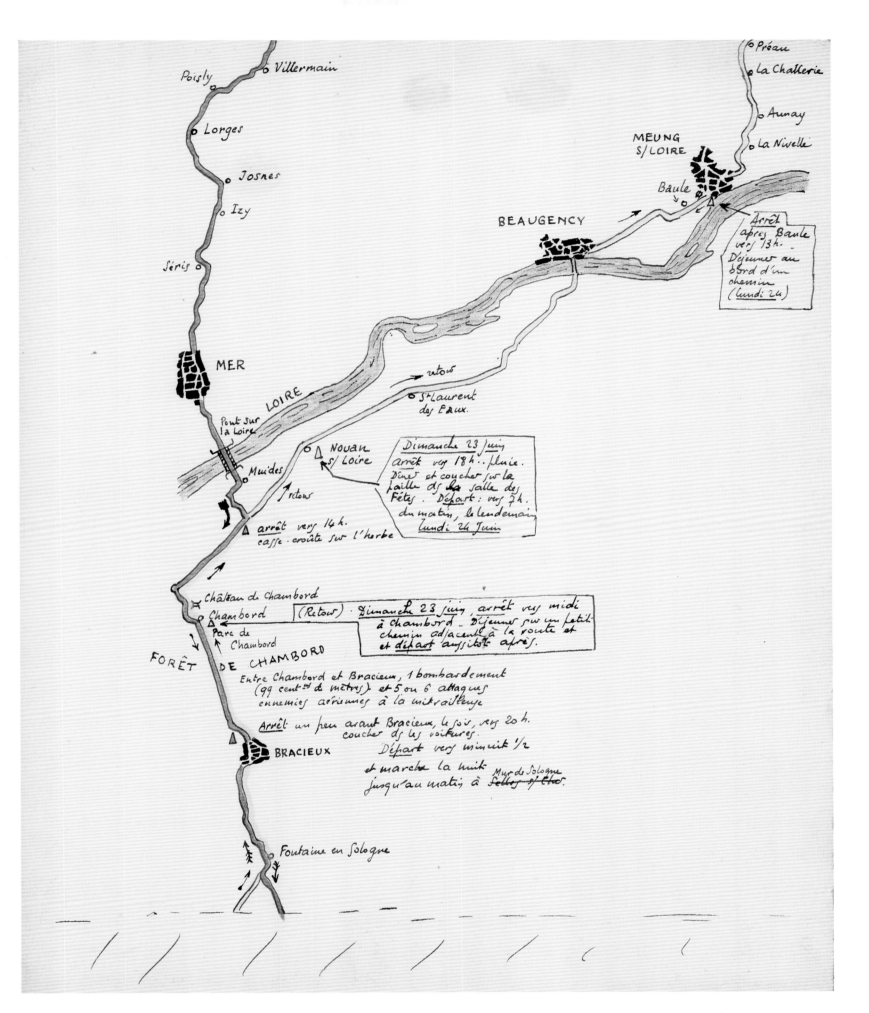

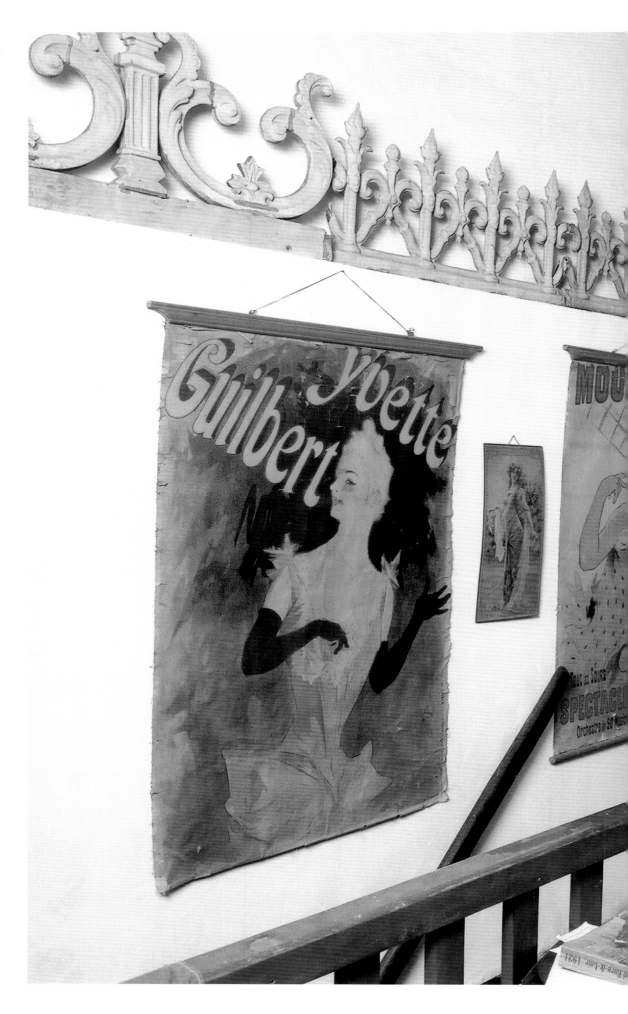

Posters by Chéret dating from the *Belle Époque* and gramophone, 1900s, on the landing leading to the studio.

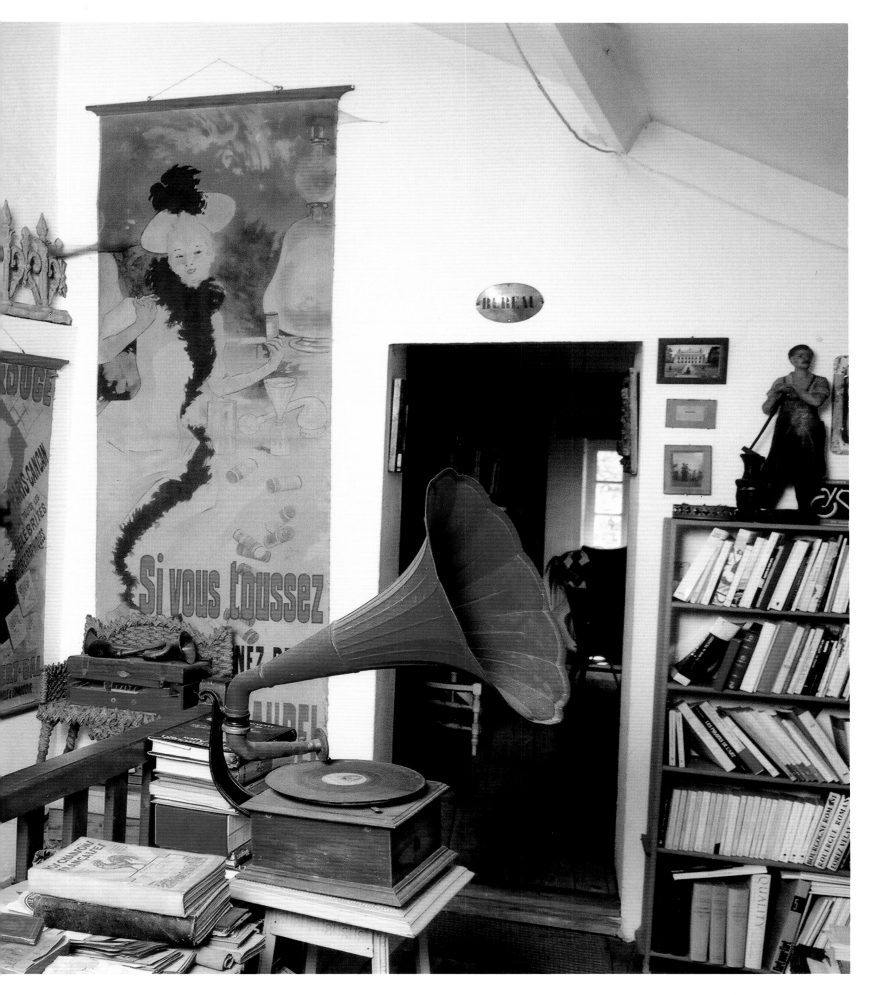

Top to bottom, left to right: covers of the monthly publication *Lectures pour tous*, 1920s; advertisement for 'Le fil au louis d'or', c.1900; 'Bitter' bottle label, 1900s.

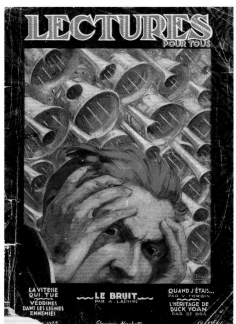

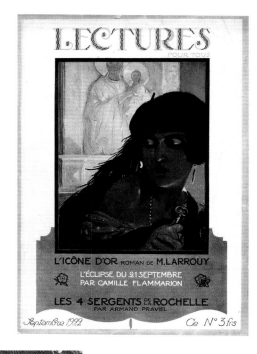

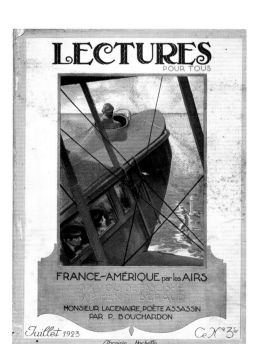

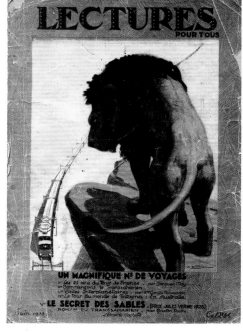

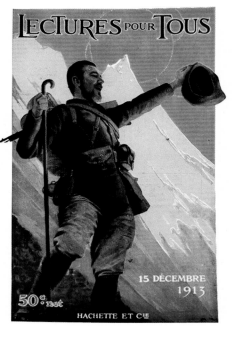

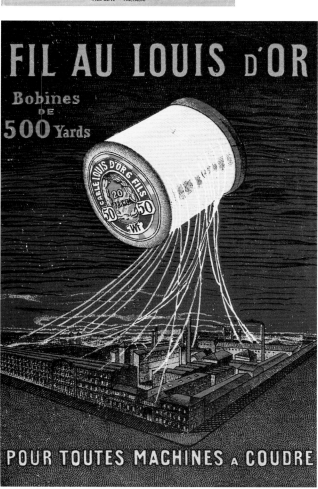

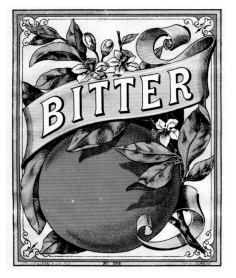

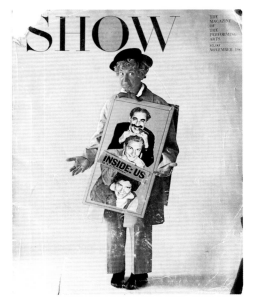

Top to bottom, left to right: covers for the magazines *Show* and *Esquire*, 1950s; headlines from newspapers (*France-Soir*, *L'Aurore*) kept by Massin for their typographical treatment of major historical events – the armistice of 8 May 1945, the death of General De Gaulle in November 1970 and the assassination of President Kennedy in 1963; calendars from *Le Petit Journal illustré*, late nineteenth century.

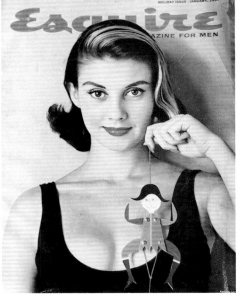

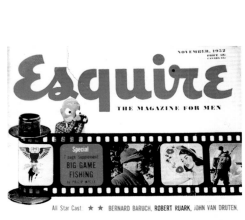

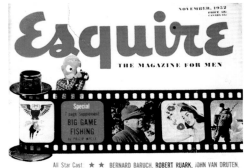

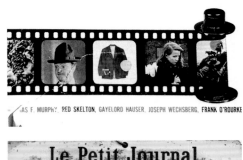

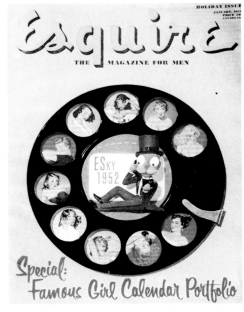

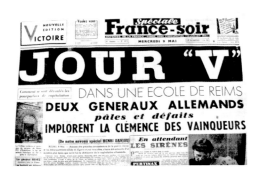

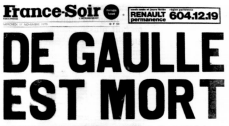

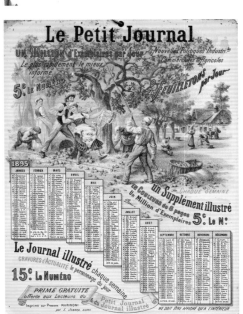

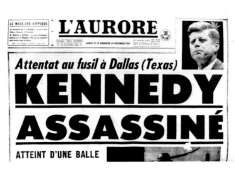

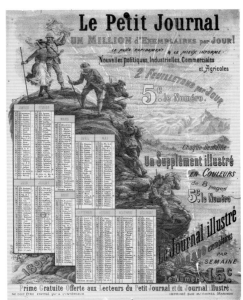

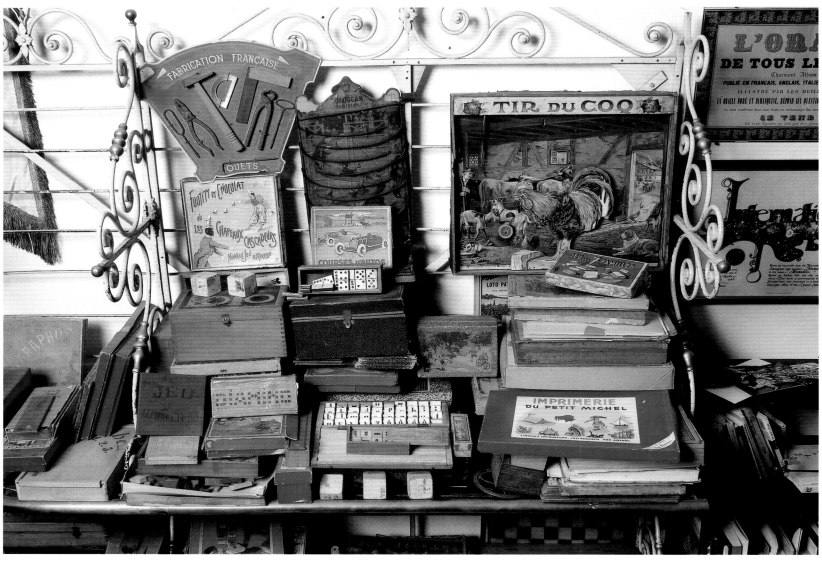

Above and right: old toys and games with their boxes, nineteenth century; reconstruction of a bar under Massin's studio.

Opposite: enamel and tin pots and stoneware bottles in the kitchen; stuffed English fighting cock, 1878.

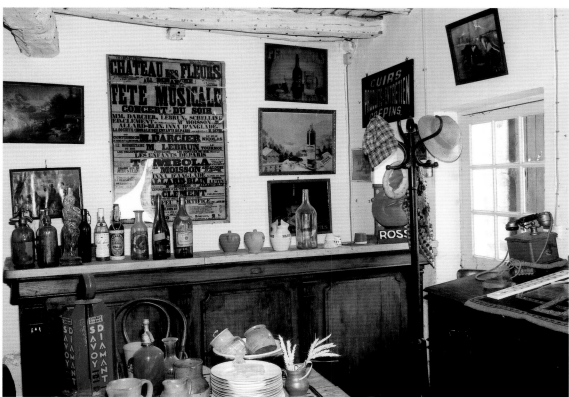

The same desire to amass and organize has led Massin to accumulate entire collections of post-war newspapers and magazines, which are now piled up in the attic or in portfolios. He has preserved the covers that inspired him at the start of his career as a young graphic artist: *Esquire* and *Harper's Bazaar* for their intelligent design, *Life Magazine* for its spectacular use of photography. As a child he had already collected and copied out newspaper headlines whose thick, bold characters announced the tragic deaths of politicians or events unleashing war, even reproducing them in his own illustrated books. As he explains, 'I began collecting newspapers when war was declared in 1939, in imitation of my mother, who used to show us in class the "historical" newspapers she had kept from the 1914–18 war, at the start of which her first husband had been killed. And I went on until the 1980s and 90s.'[17]

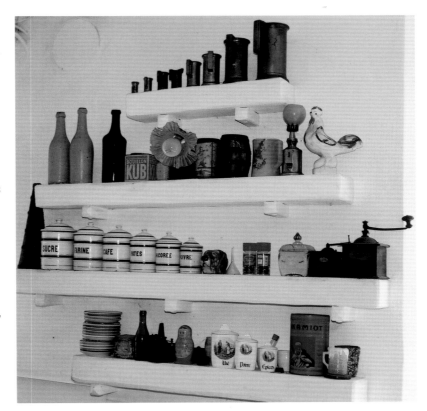

For Massin the cultural meaning of these objects is almost of a practical nature. The printed materials in particular are reproduced in his own books, either as themselves or indirectly, when one of their details or motifs has helped him to design endpapers or a cover. These objects underpin his arguments in *La Lettre et l'Image* (Paris, Gallimard, 1970), in which they appear as examples from the history of popular, expressive lettering. For instance, Marcelle Marquet's *Il était une fois* (Once upon a time), illustrated by Suza Desnoyer (Paris, L.I.E.S.A., 1952), which appears in *La Lettre et l'Image*, can be seen in his studio. Local authority notices and posters for public auctions, coloured like the posters for Bastille Day dances, inspired the decoration and choice of bold fonts for the titles of *Les Mariés de la tour Eiffel* (Paris, Hoëbeke, 1994). In addition, some of the typographical designs of these notices have more than once influenced the covers of club books, such as Cendrars' *L'Or* (Paris, Club du meilleur livre, 1956).

The boundary between collecting for its own sake and the re-use of objects in graphic designs for books seems to have become gradually blurred as the collection grew. Even if the plethora of everyday printed matter still available in the secondhand shops of the 1950s and 60s helped him create *La Lettre et l'Image*, it is hard to tell whether this research led Massin to acquire more catalogues of specimens of printing and children's alphabets or whether it was in accumulating these books that he had the idea of producing an encyclopaedic work. Massin himself confides, 'Now I usually confine myself to photographing posters and signs in the street',[18] and regularly adds

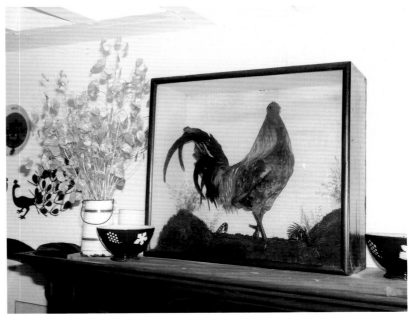

Following two pages: Camembert box lids, c.1895.

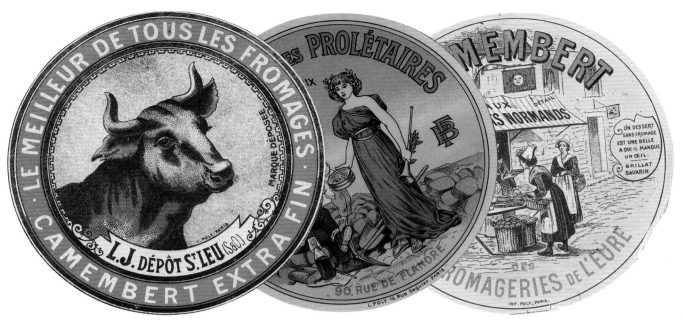

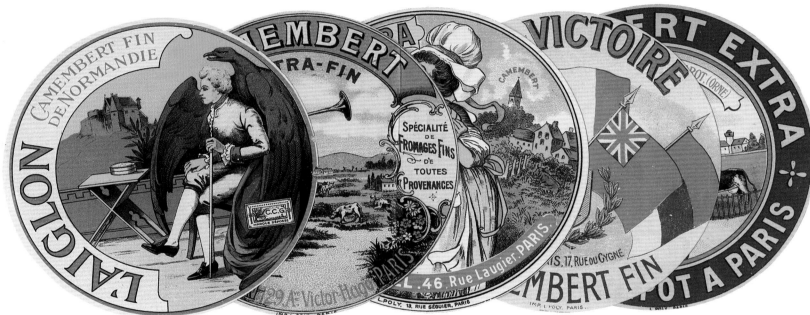

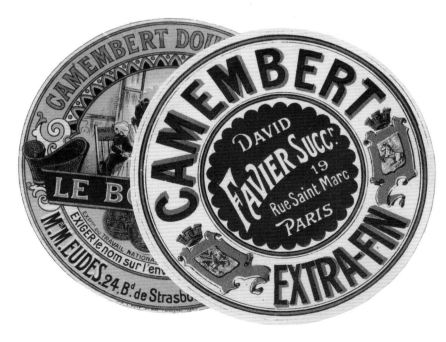

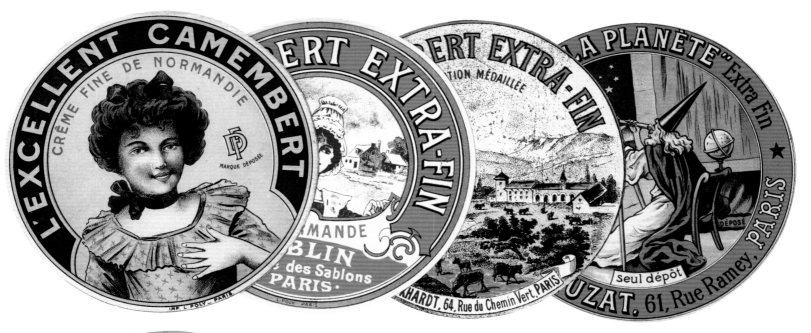

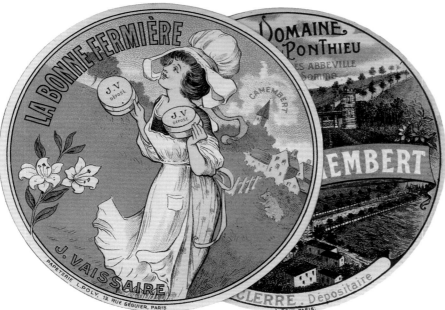

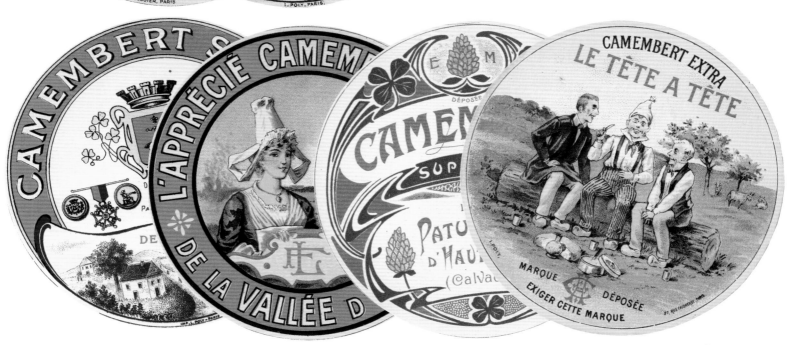

new examples of expressive typography to new editions of the book. Similarly it is hard to tell whether his collection of the monthly *Lecture pour tous* has been kept since his childhood or whether he has put it together retrospectively during his adult life for the benefit of his typographic collection. Memory has the power of resurrection: like Proust's famous little madeleine, the coincidence of a sensation in the present and the memory of that sensation brings a whole world of vanished faces, places and objects back to life.

In this respect the book project Massin is currently working on, provisionally entitled *La Curiosité* (Curiosity), is a truly Proustian enterprise. An exhaustive summation of the strange objects that surround him, this book almost certainly represents the first real meeting between reality and imagination, past and present. A magazine-book, it is a celebration and first inventory of his own collection. No longer using the objects in the house to illustrate a text, nor including them in a graphic project, the aim is to show them for what they are. Massin admits, 'I made this book for three reasons: in homage to my wife, with remorse for having sometimes met her best finds with feigned indifference; as an inventory in images which could be used for insurance purposes if something bad happened; and as an overview of my life, one of those overviews you feel like making when you get to the end of your time (let's not get ahead of ourselves!). In my view, nothing like the other books.'[19]

The classification of these posters, magazines, newspapers, educational toys, calendars, postcards, enamelled signs, signboards and notices of all kinds, from which *La Curiosité* is composed, has not been conceived with the rationality of a professional archivist or museum curator, even though the size of the collection indicates that it would be perfectly possible to set up a museum of everyday printed materials in Massin's house. The process of classifying this unusual collection has made it possible to stress at least one point: the evocative power of objects. The common denominator of all the objects Massin keeps at 'Pierrefitte' 'is that they have been handmade and remain representatives of a life that was also mine in a different time; in short, an attempt to struggle against death', he observes.[20] To this extent *La Curiosité* is a testament to his creative methodology of allowing himself to be inspired by objects, their colour, smell, graphics and cultural resonance all at once. Massin believes in the interaction between arts and sensibilities and he always operates at the meeting point of sensory influences.

This interdisciplinary approach moreover lies at the heart of the historical novels he has written, such as *Le Branle des voleurs* (The robbers' swing) and *Les Compagnons de la marjolaine* (published by La Table Ronde in 1983 and 1985, respectively), in which cultural history is combined with the history of graphics and his own imagination. But it is in socio-cultural essays such as *Les Cris de la ville, commerces ambulants et petits métiers de la rue* (Cries of the city, itinerant and street traders; Paris, Gallimard, 1978; Albin Michel, 1985) that Massin really demonstrates a synthetic approach that combines acquired, intellectual knowledge with a sensory understanding

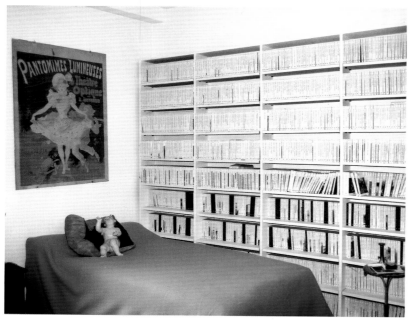

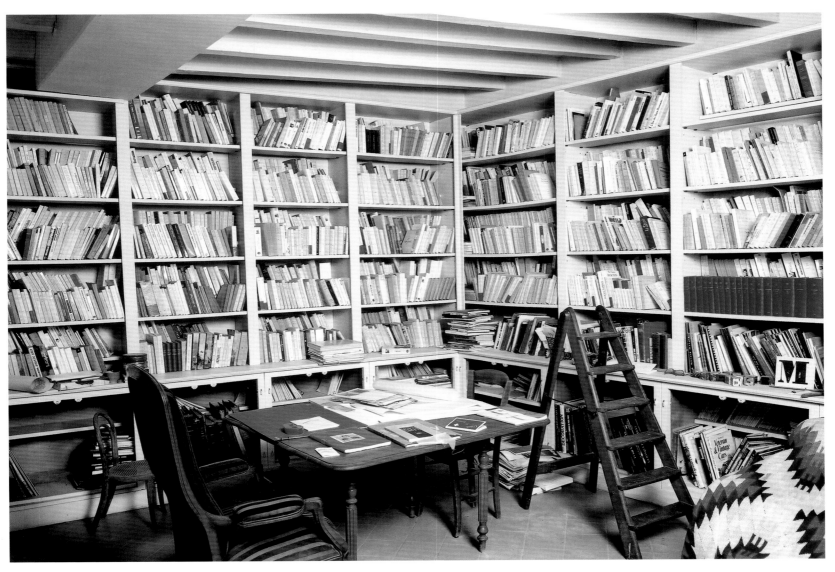

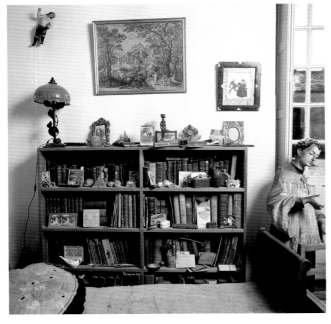

Opposite: bookshelves in Massin's bedroom containing all the books in the 'Soleil' series (Paris, Gallimard), other books published in the days of the book clubs and at the start of his career, and his complete 'Folio' collection (Paris, Gallimard).

Top to bottom: bookshelves in the annexe with several double rows of books created for Gallimard and other publishers; various other bookshelves.

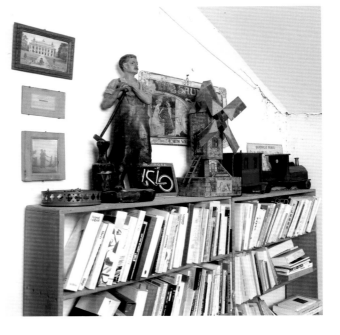

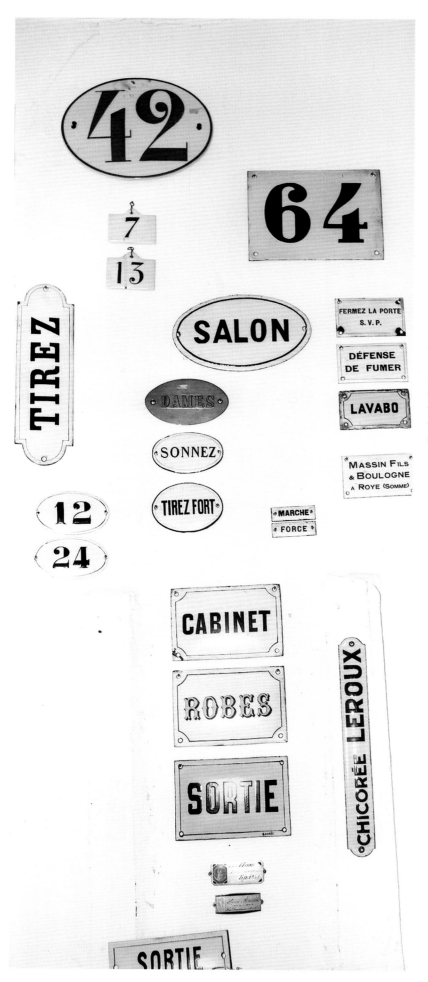

of the objects he has found while wandering through flea markets. The protagonists of the 'New History', which flourished during the 1970s with the trend for the social sciences, neglected the phenomenon of street criers – 'the cries sometimes taking the form of a tune or a song, which itinerant traders have sung out in the streets since antiquity and which you find in every city in the world'.[21] But it was a subject seized on by Massin. To assist him in his writing, his style and his responsive understanding of the subject, he combined a compilation of historical facts with the acquisition of medieval woodcuts, nineteenth-century lithographs of a basket-seller taken from *Petites Industries de Paris* (Cottage industries in Paris), eighteenth-century engravings and other popular images illustrating the lives of small-scale travelling traders. His collections of playing cards also provide classifications by trade. Massin drew heavily on these for *Les Cris de la ville*: 'I had already listened to *Les Cris de Paris* by the composer Clément Janequin, and I had looked at *La Comédie de notre temps* by Bertall (an artist almost as well-known as Honoré Daumier): his illustrations showed the costume for each trade. Every crier had their own tune to sell their products in the street – in practice, to sell to illiterate buyers. I was inspired by all this for *Les Cris*. It's a book at the intersection of the visual arts, music, cultural history and all the things I'm interested in exploring.'[22]

In this cabinet of curiosities, where letter and image meet and complement each other, Massin's fascination with rare objects is quite simply 'a reaction against the civilization of production and consumption, a distant sequel to the industrial revolution which, in the nineteenth century, deprived once handmade objects of their souls'.[23] While Massin's ultimate goal is to enjoy the resurgence of memory, his relation to writing is very similar to his relations with objects: both are symbols of a time that is past, but still imaginable.

Opposite: enamelled plates hanging in the corridor of the main building, reflecting Massin's passion for the typography of everyday objects, nineteenth and twentieth centuries.

Top to bottom, left to right: collection of objects, posters, signs and pictures made of hair, a nineteenth-century genre collected by Massin's wife, Huguette Massin.

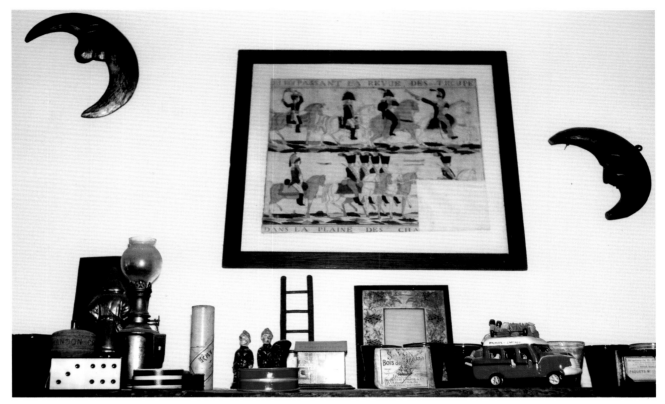

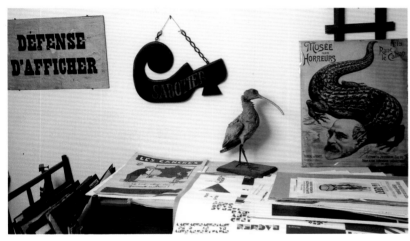

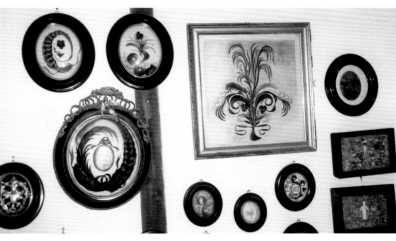

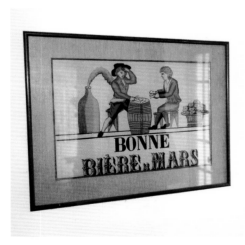

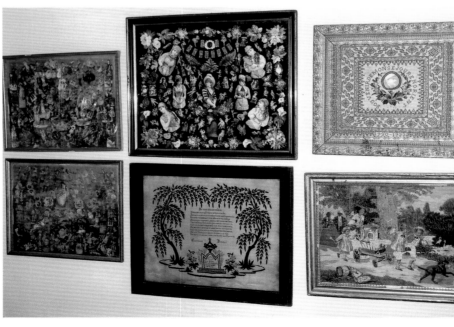

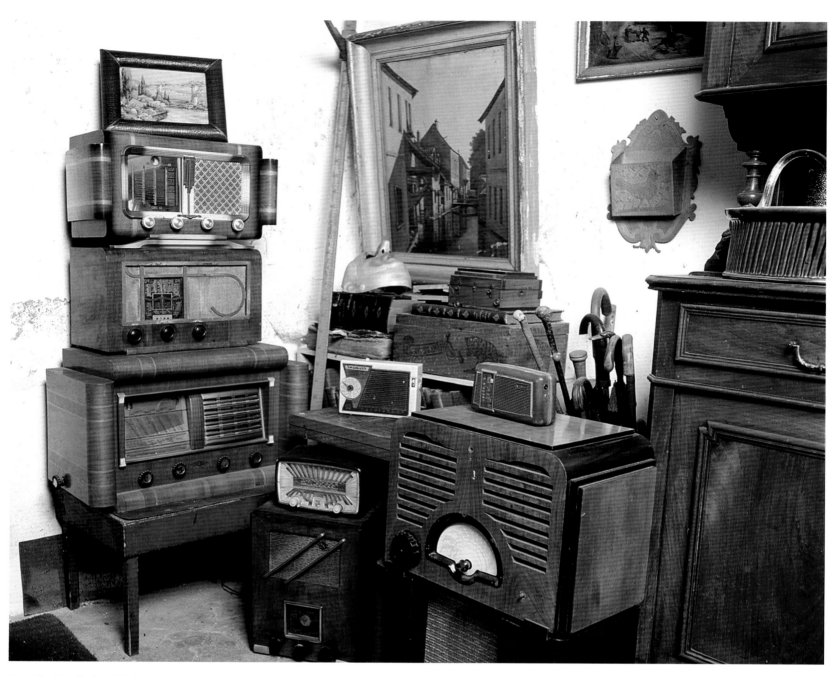

Above: Massin's collection of wireless sets, in the bar room, 1920s to 1950s.

'Proust': a book in homage to the master

Massin's many (re)readings of Marcel Proust's À la recherche du temps perdu (Remembrance of Things Past) gave him the idea for a book of literary origins, which could be seen as a personal homage to Proust. This 500-page book, printed as a unique edition (dated 1 March 1997), is bound in cork - a reference to the cork panels lining the walls and ceiling of Proust's bedroom at 102, boulevard Haussmann, Paris. The book presents Proust's correspondence and, in parallel, drafts and other versions of the printed text, including Massin's favourite passages, with notes in the margins; cultural references to the period when the book was written; extracts from correspondence relating to that period, from Proust himself and other writers, philosophers and critics (such as Henri Bergson and Jules Renard); and illustrations. 'I think I identify with

Proust, with the way he feels the world so directly. There's definitely a Balzacian side to Proust, but the sensation of the nothings which he makes into mountains by giving them extraordinary importance is fascinating. Every time I read him again I discover something new.'[24]

And the hypertext structure of the book (combining texts arranged on one page with parallels established between the main text, inserts and captions, offering a non-sequential reading) is the perfect reflection of his own creative process: Massin operates through associations of ideas and often by intuition, calling on successive, parallel layers of influences and constructing a time in which objects are a pretext for exploring memories and imagination.

Below: leather binding with cork inlay,
endpapers and inside spread from
the Proust book made by Massin, unique
edition (1997).

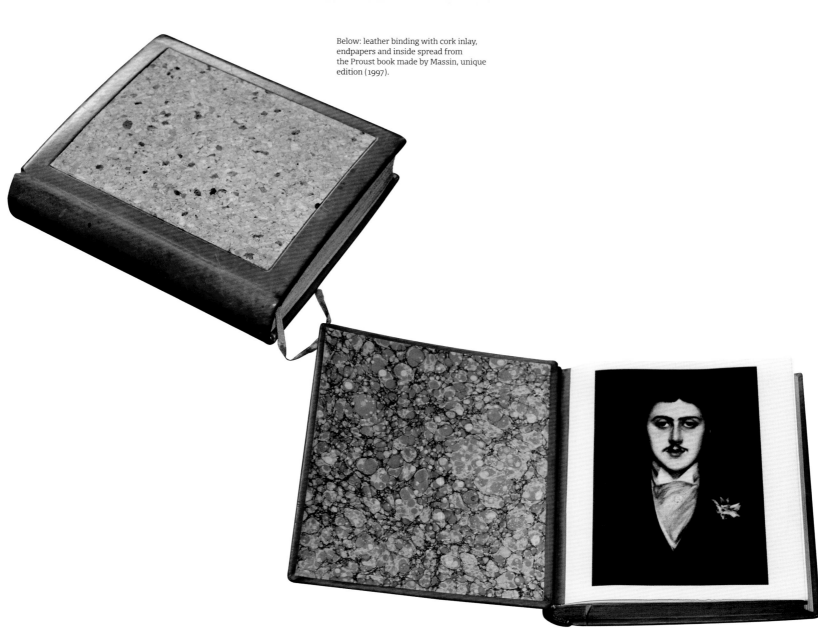

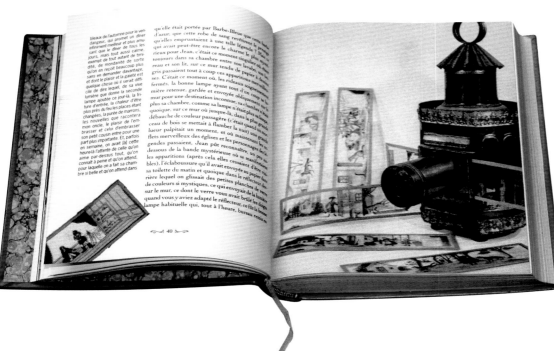

1925 Robert Massin is born at La Bourdinière, near Chartres (*département* of Eure-et-Loir), the son of Henri Massin, an engraver, sculptor and stonemason, and Palmyre Foiret, a primary school teacher.

1935– As a boy Massin creates many homemade books
1943 containing his own drawings and writings. He plays the violin and, in his teens, joins the Swingtette du Hot Club de l'Île-de-France (a jazz group modelled on the famous quintet of Django Reinhardt and Stéphane Grappelli).

1944 Leaves school and, with no technical training, becomes an author and self-taught graphic artist. Goes to Paris, intending to become a writer.

1946 As an amateur poet, becomes editor of *Proximités*, a poetry magazine whose contributors include poets Maurice Fombeure and Michel Crozier.

1946– Travels to the UK, Scandinavia and Germany.
1947 Is imprisoned for a few days in Finland by the Russians. During his travels does casual jobs of all kinds, including work as a freelance journalist.

1947 Interviews Louis-Ferdinand Céline, author of *Voyage au bout de la nuit* and other works, who is then in exile in Copenhagen.

1948 Joins the Club français du livre as editor of the monthly newsletter *Liens* (Paris).

1949 Designs his first layout, which is for Arthur Rimbaud's *Œuvres* (Paris, Club français du livre).

1951 First book cover, for William Laurence's *La Bombe H* (Paris, Corrêa).

1952 Joins the Club du meilleur livre as artistic advisor. Designs his first layout with them, for Thor Heyerdhal's *L'Expédition du Kon-Tiki* (Paris, Club du meilleur livre).

1956 Buys a Rolleiflex 2.8. Begins his photographic work.

1957 Freelance graphic designer of the 'Soleil' series for Gallimard (Paris).

1958 Designs record albums for the Club des disquaires de France (Paris).

1958– Hired as a graphic artist by Gallimard.
1979

1959– Continues to work freelance for publishers such as
1962 Corrêa and Calmann-Lévy and designs layouts for French government departments.

1960 Becomes artistic director at Gallimard. Develops the graphic design department which, in twelve years, expands its staff from one to twelve.

1961 Graphic design of Raymond Queneau's *Cent mille milliards de poèmes* (Paris, Gallimard).

1964 Graphic design of Eugène Ionesco's *La Cantatrice chauve* (Paris, Gallimard), for which he wins the Leipzig International Book Prize. Also designs two English-language editions: *The Bald Soprano* (American edition: New York, Grove Press, 1965) and *The Bald Prima Donna* (British edition: London, Calder and Boyars, 1966).

1965 Creates a typographic interpretation of Édith Piaf's song *La Foule* for *Evergreen Review* (New York, Grove Press). First trip to the United States.

1966 Graphic design of Eugène Ionesco's *Délire à deux* and Jean Tardieu's *Conversation-sinfonietta* (Paris, Gallimard). Begins work on Jean Cocteau's *Les Mariés de la tour Eiffel* (Paris, Hoëbeke, finished in 1994) and Arnold Schoenberg's *Pierrot lunaire*, still unfinished. Designs the graphic concept of the 'Poésie/Gallimard' series (Paris).

1968 Co-author of *L'Amour la ville* (Paris, Gallimard).

1970 Publishes *La Lettre et l'Image* (Paris, Gallimard), with a preface by Raymond Queneau (2nd edition 1993, revised and extended with an essay by Roland Barthes), translated into English (*Letter and Image*. British edition: London, StudioVista, 1970; American edition: New York, Van Nostrand Reinhold, 1970), German (*Buchstabenbilder und Bildalphabete*, Ravensburg, Otto Maier Verlag, 1970) and Italian (*La Lettera e l'Immagine*, Milan, A. Vallardi, 1996) as well as pirate editions in Serbo-Croat (1970) and Korean (1994). Winner of the Prix des Graphistes des Compagnons de Lure, France.

1972 Graphic design for Gallimard of the 'Folio' paperback series (Paris), publishing contemporary authors. Under the pseudonym Claude Menuet publishes *Une enfance ordinaire* (Paris, Gallimard; paperback edition: Paris, Le Seuil, 'Points Virgule' series, 1992), which wins the Prix Cazes in 1973.

1974 Under the same pseudonym publishes *Le Pensionnaire* (Paris, Gallimard; paperback edition: Paris, Le Seuil, 'Points Virgule' series, 1993), awarded the Prix Paul Flat by the Académie française.

1976 Graphic design of 'Tel', a series of books in the fields of philosophy and the social sciences, for Gallimard (Paris).

1976– Graphic design of the literary series 'L'Imaginaire'
1977 for Gallimard (Paris).

1978 Publishes his first essay, *Les Cris de la ville* (Paris, Gallimard).

1979 Leaves Gallimard. Publishes *Zola photographe* (Paris, Denoël, with François Émile-Zola).

1981 Publishes a second essay, *Les Célébrités de la rue* (Paris, Gallimard).

1980– Associate editor for Hachette through the 'Atelier
1982 Hachette/Massin'. Publishes eight titles, all inspired by the new Annales School of historians: René Nelli's *Troubadours et Trouvères* (Paris, 1979); Jean-Marie Lhôte's *Kléber et Marie-Louise* (Paris, 1979); Jean-Paul Roux's *La Chaussure* (Paris, 1980); Hubert Juin's *Le Lit* (Paris, 1980); Pierre Marly's *Les Lunettes* (Paris, 1980); François Caradec and Alain Weill's *Le Café-concert* (Paris, 1980); Pierre Gascar's *Le Boulevard du crime* (Paris, 1980); Frédérick Tristan's *Le Monde à l'envers* (Paris, 1980).

1983 Publishes his first novel, *Le Branle des voleurs* (Paris, La Table Ronde).

1984 Begins his career as a fully independent graphic artist, designing books and covers for various publishers, including Fixot, Hoëbeke, Albin Michel and Robert Laffont.

1985 Publishes his second novel, *Les Compagnons de la marjolaine* (Paris, La Table Ronde).

1986 Mounts the 'Alphabets' exhibition at the musée-galerie de la Seita, Paris, which runs in parallel with the exhibition 'Abécédaires' at the Centre Georges-Pompidou. Designs and publishes the accompanying catalogues *Alphabets* and *Abécédaires*.

1988 Publishes his third novel, *La Dernière Passion* (Paris, Albin Michel), and the first volume of his diary, *Continuo. Fragments d'un journal en désordre* (Paris, Balbec; paperback edition: Paris, Le Seuil, 'Points Virgule' series, 1992).

1988– Publishes *L'ABC du métier* (Paris, Imprimerie
1989 nationale), an autobiographical account of his career as a graphic artist.

1989 First retrospective exhibition, 'Quarante ans d'édition française. Hommage à Massin', at the musée-galerie de la Seita, Paris, with accompanying catalogue (Paris, musée-galerie de la Seita, 1989).

1990 Publication of the catalogue *Massin* (Paris, IMEC-Institut mémoire de l'édition contemporaine).

1991 Publishes *La Cour des miracles* (Paris, Payot), which wins the Bourse Goncourt for historical writing. Publishes *La Mise en pages* (Paris, Hoëbeke).

1993 Writes and designs *Le Monde sens dessus dessous* (Paris, Gallimard Jeunesse) and *Jouons avec les lettres* illustrated by Les Chats pelés (Paris, Seuil Jeunesse).

1994 Finishes *Les Mariés de la tour Eiffel, spectacle de Jean Cocteau* (Paris, Hoëbeke). Publishes *Jouons avec les chiffres*, illustrated by Les Chats pelés (Paris, Seuil Jeunesse).

1995 Triple retrospective exhibition 'On a tous un Massin chez soi: portrait d'un graphiste touche-à-tout' at La Laiterie, l'École des arts décoratifs and FNAC, Strasburg, with accompanying catalogue (Strasburg, La Laiterie, 1995).

Chronology

1996 Publishes the second volume of his diary, *Journal en désordre, 1945–1995* (Paris, Robert Laffont).

1997 Receives UNESCO's International Book Award for 'his activities on behalf of book design and culture'. Layout for Jacques Prévert 's *Dîner de têtes* (Paris, Gallimard). Donates his archives to the city of Chartres.

1998 Layout for Jacques Prévert's *Cortège* (Paris, Gallimard).

2001 Invited to join the Alliance graphique internationale (AGI). Presents works at 'Typojanchi', the exhibition of the Seoul typography biennial.

2002 Elected foreign associate member of the Académie royale de Belgique.

2001– Retrospective exhibition 'Massin in Continuo:
2003 A Dictionary' opens in New York, afterwards travelling to Boston, Montreal, Los Angeles, Baltimore, San Francisco and Istanbul.

2003 Publishes photographs of the region where he spent his childhood, *La Beauce des années cinquante* (Paris, Jacques Marseille).

2004 Publishes *Azerty, l'alphabet du monde* (Paris, Gallimard). Co-author, with his daughter Laure, of *Le Piano des couleurs* (Paris, Gallimard Jeunesse). Lectures in Beijing and Nanjing.

2005 Gives a series of lectures in Seoul. Exhibition 'Graphisme et Poésie' in Alexandria.

2006 Pursues experiments in typographical transposition with Arnold Schoenberg's *Pierrot lunaire* and other pieces of music. Establishes non-profit-making organization 'Typographies expressives', to promote works linking typography with the human voice and music.

2007 Retrospective exhibition 'Massin et le livre: la typographie en jeu' at the École nationale supérieure des arts décoratifs (ENSAD), Paris, with accompanying catalogue (Paris, ENSAD/Bookstorming, 2007).

Chapter 1
Book Clubs

1   Massin, *L'ABC du métier*, Paris, Imprimerie nationale, 1989, p. 77.
2   Interview with Laetitia Wolff, April 2005; also mentioned in 'Bref historique des clubs de livres', in Massin, *L'ABC du métier, op. cit.*, p. 208.
3   Unnamed author, 'Des "Portiques" au "Nombre d'or": la Pléiade concurrencée?', *La Lettre de la Pléiade* 14, February/March/April 2003. The 'Bibliothèque de la Pléiade' series of reference editions of the greatest works of French and world literature and philosophy were printed on bible paper and fully bound in leather with gold lettering.
4   Massin, *L'ABC du métier, op. cit.*, p. 209. Massin cites the publication, in *L'Écho de la librairie et de l'édition* (February 1952), of a conversation held in Jean-Paul Lhopital's office.
5   Massin, *Catalogue raisonné de l'œuvre typographique*, Ville de Chartres/Fonds régional d'acquisitions pour les bibliothèques de la région Centre, 1988, vol. 1 (1948–58), p. 25.
6   Interview with Laetitia Wolff, February 2005.
7   Unnamed author, 'Des "Portiques" au "Nombre d'or": la Pléiade concurrencée?', *op. cit.*
8   Cited on a poster advertising the Club du meilleur livre, reproduced in the *Catalogue raisonné de l'œuvre typographique, op. cit.*, vol. 1, p. 81.
9   *Massin* (exhibition catalogue), Paris, IMEC (Institut mémoire de l'édition contemporaine), 1990, quotation from Robert Carlier, p. 43.
10 Massin, *L'ABC du métier, op. cit.*, p. 49.
11 *Ibid.*, p. 71.
12 *Ibid.*, p. 77.
13 Massin, *op. cit.*, essay by Carlier about the book clubs, p. 45.
14 Correspondence with Laetitia Wolff, autumn 2005.
15 Pierre Faucheux, 'Graphisme et art', special issue of *Art d'aujourd'hui*, 1952.
16 Massin, *op. cit.*, p. 90.
17 Correspondence with Laetitia Wolff, autumn 2005.
18 Massin, *op. cit.*, p. 90.
19 Massin, *Journal en désordre, 1945–1995*, Paris, Robert Laffont, 1996, p. 341.
20 *Ibid.*
21 Interview with Laetitia Wolff, April 2005.
22 Unnamed author, 'Des "Portiques" au "Nombre d'or": la Pléiade concurrencée?', *op. cit.*
23 Massin, *Catalogue raisonné de l'œuvre typographique, op. cit.*, vol. 2 (1958–79) p. 18, and from interviews with Laetitia Wolff, February and April 2005.

Chapter 2
Art Direction

1   Massin, *L'ABC du métier, op. cit.*, p. 104.
2   *Ibid.*, p. 103.
3   *Ibid.*, p. 168.
4   Massin, *Catalogue raisonné de l'œuvre typographique, op. cit.*, vol. 1 (1948–1958), p. 110.
5   *Quarante ans d'édition française. Hommage à Massin* (exhibition catalogue), Paris, musée-galerie de la Seita, 1989, p. 24.
6   Éditions Gallimard grew out of La Nouvelle Revue française.
7   Interview with Laetitia Wolff, December 2005.
8   *Quarante ans d'édition française. Hommage à Massin, op. cit.*, p. 38.
9   Massin, *L'ABC du métier, op. cit.*, p. 131.

10 Interview with Laetitia Wolff, December 2005.
11 Michel Wlassikoff, *Histoire du graphisme en France*, Paris, Dominique Carré, co-published with Gingko Press for the American edition, 2005–6.
12 Correspondence with Laetitia Wolff, autumn 2005.
13 Interview with Laetitia Wolff, December 2005. Tibor Csernus (born 1927) is a painter and illustrator.
14 Interview with Laetitia Wolff, December 2005.
15 Catherine de Smet, on Robin Kinross's *Modern Typography* (Hyphen Press, 1992, 2nd edition 2004), a critical overview of the history of modern typography.
16 Interview with Laetitia Wolff, December 2005.
17 Massin, *Catalogue raisonné de l'œuvre typographique, op. cit.*, vol. 2, p. 132.
18 Correspondence with Laetitia Wolff, autumn 2005.
19 Massin, *L'ABC du métier, op. cit.*, p. 138.
20 Massin was invited to Seoul for the 50th anniversary of the Korean literary magazine *Hyundae Munhak*, for which, in 2005, he had designed a series of covers and the layout for a special issue, at the request of the Korean professor and typographer Ahn Sang Soo.
21 Interviews with Laetitia Wolff, November - December 2005.

Chapter 3
Expressive Typography

1   Massin, *L'ABC du métier, op. cit.*, p. 158.
2   Anne Ubersfeld, *Lire le théâtre I*, Paris, Belin, 1977 (2nd edition 1996), p. 113.
3   Paul Shaw, in a conversation with Laetitia Wolff in January 2002 during the retrospective exhibition 'Massin in Continuo: A Dictionary' and the 'Massin' conference curated by Laetitia Wolff with artistic direction by Philippe Apeloig, at the Herb Lubalin Study Center of Design and Typography at the Cooper Union School of Art, New York (winter 2001–2002).
4   Michel Melot, 'Le livre unique, de la religion du livre à l'idéologie du livre', lecture given at the École normale supérieure as part of the first Summer School of the Institut d'histoire du livre, 2004.
5   Interview with Laetitia Wolff, 9 December 2005.
6   Richard Hollis in the British publication *Eye Magazine* 16, 1995.
7   Massin, *Catalogue raisonné de l'œuvre typographique, op. cit.*, vol. 2 (1958–1979), p. 74.
8   Katy Lhaïk, 'La provocation typographique de *La Cantatrice Chauve*', in *Massin* (IMEC, exhibition catalogue), *op. cit.*, p. 68.
9   Massin, *La Lettre et l'Image*, Paris, Gallimard, 1970.
10 Unpublished letter to Gaston Gallimard, c.1964.
11 Interview with Laetitia Wolff, April 2006.
12 Massin, introduction to *Illustration et photographisme, 1955–1975, itinéraire graphique d'Henry Cohen*, Auxerre, bibliothèque municipale, 1992.
13 Interview with Laetitia Wolff, April 2006.
14 *Illustration et photographisme, op. cit.*
15 *Ibid.*
16 Unpublished letter to Gaston Gallimard, c.1964.
17 Eugène Ionesco, in *Massin* (IMEC, exhibition catalogue), *op. cit.*, p. 86.
18 Anne Ubersfeld, *Lire le théâtre I, op. cit.*, p. 111.
19 Marie-Laure Jaubert de Beaujeu, 'Mise en pages du théâtre, théâtre de la mise en pages', *Cahiers du musée national d'Art moderne*, Paris, autumn 2004.
20 François Caradec, 'Crû Massin 1964', *Caractère*, 1964, pp. 77–81.
21 Interview with Laetitia Wolff, February 2005.

Notes

Chapter 4
A Love of Lettering

1. Interview with Laetitia Wolff published in *Design/Issues* 18, no. 4 (autumn 2002), p. 41.
2. Massin, *L'ABC du métier, op. cit.*, p. 13.
3. *Ibid.* (title of the first chapter).
4. *Ibid.*, p. 13.
5. *Ibid.* The first chapter is devoted to these memories of graphics.
6. Philippe Schuwer, article on *La Lettre et l'Image*, *Le figaro littéraire*, 18 May 1970.
7. Preface to *Alphabets*, catalogue for the exhibition at the musée-galerie de la Seita (1987) designed by Massin using his personal collection of alphabets.
8. Hubert Juin, 'Un livre gai', *Le Monde*, 29 April 1970.
9. Katharine McCoy, 'American Graphic Design Expression: The Evolution of American Typography', *Design Quarterly* 149, Cambridge (Mass.), MIT Press, 1990, pp. 3–22.
10. Handwritten note found in the notebooks of the fonds Massin, médiathèque l'Apostrophe, Chartres, *s.d.* (c.1964–5).
11. Beatrice Warde, *The Crystal Goblet* (1932), cited in Ellen Lupton and Abbott Miller, *Design, Writing, Research*, London, Phaidon, 1999, p. 55.
12. Filippo Tommaso Marinetti, 'Destruction de la syntaxe - Imagination sans fils - Mots en liberté', *Lacerba*, Florence, 15 June 1913.
13. In August 1942, Queneau gave Noël Arnaud, who had succeeded François Le Lionnais as president of the OuLiPo (Ouvroir de Littérature Potentielle), the first manuscript of *Exercices de style* so that it could be published by La Main à plume, a surrealist group and publishing house that Arnaud headed. But censorship under the Vichy regime meant that the book was not published until 1947, by Gallimard; this edition was enhanced in 1956 (when Faucheux's version was published) and revised and corrected in 1963 (when Massin's version appeared).
14. Jacques Carelman, illustrator and painter, author of the *Catalogue des objets introuvables*, was Regent of the Collège de 'pataphysique and a founder member of the OuPeinPo (Ouvroir de Peinture Potentielle).
15. Correspondence with Laetitia Wolff, October 2005.
16. Emmanuël Souchier, Centre d'étude de l'écriture, University of Paris-VII, 'À propos d'*Exercices de style*', in *Massin* (IMEC, exhibition catalogue), *op. cit.*, p. 62.
17. Massin, *Azerty, l'alphabet du monde*, Paris, Gallimard, 2004, p. 162.
18. Cited by Marcel Brion in an article on *La Lettre et l'Image*, *Les Nouvelles littéraires*, July 1970.
19. *Ibid.*
20. Raymond Queneau, *Cent mille milliards de poèmes*, Paris, Gallimard, 1961, reprinted seven times since it was first published.
21. Claude Lebon, introduction to *Cent mille milliards de poèmes*, in Raymond Queneau, *Œuvres complètes*, Paris, Gallimard, 'Bibliothèque de la Pléiade', 1989 (revised edition 2002), p. 1318.
22. Raymond Queneau's 'instructions' for *Cent mille milliards de poèmes*, *ibid.*, p. 333.
23. In *Entretiens avec Georges Charbonnier*, Paris, Gallimard, 1962, mentioned in the 'Bibliothèque de la Pléiade' edition (cf. note 21). Queneau recalled that he had been encouraged to found this group for literary experimentation by his mathematician friend François Le Lionnais, who later wrote the postface to *Cent mille milliards de poèmes*, republished in *OuLiPo, la littérature potentielle* (Paris, Gallimard, 1973).
24. Jean Cocteau, *Les Mariés de la tour Eiffel*, Paris, Gallimard, 1921. The book designed by Massin is entitled *Les Mariés de la tour Eiffel, spectacle de Jean Cocteau*, Paris, Hoëbeke, 1994. Jean Cocteau said: 'The greatest masterpiece of literature is only ever a disordered alphabet' (cited by Massin in several works).
25. Massin, postface to *Les Mariés de la tour Eiffel, spectacle de Jean Cocteau, op. cit.*, p. 221.
26. Introduction to *Les Mariés de la tour Eiffel, spectacle de Jean Cocteau, op. cit.*, pp. 1–2.
27. Massin, postface to *Les Mariés de la tour Eiffel, spectacle de Jean Cocteau, op. cit.*
28. Massin, *L'ABC du métier, op. cit.*, p. 161.
29. Epigraph to a letter to Claude Gallimard, probably dated 7 January 1966, accompanying the design for *Les Mariés de la tour Eiffel* which Massin was sending him.
30. Massin mentions the New Dada in his letter to Claude Gallimard, *ibid.*
31. Handwritten notes by Massin, *s.d.* (1960s).
32. *Ibid.*
33. Notes on the choice of typefaces, postface to *Les Mariés de la tour Eiffel, spectacle de Jean Cocteau, op. cit.*, p. 225.
34. Introduction to *Les Mariés de la tour Eiffel, spectacle de Jean Cocteau, op. cit.*, p. 6.
35. Since the early 1990s Massin has notably designed and laid out *Doisneau, les doigts pleins d'encre* (1989; text by François Cavanna), *La Mise en pages* (1991), *Zola photographe* (1994; with François Émile-Zola) and *Picassiette* (2001; text by Michel Ragon), all for Éditions Hoëbeke.
36. Letter to Claude Gallimard, *op. cit.*
37. *Ibid.*

Chapter 5
Music

1. Massin, 'Le contrepoint', *La Mise en pages*, Paris, Hoëbeke, 1991, p. 88.
2. In 1988, Massin went to Hachette with a proposal for an 'Atelier Massin' series, inspired by the historians of Annales. The series is organized around themes that are easy to approach and whose graphic representation and cultural importance are explored in richly illustrated books (*La Chaussure, Les Lunettes, Le Boulevard du crime*, etc.). Massin had submitted the idea for this series to Claude Gallimard before he left the company.
3. Massin, *Style et écriture. Du rococo aux arts déco*, Paris, Albin Michel, 'Idées' series, 2001, p. 16.
4. Interview with Laetitia Wolff, January 2006.
5. *Ibid.*
6. 'Father Bach, "an infinitely expanding universe",' wrote Massin in *Azerty, l'alphabet du monde, op. cit.*, p. 165, citing the words of Glenn Gould.
7. Massin, *La Mise en pages, op. cit.*, pp. 81–2.
8. Massin, *De la variation*, Paris, Le Promeneur, 2000.
9. Massin, *Azerty, l'alphabet du monde, op. cit.*, p. 165.
10. Massin, *De la variation, op. cit.*, p. 46.
11. Interview with Laetitia Wolff, January 2006.
12. *Ibid.*
13. Massin, *De la variation, op. cit.*, p. 67–8.
14. *Ibid.*, p. 19.
15. *Ibid.*, p. 13–14.
16. Massin, *L'ABC du métier, op. cit.*, p. 97.
17. *Ibid.*
18. Interview with Laetitia Wolff, January 2006.
19. Massin, *L'ABC du métier, op. cit.*, p. 96.
20. Interview with Laetitia Wolff, January 2006.
21. Massin, *On a tous un Massin chez soi* (exhibition catalogue), Strasburg, La Laiterie, 1995, p. 25.
22. See *ibid.*, pp. 29–31, and also *Journal en désordre* and preparatory notes.
23. See *On a tous un Massin chez soi, op. cit.*, pp. 29–31.
24. Massin, *De la variation, op. cit.*, pp. 41–2.
25. *Viens Poupoule!*, an experiment in expressive typography, 2006, song performed by Mayol in 1902, lyrics by Trebitsch and Christiné, music by Adolph Spahn arranged by Christiné.
26. Interview with Laetitia Wolff, February 2006.
27. Massin, in a lecture on the human voice and typography given in Seoul, March 2005. Massin has written little on the *La Foule* project compared to his detailed and frequently reproduced notes on *La Cantatrice chauve*, although the typographic experimentation in *La Foule* is carried to a degree rarely reached in his work.
28. See Barney Rosset's telegram of 30 October 1964 to Massin.
29. In the lecture given in Seoul, March 2005.
30. Letter to Barney Rosset, dated 8 July 1965.
31. Seoul lecture, March 2005.
32. *Ibid.*
33. Letter to Barney Rosset, dated 17 August 1965.
34. Typed document entitled 'La Foule', *s.d.* (probably c.1965), fonds Massin, médiathèque l'Apostrophe, Chartres.

Chapter 6
The House in Étampes

1. Massin, *La Curiosité* (work in progress, started 1989).
2. Massin, *La Beauce des années cinquante* (book of photographs), Paris, Jacques Marseille, 2003.
3. Correspondence with Laetitia Wolff, April 2006.
4. *Ibid.*
5. Massin, *L'ABC du métier, op. cit.*, p. 13.
6. Interview with Laetitia Wolff on the notions of reading and writing, January 2006.
7. *Ibid.*
8. *Ibid.*
9. *Ibid.*
10. *Ibid.*
11. Massin, extract from *La Curiosité, op. cit.*
12. Interview with Laetitia Wolff on the notions of reading and writing, January 2006.
13. Massin, extract from *La Curiosité, op. cit.*
14. Massin, *L'ABC du métier, op. cit.*, 'Mythologies enfantines', pp. 9–21.
15. Massin, extract from *La Curiosité, op. cit.*
16. Correspondence with Laetitia Wolff, April 2006.
17. *Ibid.*
18. *Ibid.*
19. *Ibid.*
20. *Ibid.*
21. Massin, *On a tous un Massin chez soi* (exhibition catalogue), Strasburg, La Laiterie, 1995, p. 22.
22. Interview with Laetitia Wolff on the notions of reading and writing, January 2006.
23. *Ibid.*
24. Correspondence with Laetitia Wolff, April 2006.

Notes

Listed below are all the books designed by Massin; where Massin created the overall design of a series, the list is not exhaustive and gives only the first few titles.

Bindings, jackets and covers

1950 *Les Vrais Mémoires de Vidocq*, Paris, Corrêa.

1951 Donald Keyhoe, *Les soucoupes volantes existent*, Pierre Horay / Flore; Gerald Heard, *Les Soucoupes volantes*, Pierre Horay / Flore; Michel Crozier, *Usines et Syndicats d'Amérique*, Paris, Les Éditions ouvrières; William L. Lawrence, *La Bombe H*, Paris, Corrêa; Charles Plisnier, *Mariages*, 'Présentation spéciale' series, Paris, Corrêa; Charles Braibant, *Le roi dort*, 'Présentation spéciale' series, Paris, Corrêa; Maria Le Hardouin, *La Voile noire*, 'Présentation spéciale' series, Paris, Corrêa; Pierre Molaine, *Violences*, 'Présentation spéciale' series, Paris, Corrêa; Herman Melville, *Israël Potter*, Paris, Corrêa; Immanuel Velikovsky, *Mondes en collision*, Paris, Stock; George R. Stewart, *Maria la tempête*, Paris, le Club français du livre; Roger Vailland, *Boroboudour*, Paris, Corrêa; Ève Dessarre, *Les Vagabonds autour du clocher*, Pierre Horay / Flore; Alain Ivergny, *Les Amours brûlées*, Pierre Horay / Flore; Raoul Carson, *Les Vieilles Douleurs*, Pierre Horay / Flore; Estes Kefauver, *Le Crime en Amérique*, Pierre Horay / Flore; Henri Oberjohann, *Mon gorille et mon chimpanzé*, Paris, Corrêa; Alain Sergent, *Barnum, roi du bluff*, Paris, Pierre Horay / Flore; Guil Aumot, *Veillée de haine*, Paris, Les Éditions du Scorpion; Michel Mohrt, *Marin La Meslée*, Pierre Horay / Flore; Victor Bogomeletz, *Vivre jeune*, Paris, Pierre Horay / Flore; André Billy, *Chapelles et Sociétés secrètes*, Paris, Corrêa.

1952 Mary Jones, *Maman Jones*, Paris, Les Éditions ouvrières; Commandant Heiz Schaeffer, *U-977*, Paris, Julliard; Jean-Louis Bory, *Un noël à la tyrolienne*, Paris, Pierre Horay / Flore; Fulton-John Sheen, *La Paix de l'âme*, Paris, Corrêa; Walter Henry Thompson, *Churchill par son ombre*, Paris, Corrêa; Dorothy Caruso, *Caruso*, Paris, Corrêa; Salvador de Madariaga, *Christophe Colomb*, Paris, Calmann-Lévy; Michel Morht, *Marin La Meslée*, Paris, Pierre Horay / Flore; Henry Miller, *Le Monde du sexe*, Paris, Corrêa; Kenneth Heuer, *Les Habitants des autres planètes*, Paris, Corrêa; Michel Collinet, *L'Esprit du syndicalisme*, Paris, Les Éditions ouvrières; André de Fouquières, *La Courtoisie moderne*, Paris, Pierre Horay / Flore; Henry Miller, *Plexus*, Paris, Corrêa; Maurice Nadeau, *Littérature présente*, Paris, Corrêa; Paul Malar, *Tropique du Caducée*, I, Paris, Les Éditions du Scorpion; Robert Neuman, *Sur les pas de Morell*, Paris, Calmann-Lévy; Hans Werner Richter, *Tombés de la main de Dieu*, Paris, Pierre Horay / Flore; Georges Arnaud, *Les Oreilles sur le dos*, Paris, Les Éditions du Scorpion; Paul Malar, *Topique du Caducée*, II, Paris, Les Éditions du Scorpion; Sœur Maria del Rey, *Zigzags dans le Pacifique*, Paris, Corrêa; Jacques Danos and Marcel Gibelin, *Juin 1936*, Paris, Les Éditions ouvrières; Ferreira de Castro, Paris, *Les Brebis du Seigneur*, Paris, Pierre Horay / Flore; Louis Fischer, *La Vie de Mahatma Gandhi*, Paris, Calmann-Lévy; François de Roux, *La Jeunesse de Lyautey*, Paris, Calmann-Lévy; Anita Daniel, *Je vais à New York*, Paris, Calmann-Lévy; Peter Henn, *La Dernière Rafale*, Paris, Julliard; Herman Wouk, *Ouragan sur D. M. S. 'Caine'*, Paris, Calmann-Lévy; Noëlle Lamare, *Connaissance sensuelle de la femme*, Paris, Corrêa; Jean-Gérard Chauffeteau, *L'Affaire Villabianca*, Paris, Pierre Horay / Flore; Jeanne-Baptiste Canavaggia, *Les Bras ouverts*, Paris, Pierre Horay / Flore; Russel Grenfell, *Le Drame du Bismarck*, Paris, Julliard; Jean Lauprêtre, *Les Fugitifs de l'ennui*, Paris, Les Éditions du Scorpion; Jamblan, *Ordre alphabétique*, Paris, Les Éditions du Scorpion; Colonel Oreste Pinto, *Chasseurs d'espions*, Paris, Corrêa; Capitaine X, *2e bureau marine*, Paris, Les Éditions du scorpion; Jean Maîtron, *Paul Delesalle*, Paris, Les Éditions ouvrières; Capitaine X, *2e bureau air*, Paris, Les Éditions du Scorpion; Olga Wormser, *Les Femmes dans l'histoire*, Paris, Corrêa; Edgar Morin, *L'Homme et la Mort*, Paris, Corrêa.; Jean-Charles Pichon, *Sérum et cie.*, Paris, Corrêa; Bertrand Russell, *Les Dernières Chances de l'homme*, Paris, Pierre Horay / Flore; Hermann Gohde, *Le Huitième Jour*, Paris, Corrêa.

1953 Alain Moorhead, *Les Espions atomiques*, Paris, Calmann-Lévy; Michel Ragon, *Histoire de la littérature ouvrière*, Paris, Les Éditions ouvrières; Ferreira de Castro, *Le Renoncement de Don Alvaro*, Paris, Pierre Horay; George Woodstock and Ivan Avakoumovitch, *Pierre Kropotkine, le prince anarchiste*, Paris, Calmann-Lévy; Robert Scott, *Dieu est mon co-pilote*, Paris, Julliard; Nina Gourkinkel, *Naissance d'un monde*, Paris, Seuil; Liam O'Flaherty, *Insurrection*, Paris, Calmann-Lévy; Roger Henrard, *Un enragé du ciel*, Paris, Seuil; Arthur Koestler, *La Corde raide*, Paris, Calmann-Lévy; Salvador de Madariaga, *Hernan Cortès*, Paris, Calmann-Lévy; Victor Alba, *Le Mouvement ouvrier en Amérique latine*, Paris, Les Éditions ouvrières; Marcel Delannoy, *Honegger*, Paris, Pierre Horay; Paul Guth, *Mémoires d'un naïf*, Paris, Pierre Horay; Lion Feuchtwanger, *Le Roman de Goya*, Paris, Calmann-Lévy; André Mahé, *Le Tour de France des auberges de jeunesse*, Paris, Éditions de Paris; Robert Gaillard, *Alexandre Dumas*, Paris, Calmann-Lévy; Paul Grégor, *Vision romaine*, Paris, Les Éditions du Scorpion; Nina Gourkinkel, *L'Autre Patrie*, Paris, Seuil; Henrich Eduard Jacob, *L'Épopée du café*, Paris, Calmann-Lévy.

1954 C. V. d'Autrec, *Les Charlatans de la Médecine*, Paris, Les Éditions du Scorpion; P. M. Lambermont, *Videz vos poches*, Paris, La Table Ronde; Colonel Pinto, *Espions ou amis ?*, Paris, Corrêa; J. R Kinney and Ann Honeycutt, *Votre chien*, Paris, Calmann-Lévy; Ray Bradbury, *Chroniques martiennes*, Paris, Calmann-Lévy; Sholem Asch, *Moïse*, Paris, Calmann-Lévy; *Les Conseils pratiques du Figaro 1954*, Paris, Calmann-Lévy; Jean Davidson, *Correspondant à Washington*, Paris, Seuil; Louis Pauwels, *Monsieur Gurdjieff*, Paris, Seuil; Valérie André, *Ici, ventilateur!*, Paris, Calmann-Lévy; Lucien Dauvergne, *Louis Renault*, Paris, La Table Ronde; Pierre Humbourg, *Huitième Dernière*, Paris, Calmann-Lévy; Marie-Paule Pomaret and Hélène Cingria, *L'aventure est dans votre cuisine*, Paris, Pierre Horay; Colette Jeanson, *Principes et Pratiques de l'accouchement sans douleur*, Paris, Seuil; Léo Valentin, *Homme-Oiseau*, Paris, Éditions de Paris; Georges Houot and P. Willm, *Le Bathyscaphe*, Paris, Éditions de Paris; Maurice Dekobra, *Les femmes que j'ai aimées*, Paris, Les Éditions du Scorpion; Adolph Zukor, *Le public n'a jamais tort*, Paris, Corrêa; Robert Fabian, *Londres la nuit*, Paris, Corrêa / Buchet-Chastel; Maurice Dekobra, *L'armée rouge est à New York*, Paris, Les Éditions du Scorpion; Paul Malar, *Tropique du Caducée*, III, Paris, Les Éditions du Scorpion; Jacqueline Lenoir, *Le Tour de France par deux enfants*, Paris, La Table Ronde; Dr Bergler and Dr Kroger, *L'Erreur de Kinsey*, Paris, Pierre Horay; Jean Savant, *Napoléon raconté par les témoins de sa vie*, Paris, Corrêa / Buchet-Chastel.

1955 *Guide de Paris*, *Artes Monumentos Museos*, Paris, Artes Monumentos; Armand Gatti, *Envoyé spécial dans la cage aux fauves*, Paris, Seuil; Jacques Bergier, *Agents secrets contre armes secrètes*, Paris, Arthaud; *Picasso*, Paris, musée des Arts décoratifs; Esther Warner, *Au pays des Lomas*, Paris, Calmann-Lévy; Jean Bommard, *Celui qui va seul*, Paris, Calmann-Lévy; Salvador de Madariaga, *Bolivar*, Paris, Calmann-Lévy.

1956 Jacques Morvan, *La Belle de Monteferrare*, Paris, Robert Laffont; Raoul de Warren, *La Bête de l'Apocalypse*, Paris, Robert Laffont; Henri J. Garapon, *Vagabondages très spéciaux*, Paris, Les Éditions du Scorpion; James Ramsey Ullman, *Rivière du soleil*, Paris, Arthaud; Josef Martin Bauer, *Aussi loin que mes pas me portent*, Paris, Calmann-Lévy.

1957 Lion Feuchtwanger, *La Juive de Tolède*, Paris, Calmann-Lévy; Madeleine Fabiola Kent, *Jean Lafitte, corsaire*, Paris, Calmann-Lévy; Jean Fougère, *Voulez-vous voyager avec moi?*, Paris, Arthaud; Marianne Monestier, *La Mystérieuse Compagnie, les jésuites*, Paris, Pierre Horay; Ernst Diez, *Les Anciens Mondes de l'Asie*, Paris, Pierre Horay; Jacqueline Sneyers, *Belles demeures d'autrefois*, Paris, Pierre Horay; Tsewang Pemba, *Tibet, ma patrie*, Paris, Pierre Horay.

1958 Ernst Wiechert, *Missa sine nomine*, Paris, Calmann-Lévy; Alexandre Dumas fils, *La Dame aux camélias*, Paris, Calmann-Lévy; Anatole France, *Le Crime de Sylvestre Bonnard, Le Livre de mon ami*, Paris, Calmann-Lévy; Arthur Rimbaud, *Œuvres*, Paris, Mercure de France; Marie Dormoy, *Léautaud*, Paris, Gallimard; *Paris Lyon Côte d'Azur*, Paris, Pierre Horay; Albert Dubeux, *La Curieuse Vie de Georges Courteline*, Paris, Pierre Horay; Janine Brillet, *Le Couple*, Paris, Pierre Horay; various, *Les Jeunes Gens en colère vous parlent*, Paris, Pierre Horay; André Soubiran, *Au revoir, docteur Roch*, Paris, Kent-Segep; H. G. Wells, *Les Premiers Hommes dans la lune*, Paris, Mercure de France; Henri Raynal, *Les Pieds d'Omphale*, Paris, Jean-Jacques Pauvert.

1959 André Gide, *La Porte étroite*, Paris, Mercure de France; Claude Aveline, *Le Poids du feu*, Paris, Del Duca; Éliane Jacquet, *Quatre saisons en URSS*, Paris, Pierre Horay; Herbert George Wells, *La Machine à explorer le temps*, Paris, Mercure de France; Schichiro Fukazawa, *Étude à propos des chansons de Narayama*, Paris, Gallimard; Claude Aveline, *Lettres de la religieuse portugaise*, Paris, Mercure de France; Alain Mahé, *Colonne vertébrale, arbre de vie*, Paris, Pierre Horay; Pierre Vilar, *Historia de España*, Paris, Librería española.

List of works

1960 Jean-Paul Sartre, *Critique de la raison dialectique*, Paris, Gallimard; Jean Cassou, *Panorama des arts plastiques contemporains*, Paris, Gallimard; Arthur Koestler, *Les Somnambules*, Paris, Calmann-Lévy; André Parrot, *Sumer*, Paris, Gallimard; Claude Farrère, *Florence de Cao Bang*, Paris, Kent-Segep; Pierre Laforêt, *La Prodigieuse Aventure d'Europe, n° 1*, Paris, Pierre Horay; Yves Gandon, *L'Amérique aux Indiens!*, Paris, Kent-Segep; Alain Mahé, *Aliment normal source de santé*, Paris, Pierre Horay; Jean-Pierre Dorian, *Les Petits Mystères de Paris*, Paris, Kent-Segep; André Soubiran and Jean de Kearney, *Le Journal de la médecine*, Paris, Kent-Segep; Anne Philippe and Claude Roy, *Gérard Philippe*, Paris, Gallimard; Marguerite Duras, *Hiroshima, mon amour*, Paris, Gallimard.

1961 Robert Mallet, *Francis Jammes*, Paris, Mercure de France; Jean Cau, *Les Oreilles et la Queue*, Paris, Gallimard; Juan Goytisolo, *La Resaca*, Paris, Biblioteca Club de Bolsillo; Kurt Seligmann, *Le Miroir de la magie*, Paris, Les Éditions du Sagittaire.

1962 Victor Hugo, *Œuvres romanesques complètes*, Paris, Jean-Jacques Pauvert; Juan Goytisolo, *La Chanca*, Paris, Librería española; Jésus de Galindez, *L'Ère de Trujillo*, Paris, Gallimard; Emmanuel d'Astier de la Vigerie, *Sur Saint-Simon*, Paris, Gallimard; Roger Pillaudin, *Loin de Rueil*, Paris, Gallimard; Roger Nimier, *D'Artagnan amoureux*, Paris, Gallimard; André Brissaud, *Les Américains de Kennedy*, Paris, La Table Ronde; José Corrales Egea, *La Otra Cara*, Paris, Librería española, Manuel Tuñón de Lara, *Panorama actual de la economía española*, Paris, Librería española.

1963 Margaret Mitchell, *Autant en emporte le vent*, Paris, Gallimard; Eugène Sue, *Les Mystères de Paris*, Paris, Jean-Jacques Pauvert éditeur; Raymond Lœwy, *La laideur se vend mal*, Paris, Gallimard; Dacia Maraini, *L'Âge du malaise*, Paris, Gallimard; Antoine Dominique, *Tête-de-fer*, Paris, Gallimard; Roman Goul, *Azef*, Paris, Gallimard; Sylvain Reiner, *La Nuit à Paris*, Paris, La Table Ronde; *La Révolution russe par ses témoins*, Paris, La Table Ronde; André Soubiran, *Journal d'une femme en blanc*, Paris, Kent-Segep.

1964 Walter Umminger, *Des hommes et des records*, Paris, La Table Ronde; Hans Graf von Lehndorff, *La Mort ou l'Espérance*, Paris, La Table Ronde; Raymond Corot, *Trente ans de chiffons*, Paris, La Table Ronde; Michel Drowin, *Le Murmure des dieux*, Paris, La Table Ronde; Gérard Beaugency, *Le Fourbi*, Paris, La Table Ronde; Vladimir Volkoff, *Les Mousquetaires de la République*, Paris, La Table Ronde; William Burroughs, *Le Festin nu*, Paris, La Table Ronde; Pierre Gripari, *L'Incroyable Équipée de Phosphore Noloc et de ses compagnons racontée par un témoin oculaire et quelques détails nouveaux sur les gouvernements des îles de Budu et de Pédonisse*, Paris, La Table Ronde; Jacques Lebourgeois, *Le Pyromane*, Paris, La Table Ronde; Éric Piquet-Wicks, *Les Sables balayés*, Paris, La Table Ronde; Friedrich Deich, *Cahier d'un psychiatre*, Paris, La Table Ronde; Barry Goldwater, *Pourquoi pas la victoire?*, Paris, La Table Ronde; Jacques Laurent, *Mauriac sous de Gaulle*, Paris, La Table Ronde; Alfred Fabre-Luce, *Le Couronnement du prince*, Paris, La Table Ronde; Georges Soulié de Morant, *Précis de la vraie acupuncture*, Paris, Mercure de France.

1965 Giorgio de Chirico, *Mémoires*, Paris, La Table Ronde; Louis Mérens, *Ces Français fous, fous, fous*, Paris, La Table Ronde; Gilbert Prouteau, *Le Machin*, Paris, La Table Ronde; Marcel Montaron, *Tout ce joli monde*, Paris, La Table Ronde; Pierre Bonte, *Bonjour monsieur le maire*, Paris, La Table Ronde; Raymond de Becker, *Rêve et Sexualité*, Paris, La Table Ronde; Zoé Oldenbourg, *Les Croisades*, Paris, Gallimard; Pierre Mac Orlan, *Mémoires en chansons*, Paris, Gallimard; Pierre Frédérix, *La Millième Année*, Paris, Gallimard; Manuel Tuñon de Lara, *La España del siglo XIX*, Paris, Librería española.

1966 Marquis de Sade, *Les Infortunes de la Vertu*, Jean-Jacques Pauvert; Fulbert Youlou, *J'accuse la Chine*, Paris, La Table Ronde; Denise Legrix, *Née comme ça*, Paris, Segep-Kent.

1967 Louis Aragon, *Blanche ou L'Oubli*, Paris, Gallimard; Joseph Kessel, *Les Cavaliers*, Paris, Gallimard; André Malraux, *Antimémoires*, I, Paris, Gallimard; Jacques Laurent, *Au contraire*, Paris, La Table Ronde; Pablo Picasso, *Le Désir attrapé par la queue*, Paris, Gallimard; Eugène Ionesco, *Journal en miettes*, Paris, Mercure de France; Érasme, *Correspondance*, Paris, Gallimard.

1968 Marcel Proust, *À la recherche du temps perdu*, Paris, Gallimard; Eugène Ionesco, *Passé présent, présent passé*, Paris, Mercure de France; Julián Zugazagoitia, *Guerra y vicisitudes de los españoles*, Librería española de Paris; Jacques Laurent, *Les choses que j'ai vues au Vietnam m'ont fait douter de l'intelligence occidentale*, Paris, La Table Ronde.

1969 Willima Styron, *Les Confessions de Nat Turner*, Paris, Gallimard; Louis-Ferdinand Céline, *Rigodon*, Paris, Gallimard; Pierre Moustiers, *La Paroi*, Paris, Gallimard; Isadora Duncan, *Ma vie*, Paris, Gallimard; Emmanuel d'Astier de la Vigerie, *Portraits*, Paris, Gallimard; John Updike, *Couples*, Paris, Gallimard; John Kenneth Galbraith, *Le Triomphe*, Paris, Gallimard; *Cahiers Jean Cocteau*, Paris, Gallimard; *Cahiers André Gide*, I, Paris, Gallimard.

1970 André Malraux, *Œuvres*, Paris, Gallimard; Zoé Oldenbourg, *La Joie des pauvres*, Paris, Gallimard; Jean Cau, *Tropicanas*, Paris, Gallimard; Ernest Hemingway, *En ligne*, Paris, Gallimard; Henri Guillemin, *Jeanne dite 'Jeanne d'Arc'*, Paris, Gallimard; *Entretiens de Francis Ponge avec Philippe Sollers*, Paris, Gallimard / Seuil; Richard Wagner, *Beethoven*, Paris, Gallimard; Roger Quilliot, *La Mer et les Prisons*, Paris, Gallimard; Patricia Finaly, *Le Gai Ghetto*, Paris, Gallimard; Thérèse de Saint-Phalle, *Le Souverain*, Paris, Gallimard; Jean-Pierre Chabrol, *Le Canon Fraternité*, Paris, Gallimard; Jean-Luc Dejean, *La Feuille à l'envers*, Paris, Gallimard; Louise de Vilmorin, *Carnets*, Paris, Gallimard; *Cahiers de Marcel Proust*, Paris, Gallimard.

1971 Antoine Blondin, *Les Enfants du Bon Dieu*, Paris, La Table Ronde; Antoine Blondin, *L'Humeur vagabonde*, Paris, La Table Ronde; Bernard Barritaud, *Pierre Mac Orlan*, Paris, Gallimard; Édith Thomas, *Louise Michel*, Paris, Gallimard; Michel Déon, *Le Rendez-vous de Patmos*, Paris, La Table Ronde; Louise de Vilmorin, *Le Lutin sauvage*, Paris, Gallimard; Violette Leduc, *Le Taxi*, Paris, Gallimard; Claude Baillén and Claude Delay, *Chanel solitaire*, Paris, Gallimard; Jean-François Devay, *Trois mois pour mourir*, Paris, Gallimard.

1972 Robert Merle, *Malevil*, Paris, Gallimard; Pierrette Girault de Coursac, *L'Éducation d'un roi : Louis XVI*, Paris, Gallimard; Michel Kildaire, *La Promesse*, Paris, Gallimard; Joseph Kessel, *Des hommes*, Paris, Gallimard; Angus Calder, *L'Angleterre en guerre*, Paris, Gallimard; José Cabanis, *Charles X, roi ultra*, Paris, Gallimard; Simone de Beauvoir, *Tout compte fait*, Paris, Gallimard; Marcel Duhamel, *Raconte pas ta vie*, Paris, Mercure de France; Frédéric Forsyth, *Odessa*, Paris, Mercure de France; *Dostoïevski vivant*, Paris, Gallimard.

1973 Pierre-Jean Remy, *Une mort sale*, Paris, Gallimard; Henry de Montherlant, *Mais aimons-nous ceux que nous aimons?*, Paris, Gallimard; Michel Déon, *Un taxi mauve*, Paris, Gallimard; Romain Gary, *Les Enchanteurs*, Paris, Gallimard; Rénée Massip, *La Vie absente*, Paris, Gallimard; Sergio Vilar, *Cuba*, Paris, Librería española; Eugène Ionesco, *Le Solitaire*, Paris, Mercure de France; Vitia Hessel, *La Désaccoutumance*, Paris, Mercure de France; Joachim Fest, *Hitler*, Paris, Gallimard; Jean Giono, *Le Déserteur et autres récits*, Paris, Gallimard; Zoïa Bogouslavskaïa, *Sept cents roubles nouveaux*, followed by *Le Déménagement*, Paris, Gallimard; Suzanne Bidault, *Souvenirs de guerre et d'occupation*, Paris, La Table Ronde; Andréï Voznessenski, *Poèmes, (Skrymtymnym)*, Paris, Gallimard.

1974 Philippe Hériat, *Duel*, Paris, Gallimard; Henry de Montherlant, *Le Fichier parisien*, Paris, Gallimard; Marion Melville, *La Vie des templiers*, Paris, Gallimard; Armand Salacrou, *Dans la salle des pas perdus*, Paris, Gallimard; Michael Macdonald Monney, *Le Dirigeable 'Hindenburg'*, Paris, Gallimard; Ernst Jünger, *Le Lance-Pierres*, Paris, La Table Ronde; Pierre Moustiers, *Une place forte*, Paris, Gallimard; Noël Arnaud, *Alfred Jarry*, Paris, Gallimard; Cardinal Mindszenty, *Mémoires*, Paris, La Table Ronde.

1975 François Nourissier, *Lettre à mon chien*, Paris, Gallimard; Marie Balka, *Les Mains nues*, Paris, Gallimard; Jean-Pierre Chabrol, *Le Bouc du désert*, Paris, Gallimard; Michel de Saint-Pierre, *Je reviendrai sur les ailes de l'aigle*, Paris, La Table Ronde; Pierre Lempety, *Carnets de Jeanne*, Paris, Denoël; Claude Farragi, *Le Maître d'heure*, Paris, Mercure de France; Brassaï, *Henry Miller grandeur nature*, Paris, Gallimard; *Cahiers Valéry*, I, Paris, Gallimard; Vaslav Nijinsky, *Journal*, Paris, Gallimard.

1976 Réjean Ducharme, *Les Enfantômes*, Paris, Gallimard; Muhammad Ali and Richard Durham, *Le Plus Grand*, Paris, Gallimard; Jean Giono, *Les Terrasses de l'île d'Elbe*, Paris, Gallimard; Jean Cau, *Les Otages*, Paris, Gallimard; Philip Roth, *Ma vie d'homme*, Paris, Gallimard; Emmanuel Le Roy Ladurie, *Montaillou, village occitan de 1294 à 1324*, Paris, Gallimard; Jacques Prévert, *Grand Bal du printemps*, followed by *Charmes de Londres*, Paris, Gallimard; Gaston Vedel, *Le Pilote oublié*, Paris, Gallimard; Charles McCarry, *Les Larmes de l'automne*, Paris, Gallimard; various, *Liberté, libertés*, Paris, Gallimard; Henri Michaux, *Choix de Poèmes*, Paris, Gallimard; Georges Duby, *Le Temps des cathédrales*, Paris, Gallimard; *Œuvres d'Aldous Huxley*, Paris, La Table Ronde; Josette Clotis, *Le Temps vert*, Paris, Gallimard; Leonid Brejnev, *Le Monde et son avenir*, Paris, La Table Ronde; Rezvani, *Le Portrait ovale*, Paris, Gallimard.

List of works

1977 Félicien Marceau, *Les Personnages de la comédie humaine*, Paris, Gallimard; Eugène Ionesco, *Antidotes*, Paris, Gallimard; Claude Jamet, *Notre front populaire*, Paris, La Table Ronde; Pierre Mondet, *On a volé l'or de la Commune*, Paris, La Table Ronde; Antonin Arthaud, *Nouveaux écrits de Rodez*, Paris, Gallimard; Alphonse Boudard, *Les Combattants du petit bonheur*, Paris, La Table Ronde; Adam B. Ulam, *Staline*, Paris, Calmann-Lévy / Gallimard.

1978 Michel Déon, *Mes arches de Noé*, Paris, La Table Ronde; Gwyneth Cravens, John S. Marr, *La Peste à New York*, Paris, Gallimard; Pierre-Jean Remy, *Les Nouvelles Aventures du chevalier de La Barre*, Paris, Gallimard; Anka Muhlstein, *Victoria*, Paris, Gallimard; Anne Philippe and Claude Roy, *Gérard Philippe*, Paris, Gallimard; *Cahiers de Saint-John Perse*, I, Paris, Gallimard; *Raymond Queneau plus intime*, Paris, Gallimard.

1979 *Bibliothèque des chefs-d'œuvre*, Paris, Gallimard; Pierre Gascar, *L'Ombre de Robespierre*, Paris, Gallimard; Jeanne Bourin, *La Chambre des dames*, Paris, La Table Ronde.

1980 Jean-Paul Sartre and Simone de Beauvoir, *Œuvres romanesques*, Paris, Club de l'honnête homme; Marcel Jullian, *Le Maître de Hongrie*, Paris, La Table Ronde; Alphonse Boudard, *Le Banquet des léopards*, Paris, La Table Ronde; François Weyergans, *Les Figurants*, Paris, Balland; Victor Hugo, *Le Rhin*, Strasburg, Bueb & Reumaux.

1981 *Œuvres de Céline*, Paris, Club de l'honnête homme; Pierre Bellemare and Jacques Antoine, *Histoires vraies*, Paris, Édition°1; Jean Cau, *Réflexions dures sur une époque molle*, Paris, La Table Ronde; various, *Histoires brèves 1*, Éditions BFB; Annie Girardot, *Paroles de femmes*, Paris, Édition°1; Philippe Djian, *50 contre 1*, Paris, BFB; Jean Diwo, *Chez Lipp*, Paris, Denoël; Michel Junot, *L'Illusion du bonheur*, Paris, La Table Ronde; Régine Deforges, *La Révolte des nonnes*, Paris, La Table Ronde.

1982 Jeanne Bourin, *La Dame de beauté*, Paris, La Table Ronde; Michel Fauré, *Histoire du surréalisme sous l'occupation*, Paris, La Table Ronde; Alain Griotteray, *Le Théâtre des opérations*, Paris, La Table Ronde; Anthony Burgess, *Sur le lit*, Paris, Denoël; Donald Jackson, *Histoire de l'écriture*, Paris, Denoël; Ben Maddow, *Visages*, Paris, Denoël.

1983 Jean-Paul Picaper, *Vers le IVe Reich*, Paris, La Table Ronde; Mehdi Charaf, *Le Thé au harem d'Archi Ahmed*, Paris, Mercure de France; Jean-Pierre Monod, *La Férocité littéraire*, Paris, La Table Ronde; Fred Mayer, Helga Burger, *L'Opéra chinois*, Paris, Denoël; Alphonse Boudard, *Le Café du pauvre*, Paris, La Table Ronde; Massin, *Le Branle des voleurs*, Paris, La Table Ronde.

1984 Sacha Guitry, *La Maladie*, Paris, Club de l'honnête homme; Geneviève Carion-Machwitz, *La Wiedra*, Paris, Denoël; Jean Héritier, *La Belle Provençale*, Paris, Denoël; Nicole Gage, *La Pourpre déchirée*, Paris, La Table Ronde; Massin, *Le Branle des voleurs*, Paris, France Loisirs; Danielle de Caumon, *Les Enfants du Zodiaque*, Paris, Édition°1; Pierre Bellemare and Marie-Thérèse Cuny, *Au nom de l'amour*, Paris, Édition°1; Pierre Bellemare and Jean-François Nahmias, *Les Grands Crimes de l'histoire*, Paris, Édition°1; Jean-François Nahmias, *Exploits*, Paris, Édition°1; Marie-Thérèse Cuny, *Trésors*, Paris, Édition°1; Ronald Searle, *45 ans de dessins*, Paris, Denoël.

1985 Guy Thomas, *Au nom de la loi*, Paris, Édition°1; Jeanne Bourin, *Le Grand Feu*, Paris, La Table Ronde; Bertrand Méheust, *Soucoupes volantes et Folklore*, Paris, Mercure de France; Paul-Loup Sulitzer, *Hannah*, Paris, Édition°1 / Stock; Georges Moréas and Gilles Pudlowski, *Le Guide de l'Alsace heureuse*, Strasburg, Bueb & Reumaux; Massin, *Les Compagnons de la Marjolaine*, Paris, La Table Ronde; Édith Silve, *Paul Léautaud et le Mercure de France*, Paris, Mercure de France; Patrice Laffont and Bertrand Renard, *Voyelle consonne*, Paris, Édition° 1 / Robert Laffont; Régine, *Appelle-moi par mon prénom*, Paris, Édition°1 / Robert Laffont; René Spiess, *Le Pain de l'espoir*, Strasburg, Bueb & Reumaux; Geneviève Dormann, *Amoureuse Colette*, Paris, Albin Michel; Pierre-Jean Remy, *La Vie d'un héros* Paris, Albin Michel; *Le Livre d'or de l'humour français*, Paris, Hoëbeke; George Painter, *Marcel Proust*, Paris, Mercure de France; Gault-Millau, *Nos desserts préférés à la maison*, Paris, Édition° 1; Mireille Sorgue, *Lettres à l'amant*, II, Paris, Albin Michel; Michael Pabst, *L'Art graphique à Vienne autour de 1900*, Paris, Mercure de France.

1986 *Œuvre poétique de Paul Éluard*, Paris, Club de l'honnête homme; Nicole Calfan, *La Guerrière*, Paris, Édition°1; Florence Rémy and Patrice Bardèche, *Le SIDA*, Paris, Édition°1 / Santé Magazine; David Malouf, *Harland et son domaine*, Paris, Albin Michel; Pierre Melvine, *Le Désert des soldats perdus*, Paris, Édition n° 1; Peter Ollison and Milo Dullker, *New York, Sandra*, Paris, Newlook; Marc de Champérard and Gilles Pudlowski, *52 week-ends en France*, Paris, Albin Michel; Paul Goma, *Bonifacia*, Paris, Albin Michel; Jules Roy, *Guynemer*, Paris, Albin Michel; Ann Schlee, *Le Propriétaire*, Paris, Albin Michel; Georges Moréas, *Un solo meurtrier*, Paris, Édition°1; Roger Vadim, *D'une étoile l'autre*, Paris, Albin Michel; Michel Ragon, *Drôles de métiers*, Paris, Albin Michel; Paul-Loup Sulitzer, *L'Impératrice*, Paris, Édition°1 / Stock; Jacques Almira, *La Fuite à Constantinople*, Paris, Mercure de France; Marc de Champérard, *52 week-ends autour de Lyon*, Paris, Albin Michel; Jean-Louis Debré, *Le Curieux*, Paris, Édition°1; Jean-Pierre Dionnet and Philippe Manœuvre, *Vive la France!*, Paris, Édition°1; Alain Dugrand and Patrice Gouy, *Mexico Terremoto*, Strasburg, Bueb & Reumaux; Marquise de la Falaise, *Les Années magnifiques*, Paris, Édition°1; Muriel Cerf, *Dramma per musica*, Paris, Albin Michel; Jean-Edern Hallier, *L'Évangile du fou*, Paris, Albin Michel; Pierre-Jean Remy, *Une Ville immortelle*, Paris, Albin Michel; Pierre Serval, *Moi, la Duchesse de Berry*, Paris, Albin Michel; Alain Vircondelet, *Séraphine de Senlis*, Paris, Albin Michel; Ludmila Tcherina, *La Femme à l'envers*, Paris, Albin Michel; Dr David Elia, *50 ans vive la vie!*, Paris, Édition°1; René Nelli, *Le Roman de Ramon de Miraval, troubadour*, Paris, Albin Michel; John Rewald, *Histoire de l'impressionnisme*, Paris, Albin Michel; Charles Rozen and Henri Zerner, *Romantisme et Réalisme*, Paris, Albin Michel; Marc de Smedt, *Éloge du silence*, Paris, Albin Michel; *Vignettes*, Paris, Ramsay / Caractère; Christian Kempf and Thierry Piantanida, *Les forêts meurent aussi*, Strasburg, Bueb & Reumaux.

1987 Maryse Condé, *La Vie scélérate*, Paris, Mercure de France, Le Grand Livre du mois; Louis Pergaud, *Œuvres Complètes*, Paris, Le Grand Livre du mois; *Œuvres de Guy De Maupassant*, Paris, Club de l'honnête homme; Jean-Marie Thiveaud, *Azur*, Paris, Albin Michel; Alain Vircondelet, *Le Petit Frère de la nuit*, Paris, Albin Michel; Jacques Perry, *Oubli*, Paris, Albin Michel; Fanny Deschamps, *Louison ou l'Heure exquise*, Paris, Albin Michel; Béatrice Didier, *Le Siècle des Lumières*, Paris, MA; Jean Cocteau, *Lettres à Jean Marais*, Paris, Albin Michel; Karel Appel, *40 ans de peinture, sculpture et dessin*, Paris, Galilée; Hubert Auriol and Cyril Neveu, *Une histoire d'hommes*, Paris, Édition°1; Yves Navarre, *Fête des mères*, Paris, Albin Michel; Georges Moréas, *Amour solo*, Paris, Fixot; Jean-Luc Porquet / Dominique Pouillet, *Boomerang*, Paris, Hoëbeke; Eve Arnold, *Marilyn for ever*, Paris, Albin Michel; Emmanuel Dongala, *Le Feu des origines*, Paris, Albin Michel; Guy Hocquenghem, *Ève*, Paris Albin Michel; René-Victor Pilhes, *Les Démons de la cour de Rohan*, Paris, Albin Michel; François Liensa, *La Bague au lion*, Paris, Cie 12 / Fixot; Michel de Saint-Pierre, *Le Milieu de l'été*, Paris, Albin Michel; Jacques de Bourbon Busset, *Confession de Don Juan*, Paris, Albin Michel; Jean-Jacques Brochier, *L'Hallali*, Paris, Albin Michel; Michel Drucker, *Les n° 1*, Paris, Fixot / France Football; Françoise Parturier, *Les Chiens du Taj Mahal*, Paris, Albin Michel; Flora Groult, *Marie Laurencin*, Paris, Mercure de France; Roland Jacquard, *La Longue Traque d'Action Directe*, Paris, Albin Michel; *Guide Dussert-Gerber des vins de France 88*, Paris, Albin Michel; Michel Ragon, *Le Marin des sables*, Paris, Albin Michel; Samivel, *Bonshommes de neige*, Paris, Hoëbeke; Hubert Haddad, *Le Visiteur aux gants de soie*, Paris, Albin Michel.

1988 Andersen, *Contes*, Paris, Mercure de France; Marguerite Yourcenar, *L'Œuvre au noir*, Paris, Le Grand Livre du mois; *La Coupole*, Paris, Albin Michel; Christine Aventin, *Le Cœur en poche*, Paris, Mercure de France; Patrick Cauvin, *Werther, ce soir...*, Paris, Albin Michel; Yves Navarre, *Romans, un roman*, Paris, Albin Michel; Valéry Giscard d'Estaing, *Le Pouvoir et la Vie*, Paris, Cie 12; Massin, *La Dernière Passion*, Paris, France Loisirs; Suzanne Prou, *Le Temps des innocents*, Paris, Albin Michel; Michel Alibert, *Ballade pour un soldat perdu*, Paris, Albin Michel; Muriel Cerf, *Doux oiseaux de Galilée*, Paris, Albin Michel; Denis Desforges, *Le Pacifique*, Paris, Albin Michel; Laura Kreyder, *Thérèse Martin*, Paris, Albin Michel; Betty Mahmoody, *Jamais sans ma fille*, Paris, Fixot; René-Victor Pilhes, *L'Hitlérien*, Paris, Albin Michel; Michel Larneuil, *Si l'Adour avait voulu*, Paris, Albin Michel; Lydie Locatelli, *Cent mètres d'amour avec haies et obstacles*, Paris, Albin Michel; Auguste Scheurer-Kestner, *Mémoires d'un sénateur dreyfusard*, Strasburg, Bueb & Reumaux; Patrick Besson, *La Statue du commandeur*, Paris, Albin Michel; Jean Blot, *Sainte-Imposture*, Paris, Albin Michel; Guy Hocquenghem, *Les Voyages et Aventures extraordinaires du frère Angelo*, Paris, Albin Michel; François Liensa, *La Femme de sable*, Paris, Cie 12 / Fixot; Albert Camus, *Le Mythe de Sisyphe*, Paris, France Loisirs; Sylvie Forestier, *Les Chagall de Chagall*, Paris, Albin Michel; Ysabelle Lacamp, *La Fille du ciel*, Paris, Albin Michel; Pierre Pallardy, *Plus jamais mal au dos*, Paris, Fixot; Richard Sennett, *Palais-Royal*, Paris, Albin Michel; Douglas Skeggs, *Monet et la Seine*, Paris, Albin Michel; Chen Zhao-fu, *Découverte de l'art préhistorique en Chine*, Paris, Albin Michel;

Jean Contrucci, *Emma Calvé, la diva du siècle*, Paris, Albin Michel; Jean-Luc Hennig, *Cap Fréhel*, Paris, Albin Michel.

1989 Massin, *L'ABC du métier*, Paris, Imprimerie nationale; *Histoire économique et financière de la France*, Ministère des finances, de l'économie et du budget; Aragon, *L'Œuvre poétique*, Paris, Livre club Diderot; Ivan Cloulas, *Sur la trace des Dieux*, Paris, Albin Michel; Yves Navarre, *Hôtel Styx*, Paris, Albin Michel; Jules Roy, *Mémoires barbares*, Paris, Albin Michel; Harry F. Saint, *Mémoires d'un homme invisible*, Paris, Albin Michel; Pierre Bellemare and Jean-François Nahmias, *Les Crimes passionnels*, Paris, Edition°1/ TF1; Claude Aveline, *Histoires nocturnes et fantastiques*, Paris, Imprimerie nationale; Geneviève Dormann, *Le Bal du dodo*, Paris, Albin Michel; Claude Klotz, *Killer kid*, Paris, Albin Michel; Muriel Cerf, *La Nativité à l'Étoile*, Paris, Albin Michel; Samivel, M. *Dumollet sur le Mont-Blanc*, Paris, Hoëbeke; *Les Droits de l'homme*, Paris, Imprimerie nationale; Dr Soly Bensabat, *Le Stress, c'est la vie!*, Paris, Fixot; Dominique Cellura, *Les Voyageurs du froid*, Paris, Hoëbeke; Gilles Lapouge, *Les Folies Kœnigsmark*, Paris, Albin Michel; Jean-Maurice Rouquette and Claude Sintès, *Arles antique*, Paris, Imprimerie nationale; J. Hargrove, *Les Statues de Paris*, Paris, Fonds Mercator/Albin Michel; Charles Villeneuve, *Le Glaive et la Balance*, Paris, M6/ Cie 12; *Comédie d'amour*, Paris, Mercure de France.

1990 *L'Anthologie de Noël*, Paris, Le Grand Livre du mois; *La Bibliothèque de xxᵉ siècle*, Paris, France Loisirs; Pierre Bellemare and Jean-François Nahmias, *Nuits d'angoisse*, Paris, Édition°1/ TF1; *Chroniques d'un automne allemand*, Paris, La Nuée Bleue/ J.-C. Lattès; François Émile-Zola and Massin, *Zola photographe*, Paris, Hoëbeke / Délégation à l'Action; *Lexique des règles typographiques*, Paris, Imprimerie nationale; *Histoires d'un livre : l'Étranger d'Albert Camus*, Paris, IMEC; *Massin*, Paris, IMEC; Massin, *La Cour des miracles*, Paris, Payot.

1991 *L'Alphabet de maître E.S.*, Bibliothèque nationale and Claude Tchou and Sons; Dr David Elia, *Comment rester jeune après 40 ans*, Édition°1/ TF1 éditions; Jean-Jacques Servan-Schreiber, *Passions*, Paris, Fixot; François Nourissier, *Autos graphie*, Paris, Albin Michel; Michel Ragon, *J'en ai connu des équipages*, Paris, Hachette Littérature; Oleg Volkov, *Les Ténèbres*, Paris, J.-C. Lattès; *La Bataille des paravents*, Paris, IMEC; Henrik Ibsen, *Les Douze Dernières Pièces*, Paris, Imprimerie nationale; Anne François, *Nu-tête*, Paris, Albin Michel; Valéry Giscard d'Estaing, *Le Pouvoir et La Vie 2*. *L'Affrontement*, Paris, Cie 12; Frédéric Mitterrand, *Destins d'étoiles*, Paris, Fixot/ POL; Dr Georges Debled, *Au-delà de cette limite votre ticket est toujours valable*, Paris, Albin Michel; Jean-François Nahmias, *L'Homme à la licorne*, Paris, Cie 12/ Fixot.

1992 Jacques Vergès, *La justice est un jeu*, Paris, Albin Michel; José Luis de Vilallonga, *Le Gentilhomme européen*, Paris, Fixot; Pierre Pallardy, *Le Droit au plaisir*, Paris, Fixot; José Luis de Vilallonga, *Españas*, Paris, Fixot; Christiane Singer, *Une passion*, Paris, Le Grand Livre du mois; Pierre Bellemare and Jean-François Nahmias, *Crimes de sang*, Paris, Edition°1/ TF1; Jean-Edern Hallier, *Je rends heureux*, Paris, Albin Michel; Betty Mahmoody, *Jamais sans ma fille 2: pour l'amour d'un*

enfant, Paris, Fixot; Coluche, *Les Inoubliables*, Paris, Fixot; Martine Mauléon, *Le Guide de l'anti-galère*, Paris, Albin Michel / Canal + Éditions; G. A. Orefice, *Le Dictionnaire européen simultané en 5 langues*, Paris, Berlitz / Fixot.

1993 Jean-Jacques Servan-Schreiber, *Les Fossoyeurs*, Paris, Fixot; Sandra de Faultrier-Travers, *Le Droit d'auteur dans l'édition*, Paris, Imprimerie nationale; Jules Roy, *Amours barbares*, Paris, Albin Michel; José Luis de Vilallonga, *Le Roi*, Paris, Fixot; Eugen Drewermann, *Fonctionnaires de Dieu*, Paris, Albin Michel; Calixte Beyala, *Maman a un amant*, Paris, Albin Michel; Vadim, *Le Goût du bonheur*, Paris, Fixot; *Comment va la planète? L'Année 1993 vue par les enfants*, Paris, Calmann-Lévy / Okapi; Juan Goytisolo, *Cahier de Sarajevo*, Strasburg, La Nuée bleue; *Barcelone art nouveau*, Paris, Albin Michel; Santiago Alcolea Blanch, *Chefs-d'œuvre du Prado*, Paris, Albin Michel.

1994 Susan Herbert, *Chats de grands maîtres*, Paris, Hoëbeke; Charles Kindleberger, *Histoire mondiale de la spéculation financière*, Paris, Éditions P.A.U.; Alain Gerbault, *Un paradis se meurt*, Paris, Hoëbeke; *Rapport moral sur l'argent dans le monde 1994*, Paris, P.A.U.; Jean Bernard, *Médecin dans le siècle*, Paris, Robert Laffont; Alexandre Minkowski, *Le Vieil Homme et l'Amour*, Paris, Robert Laffont; Peynet, *L'Agenda des amoureux*, Paris, Hoëbeke; Dominique Richert, *Cahiers d'un survivant*, Strasburg, La Nuée bleue; Amélie Weiler, *Journal d'une jeune fille mal dans son siècle*, Strasburg, La Nuée bleue; René Ehni, *Vert-de-gris*, Strasburg, La Nuée bleue; Juan Goytisolo, *L'Algérie dans la tourmente*, Strasburg, La Nuée bleue; Yves-Marc Ajchenbaum, *À la vie, à la mort*, Paris, Le Monde éditions; Martin Gray, *La Prière de l'enfant*, Paris, Robert Laffont; Sélim Nassib, *Oum*, Paris, Balland; Roger Duchêne, *L'Impossible Marcel Proust*, Paris, Robert Laffont; *La CNRACL*, Paris, Éditions P.A.U; Valéry Giscard d'Estaing, *Le Passage*, Paris, Robert Laffont; Denis Lalanne, *Un long dimanche à la campagne*, Paris, Robert Laffont.

1995 Henri de Bodinat, *L'État, parenthèse de l'histoire*, Paris, P.A.U.; Jean-Claude Chesnais, *Le Crépuscule de l'Occident*, Paris, Robert Laffont; François Furet, *Le Passé d'une illusion*, Paris, Robert Laffont / Calmann-Lévy; Mark Childress, *La Tête dans le carton à chapeaux*, Paris, Robert Laffont; Peter Hamilton, *Robert Doisneau, la vie d'un photographe*, Paris, Hoëbeke; Paul Garde, *Journal de voyage en Bosnie-Herzégovine*, Paris, La Nuée bleue; Claude Imbert and Jacques Julliard, *La Droite et la Gauche*, Paris, Robert Laffont / Grasset; Carol O'Connell, *Meurtres à Gramercy Park*, Paris, Robert Laffont; Alain Gerbault, *Iles de beauté*, Paris, Hoëbeke; Jacques-Yves Le Toumelin, *Kurun autour du monde*, Paris, Hoëbeke; Jacques-Yves Le Toumelin, *Kurun aux Antilles*, Paris, Hoëbeke; Gerald Messadié, *29 jours avant la fin du monde*, Paris, Robert Laffont; Alexander Frater, *À la poursuite de la mousson*, Paris, Hoëbeke; André Gauron, *Aux politiques qui prétendent réduire le chômage*, Paris, Balland; Nicholas Negroponte, *L'Homme numérique*, Paris, Robert Laffont; Martin Veyron, *Politiquement correct*, Paris, Hoëbeke; Viviane Villamont, *Une femme irréprochable*, Paris, Le Cherche midi; Michel Field, *Le Passeur de Lesbos*, Paris, Robert Laffont; Alphonse Boudard, *Mourir d'enfance*, Paris, Robert Laffont; Michel Field, *Contes*

cruels pour Anaëlle, Paris, Robert Laffont; Vladimir Boukovsky, *Jugement à Moscou*, Paris, Robert Laffont; Valéry Giscard d'Estaing, *Dans 5 ans l'an 2000*, Paris, Cie 12; Abdulah Sidran, *Je suis une île au cœur du monde*, Strasburg, La Nuée bleue; Susan Herbert, *Chats médiévaux*, Paris, Hoëbeke; Oliviero Toscani, *La pub est une charogne qui nous sourit*, Paris, Hoëbeke; Robert Grossmann, *Comtesse de Pourtalès*, Strasburg, La Nuée bleue; Thierry Desjardins, *Lettre au Président sur le grand ras-le-bol des Français*, Fixot; Marek Halter, *La Force du bien*, Robert Laffont; Christian Bouclier, *Ma femme me trompe*, Paris, J.-C. Lattès; Bernard Clavel, *Le Carcajou*, Paris, Robert Laffont; Benjamin Rabier, *Gédéon Comédien*, *Gédéon en Afrique*, *Gédéon se marie*, *Gédéon Roi de Matapa*, *Gédéon Mécano*, Paris, Hoëbeke.

1996 Gérard Calmette, *Un Parisien à la campagne*, Paris, Hoëbeke; *Lectures de Ionesco*, Paris, L'Harmattan; Jacques Derogy and Hesi Carmel, *Ils ont tué Rabin*, Paris, Robert Laffont; Claude Gagnière, *'Entre guillemets'*, Paris, Robert Laffont; Laure Charpentier, *J'ai soif*, Paris, Fixot; Noa Ben Artzi-Pelossof, *Au nom du chagrin et de l'espoir*, Paris, Fixot; Dr Jean-Marie Andrieu, *Médecin, pour le meilleur et pour le pire*, Paris, Balland; Pierre Chaunu and Éric Mesnion-Rigau, *Baptême de Clovis, baptême de la France*, Paris, Balland; Claude Couderc, *Le Petit*, Paris, Robert Laffont; Dominique Jamet, *Carte de presse*, Paris, Balland; Massin, *Journal en désordre*, Paris, Robert Laffont; Lionel Duroy, *Mon premier jour de bonheur*, Paris, Julliard; Marie Le Drian, *Hôtel maternel*, Paris, Julliard; Leïla Marouane, *La Fille de la casbah*, Paris, Julliard; Gerald Messadié, *Tycho l'admirable*, Paris, Julliard; Fouad Laroui, *Les Dents du topographe*, Paris, Julliard; Jean-Pierre Milovanoff, *La Splendeur d'Antonia*, Paris, Julliard; Jacques Le Goff, *L'Europe racontée aux jeunes*, Paris, Seuil; Claude Michelet, *Histoires des paysans de France*, Paris, Robert Laffont; Roland Topor, *Jachère-party*, Paris, Julliard; Claude Vigée, *La Maison des vivants*, Strasburg, La Nuée bleue; John Grisham, *L'Idéaliste*, Paris, Robert Laffont; Daniel Lebard, *Engagés par l'oncle Sam des artistes engagés gravent la mémoire de la Dépression*, Paris, musée-galerie de la Seita.

1997 Daniel Goleman, *L'Intelligence émotionnelle*, Paris, Robert Laffont; *L'Appel de Strasbourg*, Strasburg, La Nuée bleue; Victoire Doutreleau, *Et Dior créa la victoire*, Paris, Robert Laffont; Robert Grossmann, *Le Choix de Malraux*, Strasburg, La Nuée bleue; Jean Mialet, *La Haine et Le Pardon*, Paris, Robert Laffont; Jean-Claude Lamy, *Prévert, les frères amis*, Paris, Robert Laffont; Dominique Abel, *Caméléone*, Paris, Robert Laffont; Misha Defonseca, *Survivre avec les loups*, Paris, Robert Laffont; Ozren Kebo, *Bienvenue en enfer*, Strasburg, La Nuée bleue; Anne Rice, *Les Infortunes de la belle au bois dormant*, Paris, Robert Laffont; André Rougeot, *La Douanière*, Strasburg, La Nuée bleue; Sylvain Bonnet, *Prof!*, Paris, Robert Laffont; Christian Jacq, *Le Pharaon noir*, Paris, Robert Laffont; Huguette Dreikaus, *Le Monde d'Huguette*, Strasburg, La Nuée bleue; *Les Lettres de Louise Jacobson et de ses proches*, Paris, Robert Laffont; Elizabeth Marshall Thomas, *Les Chats et leur nature*, Paris, Robert Laffont; Joël Robuchon, *Cuisinez comme un grand chef*, Paris, TF1 Éditions; Jean-Yves Cousteau and Yves Paccalet, *Requins*, Paris, Robert

List of works

Laffont; André Frossard, *Le Crime contre l'humanité*, Paris, Robert Laffont; Jéromine Pasteur, *Ouragan*, Paris, Fixot; Marie Sara, *La Vie pour de vrai*, Paris, Robert Laffont; Tomi Ungerer, *Mon Alsace*, Strasburg, La Nuée bleue; Jean Amadou, *De quoi j'me mêle!*, Paris, Robert Laffont; Michel Guérard, *La Cuisine gourmande des juniors*, Paris, Robert Laffont; various, *Le Livre noir du communisme*, Paris, Robert Laffont.

1998 Michael Crichton, *Voyages*, Paris, Robert Laffont; Dr Patrick Sabatier and Joël Robuchon, *Le Meilleur et le Plus Simple pour maigrir*, Paris, Robert Laffont; Georges de Caunes, *Imarra*, Paris, Hoëbeke; Max Gallo, *De Gaulle*, Paris, Robert Laffont; Ben Macintyre, *La Vie aventureuse d'Adam Worth, roi des voleurs, escroc et gentleman*, Paris, Robert Laffont; Édith Montelle, *L'Œil de la vouivre*, Strasburg, La Nuée bleue / Éditions de l'Est; Christopher Carter, *Le Cheval du crime*, Paris, Robert Laffont; Michel Déon, *Madame Rose*, Paris, Albin Michel; Michel Chaumet, *Maif, histoire d'un défi*, Paris, Le Cherche midi; Mario Puzo, *Le Parrain*, Paris, Robert Laffont; Jean-Pierre Kahane and Pierre-Gilles Lemarié-Rieusset, *Séries de Fourier et ondelettes*, Paris, Cassini; Hubert Bari, *La Bibliothèque*, Strasburg, La Nuée bleue; Roger Polvé, *En habit de soleil*, Éditions La Roudoule; Martin Graff, *Le Réveil du Danube*, Strasburg, La Nuée bleue; Muriel Amori, *Mode d'emploi*, Paris, Robert Laffont; Bertrand Blier, *Existe en blanc*, Paris, Robert Laffont; Alphonse Boudard, *L'Étrange monsieur Joseph*, Paris, Robert Laffont; Jacques Brel, *L'Œuvre intégrale*, Paris, Robert Laffont; Mark Childress, *Bienvenue au Paradis*, Paris, Robert Laffont; *La Conquête mondiale des droits de l'homme*, Paris, Le Cherche midi; Florence Daniel-Wieser, *Les Dames de Nancy*, Strasburg, La Nuée bleue; J.-L. Krivine, *Théorie des ensembles*, Paris, Cassini; Morris West, *Sa Sainteté*, Paris, Robert Laffont; David Maraniss, *Qui est vraiment Bill Clinton?*, Paris, Fixot; Olivier Todd, *Jacques Brel, une vie*, Paris, Robert Laffont; Nicolas Vanier, *Destin nord*, Paris, Robert Laffont; David Douillet, *L'Âme du conquérant*, Paris, Robert Laffont; Henri Ulrich, *Je ne fais que passer*, Strasburg, La Nuée bleue; Christina Sanchez, *Matadora*, Paris, Robert Laffont; Marek Halter, *Les Mystères de Jérusalem*, Paris, Robert Laffont; *Scandales et Affaires criminelles*, Paris, TF1 Éditions.

1999 Jean Duché, *Histoire de l'Occident*, Paris, Robert Laffont; Maïté, *C'est tout simple*, Paris, Robert Laffont; Alain Laville, *Un crime politique en Corse*, Paris, Le Cherche midi; Simone Morgenthaler, *Sonate à Catherine*, Strasburg, La Nuée bleue; Marie-Louise Roth-Zimmermann, *Je me souviens de Schelklingen*, Strasburg, La Nuée bleue; Philippe Jéhin, *Rapp*, Strasburg, La Nuée bleue; Jean Sérisé, *Mémoires d'un autre*, Paris, Éditions de Fallois; François Bon and Jérôme Schlomoff, *La Douceur dans l'abîme*, Strasburg, La Nuée Bleue / Éditions de l'Est; Olivier Larizza, *Les Nénuphars de Belgrade*, Strasburg, La Nuée bleue; Paul Mulmann, *Geneviève et les siens*, Strasburg, La Nuée bleue / Éditions de l'Est; Claude Gagnière, *Versiculets et texticules*, Paris, Robert Laffont; Jean Raspail, *Le Roi de la mer*, Paris, Albin Michel; Jean-Louis Étienne, *Le Pôle intérieur*, Paris, Hoëbeke; Alain Decaux and Alain Peyrefitte, *De Gaulle, celui qui a dit non*, Paris, TF1 Éditions / Perrin; Michel Ragon, *Georges et Louise*, Paris, Albin Michel; Jean Raspail, *Le Roi au-delà de la mer*, Paris, Albin Michel.

2000 Max Gallo, *Bleu blanc rouge Mariella*, Paris, X O Éditions; Christian Jacq, *La Pierre de lumière, Néfer le silencieux*, Paris, X O Éditions; Massin, *De la variation*, Paris, Le Promeneur; Olivier Dazat, *L'Honneur des champions*, Paris, Hoëbeke; Christiane Singer, *Éloge du mariage, de l'engagement et autres folies*, Paris, Albin Michel; René Desmaison, *Les Grimpeurs de muraille*, Paris, Hoëbeke; Paul Halmos, *Problèmes pour mathématiciens, petits et grands*, Paris, Cassini; Stéphanie Janicot, *Soledad*, Paris, Albin Michel; André Comte-Sponville, *Présentations de la philosophie*, Paris, Albin Michel; Didier van Cauwelaert, *L'Éducation d'une fée*, Paris, Albin Michel; Gisèle Loth, *Un rêve de France*, Strasburg, La Nuée Bleue / Éditions de l'Est; Simone Morgenthaler, *Un été en Californie*, Strasburg, La Nuée bleue; Thierry Roland, *Euro passionnément*, Paris, TF1 Éditions; Calixte Beyala, *Comment cuisiner son mari à l'africaine*, Paris, Albin Michel; *Le Livre mondial des inventions 2001*, Paris, Cie 12 / X O Éditions / Europe 1; Michel de Grèce, *La Nuit blanche de Saint-Pétersbourg*, Paris, X O Éditions; Philippe Olivier, *L'Horreur de l'aube*, Strasburg, La Nuée bleue; Christian Streiff, *Kriegspiel*, Strasburg, La Nuée bleue; Charles Exbrayat, *Les Parfums regrettés*, Paris, Albin Michel; *La Merveilleuse Histoire du bon Saint Florentin d'Alsace*, Strasburg, Éditions du Rhin.

2001 Nicolas Sarkozy, *Libre*, Paris, Fixot / Robert Laffont; Ingrid Betancourt, *La Rage au cœur*, Paris, X O Éditions; Michel Ragon, *Un rossignol chantait*, Paris, Albin Michel; François Moulin, *Jean Prouvé*, Strasburg, La Nuée bleue / Éditions de l'Est; Simone Morgenthaler, *Au jardin de ma mère*, Strasburg, La Nuée bleue; Savignac, *L'Affiche de A à Z*, Paris, Hoëbeke; Noël Daum, *Daum*, Strasburg, La Nuée bleue / Éditions de l'Est; Émile Jung, *Au menu de ma vie*, Strasburg, La Nuée bleue; Grégoire Gauchet, *Un siècle de ski dans les Vosges*, Strasburg, La Nuée bleue / Éditions de l'Est; André Pierre, *Peinture polychrome d'Alsace*, Strasburg, La Nuée bleue; *Regards sur la culture judéo-alsacienne*, Strasburg, La Nuée bleue; Charles Muller, *Mes rencontres avec Victor Hugo*, Strasburg, La Nuée bleue / Éditions de l'Est; *Oui aux voitures propres*, Paris, Hoëbeke; Dr Agnès Saraux, *Mes parents vieillissent*, Paris, Bonneton; *Qu'apprend-on au collège?*, Paris, X O / Centre national de documentation pédagogique.

2002 *L'Aventure de la flibuste*, Paris, Hoëbeke / Abbaye de Daoulas; Nicole-Lise Bernheim, *La Cloche de 10 heures*, Strasburg, La Nuée bleue; Martin Brem, *La Vie baroque*, Strasburg, La Nuée bleue; François Charles, *Vie et Mort de Poil de carotte*, Strasburg, La Nuée bleue; Christiane Roederer, *La Veilleuse de chagrin*, Strasburg, La Nuée bleue; Mireille Calmel, *Le Lit d'Aliénor*, Paris, X O Éditions; Max Gallo, *Victor Hugo*, Paris, X O Éditions; Henri Calet, *Poussières de la route*, Paris, Le Dilettante; Milan Dargent, *Soupe à la tête de bouc*, Paris, Le Dilettante; Janot Lamberton, *Les Moulins de glace*, Paris, Hoëbeke; *Nouvelles voix d'Afrique*, Paris, Hoëbeke; Monique Pivot, *Maggi et la magie du bouillon Kub*, Paris, Hoëbeke; Tomi Ungerer, *De père en fils*, Strasburg, La Nuée bleue; Christopher Carter, *Crimes romains*, Paris, Cie 12; Yanny Hureaux, *Nicolas Sachy*, Strasburg, La Nuée bleue / L'Ardennais; David Khayat, *Le Coffre aux âmes*, Paris, X O Éditions; Frank Deroche, *Effets secondaires*, Paris, Le Dilettante; *Carnets de Sarajevo*, I, Paris, Gallimard; José Frèches, *Les Chevaux célestes*, Paris, X O Éditions; Alexandre

Vialatte, *Au coin du désert*, Paris, Le Dilettante; *Aux knacks, citoyens!*, Strasburg, La Nuée bleue; Christian Jacq, *Champollion l'Égyptien*, Paris, X O Éditions; Christian Jacq, *Maître Hiram et le roi Salomon*, Paris, X O Éditions; *DesignIssues*, Massachusetts Institute of Technology, Cambridge; Romain Sardou, *Pardonnez nos offenses*, Paris, X O Éditions.

2003 *L'Appel de Lunéville*, Éditions de l'Est / L'Est Républicain / BNP Paribas; Jean François Deniau, *La Gloire à 20 ans*, Paris, X O Éditions; Max Gallo, *César imperator*, Paris, X O Éditions; Hansi, *Professor Knatschké*, Strasburg, Éditions du Rhin; Edmund Hillary, *Au sommet de l'Everest*, Paris, Hoëbeke; Tavae, *Si loin du monde*, Paris, Oh! Éditions; Christian Jacq, *Le Monde magique de l'Égypte ancienne*, Paris, X O Éditions; Christian Jacq, *Pouvoir et Sagesse selon l'égypte ancienne*, Paris, X O Éditions; Christian Jacq, *Trois voyages initiatiques*, Paris, X O Éditions; Christian Jacq, *Les Mystères d'Osiris*, Paris, X O Éditions; Michel Deutsch, *Alsace, terre étrangère*, Paris, X O Éditions; Jean-Noël Grandhomme, Thérèse Krempp and Charles de Roze, *Le Pionnier de l'aviation de chasse*, Strasburg, La Nuée bleue; Massin, *La Lettre et l'Image*, Paris, Gallimard; Simone Morgenthaler and Renée Roth-Hano, *À demain à New York, je porterai votre écharpe*, Strasburg, La Nuée bleue; Rosalie Firholz, *Une enfance à la ferme*, Strasburg, La Nuée bleue; Laurent Hincker, *Sectes, rumeurs et tribunaux*, Strasburg, La Nuée bleue; Raymond Matzen, Léon Daul, *Wie geht's?*, Strasburg, La Nuée bleue; Michel Paul Urban and Léon Daul, *Lieux dits*, Strasburg, Éditions du Rhin; Yanny Hureaux, *Un Ardennais nommé Rimbaud*, Strasburg, L'Ardennais / La Nuée bleue; Dr Delphine Lhuillery, *Docteur, j'ai mal*, Paris, Bonneton.

2004 Maxence Fermine, *Amazone*, Paris, Albin Michel; Gabriel Osmonde, *Les 20 000 Femmes de la vie d'un homme*, Paris, Albin Michel; Gilbert Mercier, *Femmes des Lumières à la cour de Stanislas*, La Nuée bleue / Éditions de l'Est; Sylvie Vartan, *Entre l'ombre et la lumière*, Paris, X O Éditions; Myrielle Marc, *Orfenor*, Paris, X O Éditions; Diane de Margerie, *Aurore et George*, Paris, Albin Michel; Nicolas Vanier, *L'Or sous la neige*, Paris, XO Éditions; Jean Sarenne, *Trois curés en montagne*, Paris, Hoëbeke; Jean Louis Schlienger and André Braun, *Le Buveur alsacien*, Strasburg, La Nuée bleue; Alfred Wahl, *Petites haines ordinaires*, Strasburg, La Nuée bleue; Mitch Albom, *Les cinq personnes que j'ai rencontrées là-haut*, Paris, Oh! Éditions; Jacques-Henry Gros, *Au fil du siècle*, Strasburg, La Nuée bleue; Simone Morgenthaler, *Ces années-là*, Strasburg, La Nuée bleue; Michel Breton, *Tomas Divi*, Association 'Terre de Beauce'; Marie-Joseph Bopp, *Ma ville à l'heure nazie*, Strasburg, La Nuée bleue; Dr Frédéric Chaussoy, *Je ne suis pas un assassin*, Paris, Oh! Éditions; Sandrine Dardenne, *J'avais douze ans, j'ai pris mon vélo et je suis partie à l'école*, Paris, Oh! Éditions; Michel de Grèce, *Mémoires insolites*, Paris, X O Éditions; Jacques Dutertre, *Vivez plus riche, vive les radins*, Paris, Bonneton; Tomi Ungerer, *L'Alsace côté cœur*, Strasburg, La Nuée bleue.

2005 Dominique Baudis, *Face à la calomnie*, Paris, Fixot; Jean-Claude Gall, *Alsace, des fossiles et des hommes*, Strasburg, La Nuée bleue; Tarita Tériipaia, *Marlon, mon amour, ma déchirure*, Paris, X O Éditions; Patrick Chauvel, *Sky*, Paris, Oh! Éditions;

Aude Boissaye, *Dans la jungle du Rhin*, Strasburg, Éditions du Rhin; Robert Carlier, *À la nuit la nuit*, Paris, H. C.; Aron Gabor, *Le Cri de la taïga*, Paris, Éditions du Rocher; Marie-France Hirigoyen, *Femmes sous emprise*, Paris, Oh! Éditions; Robert Steegmann, *Struthof*, Strasburg, La Nuée bleue; Sébastien Brant, *La Nef des fous*, Strasburg, La Nuée bleue; Christian and Élisabeth Busser, *Les Plantes des Vosges*, Strasburg, La Nuée bleue; Rosalie Firholz, *Rosalie, un amour pour la vie*, Strasburg, La Nuée bleue; Pierre Kretz, *Quand j'étais petit, j'étais catholique*, Strasburg, La Nuée bleue; various, *La Petite Camargue alsacienne*, Strasburg, Éditions du Rhin; Michel Caffier, *Place Stanislas*, Strasburg, La Nuée bleue; *Le Livre noir de Saddam Hussein*, Paris, Oh! Éditions; Roland Erbstein, *Racontez-moi la Lorraine*, Strasburg, La Nuée bleue; *Cavanna à Charlie Hebdo, 1969–1981*, Hoëbeke; Michel Loestcher and Jean-Charles Spindler, *Spindler*, Strasburg, La Nuée bleue; Christian Jacq, *Mozart*, Paris, X O Éditions.

2006 Jean-Noël Grandhomme, *Ultimes sentinelles*, Strasburg, La Nuée bleue; Mademoiselle de Mortemart, *Un merveilleux voyage*, Strasburg, La Nuée bleue; Michelle Maillet, *L'Étoile noire*, Paris, Oh! Éditions; Claude Muller, *Le Siècle des Rohan*, Strasburg, La Nuée bleue; *Le Livre noir de la condition des femmes*, Christine Ockrent (ed.), Paris, X O Éditions; Edmond Jung, *L'Alsadico*, Strasburg, La Nuée bleue; Philippe Bertrand, *Quand j'serai grand*, Paris, Hoëbeke / France Inter; Kamran Nazeer, *Laissez entrer les idiots*, Paris, Oh! Éditions; Jean-Marie Pontaut and Gilles Gaetner, *Règlement de comptes à l'Élysée*, Paris, Oh! Éditions; Jean-Louis Fournier, *À ma dernière cigarette*, Paris, Hoëbeke; Emmanuel Davidenkoff, *Réveille-toi Jules Ferry ils sont devenus fous!*, Paris, Oh! Éditions / France Info; Michel Caffier, *La Madeleine*, Strasburg, La Nuée bleue; Mireille Horsinga-Renno, *Cher Oncle Georg*, Strasburg, La Nuée bleue; René-Nicolas Ehni, *Chantefable*, Strasburg, La Nuée bleue; Didier Long, *Pourquoi nous sommes chrétiens?*, Paris, Oh! Éditions/Le Cherche midi; Fernand Weber, *Le Fils ingrat*, Strasburg, La Nuée bleue; Albert Ronsin, *Le nom de l'Amérique*, Strasburg, La Nuée bleue; Guy Trendel, *Racontez-moi Strasbourg*, Strasburg, La Nuée bleue.

2007 Jean-Charles Escribano, *On achève bien nos vieux*, Paris, Oh! Éditions; Luc Ferry, *Familles je vous aime*, Paris, X O Éditions; José Frèches, *Quand les Chinois cesseront de rire le monde pleurera*, Paris, X O Éditions; Jacques Frémion, *L'Histoire de la révolution écologique*, Paris, Hoëbeke.

Cover designs for series

1958 Raymond Léopold Bruckberger, *La République américaine*, 'Problèmes et documents' series, Paris, Gallimard; Alfred Einstein, *Schubert*, 'Leurs Figures' series, Paris, Gallimard; Various covers for literary publications, Paris, Mercure de France.

1959 Gabriel Casaccia, *La Limace*, 'La Croix du sud' series, Paris, Gallimard; Jacques Souniones, *Mon récit*, 'Jeune Prose' series, Paris, Gallimard; Leonard Cottrell, *La Vie au temps des pharaons*, 'Mémoire du monde' series, Paris, Pierre Horay; François Sentein, *Philippe*, 'Prénoms' series, Paris, Pierre Horay; *Cahiers Paul Claudel*, I, Paris, Gallimard; Jacques Serguine, *Les Fils de rois*, 'Le Chemin' series, Paris, Gallimard; Zoé Oldenbourg, *Le Bûcher de Montségur*, 'Trente journées qui ont fait la France' series, Paris, Gallimard.

1960 Frank Harris, *Ma vie et mes amours*, 'Les Classiques anglais' series, Paris, Gallimard; Georges Simenon, *Le Fils Cardinaud*, Paris, Gallimard; Émile Dermenghen, *Le Pays d'Abel*, 'L'Espèce humaine' series, Paris, Gallimard; Jean Dollfus, *L'Homme et le Rhin*, 'Géographie humaine' series, Paris, Gallimard; Henri Guillemin, *Le Coup du 2 décembre*, 'La Suite des temps' series, Paris, Gallimard.

1961 Mohamed Réza Pahlévi, *Mémoires d'un chah d'Iran*, 'L'Air du temps' series, Paris, Gallimard; Henri Lhote, *L'Épopée du Ténéré*, 'L'Air du temps' series, Paris, Gallimard; Lev Gourevitch, *Agents secrets contre Eichmann*, 'L'Air du temps' series, Paris, Gallimard; Professor L. Pech, *Menaces sur votre vie*, 'L'Air du temps' series, Paris, Gallimard; Nicolaï Tikhonov, *Tête brûlée*, 'Littérature soviétique' series, Paris, Gallimard; Michel Bernard, *Le Domaine du Paraclet*, 'L'Histoire fabuleuse' series, Paris, Gallimard; *Œuvres de Christophe Colomb*, 'Mémoires du passé' series, Paris, Gallimard; Roger Bordier, *Les Blés*, Paris, Calmann-Lévy; *Les Plus Belles Lettres de Voltaire*, 'Les Plus Belles Lettres' series, Paris, Calmann-Lévy; Albert Camus, *Le Mythe de Sisyphe*, 'Idées' series, Paris, Gallimard; Jean-Paul Sartre, *Réflexions sur la question juive*, 'Idées' series, Paris, Gallimard; Sigmund Freud, *Trois essais sur la théorie de la sexualité*, 'Idées' series, Paris, Gallimard.

1962 Martin Heidegger, *Chemins qui ne mènent nulle part*, 'Classiques de la Philosophie' series, Paris, Gallimard; Gaston Meyer, *L'Athlétisme*, 'Domaine du sport' series, Paris, La Table Ronde.

1963 Suétone, *La Vie des douze césars*, Paris, Le Livre de poche; Edward Atiyah, *L'Étau*, 'Panique' series, Paris, Gallimard; Yves Florenne, *Delacroix*, 'Les Plus Belles Pages' series, Paris, Mercure de France.

1964 Arthur Adamov, *Ici et maintenant*, 'Pratique du théâtre' series, Paris, Gallimard; Max Brod, *Une vie combattive*, 'La Connaissance de soi' series, Paris, Gallimard; *David de Sassoun*, 'Caucase' series, Paris, Gallimard; John Le Carré, *L'Espion qui venait du froid*, 'Le Livre du jour' series, Paris, Gallimard.

1965 Maurice Lelong O.P., *Alice*, Paris, Gallimard; Robert Mengin, *De Gaulle à Londres*, 'L'Histoire contemporaine reuve et corrigée' series, Paris,

La Table Ronde; Suzanne Pénière, *Gorge ouverte*, Paris, Gallimard; various, *Les Françaises à Ravensbrück*, Paris, Gallimard; Eugenio Montale, *Poésies*, 'Poésie du monde entier' series, Paris, Gallimard.

1966 Paul Éluard, *Capitale de la douleur*, 'Poésie Gallimard' series, Paris, Gallimard; Federico García Lorca, *Poésies*, 'Poésie Gallimard' series, Paris, Gallimard; Stéphane Mallarmé, *Poésies*, 'Poésie Gallimard' series, Paris, Gallimard; Sei Shônagon, *Notes de chevet*, 'Poésie Gallimard' series, Paris, Gallimard.

1971 Jean Sulivan, *Petite littérature individuelle*, 'Voies ouvertes' series, Paris, Gallimard; Jacques Lanzmann, *Mémoires d'un amnésique*, Paris, Denoël; André Breton, *Arcane 17*, Paris, Jean-Jacques Pauvert éditeur; James Hadley Chase, *Une manche et la belle*, 'Carré noir' series, Paris, Gallimard; Bill Pronsini, *Qui traque-t-on?*, 'Série noire' series, Paris, Gallimard; André Malraux, *La Condition humaine*, 'Folio' series, Paris, Gallimard; Albert Camus, *L'Étranger*, 'Folio' series, Paris, Gallimard; Jean-Paul Sartre, *Les Mouches*, 'Folio' series, Paris, Gallimard; Antoine de Saint-Exupéry, *Vol de nuit*, 'Folio' series, Paris, Gallimard.

1973 Pierre Gascar, *Quartier latin*, Paris, La Table Ronde; Roger Caillois, *La Pieuvre*, Paris, La Table Ronde; Joseph Kessel, *La Piste fauve*, Paris, Gallimard.

1976 Jean-Paul Sartre, *L'Être et le Néant*, 'Tel' series, Paris, Gallimard; François Jacob, *La Logique du vivant*, 'Tel' series, Paris, Gallimard; Georg Groddeck, *Le Livre du ça*, 'Tel' series, Paris, Gallimard; Maurice Merleau-Ponty, *Phénoménologie de la perception*, 'Tel' series, Paris, Gallimard; *Cahiers Céline*, I, Paris, Gallimard.

1977 Enrico Altavilla, *La Sexualité à travers le monde*, 'L'Air du temps' series, Paris, Gallimard; William Faulkner, *Les Palmiers sauvages*, 'L'Imaginaire' series, Paris, Gallimard; Raymond Queneau, *Un rude hiver*, 'L'Imaginaire' series, Paris, Gallimard; Michel Leiris, *Aurora*, 'L'Imaginaire' series, Paris, Gallimard; Henri Thomas, *La Nuit de Londres*, 'L'Imaginaire' series, Paris, Gallimard.

1980 Sylvie Caster, *Les Chênes Verts*, Paris, Éditions BFB; Michel Godet, *Demain les crises*, Paris, Hachette Littérature; Jean-Marie Chevalier, *L'échiquier industriel*, Paris, Hachette Littérature.

1982 Paul Mentré, *Gulliver enchaîné*, Paris, La Table Ronde.

1983 Covers for a series of French and foreign novels, Paris, Denoël.

1985 Serge Bernstein, *Le Nazisme*, 'Le monde de...' series, Paris, MA; Philippe Boyer, *Le Romantisme allemand*, 'Le monde de...' series, Paris, MA; Gérard de Cortanze, *Le Surréalisme*, 'Le monde de...' series, Paris, MA.

1987 Maud Marin, *Le Saut de l'ange*, Paris, Fixot; Marie-Thérèse Cuny, *Une Garce*, Paris, Fixot; *Le Mobilier domestique*, Paris, Imprimerie nationale.

1989 Franck Venaille, *Cavalier/Cheval*, 'Littératures' series, Paris, Imprimerie nationale; Mouna Pavlova, *Les Espions*, 'Le Spectateur français' series, Paris, Imprimerie nationale; *Viviers*, 'Inventaire

List of works

topographique' series, Paris, Imprimerie nationale; Jean-Claude Martel, *Le Livre des humeurs*, 'Littératures' series, Paris, Imprimerie nationale; *Orfèvrerie nantaise*, 'Cahiers de l'inventaire' series, Paris, Imprimerie nationale; *Vic-Bilh, Morlaàs et Montanarès*, 'Inventaire topographique' series, Paris, Imprimerie nationale.

1990 *Bibliothèque de france, bibliothèque ouverte*, Paris, IMEC; Glen Baxter, *Ma vie*, Paris, Hoëbeke; François Salviat, *Glanum* 'Guides archéologiques de France' series, Paris, Imprimerie nationale; Keiko Yamanaka, *L'Archipel écartelé*, 'Connaître' series, Paris, Tsuru Éditions; Pascal Dayez-Burgeon, *La Relique impériale*, 'Histoire d'histoires' series, Paris, Hatier; Grimmelshausen, *L'Aventurière courage*, Paris, Bueb and Reumaux / J.-C. Lattès; Claude Lévi-Strauss, *Tristes tropiques*, 'Littérature du xxᵉ siècle' series, Paris, France Loisirs; Henri Bergson, *Le Rire*, Paris, France Loisirs; Albin Michel, general cover for literary works.

1991 Manuel de Diéguez, *Essai sur l'universalité de la France*, 'Bibliothèque Albin Michel des idées' series, Albin Michel; various, *Lacan avec les philosophes*, 'Bibliothèque du Collège international de philosophie' series, Paris, Albin Michel; *Revue de synthèse*, Paris, Centre International de synthèse / Albin Michel; Constantin Cavafy, *Œuvres poétiques*, 'La Salamandre' series, Paris Imprimerie nationale; Alain Buisine, *Proust*, 'Une journée particulière' series, Paris, J.-C. Lattès; Richard Jorif, *Valéry*, 'Une journée particulière' series, Paris, J.-C. Lattès; Bernard Toulier, *Châteaux*, 'Cahiers de l'inventaire' series, Paris, Imprimerie nationale.

1992 *La Bhagavad Gîtâ*, 'La Salamandre' series, Paris, Imprimerie nationale; Érasme, *Colloques*, I, 'La Salamandre' series, Paris, Imprimerie nationale; Edward Abbey, *Désert solitaire*, 'Le Grand Dehors' series, Paris, Hoëbeke; Gerald Durrell, *La Forêt ivre*, 'Le Grand Dehors' series, Paris, Hoëbeke; Hassan El-Husseini, *Les Enfants du Caire*, 'Carnets de reportage' series, First; Michel Déon ed., *Stendhal*, Bibliothèque Fixot; Alain Morley and Guy Levavasseur, *Guide Seat des musées*, 'Guides' series, Le Cherche midi.

1994 Michel Grisolia, *La Petite Afrique*, 'L'Instant romanesque' series, Paris, Balland; Françoise Xenakis, *Moi j'aime pas la mer*, 'L'Instant romanesque' series, Paris, Balland; Gwenn-Aël Bolloré, *Le 6 juin 1944*, 'Documents / Histoire' series, Paris, Le Cherche midi; Jean-Luc Delblat, *Le Métier d'écrire, entretiens avec 18 écrivains*, 'Documents / Littérature' series, Paris, Le Cherche midi; Maria Jalek, *En campant sur l'Alpe* 'Retour à la montagne' series, Paris, Hoëbeke; Teresa Kennedy, *Le Stradivarius à sonnettes*, 'Nouvelles Angleterres' series, Paris, Balland; Gaston Rébuffat, *La Montagne est mon domaine*, 'Retour à la montagne' series, Paris, Hoëbeke; Edward St. Aubyn, *Peu importe*, 'Nouvelles Angleterres' series, Paris, Balland; Roger Joly, *La Libération de Chartres*, 'Documents /Histoire' series, Paris, Le Cherche midi; Ken Follett, *La Marque de Windfield*, 'Best-Sellers' series, Paris, Robert Laffont; Nicolas Saudray, *Les Mangeurs de feu*, 'Le Nadir' series, Paris, Balland; Jessie Prichard Hunter, *L'assassin habite à la maison*, 'Best-Sellers'

series, Paris, Robert Laffont; *Les Nouvelles Histoires drôles de Guy Montagné*, 'Le Sens de l'humour' series, Paris, Le Cherche midi; Philippe Val, *Allez-y vous n'en reviendrez pas*, 'Le Sens de l'humour' series, Paris, Le Cherche midi; Michel Truffaut, *La Décomposition*, Paris, Balland; Claudine Wayser, *Je ne sais rien, je me souviens de rien*, Paris, Balland.

1996 Dan Fante, *Les anges n'ont rien dans les poches*, 'Papillons' series, Paris, Robert Laffont; Primo Levi, *Si c'est un homme*, Paris, Robert Laffont.

1997 José Giovanni, *La Mort du poisson rouge*, crime novel series, Paris, Robert Laffont; Michel Demasure, *Cours d'algèbre*, 'Nouvelle Bibliothèque mathématique' series, Paris, Cassini; Michael Crichton, *Le Monde perdu*, 'Best-Sellers' series, Paris, Robert Laffont; Irving Benig, *Les Pierres du messie*, 'Les Aventures de l'esprit' series, Paris, Robert Laffont; *Rentrées des classes*, 'L'École de Brive' series, Paris, Robert Laffont.

1998 John Barnes, *La Mère des tempêtes*, Paris, Robert Laffont; Jean-Yves Ouvrard, *Probabilités 1*, Paris, Cassini.

1999 Pascal Hachet, *Le Mensonge indispensable*, Paris, Armand Colin; Annick Houel, *L'Adultère au féminin et son roman*, Paris, Armand Colin.

2001 George Steiner, *Préface à la bible hébraïque*, 'Bibliothèque Idées' series, Paris, Albin Michel; Massin, *Style et écriture*, 'Bibliothèque Idées' series, Paris, Albin Michel; Corinne Barjot, *Le Venin*, 'Un ordre d'idées' series, Paris, Stock; Régine Robin, *Berlin chantiers*, 'un Ordre d'idées' series, Paris, Stock; *Écorchés*, Paris, Albin Michel / Bibliothèque nationale de France; John Maynard Smith, *La Construction du vivant*, 'Le sel et le fer' series, Paris, Cassini.

2003 Marcel Proust, *Un amour de Swann*, 'Bibliothèque du dimanche' series, Paris, Éditions Filipacchi; Pete McCarthy, *L'Irlande dans un verre*, 'Étonnants voyageurs' series, Paris, Hoëbeke.

2004 Daniel Arsand, *Ivresses du fils*, 'Écrivains' series, Paris, Stock.

2005 Hyundae Munhak, Séoul, Corée; *Guerres et paix en Alsace-Moselle*, Strasburg, La Nuée bleue.

Book layouts

1949 Arthur Rimbaud, *Œuvres*, Paris, le Club français du livre; Erich Kästner, *Émile et les Détectives*, Paris, le Club français du livre; Joseph Peyré, *Le Mont Everest*, Paris, le Club français du livre.

1950 Georges Mikes, *Drôles de gens*, Paris, le Club français du livre; Georges Duhamel, *Les Plaisirs et les Jeux*, Paris, le Club français du livre; Franz Liszt, *Chopin*, Paris, le Club français du livre; Vidocq, *Les Vrais Mystères de Paris*, Paris, le Club français du livre; Selma Lagerlöf, *La Saga de Gösta Berling*, Paris, le Club français du livre; Pierre Lecomte de Nouÿ, *L'Homme et sa Destinée*, Paris, le Club français du livre.

1951 Jean Giono, *Un de Baumugnes*, Paris, le Club français du livre; Maurice Genevoix, *Raboliot*, Paris, le Club français du livre; Restif de la Bretonne, *Les Contemporaines*, Paris, le Club français du livre; Élisabeth Barbier, *Les Gens de Mogador*, Paris, Julliard.

1952 Nicolaï Vassiliévitch Gogol, *Les Âmes mortes*, Paris, le Club français du livre; Thor Heyerdahl, *L'Expédition du Kon Tiki*, Paris, le Club du meilleur livre; Graham Greene, *La Fin d'une liaison*, Paris, le Club du meilleur livre; Henri Calet, *Un grand voyage*, Paris, le Club français du livre.

1953 Blaise Cendrars, *Bourlinguer*, Paris, le Club du meilleur livre; Marcelle Auclair, *Sainte Thérèse d'Avila*, Paris, le Club du meilleur livre; Émile Zola, *La Bête Humaine*, Paris, le Club du meilleur livre; Benjamin Constant, *Cécile*, Paris, le Club du meilleur livre; Marcel Proust, *Un amour de Swann*, Paris, le Club du meilleur livre; Colette, *Claudine à l'école*, Paris, le Club du meilleur livre; Pierre Boulle, *Le Pont de la rivière Kwaï*, Paris, le Club du meilleur livre; Ernest Hemingway, *L'Adieu aux armes*, Paris, le Club du meilleur livre; Georges Bernanos, *L'Imposture*, Paris, le Club du meilleur livre; Jean Giono, *Colline*, Paris, le Club du meilleur livre; Louis Bromfield, *Colorado*, Paris, le Club du meilleur livre; Guillaume Apollinaire, *Alcools*, Paris, le Club du meilleur livre; Georges Arnaud, *Le Salaire de la peur*, Paris, le Club du meilleur livre; *Le Procès de condamnation de Jeanne d'Arc*, Paris, le Club du meilleur livre; Marcel Aymé, *La Vouivre*, Paris, le Club du meilleur livre; Jules Romains, *Les Copains*, Paris, le Club du meilleur livre; Antoine Blondin, *Les Enfants du Bon Dieu*, Paris, le Club du meilleur livre; Paul Claudel, *Le Soulier de satin*, Paris, le Club du meilleur livre; Louis Hémon, M. *Ripois et la némésis*, Paris, le Club du meilleur livre; Juan Ramón Jiménez, *Platero y yo*, Paris, Librería española.

1954 Albert Camus, *L'Étranger*, Paris, le Club du meilleur livre; Alphonse de Châteaubriant, *La Brière*, Paris, le Club du meilleur livre; Jean Giraudoux, *Électre*, Paris, le Club du meilleur livre; Thomas Raucat, *L'Honorable Partie de campagne*, Paris, le Club du meilleur livre; *Le Procès de réhabilitation de Jeanne d'Arc*, Paris, le Club du meilleur livre; Charles Dickens, *Notre ami commun*, Paris, le Club du meilleur livre; Jean-Paul Sartre, *La Nausée*, Paris, le Club du meilleur livre; Pierre Mac Orlan, *Sous la lumière froide*, Paris, le Club du meilleur livre; Francis Jammes, *Jeunes Filles*, Paris, le Club du meilleur livre; Jean-Paul Clébert, *Paris insolite*, Paris, le Club du meilleur livre; Maxence Van der Meersch, *Invasion 14*, Paris, le Club du meilleur livre; Louis-Ferdinand Céline, *Voyage au bout de la nuit*, Paris, le Club du meilleur livre; Molière, *Œuvres complètes*, I, Paris, le Club du meilleur livre; Jack London, *Croc blanc*, Paris, le Club du meilleur livre; Roger Martin du Gard, *Jean Barois*, Paris, le Club du meilleur livre; *Véritable Vie privée du maréchal de Richelieu*, Paris, le Club du meilleur livre; Antoine de Saint-Exupéry, *Terre des hommes*, Paris, le Club du meilleur livre.

1955   Albert Camus, *La Peste*, Paris, le Club du meilleur livre; *Le Procès des Templiers*, Paris, le Club du meilleur livre; Louis Pergaud, *La Guerre des boutons*, Paris, le Club du meilleur livre; Molière, *Théâtre*, II, Paris, le Club du meilleur livre; Léon Tolstoï, *Les Cosaques*, Paris, le Club du meilleur livre; Charles Baudelaire, *Œuvres complètes*, I, Paris, le Club du meilleur livre; André Malraux, *L'Espoir*, Paris, le Club du meilleur livre; Paul Claudel, *L'Annonce faite à Marie*, Paris, le Club du meilleur livre; Remy de Gourmont, *Esthétique de la langue française*, Paris, Le Club du meilleur livre; Ernest Hemingway, *Le Vieil Homme et la Mer*, Paris, le Club du meilleur livre; *Napoléon et Joséphine*, Paris, le Club du meilleur livre; Victor Segalen, *Stèles et Peintures*, Paris, le Club du meilleur livre; Antoine Furetière, *Le Roman Bourgeois*, Paris, le Club du meilleur livre; André Maurois, *Olympio ou la vie de Victor Hugo*, Paris, le Club du meilleur livre; Charles Baudelaire, *Œuvres complètes*, II, Paris, le Club du meilleur livre; *Le Cabinet des fées*, Paris, le Club du meilleur livre; G. de Santillana, *Le Procès de Galilée*, Paris, le Club du meilleur livre; Guillaume Apollinaire, *Calligrammes*, Paris, le Club du meilleur livre.

1956   André Malraux, *Les Conquérants*, Paris, le Club du meilleur livre; Molière, *Théâtre*, III, Paris, le Club du meilleur livre; Léon Tolstoï, *Le Père Serge*, Paris, le Club du meilleur livre; Jean Giono, *Le Hussard sur le toit*, Paris, le Club du meilleur livre; *Le Procès de Marie Stuart*, Paris, le Club du meilleur livre; William Faulkner, *Jefferson, Mississippi*, Paris, le Club du meilleur livre; Alain, *Minerve ou de la sagesse*, Paris, le Club du meilleur livre; Blaise Cendrars, *L'Or*, Paris, le Club du meilleur livre; Françoise Sagan, *Bonjour tristesse*, Paris, le Club du meilleur livre; *Le Procès de Vidocq*, Paris, le Club du meilleur livre; Jules Roy, *La Vallée heureuse*, Paris, le Club du meilleur livre; Erskine Caldwell, *Le Petit Arpent du Bon Dieu*, Paris, le Club du meilleur livre; Léon Tolstoï, *La Guerre et la Paix*, Paris, le Club du meilleur livre; Jean Cocteau, *Thomas l'imposteur*, Paris, le Club du meilleur livre; Alphonse Daudet, *Les Lettres de mon moulin*, Paris, le Club du meilleur livre; Marcel Pagnol, *Marius, Fanny, César*, Paris, le Club du meilleur livre; Charles Péguy, *Le Mystère de la charité de Jeanne d'Arc*, Paris, le Club du meilleur livre; Marcel Aymé, *La Jument verte*, Paris, le Club du meilleur livre; Kurt Seligmann, *Le Miroir de la magie*, Paris, le Club du meilleur livre.

1957   Erskine Caldwell, *La Route du tabac*, Paris, le Club du meilleur livre; Henry de Montherlant, *La Reine morte*, Paris, le Club du meilleur livre; Michel de Saint Pierre, *Les Écrivains*, Paris, Calmann-Lévy; Albert Camus, *L'Exil et le Royaume*, Paris, Gallimard; Henry de Montherlant, *Carnets 1930 à 1944*, Paris, Gallimard; Philippe Hériat, *Les Grilles d'or*, Paris, Gallimard; Jean Giono, *Le Bonheur fou*, Paris, Gallimard; Ernest

Hemingway, *Les Neiges du Kilimanjaro*, Paris, le Club du meilleur livre; Jean Giono, *Le Chant du monde*, Paris, le Club du meilleur livre; Jean Anouilh, *Pièces roses pièces noires*, Paris, Calmann-Lévy; John Steinbeck, *Les Raisins de la colère*, Paris, le Club du meilleur livre; Albert Vidalie, *Les Bijoutiers du clair de lune*, Paris, le Club du meilleur livre; Louise de Vilmorin, *Le Retour d'Érica*, Paris, le Club du meilleur livre; Thomas Mann, *Les Confessions du chevalier d'industrie Félix Krüll*, Paris, le Club du meilleur livre; *Six comédies de Labiche*, Paris, le Club du meilleur livre; *Le Procès de Savanarole*, Paris, le Club du meilleur livre; Luc Estienne, *L'Art du contrepet*, Paris, Jean-Jacques Pauvert; Charles Nodier, *Contes fantastiques*, I, Paris, Jean-Jacques Pauvert; Paul Valéry, *La Jeune Parque*, Paris, le Club du meilleur livre; Charles Nodier, *Contes fantastiques*, II, Paris, Jean-Jacques Pauvert; Christophe, *La Famille Fenouillard*, Paris, le Club du meilleur livre; Herman Wouk, *Ouragan sur le 'Caine'*, Paris, Calmann-Lévy; Albert Simonin, *Ne touchez pas au grisbi, Grisbi or not grisbi, Le cave se rebiffe*, Paris, Gallimard.

1958   Noël Ballif and Georges Bourdelon, *La Perse millénaire*, Paris, Arthaud; Claude Arthaud and François Hébert-Stevens, *Mongolie, dans les steppes de Gengis Khan*, Paris, Arthaud; Robert Brasillach, *Comme le temps passe*, Paris, le Club du meilleur livre; Henry de Montherlant, *Port-Royal*, Paris, le Club du meilleur livre; Françoise Sagan, *Bonjour Tristesse*, Paris, le Club du meilleur livre; Jean-Paul Sartre, *Le Mur*, Paris, le Club du meilleur livre; Christophe, *L'Idée fixe du savant Cosinus*, Paris, le Club du meilleur livre; Albert Camus, *La Chute*, Paris, le Club du meilleur livre; Ernest Hemingway, *Cinquante mille dollars*, Paris, le Club du meilleur livre; Émile Zola, *Nana*, Paris, le Club du meilleur livre; Alfred Jarry, *Ubu roi ou les Polonais*, Paris, le Club du meilleur livre; Émile Zola, *Germinal*, Paris, le Club du meilleur livre; Jean Giono, *Le Moulin de Pologne*, Paris, le Club du meilleur livre; Marcel Thomas, *L'Affaire du Bounty*, Paris, le Club du meilleur livre; Christophe, *Les Facéties du sapeur Camenber*, Paris, le Club du meilleur livre; Jacob Burkhardt, *La Civilisation de la Renaissance en Italie*, Paris, le Club du meilleur livre; *La Chasse*, Paris, Gallimard; Juan Goytisolo, *La Resaca*, Librería española; Nicolas Gogol, *Récits de Saint-Pétersbourg*, Paris, le Club du meilleur livre.

1959   Federico García Lorca, *Poésies*, Paris, le Club du meilleur livre; Louis Aragon, *Les Beaux Quartiers*, Paris, le Club du meilleur livre; Jean Rostand, *Espoirs et Inquiétudes de l'homme*, Paris, Le Club du meilleur livre; Georges Feydeau, *Du mariage au divorce*, Paris, le Club du meilleur livre; Paul Éluard, *Poésies*, Paris, le Club du meilleur livre; Edmond Rostand, *Cyrano de Bergerac*, Paris, le Club du meilleur livre; Guillaume Apollinaire, *Le Poète assassiné*, Paris, Gallimard; Robert Mallet, *Jardins et Paradis*, Paris, Gallimard; *Journal d'Anne Franck*, Paris, Calmann-Lévy / Comité parisien de l'Alliance israélite universelle; *Petit Littré*, Paris, Gallimard / Hachette; Restif de la Bretonne, *Monsieur Nicolas ou le Cœur humain dévoilé*, Paris, Jean-Jacques Pauvert.

1960   Billie Holiday, *Lady sings the blues*, Paris, le Club du meilleur livre; Louis Aragon, *Poésies*, Paris, le Club du meilleur livre; Marcel Pagnol, *La Gloire de mon*

père, Paris, le Club du meilleur livre; *Dictionnaire des auteurs de la Pléiade*, Paris, Gallimard; Marcel Pagnol, *Le Château de ma mère*, Paris, le Club du meilleur livre; Paul Verlaine, *Œuvres complètes*, I, Paris, le Club du meilleur livre; Blaise Cendrars, *Rhum*, Paris, le Club du meilleur livre; Vincent Van Gogh, *Correspondance complète*, Paris, Gallimard / Hachette; Maurice Leblanc, *Les Aventures d'Arsène Lupin, gentleman-cambrioleur*, Paris, Gallimard / Hachette; *Lettres de Saint-Exupéry*, Paris, le Club du meilleur livre; André Breton, *Poésie et Autre*, Paris, le Club du meilleur livre; Stéphane Mallarmé, *Madrigaux*, Cercle du Livre précieux; Jacques Casanova de Seingalt, *Histoire de ma vie*, Paris, Gallimard / Hachette.

1961   Raymond Queneau, *Pierrot mon ami*, Paris, le Club du meilleur livre; Henri Pichette, *Odes à chacun*, Paris, Gallimard; Alain, *Les Idées et les Âges*, Paris, le Club du meilleur livre; Max Aub, *Jusep Torres Campalans*, Paris, Gallimard; Jean Giono, *Les Grands Chemins*, Paris, le Club du meilleur livre; *Lettres de Madame Palatine*, Paris, le Club du meilleur livre; Jean Rostand, *L'Homme*, Paris, le Club du meilleur livre; Effe Geache, *Une nuit d'orgie à Saint-Pierre Martinique*, Paris, Le Cercle du livre précieux; Raymond Queneau, *Cent mille milliards de poèmes*, Paris, Gallimard; *Les Mémoires d'une chanteuse allemande*, Paris, Le Cercle du livre précieux; *Florilège de la poésie sacrée*, Paris, le Club du meilleur livre; Lionel Terray, *Les Conquérants de l'inutile*, Paris, Gallimard; Maurice Hollande, *Trésors de Reims*, Reims, Michaud S.A.; Arthur Rimbaud, *Album zutique*, Paris, Le Cercle du livre précieux; *Les Estampes érotiques japonaises*, Paris, Le Cercle du livre précieux.

1962   Simone de Beauvoir and Gisèle Halimi, *Djamila Boupacha*, Paris, Gallimard; Michel Butor, *Mobile*, Paris, Gallimard; Janis Bogdanov, *Ceux de Kronsdadt*, Paris, Gallimard; Antoine de Saint-Exupéry, *Pages choisies*, Paris, Gallimard; Jean Paulhan, *L'Art informel*, Paris, Gallimard; Marcel Pagnol, *Le Temps des secrets*, Paris, Gallimard; Michel Butor, *Réseau aérien*, Paris, Gallimard.

1963   Robert Brasillach, *Œuvres complètes*, Paris, le Club de l'honnête homme; Raymond Queneau, *Exercices de style*, Paris, Gallimard; Juan Goytisolo, *Pueblo en marcha*, Paris, Librería española; Marcel Aymé, *Les Contes bleus du chat perché*, Paris, Gallimard; Herbert George Wells, *Œuvres*, Paris, Mercure de France; Louis Pergaud, *Romans et Récits*, Paris, Mercure de France; René Gimpel, *Journal d'un collectionneur*, Paris, Calmann-Lévy.

1964   Comtesse de Ségur, *Un Bon Petit Diable*, Paris, Jean-Jacques Pauvert éditeur; Alphonse Allais, *Tout Allais*, Paris, La Table Ronde; Saint-Simon, *Œuvres complètes*, Paris, Jean-Jacques Pauvert; John Buchan, *Les Aventures de Richard Hannay*, I and II, Paris, Gallimard; Charles Baudelaire, *Les Fleurs du mal*, Paris, Le Cercle précieux du livre; Eugène Ionesco, *La Cantatrice chauve*, Paris, Gallimard; *Simenon*, I, Paris, Gallimard; Brassaï, *Conversations avec Picasso*, Paris, Gallimard. Paul Claudel, *L'œil écoute*, Paris, Gallimard; *Dictionnaire ou Recueils alphabétiques des opinions et jugements de Napoléon Ier*, Club de l'honnête homme.

List of works

1965 Heimito von Doderer, *Les Démons*, Paris, Gallimard; Jack London, *Œuvres*, Paris, Gallimard / Hachette; Roger Caillois, *Au cœur du fantastique*, Paris, Gallimard; *Almanach du farceur français*, Éditions Rabelais; Michel Butor, *6 810 000 litres d'eau par seconde*, Paris, Gallimard; 'La Foule', *Evergreen Review*, New York, Grove Press; Eugène Ionesco, *The Bald Soprano*, New York, Grove Press; *L'Œuvre de Maurice Barrès*, Paris, Club de l'honnête homme; Lionel Terray, Jean Franco, *Bataille pour le Jannu*, Paris, Gallimard; Béatrice Beck, *Contes à l'enfant né coiffé*, Paris, Gallimard; Henri Bosco, *Le Renard dans l'île*, Paris, Gallimard; Jacques Demange, *Le Monde enchanté des Pink Lodge*, Paris, Gallimard; André Breton, *Le Surréalisme et la Peinture*, Paris, Gallimard.

1966 George Duncan Painter, *Marcel Proust*, Paris, Mercure de France; Marie-Jeanne Gillet-Maudot, *Paul Claudel*, Paris, Gallimard; Agathe Rouart-Valéry, *Paul Valéry*, Paris, Gallimard; Violette Leduc, *Thérèse et Isabelle*, Paris, Gallimard; Eugène Ionesco, *Délire à deux*, Paris, Gallimard; Jean Tardieu, *Conversation-sinfonietta*, Paris, Gallimard; James Joyce, *Le Chat et le Diable*, Paris, Gallimard; Raymond Queneau, *Zazie dans le métro*, Paris, Gallimard; Jean Arp, *Jours effeuillés*, Paris, Gallimard; William Faulkner, *Proses, Poésies et Essais critiques de jeunesse*, Paris, Gallimard; Joseph Kessel, *Mermoz*, Paris, Gallimard; *Œuvres complètes de Labiche*, Paris, Club de l'honnête homme; Eugène Ionesco, *The Bold Prima Donna*, London, Calder and Boyars; Manuel Tuñon de Lara, *La España del siglo xx*, Paris, Librería española; José Corrales Egea, Pierre Darmangeat, *Poesía española*, Paris, Librería española.

1967 various, *A. de Luze & fils*, Bordeaux; Simone de Beauvoir, *La Femme rompue*, Paris, Gallimard; Honoré de Balzac, *Lettres à Madame Hanska*, Paris, Éditions du Delta; Jacques Roubaud, *E*, Paris, Gallimard; Jean Dubuffet, *Propectus et tous Écrits suivants*, Paris, Gallimard; Jean-Claude Grosjean, *Poésie*, Paris, Gallimard.

1968 Pierre Garnier, *Spatialisme et Poésie concrète*, Paris, Gallimard; Albert Aycard, Jacqueline Franck, *Comic-Mac*, Paris, Gallimard; Jacques Salomon, *Vuillard*, Paris, Gallimard; François Guiot, Massin, Maurice Pech et Marcel Viguier, *L'Amour la ville*, Paris, Gallimard; Victor Chklovski, *Capitaine Fédotov*, Paris, Gallimard; Elsa Triolet, *Écoutez voir*, Paris, Gallimard; Panaït Istrati, *Œuvres*, Paris, Gallimard.

1969 Georges Sadoul, *Jacques Callot miroir de son temps*, Paris, Gallimard; *Présentation critique d'Hortense Flexner*, Paris, Gallimard.

1970 Massin, *La Lettre et l'Image*, Paris, Gallimard; André Malraux, *Le Triangle noir*, Paris, Gallimard; Thomas Browne, *Les Urnes funéraires*, Paris, Gallimard; Philippe Hériat, *Les Boussardel*, Paris, Gallimard.

1971 *Album Apollinaire*, Paris, Gallimard; Louis Aragon, *Henri Matisse, roman*, Paris, Gallimard; Jean Effel, *Ce crapaud de granit bavant du goémon*, Paris, Gallimard; Marguerite Yourcenar, *Mémoires d'Hadrien*, Paris, Gallimard.

1972 *Album Flaubert*, Paris, Gallimard; Lucette Finas, *La Crue*, Paris, Gallimard.

1973 *Album George Sand*, Paris, Gallimard; Jean Marie Gustave Le Clézio, *Les Géants*, Paris, Gallimard; Henry de Montherlant, *Les Garçons*, Paris, Gallimard; Bella Chagall, *Lumières allumées*, Paris, Gallimard.

1974 *Album Baudelaire*, Paris, Gallimard.

1975 *Album Dostoïevski*, Paris, Gallimard; Michel Déon, *Thomas et l'Infini*, Paris, Gallimard; *Œuvres complètes de Louis Pergaud*, Paris, Club de l'honnête homme.

1976 *Album Rousseau*, Paris, Gallimard; Brassaï, *Le Paris secret des années trente*, Paris, Gallimard; *Œuvres complètes de Saint-Exupéry*, Paris, Club de l'honnête homme; Jacques Prévert, *Arbres*, Paris, Gallimard.

1977 *Album Céline*, Paris, Gallimard; Jean-Louis Rabeux, *Aragon ou les Métamorphoses*, Paris, Gallimard; *Œuvres complètes de Marcel Pagnol*, Paris, Club de l'honnête homme; Henri Pourrat, *Le Diable et les Diableries*, Paris, Gallimard.

1978 Liliane Sendyck-Siegel, *Sartre*, Paris, Gallimard; *Album Pascal*, Paris, Gallimard; Massin, *Les Cris de la ville*, Paris, Gallimard; Michel Butor, *Boomerang*, Paris, Gallimard.

1979 François Émile-Zola and Massin, *Zola photographe*, Paris, Denoël; *Coucou la fourmi*, Paris, Hachette.

1980 Daniel Cordier and Alfred Pacquement, *Les Années soixante*, Paris, Hachette; Henri Vincenot, *l'âge du chemin de fer*, Paris, Denoël; Philippe Chatel, *Émilie jolie*, Édition°1.

1981 Massin, *Les Célébrités de la rue*, Paris, Gallimard; René Fallet, *Les Pieds dans l'eau*, Paris, Denoël / Mercure de France; Cécile Philippe and Patrice Tourenne, *Les Frères Jacques*, Paris, Balland; John Humbley, Mary Martinez Rosselin and Claude Vollaire, *Highway*, Paris, Classiques Hachette.

1984 Laure Beaumont-Maillet, *La Guerre des sexes*, Paris, Albin Michel; Laure Beaumont-Maillet, *Paris inconnu*, Paris, Albin Michel; Marianne Grivel, *Hiroshige*, Paris, Albin Michel.

1985 *Les Artistes indépendants*, Paris, Société des artistes indépendants; Gisèle Freund, *Itinéraires*, Paris, Schirmer / Mosel; Michel Melot, *Les Femmes de Toulouse-Lautrec*, Paris, Albin Michel; Charles Rodat and Jean Cazelles, *Toulouse-Lautrec*, Paris, Hatier; Nadine Haim, *Les Peintres aux fourneaux*, Paris, Flammarion; Floc'h, *Un homme dans la foule*, Paris, Albin Michel / Groupe Graphique d'expression française; *Le Roman d'Hernani*, Paris, Comédie française / Mercure de France; *Samivel des cimes*, Paris, Hoëbeke.

1986 Theodor Fontane, *Journal de captivité*, Strasburg, Bueb & Reumaux; Nina Sutton, *Les Mamandises ou Ma mère me l'avait bien dit*, Paris, Albin Michel; Jean-Marie Drot, *Voyage au pays des naïfs*, Paris, Hatier; Régine Deforges and Geneviève Dormann, *Le Livre du point de croix*, Paris, Albin Michel / Régine Deforges; Jacques Marseille, *L'âge d'or de la France coloniale*, Paris, Albin Michel; Jean Rolin, *Vu sur la mer*, Strasburg, Bueb & Reumaux; *Le Musée d'Orsay*, Paris, Réunion des musées nationaux; *Samivel des rêves*, Paris, Hoëbeke; Alain Weil, *Brenot*, Paris, Hoëbeke; Massin and Ségolène Le Men, *Alphabets / abécédaires*, musée-galerie de la Seita / Centre Georges-Pompidou.

1987 Dubout, *Les Chats*, Paris, Hoëbeke; Jean-Jacques Brochier, *Anthologie de la bécasse*, Paris, Hatier; Siné, *Droit de réponse*, Paris, Albin Michel; Peynet, *De tout cœur*, Paris, Hoëbeke; Savignac, Paris, Hoëbeke; Massin and François Émile-Zola, *Zola Photographe*, Paris, musée-galerie de la Seita.

1988 Cabu, *Le Gros Blond avec sa chemise noire*, Paris, Albin Michel; Cabu, *Tonton accroc*, Paris, Albin Michel; Martin Veyron, *Vite!*, Paris, Albin Michel; Massin, *Continuo*, Paris, Balbec [IMEC]; Bernard Pivot, *La Bibliothèque idéale*, Paris, Albin Michel; Michel Ragon, *Karel Appel*, Paris, Editions Galilée; Dubout, *Locomobiles*, Paris, Hoëbeke; Jean Jenger, *Souvenirs de la gare d'Orsay*, Paris, Réunion des musées nationaux; Jean-Jacques Brochier, *Anthologie du sanglier*, Paris, Hatier; Léo Malet, *La Vache enragée*, Paris, Hoëbeke; Jean Durry, *Le Sport à l'affiche*, Paris, Hoëbeke; *Le Quartier François Ier*, Paris, Auguste Thouard dans la ville / Albin Michel; François-Émile Zola and Massin, *Zola : Photographer*, New York, Seaver Books.

1989 Marcel Brion, *L'Art fantastique*, Paris, Albin Michel; Robert Doisneau et Cavanna, *Les Doigts pleins d'encre*, Paris, Hoëbeke; *Les Plus Beaux Poèmes d'amour de la poésie française*, Paris, Le Grand Livre du mois; *Ubu cent ans de règne*, Paris, musée-galerie de la Seita.

1990 Bovis and Mac Orlan, *Fêtes foraines*, Paris, Hoëbeke; *La Science de Doisneau*, Paris, Hoëbeke; Yves Simon, *La Movida*, Paris, Barclay; Juliette Gréco, Paris, Imprimerie nationale; Jacques Séguéla, *C'est gai, la pub!*, Paris, Hoëbeke; *Les Ateliers de Soulages*, Paris, Albin Michel; Brassaï and Modiano, *Paris Tendresse*, Paris, Hoëbeke; *Le Livre d'or du compagnonnage*, Paris, Jean-Cyrille Godefroy.

1991 Pascal Ory, *La Légende des airs*, Paris, Hoëbeke; Geneviève Dormann, *Paris est une ville pleine de lions*, Paris, Albin Michel; Massin, *La Mise en pages*, Paris, Hoëbeke; Guillaume Villemot and Vincent Vidal, *La Chevauchée de la Vache qui rit*, Paris, Hoëbeke; Robert Doisneau and Daniel Pennac, *Les Grandes Vacances*, Paris, Hoëbeke; Michel Ragon, *La Voie libertaire*, Paris, Plon; Daniel Challe and Bernard Marbot, *Les Photographes de Barbizon*, Paris, Hoëbeke / Bibliothèque nationale; Robert Sabatier, *Le Livre de la déraison souriante*, Paris, Albin Michel.

1992 Michel Tournier, *Le crépuscule des masques*, Paris, Hoëbeke; Robert Doisneau, *Rue Jacques Prévert*, Paris, Hoëbeke; Jacques Lanzmann and Pierre Ripert, *Cent ans de prêt-à-porter*, Editions P. A. U.; Michel Ragon, *L'Insurrection vendéenne et les malentendus de la liberté*, Albin Michel; Michel Poivert, *Le Pictoralisme en france*, Hoëbeke / Bibliothèque Nationale; Muriel Lapidus, *Lapidaires*, Le Bel Atelier; Willy Ronis and Régine Deforges, *Toutes belles*, Paris, Hoëbeke; *Figures de pierre*, Paris, musée-galerie de la Seita; *Le Musée Jeannette Matossian*, as yet unpublished.

1993 Massin, *La Lettre et L'Image*, Paris, Gallimard; André François and François David, *Le Fils de l'ogre*, Paris, Hoëbeke / Møtus: Olivier Darmon, Rémi Noël and Éric Holden, *30 ans de publicité Volkswagen*, Paris, Hoëbeke; Jean Bourdeaux, *Le Roman d'un fabricant*, Paris, Albino Micheli; *Voyage en douce France*, Paris, Albin Michel; Françoise Sagan, *... Et toute ma sympathie*, Paris, FNAC / Julliard; Benoît Barbier, *Germinal blues*, Paris, Hoëbeke; Cavanna, *Les Enfants de germinal*, Paris, Hoëbeke; Jérôme Peignot, *Typoésie*, Paris, Imprimerie nationale; François Robichon, *Benjamin Rabier, l'homme qui fait rire les animaux*, Paris, Hoëbeke; Alain Cavalier, *Libera me*, Paris, Les Rencontres culturelles de la FNAC; Olivier Rolin, *L'Invention du monde*, Paris, FNAC / Seuil; Robert Doisneau and Daniel Pennac, *La Vie de famille*, Paris, Hoëbeke; *Figures de la BD*, Paris, Hoëbeke; Karel Kosik, *Le Printemps de Prague*, Paris, Gallimard / FNAC; Abdulah Sidran, *Cercueil de Sarajevo*, Paris, Les Rencontres culturelles de la FNAC / Sarajevo, capitale culturelle de l'Europe / Arte; Juan Goytisolo, *Sarajevo, deuxième hiver*, Paris, Les Rencontres culturelles de la FNAC; Ernest Breleret Milan Kundera, *D'en bas tu humeras des roses*, Strasburg, La Nuée bleue; Jorge Semprun, *Federico Sánchez vous salue bien*, Paris, Les Rencontres culturelles de la FNAC / Grasset / Bouillon de culture; Moisan, *Histoire d'une République de De Gaulle à Mitterrand*, Paris, musée-galerie de la Seita.

1994 Pascal Ory, *Doisneau 40/44*, Paris, Hoëbeke / Centre d'histoire de la résistance et de la déportation; *Chaque jour pour Sarajevo*, Paris, Arte / FNAC / Point du jour / Reporters sans frontières / Saga Production; André Malraux, *Esquisse d'une psychologie du cinéma*, Paris, FNAC / Gallimard / Lire; *Bosna!*, Paris, Les Rencontres culturelles de la FNAC; *La Reine Margot, un film de Patrice Chéreau d'après le roman d'Alexandre Dumas*, Paris, Grasset; *Musiques au Louvre*, Paris, Réunion des Musées Nationaux; Jacques Séguéla, *Pub story*, Paris, Hoëbeke; Jean Cocteau, *Les Mariés de la tour Eiffel*, Paris, Hoëbeke; *Comment Pantagruel monta sur mer*, Paris, Hatier; François Robichon, *Poulbot, le père des gosses*, Paris, Hoëbeke; *Mariscal à Paris*, Paris, musée-galerie de la Seita.

1995 Peter Hamilton, *Robert Doisneau la vie d'un photographe*, Paris, Hoëbeke; *Baroque du Paraguay*, musée-galerie de la Seita.

1996 Willy Ronis and Didier Daeninckx, *À nous la vie!*, Paris, Hoëbeke; Yves Ballu, *Gaston Rébuffat*, Paris, Hoëbeke; Daniel Picouly, *Vivement noël!*, Paris, Hoëbeke; Paul Éluard, *Corps mémorable*, Paris, Seghers; *Cathelin*, Paris, musée-galerie de la Seita; *Agenda Gédéon 1997*, Paris, Hoëbeke; *Signes de terre*, Paris, musée-galerie de la Seita; *L'Amérique de la dépression*, Paris, musée-galerie de la Seita.

1997 *Proust*, Paris, À telle enseigne; Gérard Rondeau and Bernard Franck, *Strasbourg*, Strasbourg, La Nuée bleue; Olivier Darmon, *Le Grand Siècle de bibendum*, Paris, Hoëbeke; Jacques Péron, *La Bretagne dans tous ses objets*, Paris, Hoëbeke; Philippe Delerm, *Les chemins nous inventent*, Paris, Stock; *Bellmer graveur*, Paris, musée-galerie de la Seita; Dominique and Michèle Frémy, *Quid98*, Paris, Robert Laffont; Alfred Hrdlicka, Paris, musée-galerie de la Seita; Hugh Johnson, *Guide poche du vin 1998*, Paris, Robert Laffont; Thierry Crouzet, *Word en un clin d'œil*, Paris, Microsoft; *Le Guide Lebey 1998 des restaurants de Paris*, Paris, Robert Laffont; *Spilliaert*, Paris, musée-galerie de la Seita.

1998 Jacques Prévert and Massin, *Cortège*, Paris, Gallimard; Michel Picouly, *Le 13e but*, Paris, Hoëbeke; *30 ans dans l'impasse*, Paris, Le Récamier; *Le Bonheur de l'enfance*, Paris, Hoëbeke; Pierre Tairraz, *Montagnes de lumières*, Paris, Hoëbeke; *Catalogue raisonné de l'œuvre typographique de Massin, I (1948–1958)*, Ville de Chartres; *Réalistes des années vingt*, Paris, musée-galerie de la Seita; *Ludwika Ogorzelec*, Paris, musée-galerie de la Seita; *Kokoschka*, Paris, Paris, musée-galerie de la Seita; Hugh Johnson, *Guide de poche du vin 1999*, Paris, Robert Laffont.

1999 *200 ans de prières*, Paris, Éditions du Signe; Gérard Rondeau, *C'est écrit*, Strasburg, L'Union / La Nuée bleue; Jacques Séguéla, *80 ans de publicité Citroën et toujours vingt ans*, Paris, Hoëbeke; *Du côté de chez Gaston, catalogue raisonné de l'œuvre typographique de Massin, 2 (1959–1979)*, Ville de Chartres; *Photographes en Algérie au XIXe siècle*, Paris, musée-galerie de la Seita; *Sécession l'art graphique à Vienne autour de 1900*, Paris, musée-galerie de la Seita.

2000 Gérard Dalmaz, *De Gaulle à la une*, Paris, Hoëbeke; Jean-Claude Izzo et Daniel Mordzinski, *Marseille*, Paris, Hoëbeke; *Le Mangeur alsacien*, Strasburg, La Nuée bleue; Robert Wagner et Bernard J. Naegelen, *Magie de noël en Alsace*, Strasburg, La Nuée bleue; *Haïti*, Paris, Hoëbeke /La Halle Saint-Pierre; *Jawlensky et Werefkin*, Paris, musée-galerie de la Seita.

2001 Nicolas Bouvier, *L'Œil du voyageur*, Paris, Hoëbeke / Musée de l'Élysée, (Lausanne); Noël Daum, *Daum art déco*, Strasburg, La Nuée bleue / Éditions de l'Est; Massin/Ragon, *Picassiette*, Paris, Hoëbeke; Cabu, *Ma Ve République*, Paris, Hoëbeke; François Cheng, *Et le souffle devient signe*, Paris, L'Iconoclaste; Roger Forst, *Strasbourg disparu*, Strasburg, La Nuée bleue / Éditions de l'Est; Émile Jung, *À la table du crocodile*, Strasburg, La Nuée bleue; *Cavalier seul, catalogue raisonné de l'œuvre typographique de Massin (1979–2000)*, Ville de Chartres; *Tomi Ungerer et New York*, Strasburg, Musées de Strasbourg / La Nuée bleue.

2002 *Le Japon de Nicolas Bouvier*, Paris, Hoëbeke; *La Caravane de sel*, Paris, Hoëbeke / France 3; *La Chevauchée des kids*, Paris, Hoëbeke / France 3; *Les Hommes des rochers*, Paris, Hoëbeke / France 3; *Le Réveil des géants*, Paris, Hoëbeke / France 3; René Koechlin, *Voyage en Asie centrale*, Strasburg, La Nuée bleue; *Sculpture romane en Alsace*, Strasburg, La Nuée bleue.

2003 Massin, *La Beauce des années cinquante*, Paris, Éditions Jacques Marseille; Marie-Christine Périllon, *Strasbourg*, Paris, Hoëbeke; Cavanna, *Sur les murs de la classe*, Paris, Hoëbeke.

2004 Marcel Proust, *La Petite Phrase*, Paris, À telle enseigne; *Viens poupoule!*, Paris, À telle enseigne; François Cavanna and Philippe Val *Les Années Charlie*, Paris, Hoëbeke; Yves Paccalet, *L'École de la nature*, Paris, Hoëbeke; Bernard Pivot, *100 mots à sauver*, Paris, Albin Michel.

2005 *50 years Hunhae Munhak*, Séoul, Corée; Guillaume Villemot, *Villemot*, Paris, Hoëbeke; *Charlie Hebdo présente les années Jean-Paul II*, Paris, Hoëbeke.

2006 *Albert Dubout, le fou dessinant*, Paris, Bibliothèque nationale de France / Hoëbeke; Abbé Pierre, *Images d'une vie*, Paris, Hoëbeke; Daniel Pennac, *Nemo*, Paris, Hoëbeke; *La Success story du Président*, Paris, Hoëbeke.

List of works

Listed below are all the books written by Massin.

1968   *L'Amour la ville*, Paris, Gallimard (collective work).

1970   *La Lettre et l'Image*, Paris, Gallimard.

1972   *Une enfance ordinaire*, Paris, Gallimard (pocket edition, Paris, Éditions du Seuil, 'Points Virgule' series, 1992).

1974   *Le Pensionnaire*, Paris, Gallimard (pocket edition, Paris, Éditions du Seuil, 'Points Virgule' series, 1993).

1978   *Les Cris de la ville, commerces ambulants et petits métiers de la rue*, Paris, Gallimard (re-published Paris, Albin Michel, 1985).

1981   *Les Célébrités de la rue*, Paris, Gallimard.

1983   *Le Branle des voleurs*, Paris, La Table Ronde.

1985   *Les Compagnons de la marjolaine*, Paris, La Table Ronde.

1987   *Alphabets*, exhibition catalogue, musée-galerie de la Seita, Paris.

1988   *La Dernière Passion*, Paris, Albin Michel; *Continuo. Fragments d'un journal en désordre*, Paris, Balbec (pocket edition, Paris, Éditions du Seuil, 'Points Virgule' series, 1992).

1989   *Quarante ans d'édition française. Hommage à Massin*, Paris, musée-galerie de la Seita; *L'ABC du métier*, Paris, Imprimerie nationale.

1991   *La Mise en pages*, Paris, Hoëbeke; *La Cour des miracles*, Paris, Payot.

1992   *Jouons avec les lettres*, Paris, Seuil Jeunesse.

1993   *Jouons avec les chiffres*, Paris, Seuil Jeunesse.

1995   *On a tous un Massin chez soi, portrait d'un graphiste touche-à-tout*, exhibition catalogue for La Laiterie, FNAC and the École des arts décoratifs de Strasbourg, Strasburg.

1996   *Journal en désordre, 1945–1995*, Paris, Robert Laffont.

2000   *De la variation*, Paris, Le Promeneur.

2001   *Style et écriture. Du rococo aux arts déco*, Paris, Albin Michel, 'Idées' series.

2002   *'L'interaction des arts'*, discussion at the Royal Academy, Belgium.

2003   *La Beauce des années cinquante*, Paris, Éditions Jacques Marseille.

2004   *Azerty, l'alphabet du monde*, Paris, Gallimard.

To be published : *La Curiosité* (started in 1989).

Listed below are all the books published by Massin.

1979   Réné Nelli, *Troubadours et trouvères*, Paris, Hachette / Massin; Jean-Marie Lhôte, Klébar and Marie-Louise, Paris, Hachette / Massin; Anne Gaël and Serge Chirol, *Châteaux et sites de la France médiévale*, Hachette Réalités; *Au donjon des Aigles*,Joël Cuénot / Hachette Réalités.

1980   Jean-Paul Roux, *La Chaussure*, Paris, Atelier Hachette / Massin; François Caradec and Alain Weill, *Le Café-concert*, Paris, Atelier Hachette / Massin; Frédérick Tristan, *Le Monde à l'envers*, Paris, Atelier Hachette / Massin; Pierre Gascar, *Le Boulevard du crime*, Paris, Atelier Hachette / Massin; Hubert Juin, *Le Lit*, Paris, Atelier Hachette / Massin; Pierre Marly, *Les Lunettes*, Paris, Atelier Hachette / Massin.

1981   Frédérick Tristan, *Les Tentations de Jérôme Bosch à Salvador Dalí*, Paris, Balland / Massin.

1982   Claire Krafft Pourrat, *Le Colporteur et la Mercière*, Paris, Denoël; Georges Perec, *Quel petit vélo à guidon chromé au fond de la cour?*, Paris, Denoël; Gisèle Freund, *Trois jours avec Joyce*, Paris, Denoël; Alain Barandard, *La Cathédrale de Chartres dans tous ses états*, Paris, Denoël; Alain René Girard and Claude Quétel, *L'Histoire de France racontée par le jeu de l'Oie*, Paris, Balland / Massin.

1983   Antoine Terrasse, *Degas et la Photographie*, Paris, Denoël; Blaise Cendrars and Robert Doisneau, *La Banlieue de Paris*, Paris, Denoël; Robert Giraud, *Le Vin des rues*, Paris, Denoël; Régine Pernoud and Jean Vigne, *La Plume et le Parchemin*, Paris, Denoël; Serge Fauchereau, *La Révolution cubiste*, Paris, Denoël; Claire Brétécher, *Portraits*, Paris, Denoël.

1984   *Un siècle d'art moderne*, Paris, Denoël; *Jérusalem, Photographies de Frédéric Brenner*, Paris, Denoël; Desclozeaux, *Mine de rien*, Paris, Denoël.

1990   *La Pieuse Orpheline*, Paris, À telle enseigne.

1991   Mope, *Une chanson savante*, Paris, À telle enseigne; *Le Professeur de silence*, Paris, À telle enseigne; Victor Hugo, *Ce que contient l'alphabe*, Paris, À telle enseigne; Massin, *Le Monde à l'envers*, Paris, À telle enseigne; Massin, *Le Vent*, Paris, À telle enseigne; Courteline, *Panthéon-Courcelles*, Paris, À telle enseigne; René Ghil, *Traité du verbe*, Paris, À telle enseigne; *Cinq lettres de Reynaldo Hahn à Marcel Proust*, Paris, À telle enseigne; Massin, *Un monsieur pressé*, Paris, À telle enseigne; Adrienne Monnier, *Éloge du livre pauvre*, Paris, À telle enseigne; Paul Valéry, *Les deux vertus d'un livre*, Paris, À telle enseigne; Massin, *La Danse du feu*, Paris, À telle enseigne; Massin, *Des gens célèbres*, Paris, À telle enseigne; Massin, *Il pleut*, Paris, À telle enseigne; Massin, *Jouons avec les lettres*, Paris, À telle enseigne; Claude Moatti, *L'Invention de Rome*, Paris, À telle enseigne; Massin, *Jouons avec les chiffres*, Paris, À telle enseigne; Massin, *Les Murmures de la forêt*, Paris, À telle enseigne; André Suarès, *Art du livre*, Paris, À telle enseigne; Massin, *L'Arche de Noé*, Paris, À telle enseigne; Massin, *Un gros mangeur*, Paris,

À telle enseigne; Massin, *Le Monde à l'endroit*, Paris, À telle enseigne; Massin, *La Part de l'ombre*, Paris, À telle enseigne; *Lettre d'aliéné*, Paris, À telle enseigne.

1992   Blaise Cendrars, *Publicité = Poésie*, Paris, À telle enseigne; Léon-Paul Fargue, *Salut à la publicité*, Paris, À telle enseigne; *Là ci darem la mano*, Paris, À telle enseigne; *Da capo*, Paris, À telle enseigne; F. Scott Fitzgerald, *Une fête chez Gatsby*, Paris, À telle enseigne.

1993   Thierry Mignon, *La Belle Champenoise*, Paris, À telle enseigne; Massin, *La Maison du docteur Enfoirus*, Paris, À telle enseigne.

2000   Massin, *L'Aïr*, Paris, À telle enseigne; *La Fausse Ignorante*, Paris, À telle enseigne; *Eulalie ou La Pension*, Paris, À telle enseigne; *Mademoiselle de Bocey*, Paris, À telle enseigne.

2002   Arnold Schönberg, *Pierrot lunaire op.21*, Paris, À telle enseigne; Blaise Cendrars, *Les Pâques à New York*, Paris, À telle enseigne.

General works

Roxane Jubert, *Graphisme, typographie, histoire*, Paris, Flammarion, 2005.

Filippo Tommaso Marinetti, 'Destruction de la syntaxe – Imagination sans fils – Mots en liberté', *Lacerba* (Florence), 15 June 1913.

Raymond Queneau, *Entretiens avec Georges Charbonnier*, Paris, Gallimard, 1962.

Raymond Queneau, *Œuvres complètes*, Paris, Gallimard, 'Bibliothèque de la Pléiade', 1989 (revised edition 2002).

Catherine de Smet, 'Notre livre (France)', *Graphisme en France 2003*, Paris, Délégation aux arts plastiques, ministère de la Culture, January 2003.

Anne Ubersfeld, *Lire le théâtre I*, Paris, Belin, 1977 (new edition 1996).

Beatrice Warde, *The Crystal Goblet* (1932), cited in Ellen Lupton and Abbott Miller, *Design, Writing, Research*, London, Phaidon, 1999, p. 55.

Alain Weill, *Le Graphisme*, Paris, Gallimard, 'Découvertes' series, 2004.

Michel Wlassikoff, *Histoire du graphisme en France*, Paris, éditions Dominique Carré, 2005.

Cited articles and books on Massin

Unamed author, 'Des "Portiques" au "Nombre d'or" : La Pléiade concurrencée?', *La Lettre de la Pléiade*, no. 14, February/March/April 2003.

Unamed author, 'Massin', in catalogue for the International Graphic Design Exhibition, Istanbul, 2003.

Unamed author, *Massin*, collection 'The Great Masters of the International Design', Peking.

Unamed author, 'L'Œuvre typographique de Massin', in *Hyundae Munhak*, Seoul, 2001.

Unamed author, 'Robert Massin', in *New AGI Members*, Peking, 2002.

Philippe Apeloig, *Massin*, Paris, Pyramyd, 2005.

Roland Barthes, 'L'Esprit et la Lettre', in *La Quinzaine des Lettres*, 1970 '; in *L'Obvie et l'Obtus, Essais critiques III*, 'Tel Quel' series, 1982, Paris, Seuil; in *La Lettre et l'Image*, postface, Paris, Gallimard, 1993.

Marcel Brion, 'Honneur de la lettre sainte image', *Les Nouvelles littéraires*, 2 July 1970.

François Caradec, 'Crû Massin 1964', *Caractère*, 1964, pp. 77–81.

Kim Chang-Sik, 'Massin – The Alchemist of Characters and Image', in the 'Typojanchi' exhibition catalogue, Seoul, 2001.

Various, *Massin*, IMEC catalogue (Institut mémoires de l'édition contemporaine), Paris, 1990.

Jean-Luc Dusong and Fabienne Siegwart, 'Massin', in *Typographie, du plomb au numérique*, Paris, Dessain et Tolra, 1996.

Friedrich Friedl, Nicolaus Ott and Bernard Stein, 'Massin', in *Typo*, Cologne, Könemann, 1998.

John Gall and Steven Brower, 'Massin Ahead of Time', in *Graphic Design History*, New York, Allworth Press, 2001.

Richard Hollis, 'Massin: Language unleashed', *Eye Magazine* (London), no. 16, 1995, pp. 67–77.

Marie-Laure Jaubert de Beaujeu, 'Mise en pages du théâtre, théâtre de la mise en pages', *Cahiers du musée national d'Art moderne*, Centre Georges-Pompidou, Paris, Autumn 2004, pp. 70–93.

Hubert Juin, 'Un livre gai', *Le Monde*, 29 April 1970, 'Littérature' section, pp. 4–5.

Anne-Marie Koenig, 'L'Œil et la Lettre', in *Magazine littéraire*, no. 365, Paris, May 1998.

Gilbert Lascault, 'Lettres figurées, alphabet fou', in *Critique*, no. 285, Paris, February 1971.

Patrick Lesort, 'La Lettre et le Musicien', in *Grafika*, Montreal, 2003.

Katy Lhaïk, 'La provocation typographique de La Cantatrice chauve', cited in *Massin*, IMEC catalogue, op. cit. (Original title: *Étude d'une mise en pages, La Cantatrice chauve*, master's paper, université Paris-XIII, 1983.)

Katherine McCoy, 'American Graphic Design Expression: The Evolution of American Typography', *Design Quarterly*, no. 149, 1990, pp. 3–22, MIT Press, Cambridge (Mass.), © 1998 High Ground Design.

Massin, *Catalogue raisonné de l'œuvre typographique 1948–1958* (1998), *Catalogue raisonné de l'œuvre typographique 1958–1979 : Du côté de chez Gaston* (1999), *Catalogue raisonné de l'œuvre typographique 1979–2000 : Cavalier seul* (2001), Ville de Chartres, avec le concours du Fonds régional d'acquisitions pour les bibliothèques de la région Centre.

Philip Meggs, 'The Bald Soprano', in *Graphic Design History*, New York, Allworth Press, 2001.

Michel Melot, 'Le livre unique, de la religion du livre à l'idéologie du livre', conference given at the École normale supérieure, Paris, published in the first edition of the 'École d'été' for the Institut d'histoire du livre, 2004.

Michel Olyff, *Conversation avec Massin*, Brussels, Éditions Tandem, 2006.

Vanina Pinter, 'L'histoire vaut d'être racontée...', in *Étapes Graphiques*, Paris, Pyramyd, no. 115, 2004.

Michel Ragon, 'Massin graphiste et génie', in *Beaux Arts Magazine*, no. 212, Paris, January 2002.

Da Redação (after texts by Laetitia Wolff) 'Robert Massin, ação na página impressa', in *Arc Design*, São Paulo, 2003.

Gabrielle Rolin, 'L'homme qui vous fait les poches', in *Lire*, no. 287, Paris, Summer 2000.

Philippe Schuwer, 'L'écriture au pied de la lettre, treize fois deux', *Le Figaro littéraire*, 18 May 1970.

Emmanuël Souchiez, 'À propos d'Exercices de style', in *Massin*, IMEC catalogue, op. cit., p. 62.

Laetitia Wolff, 'Massin in Continuo: A Dictionary', *Design Issues*, vol. 18, no. 4, Autumn 2002, MIT Press, Cambridge (Mass.).

Laetitia Wolff, *Massin in Continuo: A Dictionary*, Milan, Abitare, 2002.

University papers

Sylvie Deroure, *Les Calligrammes d'Apollinaire ou Vers un renouveau typographique et poétique*, final year thesis, ICART, 1968.

Noémi Goldstein, *La Réappropriation du visuel dans l'œuvre typographique de Massin*, master's thesis in modern literature, université Paris VI, 2001.

Laure Lacombe, *Les Collaborations entre écrivains et photographes. Doisneau/Pennac : 'Les Grandes Vacances'*, master's thesis, université Paris III-Sorbonne Nouvelle, 1993.

Anne-Marie Lereboullet, *Les Calligrammes dans l'expression littéraire*, dissertation for diploma, under the direction of Étiemble, université de Paris, 1966–1967.

So-hyoun Park, *Research into the Narrative Structure Immanent in Editorial Space of a Book-focus on 'La Cantatrice chauve' designed by R. Massin*, Department of visual communication design, Graduate School of Hong-ik University, Seoul, 2003.

Daniel Truong, *Massin et la Typographie expressive. Leur place dans l'évolution de la typographie*, Paris, Estienne technical college, 1968.

Bibliography

Index

To my mother, Claude Toselli Wolff (1937–2000), graphic artist and artist.

This book could not have been written without the generous help and inspiration of Massin himself. Through him I have learnt so much, not just about his own life and work, but also about the salutary powers of art, graphic design and culture in general. His role as editorial and artistic advisor and his openness in all the interviews I have conducted with him have been absolutely invaluable, enabling me to bring authenticity to my research and sincerity to my writing.

I should also like to thank my dear husband Harvey Tulcensky for his moral support throughout the years I have spent researching and writing this book, and above all for his belief in what I was doing. Thanks to my mentor Mirko Ilić for giving me the idea for this project, six or seven years ago now, for the magnificent poster he created for the opening of the retrospective 'Massin in Continuo: A Dictionary' at the Cooper Union, New York, in December 2001, for his support, advice and generosity in sharing his knowledge of graphic art and artists. Thanks to Corinne Brivot for her precious help in reading some of the pieces. Thanks to all those who have supported my project for a travelling exhibition in North America and who invited Massin and me to take part in conferences, debates and workshops with students, including Milton Glaser of the Cooper Union, Steven Heller and Steven Guarnaccia of the School of Visual Arts, Peggy Re of Maryland University, Baltimore, Elizabeth Resnick of Massachusetts College of Art, Boston, Marc Choko of the Centre de Design at UQAM, Montreal, Laurent Deveze, who was then cultural attaché at the French Consulate in Los Angeles, typographer and UCLA professor Joe Molloy, freelance graphic artist Kaly Nikitas, who was then head of the Department of Design at the University of Minneapolis, Steve Woodall, Director of the San Francisco Center for Book Art, typographer and critic John Berry and Antoine Vigne, former head of Visual Arts at the Culture Department of the French embassy.

Thanks to Jean-Pierre Dauphin and Laurent Graff at Gallimard for their logistical help, to photographers Louis Monier and Henry Cohen and to illustrators Jean Alessandrini, Jacques Carelman, Étienne Delessert, Jean-Olivier Héron, Jean Lagarrigue, Georges Lemoine and Jean-Michel Nicollet for their respective contributions.

Finally my thanks go to Julia Hasting for encouraging me to submit the idea for this book to Phaidon, to the great Alan Fletcher for believing in it and to Valerie Buffet, Hélène Gallois Montbrun and Amélie Despérier for their patient encouragement and the quality of their editorial input.

All the illustrations in this book are reproduced courtesy of Robert Massin, with the exception of the following photographs:
page 8 and page 10 © Roger Roche;
page 17, bottom left © Philippe Lavieille;
page 52 © Jacques Robert;
pages 76 and 142 : © Yan;
pages 78 to 87, pages 96 to 98 and pages 102 to 109 : © Henry Cohen.
pages 110, 150, 166, pages 168 to 169, page 170, bottom, and pages 171 to 195 : © Louis Monier.

Acknowledgements and photographic credits